Atlas of Pediatric
Emergency
THIRD EDITION
Medicine

Editor-in-Chief

Binita R. Shah, MD, FAAP

Distinguished Professor of Emergency Medicine and Pediatrics
SUNY Downstate Medical Center
Director Emeritus, Pediatric Emergency Medicine
Kings County Hospital Center
Brooklyn, New York

Associate Editors

Prashant Mahajan, MD, MPH, MBA

Professor of Emergency Medicine and Pediatrics
Vice-Chair, Department of Emergency Medicine
Section Chief, Pediatric Emergency Medicine
University of Michigan and CS Mott Children's Hospital
Ann Arbor, Michigan

John Amodio, MD, FACR

Chief, Pediatric Radiology
Cohen Children's Medical Center
System Chief, Pediatric Radiology
Northwell Health System
Professor of Radiology
Zucker/Hofstra School of Medicine
Hempstead, New York

Michael Lucchesi, MD, MS

Professor and Chairman
Department of Emergency Medicine
Interim Dean, College of Medicine
SUNY Downstate Medical Center
Chief Medical Officer
University Hospital of Brooklyn
Brooklyn, New York

New York   Chicago   San Francisco   Athens   London   Madrid   Mexico City
Milan   New Delhi   Singapore   Sydney   Toronto

Atlas of Pediatric Emergency Medicine, Third Edition

3 4 5 6 7 8 9   LKV   28 27 26 25 24

ISBN 978-1-259-86338-7
MHID 1-259-86338-7

This book was set in Times LT Std by Cenveo® Publisher Services.
The editors were Amanda Fielding, Kay Conerly, and Christie Naglieri.
The production supervisor was Catherine H. Saggese.
Project management was provided by Revathi Viswanathan, Cenveo Publisher Services.

Library of Congress Cataloging-in-Publication Data

Names: Shah, Binita R., editor. | Mahajan, Prashant, editor. |
  Amodio, John, editor. | Lucchesi, Michael, editor.
Title: Atlas of pediatric emergency medicine / editor, editor-in-chief,
  Binita R. Shah ; associate editors, Prashant Mahajan, John Amodio, Michael
  Lucchesi.
Description: Third edition. | New York : McGraw-Hill Companies, Inc., [2019]
  | Includes index.
Identifiers: LCCN 2018044207| ISBN 9781259863387 (hardcover) | ISBN
  1259863387 (hardcover) | ISBN 9781259863394
Subjects: | MESH: Emergencies | Child | Child Abuse | Infant | Wounds and
  Injuries | Emergency Treatment | Atlases
Classification: LCC RJ370 | NLM WS 17 | DDC 618.92/0025—dc23 LC record available at
  https://lccn.loc.gov/2018044207

McGraw-Hill books are available at special quantity discounts to use as premiums and sales promotions, or for use in corporate training programs. To contact a representative please visit the Contact Us pages at www.mhprofessional.com.

To my grandchildren Roshni, Saachiv, Kailen and Ariya
For bringing Heaven on Earth to my life.

To my children Toral & Vikas and Ronak & Kunal
For carrying the torch of serving humanity through the practice of medicine.

To my husband Rajni P. Shah, MD
For serving as my backbone during the pursuit of my professional career for the past 47 years!

To my mother Chanchalben
For your perseverance and intense desire that I become a physician.

To my father Ratilal P. Patel, MD
You were my greatest inspiration and inner strength.
Everything I have become is because of you!

Binita R. Shah, MD, FAAP

To my parents, Vithal and Geeta Mahajan, who have taught me the value of education.

To my wife Jayashree and my two daughters Arushi and Aditi whose selfless support and love keep me grounded and humble.

To my brothers Arun and Ravi whom I can only hope to emulate.

To my friend and mentor Binita, whose vision about the global impact of this book on diagnostic decision making is my primary driver to learn and collaborate on this endeavor.

Prashant Mahajan, MD, MPH, MBA

To my parents Ann and John: A day doesn't go by that I don't think about you and realize how important you were to my career and my life.

To my children Mike, Jess, and John: Who make me proud every day and have turned my house into a home.

To Mason and The Chief: Who's unconditional love is testament to the fact that I live with my five best friends.

Michael Lucchesi, MD, MS

About the Cover Images

Front Cover, from left to right
Subgaleal Hematoma From Forceful Hair Pulling
Raynaud Phenomenon; Systemic Lupus Erythematosus
Herpes Simplex Virus Periorbital Infection

Back Cover, from left to right
Annular Psoriasis (Misdiagnosed as Tinea Corporis)
Elbow Dislocation
Hair-Tourniquet Syndrome
Reactivation Pulmonary Tuberculosis with Lung Abscess and a Bullet in the Neck

Contributing Authors xv
Photography Credits xix
Radiography Credits xxviii
Foreword xxx
Preface xxxi
Acknowledgments xxxii

Chapter 1
NONACCIDENTAL TRAUMA 1
Earl R. Hartwig

CHILD ABUSE 2
CUTANEOUS MANIFESTATIONS OF CHILD ABUSE 8
OROFACIAL TRAUMA 13
INFLICTED BURNS 18
SKELETAL MANIFESTATIONS OF CHILD ABUSE 23
FEMUR FRACTURES 28
RIB FRACTURES DUE TO ABUSE 30
SKULL FRACTURES DUE TO ABUSE 32
ABUSIVE HEAD TRAUMA 35
ABUSIVE THORACOABDOMINAL TRAUMA 39
INFANTICIDE VERSUS SUDDEN UNEXPLAINED
 INFANT DEATH SYNDROME 43

Chapter 2
CONDITIONS MISTAKEN FOR PHYSICAL AND SEXUAL ABUSE 47
Allison M. Jackson ■ Tanya S. Hinds

CONGENITAL DERMAL MELANOCYTOSIS 48
FOLK HEALING PRACTICES 50
COLD PANNICULITIS 53
NEVI OF OTA AND ITO 55
PORT-WINE STAIN 57
PHYTOPHOTODERMATITIS 59
CONTACT DERMATITIS FROM SENNA 61
ACUTE HEMORRHAGIC EDEMA OF INFANCY 63
IMPETIGO 65
POSTINFLAMMATORY HYPERPIGMENTATION 68
RACCOON EYE 69
HAIR-TOURNIQUET SYNDROME 72
MENKES DISEASE 74
VITAMIN D INSUFFICIENCY, VITAMIN D
 DEFICIENCY, AND RICKETS 76
OSTEOGENESIS IMPERFECTA 79
LICHEN SCLEROSUS ET ATROPHICUS 82
PERIANAL BACTERIAL DERMATITIS 84
LABIAL ADHESION 86
URETHRAL PROLAPSE 88
STRADDLE INJURY 90

Chapter 3
INFECTIOUS DISEASES 93
Michelle W. Parker ■ Samir S. Shah

STREPTOCOCCAL PHARYNGITIS
 AND SCARLET FEVER 94
IMPETIGO 98
ECTHYMA 101
ERYSIPELAS 103
NECROTIZING FASCIITIS 105
ECTHYMA GANGRENOSUM 108
TOXIC SHOCK SYNDROME 110
STAPHYLOCOCCAL SCALDED SKIN SYNDROME 114
MENINGOCOCCEMIA 118
ROCKY MOUNTAIN SPOTTED FEVER 121
CAT-SCRATCH DISEASE 124
LYMPHADENITIS 126
CHICKENPOX 129
HERPES ZOSTER 131
OROPHARYNGEAL HERPES SIMPLEX
 VIRUS INFECTION 134
HERPETIC WHITLOW 136
MUMPS 137
ROSEOLA INFANTUM 138
MEASLES 140
RUBELLA 142
INFECTIOUS MONONUCLEOSIS 144
ERYTHEMA INFECTIOSUM 147
HAND-FOOT-AND-MOUTH DISEASE 149
HERPANGINA 152
CUTANEOUS LARVAE MIGRANS 153
ASCARIASIS 155
MALARIA 157

Chapter 4
SEXUAL ABUSE, GYNECOLOGY, AND SEXUALLY TRANSMITTED INFECTIONS 159
Tanya S. Hinds ■ Angela Lumba-Brown

OVERVIEW OF CHILD SEXUAL ABUSE
 AND ASSAULT 160

SEXUAL ABUSE AND SEXUALLY TRANSMITTED
   INFECTIONS 163
CONDYLOMATA ACUMINATA................... 168
TRICHOMONIASIS 170
CONGENITAL SYPHILIS 171
PRIMARY AND SECONDARY SYPHILIS 174
GONORRHEA 177
GENITAL HERPES 179
PELVIC INFLAMMATORY DISEASE 182
ABNORMAL UTERINE BLEEDING.............. 184
ECTOPIC PREGNANCY 187

Chapter 5
CARDIOLOGY 189

Shyam K. Sathanandam ■ Sushitha Surendran

BRADYCARDIA 190
FIRST-DEGREE ATRIOVENTRICULAR BLOCK ... 193
SECOND-DEGREE ATRIOVENTRICULAR BLOCK ... 195
THIRD-DEGREE ATRIOVENTRICULAR BLOCK... 197
LONG QT SYNDROME 200
SYNCOPE 204
SINUS TACHYCARDIA.................................. 208
SUPRAVENTRICULAR TACHYCARDIA.......... 210
ATRIAL FLUTTER 217
PREMATURE VENTRICULAR CONTRACTIONS.............. 219
HYPERCYANOTIC SPELL OF TETRALOGY
   OF FALLOT... 222
DUCTAL-DEPENDENT CARDIAC LESIONS/
   HYPOPLASTIC LEFT HEART SYNDROME 226
INFECTIVE ENDOCARDITIS 229
CHEST PAIN 232
ACUTE PERICARDITIS 236
ACUTE MYOCARDITIS 239
CONGESTIVE HEART FAILURE 243
ACUTE RHEUMATIC FEVER 247
PULMONARY HYPERTENSIVE CRISES.......... 249

Chapter 6
RESPIRATORY DISORDERS 253

Todd A. Florin ■ Andrea T. Cruz

TRACHEOBRONCHIAL FOREIGN BODIES 254
PERTUSSIS... 258
CROUP 259
BACTERIAL TRACHEITIS 261
EPIGLOTTITIS... 263
BRONCHIOLITIS 265
COMMUNITY-ACQUIRED PNEUMONIA...... 268
INTRATHORACIC TUBERCULOSIS 273
MILIARY TUBERCULOSIS 278
OBSTRUCTIVE SLEEP APNEA SYNDROME 280
ASTHMA 283
PRIMARY SPONTANEOUS PNEUMOTHORAX 287
PULMONARY EMBOLISM 291

Chapter 7
DERMATOLOGY 293

Sharon A. Glick ■ Jeannette Jakus ■ Julie Cantatore-Francis
■ Kunal M. Shah
Edited by Sharon A. Glick

URTICARIA.. 294
ANGIOEDEMA... 296
SERUM SICKNESS/SERUM SICKNESS–LIKE
   REACTIONS 298
URTICARIA MULTIFORME........................... 300
ERYTHEMA MULTIFORME 302
STEVENS-JOHNSON SYNDROME AND
   TOXIC EPIDERMAL NECROLYSIS................ 305
DRUG REACTIONS 310
HENOCH-SCHÖNLEIN PURPURA................. 314
ACNE FULMINANS 317
SEBORRHEIC DERMATITIS 318
ALLERGIC CONTACT DERMATITIS 320
ATOPIC DERMATITIS................................... 323
ECZEMA HERPETICUM 327
PSORIASIS 329
GUTTATE PSORIASIS 332
PITYRIASIS ROSEA 335
GRANULOMA ANNULARE 337
SCABIES 339
TINEA VERSICOLOR 342
TINEA CAPITIS 345
TINEA CORPORIS....................................... 348
TINEA CRURIS... 350
TINEA PEDIS 352
TINEA UNGUIUM 354
WARTS 356
MOLLUSCUM CONTAGIOSUM 358
ACROPUSTULOSIS OF INFANCY.................. 360
ERYTHEMA TOXICUM NEONATORUM 362
EPIDERMOLYSIS BULLOSA 363

INFANTILE HEMANGIOMA 366

MASTOCYTOSIS...370

CAFÉ-AU-LAIT SPOTS 373

ERYTHEMA NODOSUM 375

ACANTHOSIS NIGRICANS 376

HIDRADENITIS SUPPURATIVA 378

TRANSIENT NEONATAL PUSTULAR MELANOSIS............380

SUBCUTANEOUS FAT NECROSIS OF
    THE NEWBORN 382

CANDIDAL DIAPER DERMATITIS 384

PERIORAL DERMATITIS 386

INCONTINENTIA PIGMENTI 387

Chapter 8
OPHTHALMOLOGY..................................389

Suzanne M. Schmidt ▪ Steven E. Krug

ORBITAL CELLULITIS 390

PRESEPTAL CELLULITIS 394

HORDEOLUM AND CHALAZION 396

ACUTE CONJUNCTIVITIS 398

OPHTHALMIA NEONATORUM
    (NEWBORN CONJUNCTIVITIS) 400

LEUKOCORIA 402

INFANTILE GLAUCOMA 404

CORNEAL FOREIGN BODY 406

CORNEAL ABRASION 407

CORNEAL ULCER...408

HYPOPYON 410

HYPHEMA 411

SUBCONJUNCTIVAL HEMORRHAGE 413

EYELID LACERATION 414

TRAUMATIC GLOBE RUPTURE 416

ORBITAL FRACTURE 419

RETROBULBAR HEMORRHAGE 420

CHEMICAL BURNS 422

Chapter 9
OTOLARYNGOLOGY 425

Sydney C. Butts ▪ Nira A. Goldstein ▪ Richard M. Rosenfeld
▪ Aaron L. Thatcher ▪ David J. Brown ▪ Christopher Discolo
▪ Jennifer H. Chao
Edited by Sydney C. Butts

ACUTE OTITIS MEDIA..426

COMPLICATIONS OF OTITIS MEDIA 429

OTITIS EXTERNA...432

PERICHONDRITIS...434

AURICULAR FOREIGN BODY 437

AURICULAR HEMATOMA 439

EPISTAXIS 441

NASAL FOREIGN BODIES 444

ACUTE SINUSITIS 447

CHRONIC SINUSITIS 451

POTT PUFFY TUMOR 454

DEEP NECK SPACE INFECTION 456

PERITONSILLAR ABSCESS 460

LEMIERRE SYNDROME 462

Chapter 10
SURGICAL AND GENITOURINARY 465

Neil G. Uspal ▪ Vincent J. Wang

INTUSSUSCEPTION 466

HYPERTROPHIC PYLORIC STENOSIS 471

ACUTE NONPERFORATED APPENDICITIS 473

PERFORATED APPENDICITIS.................................476

INCARCERATED INGUINAL HERNIA.................478

TESTICULAR TORSION 480

TESTICULAR TRAUMA 485

EPIDIDYMO-ORCHITIS 487

TORSION OF THE APPENDIX TESTIS 490

VAGINAL FOREIGN BODY IN A
    PREPUBERTAL CHILD 491

CONGENITAL IMPERFORATE HYMEN WITH
    HEMATOMETROCOLPOS.....................................493

BARTHOLIN GLAND ABSCESS 496

PARAPHIMOSIS 497

OVARIAN TORSION 501

INTESTINAL MALROTATION AND VOLVULUS 504

UMBILICAL GRANULOMA 506

UMBILICAL HERNIA 508

Chapter 11
HEMATOLOGY AND ONCOLOGY 509

Scott T. Miller ▪ Kusum Viswanathan

SICKLE CELL ANEMIA WITH FEVER 510

SICKLE CELL ANEMIA WITH ACUTE PAIN 512

SICKLE CELL ANEMIA WITH ACUTE CHEST
    SYNDROME 516

SICKLE CELL ANEMIA AND CEREBROVASCULAR
    DISEASE..519

SICKLE CELL ANEMIA WITH PRIAPISM 522

SICKLE CELL ANEMIA WITH RIGHT UPPER
   QUADRANT SYNDROME 524

SICKLE CELL ANEMIA AND TRANSIENT
   APLASTIC CRISIS 527

SICKLE CELL ANEMIA AND ACUTE SPLENIC
   SEQUESTRATION CRISIS 529

NEWLY DIAGNOSED IMMUNE
   THROMBOCYTOPENIA 531

HEMOPHILIA 534

LYMPHADENOPATHY 537

ACUTE LYMPHOBLASTIC LEUKEMIA............539

HODGKIN LYMPHOMA 541

ABDOMINAL MASS 543

NEUROBLASTOMA 546

OVARIAN TUMORS 549

OSTEOSARCOMA 553

EWING SARCOMA 558

Chapter 12
RHEUMATOLOGY 561
Julie Cherian ■ Farzana Nuruzzaman ■ Sarah F. Taber

KAWASAKI DISEASE 562

INCOMPLETE KAWASAKI DISEASE 567

SYSTEMIC LUPUS ERYTHEMATOSUS 570

NEONATAL LUPUS 574

RAYNAUD PHENOMENON 576

JUVENILE DERMATOMYOSITIS 579

JUVENILE IDIOPATHIC ARTHRITIS 582

GRANULOMATOSIS WITH POLYANGIITIS 587

MACROPHAGE ACTIVATION SYNDROME........589

LYME DISEASE 591

Chapter 13
NEUROLOGY 595
Geetha Chari ■ Vikas S. Shah

BACTERIAL MENINGITIS........................596

RAISED INTRACRANIAL PRESSURE 601

ALTERED MENTAL STATUS........................605

FEBRILE SEIZURES 609

SEIZURES AND EPILEPSY 611

STATUS EPILEPTICUS 614

STROKE IN CHILDREN 617

NEUROCYSTICERCOSIS 621

BELL PALSY 624

HEADACHE 626

BRAIN TUMORS........................629

HYDROCEPHALUS........................632

SPINAL CORD LESIONS (NONTRAUMATIC) 637

GUILLAIN-BARRÉ SYNDROME........................640

MYASTHENIA GRAVIS 642

INFANTILE BOTULISM 644

Chapter 14
ENDOCRINOLOGY 647
Glenn D. Harris ■ Irma Fiordalisi ■ Scott M. Thomas

DIABETIC KETOACIDOSIS........................648

ADDISON DISEASE 654

CONGENITAL ADRENAL HYPERPLASIA............656

HYPOTHYROIDISM AND MYXEDEMA 658

HYPERTHYROIDISM AND THYROID STORM 661

Chapter 15
GASTROINTESTINAL DISORDERS 665
Sandra Herr ■ Cole Condra

ESOPHAGEAL FOREIGN BODIES 666

FOREIGN BODIES DISTAL TO ESOPHAGUS........671

ANORECTAL FOREIGN BODIES..................673

BATTERY INGESTIONS 675

RETAINED BONES 679

SHARP OBJECTS........................681

MAGNET INGESTIONS 683

HEMATEMESIS 684

PANCREATITIS 687

BILIARY COLIC 689

INFLAMMATORY BOWEL DISEASE EXACERBATIONS 690

CONSTIPATION 692

RECTAL BLEEDING 695

Chapter 16
NEPHROLOGY 699
Anil K. Mongia ■ Manju Chandra

PROTEINURIA 700

HEMATURIA 702

MINIMAL CHANGE NEPHROTIC SYNDROME....707

ACUTE POSTSTREPTOCOCCAL
   GLOMERULONEPHRITIS 711

URINARY TRACT INFECTION.............................713

HEMOLYTIC UREMIC SYNDROME 716

OBSTRUCTIVE UROPATHY...............................718

HYPERTENSIVE EMERGENCIES 720

NEPHROLITHIASIS...722

HYPOCALCEMIA..725

HYPERCALCEMIA 728

HYPOKALEMIA..731

HYPERKALEMIA..733

Chapter 17
TOXICOLOGY 737

Mark K. Su ■ Madeline H. Renny

THE EVALUATION AND MANAGEMENT
OF POISONING IN CHILDREN: GENERAL
APPROACH AND GI DECONTAMINATION 738

ACUTE ACETAMINOPHEN TOXICITY.............746

ACUTE SALICYLATE TOXICITY.........................749

IRON TOXICITY 752

OPIOID TOXICITY 754

COCAINE TOXICITY 757

METHEMOGLOBINEMIA 760

ORGANOPHOSPHATE AND CARBAMATE
INSECTICIDE TOXICITY 762

CASTOR BEAN AND ROSARY PEA INGESTION 764

PHENOTHIAZINE TOXICITY 766

ANTICHOLINERGIC DRUG AND PLANT
TOXICITY 768

ACUTE ISONIAZID TOXICITY...........................770

CAMPHOR TOXICITY 772

HYDROCARBON AND NAPHTHALENE TOXICITY.........773

ECSTASY/MOLLY TOXICITY 776

KETAMINE TOXICITY..778

DEXTROMETHORPHAN TOXICITY 779

MARIJUANA TOXICITY.......................................780

ETHYLENE GLYCOL TOXICITY.........................782

METHANOL TOXICITY 784

ETHANOL TOXICITY 786

PRESCRIPTION DRUGS OF ABUSE...................788

β-BLOCKER AND CALCIUM CHANNEL
BLOCKER TOXICITY 790

CLONIDINE TOXICITY 792

CYCLIC ANTIDEPRESSANT TOXICITY...............794

LEAD TOXICITY...796

CAUSTICS 798

NICOTINE 802

CAFFEINE 804

Chapter 18
ENVIRONMENTAL EMERGENCIES 807

Jeanine E. Hall ■ Christine S. Cho

THERMAL BURNS...808

PERIPHERAL COLD INJURIES 814

ANAPHYLAXIS 817

BROWN RECLUSE SPIDER ENVENOMATION 820

BLACK WIDOW SPIDER ENVENOMATION.......823

SCORPION ENVENOMATION 824

DOG BITES...826

RABIES EXPOSURE AND VACCINE PROPHYLAXIS 829

CAT BITES 831

HUMAN BITES...833

VENOMOUS MARINE ANIMALS: STINGING
MARINE ANIMALS—CORALS, SEA ANEMONES,
HYDROIDS, AND FIRE CORAL.......................835

STINGING MARINE ANIMALS: BOX JELLYFISH,
TRUE JELLYFISH, AND PORTUGUESE
MAN-OF-WAR 837

STINGING MARINE ANIMALS: SPONGES
(PHYLUM PORIFERA) 840

STABBING MARINE ANIMALS: STARFISH,
SEA URCHINS, AND CROWN-OF-THORNS
STARFISH 842

STABBING MARINE ANIMALS: STONEFISH AND
SCORPIONFISH (FAMILY SCORPAENIDAE) 844

STABBING MARINE ANIMALS: STINGRAY 846

STABBING MARINE ANIMALS: CONE SHELLS
(FAMILY CONIDAE) 847

BITING MARINE ANIMALS: BLUE-RINGED
OCTOPUS 848

LIGHTNING INJURIES 849

SNAKE ENVENOMATIONS 850

HIGH-ALTITUDE ILLNESS 854

Chapter 19
ORTHOPEDICS 857

Konstantinos Agoritsas ■ Ameer Hassoun ■ Jennifer H. Chao
■ Sathyaseelan Subramaniam ■ Andrea T. Cruz ■ Ryan Logan Webb
■ Josh Greenstein

FRACTURES AND FRACTURE CLASSIFICATION 858

TUFT FRACTURES 867

PHALANX FRACTURES 868

MALLET FINGER..870

BENNETT FRACTURE AND ROLANDO FRACTURE.........871

BOXER'S FRACTURE...872

FRACTURES OF CARPAL BONES
(SCAPHOID FRACTURE) 873

FOREARM FRACTURES...874

GALEAZZI FRACTURE DISLOCATION AND
MONTEGGIA FRACTURE DISLOCATION..................876

OLECRANON FRACTURE.......................................877

RADIAL HEAD AND NECK FRACTURES 878

SUPRACONDYLAR FRACTURE................................880

HUMERUS FRACTURE..882

CLAVICLE FRACTURE..884

SCAPULAR FRACTURE...886

FEMUR FRACTURE...888

PATELLA FRACTURES..890

MAISONNEUVE FRACTURE....................................891

ANKLE FRACTURE AND SPRAIN 892

CALCANEAL FRACTURE.......................................894

JONES FRACTURE..895

LISFRANC FRACTURE...897

STRESS FRACTURE...898

DISLOCATIONS: INTERPHALANGEAL JOINT
DISLOCATION 899

LUNATE AND PERILUNATE DISLOCATIONS....................901

ELBOW DISLOCATION 903

ANTERIOR AND POSTERIOR GLENOHUMERAL
JOINT DISLOCATIONS...................................904

HIP DISLOCATION 907

KNEE DISLOCATION..909

ANKLE DISLOCATION 911

PATELLA DISLOCATION.......................................913

PELVIC AVULSION FRACTURES 914

TIBIAL TUBERCLE AVULSION FRACTURE 915

MUSCULOSKELETAL INJURIES:
GAMEKEEPER'S THUMB 916

NURSEMAID'S ELBOW.......................................917

ACROMIOCLAVICULAR INJURIES...........................919

SLIPPED CAPITAL FEMORAL EPIPHYSIS 920

LEGG-CALVÉ-PERTHES DISEASE............................922

ANTERIOR CRUCIATE LIGAMENT TEAR....................923

OSGOOD-SCHLATTER DISEASE 924

ACHILLES TENDON RUPTURE...............................925

FOREIGN BODIES AND PENETRATING INJURIES 927

HAND INFECTIONS: PARONYCHIA 928

FLEXOR TENOSYNOVITIS 929

BONE AND JOINT INFECTIONS: ACUTE
OSTEOMYELITIS 930

CHRONIC OSTEOMYELITIS 933

OSTEOMYELITIS IN SICKLE CELL DISEASE 935

SEPTIC ARTHRITIS..937

NEONATAL OSTEOMYELITIS AND
SEPTIC ARTHRITIS 942

POTT DISEASE...944

Chapter 20
TRAUMA......................................947

Joshua Nagler ■ Caitlin A. Farrell ■ Marc Auerbach
■ Sydney C. Butts ■ Roman Shinder ■ Ilaaf Darrat
■ Lamont R. Jones

HEAD TRAUMA 948

SKULL FRACTURES 951

BASILAR SKULL FRACTURE 953

ACUTE SUBDURAL HEMATOMA 955

EPIDURAL HEMATOMA.......................................957

CEREBRAL CONTUSION 959

CEREBRAL CONCUSSION 960

NASAL SEPTAL HEMATOMA 961

NASAL FRACTURES 963

MANDIBLE FRACTURES.......................................965

MIDFACIAL FRACTURES (MAXILLARY/LE FORT,
FRONTAL SINUS, NASOORBITOETHMOID) 968

ORBITAL TRAUMA..972

FRACTURES OF THE ZYGOMATIC COMPLEX
AND ZYGOMATIC ARCH 975

SOFT TISSUE TRAUMA.......................................978

LIP LACERATION INVOLVING THE
VERMILION BORDER....................................981

TONGUE LACERATION 982

TRAUMATIC TEMPOROMANDIBULAR JOINT
DISLOCATION 983

PENETRATING NECK INJURY 984

CERVICAL SPINE INJURIES 986

JEFFERSON (4-PART) BURST FRACTURES 988

ODONTOID FRACTURES......................................989

TRAUMATIC SPONDYLOLISTHESIS OF C2 990

EXTENSION TEARDROP FRACTURE 991

ANTERIOR FLEXION FRACTURES
(FLEXION TEARDROP)..................................992

ATLANTO-OCCIPITAL DISLOCATION...............................994

SPINAL CORD INJURY WITHOUT RADIOGRAPHIC
 ABNORMALITY 996
BILATERAL FACET DISLOCATION 998
UNILATERAL FACET DISLOCATION 999
ANTERIOR SUBLUXATION 1001
SPINAL PROCESS (CLAY SHOVELER'S) FRACTURE 1002
DENTAL TRAUMA 1003
PULMONARY CONTUSION 1006
RIB FRACTURES AND FLAIL CHEST 1008
PNEUMOTHORAX AND TENSION
 PNEUMOTHORAX 1010
HEMOTHORAX 1012
TRAUMATIC AIRWAY OBSTRUCTION 1013
AORTIC DISRUPTION 1014
TRAUMATIC DIAPHRAGM RUPTURE 1015
TRACHEOBRONCHIAL TREE INJURY 1017
ABDOMINAL TRAUMA 1019
SPLENIC INJURIES 1022
HEPATIC INJURIES 1024
OTHER INTRA-ABDOMINAL TRAUMA
 INCLUDING SEATBELT INJURIES 1025
PELVIC FRACTURES 1027
RING INCARCERATION 1029
NAIL BED INJURY 1030
SUBUNGUAL HEMATOMA 1032

DIGITAL AMPUTATION 1034
DEGLOVING INJURY 1036
PENETRATING HAND OR FOOT INJURY 1038
TRAUMATIC EXTREMITY AMPUTATION 1040
FISHHOOK REMOVAL 1042
ZIPPER INJURY 1043

Chapter 21
EMERGENCY ULTRASOUND 1045

Jay Pershad ■ John P. Gullett

EMERGENCY ULTRASOUND 1046
APPENDICITIS 1050
INTUSSUSCEPTION 1052
PYLORIC STENOSIS 1053
BILIARY ULTRASOUND 1054
FIRST-TRIMESTER PREGNANCY 1056
PEDIATRIC LUNG ULTRASOUND 1058
ABSCESSES AND CELLULITIS 1060
PEDIATRIC HIP ULTRASOUND 1062
PEDIATRIC FRACTURES 1063
POINT-OF-CARE CARDIAC ULTRASONOGRAPHY
 AND ASSESSMENT OF VOLUME STATUS 1064

Index 1067

Konstantinos Agoritsas, MD, MBA

Associate Chief, Emergency Medicine
Director, Pediatric Emergency Medicine
Department of Emergency Medicine
NYC Health + Hospitals/Kings County
Clinical Assistant Professor
SUNY Downstate Medical Center
Brooklyn, New York
Chapter 19

Marc Auerbach, MD, MSCi, FAAP

Associate Professor, Pediatrics and Emergency Medicine
Yale University School of Medicine
New Haven, Connecticut
Chapter 20

David J. Brown, MD

Associate Vice President and Associate Dean
Health Equity and Inclusion
Associate Professor Pediatric Otolaryngology
Michigan Medicine
Ann Arbor, Michigan
Chapter 9

Sydney C. Butts, MD, FACS

Vice Chair and Associate Professor
Chief, Facial Plastic and Reconstructive Surgery
Department of Otolaryngology
SUNY Downstate Medical Center
Brooklyn, New York
Chapters 9 and 20

Julie Cantatore-Francis, MD

Dermatology Physicians of Connecticut
Norwalk, Connecticut
Yale New Haven Hospital
Assistant Clinical Professor
Department of Dermatology
New Haven, Connecticut
Chapter 7

Manju Chandra, MD

Director, Division of Pediatric Nephrology
NYU Winthrop Hospital
Mineola, New York
Professor of Clinical Pediatrics
Stony Brook University School of Medicine
Stony Brook, New York
Chapter 16

Jennifer H. Chao, MD, FAAP

Clinical Associate Professor
Fellowship Director, Pediatric Emergency Medicine
SUNY Downstate Medical Center
NYC Health + Hospitals/Kings County
Brooklyn, New York
Chapters 9 and 19

Geetha Chari, MD

Clinical Professor of Neurology and Pediatrics
Clinical Neurophysiology Program Director
SUNY Downstate Medical Center
NYC Health + Hospitals/Kings County
Brooklyn, New York
Chapter 13

Julie Cherian, MD, FACR

Assistant Professor of Pediatrics
Chief, Division of Pediatric Rheumatology
Stony Brook University Medical Center
Stony Brook Children's Hospital
Stony Brook, New York
Chapter 12

Christine S. Cho, MD, MPH, MEd

Associate Professor of Pediatrics
USC Keck School of Medicine
Children's Hospital Los Angeles
Los Angeles, California
Chapter 18

Cole Condra, MD, MSc, FAAP, FACEP

Assistant Professor of Pediatrics
Division of Pediatric Emergency Medicine
University of Louisville
Louisville, Kentucky
Chapter 15

Andrea T. Cruz, MD, MPH

Associate Professor of Pediatrics
Sections of Pediatric Emergency Medicine and Pediatric
  Infectious Diseases
Baylor College of Medicine
Texas Children's Hospital
Houston, Texas
Chapters 6 and 19

Ilaaf Darrat, MD, MBA

Division Head, Pediatric Otolaryngology
Henry Ford Health System
Department of Otolaryngology Head & Neck Surgery
Clinical Assistant Professor of Otolaryngology
Wayne State University College of Medicine
Detroit, Michigan
Chapter 20

Christopher Discolo, MD, MSCR

Associate Professor
Department of Otolaryngology—Head & Neck Surgery
Director, Craniofacial Anomalies and Cleft Palate Team
Medical University of South Carolina
Charleston, South Carolina
Chapter 9

Caitlin A. Farrell, MD

Instructor of Pediatrics, Harvard Medical School
Division of Emergency Medicine
Boston Children's Hospital
Boston, Massachusetts
Chapter 20

Irma Fiordalisi, MD

Professor of Pediatrics
Professor Emerita, Pediatrics
Pediatric Critical Care
East Carolina University, Brody School of Medicine
Greenville, North Carolina
Chapter 14

Todd A. Florin, MD, MSCE

Associate Professor of Pediatrics
Northwestern University Feinberg School of Medicine
Division of Emergency Medicine
Ann and Robert H. Lurie Children's Hospital of Chicago
Stanley Manne Children's Research Institute
Chicago, Illinois
Chapter 6

Sharon A. Glick, MD, MS

Professor, Clinical Dermatology and Pediatrics
SUNY Downstate Medical Center
Director of Pediatric Dermatology
SUNY Downstate, NYC Health + Hospitals/Kings County and
  Maimonides Medical Center
Brooklyn, New York
Chapter 7

Nira A. Goldstein, MD, MPH

Professor of Clinical Otolaryngology
SUNY Downstate Medical Center
NYC Health + Hospitals/Kings County
Brooklyn, New York
Chapter 9

Josh Greenstein, MD

Director of Ultrasound Division
Associate Research Director
Department of Emergency Medicine
Staten Island University Hospital/Northwell
Assistant Professor
Zucker School of Medicine at Hofstra/Northwell
Staten Island, New York
Chapter 19

John P. Gullett, MD

Associate Professor
Co-Director of Emergency Ultrasound
Department of Emergency Medicine
University of Alabama at Birmingham School of Medicine
Birmingham, Alabama
Chapter 21

Jeanine E. Hall, MD, FAAP

Assistant Professor of Pediatrics
USC Keck School of Medicine
Division of Emergency Medicine and Transport Medicine at
  Children's Hospital Los Angeles
Los Angeles, California
Chapter 18

Glenn D. Harris, MD

Professor Emeritus, Pediatrics
Pediatric Endocrinology and Diabetes
East Carolina University, Brody School of Medicine
Greenville, North Carolina
Chapter 14

Earl R. Hartwig, MD, FAAP

Education Director
Pediatric Emergency Medicine
Clinical Associate Professor of Pediatrics and Emergency Medicine
Wayne State University School of Medicine
Children's Hospital of Michigan
Detroit, Michigan
Chapter 1

Ameer Hassoun, MD

Director
Pediatric Emergency Medicine
Department of Emergency Medicine
New York-Presbyterian Queens
Clinical Assistant Professor
Weill Cornell Medical College
New York, New York
Chapter 19

Sandra Herr, MD

Professor of Pediatrics
University of Louisville School of Medicine
Director, Pediatric Emergency Department
Norton Children's Hospital
Louisville, Kentucky
Chapter 15

Tanya S. Hinds, MD, FAAP

Child Abuse Pediatrician
Child and Adolescent Protection Center
Children's National Health System
Assistant Professor of Pediatrics
The George Washington University School of Medicine and
  Health Sciences
Washington, DC
Chapters 2 and 4

Allison M. Jackson, MD, MPH, FAAP

Division Chief, Child & Adolescent Protection Center
Children's National Health System
Washington Children's Foundation Professor of Child &
  Adolescent Protection
Associate Professor of Pediatrics
The George Washington University School of Medicine and
  Health Sciences
Washington, DC
Chapter 2

Jeannette Jakus, MD, MBA, FAAP, FAAD

Director of Clinical Research
Clinical Assistant Professor
Department of Dermatology
SUNY Downstate Medical Center
Brooklyn, New York
Chapter 7

Lamont R. Jones, MD, MBA

Vice Chair
Department of Otolaryngology Head and Neck Surgery
Facial Plastic and Reconstructive Surgery
Director, Cleft and Craniofacial Clinic
Henry Ford Hospital
Detroit, Michigan
Chapter 20

Steven Krug, MD

Professor of Pediatrics
Northwestern University Feinberg School of Medicine
Division of Emergency Medicine
Ann & Robert H. Lurie Children's Hospital of Chicago
Chicago, Illinois
Chapter 8

Angela Lumba-Brown, MD
Clinical Assistant Professor
Department of Emergency Medicine and Pediatrics
Stanford University School of Medicine
Co-Director of Stanford Brain Performance Center
Stanford, California
Chapter 4

Scott T. Miller, MD
Professor Emeritus of Clinical Pediatrics
Director Emeritus, Division of Pediatric Hematology/Oncology
SUNY Downstate Medical Center
Brooklyn, New York
Chapter 11

Anil Mongia, MD, DCH, FAAP
Associate Professor
Fellowship Director, Pediatric Nephrology
Department of Pediatrics
SUNY Downstate Medical Center
Brooklyn, New York
Chapter 16

Joshua Nagler, MD, MHPEd
Fellowship Director
Associate Division Chief
Division of Emergency Medicine
Boston Children's Hospital
Assistant Professor of Pediatrics and Emergency Medicine
Harvard Medical School
Boston, Massachusetts
Chapter 20

Farzana Nuruzzaman, MD, FACR
Assistant Professor of Clinical Pediatrics
Stony Brook University School of Medicine
Division of Pediatric Rheumatology, Department of Pediatrics
Stony Brook Children's Hospital
Stony Brook, New York
Chapter 12

Michelle W. Parker, MD
Assistant Professor
Department of Pediatrics
University of Cincinnati College of Medicine
Division of Hospital Medicine
Cincinnati Children's Hospital Medical Center
Cincinnati, Ohio
Chapter 3

Jay Pershad, MD, MMM
Clinical Chief, Emergency Medicine
Children's National Medical Center
Professor of Pediatrics & Emergency Medicine
George Washington University
Washington, DC
Chapter 21

Madeline H. Renny, MD
Medical Toxicology Fellow
Division of Medical Toxicology
Ronald O. Perelman Department of Emergency Medicine
New York University School of Medicine
New York, New York
Chapter 17

Richard M. Rosenfeld, MD, MPH, MBA
Distinguished Professor and Chairman
Department of Otolaryngology
SUNY Downstate Medical Center
Brooklyn, New York
Chapter 9

Shyam K. Sathanandam, MD, FSCAI
Associate Professor of Pediatrics
Director of Large Animal Cardiovascular Research
University of Tennessee Health Science Center
Medical Director, Invasive Cardiovascular Imaging and
  Interventional Catheterization Laboratory
LeBonheur Children's Hospital
Memphis, Tennessee
Chapter 5

Suzanne M. Schmidt, MD
Assistant Professor of Pediatrics
Northwestern University Feinberg School of Medicine
Ann & Robert H. Lurie Children's Hospital of Chicago
Chicago, Illinois
Chapter 8

Kunal M. Shah, MD
Allergist/Immunologist
Allergy, Asthma & Sinus Center
Leesburg, Virginia
Chapter 7

Samir S. Shah, MD, MSCE
Director, Division of Hospital Medicine
James M. Ewell Endowed Chair
Attending Physician in Hospital Medicine & Infectious Diseases
Cincinnati Children's Hospital Medical Center
Professor, Department of Pediatrics
University of Cincinnati College of Medicine
Cincinnati, Ohio
Chapter 3

Vikas S. Shah, MD
Director, Pediatric Intensive Care
New York Health + Hospitals/Kings County
Assistant Professor of Pediatrics
SUNY Downstate Medical Center
Brooklyn, New York
Chapter 13

Roman Shinder, MD, FACS
Professor of Ophthalmology and Otolaryngology
Director of Oculoplastics
SUNY Downstate Medical Center
Brooklyn, New York
Chapter 20

Mark K. Su, MD, MPH
Clinical Associate Professor
The Ronald O. Perelman Department of Emergency Medicine
New York University School of Medicine
Director, New York City Poison Control Center
New York, New York
Chapter 17

Sathyaseelan Subramaniam, MD, FAAP
Pediatric Emergency Medicine Attending
Summerlin Hospital Medical Center
Children's Medical Center
Emergency Department
Las Vegas, Nevada
Chapter 19

Sushitha Surendran, MD
Assistant Professor of Pediatrics & Pediatric Cardiology
University of Tennessee Health Science Center
LeBonheur Children Hospital
Memphis, Tennessee
Chapter 5

Sarah F. Taber, MD
Assistant Attending Physician
Pediatric Rheumatology
Hospital for Special Surgery
Assistant Professor of Pediatrics
Weill Cornell Medical College
New York, New York
Chapter 12

Aaron L. Thatcher, MD
Assistant Professor
Department of Otolaryngology—Head & Neck Surgery
Division of Pediatric Otolaryngology
University of Michigan
Ann Arbor, Michigan
Chapter 9

Scott M. Thomas, MD, FAAP
Assistant Professor of Pediatrics
Department of Pediatrics
Saint Louis University School of Medicine
St. Louis, Missouri
Chapter 14

Neil G. Uspal, MD
Associate Professor
Department of Pediatrics, Division of Emergency Medicine
University of Washington
Attending Physician
Seattle Children's Hospital
Seattle, Washington
Chapter 10

Kusum Viswanathan, MD, FAAP
Chair, Department of Pediatrics
Director, Division of Pediatric Hematology/Oncology
Brookdale University Hospital & Medical Center
Professor of Clinical Pediatrics
New York Medical College
Brooklyn, New York
Chapter 11

Vincent J. Wang, MD, MHA
Seay Distinguished Chair in Pediatric Medicine
Professor of Pediatrics and Emergency Medicine
Division Chief, Pediatric Emergency Medicine
UT Southwestern Medical Center
Director of Emergency Services
Children's Health
Dallas, Texas
Chapter 10

Ryan Logan Webb, MD
Assistant Professor of Radiology
Zucker School of Medicine at Hofstra/Northwell
Staten Island University Hospital
Staten Island, New York
Chapter 19

Konstantinos Agoritsas, MD, MBA

Associate Chief, Emergency Medicine
Director, Pediatric Emergency Medicine
Department of Emergency Medicine
NYC Health + Hospitals/Kings County
Clinical Assistant Professor
SUNY Downstate Medical Center
Brooklyn, New York

Tahmeena Ahmed, MBBS

Assistant Professor, Department of Pathology
Stony Brook University Hospital
Stony Brook, New York

Angela C. Anderson, MD

Director, Pediatric Pain and Palliative Care
Hasbro Children's Hospital
Associate Professor of Pediatrics and Emergency Medicine
The Warren Alpert School of Medicine at Brown University
Providence, Rhode Island

Falguni Asrani, MD, FAAD

Clinical Assistant Professor of Dermatology
NYU Langone Health
Chief of Dermatology
Woodhull Hospital and Medical Center
Brooklyn, New York

Anika Backster, MD, MSCR

Department of Emergency Medicine
Emory University
Atlanta, Georgia

Carlos Barahona, MD

Attending, Pediatric Emergency Medicine
Holtz Children's Hospital
University of Miami/Jackson Memorial Medical Center
Miami, Florida

Marc N. Baskin, MD

Assistant Professor of Pediatrics
Harvard Medical School
Senior Physician in Medicine
Division of Emergency Medicine
Boston Children's Hospital
Boston, Massachusetts

Prerna Batra, MD

Professor of Pediatrics
University College of Medical Sciences
Guru Tegh Bahadur Hospital
New Delhi, India

Kirsten Bechtel, MD

Associate Professor Pediatrics and Emergency Medicine
Yale School of Medicine
New Haven, Connecticut

Christy Beneri, DO

Associate Professor of Pediatrics
Program Director, Pediatric Infectious Diseases
Stony Brook Children's Hospital
Stony Brook, New York

Cynthia L. Benson, DO, MPH, MBA

Assistant Medical Director, Emergency Department
Overlook Medical Center
Summit, New Jersey

Amrit P. Bhangoo, MD

Pediatric Endocrinologist
Children Hospital of Orange County
Assistant Clinical Professor of Pediatrics
University of California, Irvine
Irvine, California

Loring Bjornson, PhD, DABCC, FACB

Technical Director
Laboratory Operations
Northwell Health
Manhasset, New York

Stuart A. Bradin, DO, FAAP, FACEP

Associate Professor of Pediatrics and Emergency Medicine
Children's Emergency Services
The University of Michigan Health System
Ann Arbor, Michigan

David J. Brown, MD

Associate Vice President and Associate Dean for Health Equity
   and Inclusion
Associate Professor, Pediatric Otolaryngology
Michigan Medicine
Ann Arbor, Michigan

David H. Burstein, MD

Attending Physician
Summit Medical Group
Livingston, New Jersey

Sydney C. Butts, MD, FACS

Vice Chair and Associate Professor
Chief, Facial Plastic and Reconstructive Surgery
Department of Otolaryngology
SUNY Downstate Medical Center
Brooklyn, New York

Julie Cantatore-Francis, MD

Dermatology Physicians of Connecticut
Norwalk, Connecticut
Yale New Haven Hospital
Assistant Clinical Professor
Department of Dermatology
New Haven, Connecticut

Arnold Carlson Merrow, Jr., MD, FAAP

Corning Benton Chair for Radiology Education
Cincinnati Children's Hospital Medical Center
Associate Professor of Clinical Radiology
University of Cincinnati College of Medicine
Cincinnati, Ohio

Charles A. Catanese, MD

Forensic Pathologist of Ulster County New York
Department of Pathology
Westchester County Medical Center
Valhalla, New York

Praneetha Chaganti, MD, FAAP

Fellow, Pediatric Emergency Medicine
SUNY Downstate/NYC Health + Hospitals/Kings County
Brooklyn, New York

Haamid S. Chamdawala, MD, MPH

Pediatric Emergency Medicine Attending
NYC Health + Hospitals/Jacobi Medical Center
Albert Einstein College of Medicine
Bronx, New York

Jennifer H. Chao, MD, FAAP

Clinical Associate Professor
Fellowship Director, Pediatric Emergency Medicine
SUNY Downstate Medical Center
NYC Health + Hospitals/Kings County
Brooklyn, New York

Geetha Chari, MD

Clinical Professor of Neurology & Pediatrics
Clinical Neurophysiology Program Director
SUNY Downstate Medical Center
NYC Health + Hospitals/Kings County
Brooklyn, New York

Kanwal S. Chaudhry, MD

Department of Emergency Medicine
Carle Foundation Hospital
Urbana, Illinois

Susan H. Cheng, MD, MPH

Assistant Professor of Emergency Medicine
Assistant Professor of Critical Care Medicine
New York University (NYU) School of Medicine
NYU Langone-Tisch Medical Center
NYU Langone-Brooklyn Medical Center
Brooklyn, New York

Julie Cherian, MD, FACR

Assistant Professor of Pediatrics
Chief, Division of Pediatric Rheumatology
Stony Brook University Medical Center
Stony Brook Children's Hospital
Stony Brook, New York

Maria Chitty Lopez, MD

Pediatric Chief Resident
Department of Pediatrics
SUNY Downstate Medical Center
Brooklyn, New York

Jonathan Cohen, MD

Attending
Sioux Falls, North Dakota

Andrea T. Cruz, MD, MPH

Associate Professor of Pediatrics
Sections of Pediatric Emergency Medicine and Pediatric Infectious
  Diseases
Baylor College of Medicine
Texas Children's Hospital
Houston, Texas

Jeanine Daly, MD

Practicing Dermatologist
Mount Sinai Doctors Long Island
Greenlawn, New York

Ilaaf Darrat, MD, MBA

Division Head General and Pediatric Otolaryngology and
  Neurotology
Henry Ford Health System
Department of Otolaryngology Head and Neck Surgery
Clinical Assistant Professor of Otolaryngology
Wayne State University College of Medicine
Detroit, Michigan

Dawn Davis, MD

Associate Professor of Dermatology and Pediatrics
Section Head, Pediatric Dermatology
Mayo Clinic
Rochester, Minnesota

Mae De La Calzada-Jeanlouie, DO

Clinical Instructor
Department of Emergency Medicine
VA New Jersey Health Care System
Rutgers University
East Orange, New Jersey

Silvia Delgado-Villalta, MD

Assistant Professor
University of Florida
Pediatric Pulmonary Division
Gainesville, Florida

Christopher Discolo, MD, MSCR

Associate Professor
Department of Otolaryngology–Head and Neck Surgery
Director, Craniofacial Anomalies and Cleft Palate Team
Medical University of South Carolina
Charleston, South Carolina

Anastasios Drenis, MD, FAAP

Fellow, Pediatric Emergency Medicine
Cohen Children's Medical Center
New Hyde Park, New York

Donita Dyalram, DDS, MD, FACS

Assistant Professor
Associate Program Director
  Oral Maxillofacial Surgery Residency Program
Associate Fellowship Director
  Head and Neck Surgery/Microvascular Fellowship Program
University of Maryland Medical Center
R. Adams Cowley Shock Trauma Center
Baltimore, Maryland

Richard A. Falcone, Jr, MD, MPH

Associate Chief of Staff, Surgical Services
Director, Trauma Services
Professor of Surgery
Cincinnati Children's Hospital Medical Center
Cincinnati, Ohio

Yusra Farooqui, MD, FACEP

Assistant Professor
Department of Emergency Medicine
Hofstra School of Medicine
Staten Island University Hospital/Northwell Health
Staten Island, New York

Caitlin A. Farrell, MD

Instructor of Pediatrics, Harvard Medical School
Division of Emergency Medicine
Boston Children's Hospital
Boston, Massachusetts

Caitlin Feeks, DO, FAAP

Clinical Assistant Professor
Pediatric Emergency Medicine
Stony Brook Children's Hospital
Stony Brook, New York

David Fernandez, MD, PhD

Assistant Attending Physician
Hospital for Special Surgery
New York, New York

Todd A. Florin, MD, MSCE

Associate Professor of Pediatrics
Northwestern University Feinberg School of Medicine
Division of Emergency Medicine
Ann and Robert H. Lurie Children's Hospital of Chicago
Stanley Manne Children's Research Institute
Chicago, Illinois

Erin Gilbert, MD, PhD

Practicing Dermatologist
Brooklyn, New York

M.G.F. Gilliland, MD

Professor of Pathology
Department of Pathology
Brody School of Medicine
Greenville, North Carolina

Radha Giridharan, MD

Clinical Associate Professor of Neurology and Pediatrics
SUNY Downstate Medical Center
Brooklyn, New York

Yvonne P. Giunta, MD, FAAP

Division Director, Pediatric Emergency
Assistant Professor
Hofstra Northwell School of Medicine
Staten Island University Hospital/Northwell Health
Staten Island, New York

Sharon A. Glick, MD, MS

Professor of Clinical Dermatology and Pediatrics
SUNY Downstate Medical Center
Director, Pediatric Dermatology
SUNY Downstate, NYC Health + Hospitals/Kings County and
   Maimonides Medical Center
Brooklyn, New York

Nira A. Goldstein, MD, MPH

Professor of Clinical Otolaryngology
SUNY Downstate Medical Center
NYC Health + Hospitals/Kings County
Brooklyn, New York

Samridhi Goyal, MD

Senior Resident
Department of Pediatrics
Lady Hardinge Medical College and Kalawati Saran Children
   Hospital
New Delhi, India

Howard A. Greller, MD, FACEP, FACMT

Affiliated Medical Professor
Department of Clinical Medicine
CUNY School of Medicine
Director of Research
Director of Medical Toxicology
Department of Emergency Medicine
SBH Health System
Bronx, New York

Raavi Gupta, MD

Associate Professor
Department of Pathology
SUNY Downstate Medical Center
Brooklyn, New York

Allysia Guy, MD, RDMS, FACEP

Director of Emergency Ultrasonography, Littleton Regional
   Hospital
Consulting Director of POCUS at North Country Healthcare
   Systems
Littleton Regional Hospital–North Country Healthcare
Littleton, New Hampshire

Barry Hahn, MD, FACEP

Department of Emergency Medicine
Staten Island University Hospital/Northwell Health
Staten Island, New York

Jeanine E. Hall, MD, FAAP

Associate Director of Process Improvement
Division of Emergency Medicine
Children's Hospital Los Angeles
Assistant Professor of Pediatrics
University of Southern California Keck School of Medicine
Los Angeles, California

Karen Hammerman, MD

Practicing Dermatologist
Forest Hills, New York

Earl R. Hartwig, MD, FAAP

Education Director, Pediatric Emergency Medicine
Clinical Associate Professor of Pediatrics and Emergency Medicine
Wayne State University School of Medicine
Children's Hospital of Michigan,
Detroit, Michigan

Amanda Hassler, MD, FAAD

Practicing Dermatologist
Houston, Texas

Ameer Hassoun, MD

Director, Pediatric Emergency Medicine
Department of Emergency Medicine
New York-Presbyterian Queens
Clinical Assistant Professor
Weill Cornell Medical College
New York, New York

Sarah Hilkert Rodriguez, MD, MPH

Department of Ophthalmology and Visual Science
The University of Chicago Medicine and Biological Sciences
Chicago, Illinois

Tanya S. Hinds, MD, FAAP
Child Abuse Pediatrician
Child and Adolescent Protection Center
Children's National Health System
Assistant Professor of Pediatrics
The George Washington University School of Medicine and
  Health Sciences
Washington, DC

Robert J. Hoffman, MD, MS
Medical Director, Qatar Poison Center
Program Director, Medical Toxicology
Department of Emergency Medicine
Sidra Medicine
Doha, Qatar

Robert S. Hoffman, MD, FAACT, FACMT
Director, Division of Medical Toxicology
Ronald O. Perelman Department of Emergency Medicine
NYU School of Medicine
New York, New York

Mark Horowitz, MD, FACS, FAAP
Associate Professor of Urology, Northwell Health
Chief, Division of Pediatric Urology
Staten Island University Hospital
Attending Pediatric Urology
Cohen Children's Medical Center

Allison M. Jackson, MD, MPH, FAAP
Division Chief, Child & Adolescent Protection Center
Children's National Health System
Washington Children's Foundation Professor of Child and
  Adolescent Protection
Associate Professor of Pediatrics
The George Washington University School of Medicine and Health
  Sciences
Washington, DC

Jeannette Jakus, MD, MBA, FAAP, FAAD
Director of Clinical Research
Clinical Assistant Professor
Department of Dermatology
SUNY Downstate Medical Center
Brooklyn, New York

Aditi Jayanth, MD, FAAP
Clinical Assistant Professor
SUNY Downstate Medical Center
NYC Health + Hospitals/Kings County
Brooklyn, New York

Angela Jeffries, MD, MSc
Assistant Professor
University of Louisville
Pediatric Gastroenterology
Department of Pediatrics
Louisville, Kentucky

Lamont R. Jones, MD, MBA
Vice Chair
Department of Otolaryngology–Head and Neck Surgery
Facial Plastic and Reconstructive Surgery
Director, Cleft and Craniofacial Clinic
Henry Ford Hospital
Detroit, Michigan

Majo Joseph, MD, FAAP
Associate Director, Pediatric Emergency Department
The Brooklyn Hospital Center
Brooklyn, New York

Nikita Joshi, MD
Assistant Professor
Alameda Health System
Oakland, California

Ernesto Jose Jule, MD
Associate Director Emeritus
Pediatric Emergency Medicine
NYC Health + Hospitals/Kings County
Brooklyn, New York

Raffi Kapitanyan, MD, FACEP
Brunswick Urgent Care
Franklin Park, New Jersey

Vania L. Kasper, MD
Assistant Professor of Pediatrics, Clinician Educator
Warren Alpert Medical School of Brown University
Director of the Children's Center for Liver Disease
Medical Director of the CHANGES Program
Department of Pediatric Gastroenterology, Nutrition, and Liver
  Disease
Hasbro Children's Hospital
Providence, Rhode Island

Gurpreet Kaur, MD
Pediatric resident
SUNY Downstate Medical Center
Brooklyn, New York

Viktoryia Kazlouskaya, MD, PhD
Dermatology Resident
SUNY Downstate Medical Center
Brooklyn, New York

Maria C. Kessides, MD
The Permanente Medical Group
Oakland, California

Ambreen S. Khan, MD
Assistant Professor, Department of Emergency Medicine
Associate Director, Pediatric Emergency Medicine Fellowship
Director, Pediatric Emergency Medicine Elective MS 3 and MS 4
Clinical Skills Instructor, MS 1 and MS 2
SUNY Downstate Medical Center
NYC Health + Hospitals/Kings County
Brooklyn, New York

Smita N. Kumar, MD, MPH
Senior Newborn Advisor with USAID
Washington, District of Columbia

Moshe Kupferstein, DO
Practicing Pediatrician, Brooklyn
Attending, Department of Pediatrics
Good Samaritan Hospital
Suffern, New York

Karen Kwan, MD

Resident and Medical Student Director
Emergency and Transport Medicine
Children's Hospital Los Angeles
Assistant Professor of Pediatrics
Keck School of Medicine/University of Southern California
Los Angeles, CA

Brian I. Labow, MD, FACS, FAAP

Associate Professor of Surgery
Harvard Medical School
Department of Plastic and Oral Surgery
Boston Children's Hospital
Boston, Massachusetts

Douglas R. Lazzaro, MD, MBA, FACS

Professor and Vice Chairman of Operations, Clinical Affairs and
    Business Development
Department of Ophthalmology
Physician Director of Brooklyn Network Development, NYU
    Langone Health
NYU School of Medicine
New York, New York

Alexandra Leonard, MSIV

Albany Medical College
Albany, New York

Rachel Levene, MD, MEd

Pediatric Chief Resident
SUNY Downstate Medical Center
Brooklyn, New York

Michael D. Levine, MD

Associate Professor of Emergency Medicine
Chief, Division of Medical Toxicology
Department of Emergency Medicine
University of Southern California
Los Angeles, California

Tian Liang, MD

Fellow, Pediatric Emergency Medicine
Department of Emergency Medicine
SUNY Downstate Medical Center
Brooklyn, New York

Miriam R. Lieberman, MD

Dermatology Resident
SUNY Downstate Medical Center
Brooklyn, New York

Jessyka G. Lighthall, MD

Director, Facial Plastic and Reconstructive Surgery
Assistant Professor, Otolaryngology-Head and Neck Surgery
Penn State Health-Milton S. Hershey Medical Center
Hershey, Pennsylvania

James G. Linakis, PhD, MD

Associate Director for Academics, Pediatric Emergency Medicine
Hasbro Children's Hospital/Rhode Island Hospital
Professor of Emergency Medicine and Pediatrics
The Alpert Medical School of Brown University
Providence, Rhode Island

David B. Liss, MD

Assistant Professor of Emergency Medicine
Section of Medical Toxicology
Division of Emergency Medicine
Washington University School of Medicine
St. Louis, Missouri

Deborah R. Liu, MD

Associate Division Head
Division of Emergency Medicine
Children's Hospital Los Angeles
Associate Professor of Pediatrics
Keck School of Medicine/University of Southern California
Los Angeles, California

Julia K. Lloyd, MD

Assistant Professor
The Ohio State University
Department of Pediatrics
Nationwide Children's Hospital
Columbus, Ohio

Eve Lowenstein, MD, PhD, FAAD

Director, Medical Dermatology
Clinical Professor of Dermatology
SUNY Downstate Medical Center/Kings County Hospital
Associate, South Nassau Dermatology PC
Oceanside and Long Beach, New York

Michael Lucchesi, MD, MS

Professor and Chairman
Department of Emergency Medicine
Interim Dean, College of Medicine
SUNY Downstate Medical Center
Chief Medical Officer
University Hospital of Brooklyn
Brooklyn, New York

Rabia Malik, MD

Pediatric Emergency Medicine Fellow
Yale-New Haven Hospital
New Haven, Connecticut

Andrea Marmor, MD, MSEd

Professor of Pediatrics
University of California, San Francisco
Zuckerberg San Francisco General Hospital
San Francisco, California

Brian P. Marr, MD

Director of Ophthalmic Oncology
NewYork-Presbyterian/Columbia University Medical Center
New York, New York

Daniel R. Mazori, MD

Dermatology Resident
SUNY Downstate Medical Center
Brooklyn, New York

Swati Mehta, MD

Clinical Assistant Professor of Pediatrics
SUNY Downstate Medical Center
NYC Health + Hospitals/Kings County
Brooklyn, New York

Dimpy Mody, MD
Pediatric Chief Resident
SUNY Downstate Medical Center
Brooklyn, New York

Anil Mongia, MD, DCH, FAAP
Associate Professor of Pediatrics
Fellowship Director, Division of Pediatric Nephrology
SUNY Downstate Medical Center
Brooklyn, New York

Shella K. Mongia, MD
Laboratory Medical Director
ICON Laboratories
Farmingdale, New York

Cindy Moran, BS
Scientific Operations Director
Arkansas State Crime Laboratory
Little Rock, Arkansas

Joshua Nagler, MD, MHPEd
Fellowship Director
Associate Division Chief
Division of Emergency Medicine
Boston Children's Hospital
Assistant Professor of Pediatrics and Emergency Medicine
Harvard Medical School
Boston, Massachusetts

Trushar Naik, MD, MBA
Attending Physician, Advocate Medical Group
Department of Emergency Medicine and Internal Medicine
Advocate Christ Medical Center
Oak Lawn, Illinois

Stephen E. Nanton, MD
Clinical Associate Professor of Pediatrics and Internal Medicine
Sanford School of Medicine
The University of South Dakota
Director, Pediatric Gastroenterology
Avera Children's Hospital
Sioux Falls, South Dakota

Rita Nathawad, MD, MSc-GHP, FAAP
Assistant Professor of Pediatrics
Medical Director, Jacksonville Health and Transition Services
University of Florida, College of Medicine
Jacksonville, Florida

Farzana Nuruzzaman, MD, FACR
Assistant Professor of Clinical Pediatrics
Stony Brook University School of Medicine
Division of Pediatric Rheumatology, Department of Pediatrics
Stony Brook Children's Hospital
Stony Brook, New York

Daniel Ostro, MD, FAAP
Mackenzie Health Hospital
Richmond Hill, Ontario, Canada

Kathryn H. Pade, MD
Assistant Professor of Pediatrics
Rady Children's Hospital
University of California San Diego
San Diego, California

Bipin Patel, MD, FAAP
Chairman, Department of Pediatrics
Physician-in-Chief, The Children's Hospital
Saint Peter's University Hospital
New Brunswick, New Jersey

Mario Peichev, MD
Attending Hematologist
Department of Pediatrics
Brookdale University Hospital Medical Center
Brooklyn, New York
Richmond University Medical Center
Staten Island, New York

Shahina Qureshi, MD
Practicing Pediatrician and Hematologist
Queens, New York

Morgan Rabach, MD
Assistant Professor of Dermatology
The Icahn School of Medicine at Mount Sinai
New York, New York

Bahram Rahmani, MD, MPH
Ann & Robert H. Lurie Children's Hospital of Chicago
Associate Professor of Ophthalmology
Feinberg School of Medicine, Northwestern University
Chicago, Illinois

Chandrakant Rao, MD
Clinical Associate Professor Emeritus
Department of Pathology
SUNY Downstate Medical Center
NYC Health + Hospitals/Kings County
Brooklyn, New York

Sudha M. Rao, MD
Director, Pediatric Cardiology
NYC Health + Hospitals/Kings County
Clinical Associate Professor of Pediatrics
NYU Langone Health
New York, New York

Shashidhar Rao Marneni, MD
Clinical Assistant Professor
University of Texas Southwestern Medical Center
Dallas, Texas

Yagnaram Ravichandran, MD, FAAP
Fellow, Pediatric Emergency Medicine
Children's Hospital of Michigan/Detroit Medical Center
Detroit, Michigan

Madeline H. Renny, MD
Medical Toxicology Fellow
Division of Medical Toxicology
Ronald O. Perelman Department of Emergency Medicine
New York University School of Medicine
New York, New York

Daniel J. Repplinger, MD
Assistant Clinical Professor
Department of Emergency Medicine
University of California, San Francisco
Zuckerberg San Francisco General Hospital
San Francisco, California

Christy Riley, MD
Practicing Pediatrician
Coeur D Alene, Idaho

Richard M. Rosenfeld, MD, MPH, MBA
Distinguished Professor and Chairman
Department of Otolaryngology
SUNY Downstate Medical Center
Brooklyn, New York

Mandakini Sadhir, MD FAAP
Assistant Professor of Pediatrics
Division of Adolescent Medicine
University of Kentucky
Lexington, Kentucky

Abhijeet Saha, MD
Professor of Pediatrics
Fellow, International Pediatric Nephrology Association
Fellow, International Society of Peritoneal Dialysis
Lady Hardinge Medical College and Kalawati Saran Children's
    Hospital
New Delhi, India

Shyam K. Sathanandam, MD, FSCAI
Associate Professor of Pediatrics
Director of Large Animal Cardiovascular Research
University of Tennessee Health Science Center
Medical Director, Invasive Cardiovascular Imaging and
    Interventional Catheterization Laboratory
LeBonheur Children's Hospital
Memphis, Tennessee

Heather Schultz, MD, FAAD
Practicing Dermatologist
Yonkers, New York

Janet Semple-Hess, MD
Attending Physician
Division of Emergency Medicine
Children's Hospital Los Angeles
Assistant Professor of Pediatrics
Keck School of Medicine/University of Southern California
Los Angeles, California

Binita R. Shah, MD, FAAP
Distinguished Professor of Emergency Medicine and Pediatrics
SUNY Downstate Medical Center
Director Emeritus, Pediatric Emergency Medicine
Kings County Hospital Center
Brooklyn, New York

Kunal M. Shah, MD
Allergist/Immunologist
Allergy, Asthma, and Sinus Center
Leesburg, Virginia

Rajni P. Shah, MD
Rheumatologist
New Hyde Park, New York

Ronak R. Shah, MD
Attending Physician of Emergency Medicine
Winchester Medical Center
Winchester, Virginia

Samir S. Shah, MD, MSCE
Director, Division of Hospital Medicine
James M. Ewell Endowed Chair
Attending Physician in Hospital Medicine and Infectious Diseases
Cincinnati Children's Hospital Medical Center
Professor, Department of Pediatrics
University of Cincinnati College of Medicine
Cincinnati, Ohio

Toral Shah, BS, PA-C
Division of Gastroenterology
NYU Langone Health/Bellevue Hospital Center
New York, New York

Vikas S. Shah, MD
Director, Pediatric Intensive Care
New York Health + Hospitals/Kings County
Assistant Professor of Pediatrics
SUNY Downstate Medical Center
Brooklyn, New York

Joanne Sheu, MD
Clinical Assistant Instructor
Department of Obstetrics and Gynecology
SUNY Downstate Medical Center
Brooklyn, New York

Roman Shinder, MD, FACS
Professor of Ophthalmology and Otolaryngology
Director of Oculoplastics
SUNY Downstate Medical Center
Brooklyn, New York

Haseeb A. Siddiqi, PhD
Director, Diagnostic Immunology and Clinical Parasitology
    Laboratories
NYC Health + Hospitals/Kings County
Professor
Departments of Medicine, Pathology, and Cell Biology
SUNY Downstate Medical Center
Brooklyn, New York

Sadie De Silva, MSIV
St. George's University School of Medicine
St. George's, Grenada

Lawrence Silverberg, DPM
Beth Israel Medical Center
New York, New York

Mark Silverberg, MD, MMB, FACEP
Associate Professor of Emergency Medicine
Associate Residency Director
Department of Emergency Medicine
SUNY Downstate Medical Center
New York Health + Hospitals/Kings County
Brooklyn, New York

Anup Singh, MD
Chief, Division of Pediatric Nephrology
The Children's Hospital at Saint Peter's University Hospital
Clinical Associate Professor
Rutgers Robert Wood Johnson Medical school
New Brunswick, New Jersey

Bhuvanesh Singh, MD, PhD

Attending Surgeon
Memorial Sloan-Kettering Cancer Center
New York, New York

Deeptej Singh, MD, FAAD

Clinical Assistant Professor of Dermatology
University of New Mexico School of Medicine
Albuquerque, New Mexico

Raj Pal Singh, MD

Senior Specialist, Pediatrics
Vindhya Hospital
NTPC Vindhyanagar
Singrauli, India

Arpan Sinha, MBBS, MD

Assistant Professor
Division of Pediatric Hematology/Oncology
The Jimmy Everest Center for Cancer and Blood Disorders in
  Children
University of Oklahoma Health Sciences Center
Oklahoma City, Oklahoma

Virteeka Sinha, MD, FAAP

Assistant Professor
Pediatric Emergency Medicine
Department of Emergency Medicine
Rutgers New Jersey Medical School
Newark, New Jersey

Mark Spektor, DO, MBA, FACEP

Chief Medical Officer of Clover Health
Jersey City, New Jersey & San Francisco, California

Neil Sperling, MD

Assistant Attending Otolaryngologist
New York Presbyterian Hospital
Adjunct Associate Professor of Otolaryngology
SUNY Downstate Medical Center
Brooklyn, New York

Jessica Stetz, MD MS

Associate Professor of Clinical Emergency Medicine
Department of Emergency Medicine
SUNY Downstate Medical Center
Brooklyn, New York

Michael Stracher, MD

New York Surgical Specialists
Fresh Meadows, New York
Attending Physician, Orthopaedic Surgery
Jamaica Hospital Medical Center
Jamaica, New York

Mark K. Su, MD, MPH

Clinical Associate Professor
The Ronald O. Perelman Department of Emergency Medicine
New York University School of Medicine
Director, New York City Poison Control Center
New York, New York

Sathyaseelan Subramaniam, MD, FAAP

Pediatric Emergency Medicine Attending
Summerlin Hospital Medical Center
Children's Medical Center
Las Vegas, Nevada

Sushitha Surendran, MD

Assistant Professor of Pediatrics and Pediatric Cardiology
University of Tennessee Health Science Center
Le Bonheur Children's Hospital
Memphis, Tennessee

TK Susheel Kumar, MD

Associate Professor
Congenital Cardiothoracic Surgery
New York University Medical Center
New York, New York

Darien Sutton-Ramsey, MD, MBA

Emergency Medicine Resident
Ronald O. Perelman Department of Emergency Medicine
NYU Langone Health/Bellevue Hospital Center
New York, New York

Amir H. Taghinia, MD, MPH, MBA

Staff Surgeon, Department of Plastic and Oral Surgery
Boston Children's Hospital
Assistant Professor of Surgery
Harvard Medical School
Boston, Massachusetts

Ee Tein Tay, MD

Assistant Professor of Emergency Medicine and Pediatrics
Clinical Site Director, Bellevue Hospital Pediatric Emergency
  Services
NYU Langone Health/Bellevue Hospital Center
New York, New York

Nooruddin Tejani MD, FAAP

Director, Pediatric Emergency Medicine
Assistant Professor, Department of Emergency Medicine
SUNY-Downstate Medical Center
Brooklyn, New York

Svetlana Ten, MD

Pediatric Endocrinologist
Brooklyn, New York

Mihir M. Thacker, MD

Associate Professor of Orthopedics and Pediatrics
Thomas Jefferson University Philadelphia, Pennsylvania
Attending, Pediatric Orthopaedic Surgeon and Orthopedic
  Oncologist
Nemours Alfred I. duPont Hospital for Children
Wilmington, Delaware

Jonathan Thackeray, MD

Chief Medical Community Health Officer
Professor and Vice-Chair, Department of Pediatrics
Wright State University Boonshoft School of Medicine
Dayton Children's Hospital
Dayton, Ohio

Aaron L. Thatcher, MD

Assistant Professor
Department of Otolaryngology–Head and Neck Surgery
Division of Pediatric Otolaryngology
University of Michigan
Ann Arbor, Michigan

Mark K. Thompson, MD, FAANS, FACS
President, Cerebrospinal Neurosurgical Specialties
New York, New York

Matthew T. Timberger, MD
Attending, Department of Emergency Medicine
Falmouth Hospital
Cape Cod Healthcare
Falmouth, Massachusetts

Chika Ugorji, MD
Pediatric Dermatology Research Fellow
Department of Dermatology
SUNY Downstate Medical Center
Brooklyn, New York

Neil G. Uspal, MD
Associate Professor
Department of Pediatrics, Division of Emergency Medicine
University of Washington
Attending, Seattle Children's Hospital
Seattle, Washington

Kusum Viswanathan, MD, FAAP
Chair, Department of Pediatrics
Director, Division of Pediatric Hematology/Oncology
Brookdale University Hospital & Medical Center
Professor of Clinical Pediatrics
New York Medical College
Brooklyn, New York

Kathleen E. Walsh-Spoonhower, MD
Assistant Professor of Clinical Pediatrics
Division of Pediatric Cardiology
Stony Brook Children's Hospital
Stony Brook, New York

Diana E. Weaver, MD, FAAP
Assistant Professor of Pediatrics
SUNY Downstate Medical Center
Director, Pediatric Pulmonology and Asthma Service
NYC Health + Hospitals/Kings County
Brooklyn, New York

Rachel Weiselberg, MD
Attending, Department of Emergency Medicine
Northwell Health at Syosset Hospital
Syosset, New York

David P. Witte, MD
Professor of Pathology
University of Cincinnati College of Medicine
Division Director, Division of Pathology and Laboratory Medicine
Children's Hospital Medical Center
Cincinnati, Ohio

RADIOGRAPHY CREDITS

John Amodio, MD, FACR

Chief, Pediatric Radiology
Cohen Children's Medical Center
System Chief, Pediatric Radiology
Northwell Health System
Professor of Radiology
Zucker/Hofstra School of Medicine
New Hyde Park, New York

Jesse Chen, MD

Radiology Resident
Staten Island University Hospital/Northwell Health
Staten Island, New York

Thomas J. Chi, MD, FACEP

Director Emergency Ultrasound, Middlesex Health
Middletown, Connecticut

Danielle Del Re, DO

Radiology Resident
Staten Island University Hospital/Northwell Health
Staten Island, New York

David S. Dinhofer, MD

Chief Executive Officer, Advanced Medical Imaging and
    Informatics
Paramus, New Jersey

Philip Dydynski, MD

Chief Radiologist
Norton Children's Hospital
Assistant Professor
University of Louisville
Louisville, Kentucky

Daniel M. Eisman, MD

Radiology Resident
Staten Island University Hospital/Northwell Health
Staten Island, New York

Gregory N. Emmanuel, MD

Radiology Resident
Staten Island University Hospital/Northwell Health
Staten Island, New York

Ami Gokli, MD

Associate Program Director
Radiology Residency and Fellowship Program
Children's Hospital of Philadelphia
Instructor of Clinical Radiology
Perelman School of Medicine at the University of Pennsylvania
Philadelphia, Pennsylvania

Rachelle Goldfisher, MD

Assistant Professor of Radiology
Cohen Children's Medical Center/Northwell Health
New Hyde Park, New York

Josh Greenstein, MD

Director of Ultrasound Division
Associate Research Director
Department of Emergency Medicine
Assistant Professor
Zucker School of Medicine at Hofstra/Northwell Health
Staten Island University Hospital/Northwell Health
Staten Island, New York

John P. Gullett, MD

Associate Professor
Co-Director of Emergency Ultrasound
Department of Emergency Medicine
University of Alabama at Birmingham School of Medicine
Birmingham, Alabama

Richard Hong, MD

Assistant Professor of Radiology
Cohen Children's Medical Center/Northwell Health
New Hyde Park, New York

Marlena Jbara, MD

Attending Faculty, Musculoskeletal Radiology
Assistant Professor of Radiology
Zucker School of Medicine at Hofstra/Northwell Health
Staten Island University Hospital/Northwell Health
Staten Island, New York

Dan Klein, MD

Attending Faculty, Neuroradiology
Assistant Professor of Radiology
Zucker School of Medicine at Hofstra/Northwell Health
Staten Island University Hospital/Northwell Health
Staten Island, New York

Brandon Z. Lei, MD

Radiology Resident
Staten Island University Hospital/Northwell Health
Staten Island, New York

Cheryl H. Lin, MD

Section Chief, General Ultrasonography
Attending faculty, Musculoskeletal Radiology
Assistant Clinical Professor of Radiology
Zucker School of Medicine at Hofstra/Northwell Health
Staten Island University Hospital/Northwell Health
Staten Island, New York

Berenice Lopez Leal, MD

Radiology Resident
Staten Island University Hospital/Northwell Health
Staten Island, New York

Daniel Luu, MD

Radiology Resident
Staten Island University Hospital/Northwell Health
Staten Island, New York

Varun Mehta, MD

Radiology Resident
Staten Island University Hospital/Northwell Health
Staten Island, New York

Eric Minkin, MD

Department of Radiology
Brookdale University Hospital Medical Center
Brooklyn, New York

Jeremy Neuman, MD

Director of Pediatric Radiology
Staten Island University Hospital/Northwell Health
Staten Island, New York

Dimitrios Papanagnou, MD, MPH
Associate Professor and Vice Chair for Education
Department of Emergency Medicine
Associate Dean for Faculty Development
Sidney Kimmel Medical College at Thomas Jefferson University
Philadelphia, Pennsylvania

Jay Pershad, MD, MMM
Clinical Chief, Emergency Medicine
Children's National Medical Center
Professor of Pediatrics & Emergency Medicine
George Washington University
Washington, DC

Daniel Portal, MD
Radiology Resident
Department of Radiology
Staten Island University Hospital/Northwell Health
Staten Island, New York

Steven Pulitzer, MD
Chief Medical Officer
NYC Health + Hospitals/Kings County
Assistant Professor of Radiology
SUNY Downstate Medical Center
Brooklyn, New York

Mark Raden, MD
Chairman, Department of Radiology
Director of Neuroradiology
Assistant Professor of Radiology
Zucker School of Medicine at Hofstra/Northwell
Staten Island University Hospital/Northwell Health
Staten Island, New York

Amit Ramjit, MD
Radiology Resident
Staten Island University Hospital/Northwell Health
Staten Island, New York

Mantosh S. Rattan, MD
Assistant Professor of Radiology
Cincinnati Children's Hospital Medical Center
Cincinnati, Ohio

Rafael Rivera, MD, MBA
Assistant Professor of Radiology
Associate Dean for Admissions and Financial Aid
NYU Langone Health
New York, New York

David Sarkany, MD, MS-HPEd
Program Director of Radiology Residency
Associate Professor
Zucker School of Medicine at Hofstra/Northwell Health
Staten Island University Hospital/Northwell Health
Staten Island, New York

Michael Secko, MD, RDMS, FACEP
Clinical Associate Professor of Emergency Medicine
Division Chief, Emergency Ultrasound
Stony Brook University Hospital
Stony Brook, New York

Michael H. Siegel, MD
Emeritus Clinical Assistant Professor
Department of Radiology
SUNY Downstate Medical Center
Brooklyn, New York

Jonathan N. Stern, MD
Radiology Resident
Staten Island University Hospital/Northwell Health
Staten Island, New York

Michael Stone, MD
Northwest Acute Care Specialists
Legacy Emanuel Medical Center
Portland, Oregon

James W. Tsung, MD, MPH
Professor of Emergency Medicine and Pediatrics
Icahn School of Medicine at Mount Sinai
New York, New York

Vinodkumar Velayudhan, DO
Radiology Residency Associate Program Director
Clinical Associate Professor of Radiology and Neurology
SUNY Downstate Medical Center
Director of Neuroradiology, NYC Health + Hospitals/Kings County
Brooklyn, NY

Ryan Logan Webb, MD
Assistant Professor of Radiology
Zucker School of Medicine at Hofstra/Northwell Health
Staten Island University Hospital/Northwell Health
Staten Island, New York

Sharon Yellin, MD, FAAP
Pediatric Emergency Ultrasound Director
Pediatric Emergency Medicine
Department of Emergency Medicine
New York Presbyterian
Brooklyn Methodist Hospital
Brooklyn, New York

Daniel Zinn, MD
Assistant Professor of Radiology
SUNY Downstate Medical Center
Brooklyn, New York

FOREWORD

This masterpiece marks two landmark events. First, the formulation of a collection of over 40 years of Pediatrics and Pediatric Emergency Medicine captured poignantly in patient photographs, coupled in a complementary fashion with pearls of wisdom that are sure to enlighten, educate and rejuvenate even the most accomplished clinician. Second, the culmination of a remarkable career spanning more than four decades. Doctor Binita R. Shah positively influenced the lives of hundreds of thousands of children and their families. She did so in a seemingly effortless and fluid fashion that at times could only be described as magical, while teaching thousands of residents and faculty including me, the true art of medicine and healing.

In every one of the 1136 pages of this *Atlas*, you can feel Dr. Shah's passion for teaching, incomparable enthusiasm, energy and zeal coupled with her unparalleled love and respect for her patients and her students. As her final contribution to the medical field just before her retirement, Dr. Shah has assembled national and international experts to join her in presenting this work of art to you. She has collaborated with seasoned co-editors and co-authors to brilliantly and methodically compile decades of collective bedside clinical expertise into one easily accessible reference.

In an era when so much is "on-line" or electronically accessed, discriminating healthcare providers will surely embrace these dynamic pages, the human stories they tell, the medical lessons they convey, and the pearls of wisdom they impart.

Karen Santucci, MD FAAP
Professor of Pediatrics and Emergency Medicine
Vice Chair for Clinical Affairs, Department of Pediatrics
Yale University School of Medicine
Chief, Pediatric Emergency Medicine
Yale New Haven Children's Hospital
New Haven, Connecticut
and
Forever a grateful student of Dr. Binita R. Shah

Emergency care is a highly complex, cognitively demanding specialty that is often challenging because providers work in time-, resource-, and information-constrained settings while caring for patients whose illnesses are still evolving. In the United States alone, there are approximately 145 million annual visits to EDs and many more to urgent care settings. The pressures of clinical practice continue to increase with demands on productivity in the face of decreasing reimbursement and a steadily rising volume of patients. All these factors unfortunately have "contaminated" the "art" of medicine (ie, arrival at a diagnosis after careful and comprehensive clinical examination) with the "knee jerk" aspect of indiscriminate ordering of tests to arrive at the diagnosis. The diagnostic process is even more complex in the context of pediatric emergency care not only because of the spectrum of physiological, anatomical, and psychological differences compared with adults but also because many clinicians are uncomfortable with pediatric patients, are inadequately trained, or work in settings that do not have population-specific management resources. The dangers of over- or under-diagnosis, over- or under-testing, or over- or under-treatment is the risk of patient harm. Injury to patients due to diagnostic mishaps is currently recognized as the most important yet understudied aspect of patient safety (ie, "the blind spot" in the patient safety movement.) The National Academies of Science, Engineering, and Medicine has highlighted the importance of making a timely and accurate diagnosis.

The endeavour of my co-editors and me in revising the *Atlas of Pediatric Emergency Medicine* is to continue to empower the clinician with a readily accessible and highly relevant resource to make a timely and accurate diagnosis.

Instead of the dense prose of traditional textbooks, this *Atlas* features a consistent format organized as a *Clinical Summary, Emergency Department Treatment and Disposition*, and *Pearls* ("must-know" clinical essentials) for each topic. Side by side with this easy-to-read text is a wealth of images illustrating how these clinical problems look in real life in an emergency setting. By using a high-yield text, we have been fortunate to include more than 2000 images in this edition, greatly enhancing the original work. All 21 sections have been updated with many newly added entities that are applicable to the practice of pediatric emergencies. We have updated the *Atlas* with the most current imaging techniques available in the emergency setting. Chapter 21 on emergency ultrasound as well as other sections where point-of-care ultrasound (PoCUS) is applicable have been updated because the impact of ultrasound in pediatric emergency medicine care delivery has exponentially increased since the second edition of our *Atlas*. While PoCUS helps answer a focused clinical question, our reliance on additional imaging remains a crucial part of arriving at the most likely diagnosis. Thus, many entities are presented with CT and/or MRI images. We continue to remain cognizant and enthusiastically supportive of the medical and lay communities who are radiation conscious and cautious. Hopefully, advances in ultrasound technology, such as contrast-enhanced sonography and elastography, will play greater roles in the pediatric ED in the future.

Working in the environment of the ED, we have accumulated a plethora of clinical pathology that enhances and finely tunes our visual diagnostic skills. Armed with a camera and a consent form, we were able to build a library of educational material in the form of clinical pictures, radiographic images, and fascinating stories. With these assets, we prepared the first edition of the *Atlas of Pediatric Emergency Medicine* (2006) and have been humbled and extremely pleased by the enthusiastic response of our readers. Based upon that response, we published the second edition (2013), also translated into Spanish (2014). Nationally and internationally known experts in pediatric emergency care have contributed their expertise to enhance the impact of this third edition.

This *Atlas* is written for anyone who has the privilege of taking care of acutely ill and/or injured children. It is designed with the end-user in mind. We hope our experience and images will aid all dedicated practitioners in their efforts to hone their visual diagnostic and differential diagnosis skills and help clinicians to avoid the pitfalls that occur when the "art" is lost.

We are committed to keeping the art of visual diagnosis off the endangered species list and keeping it as the highlight of our clinical day. Our trainees are being schooled in processing flow and survival mode ideation. The following quotation by Sir William Osler has always influenced our approach at the bedside while caring for patients: "*Don't touch the patient . . . state first what you see; cultivate your powers of observation.*"

The familiar old adages "*A picture is worth a thousand words*" and "*I cannot define an elephant but I know one when I see one*" underscore the benefits of learning from photographs. The student of visual diagnosis is not only more likely to make the right diagnosis but is also more likely to avoid costly errors. We urge our fellow physicians to treasure this art.

Ars longa vita brevis (Art is long while life is short). With this quote, Hippocrates reminds us how much there is to learn in a short period and thereby (hopefully) inspires us to be humble, scholarly, and better clinicians.

Binita R. Shah, MD, FAAP
Prashant Mahajan, MD, MPH, MBA
John Amodio, MD, FACR
Michael Lucchesi, MD, MS

ACKNOWLEDGMENTS

First and foremost, we are indebted to our patients and their families. In spite of their sufferings, they gave us permission to take their photographs without any reservations. *They are the unsung heroes of this book.* We salute them for giving us the privilege of taking care of them and for their kindness in allowing us to learn from them and teach others. We trust that with this *Atlas* we are in some way repaying the great debt we owe to our patients.

Next, we express our deepest gratitude to all the contributing authors and photography and radiography contributors for making this *Atlas* an enormous encyclopedia of pathology. Their untiring efforts and dedication to this *Atlas* and its previous editions (for many) are responsible for this *Atlas*. We have learned so much from all of you during this collaboration—*thank you*! In addition, we are grateful to all the fellows, residents, and medical students who rotate through emergency and radiology departments, and to our colleagues and nursing staff of the emergency and radiology departments. They have constantly stimulated us by challenging us. Learning from each other as we work together has been a privilege and very rewarding. *We thank you all.*

We express our heartfelt gratitude to Amanda Fielding and Kay Conerly (Senior Editors) and Christie Naglieri (Senior Project Development Editor) for their countless hours in helping us in the creation of this revised edition of the *Atlas*. Their unflinching encouragement and inspiring phone calls were a big motivation (at first dreaded, and then understood as a shared commitment to producing the best revision possible). Without their help, this *Atlas* would not have come to fruition. We also extend our sincere appreciation to Leah Carton (Editorial Assistant), Sheryl Krato (Permissions Coordinator), Catherine Saggese (Senior Production Supervisor), and Jeffrey Herzich (Director of Production) for shepherding the manuscript through the production process.

I extend my gratitude also to Brian Belval (Ex-Executive Editor) for his perseverance in convincing me to continue serving as an editor-in-chief for this edition and mentoring contributors for the challenging endeavor of serving as future editors for this *Atlas*, so that even after my retirement, this legacy continues!

Our heartfelt gratitude goes to Revathi Viswanathan (Senior Project Manager; Cenveo Publisher Services) and her entire team for doing an extraordinary job. All our editorial suggestions in the page proofs were welcomed with one expression "Sure thing!" We could feel Revathi's willingness "to walk an extra mile," handling a complex manuscript incorporating more than 2000 figures and turning it into an elegant book. *Revathi, we salute you and your entire team!*

Last but not the least, we thank the thousands of readers who have found the previous editions of the *Atlas* a very valuable resource, for their suggestions and praise inspiring us to take on the challenge of a third edition. The Spanish translation of the second edition also became a driving force for us. We hope that you will find this edition equally valuable.

Binita R. Shah, MD, FAAP
Prashant Mahajan, MD, MPH, MBA
John Amodio, MD, FACR
Michael Lucchesi, MD, MS

Chapter 1

NONACCIDENTAL TRAUMA

Earl R. Hartwig

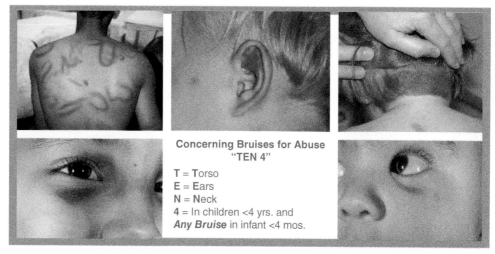

Concerning Bruises for Abuse
"TEN 4"

T = **T**orso
E = **E**ars
N = **N**eck
4 = In children <4 yrs. and
Any Bruise in infant <4 mos.

(Photo contributors: Smita Kumar, MD, Earl R. Hartwig, MD,
Jonathan Thackeray, MD, and Binita R. Shah, MD)

The author acknowledges the special contributions of Konstantinos Agoritsas, MD, and Mary Birmingham, MD, to prior edition.

Clinical Summary

In the United States, child abuse is defined as "any act or failure to act on the part of a parent or caretaker which results in death, serious physical or emotional harm, sexual abuse or exploitation" or "an act or failure to act which presents an imminent risk of serious harm." The key aspect of child abuse is maltreatment by someone who at the time of the incident has a duty to supervise and provide a safe environment for the child or an obligation to provide for the child's well-being. Risk factors for child abuse include families with a history of substance abuse, single-parent households, young parental age, lack of parental education, previous incidents of domestic violence, socioeconomic constraints, and mental health problems. Mechanisms of inflicted injuries include direct impact (eg, punch, slap, kick, or strike with or against an object), violent shaking, penetrating injuries, and injuries related to asphyxiation. Abused children can have variable presentations; some may be completely asymptomatic while others have a range of signs and symptoms spanning minor bruises and contusions, to critically ill manifestations including respiratory distress, seizures, coma, or death, with the latter usually being associated with abusive head or blunt abdominal trauma. While inflicted abdominal injuries may present early with minimal findings such as vomiting alone, some children may progress to hypovolemic or even septic shock secondary to solid organ injury or a perforated viscus. Skeletal injuries, burns, poisoning, and Munchausen syndrome by proxy are all possible presentations for child abuse. Abused children are also often subject to a variety of forms of neglect, such as nutritional neglect, medical neglect, and lack of appropriate clothing, proper hygiene, or supervision, which may lead to injuries as well.

Emergency Department Treatment and Disposition

The approach to a child who has been abused or neglected is not significantly different from the standard evaluation and management of any child in the ED. Stabilize the patient and perform a thorough evaluation to exclude immediate life- or limb-threatening injuries. Next, obtain a detailed account of the mechanism of injury with clarification of events, timing, treatments, and who may have been present. Past medical history (eg, prior hospitalizations, injuries, co-morbid conditions such as other illnesses), family history, child temperament,

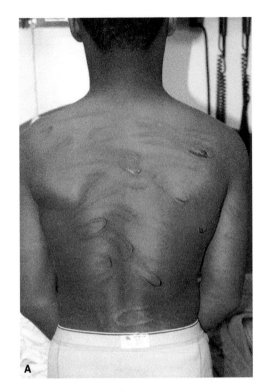

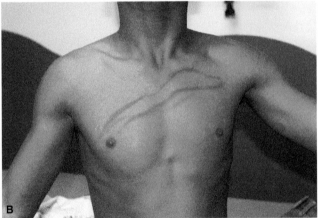

FIGURE 1.1 ■ "Loop Marks"; Inflicted Bruises and Abrasions. (**A, B**) An extension cord is a common instrument used to inflict injury. Such a whipping or beating can cause "loop marks," which commonly have a "U" or "C" shape, often with parallel "train track" linear marks. With greater force, deeper abrasions are seen. This 12-year-old boy was struck by his mother over 50 times in the head, trunk, and extremities after allegedly molesting his 5-year-old sister. (Photo contributor: Earl R. Hartwig, MD.)

developmental delay, caregiver's substance abuse, caregiver's details such as single parent, and socioeconomic constraints can add much to your overall impression as to whether or not the presentation represents abuse. The electronic medical record has become an invaluable tool for reviewing prior visits to a medical facility and should be examined for past

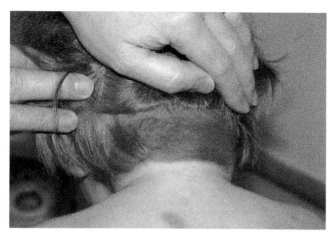

FIGURE 1.2 ■ Subgaleal Hematoma. Child's mother admitted to forcefully pulling her hair. (Photo contributor: Jonathan Thackeray, MD.)

presentations that may suggest abuse or neglect. Plot growth parameters of height, weight, and head circumference to exclude failure to thrive. Perform a complete (literally head to toe) physical examination including scalp, ears, frenulum of the lip, and tongue as these are uncommon locations for accidental trauma. Complete a formal retinal examination in all suspected cases of abuse in patients <2 years of age and in older children if brain injury is suspected.

Diagnostic evaluation depends on the severity and type of injury, age of patient, and examination; it may include CBC (screening for anemia and platelet count), lipase (for pancreatic injury), liver enzymes (elevation of transaminase seen with liver injury), urine analysis (hematuria with renal injury), and coagulation profile (to exclude bleeding disorders).

Order a radiographic skeletal survey for occult fractures in all suspected cases of abuse in children <2 years of age and consider one in children in whom an accurate history and physical examination cannot be obtained (eg, developmentally delayed). A skeletal survey can be repeated in 2 weeks to increase diagnostic yield, especially when abnormal or equivocal findings are found on initial study or when abuse is highly suspected. Nondisplaced fractures, especially rib and metaphyseal corner fractures (the classic metaphyseal lesion [CML]), are easily missed initially but will be better identified when periosteal reaction has begun. A single x-ray (body gram) is unacceptable. Obtain posteroanterior and oblique views of the ribs and an anteroposterior and lateral view of each bone. The yield from the skeletal survey decreases with increasing age, as the frequency of occult fractures decreases

in older children (between 2 and 5 years of age). Instead, order appropriate radiographs based on physical examination and any complaints of pain.

Consider radionuclide bone scans, which identify most fractures within 48 hours of injury and are helpful in infants and young children with suspected abuse and a negative skeletal survey. Bone scans can increase the detection of fractures in locations that are difficult to visualize radiographically (eg, hands, feet, or ribs) and are helpful for detecting recent fractures (<7- to 10-day-old rib fractures or subtle diaphyseal fractures). They serve as a complementary test to radiography when additional evidence of abusive injuries is required to establish the diagnosis. It should be noted that the common fracture of abuse, the CML, may be missed on bone scan because the rapidly growing metaphyses typically light up strongly and can mask this subtle injury.

Order a head CT scan and/or consider brain MRI for all patients younger than 2 years old and for all children with suspected intracranial injury. CT is highly sensitive and specific for brain injuries, especially those that require emergent intervention; it is readily available and better for the evaluation of acute hemorrhage. Brain MRI is best for fully assessing intracranial injury, including contusions, shear injuries, cerebral edema, and intraparenchymal hemorrhages. Obtain MRI whenever it can be readily obtained and when there are positive head CT findings and consider in selected cases with a normal CT but with high clinical concern for intracranial injury. MRI is also used to evaluate for subacute or chronic injuries that may be missed on a head CT and can sometimes provide better identification and dating of injuries.

Carefully document all visible findings both in the medical record and supplement the findings with pictures. First take a picture of the patient's identifying information (eg, name, date of birth, medical record number), and then photograph the patient's face and other areas. Clearly label all pictures, documenting the photographer's name, date, and time in the chart. Obtain a minimum of 2 views of each skin finding, first showing the injury in the context of the body region involved and then showing a close-up of the injury with a scale (such as a coin or a tape ruler). Body diagrams can be useful to clarify location and further describe findings, such as swelling and subtle bruising, that may not photograph well. Use of camera settings without a flash (or zooming from a further distance from the child) may reduce glare for these subtle findings as well. Take pictures early on in the course of admitted patients to capture findings that may resolve quickly with time.

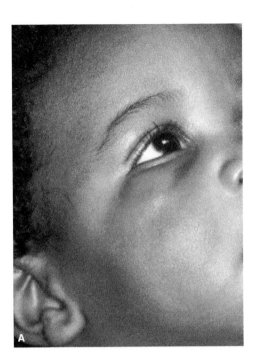
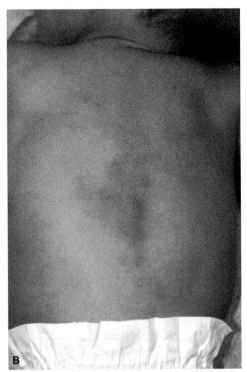
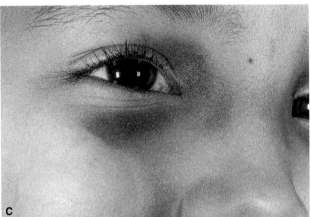

FIGURE 1.3 ■ Inflicted Bruises. (**A, B**) An 8-month-old infant with facial and back bruises. Bruises, often subtle, are the most common injuries of NAT and serve as a reminder to the clinician to consider abuse in the differential diagnosis. This infant also had multiple bilateral rib fractures seen on the skeletal survey. (**C**) Simple falls usually injure the more prominent forehead, nose, and cheek. Bruises on relatively well-protected areas (eg, periorbital bruising) should be looked at with suspicion. Dating of bruises based on color is imprecise: purple, blue or black bruises may all be from the same or a different time period. One cannot "date bruises" based on these colors. The yellowish coloration seen here is not consistent with recent (<18 hours) mechanism. (Photo contributors: Earl R. Hartwig, MD [A, B], and Binita R. Shah, MD [C].)

For children old enough to describe what happened, conduct the interview in a closed environment using questions that are developmentally appropriate and open ended (eg, "Can you tell me what happened to your arm?"), rather than asking leading questions (eg, "Did your mommy hit you?"). Document the child's and caregiver's exact statements about the injuries verbatim, as the child's statements are often allowed in court as an exception to the "hearsay rule." When available, perform a limited interview of the child in a general, age-appropriate manner and arrange for forensic interviewing by experts after the ED evaluation. Consult with a multidisciplinary team, including a pediatrician, child abuse consultant, social worker, and specialists in pediatric radiology, orthopedics, neurosurgery, surgery, and ophthalmology as indicated.

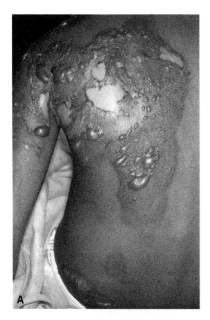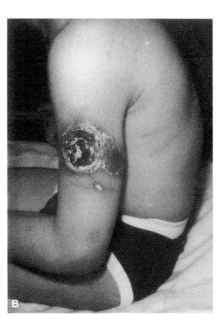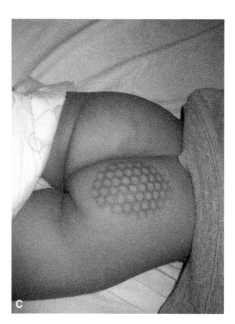

FIGURE 1.4 ■ Inflicted Burns. (**A**) Hot coffee was thrown on this girl by her mother during an argument. (**B**) Necrotic ulcerated lesion following a neglected burn and multiple bruises were seen on this child. (**C**) Inflicted burn from a space heater. (Photo contributors: Binita R. Shah, MD [A, B], and Barry Hahn, MD [C].)

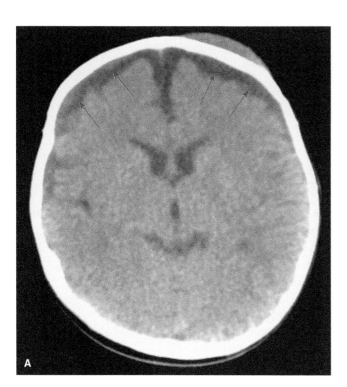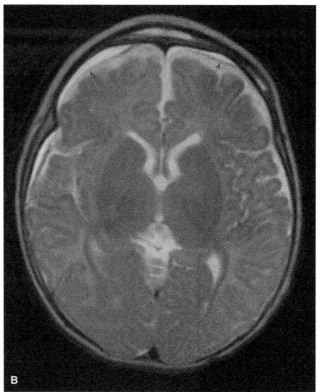

FIGURE 1.5 ■ Abusive Head Trauma. (**A**) Bilateral subdural hematomas. A noncontrast CT image shows a subtle increased attenuation (density) along the inner table of the right and left frontal bones representing acute hematoma (arrows). (**B**) MRI shows bilateral crescentic collections of high signal (white) along the frontal bones, with right greater than left (arrows). Extracranial hematomas along the frontal bone are also noted in both CT and MRI images. This 5-month-old infant was reported as "falling off the bed" by mother's boyfriend. (Photo contributor: David S. Dinhofer, MD.)

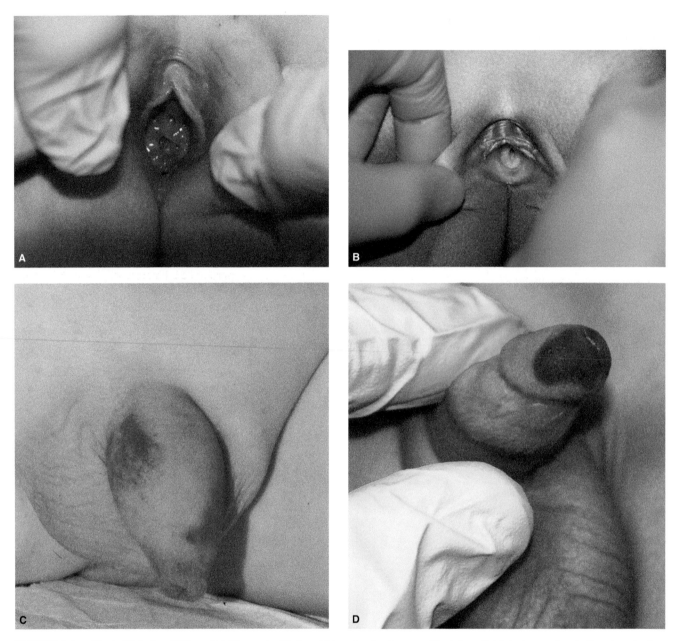

FIGURE 1.6 ■ Genital Injuries: Differential Diagnosis. Distinguishing abusive from accidental genital injuries can be challenging. A plausible history and associated physical findings may help, as mentioned in these examples. (**A**) A 2-year-old girl wearing a diaper and clothes was brought with a complaint of "falling in a boat." She presented with persistent genital bleeding. Such a focal injury in a diapered child would be highly unlikely after an accidental fall. (**B**) A 3-year-old girl stated that her 11-year-old cousin poked her with his finger. A small abrasion with a bruise to the introitus corroborates her history. (**C**) Penile bruises seen in an 18-month-old child left with his grandparents for a few hours. Pinches to the penis are occasionally seen as a punishment for "toileting accidents" in toddlers, an example of nonaccidental trauma with unrealistic expectations in a child. (**D**) A 33-month-old child who was standing to urinate when the toilet seat fell down presented with ecchymosis of the glans penis, which corroborates the history. (Photo contributor: Earl R. Hartwig, MD.)

Reporting all suspected abuse to the local Child Protective Services (CPS) agency is a legal mandate in the United States. This requirement includes the reporting of all suspected (not necessarily proven) cases of physical or sexual child abuse.

Mandated reporters are individuals routinely responsible for a child's health or well-being, including medical personnel, teachers, day care workers, and law enforcement professionals. Mandated reporters who report their suspicions in good faith are protected from lawsuits. However, a mandated reporter may be prosecuted for failing to report abuse, and civil malpractice litigation may be brought against a physician or other health care provider for failure to recognize or diagnose child physical or sexual abuse in a timely manner. Document in the medical record a clear, concise, and legible history and the examination, laboratory, and radiologic findings. These records may become evidence in a criminal proceeding and will be invaluable if there is considerable (sometimes months to years) time delay in testifying.

If abuse is considered likely, consult CPS workers and together decide about the safe disposition of the child and the possibility of further harm if the child (or siblings) remains in the custody of the caregiver in question. Options include immediate placement in foster care (either with a relative or designated foster parent) or, rarely, temporary hospitalization while awaiting arrangements for transport to a safe environment.

Refer the victim and his or her innocent relatives or caregivers to mental health services to help them cope with the emotional trauma of abuse. Request evaluation of all siblings and other minors in the household if they may have been in contact with the alleged perpetrator.

Pearls

1. Child abuse has myriad presentations and should be one of the differential diagnosis during the evaluation of a child with injuries.

2. Undress the child completely so that a thorough examination may be carried out to evaluate for unusual bruises, marks, burns, and areas of swelling or tenderness. A toddler with a minor bruise and clavicular fracture will likely not be considered to have been abused until you discover the old immersion burn scars hiding under his socks!

3. Some children who are physically abused may also be sexually abused. Exclude sexual abuse by taking a thorough history, always performing a thorough examination, and ordering appropriate laboratory studies as indicated.

4. Red flags for child abuse include inconsistent, unexplained, and implausible history; delays in seeking treatment; and repeated "accidents." Obtaining an accurate history is essential.

Clinical Summary

Bruising, often the first and sometimes the only manifestation, is one of the most common signs, estimated to be seen in approximately 90% of child abuse cases. Bruises may be accidental or inflicted. Consider physical abuse whenever the history is lacking, changes over time, or is inconsistent with the injury or developmental stage of the child. It is important to remember that bruises may be hidden by clothing, and it is imperative to examine the child fully undressed. In cases of excessive corporal punishment, bruising may be present in the pattern of the inflicting object. There is a long-held belief that bruises of different color represent injuries of different ages.

More recent studies, involving solely Caucasian patients, have shown that several different colors can be present at the same time within one bruise and that red, purple, blue, and brown may be seen from the onset of injury up to 2 weeks later. Of note, yellow coloration was only seen in bruises older than 18 to 24 hours in 2 studies. Until further studies are performed in children of all race and ethnicities, caution should be used in attempting to determine the age of a bruise by its color. A Wood's lamp with digital camera may improve the visualization of faint bruises that otherwise might be missed. Photo-documentation with an alternative light source and no flash may allow better depiction of subtle bruises and areas

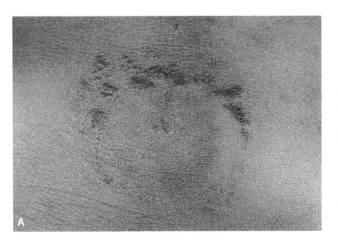
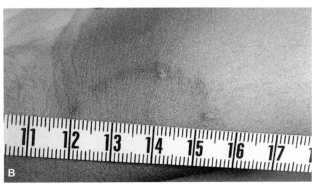
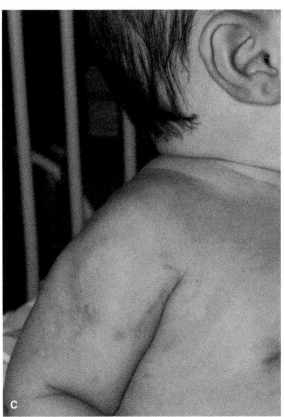

FIGURE 1.7 ■ Inflicted Bites. (**A, B**) Bite marks lead to distinctive patterns of bruises and should be suspected when ecchymosis, lacerations, or abrasions are elliptical or oval (two arched patterns as mirror images if both mandibular and maxillary teeth are used to bite). Canine marks are the most prominent (or deep) part of the bite. The normal distance between maxillary canines in adult humans is 2.5 to 4 cm, and in a child, it is <3 cm. (**C**) A 4-month-old infant allegedly bitten by his 19-month-old sister. When asked about further bruising found to the infant's body, mom stated "he must have done it to himself." In addition, the sibling was present and did not have full dentition. Self-inflicted injuries in an infant and alleged "sibling-inflicted" injuries should always be regarded with a high degree of suspicion. (Photo contributors: Binita R. Shah, MD [A, B], and Earl R. Hartwig, MD [C].)

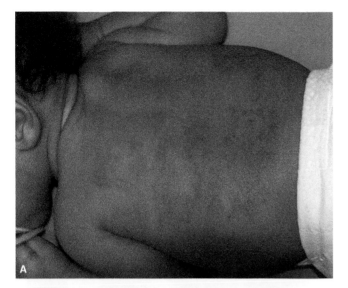

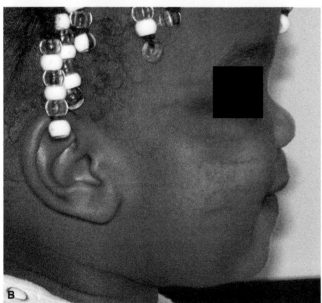

FIGURE 1.8 ■ Inflicted Bruises. (**A**) A 2-month-old infant presented with mom for a "rash." The mother had left the child with the father while going to school. The father later admitted that the infant was crying, so he "flicked him" with his finger. He continued to "thump him" several times as the infant kept crying. (**B**) Slap marks. An 18-month-old girl was picked up by her foster mother from a weekend visit with the biological family who said she developed "a rash." Pattern is consistent with a negative imprint of hand with repeated slaps. (Photo contributor: Earl R, Hartwig, MD.)

of swelling. Differential diagnoses include accidental trauma, infections associated with petechiae or purpura, Henoch-Schönlein purpura, folk healing practices (eg, cupping), and dermatologic conditions such as hypersensitivity reactions, cold panniculitis, and phytophotodermatitis.

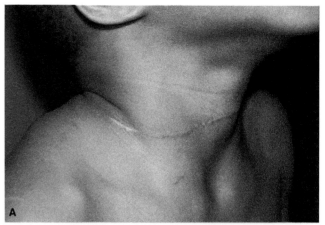

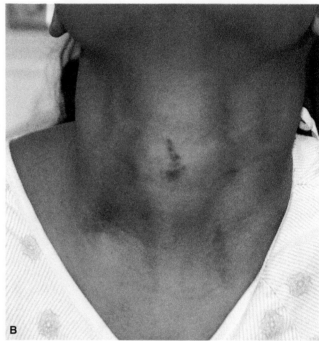

FIGURE 1.9 ■ Inflicted Neck Injuries. (**A**) A 5-year-old reportedly "playing with blinds" 1 week ago with younger sister. His circumferential deep linear scar to the neck and scattered linear scars and loop marks (not shown) to the body were consistent with abuse. (**B**) A 15-year-old girl presenting with these neck bruises reportedly came home late at night and stated that her "stepfather angrily grabbed her by the neck and choked her." After similar bruises were found on her breasts, she recanted her history and admitted these were suction bruises ("hickeys") from making out with her boyfriend. (Photo contributor: Earl R. Hartwig, MD.)

Emergency Department Treatment and Disposition

Since bruises that are not over bony prominences require substantial force/trauma, the provider should always consider the

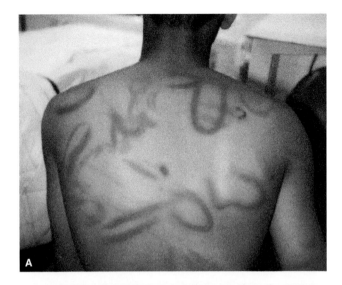

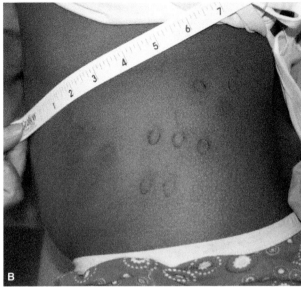

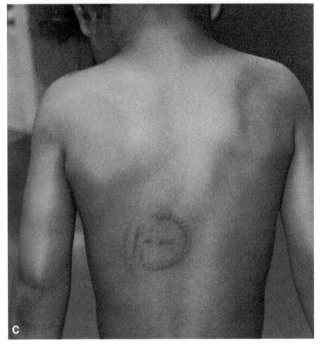

FIGURE 1.10 ■ Abusive Pattern Marks. (**A**) Loop and linear marks from an electrical cord. (**B**) A 6-year-old child was brought in for CPS exam on referral from school. Mom states that she hit the child yesterday with a belt that had buttons on it. His prior ED visits included a fractured toe ("table fell on it" at age 2 years) and nail primer ingestion (at age 20 months). (**C**) A 3-year-old boy was noted to have a belt mark on his back while being examined in the ED for acute gastroenteritis. (Photo contributors: Smita Kumar, MD [A], and Earl R. Hartwig, MD [B, C].)

potential for more severe underlying injuries such as head injury, abdominal trauma, or fractures and investigate as appropriate. Document skin findings (eg, swelling, bruises, burns, abrasions, lacerations) on initial presentation with photographs and a body diagram if needed and include the shape, pattern, location, and size of each lesion. Involve CPS in any suspected case of abuse. Pattern bruises are frequently indicative of abuse. When multiple bruises are found without a discreet pattern and there is no clear explanation, obtain a CBC and coagulation studies to rule out underlying bleeding disorders.

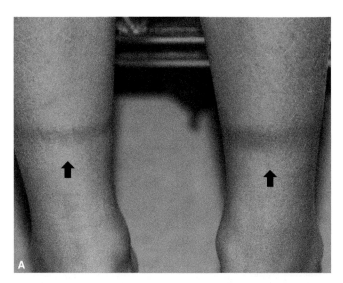
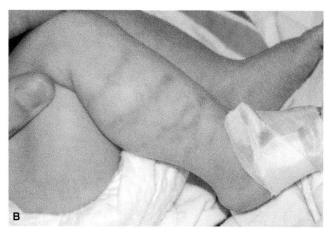

FIGURE 1.11 ■ Abusive Linear Marks. (**A**) An 8-year-old punished for "stealing" and hit with a belt by father. Numerous linear marks to body were seen, and shown here are old healed hyperpigmented scars to the ankles concerning for "ligature marks." (**B**) Patterned bruising inflicted by a hand. (Photo contributors: Earl R. Hartwig, MD [A], and Jonathan Thackeray, MD [B].)

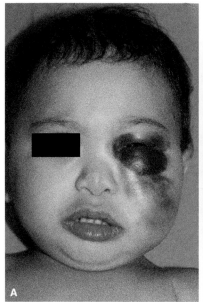
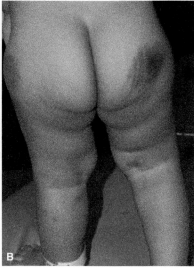
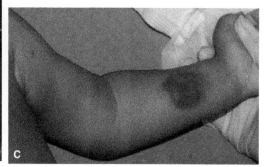

FIGURE 1.12 ■ Coagulopathy: Differential of Abusive Bruises. (**A**) A 17-month-old boy presented for evaluation of left-sided facial swelling. The child reportedly "fell" 2 days prior, hitting his left eye against a door knob. By history, initially there was a small amount of bruising that had considerably progressed. (**B, C**) Numerous other bruises were noted on exam. Even though some bruises (eg, over the buttocks) were concerning, there were no patterned bruises, and many bruises were over expected bony prominences. His coagulation profile was abnormal (prolonged partial thromboplastin time and prothrombin time and increased international normalized ratio), leading to a previously undiagnosed coagulation disorder. Extensive bruising without pattern requires a comprehensive evaluation to exclude a bleeding disorder. (Photo contributor: Earl R. Hartwig, MD.)

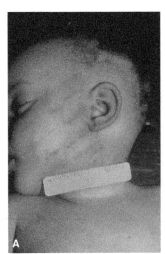 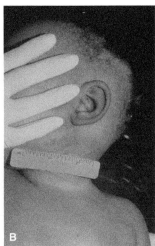 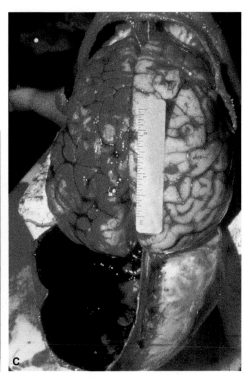

FIGURE 1.13 ■ Slap Marks and Abusive Head Trauma. (**A, B**) Finger patterns seen on the face of the infant brought to the ED in cardio-pulmonary arrest. Gloved fingers corresponding to the finger patterns. (**C**). Subarachnoid hemorrhage (SAH) and subdural hemorrhage (SDH). An autopsy photograph taken just prior to brain removal shows a SAH on the upper left-hand side and SDH in the lower left-hand side. This 8-month-old infant was seen 4 weeks earlier because of bleeding from the ear and was sent home with a diagnosis of otitis externa. Subsequently, he was seen for facial palsy on the same side as the bloody otorrhea. He was treated with antibiotics with a clinical diagnosis of otitis media with facial palsy. A few days later, he was brought to the ED in cardiopulmonary arrest. He was also found to have skull and multiple rib fractures. (Otorrhea and facial palsy were due to a basal skull fracture. *Clinical Pearls*: Otitis externa is an exceedingly uncommon diagnosis in infancy, and bloody ear discharge is seen in neither otitis media nor otitis externa.) (Photo contributor: Binita R. Shah, MD.)

Pearls

1. Age of a bruise is indeterminate; location, type of impact inflicted, and skin color all may affect bruise appearance. In Caucasian children, yellow coloration is not expected in the first 18 hours.
2. It is extremely uncommon for preambulatory children to bruise. "Those who can't cruise don't bruise."
3. Bruises from normal activity occur more commonly on bony prominences of the anterior surfaces (eg, forehead, shins, elbows, knees, lower arms, and dorsum of hands).
4. Bruises on fleshy or well-protected areas such as the ears, cheeks, frenulum, neck, upper arms and trunk, flanks, thighs, and buttocks suggest inflicted injuries.

Clinical Summary

It is estimated that approximately half of all child abuse injuries involve the head and orofacial region. Mechanisms range from blunt trauma such as punching and slapping to inflicted bites, forced sexual abuse, and abusive head trauma. Findings in abused children include fractures to the maxilla, mandible, and facial bones and fractures or avulsions of the teeth. Further injuries include facial bruises, such as the classical slap

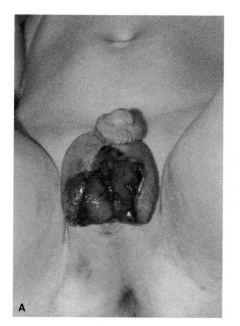

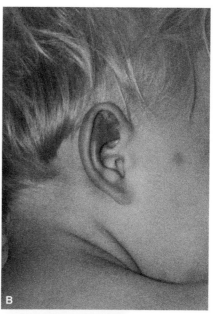

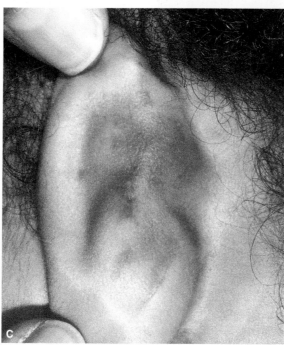

FIGURE 1.14. ■ Ear Bruises. (**A, B**). A 2-year-old child who reportedly awakened with crying and blood in his bed. Deep scrotal laceration (**A**) initially attributed to "eczema" and later to a "self-inflicted injury" was the history given by the parents. Later, the mother added that he slept in his bed with his cars and books and "may have cut himself on them." Bilateral ear bruising (**B**; shown here on right ear) and subgaleal hematoma were also noted. Even though the exact mechanism of his scrotal injury could not be determined, the combination all these findings was highly concerning for abuse. (**C**). Inflicted ear bruising in another child. Ears are not frequently injured accidentally, and bruises are strong indicators of abuse. Ears can be bruised by pulling, pinching, or grabbing. (Photo contributors: Earl R. Hartwig, MD [A, B], and Binita R. Shah, MD [C].)

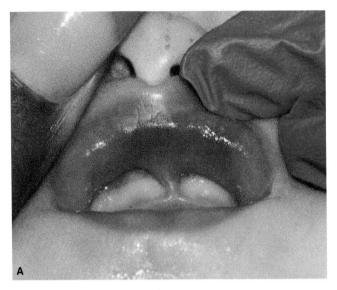

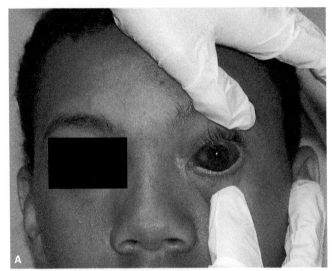

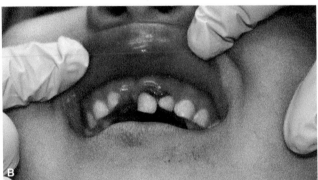

FIGURE 1.15 ■ Intraoral Injuries: Differential Diagnosis. (**A**) Abusive injuries. A 5-month-old infant with frenulum bruising and lacerations secondary to forced feeding with a spoon or bottle or excessive force with a pacifier. Such injuries are often seen in young infants. (**B**) Accidental injuries. Toddlers and children may sustain intraoral injuries (eg, lip mucosa bruising and tooth subluxation, as seen here) with a simple fall. A complete history, examination, and review of available records should always be done to exclude concerns of abuse. (Photo contributor: Earl R. Hartwig, MD.)

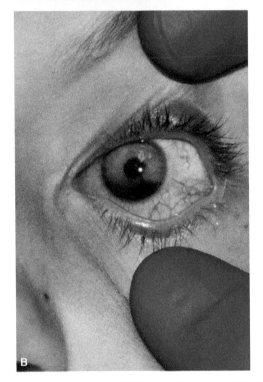

FIGURE 1.16 ■ Eye Injuries: Differential Diagnosis. (**A**) Abusive injury. Digital retraction of the eyelids shows 360-degree subconjunctival hemorrhage in this 15-year-old boy "punched in the eye by his stepfather." Although subconjunctival hemorrhages can often be seen with benign mechanisms such as forceful sneezing or vomiting, one should not assume "benign" etiology without further inquiry. (**B**) Accidental injury. Digital retraction of the eyelids shows hyphema in an 11-year-old boy accidently shot in the eye with a pellet gun. (Photo contributor: Earl R. Hartwig, MD.)

mark; burns; lacerations to the lips, tongue, and lingual frenulum; and bite marks to the neck and face. Forced feeding with a bottle, spoon, or fork and forceful pacifier insertion may lead to bruises or tears to the frenulum or fractured teeth.

Forced fellatio leads to intraoral bruising, typically at the junction of the hard and soft palate. Intraoral bruising or erythema is typically midline or bilateral, often spares the posterior uvula and tonsils and tends to be asymptomatic. This is in contrast to pharyngitis, which will be painful and consistently involves the tonsils and posterior pharynx. Other evidence of

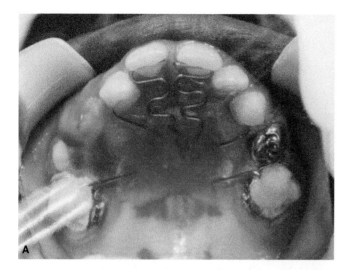

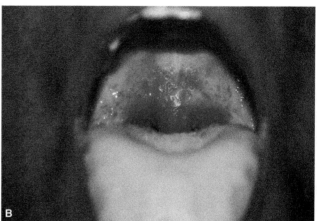

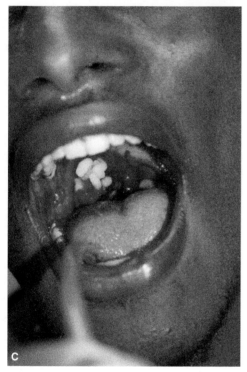

FIGURE 1.17 ■ Oral Bruising: Differential Diagnosis. Oral bruising can have varied etiologies as shown here in 3 different patients. (**A**) Oral sexual abuse. A 10-year-old boy with a retainer who had a routine dental visit and was then referred to the ED with concerns of "forced sexual abuse." He was noted to have painless "scratches" in his hard palate per the mom. Bruising extended beyond the retainer but did not involve uvula or tonsillar pillars. Although the patient denied any inappropriate sexual contact, his urine DNA amplification was positive for gonorrhea, and a 2-year-old sister was subsequently found to have gonococcal vaginitis. (**B**) Streptococcal pharyngitis. Palatal petechiae extending to the uvula and tonsillar pillars are seen in this child diagnosed with streptococcal pharyngitis. Other associated findings may include exudates and tender cervical lymphadenopathy. (**C**) Coagulopathy. Oral bleeding with bruising is seen in this patient after an attempted drainage of peritonsillar abscess. He was found to have thrombocytopenia (and a prior history of aplastic anemia with poor follow-up!). Coagulopathy needs to be excluded whenever oral bruising is encountered, and a history of coagulopathy should also be sought prior to undergoing any surgical procedures! (Photo contributor: Earl R. Hartwig, MD.)

oral sexual abuse involves ulcerative, vesiculopustular, pseudomembranous, and condylomatous lesions within the oral cavity. A positive finding of gonorrhea in prepubertal children is diagnostic of sexual abuse. However, human papillomavirus and herpes infections can be transmitted via sexual or nonsexual means, and a careful history must be obtained.

Dental neglect is also commonly seen and frequently occurs secondary to lack of knowledge of dental hygiene in young children and/or lack of resources. It is important to establish a dental home for children early so that proper oral care and anticipatory guidance can be provided. Subsequent to elimination of these considerations during the history taking, oral neglect should be suspected if significant caries, oral infections, or untreated trauma persists on follow-up. As with any traumatic injuries in children, a careful history and complete physical exam are necessary to determine feasibility of the physical findings encountered. Many oral injuries are accidental, as a result of a simple fall, but the history and

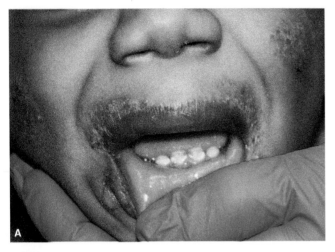

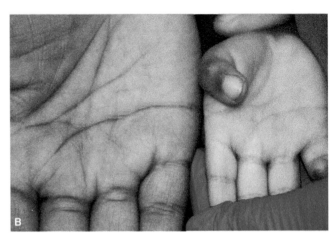

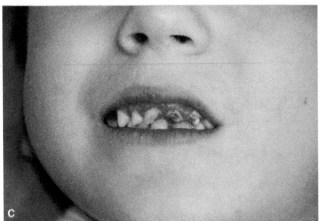

FIGURE 1.18 ■ Dental Neglect: A Form of Child Maltreatment. (**A**) A 22-month-old boy who presented to the ED was found to have numerous dental caries. Neglect of proper oral care should prompt a further look into the overall care of the child. (**B**) This child also had pallor (shown against mother's hand) and severely neglected eczema. A hemoglobin of 5 g/dL was found, likely due to his diet, which consisted solely of milk and applesauce. (**C**) A 6-year-old boy with known developmental delay presented with oral pain and dental carries. Delayed children, in particular, often experience complications secondary to challenges in oral care and may require assistance in securing an appropriate "dental home" to ensure appropriate treatment and adequate follow-up care. (Photo contributor: Earl R. Hartwig, MD.)

developmental stage of the child need to be considered in determining the likelihood of each scenario. Similar to with other routine or urgent medical care visits, dental care visits and visits to the ED for dental complaints may provide an opportunity to identify possible abuse and provide potentially lifesaving interventions with reports to CPS. Although a child may be presenting for oral trauma, one should consider injuries to the scalp, face, ears, and neck, as well as lack of proper hygiene, failure to thrive, and other concerns for abuse or neglect.

Emergency Department Treatment and Disposition

The initial management includes identification and management of any potential life-threatening injuries. Any trauma to the oral cavity implies the potential for head injury, and the child's mental status and risk for CNS injury must be

addressed. Although the likelihood is low, the cervical spine should be assessed and injury excluded. Following stabilization, a thorough history and head-to-toe examination are indicated to evaluate and exclude other possible injuries. A review of the medical record should be conducted to assess for prior visits that may be related to abuse or neglect. The entire history and constellation of findings may make the difference between the diagnosis of a seemingly benign injury and concern for abuse. Minor injuries are documented and treated with consultation with dental, ophthalmology, and otorhinolaryngology services, as necessary, for special situations.

Suspicion of abuse or neglect should be reported to CPS with reasons substantiating your concerns. Good-quality photographs are helpful early on in documenting any positive findings, particularly bruises and intraoral lesions that may heal quickly. An external light source and camera with manual focus are essential in photographing lesions of the oral cavity because autofocus cameras will likely focus on the lips or teeth while blurring inner lesions. With suspicion of oral sexual abuse, a workup should include oral samples standard for rape kit testing and cultures for gonorrhea and chlamydia. A head-to-toe exam with detailed anogenital exam with cultures and blood collection for sexually transmitted infections (STIs) including but not limited to HIV and syphilis testing is also indicated.

Pearls

1. A careful examination of the face must always be carried out, and injuries must be documented along with pictures because, in many instances, the patterns are recognizable and pathognomonic (eg, slap marks) but could be insidious (eg, frenulum tears).

2. Evidence of STIs such as gonorrhea is always due to abuse; however, human papillomavirus and herpetic lesions can result from nonsexual contact, so clinicians need to be very meticulous in their history taking.

Clinical Summary

Although burn injuries may be inflicted or accidental, up to 40% of admitted patients to pediatric burn centers are believed to have experienced abuse. Accidental splash burns commonly occur on the face, neck, and chest when ambulating toddlers pull hot liquid or objects onto themselves. Usually the most severe burns are seen on the face and shoulder, where the liquid hits first, with splash marks away from the

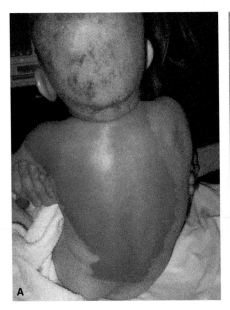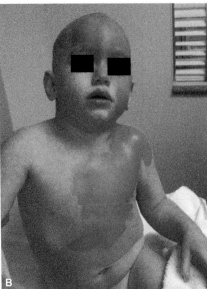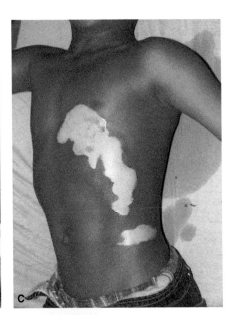

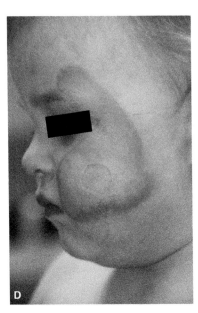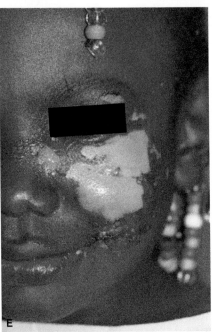

FIGURE 1.19 ■ Accidental Scald Burns. (**A, B**) A 3-year-old child suffered extensive burns as he tipped a pot of water from the stove on top of himself. The scalp, chest, and back were involved. Typical splash configuration seen on back and chest. (**C**) A 7-year-old boy sustained a burn to his chest and abdomen with hot water while "making noodles" in the microwave. Typical splash pattern is anterior and trails off in a "V" configuration due to cooling as it runs down the body. (**D**) A 20-month-old who ran into the grill at a family picnic. There is asymmetry and varying depth noted to the burn. (**E**) A 4-year-old child who reportedly "ran into a pot of hot noodles yesterday." Although the injury itself may have been accidental, the delay in seeking care is of concern. Even "accidental burns" often involve a lack of supervision and protection of young children and may constitute neglect. A fluorescein stain is necessary to exclude corneal involvement. (Photo contributor: Earl R. Hartwig, MD.)

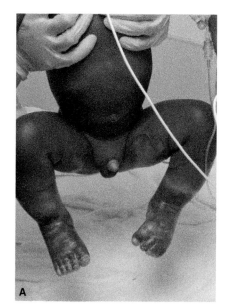

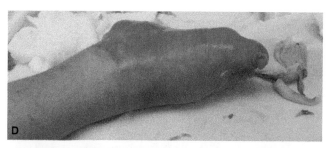

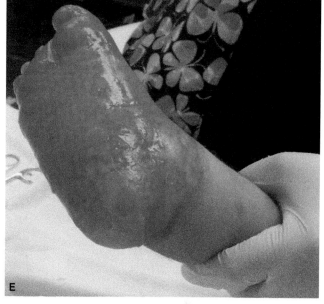

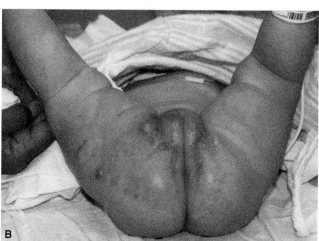

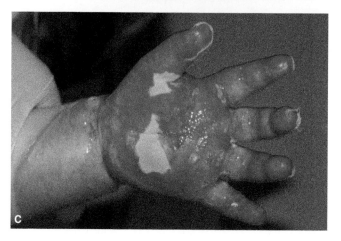

FIGURE 1.20 ■ Immersion Burns. (**A**) An 11-month-old infant whose mother "heard him crying and found him in the bathtub with hot water running." This stocking-and-glove pattern requires an immersion in deeper water and is often seen with areas of sparing as seen here in the dorsal crease of the foot. (**B**) A 5-month-old infant was "bathed at her baby sitter's home." Note the spared creased areas as the infant flexed her legs (in pain) during the incident. (**C**) A 14-month-old toddler was "near a stove and reached into a boiling pot of water." However, it is highly unlikely for a toddler to position himself up on a stove to sustain such a burn. (**D, E**) A 6-year-old child with a history of meningomyelocele, with insensate lower extremities. Father bathed her in a bathtub seat with her right foot sitting in the hot water. The subsequent burn has the appearance of a typical abusive immersion burn with a clear demarcation line and no splashes. (Photo contributor: Earl R. Hartwig, MD.)

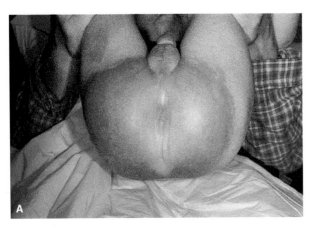

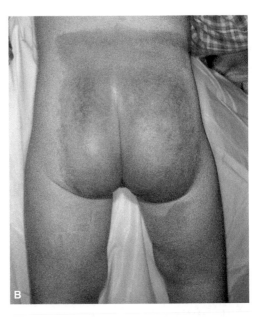

FIGURE 1.21 ■ Chemical Burns. (**A, B**) Burn caused by chlorine bleach accidentally spilled in this infant's diaper that served as an occlusive dressing. The incident was reported to Child Protective Services. After a thorough investigation, this injury was considered to be accidental. (Photo contributor: Binita R. Shah, MD.)

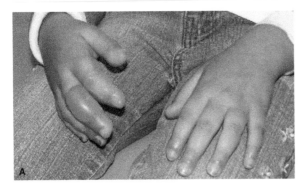

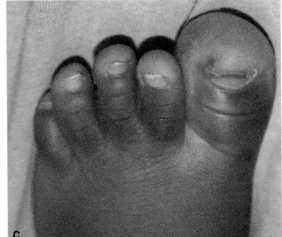

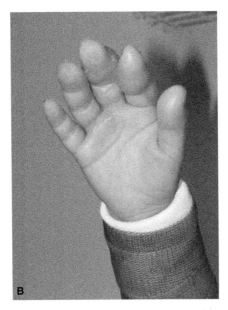

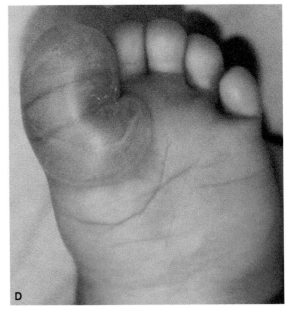

FIGURE 1.22 ■ Immersion Burns: Differential Diagnosis. Several conditions may mimic immersion burn injuries, as shown here. (**A, B**) Bullous contact dermatitis, as seen in this child with poison ivy exposure. (**C, D**) Bullous staphylococcal toe abscess (see also Figure 2-29). (Photo contributor: Earl R. Hartwig, MD.)

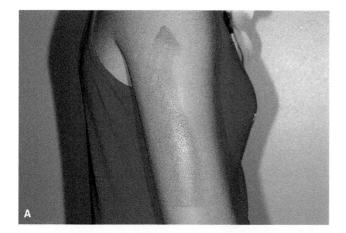

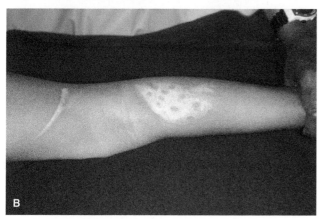

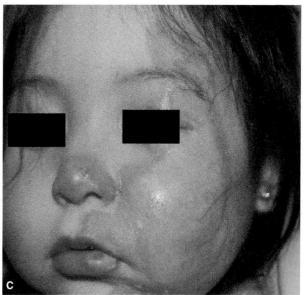

FIGURE 1.23 ■ Iron Burns: Inflicted Versus Accidental. (**A**) Burn from iron inflicted on the upper arm. (**B**) A healed iron burn inflicted to the forearm. (**C**) A toddler who pulled an iron down onto her face. The less distinct margins and more superficial burn depth suggest an accidental injury. (Photo contributors: Binita R. Shah, MD [A, B], and Kirsten Bechtel, MD [C].)

point of maximal contact. Infants and toddlers may also be victims of forced immersion burns, which often present as a well-demarcated burn injury on the perineum, buttocks, and/ or extremities. At times, there is an area of sparing either on the buttocks or feet where the child is held against the cooler surface of the tub. Children who accidentally come in contact with a hot liquid will usually present with a lesser degree of burn, an indistinct burn margin, and splash marks as the child reflexively tries to move away. Inflicted burns generally do not have splash marks because the child is held in position.

Abusive contact burns result from a hot object being held against the child's skin. On physical examination, there will usually be a distinct outline that may be helpful in distinguishing the object used. Burns may occur accidentally when children run into or pull a hot object onto themselves; here, the outline of the object will usually be asymmetric and less distinct and burns more superficial than with abusive burn injuries. Differential diagnosis includes chemical burns, infections, arthropod bites, and bullous or blistering dermatologic conditions.

Emergency Department Treatment and Disposition

Patients should be initially managed and resuscitated as any other burn patient, with careful attention to airway, fluid resuscitation, pain management, and infection control. While burn injuries are frequently visibly dramatic and may serve as a distraction, a complete exam should be performed so that potentially serious nonburn injuries are not overlooked. Take a careful history with attention to whether the type and degree of burn are consistent with the history provided. Document the initial presentation of the burn; undress and look for other signs of abuse or neglect in any pediatric burn victim. Review the available medical record for prior visits concerning for abuse or neglect. As with other mechanisms of injury, consider a laboratory workup and skeletal survey in infants and toddlers with suspicion of abuse. If abuse is suspected, a report should be made to CPS.

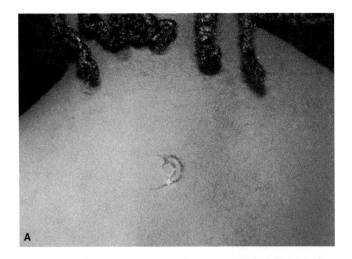

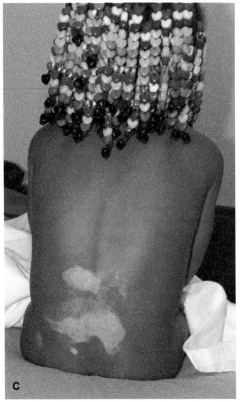

FIGURE 1.24 ■ Abusive Burns. (**A**) A 2-year-old child with a well-demarcated burn pattern on the upper back. As with bruises, well-demarcated burns, particularly when on the back, are very concerning for nonaccidental trauma (NAT). (**B**) A 19-month-old child presenting with a well-demarcated burn in the shape of a lighter is consistent with contact burn from NAT. (**C**) A 2-year-old with several burn scars on the buttocks from contact burns (an unusual area for an accidental burn). (Photo contributor: Earl R. Hartwig, MD.)

Pearls

1. Evaluate carefully every pediatric burn for possible abuse. Obtain a thorough history and examine the burn closely to determine plausibility of the history.

2. Stocking-and-glove distribution and any pattern burn are highly suspicious for child abuse. Small circular burns, especially if multiple, should be examined closely for the potential of cigarette burns.

3. Abusive immersion burns are more common in infants and toddlers. Scald burn is the most common mechanism of burn injury in both abused and nonabused children.

4. Accidental burns may also be the result of poor supervision, so pay careful attention to the social situation in every child who presents with a burn.

Clinical Summary

Skeletal fractures related to child abuse are rarely life threatening; however, they may be the first indication of child abuse and thus are an important diagnostic tool. Inflicted skeletal injures may involve any part of the axial and appendicular skeleton and occur in up to 55% of physically abused children. Age is the single most important risk factor for abusive skeletal injuries, and 55% to 70% of skeletal injuries are seen in infants <1 year of age. Intracranial and thoracoabdominal

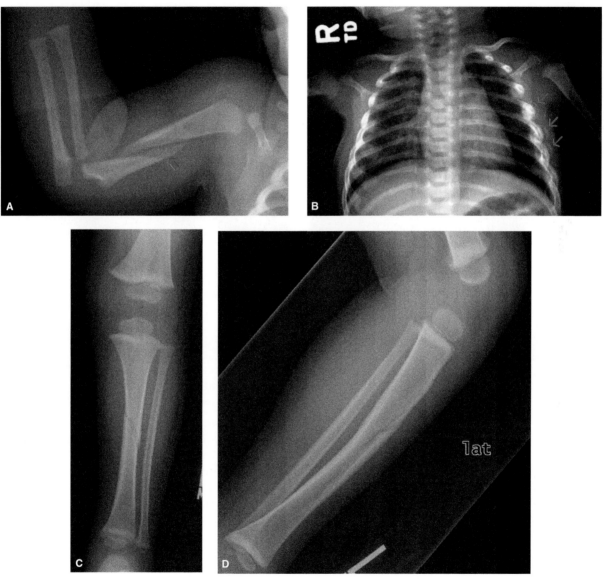

FIGURE 1.25 ■ Inflicted Versus Accidental Fractures. (**A, B**) Lateral view of right arm showing an acute oblique displaced fracture of the humerus (arrow; **A**) in a 5-month-old infant who was "being carried against the father's chest when dad tripped over something" and fell on the baby. The baby's right arm "snapped" when it hit the floor. (**B**) Given the concerning history, a skeletal survey was performed. Anteroposterior view of the chest reveals multiple healing left lateral rib fractures with callus formation (arrows). Although the humerus fracture may have been sustained in the manner described, the healed ribs fractured were not from the current fall. (**C, D**) Toddler's fracture. Anteroposterior and lateral views of left leg demonstrate acute oblique nondisplaced fracture of the mid-tibial shaft in a 2-year-old toddler who was playing in an inflatable bounce house when he began to have a limp. The remainder of history, exam, and record review were normal. Toddler's fractures usually occur in the distal half to distal third of the tibia in an active toddler. The appearance may mimic spiral fracture from nonaccidental trauma, but given an appropriate history in an ambulatory toddler with no other injuries or red flags, accidental trauma is the most likely etiology. Fractures of the more proximal tibia may be suspicious for nonaccidental trauma. (Photo/legend contributors: Earl R. Hartwig, MD [A, B], Tian Liang, MD, and Ryan Logan Webb, MD [C, D].)

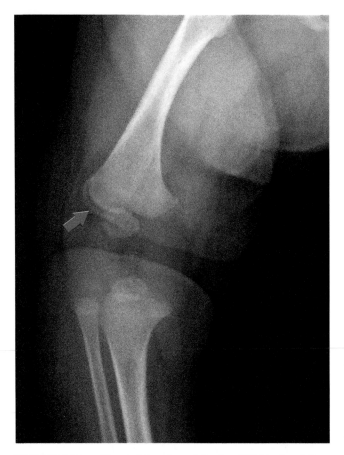

FIGURE 1.26 ■ Classic Metaphyseal Lesion (CML). An oblique view of the right lower extremity showing a bucket handle fracture of the femoral metaphysis (arrow) in a 4-month-old infant who presented with crying when the right knee was touched. No history of injury was given. Skeletal survey also revealed CMLs of the right and left tibia. (Photo/legend contributors: Earl R. Hartwig, MD, and Ryan Logan Webb, MD.)

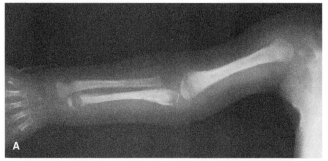

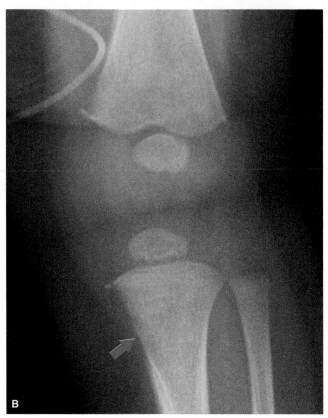

FIGURE 1.27 ■ Congenital Syphilis: Differential of Classic Metaphyseal Lesions. (A) Frontal view of the upper extremity demonstrates areas of bone destruction in the metaphyses of the humerus, radius, and ulna, compatible with congenital syphilis. (B) Wimberger sign. This infant presented with pain and guarding of his extremities (pseudoparalysis). Note metaphyseal lesion along the medial surface of the tibia (arrow). These lesions are seen bilaterally and are highly suggestive of congenital syphilis. (Photo contributors: Lynne Pinkney, MD [A], and Earl R. Hartwig, MD [B].)

injures often coexist with abusive skeletal injuries; the presence of one indicates the need to evaluate for the other. Suspect child abuse when fractures occur in preambulatory children, particularly in patients <6 months of age, those with an inconsistent history, or those with multiple or repeat injuries. A review of the medical record is important because prior visits may reveal additional concern for abuse. Certain fractures such as CML, posterior rib fractures, scapular fractures, spinous process fractures, and sternal fractures have the highest specificity for abuse. These generally require a unique mechanism (eg, pull, twist, torque, or squeeze) or forces greater than what is produced by usual accidental trauma of infancy. Fractures with moderate specificity include multiple fractures, fractures of different ages, epiphyseal separations, vertebral body fractures, digital fractures, and complex skull fractures. Fractures with lower specificity include clavicular fractures, isolated long bone shaft fractures (femur, humerus, and tibia), linear skull fractures in children older

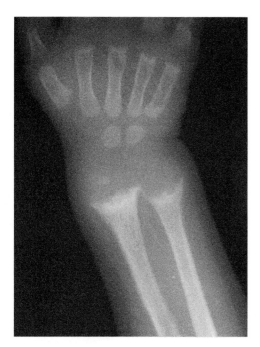

FIGURE 1.28 ▪ Rickets: Differential of Classic Metaphyseal Lesions (CMLs). Although rickets may sometimes be confused with CMLs, the more rapid growth areas of the wrists and knees show the obvious demineralization, cupping, and fraying of the metaphyses classically seen in rickets. Typically, rachitic changes are also seen bilaterally, and nutritional history or underlying metabolic bone disease will also aid in the further differentiation. (Photo contributor: Earl R. Hartwig, MD.)

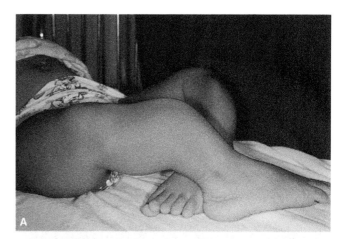

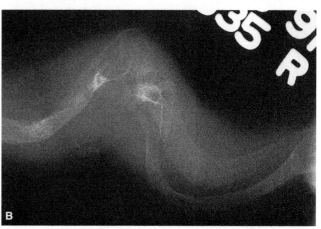

FIGURE 1.29 ▪ Osteogenesis Imperfecta (OI): Differential of Nonaccidental Trauma (NAT). (**A**) Severe deformities of both upper and lower extremities are seen in this girl with OI. She had severe bone fragility leading to multiple fractures from early infancy. (**B**) Radiograph of lower extremity shows severe generalized osteopenia, thinned cortices, and marked angular deformities of the bones. (See also Figures 2-46 to 2-49). The differentiation of OI from NAT can be complex and challenging. A multidisciplinary team including a child abuse specialist and pediatric radiology consultations may be warranted in such cases. (Photo contributor: Binita R. Shah, MD.)

than 18 months of age, and supracondylar fractures. Realize that most fractures seen in abused children are the same common fractures that are seen in the nonabused children. Subtle (hairline) tibial spiral fractures, or toddler's fractures, may be due to accidental trauma unless they occur in preambulatory young infants. The differential diagnosis of abusive fractures includes conditions with increased tendency to fracture (eg, cystic bone lesions, osteogenesis imperfecta, rickets), infections with metaphyseal lesions (eg, osteomyelitis, congenital syphilis), and malignancy (eg, Ewing sarcoma, leukemia).

Emergency Department Treatment and Disposition

Although fractures may present with limb-threatening potential, even the most gruesome fractures are rarely life threatening. Significant force is required to cause most fractures, and focus should be turned to head, chest, and abdominal injuries that may be life threatening. Initial focus should be on rapid assessment of these more significant injuries with transition

to fracture management when the patient is stable. A multidisciplinary team approach including consultations with pediatric orthopedics and surgery, child abuse consultant, social worker, and a specialist in pediatric radiology is often the optimal approach in managing such patients. In long bones, a rough estimate of age of injury may be possible based on evidence of healing such as periosteal reaction and callous formation. In an unstable patient, admission may need to occur prior to completion of radiographic diagnostic evaluation; however, a complete skeletal survey should be performed as soon as medically stable or postmortem. Order a full

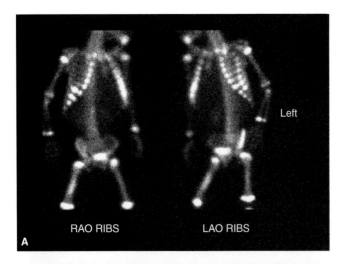

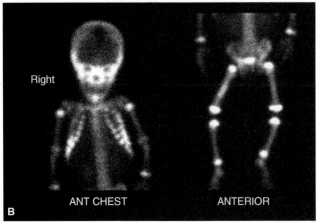

FIGURE 1.30 ■ Radionuclide Bone Scan. A 2-month-infant was brought to the ED for CPS evaluation after twin sister was found to have abusive head trauma. This infant was seen in the ED 2 weeks earlier, and a history provided by dad (and corroborated by mother) at that time was that dad "slipped on ice and fell with the twins." Questionable rib fractures were seen on a skeletal survey. (**A, B**) Whole-body images from a radionuclide bone scan demonstrate multiple adjacent areas of increased activity within the ribs bilaterally, compatible with multiple rib fractures and a questionable right femur fracture. Nondisplaced fractures, especially rib fractures, can easily be missed on radiographs prior to developing periosteal reaction or callous formation. LAO, left anterior oblique; RAO, right anterior oblique. (Photo contributor: Earl R. Hartwig, MD.)

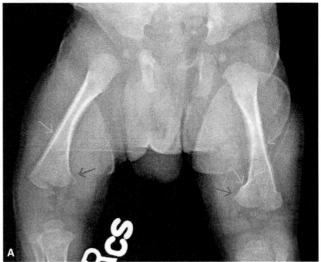

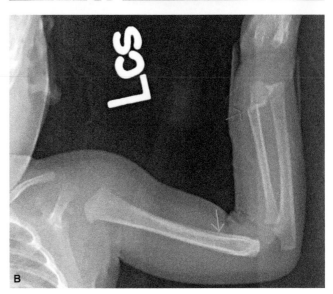

FIGURE 1.31 ■ Multiple Fractures: An 8-week-old Infant Presenting with "irritability for few hours." (**A**) Anteroposterior view of both femurs showing bilateral metaphyseal corner fractures (red arrows) and angulation of the left femoral cortex representing fracture (blue arrow). Periosteal reaction along both femoral cortices (green arrows) indicates a subacute component of injury, as this finding takes time to develop following the acute injury. (**B**) Lateral view of left arm showing displaced fracture of the distal radial diaphysis (red arrow). There is also periosteal reaction along the distal humeral cortices (blue arrows) indicating a healing fracture. (Photo/legend contributors: Earl R. Hartwig, MD, and Ryan Logan Webb, MD.)

skeletal survey, including complete views of any injuries that require orthopedic management. Review the medical record for previous visits of concern, and complete a head-to-toe evaluation for additional injuries. Laboratory and genetics examination should be considered in patients with multiple fractures to exclude metabolic disease. Despite this

possibility, children with metabolic bone disease generally have obvious past (or family) history or obvious physical or skeletal findings consistent with their diagnosis. In addition, children with metabolic bone diseases typically present with common fractures and typically not those (eg, ribs, CMLs) that are known to have higher specificity for abuse. Report suspected cases of physical abuse to CPS. Manage fractures as described in Chapter 19. Some specific fractures are discussed further in the following sections.

Pearls

1. Skull fractures, rib fractures, and CMLs are the predominant types of abusive injuries seen during infancy; long bone fractures are the most common abusive skeletal injury after 1 year of age.

2. Even though diaphyseal fractures are the most common type of fracture seen in child abuse, they can also often result from accidental injuries.

3. The hallmark characteristic in fractures caused by abuse is lack of a plausible explanation.

4. A follow-up skeletal survey 2 weeks after the initial study is helpful in identifying missed fractures. It may also confirm normal anatomic variants and metabolic bone diseases that mimic abusive injuries.

Clinical Summary

Femoral shaft fractures are common diaphyseal fractures in children that result from falls, motor vehicle accidents (MVAs), and sporting injuries. In infants, they are more likely due to nonaccidental injury. Distinguishing abuse from accidental trauma can be difficult and is often based on clinical suspicion. A history suspicious for abuse, physical or radiographic evidence of prior injury, and age <18 months are risk factors. An infant who is completely nonambulatory (especially if unable to crawl or roll) is much more likely to have sustained abuse. Associated injuries (eg, head injuries, bruises) need to be sought. After the first year of life, as an infant becomes more mobile, the likelihood of accidental as

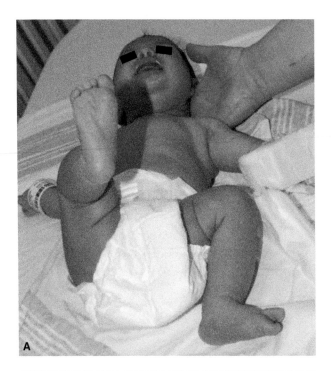

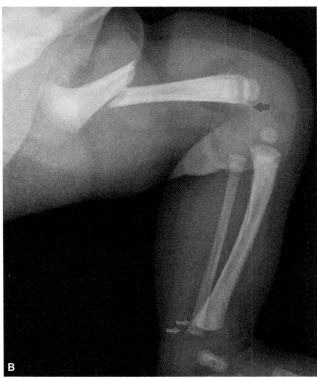

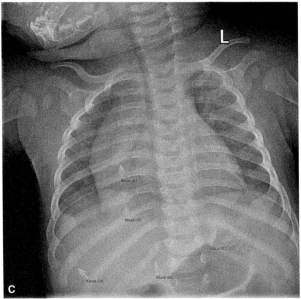

FIGURE 1.32 ■ Multiple Fractures of Nonaccidental Trauma (NAT). (**A**) This was a 3-week-old neonate who "fell from the father's shoulder to the carpeted floor" after father fell asleep on the couch while burping the neonate. This clinical picture shows neonate not moving the left extremity. (**B**) Frog leg lateral view of the left femur shows a complete femur fracture with overriding of fracture fragments. Also notice corner fractures of the distal tibia, fibula, and distal femur (arrows; the classic metaphyseal lesions [CMLs]). (**C**) Rib fractures. AP projection of chest shows multiple healing posterior and anterior rib fractures (arrows). The femur fracture was unlikely to have occurred with such a short fall but is often the impetus for further workup leading to the confirmatory diagnosis of NAT. The classic CMLs and rib fractures seen in this neonate are also highly specific for NAT. (Photo/legend contributors: Earl R. Hartwig, MD, and John Amodio, MD.)

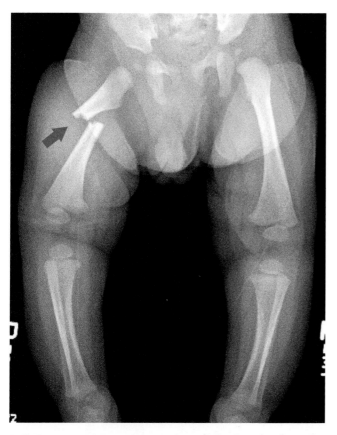

FIGURE 1.33 ■ Femur Fracture. Acute oblique displaced fracture of the right femoral diaphysis (arrow) is seen in this 3-month-old infant brought in with a history of "favoring the right leg and seemed to be in pain." His 16-year-old babysitter stated that the infant had been "in the crib all day." Skeletal survey also showed a healed fracture of the left 4th and 5th ribs anterolaterally. Lack of any history for such injury and fractures of different ages are indicative of nonaccidental trauma. (Photo/legend contributors: Earl R. Hartwig, MD, and Ryan Logan Webb, MD.)

opposed to nonaccidental injury increases. In an active toddler, an isolated femur fracture is more likely to be accidental than nonaccidental.

Emergency Department Treatment and Disposition

Femoral shaft fractures in infancy rarely require operative intervention. Consult orthopedics for treatment with traction, spica casting, or a combination of both. Skeletal traction with delayed spica casting and early and immediate spica casting have all been advocated. Admit young children with femur fractures for further management, including serial exams for occult injuries and evaluation for possible abuse. Great force is required to cause a femur fracture, and other possibly life-threatening injuries should be considered and excluded.

Pearls

1. Have a high index of suspicion for NAT when children <3 years of age (especially those <18 months) are evaluated for a femur fracture.
2. Spiral femur fractures are concerning for nonaccidental injury, particularly in children who are preambulatory.
3. Proximal epiphyseal fractures and CMLs involving the femur have a high specificity for abuse.

Clinical Summary

Rib fractures account for up to approximately 30% of all fractures found in abused children, and a higher incidence of rib fractures is reported in autopsy findings. Ribs of infants and young children are pliable and difficult to fracture by accidental means, and there are several reports of severe crush mechanisms (roll over by a car!) without any evidence of ribs being fractured. Rib fractures are usually seen with violent shaking, with anteroposterior thoracic compression in infants, and with direct blows to the chest in older children. Involvement of the posterior arc of a rib is most common; however, rib fractures can be seen at any location in abuse. Posterior rib fractures are due to levering of the posterior neck over the transverse spinous process as the rib cage is vigorously squeezed or as the perpetrators' fingers serve as a fulcrum against which the rib is stressed. There may be associated anterior and costochondral junction fractures as well. Clinically significant injury to the lungs and heart is uncommon despite the high frequency of rib fractures seen in abused children. Other thoracic injuries that are encountered with rib fractures include cardiac contusions, pulmonary contusions, hemo- and pneumothoraces, and pleural effusions.

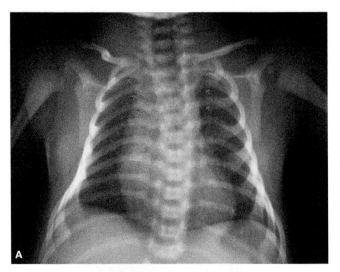

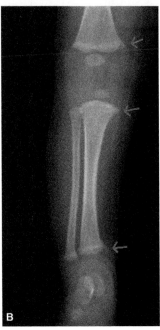

FIGURE 1.35 ■ Rib Fractures and Abusive Head Trauma. A 7-week-old infant presented with multiple bruises and leg swelling. As shown in this case, rib fractures and classic metaphyseal lesions are often a harbinger of shaking and abusive head trauma. (**A**) Anteroposterior (AP) view of the chest showing fractures of the bilateral posterior second, third, and fourth ribs (red arrows). Absence of callus formation indicates that the fractures are acute. Posterior rib fractures are highly specific for nonaccidental trauma. (**B**) AP view of right tibia and fibula showing metaphyseal corner fractures of femur and tibia (arrows). (Photo/legend contributors: Earl R. Hartwig, MD, and Ryan Logan Webb, MD.)

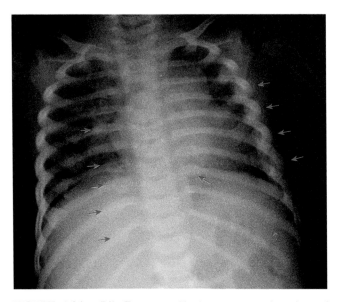

FIGURE 1.34 ■ Rib Fractures. Single anteroposterior view of the chest demonstrates multiple posterior and lateral rib fractures (arrows) with surrounding callus in the classic "rosary beads" appearance in an infant with bilateral subdural hematomas. (Photo/legend contributors: Manadakini Sadhir, MD, and Rachelle Goldfisher, MD.)

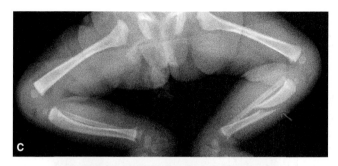

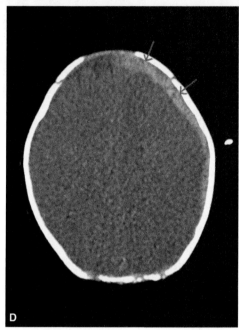

FIGURE 1.35 ■ (*Continued*) (**C**) Acute oblique displaced fracture of left tibia (arrow). (**D**) Axial head CT reveals acute subdural hemorrhage along the left frontal and parietal convexities (arrows). (Photo/legend contributors: Earl R. Hartwig, MD, and Ryan Logan Webb, MD.)

Emergency Department Treatment and Disposition

As part of a routine skeletal survey, AP and lateral chest radiographs and right and left posterior oblique views will further delineate rib fractures that may be missed on an initial posteroanterior chest radiograph. Admit all patients with rib fractures due to child abuse for serial exams and additional tests for other injuries as indicated. Pulmonary contusion should be sought with pulse oximetry and attention to exam changes (eg, tachypnea, rales). Pay particular attention to upper rib fractures that may be associated with cervical spine injuries and lower rib fractures that may portend significant abdominal injury. Child protective services investigation should be initiated. Rib fractures heal rapidly and do not require any specific therapy beyond pain management to allow adequate ventilation and prevention of atelectasis or pneumonia.

Pearls

1. Rib fractures are the most common type of thoracic trauma in physically abused children. These injuries are rare even in the setting of severe accidental trauma in infants.
2. Rib fractures are often bilateral, involve multiple levels, and frequently involve posteromedial ribs.
3. In contrast to adults, rib fractures are NOT a complication of cardiopulmonary resuscitation in infants and young children.
4. The presence of rib fractures in the absence of any clear etiology (eg, severe MVA or obvious metabolic bone disease) should be considered evidence of child abuse until proven otherwise.
5. Children with rib fractures from accidental injuries are significantly older with a plausible mechanism (eg, MVA) than children with rib fractures related to abuse.

Clinical Summary

Child abuse is the most common cause of severe head injury in children <1 year of age, and skull fractures are the second most common form of abusive skeletal injuries, accounting for 7% to 30% of all fractures in abused children. An abusive

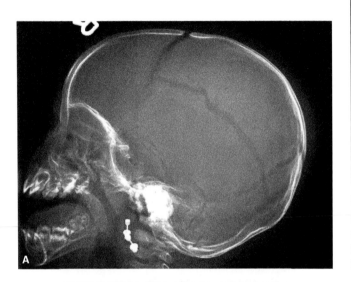

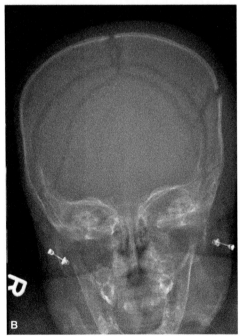

FIGURE 1.36 ■ Diastatic Skull Fracture. (**A, B**) Lateral and antero-posterior views of the skull show diastatic fracture extending over parietal region with widening of the coronal and lambdoid sutures in a 9-month-old infant brought in with bilateral eye swelling and vom-iting. Grandmother then reported that he was "standing up and hit his head on a shelf earlier in the day." A diastatic fracture in an infant without significant mechanism is highly suspect for nonaccidental trauma. (Photo contributor: Earl R. Hartwig, MD.)

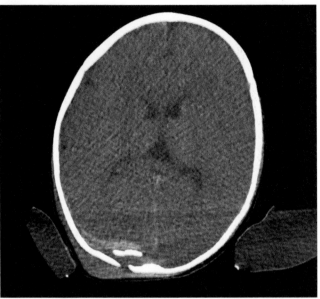

FIGURE 1.37 ■ Depressed Skull Fracture With Subdural Hematoma. Axial CT scan of the brain demonstrates occipital depressed fracture with subdural hematoma in an 8-month-old infant brought to the ED for altered mental status. (Photo contributor: Earl R. Hartwig, MD.)

skull fracture is caused by a forceful blow to the head with a solid object or being forcefully thrown or dropped onto a hard surface. The absence of a skull fracture does not exclude the possibility of intracranial injury. Dating of skull fractures is difficult because they do not heal with the evident callus formation that is seen with long bone fractures.

Emergency Department Treatment and Disposition

Plain skull radiographs, including AP and lateral views, should be considered to identify suspected skull fractures even when cranial CT has been performed, because skull frac-tures coursing in the axial plane may be missed with axial CT. Bone scans are not helpful in identifying skull fractures. MRI or head CT without contrast is indicated for initial evaluation of all suspected inflicted head injuries. Isolated skull fractures require no specific therapy beyond pain control and heal well in the majority of cases. Depressed skull fractures will require neurosurgical evaluation to determine if elevation may be necessary. Underlying intracranial bleeds should always be considered, and appropriate workup performed. Patients need continuing follow-up by their primary care provider due to risk for development of a leptomeningeal cyst.

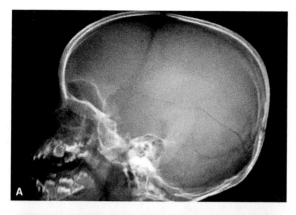

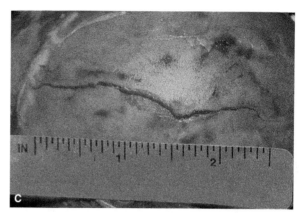

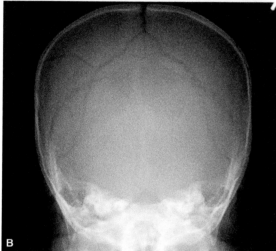

FIGURE 1.38 ■ Linear Skull Fracture. (**A, B**). A simple linear fracture in the right parietal bone with associated soft tissue swelling was seen in this active and playful 12-month-old infant presenting to the ED for a swelling to the right scalp without any history of trauma. His exam, medical record review, and skeletal survey were unremarkable. Given no history provided, this is still suspicious for a nonaccidental trauma (NAT). (**C**). An autopsy finding of the scalp in an infant brought to the ED in cardiopulmonary arrest shows a linear skull fracture of the parietal bone. There was brain injury with swelling, but no intracranial hemorrhage was noted. Although bilateral, depressed, and diastatic fractures are more specific for NAT, the most commonly seen skull fracture in NAT is a simple linear fracture such as this. (Photo contributors: Earl R. Hartwig, MD [A, B], and Binita R. Shah, MD [C].)

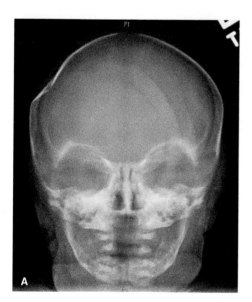

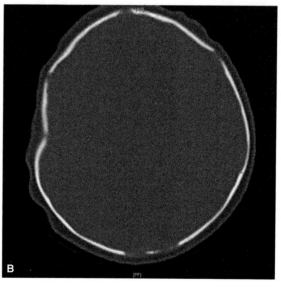

FIGURE 1.39 ■ Ping Pong Fracture. (**A**) Frontal view of the skull demonstrates right "ping pong" fracture of parietal bone in a neonate who was brought in for "a deformity in his scalp since birth." He was born via vaginal delivery, and as per mom, "it was a difficult delivery." (**B**) Axial CT image of the head; the bone window shows depressed and angulated fracture of the right parietal bone, resembling a crushed ping pong ball. Child Protective Services was consulted as this story was "very suspicious" mandating a thorough evaluation including birth records and ensuring a very close follow-up. (Photo/legend contributors: Earl R. Hartwig, MD, and Ryan Logan Webb, MD.)

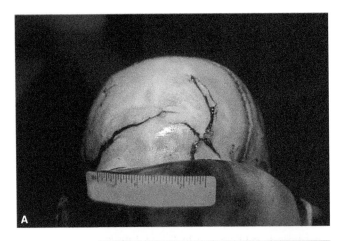

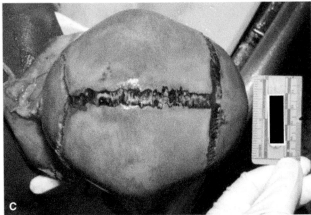

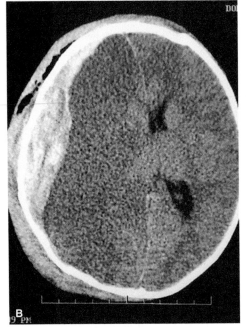

FIGURE 1.40 ■ Abusive Head Trauma. (**A, B**) Comminuted skull fractures (**A**) can be seen radiating from areas subjected to traumatic force in a toddler presenting with signs of herniation due to increased intracranial pressure from an epidural hematoma (**B**). A fracture of this nature would take tremendous force to produce. This patient's head was slammed against the kitchen counter. (**C**) Autopsy photograph in a different toddler depicting diastasis of cranial sutures (not skull fractures) from the brain swelling in a fatal case of abusive head trauma. (Photo contributors: Binita R. Shah, MD [A, B], and Earl R. Hartwig, MD [C].)

Pearls

1. No pattern of skull fracture is pathognomonic of child abuse; however, skull fractures that are multiple, bilateral, diastatic, or depressed and those that cross suture lines are more likely due to abuse rather than accidental.

2. Skull fractures that occur in children after simple accidental falls (eg, falls <4 feet, falling off of a bed or table) are unusual and are seen in only a small percentage of children with this mechanism. When accidental, they are typically single, linear, and nondiastatic and most commonly involve the parietal bone. Fractures associated with simple accidental falls are also not associated with intracranial injury.

3. Suspect abuse in a child presenting with a history of minor trauma with depressed, diastatic, complex, or multiple fractures, particularly those involving the occipital bone.

Clinical Summary

Abusive head trauma (AHT) is a leading cause of death in infants and often causes long-term neurologic disabilities in survivors. Shaken impact syndrome (violent shaking of an infant often in combination with blunt impact) is one of the important mechanisms of AHT. Cardinal signs of shaken impact syndrome include brain injury (subdural hematomas and cerebral edema), retinal hemorrhages, and skeletal injuries (specifically rib fractures and classic metaphyseal lesion [CML]). Cervical spine injuries may be seen in severe cases. However, because blunt impact trauma may occur alone or in combination with shaking, the more inclusive term *abusive head trauma* is preferred when describing these injuries. Because there is often no history of trauma or only a vague history of minor trauma (eg, fall from caretaker's arms or from a changing table), a high degree of suspicion is necessary when assessing the need for imaging in an infant or very young child suspected of having AHT. Victims may present with respiratory distress, apnea, seizures, altered mental status, or cardiac arrest, but also may present with subtle or nonspecific symptoms, such as irritability, vomiting, or sleepiness. Focal neurologic signs may or may not be present; thus, it may be very easy to incorrectly confuse these patients as having common pediatric illnesses. In addition, there are often no other signs of external trauma on examination or very subtle bruising that is initially overlooked.

Emergency Department Treatment and Disposition

With AHT, perform initial stabilization and resuscitation as indicated, with initial focus on maintaining adequate ventilation, hemodynamic stability, and temperature control. Many head-injured patients will never require neurosurgical intervention, but their outcome may be greatly improved with careful attention to these factors. These patients should be admitted for close monitoring and management to a pediatric intensive care unit. Depending on stability of the patient and urgency, order a head CT or MRI for the evaluation of possible subdural or subarachnoid hematomas or subdural hematohygromas representing bleeds of different ages. Consider plain films to evaluate for skull fractures, which may or may not be seen depending on the type of force inflicted and can be missed by a CT scan. MRI is a superior tool to CT to

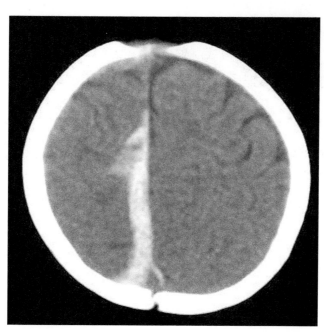

FIGURE 1.41 ■ Abusive Head Trauma. A noncontrast CT scan of the brain shows hyperdense area along the right tentorium extending into the posterior interhemispheric fissure, along the falx, and over the convexity, suggestive of an acute subdural hematoma. This 3-month-old infant was brought to the ED with lethargy and signs of Cushing triad with bulging anterior fontanelle and absence of any external injuries. Subsequently, the father confessed to "shaking the infant." (Photo contributor: Binita R. Shah, MD.)

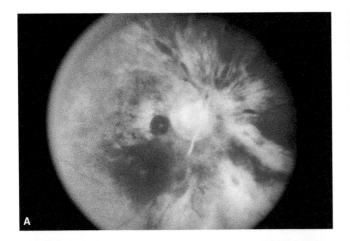

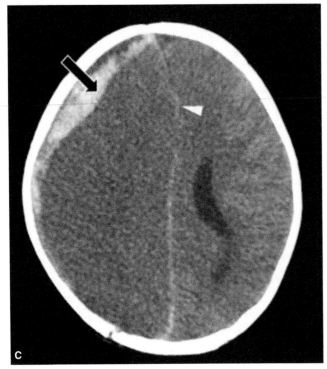

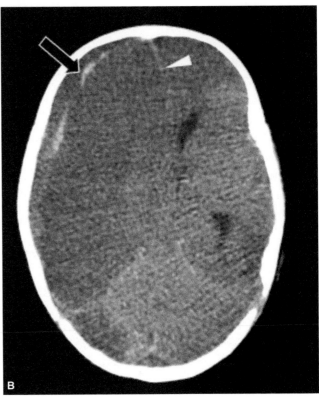

FIGURE 1.42 ■ Abusive Head Trauma. (**A**) Diffuse retinal hemorrhages seen in a 6-month-old infant brought to the ED receiving bag-valve-mask resuscitation by emergency medical services. He had bruises in the right periorbital area and on the trunk. (**B, C**) Axial CT images demonstrate a large right-sided, mixed-density subdural hematoma (black arrow). There is significant mass effect, including leftward midline shift (arrowhead) with complete effacement of the right lateral ventricle, sulci, and cisterns. Diffuse edema is seen throughout the right cerebral hemisphere and medially on the left. (Photo/Legend contributors: Earl R. Hartwig, MD, and Vinodkumar Velayudhan, DO.)

assess for diffuse axonal injury but is often not easily accessible in the emergency setting. Consult a multidisciplinary team, including ophthalmology (eye examination for retinal hemorrhages) and neurosurgery, as indicated. Obtain a full skeletal survey including skull films to evaluate for other injuries. Obtain tests to evaluate for internal organ injury, including CBC; liver, pancreatic, and renal screens; and creatine phosphokinase, urinalysis, and coagulation studies. From a legal standpoint, it is helpful to obtain coagulation studies early in the course because a coagulopathy may also develop secondary to severe head injury. A normal coagulation profile at the onset of presentation will help exclude a preexisting coagulopathy as a contributor (or legal defense) to the child's intracranial bleed.

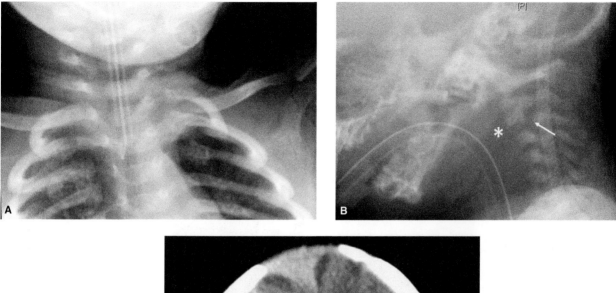

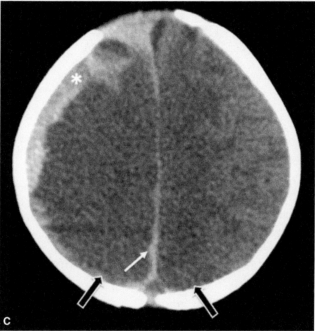

FIGURE 1.43 ▪ Nonaccidental Trauma with Traumatic Brain Injury. A 6-week-old infant presented with decrease in oral intake, staring episodes, and bulging fontanel. (**A**) Frontal view of the clavicles demonstrates a fracture of the left acromion. (**B**) Hangman's (C2 pars) fracture. Lateral radiograph of neck demonstrates a displaced fracture through the pars interarticularis of C2 with anterior subluxation of C2 on C3. Note the marked prevertebral soft tissue swelling with displacement of the endotracheal tube anteriorly (asterisk). (**C**) Axial CT demonstrates a large right-sided subdural hematoma adjacent to the right frontal and parietal lobes (asterisk) and tracking along the posterior falx (white arrow) with trace subarachnoid hemorrhage in the adjacent sulci. There is edema with loss of gray-white differentiation involving the entire right and medial left cerebral hemispheres (black arrows). (Photo/legend contributors: Earl R. Hartwig, MD, and Vinodkumar Velayudhan, DO.)

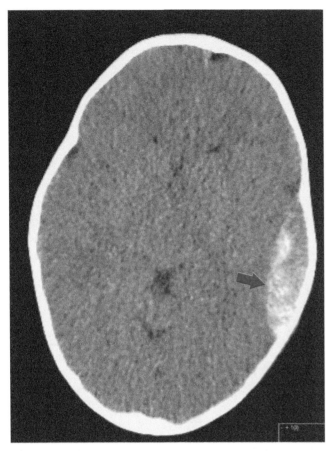

FIGURE 1.44 ■ Epidural Hematoma. Axial CT of the brain demonstrates a lenticular-shaped area of high attenuation over the left parietal lobe consistent with an epidural hematoma (arrow) in an infant presenting with lethargy and vomiting. He also had multiple bruises. (Photo contributor: Rachelle Goldfisher, MD.)

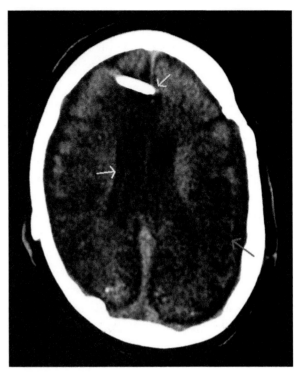

FIGURE 1.45 ■ Abusive Head Trauma (AHT). A follow-up CT scan in a different infant with AHT shows diffuse gray and white matter hypoattenuation and diffuse encephalomalacia (red arrow). There is associated ventricular enlargement (ex vacuo dilation, yellow arrow) and prominent extra-axial fluid. Patient is postplacement of intracranial shunt catheter (blue arrow). The impact of the shearing forces, increased intracranial pressure, and hypoxic changes associated with AHT are devastating. (Photo/legend contributors: Earl R. Hartwig, MD, and Ryan Logan Webb, MD.)

Pearls

1. Minor falls rarely result in life threatening injuries. Maintain a high index of suspicion for patients who present with a history of fall from low height with multiple or complex skull fractures or intracranial bleeds, particularly subdural hemorrhage.

2. The classic triad of subdural hematoma, retinal hemorrhages, and posterior rib fractures is present in only a minority of abused patients. Shaken impact syndrome may present initially with a normal head CT and with unilateral or no retinal hemorrhages.

3. Every infant with nonspecific symptoms (eg, irritability, vomiting) should be carefully examined for alertness, bruising in hidden areas, bulging fontanelle, or long bone tenderness to rule out a subtle presentation of AHT, realizing however, that often there are no signs of external trauma.

4. Consult ophthalmology for a dilated eye examination in every suspected victim of AHT. Documentation of the type, extent, and location of retinal hemorrhages can be helpful in confirming the diagnosis of AHT.

Clinical Summary

Studies of blunt abdominal trauma in children show that child abuse represents approximately 11% of all pediatric blunt trauma cases. Estimated rates of thoracoabdominal "visceral" injuries in abuse range from 2% to 20%. However, this is likely a significant underestimate secondary to lack of recognition of these injuries. Inflicted abdominal presentations may include hypovolemic or septic shock from ruptured organs or intestinal perforation, duodenal hematoma, or pancreatic, renal, or vascular injuries. Many of these infants and young children present early with vague symptoms or present later in their course and cannot verbalize their discomfort. Thoracic injuries such as hemothorax and pulmonary and cardiac injuries have been reported but are quite rare.

Although many abused infants and children undergo chest radiography, full evaluation for abdominal trauma has generally been limited to children with abnormal laboratory values and those with clinical evidence of injuries such as bruising, pain, distension, and/or vomiting. Associated injuries such as CNS and skeletal injuries also distract from the ability to fully assess the abdomen or may delay the full evaluation. Hemodynamic instability should call attention to the thorax and abdomen as potential sources. Observation of the patient with significant organ injury with serial examinations, without the need for surgical intervention, is the recommended practice. There is also a strong desire to reduce radiation exposure due to potential future health risk, all of which increases the likelihood of missing thoracic and abdominal trauma in abused children.

The mechanism of most thoracoabdominal injuries in abuse is due to focal blunt force, such as a direct blow from a punch or kick. When compared with children who sustain accidental abdominal trauma, abused children tend to be younger, with a mean age of approximately 2 to 3 years compared with 7 to 10 years for nonabused children with abdominal trauma. In

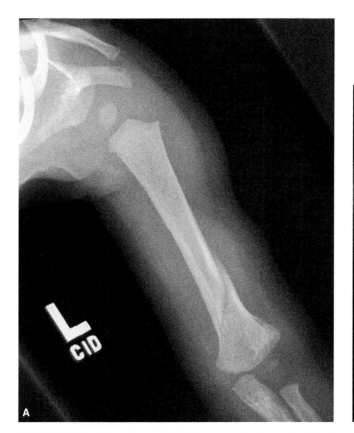
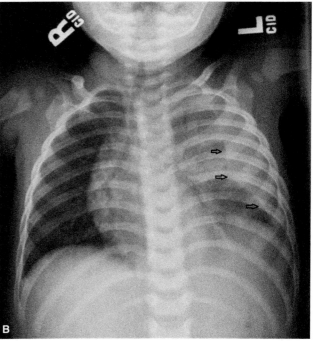

FIGURE 1.46 ■ Hemothorax With Fractures. An 8-month-old infant was brought to the ED favoring his left arm. There was no history of trauma. (**A**) Anteroposterior view of the left humerus demonstrates a spiral fracture. (**B**) Frontal view of the chest demonstrates large left pleural collection (hemothorax, black arrows) and subacute right clavicle fracture. Due to the impressive pliability of the ribs in children, it is not uncommon to see intrathoracic trauma such as pulmonary contusion and hemothorax without overlying rib fractures. (Photo/legend contributors: Earl R. Hartwig, MD, and John Amodio, MD.)

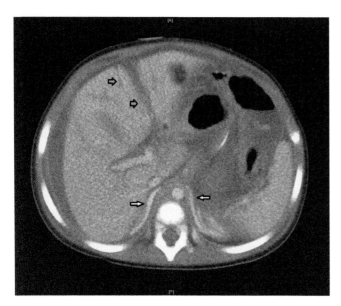

FIGURE 1.47 ■ Blunt Abdominal Trauma. A 19-month-old toddler with a history of vomiting and refusal to feed became progressively more lethargic and presented to the ED in shock. She was resuscitated and found to have elevated liver enzymes, azotemia, and metabolic acidosis. Axial CT scan view through upper abdomen demonstrates liver lacerations (black arrows), hemoperitoneum, and hyperenhancement of the adrenal glands (white and black arrows), compatible with shock (CT hypotension complex). (Photo/legend contributors: Earl R. Hartwig, MD, and John Amodio, MD.)

addition, vague, inconsistent or inadequate histories are often provided in the abused children, whereas clear mechanisms (such as MVA or significant fall) are identified in those with accidental trauma. Children in the accidental group tend to receive prompt medical care, whereas we often see significant delays in presentation with abused children. Finally, abused children have a much higher mortality than the accidental group (estimated at 50% versus 20%, respectively). Despite the low rates of abdominal injuries in abuse, this is the second most common cause of death in abused children.

In contrast to those who sustain accidental injuries, abused infants and children are often subject to a more focal blunt force mechanism. Children inherently have less protective abdominal musculature and the smaller AP diameter of the abdomen leads to injuries from compression and shearing against the spine. Compressed bowel and increases in pressure result in hollow viscus rupture. Shearing forces in areas of fixed mesentery result in avulsion of the bowel from its mesentery with resultant injury to the vascular supply. Fixed structures such as the duodenum, proximal jejunum, pancreas, and left lobe of the liver are most commonly injured

in abuse. Solid organs and colonic injuries (related to seatbelt compression) are seen in accidental trauma. The frequency of solid organ injury in abuse is actually similar to that of accidental trauma, but hollow viscus rupture or a combination of the two is much more likely in abuse. By some estimates, about 39% of abused children had both solid organ and hollow viscus injury, whereas that combination was not present in any patients in the accidental group. Of the solid organs, abusive injuries to the liver predominately involve the left lobe, reflective of a midline upward punch or kick mechanism; in accidental injuries (mostly MVAs), a more lateral blunt force is seen. Injuries involving the spleen, kidneys, and adrenals are encountered but to a much lesser degree. A high index of suspicion is needed in any infant or child presenting with abdominal complaints, particularly if associated with abdominal bruising, and in those with altered mental status, shock, cardiac arrest, or other suspicious signs (eg, skin, skeletal, CNS) of abuse. Due to delays in presentation, there should be a lower threshold for imaging (focused assessment with sonography for trauma [FAST] and CT) and laboratory evaluation in these children.

Emergency Department Treatment and Disposition

Children with abusive thoracoabdominal trauma should receive resuscitation and stabilization per trauma surgery protocols. Providers should recognize that altered mental status may be a result of hemodynamic instability, and fluid and blood resuscitation may be required. Consideration should be given for transfer to a pediatric trauma center early in the patient's course if possible. Although surgical management is often expectant, patients with continued blood loss or evidence of viscus rupture require laparotomy. Symptoms related to hollow viscus injury often progress and require vigilance with frequent serial examinations. Often, other significant injuries, such as CNS injuries, are coexistent and require a multidisciplinary approach. A history of the mechanism of injury, or lack thereof, should be sought and documented with attention to timing of signs and symptoms. The findings of significant thoracoabdominal injuries with report of a short-distance or "stair" fall mechanism in an infant or young child are red flags to the likelihood of abuse.

Along with hemodynamic stabilization, any patient with suspicion of abdominal trauma should receive a FAST US in the ED with laboratory evaluation of urine and pancreatic and

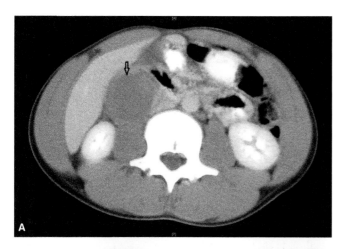

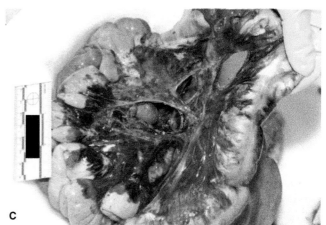

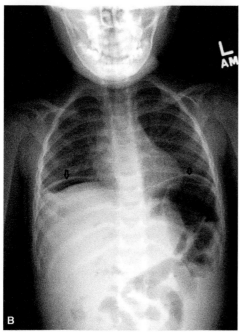

FIGURE 1.48 ■ Blunt Abdominal Trauma. (**A**) A 13-year-old child was repeatedly punched in the stomach by the stepfather during an argument. Axial CT scan view of abdomen shows intramural duodenal hematoma (arrow). (**B, C**) A 22-month-old toddler was left with mother's cousin because "her house was on fire." Two days later, the baby presented with fever and bilious emesis. (**B**) Erect view of abdomen shows free intraperitoneal air (arrows). Laparotomy revealed a large hematoma within the mesentery of the small bowel as well as a hematoma involving the hepatic flexure of the colon. There was a significant amount of inflammatory exudate and biliary drainage from a duodenal laceration, which was repaired. (**C**) Mesenteric tears with subsequent avascular compromise to the bowel. (Photo/legend contributors: Earl R. Hartwig, MD, and John Amodio, MD.)

liver enzymes. A chest radiograph may reveal rib fractures and associated injuries such as pulmonary contusions and hemothorax, which may require chest tube placement if present. Lower rib injuries should alert clinicians to potential for underlying abdominal injuries. Monitoring of ECG, serial cardiac enzymes (eg, troponin) along with echocardiograms may be helpful in identifying suspected cardiac injuries. Hemodynamically unstable patients will likely undergo urgent surgical exploration, whereas more stable patients with laboratory or clinical evidence of abdominal trauma will likely undergo CT evaluation for diagnosis. Although some use specific cutoff laboratory values for imaging in pediatric abdominal trauma, considerations should be made for a lower threshold

to image with concerns of abuse. Liver enzymes, in particular, may return to baseline quickly, and the time delay seen with abuse should be considered as a factor. The risk of radiation must be balanced with the importance of missing a diagnosis of abuse with potential for subsequent injury and death. In regard to time delay, intraoperative biopsies or postmortem specimens may allow dating of severe abdominal injuries as well. A full skeletal survey is indicated in younger children with suspicion of abuse. Stable children found to have intra-abdominal solid organ injuries (eg, liver, splenic, or renal lacerations and contusions) are best treated in conjunction with pediatric surgical specialists in a pediatric intensive care unit setting. A multidisciplinary approach is often indicated.

Pearls

1. Household falls such as stair injuries rarely result in significant thoracoabdominal injuries. Maintain a high index of suspicion for abuse when these injuries are encountered with a history of minor trauma.
2. Abdominal injuries seen in abuse include solid organ, mostly medial liver injury, with a much higher incidence of hollow viscus injury. Upper mid-abdomen injuries such as duodenal and jejunal viscus injury (hematomas, perforations) should alert you to potential of abuse.
3. Although the incidence of rib fractures is high in abused infants and children, underlying pleural, pulmonary, and cardiac injuries are unlikely.

Clinical Summary

Sudden unexplained infant death syndrome (SUIDS) is the sudden death of an infant <1 year of age that remains unexplained after a thorough case investigation, including performance of a complete autopsy, examination of the crime scene, and review of the clinical history. The incidence of SUIDS is more common in non-Hispanic black and American Indian/ Native American infants than non-Hispanic white infants. Although it was thought to rarely occur in the first month of life, approximately 10% of cases occur in the first month of life, and incidence peaks between 3 and 4 months of age. Up to 90% of cases occur in infants <6 months of age.

Contributory factors for SUIDS include sleeping in a prone position or sleeping on soft material or a soft surface, young maternal age, maternal smoking, lack of prenatal care, prematurity, low birth weight, male sex, overheating, and overwrapping. Infanticide is an incident of nonaccidental trauma that is fatal during infancy. Estimates of the incidence of infanticide among cases diagnosed as SUIDS range from <1% to 5%. It is difficult to distinguish at autopsy between SUIDS and accidental or intentional suffocation with a soft object.

Postmortem studies performed by the medical examiner include radiographic skeletal survey, toxicology screening, metabolic screening for inborn errors of metabolism, and

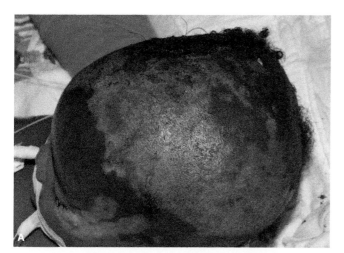

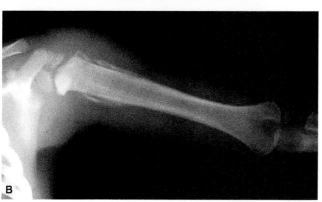

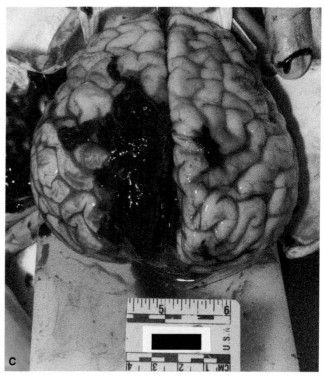

FIGURE 1.49 ■ Multiple Trauma. (**A**) A 16-month-old boy presented unconscious with posturing. He was noted to have a partial-thickness burn to the scalp and face with multiple bruises. When questioned, mom stated that he was burned by hot water "in a shower 2 days ago." He was seen 2 weeks earlier in the ED with a history of unwitnessed fall and shoulder injury. He was sent home with a diagnosis of "contusion vs. Salter I fracture to the proximal humerus." Despite aggressive management, the patient died from progressive increased intracranial edema and herniation. (**B**) Postmortem skeletal survey revealed occipital fracture and a healing fracture of the proximal left humerus. (**C**) Autopsy photo depicting subdural hemorrhage. (Photo contributor: Earl R. Hartwig, MD.)

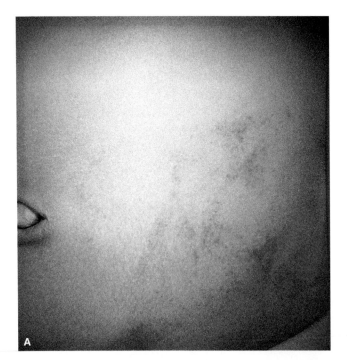

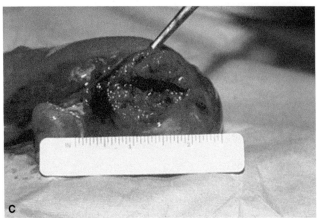

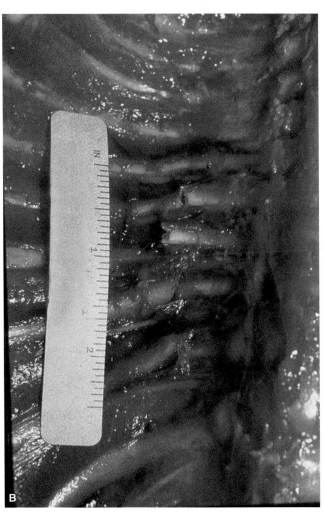

FIGURE 1.50 ■ Infanticide. (**A**) Abdominal bruise. An infant brought in with cardiopulmonary arrest was found to have this bruise on the abdominal wall. The mother gave a history of finding the baby "not breathing" 4 hours after she had fed the baby. (**B**) Multiple rib fractures (ribs 5 through 11) were seen at autopsy. Rib fractures are highly unlikely in the setting of cardiopulmonary resuscitation even with inexperienced providers. (**C**) Liver laceration found at autopsy. Other injuries included laceration of the lung and heart. (Photo contributor: Binita R. Shah, MD.)

tissue analysis of the brain, liver, kidney, heart, muscle, adrenal glands, and pancreas.

Emergency Department Management

Once the infant is pronounced dead, approach the family with an empathetic, compassionate, supportive, and nonaccusatory manner while attempting to learn more about the circumstances surrounding the infant's death. Note the reaction of

the caregivers or parents and try to obtain any observations made by the first-response teams and document them in the medical record (eg, position of the infant, body temperature, rigor or lividity, the presence of any marks on the body prior to transport). Other factors to consider are the type of crib or bed and any defects, the type of mattress (firm versus a water bed), the presence of a blanket or comforter, soft stuffed toys or pillows in the crib, amount of clothing on the baby, room temperature, and type of ventilation and heating. The

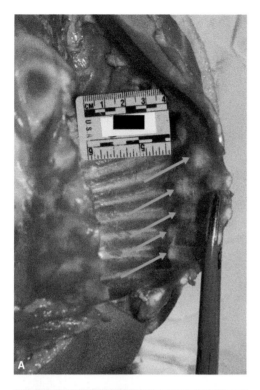
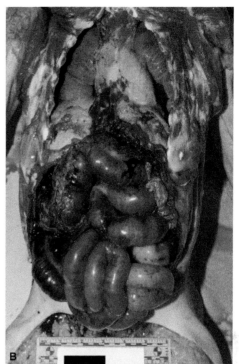
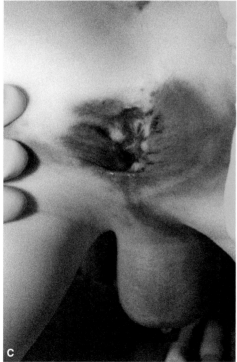

FIGURE 1.51 ■ Autopsy Findings Seen in Fatal Abdominal Trauma. An infant presented in cardiopulmonary arrest. Every sudden unexplained infant death (SUID) should be followed by a scene investigation and autopsy, as shown in this example. (**A**) Rib fracture callus formation. (**B**) Necrotic right colon secondary to mesenteric tears and subsequent ischemia. (**C**) Perianal contusion; forced anal penetration may sometimes lead to rectal perforation and subsequent intraperitoneal bleed or infection. (Photo contributor: Earl R. Hartwig, MD.)

history and exam findings along with the clinician's overall impression are important to convey to the medical examiner after fully interviewing the caretaker and family members who were present at the scene. Even though a thorough

investigation of the death scene will be done by law enforcement officers, the information obtained in real time may be more accurate and the death scene may quickly be altered. A thorough examination of the dead infant should be done

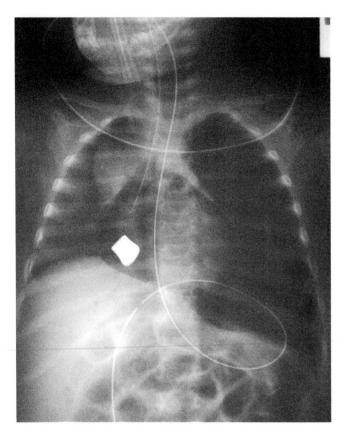

FIGURE 1.52 ▪ Fatal Gun Shot Wound. An 8-month-old infant shot in the chest with a bullet lodged in the right ventricle. Frontal view of the chest shows bullet overlying the heart. There is pneumopericardium, pneumomediastinum, and left tension pneumothorax. Endotracheal tube is also in right bronchus intermedius. This is a stark reminder of the extremely dangerous world so many young children live in. (Photo/legend contributors: Earl R. Hartwig, MD, and John Amodio, MD.)

by either a child maltreatment specialist or pediatrician with expertise in child maltreatment. Photographs taken in the ED are valuable to document any lesions, especially prior to the development of lividity.

Suspect possible intentional suffocation or infanticide with any of the following: a previous history of recurrent episodes of cyanosis, apnea, or brief resolved unexplained events (BRUE) while under the care of the same person; age >6 months; previous unexplained and unexpected death of one or more siblings; simultaneous or nearly simultaneous death of twins; previous death of infants under the care of the same unrelated person; or discovery of blood on the infant's nose or mouth in association with BRUEs.

In the absence of any external evidence of trauma, a preliminary diagnosis of "probable SUIDS" can be given to a previously healthy infant who has died suddenly and without any explainable cause. Postmortem findings in fatal child abuse most often reveal intracranial injuries (eg, subdural hematoma, intracerebral hemorrhage), intra-abdominal trauma (eg, liver laceration, hollow viscus perforation, intramural hematoma), burns, and drowning or toxic exposure.

Pearls

1. An autopsy must be performed on any infant who dies suddenly and unexpectedly. Infant deaths without postmortem examination should not be attributed to SUIDS.
2. Excluding child abuse through a thorough investigation in every sudden and unexplained death can help protect surviving and subsequent siblings.
3. Suspect SUIDS when a previously healthy infant apparently dies during sleep, prompting an urgent call for emergency services. Often the history reveals that the infant fed appropriately before going to sleep, and the infant was found in the same position in which he or she had been placed at bedtime.

Chapter 2

CONDITIONS MISTAKEN FOR PHYSICAL AND SEXUAL ABUSE

Allison M. Jackson
Tanya S. Hinds

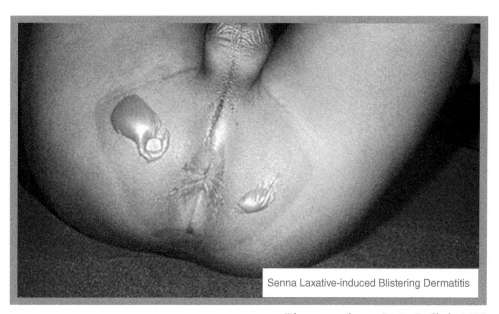

Senna Laxative-induced Blistering Dermatitis

(Photo contributor: Binita R. Shah, MD)

The authors acknowledge the special contributions of Binita R. Shah, MD, to prior edition.

Clinical Summary

Congenital dermal melanocytosis (also referred to as Mongolian spots or blue-gray macules of infancy) is the most frequently encountered birthmark in neonates. Melanin-containing melanocytes in the dermis are present (migrational arrest), and the distinctive blue color, characteristic of dermal melanin, occurs as a result of the Tyndall effect (when light strikes the surface of the lesion, red wavelengths of light are absorbed and blue wavelengths are reflected back from the brown melanin pigment from the dermis). Mongolian spots are more prevalent in Asian (40% to >80%), African American (30% to >60%), Hispanic (25%–70%), and Native American

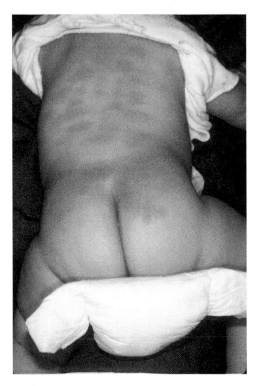

FIGURE 2.2 ■ Congenital Dermal Melanocytosis (Mongolian Spot). Multiple areas of bluish discoloration are seen on the back and buttocks in a Caucasian infant, in whom the incidence of Mongolian spots is uncommon (<10%), and these lesions may be mistakenly attributed to inflicted bruises. (Photo contributor: Binita R. Shah, MD.)

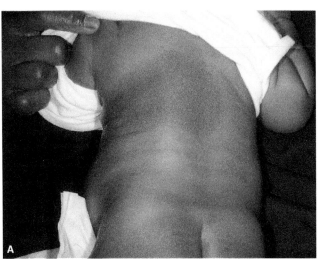

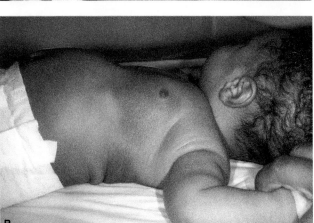

FIGURE 2.1 ■ Congenital Dermal Melanocytosis (Mongolian Spots). (A) Bluish-gray macular lesions, present since birth, are seen on the back and buttocks (the most common location) of an otherwise healthy African American infant. (B) Lesion on the anterior chest wall in the same infant. (Photo contributor: Binita R. Shah, MD.)

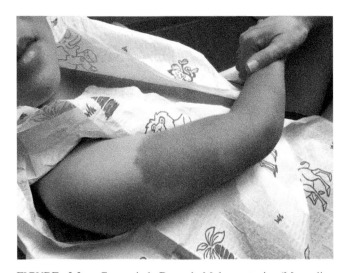

FIGURE 2.3 ■ Congenital Dermal Melanocytosis (Mongolian Spot). A 4-year-old child with bruise-like discoloration on his right forearm. He also had several similar blue-gray lesions on his lower sacral area (typical distribution). These lesions have been present since birth. (Photo contributor: Julie Cantatore-Francis, MD.)

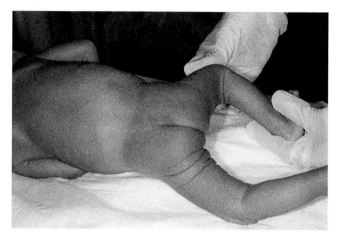

FIGURE 2.4 ■ Congenital Dermal Melanocytosis (Mongolian Spot). An infant brought to the ED in cardiopulmonary arrest had these lesions thought to be Mongolian spots; however, inflicted bruises from child abuse were in the differential diagnosis. The medical examiner would typically incise areas of skin discoloration to exclude underlying contusions from inflicted injuries. (Photo contributor: Binita R. Shah, MD.)

infants than in white infants (<10%). The skin lesion is flat (macular), slate-gray, greenish-blue or brown, and consists of poorly circumscribed, single or multiple lesions ranging in size from a few millimeters to several centimeters. The most common location are the sacrum and buttocks (90%), but lesions may occur anywhere, including the back, shoulders, or flank. Mongolian spots fade gradually and resolve by age 5 to 6 years in about 96% of cases. Differential diagnosis of Mongolian spots includes accidental or inflicted injury and other forms of dermal melanocytosis (eg, nevus of Ito or Ota; See Figures 2.13 to 2.15).

Emergency Department Treatment and Disposition

Mongolian spots do not lead to any symptoms and require no treatment. Family needs to be reassured about the benign nature of these lesions. Documenting their presence in the medical record can alleviate future confusion with bruises.

Pearls

1. Mongolian spots can be mistaken for contusions resulting from inflicted injuries. Mongolian spots are nontender unlike contusions, which may be tender.
2. A contusion from inflicted injuries undergoes sequential color changes and resolves within a few days, whereas Mongolian spots *do not undergo similar color changes* and fade spontaneously over a period of years.

Clinical Summary

Folk healing practices are used by various cultures to treat illness. Coin rubbing (also known as Cao Gio, scratch the wind, or coining) is practiced among Southeast Asians (Vietnamese and Cambodians) when a child is sick. Warm oil (eg, tiger balm or mentholated oil) is applied over the affected region of the body, and then it is vigorously rubbed in with the edge of a coin. This is an attempt to rid the body of "ill wind" to reduce fever and chills. Cupping (ventosa) is used in some Eastern European, Latin American, and Russian cultures to reduce congestions. Alcohol is applied to the inner rim of the cupping glass and ignited with cotton soaked in alcohol. The cup is applied to the skin after the flame is extinguished. As it cools, a vacuum forms in the cup, causing an ecchymotic lesion at the site. Spooning (spoon rubbing or quat sha) is used among the Chinese to relieve pain and headache. The skin is scratched with a porcelain spoon until ecchymotic lesions appear. Garlic is used orally and topically for medicinal

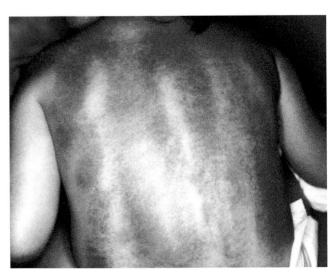

FIGURE 2.6 ■ Coin Rubbing. Purpura from "coining," a cultural practice for fever management. (Reproduced with permission from Tenenbein M, Macias CG, Sharieff GQ, et al. *Strange and Schafermeyer's Pediatric Emergency Medicine.* 5th ed. McGraw-Hill Education; New York, 2019.)

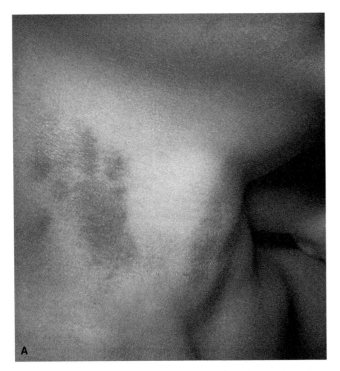

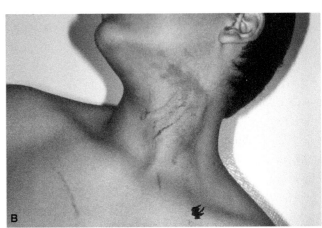

FIGURE 2.5 ■ Coin Rubbing (Cao Gio) versus Inflicted Child Abuse Bruises. (**A**) This Cambodian boy with linear patterns of petechiae and purpura on the neck was referred by the school nurse to "rule out" child abuse. The common sites in coin rubbing are along bony prominences and include spine, neck, and intercostal spaces. (**B**) Bruises inconsistent with the stated history or multiple bruises in different stages of healing (suggestive of repeated abuse) or in unusual locations (eg, genitalia, buttocks, neck) suggest child abuse. (Photo contributor: Binita R. Shah, MD.)

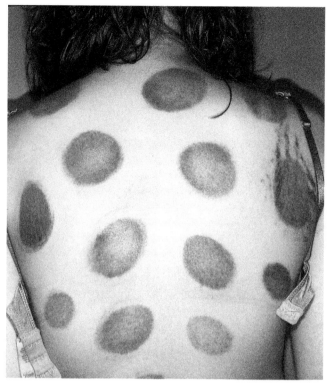

FIGURE 2.7 ▪ Cupping (Ventosa). Several round identical purpuric lesions are seen on the back from cupping that was used to relieve back pain. First- or second-degree burns may also be seen in cupping. The common sites are back, abdomen, and chest. (Photo contributor: Binita R. Shah, MD.)

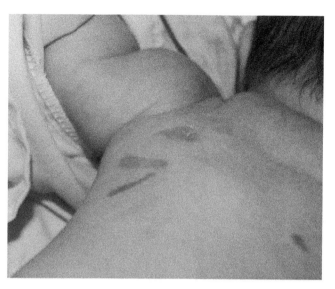

FIGURE 2.8 ▪ Garlic Burn. This previously healthy Hispanic infant with pyelonephritis was noted to have multiple linear and loop-shaped and irregularly shaped cutaneous lesions, some of which had bullae, on his torso consistent with burns. These lesions were not consistent with any infectious or dermatologic condition. No explanation was provided for the injuries, prompting a Child Protective Services report. On investigation, the detective learned that the grandmother used a mixture of tequila, herbs, and garlic and rubbed it on the infant followed by wrapping in a warm blanket and putting him in a hot room. This was done to get rid of the evil eye (mal de ojo), which was suspected due to fever. (Photo contributor: Allison M. Jackson, MD, MPH.)

purposes in a number of cultural communities for a variety of health conditions, including fever, respiratory and gastrointestinal illnesses. Topical application may involve placing garlic cloves on the skin and then wrapping the area for a period of time. This may result in partial-thickness chemical burns of the skin. Moxibustion is also practiced among the Chinese. It is a form of acupuncture. Burning sticks of incense, yarn, cigarettes, or cones of the herb *Artemisia* are used to make small circular burns on the skin at therapeutic points. Maquas is used by Arabs, Jews, and Bedouins. Hot metal spits or coals are applied to areas of disease or over a traditional "draining point" to produce burns. Caida de mollera (fallen fontanelle) may prompt a range of Latino folk remedies that use physical force and gravity to restore the fontanelle. Subdural and retinal hemorrhaging, resembling abusive head trauma, is possible in the few instances when physical force is significant.

Emergency Department Treatment and Disposition

These practices are not followed to injure the child, but rather are performed with the belief that they will help the child heal or recover from an illness. Ignorance of these folk healing practices on part of the medical team results in allegations of physical abuse, and trust between the medical team and the family may be irrevocably damaged. Consultation with a child abuse specialist may help in difficult cases. Educate parents about the injurious nature of these practices and suggest alternative approaches to treating illness. Performing a thorough review of systems is important to determine the symptoms that led to the cultural intervention, so that the patient's primary illness can be diagnosed and appropriately treated.

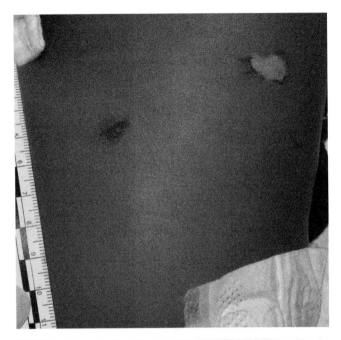

FIGURE 2.9 ■ Garlic Burn. Oval partial-thickness burns in the mid torso are seen on this infant, prompting a Child Protective Services report. Grandmother reported placing garlic on infant's skin and dressing and wrapping him in blankets overnight so warmth and garlic might relieve cold symptoms. Garlic remnants were found in a soiled undergarment. Chemical burns were deemed accidental. (Photo contributor: Tanya S. Hinds, MD.)

Pearls

1. Folk healing practices (also known as pseudo-battering) may be mistaken for inflicted injuries from child abuse.
2. Healthcare providers should become familiar with folk healing practices in their community.

Clinical Summary

Cold panniculitis is an inflammation of subcutaneous fat after prolonged exposure to cold or prolonged application of a cold object to any area of the skin (eg, ice packs applied to the face of an infant to control supraventricular tachycardia or ice packs applied to the lower extremities after vaccination). It is believed to occur solely because of the inherent properties of infant body fat with a higher percentage of saturated fatty acids (compared with older children and adults) and an increased propensity to solidify with prolonged exposure to a cold object. The degree of fat necrosis is inversely related to the age of the patient. Popsicle panniculitis is caused by sucking on ice, seen especially in infants who while sucking on the popsicles or ice cubes do not move them around in the mouth (as done by adults), keeping the cold object in contact with buccal fat for a prolonged period.

Popsicle panniculitis is commonly seen in the summer. Typically there are no systemic signs such as fever or leukocytosis. The skin lesions are red to purplish, indurated, discrete nodules or plaques with mild tenderness and sometimes itching. Lesions are seen in the perioral area (adjacent to the

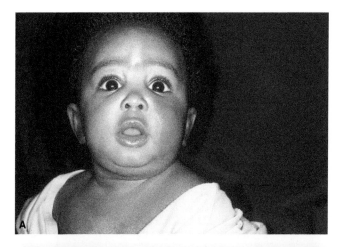

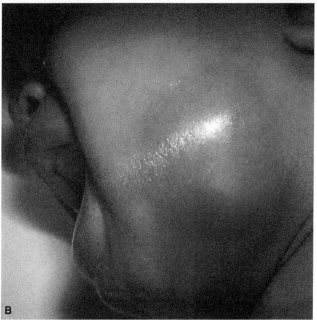

FIGURE 2.11 ■ Cold Panniculitis Versus Buccal Cellulitis. (**A**) An afebrile, very playful infant with an erythematous, indurated, and mildly tender lesion on the cheek was admitted with a diagnosis of child abuse versus buccal cellulitis. A history of putting ice packs on his cheeks because of an extreme heat wave 2 days prior to appearance of the rash was obtained subsequently. (**B**) Erythematous, indurated, and tense swelling with severe tenderness was seen in this highly febrile and irritable child. Blood culture was positive for *Streptococcus pneumoniae*. (Photo contributor: Binita R. Shah, MD.)

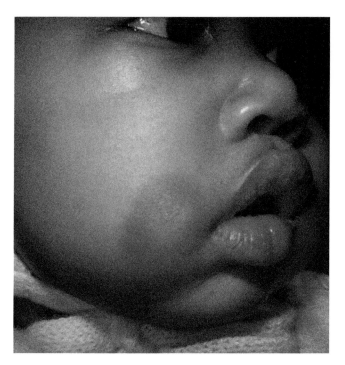

FIGURE 2.10 ■ Cold Panniculitis. This infant was referred to "rule out" child abuse when this erythematous and indurated lesion near the corner of the mouth was seen during a well-baby visit. It was thought to be a red bruise produced by pinching. A history of sucking on an ice cube 2 days prior to appearance of this lesion was subsequently obtained. (Photo contributor: Binita R. Shah, MD.)

corners of the mouth) and may be unilateral or bilateral. Panniculitis lesions resolve spontaneously in 2 to 3 weeks without scarring. Differential diagnosis includes child abuse, subcutaneous fat necrosis from other etiology (eg, hypercalcemia, trauma), buccal cellulitis, giant urticaria, contact dermatitis, or frostbite.

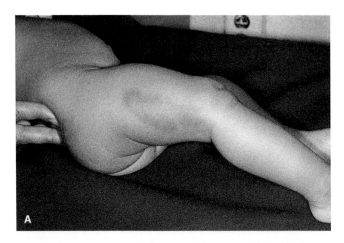

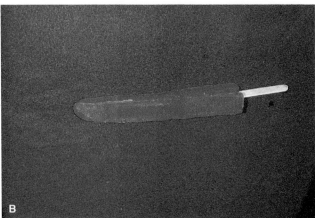

FIGURE 2.12 ■ Cold Panniculitis. (**A**) This young infant with an erythematous, indurated, linear "skin rash" was thought to have a bruise inflicted by a long object (eg, a ruler or belt) prompting a Child Protective Services report. The mother said that her 6-year-old son was eating a popsicle (like one shown in **B**) and had placed the popsicle on the thigh of the infant. A skin biopsy confirmed the diagnosis of cold panniculitis, and charges were subsequently dropped against the family. (Photo contributor: Binita R. Shah, MD.)

Emergency Department Treatment and Disposition

Cold panniculitis is self-limiting and does not require specific therapy except reassuring caregivers. Recurrence is common, and parents must be educated about the condition. Dermatology consultation and a skin biopsy (nonspecific lobular adipocyte necrosis at the dermal–epidermal junction with a surrounding mixed inflammatory infiltrate seen) may aid in doubtful cases.

Pearls

1. A history of skin exposure to a cold object followed by a skin lesion supports the diagnosis of cold panniculitis. (*Important: Panniculitis arises within hours to 1–2 days after the exposure to a cold object.*)
2. Popsicle panniculitis lesions due to sucking on ice are seen adjacent to the corners of the infant's mouth.

Clinical Summary

Nevi of Ota and Ito arise from dermal melanocytes and are present at birth in about 50% of cases. A second peak occurs during puberty. The skin lesion is a light to dark brown, blue-black, or bluish-gray macule with a mottled or specked appearance. It increases in intensity and size with time and persists for life. They are more common in Asians (about 75% of cases; most commonly found in the Japanese), in African Americans, and in girls. Nevi of Ota occur on the face, forehead, zygomatic region, periorbital area, cheek, nose, or eye. Ipsilateral eye involvement (ocular melanosis) is commonly seen in moderate to severe cases and may involve the sclera (most common), conjunctiva, cornea, iris, retina, and optic nerve. Other mucous membranes and tissues (ear canal, tympanic membrane, pharynx, hard palate, nasal mucosa, buccal mucosa) may be rarely involved. Nevi of Ito occur on the supraclavicular region, shoulder, upper arm, and neck. Differential diagnosis of these nevi includes postinflammatory hyperpigmentation, café-au-lait spot, or Mongolian spots.

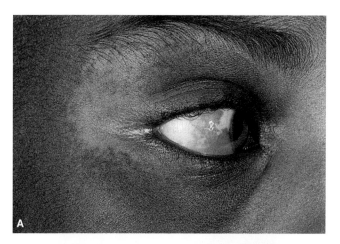

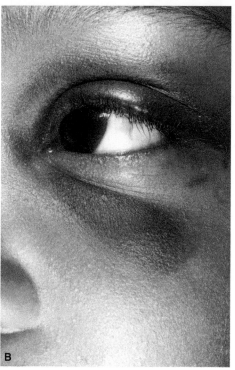

FIGURE 2.14 ■ Nevus of Ota Versus Inflicted Bruise From Child Abuse. (**A**) Close-up of patient in Figure 2.13 showing blue-gray pigmentation with a specked appearance and involvement of the sclera. (**B**) Bluish and red areas of discolorations are seen around the eye of a patient who was punched in both eyes by her stepmother. She also had subconjunctival hemorrhage in her other eye and numerous bruises in different stages of healing. (Photo contributor: Binita R. Shah, MD.)

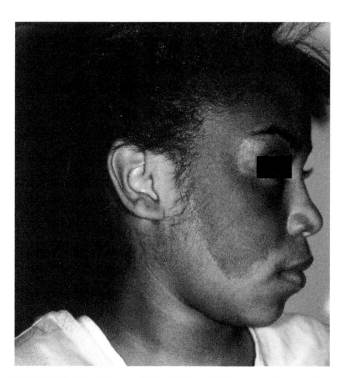

FIGURE 2.13 ■ Nevus of Ota. Unilateral blue-gray pigmentation involving the face and periorbital area (ophthalmic and maxillary divisions of the trigeminal nerve). (Photo contributor: Binita R. Shah, MD.)

Emergency Department Treatment and Disposition

The diagnosis is made by typical clinical appearance. These nevi do not require any intervention in the ED. Patient can be

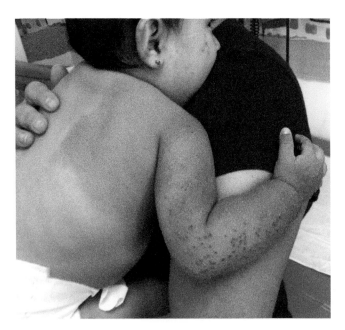

FIGURE 2.15 ■ Nevus of Ito. An incidental finding of blue-gray pigmentation involving the scapular and deltoid region in a child with Gianotti Crosti syndrome. (Photo contributor: Sharon A. Glick, MD.)

referred to a dermatologist for evaluation and therapies that may include laser surgery or masking with cosmetics. If ocular melanosis is present, glaucoma may occur (melanocytes in the ciliary body of the anterior chamber may impede normal flow of fluid), and patients also need periodic funduscopic examinations by an ophthalmologist.

Pearls

1. Nevi of Ota and Ito may be mistaken for ecchymoses due to inflicted child abuse injuries. However, these nevi are nontender unlike ecchymoses, which may be tender.
2. An ecchymotic lesion undergoes sequential color changes and resolves within a few days. These nevi *do not undergo similar color changes* and are permanent lesions.
3. The majority of these nevi are unilateral, present in a specific anatomic location, and have a speckled or mottled appearance, unlike Mongolian spots, which are uniform in appearance and fade spontaneously over the years.

Clinical Summary

A port-wine stain (PWS), also known as nevus flammeus, is a congenital vascular malformation (capillary ectasias) of dermal capillaries present at birth. Most commonly, they are seen on the face or neck but may occur anywhere. The lesion is pink to purple, varied in size and shape, and sharply circumscribed. Large lesions follow a dermatomal distribution and rarely cross the midline. During infancy and childhood, the lesion is macular; as age increases, it may become darker in color, papular, or nodular, causing disfigurement. Elevated skin lesions may bleed spontaneously.

PWS may occur as an isolated birthmark (majority of patients) or be associated with a syndrome, including Sturge-Weber syndrome (eg, PWS in the distribution of the ophthalmic (V1) and maxillary (V2) branch of the trigeminal nerve, intracranial calcifications, seizures, glaucoma) and Klippel-Trenaunay syndrome (PWS over an extremity, hemangiomas, varicosities, and limb hypertrophy of the involved extremity). Differential diagnosis includes capillary hemangioma and other vascular malformations (eg, salmon patch).

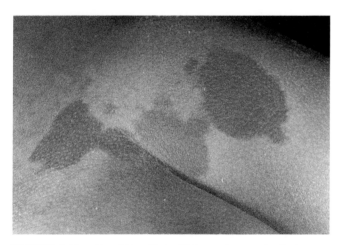

FIGURE 2.16 ■ Port-Wine Stain. Pink-purple macular lesions on the buttocks led to referral of this infant to "rule out" child abuse. These lesions were present since birth. Location of these lesions can mimic abuse because one of the typical sites for inflicted bruises are buttocks and lower back. (Photo contributor: Binita R. Shah, MD.)

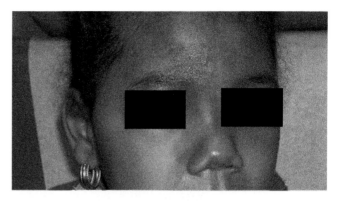

FIGURE 2.17 ■ Port-Wine Stain (PWS) in Sturge-Weber Syndrome. Most common location of PWS is the face. It may be confused with a red or purple bruise inflicted by abuse, especially when it is very extensive as shown. When a PWS is localized to the trigeminal area of the face (especially around the eyelids), a diagnosis of Sturge-Weber syndrome must be considered. (Photo contributor: Sharon A. Glick, MD.)

Emergency Department Treatment and Disposition

PWS is diagnosed clinically and does not require any intervention in the ED. Because PWSs do not involute, they may represent a significant, lifelong cosmetic problem. Refer the patient to a dermatologist for evaluation for laser therapy. Radiologic studies (as clinically indicated) may be ordered to evaluate patients with Sturge-Weber syndrome presenting to the ED with seizures and may include CT scan and/or MRI. Such patients will need appropriate referrals to neurology and ophthalmology.

Pearls

1. PWS can be confused with inflicted bruises from child abuse.
2. An ecchymotic skin lesion undergoes sequential color changes and resolves within a few days. PWS *does not undergo similar color changes*; however, PWS may become darker in color and more nodular over the years.
3. PWS does not regress spontaneously and *persists for a lifetime.*

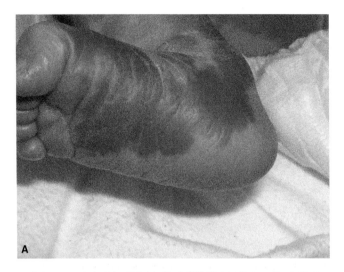

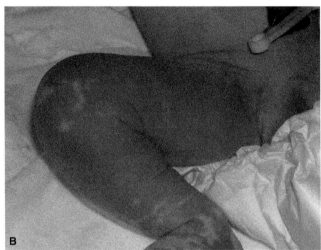

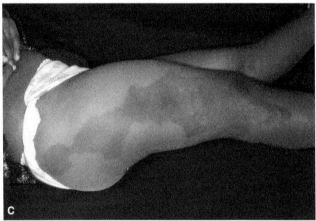

FIGURE 2.18 ■ Port-Wine Stain (PWS); Klippel-Trenaunay Syndrome (KTS). PWS on the foot and extending onto the leg and thigh in an infant with KTS. (**A, B**). PWS associated with hemihypertrophy of the extremity in a child with KTS. Skin discoloration and "swollen" (hypertrophied) extremity may be mistaken for inflicted injuries (**C**). (Photo contributors: Sharon A. Glick, MD [A, B], and Binita R. Shah, MD [C].)

Clinical Summary

Phytophotodermatitis (PPD) is an acute phototoxic eruption following contact with certain plants, fruits, or vegetables containing photosensitizing compounds and exposure to sunlight. Examples of plants causing phototoxic reactions include limes, lemons, celery, parsnip, fig, fennel, parsley, dill, mangoes, carrots, and meadow grass. PPD occurs only with contact with a photosensitizing furocoumarin (psoralens) compound that readily penetrates the epidermis *and* subsequent exposure to ultraviolet (UV) radiation (wavelengths >320 nm). PPD is common among food handlers (eg, salad makers and grocery workers), and the most common compounds are limes and lemons used in mixing drinks or making lemonade. A history of helping parents to make such drinks or spilling juice on the body during outdoor activities may be present. Other means of exposure may be landscaping or gardening. In temperate countries, cases are often seen among children playing outdoors during summer, when psoralens are most abundant in wild and garden plants.

Berloque dermatitis refers to dermatitis that results from application of a psoralen-containing perfume (eg, oil of bergamot), followed by UV exposure. The patient develops a rash at the exact areas where the perfume was applied.

Acute presentation of PPD after inflammation can be a mild reaction with erythema or a severe reaction that includes

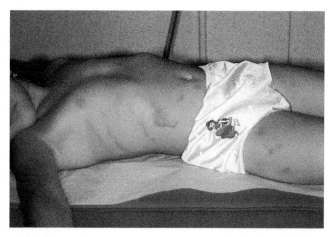

FIGURE 2.20 ■ Phytophotodermatitis (PPD). Bizarre streaky hyperpigmentation on the torso can be mistaken for resolving bruises. A history of mixing lemonade at the beach confirmed the impression of PPD. (Photo contributor: Binita R. Shah, MD.)

tingling of exposed skin and erythema followed by edema and vesiculation (after 24 hours; similar to severe sunburn). Bullous formation lasting for days may occur. Presentation after resolution of inflammation includes desquamation followed by hyperpigmentation. Configuration of lesions may be puzzling or unusual patterns such as streaks (eg, from brushing against a plant), drip marks or haphazard lines (eg, from spilling celery juice), hand prints (eg, child touched with hands soaked with lemon juice), or crisscrossing linear streaks of erythema, vesicles, and bullae (eg, due to meadow grass rubbing on the skin). The lesions of PPD are sharply limited to areas of sun exposure and at the sites of contact (eg, mouth, face, arms, legs) and seen during hot and humid sunny days. Ecchymosis from inflicted bruises due to child abuse is an important differential diagnosis.

Emergency Department Treatment and Disposition

Symptomatic relief may be required for acute presentations, including baths with colloidal oatmeal (eg, Aveeno), emollients (eg, Aquaphor or Vaseline), and topical steroids. Systemic therapy as indicated may include analgesics, antihistamines (eg, hydroxyzine), and systemic steroids (eg, prednisone for 5–14 days). Patients presenting with hyperpigmentation do not require any treatment, and it will fade over a period of weeks to months.

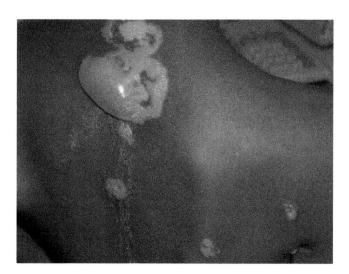

FIGURE 2.19 ■ Phytophotodermatitis. A blistering rash is seen on the back of the trunk this child who had applied topical psoralen prescribed for a family member. Subsequently, playing outdoors without a shirt on a very hot sunny day resulted in this rash. (Photo contributor: Sharon A. Glick, MD.)

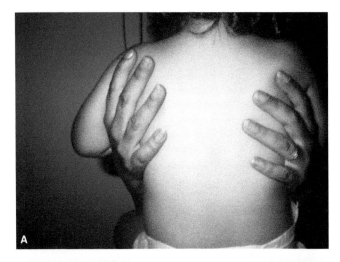

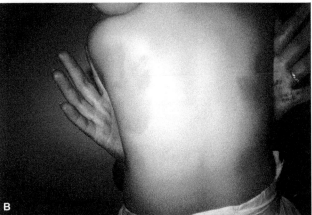

FIGURE 2.21 ■ Phytophotodermatitis. (**A**) An infant with hyperpigmentation that corresponds to mother's hands is seen. (**B**) The mother, whose hands were wet mixing the lime juice, picked up the unclothed infant on a hot, humid sunny day. (Photo contributor: Binita R. Shah, MD [A] and Reproduced with permission from: Shah BR, Laude TL: Atlas of Pediatric Clinical Diagnosis. WB Saunders; Philadelphia, PA, 2000 [B].)

Pearls

1. PPD is an example of photo-irritant contact dermatitis.
2. The most common produce containing the offending compounds are limes and lemons used in mixing drinks or in making lemonade (hence often referred as "lime disease").
3. PPD may be easily overlooked when a patient presents with erythema and vesicles following contact with plants or foods thought by parents to be irrelevant. Diagnosis can be easily made by taking a thorough history.
4. PPD may be mistaken for child abuse because of its unusual patterns of cutaneous lesions.

Clinical Summary

Senna is an anthraquinone-based laxative. Ingestion of senna-containing laxatives by young children (either accidentally or given therapeutically for constipation) may result in an irritant contact dermatitis. Dermatitis is caused by repeated and/or prolonged close contact with stool containing senna. Pathogenesis is not certain; it is likely related to interaction among senna, intestinal bacteria, and/or digestive enzymes. The typical patient is a 2- to 3-year-old child who is in diapers at least part time and who accidentally self-ingests between 15 and 375 mg of senna, usually as chocolate-flavored senna-based laxative tablets or squares. Onset of diarrhea is approximately 6 hours after ingestion, with blistering recognized by caregivers approximately 14 to 15 hours after onset of loose stool. Diarrhea typically lasts around 24 hours or longer. There does not appear to be a dose-dependent relationship between amount of ingested senna and severity of skin symptoms. On anogenital examination, erythema, blistering, and sloughing classically occur in a triangular or pear-shaped distribution on buttocks. There may be linear demarcation between affected and unaffected gluteal skin that aligns with the inner absorbent liner of a child's diaper. These partial-thickness burns on buttocks often extend toward the child's back and downward toward the perineum, with frequent sparing of the perianal skin. The usually sharp borders between affected and unaffected skin may raise concern for an inflicted partial-thickness scald burn in children with severe skin breakdown, blistering, and sloughing. Similar, severe irritant contact dermatitis has not been widely reported in children who have ingested phenolphthalein-containing laxatives.

Emergency Department Treatment and Disposition

Caregivers should be counseled that soiled diapers should be promptly removed, and anogenital skin should be frequently cleansed, followed by barrier cream. Caregivers should also be counseled about fluid replacement.

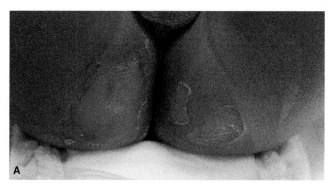

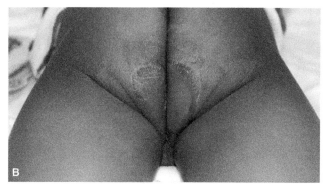

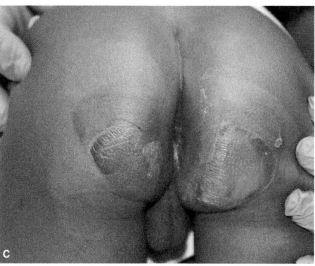

FIGURE 2.22 ■ Laxative-Induced Dermatitis. (**A, B, C**) A 3-year-old boy with a history of chronic constipation was given a senna-containing laxative, resulting in diarrhea the following day. Three days later, he was noted to have "peeling skin." A 4 cm × 2 cm well-demarcated area of centrally denuded skin with peripheral peeling is seen on the right buttock. Two areas of denuded skin with peripheral peeling are also seen on the left buttock. Note sparing of the perianal region and scrotum. (Photo contributor: Tanya S. Hinds, MD.)

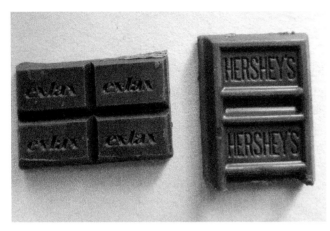

FIGURE 2.23 ■ Look-alikes. Senna-Containing Laxative and Hershey's Chocolates. Accidental ingestion of senna-containing chocolate laxatives is also seen in young children as they appear similar to Hershey's chocolates and who doesn't like Hershey's? (Photo contributor: Tanya S. Hinds, MD.)

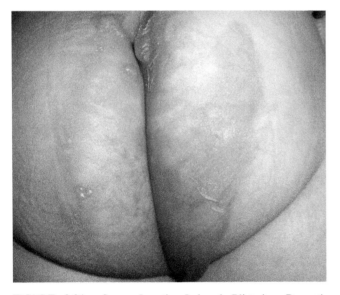

FIGURE 2.24 ■ Senna Laxative–Induced Blistering Dermatitis. Infants and toddlers ingesting senna-based laxatives may rarely develop a burn-like eruption on the buttocks. The eruption tends to occur after the buttock has been exposed to a loose stool for a few hours in a patient given this medication. It is important to differentiate this from a scald from hot water immersion (as seen in Figure 1.20.) (Reproduced with permission from Prose NS, Kristal L. *Weinberg's Color Atlas of Pediatric Dermatology*, 5th ed. McGraw-Hill Education; New York, 2017.)

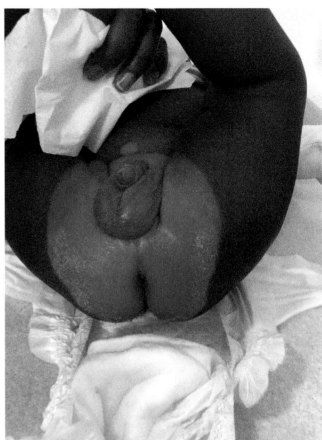

FIGURE 2.25 ■ Napkin Psoriasis: Differential Diagnosis of Scald Burns. Note the overlying scale and sharp demarcation seen in napkin psoriasis in an infant. This sharp demarcation can be mistakenly attributed to inflicted scald burn. Typical sparing of the creases between the thigh and abdomen that is seen in forced immersion burn (secondary to instinctive flexion of hips while child's buttocks are forcefully plunged into hot water) is not seen here. (Photo contributor: Sharon A. Glick, MD.)

Pearls

1. A careful history is needed to differentiate between an abusive scald burn and laxative-induced diaper dermatitis.
2. A history that diarrhea preceded skin changes and/or the possibility of ingestion of senna-containing laxatives may lessen concern for an abusive scald burn.
3. Senna-induced contact dermatitis is most likely to occur in children wearing diapers compared with toilet-trained children but has occurred in a minority of toilet-trained children.

Clinical Summary

Acute hemorrhagic edema of infancy (AHEI), also referred to as Finkelstein disease or Seidlmayer syndrome, is a benign self-limited condition characterized by a characteristic purpuric rash. First described as a cutaneous variant of Henoch-Schönlein purpura (HSP), it is now considered a separate entity. Leukocytoclastic vasculitis and fibrinoid necrosis are seen in patients with AHEI as well as HSP. However, patients with HSP usually have immunoglobulin [Ig] A deposition, whereas IgA deposition is demonstrable in only about one-third of patients with AHEI. Other differentiating features between the 2 conditions include lack of visceral involvement and a better prognosis in AHEI.

Unlike HSP, AHEI occurs most frequently in infants and toddlers (usually children <2 years old). Patients often have a history of a preceding respiratory illness or medication exposure (eg, penicillin, cephalosporin). The rash occurs on nonmucosal cutaneous surfaces involving face, ears, and extremities. It starts as annular erythematous patches that may coalesce and become purpuric assuming a classic rosette or target shape. In addition to the purpuric rash, physical exam is also notable for edema of the face, extremities, hands, or feet. Edema typically begins distally and progresses proximally.

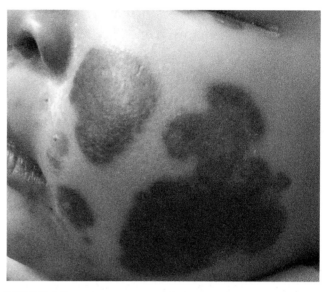

FIGURE 2.27 ■ Acute Hemorrhagic Edema of Infancy. Biopsy of an active lesion reveals an intense leukocytoclastic vasculitis. However, in contrast to Henoch-Schönlein purpura, systemic symptoms are rare. There may be several outbreaks of new lesions, but the entire process generally resolves in approximately 2 weeks. (Reproduced with permission from Prose NS, Kristal L. *Weinberg's Color Atlas of Pediatric Dermatology*, 5th ed. McGraw-Hill Education; New York, 2017.)

Whereas HSP is associated with systemic involvement manifesting as arthritis or affecting gastrointestinal or renal systems, AHEI does not have significant systemic involvement. Patients may have a low-grade fever. Because any

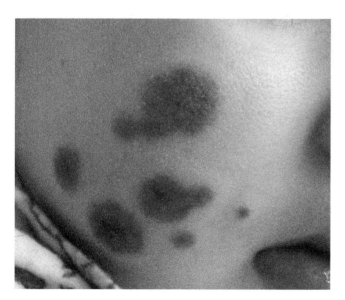

FIGURE 2.26 ■ Acute Hemorrhagic Edema of Infancy. This striking disorder occurs in infants between 4 months and 2 years of age. The sharply circumscribed lesions favor the extremities and are edematous, ecchymotic, and purpuric. Edema of the ears and eyelids may also be noted. (Reproduced with Permission from Prose NS, Kristal L. *Weinberg's Color Atlas of Pediatric Dermatology*, 5th ed. McGraw-Hill Education; New York, 2017.)

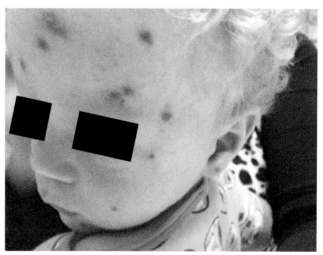

FIGURE 2.28 ■ Acute Hemorrhagic Edema of Infancy. A 2-year-old well-appearing toddler presented with purpuric lesions on face, ear, and distal extremities associated with edema of the forehead. These lesions self-resolve within 5 days. (Photo contributor: Sharon A. Glick, MD.)

bruise in an infant should raise concerns for inflicted trauma, providers may interpret the purpuric rash of AHEI as inflicted bruises. The medical history and accompanying edema should allow the provider to differentiate AHEI from physical abuse. Similarly, the purpuric lesions of HSP that tend to occur on dependent areas including the buttocks (a high-target area for corporal punishment) may be confused with bruises from physical abuse. Again, eliciting history of a recent upper respiratory illness, recent or current abdominal pain, signs or symptoms of a migratory arthritis, or hematuria should help the provider distinguish HSP from physical abuse.

Emergency Department Treatment and Disposition

AHEI is a benign and self-limited condition in the vast majority of the children and resolves within 1 to 3 weeks. Such children do not require hospitalization and can be followed by the primary care physician with symptomatic treatment as indicated. A thorough review of systems should yield symptoms that correlate with a diagnosis of AHEI (or HSP).

Pearls

1. Typical triad of AHEI is fever, edema, and annular or targetoid-shaped purpura. The co-occurrence of such signs should help differentiate AHEI from physical child abuse.
2. The most common locations of AHEI rash are the face, ears, and extremities (symmetrically distributed), whereas it spares the trunk and mucous membranes.
3. When acute, bruises are tender, whereas the purpuric lesions of AHEI (and HSP) are not tender and may, in fact, be pruritic.

Clinical Summary

Skin infections, such as impetigo and erysipelas (see also pages 98–104), may have clinical features that resemble burns, thereby raising suspicion for physical abuse. Impetigo is a

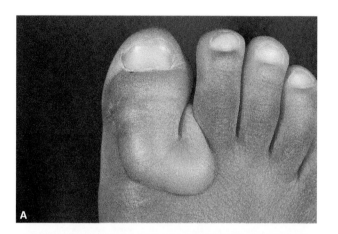

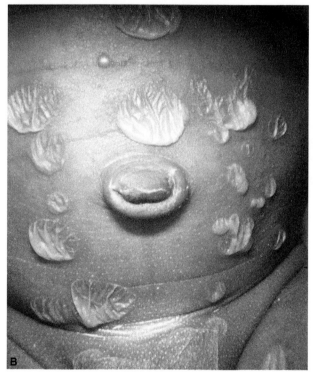

FIGURE 2.29. ■ Bullous Impetigo. (A) This lesion was thought to be an inflicted burn injury for which this infant was referred to the ED. Aspiration of the lesion showed gram-positive cocci in clusters on Gram stain and culture was positive for *S aureus*. Posttraumatic paronychia due to *S aureus* should also be considered in the differential diagnosis. (B) An infant with numerous flaccid bullae filled with pus. This can be also mistaken for inflicted burn injury, (Photo contributor: Binita R. Shah, MD [A], and [B] reproduced with permission from Shah BR, Laude TL. *Atlas of Pediatric Clinical Diagnosis.* WB Saunders; Philadelphia, PA, 2000.)

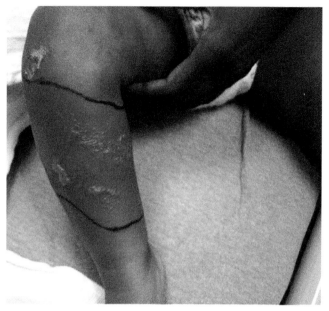

FIGURE 2.30 ■ Erysipelas. A 19-month-old girl presented with fever and rapidly progressing indurated and circumferential area of the upper right leg with bullae and erythema responding to antibiotic therapy. Macular areas of purple and red discoloration to medial right thigh and a healing wound on the knee were also seen. The erythema progressed beyond the lines of demarcation marked (as seen). The rapid progression of involvement, fever, and improvement with antibiotic treatment was consistent with erysipelas. (Photo contributor: Allison M. Jackson, MD, MPH.)

superficial localized skin infection most commonly caused by *Staphylococcus aureus*, but it can also be caused by group A β-hemolytic *Streptococcus*. It tends to occur in young children between the ages of 2 and 5 years old. Impetigo can occur with or without bullae. Nonbullous impetigo is the most contagious and is characterized by papules that first develop into vesicles with surrounding erythema with subsequent pustule development. When ruptured, a golden or honey-colored crust is present. With bullous impetigo, the vesicles enlarge, becoming flaccid bullae that resemble partial-thickness burns. When ruptured, a thin brown crust and collaret of scale are present. If involvement is extensive, patients may also have systemic symptoms such as fever and malaise. Bullous impetigo results from toxin-producing strains of *S aureus*. Erysipelas is an infection of the upper dermis with lymphatic involvement characterized by warmth, erythema, and edema. Patients usually have fever and chills and may also develop vesicles, bullae, and ecchymosis. The involvement is unilateral and usually involves lower extremities; however, bilateral involvement may be seen with erysipelas involving

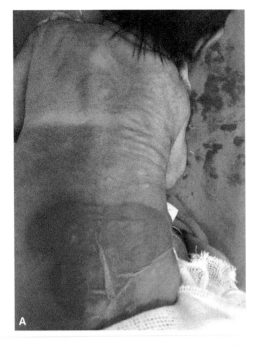
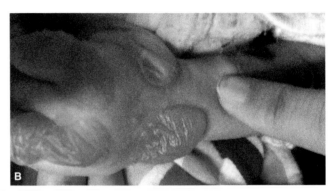
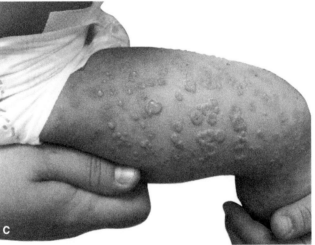

FIGURE 2.31 ■ Conditions Presenting With Bullous Lesions: Differential Diagnosis of Inflicted Burns. (**A, B**) Epidermolysis bullosa (EB). Blisters in the areas of trauma are characteristic of patients with EB. Seen here is a neonate with a blister on the back and a deep scarring ruptured blister and intact blisters on the hand. (**C**) Linear immunoglobulin A bullous dermatosis. Tense bullae along with annular vesiculobullous lesions on the thigh of a child, characteristic of this disorder, are shown. (Photo contributors: Prerna Batra, MD [A, B], and Sharon A. Glick, MD [C].)

the face. These bullous skin infections may mimic scald burns resulting from child abuse. Intentional scald burns can result from immersion or splash. The distribution of immersion burns tends to be clearly demarcated, circumferential bilateral involvement of the upper or lower extremities and buttocks/perineum. The differential diagnosis of bullous skin conditions includes but is not limited to epidermolysis bullosa, staphylococcal scalded skin syndrome, necrotizing

fasciitis, contact dermatitis, and accidental or inflicted partial-thickness burns.

Emergency Department Treatment and Disposition

Although the diagnosis of impetigo is clinical, obtaining a Gram stain and culture of pus, exudate, or debrided material and/or consultation with dermatologist may be beneficial, particularly if the diagnosis is uncertain. Impetigo is a minor skin infection that is treated with topical antibiotics. Oral antibiotic therapy is recommended for methicillin-resistant *S aureus* or *Streptococcus* or for more extensive bullous impetigo. An ill-appearing patient with erysipelas will require hospitalization and parenteral antibiotics and may require wound debridement (see also Figures 3.15 to 3.17). Patients should be appropriately managed for fever and pain.

Pearls

1. Bullous skin infections can be mistaken for inflicted scald burns.
2. Inflicted scald burns tend to involve the extremities, buttocks, and/or perineum, and be bilateral.
3. Bullous skin infections respond to antibiotic treatment; burns do not.

Clinical Summary

Postinflammatory hyperpigmentation can occur in individuals of any age and gender. Individuals with brown skin are, however, most susceptible to postinflammatory hyperpigmentation. The causes of the inflammation can vary from an allergic reaction to traumatic cutaneous injuries that may be accidental, intentional, or therapeutic in origin. Obtaining a history from the parent or from a verbal child about the cause can help identify the cause. Through a number of mediators, the inflammatory response can stimulate melanocytes, resulting in increased production or abnormal distribution of melanin. On exam, patients may have areas of increased pigmentation that may be irregularly shaped or patterned. Differential diagnosis includes café-au-lait macules, bruises, or PPD.

Emergency Department Treatment and Disposition

Postinflammatory hyperpigmentation does not require emergency management, although daily use of sunscreen (SPF ≥15) can prevent increasing hyperpigmentation of the affected area.

Pearls

1. Postinflammatory hyperpigmentation can be a residual finding from a variety of causes that may include allergic reactions, insect bites, accidental injury, inflicted injury, or therapeutic interventions.

2. Getting a history of the source of the hyperpigmentation may help differentiate other causes from prior physical abuse.

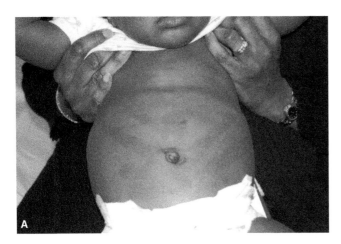

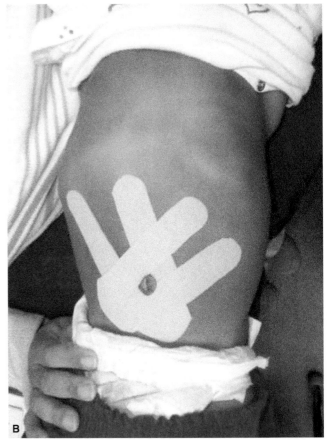

FIGURE 2.32 ■ Postinflammatory Hyperpigmentation. (**A**) A 3-year-old girl with developmental delay and failure to thrive living in a foster home was referred for child abuse assessment due to a recent right distal femur buckle fracture sustained after a fall. Her right lower extremity was casted, and broad linear hyperpigmented macules with curved edges converging at the mid-abdomen were observed. The Child Protective Services staff member accompanying the patient was not aware of this aspect of her physical therapy or marks on her abdomen. (**B**) After calling multiple providers, the physical therapist explained that the patient had been reacting to the tape (applied as shown here) used for her kinesiotaping. She receives physical therapy that includes kinesiotaping at home to help her with the awareness that she is full when eating. (Photo contributor: Allison M. Jackson, MD, MPH.)

Clinical Summary

"Raccon" eye refers to periorbital ecchymosis and results from subgaleal bleeding, bleeding from a fracture site in the anterior portion of the base of skull (basilar skull fracture [BSF]) or from a blow to the forehead. In an upright child, bleeding from the subgaleal space or forehead leaks ventrally into the facial soft tissues alongside of the nose and into the periorbital space. Darkening of the soft tissue swelling and eyes (ecchymosis) is seen about 1 to 3 days after the trauma because of degradation of blood products. Because of the loose connection of the eyelid skin and underlying subcutaneous tissues, dramatic ecchymosis can be seen with mild blunt trauma. The initial subgaleal hematoma may be masked by the child's hair, while a forehead hematoma may be seen or palpated. Raccoon eyes from BSF are usually seen 4 to 6 hours after the traumatic event. The other signs of BSF that may be seen are retroauricular ecchymosis (Battle's sign; see Figure 20.7), hemotympanum, CSF leaks (rhinorrhea or otorrhea; see Figure 20.6), or VII nerve palsy. Raccoon eye can be bilateral (eg, forehead hematoma, subgaleal bleeding, BSF, LeFort II and III fractures) or unilateral or bilateral (eg, direct eye trauma). Other differential diagnosis of raccoon eye includes coagulopathy and metastatic neuroblastoma with orbital involvement (see Figure 8.5). Subgaleal hematoma can result from inflicted hair pulling (see Figure 1.2) or tight hair braiding in children with a coagulopathy.

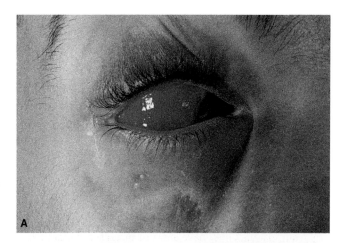

A

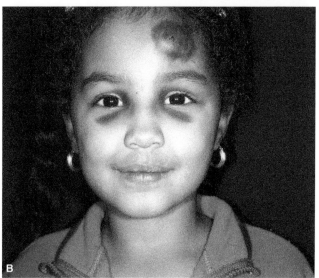

B

FIGURE 2.34 ■ Inflicted Eye Trauma Due to Child Abuse Versus Raccoon Eyes Due to Accidental Trauma. (**A**) Subconjunctival hemorrhage with periorbital ecchymosis and abrasion of the lower eyelid in a patient who was punched in the eye by his father. Other signs of trauma such as laceration, eyelid swelling, tenderness, or hyphema may also be seen with direct eye trauma. (Photo contributor: Binita R. Shah, MD.) (**B**) Raccoon eyes 3 days after patient hit her forehead against the bed railing while jumping. Note the absence of subconjunctival hemorrhage or other signs of direct eye trauma. (Reproduced with permission from Shah BR, Laude TL. *Atlas of Pediatric Clinical Diagnosis.* WB Saunders; Philadelphia, PA 2000.)

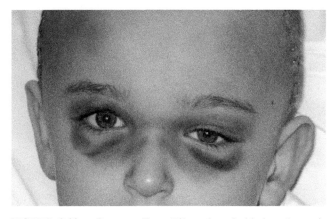

FIGURE 2.33 ■ Raccoon Eyes. Bilateral periorbital ecchymosis (raccoon eyes) are seen in this a child after being involved in a motor vehicular accident. He had sustained epidural hematoma requiring evacuation (staples seen on the scalp). Note the absence of any other injuries in the periorbital region or subconjunctival hemorrhage. (Photo contributor: Ronak R. Shah, MD.)

Emergency Department Treatment and Disposition

A raccoon eye due to accidental forehead hematoma or subgaleal bleeding is usually a benign finding and only requires reassurance. Neurosurgery consultation will be required for raccoon eye due to BSF. Laboratory evaluation for a bleeding

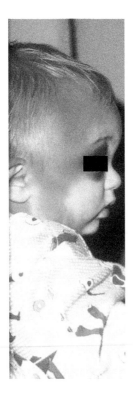

FIGURE 2.35 ■ Raccoon Eye. Extensive subgaleal bleeding and unilateral raccoon eye are seen in a toddler after an accidental fall while running and hitting right side of the scalp. Severity of such bleeding can be easily mistaken for inflicted injuries. Bleeding disorders also need to be excluded in such cases. (Photo contributor: Bipin Patel, MD.)

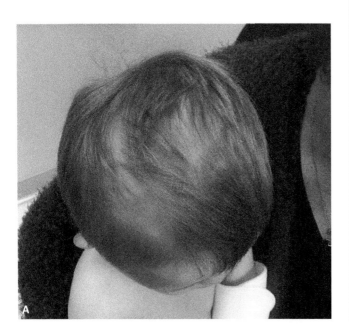

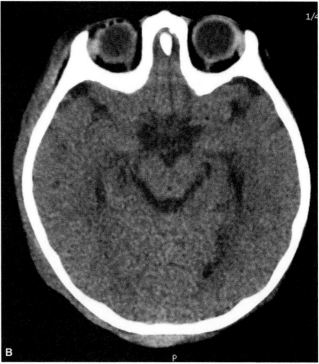

FIGURE 2.36 ■ Diffuse Subgaleal Hematoma. (**A**) This previously healthy 14-month-old toddler presented with patches of alopecia, extensive right-sided subgaleal hemorrhage, right facial ecchymosis, and a bruise to his posterior right thigh without any prior history of trauma. The presence of alopecia and subgaleal hemorrhage was concerning for hair traction. A skeletal survey and comprehensive evaluation for a coagulopathy was negative. Traumatic alopecia can cause subgaleal hemorrhage in patients without an underlying coagulopathy. (**B**) A noncontrast axial head CT scan demonstrates an extensive subgaleal hematoma overlying the right convexity without underlying fracture or intracranial haemorrhage. (Photo contributor: Allison M. Jackson, MD, MPH.)

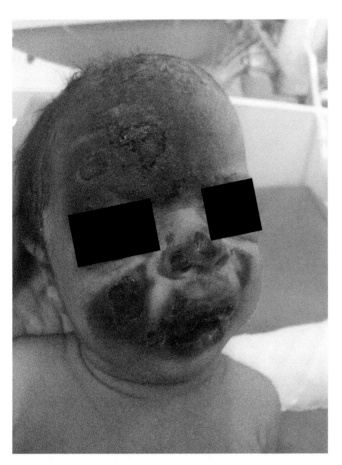

FIGURE 2.37 ■ Traumatic Purpura with Abrasions. Extensive facial purpura and superficial abrasions with edema were seen in this neonate with face presentation through the birth canal in a prolonged spontaneous delivery. All these lesions completely healed in a week with supportive wound care. (Photo contributor: Prerna Batra, MD.)

diathesis may be required. In the ED setting, a CBC with platelets, prothrombin time, and partial thromboplastin time should be obtained. Further evaluation by a hematologist may be indicated.

Pearls

1. Raccoon eye of accidental trauma can be mistaken for inflicted trauma from child abuse. The orbital rim and ecchymotic shiner is nontender in a raccoon eye from etiologies such as forehead trauma or BSF.
2. Identifying pulled hairs or traction alopecia in patients with subgaleal hematomas and no evidence of skull fracture may be indicative of intentional trauma or an underlying coagulopathy.

HAIR-TOURNIQUET SYNDROME

Clinical Summary

Hair-tourniquet syndrome (HTS) occurs when fibers of hair or thread are wrapped around an appendage producing tissue necrosis. HTS is frequently an accidental injury. A constricting hair or thread decreases lymphatic drainage, and lymphedema subsequently impedes venous drainage, leading to more edema and eventually preventing arterial flow to the appendage. This obstruction leads to necrosis and tissue loss if not promptly relieved.

Common sites of HTS include toes, fingers, penis, clitoris, and labia. Involvement of toes or fingers is seen in young infants (birth to 2 years). Penile-tourniquet syndrome is seen in infancy up to age 6 years, and clitoral-tourniquet syndrome is seen in older girls (8 years to adolescence). Symptoms may include inconsolable crying or irritability (young infants) and odd gait or genital pain (older children). The physical exam may show erythema and swelling of the involved area (early presentation) or gangrene and amputation (late presentation). Complications are variable depending on duration of strangulation and include amputation of the digit, clitoris, or penis and partial or complete transection of the urethra. Differential diagnosis of HTS includes child abuse or self-inflicted injury (eg, older girls with clitoral-tourniquet syndrome).

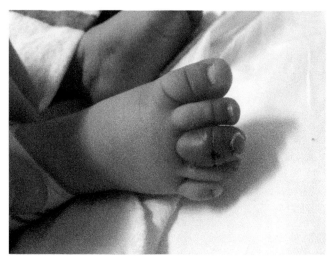

FIGURE 2.39 ■ Hair-Tourniquet Syndrome. A 2-month-old infant with inconsolable crying for the past few hours was brought to the ED. Her right third toe was edematous and purple without circulation distally. Some tissue breakdown on the plantar portion of the toe with a foul smell was also noted. With a digital block, hair tourniquet was incised and circulation was restored to the distal portion of the toe. She received IV antibiotic therapy in the ED followed by hospitalization. (Photo contributor: Daniel Ostro, MD.)

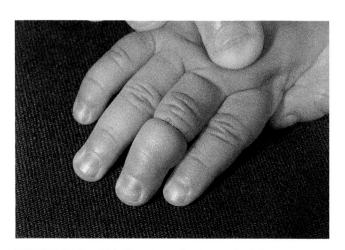

FIGURE 2.38 ■ Hair-Tourniquet Syndrome. An infant presenting with inconsolable crying was found to have a hair wrapped around a digit that was erythematous and edematous. One or more hairs may be wrapped around one or more times, so a thorough inspection is required after removal of hair to be sure no strands remain. (Photo contributor: Binita R. Shah, MD.)

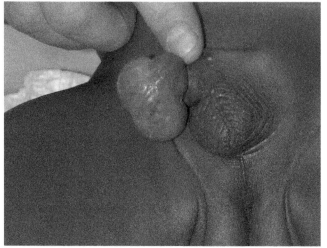

FIGURE 2.40 ■ Penile-Tourniquet Syndrome. Erythema and edema of the glans penis was produced by a hair wrapped around the glans. With extreme swelling of the glans and edema of the coronal sulcus as a result of venous and arterial occlusion, constricting strands of hair may be difficult to see (as in this photo). Hair was deliberately wrapped around the penis to stop bedwetting in this patient as a punishment by his mother. (Photo contributor: Michael Stracher, MD.)

Emergency Department Treatment and Disposition

As the encircling hair dries out, it shrinks, cutting through the skin and becoming enveloped, making diagnosis difficult. Prompt removal of the constricting hair or fibers is required to prevent tissue loss. Sometimes the end of the hair or fiber is visible and can be used to facilitate its removal; otherwise the wound needs exploration to dissect and remove all the strands. A meticulous hunt to remove every single strand is required before discharging the patient.

Pearls

1. Consider HTS in any infant presenting with irritability or inconsolable crying or swelling of an appendage including the penis or clitoris.

2. Even though most cases of HTS are unintentional, the possibility of child abuse must be considered, especially if there is a delay in seeking medical care.

3. Deliberate wrapping of hair around the penis to stop wetting has been reported to be a form of punishment used by some caretakers.

4. A cursory examination of digits or other appendages may fail to identify the problem in an infant presenting with irritability or inconsolable crying. A thorough physical examination of all digits (after removal of the socks and mittens) and genitalia is required.

5. Evaluate thoroughly including examining all digits and genitalia in any infant presenting with irritability or inconsolable crying before any sepsis workup!

Clinical Summary

Copper deficiency may result from inadequate dietary intake (nutritional copper deficiency) or a fatal X-linked disorder in which there is defective gastrointestinal absorption of copper (Menkes disease or Menkes kinky hair syndrome). Healthy,

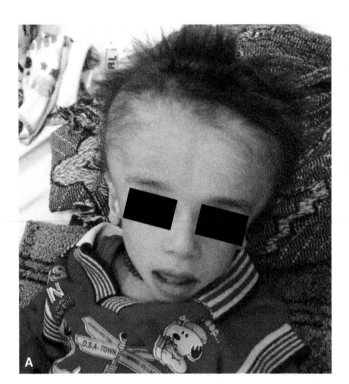

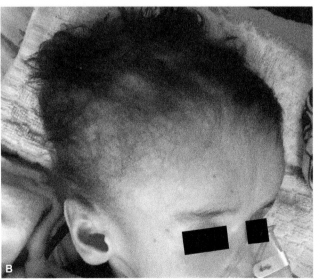

FIGURE 2.41 ■ Menkes Disease. (**A**) A 15-month-old boy with Menkes disease with macrocephaly, hypopigmented pale skin, and pudgy, sagging cheeks. (**B**) Close-up showing typical sparse, short, brittle, kinky, steel wool–like hypopigmented hair. (Photo contributor: Samridhi Goyal, MD.)

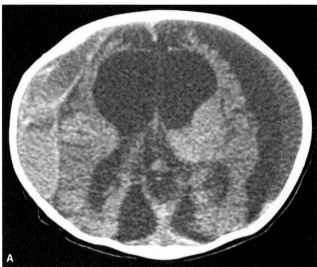

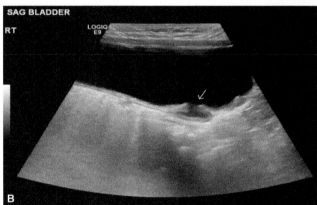

FIGURE 2.42 ■ Menkes Disease. (**A**) A CT scan of the brain demonstrates bilateral subdural hemorrhages of different ages (raising concerns for abusive head trauma), hydrocephalus, and left intraventricular hemorrhage in a 13-month-old toddler presenting with seizures (beginning at age 2 months), hypothermia, and bradycardia. His exam was also notable for sparse "kinky hair" particularly on sides, a high arched palate, no teeth, and profound truncal hypotonia. Laboratory evaluation was notable for low ceruloplasmin and low copper values. Molecular testing confirmed a pathogenic variant on the *ATP7A* gene. (**B**) Sonogram of the bladder shows posterior diverticulum (arrow). (Photo/legend contributors: Tanya S. Hinds, MD, and John Amodio, MD.)

term infants are born with adequate liver stores of copper for 4 to 5 months. Low birth weight, exclusive exposure to copper-deficient total parenteral nutrition or copper-deficient cow's milk, and chronic malabsorption are risk factors for inadequate dietary intake (nutritional copper deficiency). Nutritionally deficient infants have suboptimal weight gain, hypopigmented pale skin, neurodevelopmental (usually motor) deficits, neutropenia, hypochromic anemia (resistant to treatment with iron), low plasma copper, low ceruloplasmin, and skeletal changes (metaphyseal cupping, metaphyseal spurs, epiphyseal fractures, and osteopenia). Menkes disease, an infantile-onset, X-linked, recessive neurodegenerative disorder caused by dysfunction of a copper-transporting ATPase (ATP7A), occurs in approximately 1 in 250,000 live-born males in many Western countries. Patients with Menkes disease have a similar but not identical spectrum of findings compared with patients with inadequate dietary copper intake. Anemia and neutropenia are not seen in Menkes disease; intracranial pathology is reported in Menkes disease but not in nutritional copper deficiency. Patients with Menkes disease generally are in good health as a newborn, although nonspecific hypothermia, cephalohematomas, persistent hyperbilirubinemia, feeding difficulties, and minor facial dysmorphisms may occur. At 2 to 3 months, Menkes disease patients have neurodevelopmental deficits. Deficits are accompanied by impaired growth in head circumference and weight, seizures, and characteristic clinical and radiologic features, including pili torti (microscopic hair shaft flattening and twisting), tortuous intracranial and abdominal blood vessels, and bladder diverticula. Neurodegeneration, feeding difficulties, and respiratory infections usually contribute to death between 6 months and 3 years.

Emergency Department Treatment and Disposition

A patient with a copper deficiency may present with fracture(s). When fracture(s) occur because of copper deficiency, there are coexisting clinical features (eg, a history that the low-birth-weight infant's copper supplementation was reduced due to cholestasis) and laboratory and/or radiologic changes compatible with copper deficiency. A skeletal survey (to look for additional fractures and stigmata of disease) should be obtained in the absence of historical and physical examination findings compatible with a copper deficiency. Classic metaphyseal lesions (subepiphyseal fractures through immature metaphyseal bone) and other inflicted fractures will typically occur in the setting of radiologically normal bones. Fracture(s) due to copper deficiency are usually accompanied by symmetric skeletal changes and stigmata of compromised bone health such as excess wormian bones (skull), metaphyseal spurring (long bones), and flaring of the anterior rib ends. Menkes disease patients and those with abusive trauma may both present with subdural hemorrhage and metaphyseal fractures. In this setting, clinical, laboratory, and nonskeletal findings that are characteristic of Menkes disease help with the distinction. Widespread, multilayered retinal hemorrhaging has not been described in Menkes disease, further aiding the distinction between Menkes disease and abuse.

Pearls

1. Distinction must be made among classic metaphyseal lesions (eg, abusive fractures) and metaphyseal cupping, fraying, or spurs. This distinction is best made by an experienced pediatric radiologist.
2. Retinal degeneration has been described in Menkes disease. Widespread, multilayered retinal hemorrhaging (typical of child abuse) has not been described. A dilated fundoscopic examination by a pediatric ophthalmologist is warranted.
3. When Menkes disease is suspected, consultation with a geneticist and molecular analysis are ideal. When child abuse is suspected, a psychosocial assessment by Child Protective Services and law enforcement investigation are standard of care.

VITAMIN D INSUFFICIENCY, VITAMIN D DEFICIENCY, AND RICKETS

Clinical Summary

Rickets is caused by undermineralization and abnormal organization of the cartilaginous epiphyseal growth plate (present only in childhood). In a vitamin D insufficient (12–20 ng/mL; 30–50 nmol/L) or deficient (<12 ng/mL; <30 nmol/L) state, there can be impaired absorption of calcium and phosphorus and elevations in bone turnover markers (such as alkaline phosphatase). Decreased levels of calcium and phosphorus and decreased calcium × phosphorus product may ultimately result in radiologic rickets; radiologic rickets generally occurs only in moderate to severe vitamin D deficiency. A deficiency of vitamin D metabolites can be multifactorial, including "sunshine deficiency" (inadequate exposure to sunlight or factors preventing UV light penetration such as industrial pollution, darkly pigmented skin, abundant clothing), dietary vitamin D deficiency (eg, exclusive breastfeeding without vitamin D supplementation, strict vegan diet), and/or deficiency due to fat malabsorption (eg, celiac disease, extrahepatic biliary atresia).

Rachitic deformities that are seen on physical examination include prominent widening of wrists and ankles, rachitic rosary (prominence of costochondral junctions), Harrison groove (weakened ribs pulled by muscles, producing flaring over the diaphragm), craniotabes (softening of the skull), frontal bossing (with craniosomatic disproportion), genu varum (bow legs), genu valgum (knock-knees), and/or kyphoscoliosis. Varying degrees of irritability (bone pain), generalized muscular hypotonia, gross motor delay, failure to thrive, hypocalcemic seizures or tetany (latent or manifest), and increased risk of infections are other features of rickets.

Emergency Department Treatment and Disposition

Laboratory tests suggestive of vitamin D deficiency include either low (in early stage) or normal ionized serum calcium, secondary hyperparathyroidism, low phosphate, and elevated alkaline phosphatase values. A decreased serum 25(OH)-vitamin D (calcidiol) value is confirmatory. Liver enzymes, serum albumin, BUN, and creatinine values help in excluding underlying liver or kidney disease as a cause of rickets. Vitamin D insufficiency or deficiency based on laboratory indices is more common than radiologic rickets (radiologically apparent bone changes) in a given population of infants and children.

Plain film is used to diagnose rickets and to screen for occult fractures. A single anteroposterior (AP) view of the knee in children <3 years of age (femur and tibia being the most rapidly growing bones in infants leading to accentuated rachitic changes) or a single AP view of the wrist in older children can be obtained when child physical abuse is not suspected. Radiographic changes suggestive of rickets include cupping of metaphyses (concave deformity of end of long bone shaft, instead of normal convex or flat appearance), fraying of metaphyses (indistinct, shaggy borders), widening of metaphyses, apparent widening of growth plate (increased distance between the epiphysis and metaphysis), generalized osteopenia, thinning of cortex, pseudofractures, and bowing deformities of long bones. When child physical abuse is suspected, a skeletal survey (typically 21 radiographs) of children <24 months old is obtained. Consultation with a child abuse pediatrician, endocrinologist, and/or pediatric radiologist may be requested, if diagnosis is uncertain.

Patients presenting with symptomatic or asymptomatic hypocalcemia require hospitalization for correction of hypocalcemia and initiation of vitamin D therapy. Asymptomatic normocalcemic patients can be referred to a primary care physician or endocrinologist for the treatment of vitamin D insufficiency, deficiency, or rickets. It is important that those at risk for vitamin D insufficiency take a daily maintenance dose of vitamin D. Once vitamin D deficiency or radiologic rickets is diagnosed, therapeutic doses of vitamin D with adequate concurrent calcium are initiated.

Pearls

1. Metaphyseal changes of rickets can be mistaken for skeletal injuries of abuse. Presence of rachitic changes seen either on physical examination or radiographically and/or lack of coincident abusive brain, eye, abdominal, or cutaneous injuries will help differentiate rickets from abusive skeletal trauma.
2. Lucent epiphyseal-metaphyseal junctions seen in rickets may resemble the "bucket-handle" fractures of child abuse. However, widening of the metaphyseal plates distinguishes rickets radiographically from abuse-related fractures.
3. In the absence of radiologic rickets, inflicted trauma and abuse should be suspected when an infant presents with unexplained fracture(s).

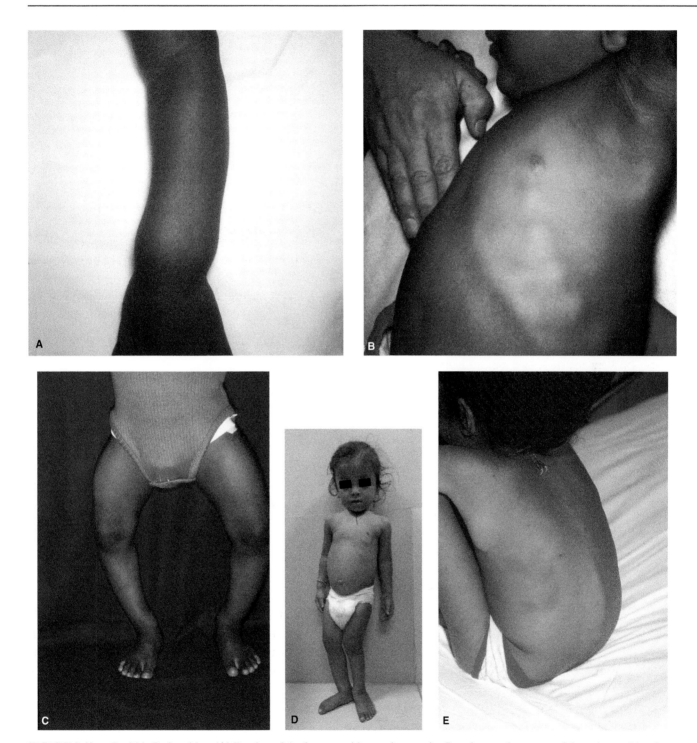

FIGURE 2.43 ■ Rachitic Deformities. (**A**) Bowing of the forearm with prominent wrist. Prominent enlargement of the wrist resulting from excessive accumulation of osteoid is seen in this African American infant who was exclusively breastfed without any vitamin D supplementation. This finding can be mistaken for abusive injury (eg, swelling due to fracture). (**B**) Rachitic rosary (enlargement of costochondral junctions). (**C**) Bow legs (genu varum). (**D**) Knock-knees (genu valgum) with prominent wrists and ankles. (**E**) Kyphosis. Vertebral softening due to rickets leading to kyphosis is seen in a malnourished child who was fed a strict vegan diet (boiled vegetables and rice) with no dairy products. Child abuse/neglect needs to be excluded in such patients. (Photo contributors: Binita R. Shah, MD [A, C, E], and Abhijeet Saha, MD [D], and [B] reproduced with permission from Shah BR, Laude TL. *Atlas of Pediatric Clinical Diagnosis.* WB Saunders; Philadelphia, PA, 2000.)

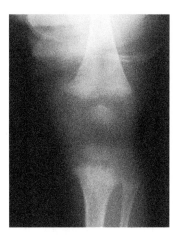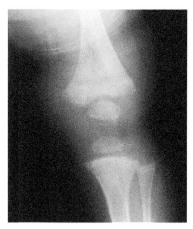

FIGURE 2.44 ■ Rickets. Anteroposterior view of the knee (left; pretreatment) shows metaphyseal widening, cupping, and fraying of the distal femur and proximal tibia and fibula. Normally the epiphyses should be "hugging" the metaphyses; the increased distance seen between the metaphyses and epiphyses (radiolucent zone) is due to the presence of radiolucent osteoid. A repeat radiograph (right) 2 weeks after vitamin D therapy shows healing rickets. (Photo contributor: Binita R. Shah, MD.)

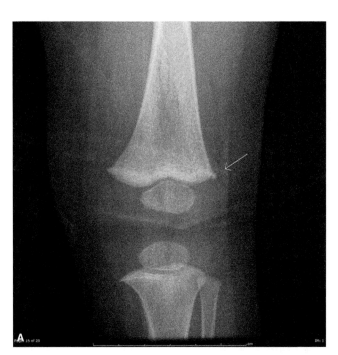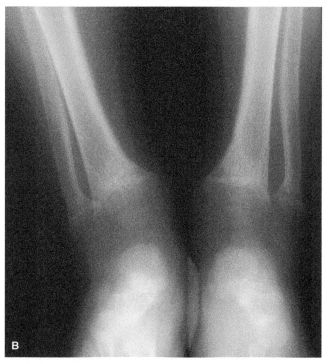

FIGURE 2.45 ■ Differential of Child Abuse and Rickets. (A) Anteroposterior view of the knee demonstrates a corner fracture of the distal portion of the femur, along the lateral aspect (pathognomic for abusive injuries). (B) Rickets. Bilateral and usually symmetrical pattern of skeletal involvement with diffuse osteopenia, widening of physis, and metaphyseal fraying distinguishes rickets radiographically from abuse-related fractures. (Photo contributors: Allison M. Jackson, MD, MPH [A], and Binita R. Shah, MD [B].)

Clinical Features

Osteogenesis imperfecta (OI) is a genetic disorder of connective tissue seen in all racial and ethnic groups. It results from an abnormal quantity or quality of type I collagen, a primary component of the extracellular matrix of the bone and skin. Eight clinical subtypes of OI (type I to VIII) are seen with variable manifestations. Genetic inheritance is autosomal dominant in the majority of the subtypes, although spontaneous mutations can occur. The features of OI often include a triangular face, fragile bones, blue sclerae, and

deafness (conductive hearing loss seen in adolescents and adults). Other characteristics include easy bruising, fragile skin, growth retardation with short stature, defective dentinogenesis, joint laxity, wormian bones (small, irregular bones seen along the cranial sutures), and spine changes (scoliosis, kyphosis, codfish vertebrae). Fractures in OI occur after a slight trauma or spontaneously in an ambulatory child.

Emergency Department Treatment and Disposition

Serum calcium, phosphorus, and alkaline phosphatase values and coagulation profile tests are normal in a child with OI. Radiographic features of OI include osteopenia, wormian bones, thin cortices, bowing, angulation of healed fractures, and excessive callus formation at the sites of recent fractures. Most fractures in OI are situated in the diaphysis. Posterior

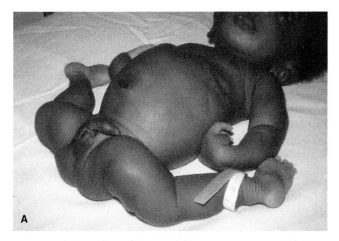

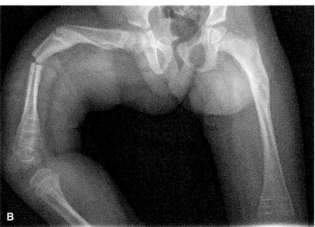

FIGURE 2.46 ■ Osteogenesis Imperfecta (OI). (**A**) An infant with multiple angular deformities with OI, type I (the most common type of OI). (**B**) Anteroposterior view of the lower extremity in a different patient with OI, type I, demonstrates diffuse osteopenia, bowing deformity of right femur, and fractures in different stages of prolonged healing. Note the multiple growth arrest lines of the distal femora, frequently seen in OI. (Photo contributors: [A] Reproduced with permission from Shah BR, Laude TL. *Atlas of Pediatric Clinical Diagnosis.* WB Saunders; Philadelphia, PA, 2000, and John Amodio, MD [B].)

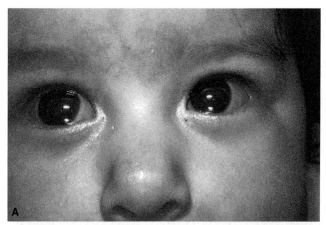

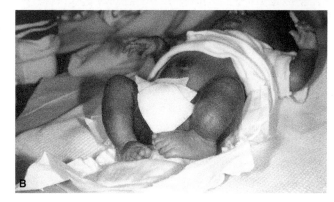

FIGURE 2.47 ■ Osteogenesis Imperfecta (OI). (**A**) Bilateral blue sclera noted at birth in a patient with OI, type II. (**B**) An infant with OI, type II, with deformities noted at birth (type II presents with multiple fractures in utero and in the perinatal period).

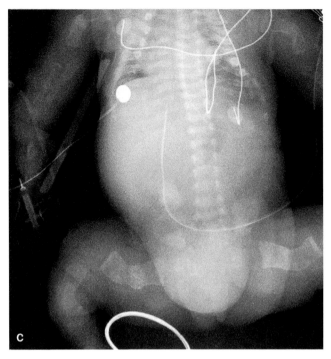

FIGURE 2.47 ■ (*Continued*) (**C**) Anteroposterior view of an infant with OI, type II, shows multiple congenital fractures involving the upper and lower extremities and ribs, with small lung capacity. (Photo contributors: [A] Reproduced with permission from Shah BR, Laude TL. *Atlas of Pediatric Clinical Diagnosis.* WB Saunders; Philadelphia, PA, 2000, and Binita R. Shah, MD [B], and John Amodio, MD [C].)

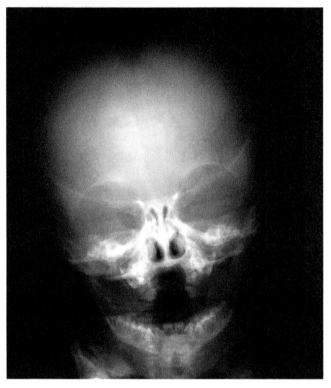

FIGURE 2.48 ■ Osteogenesis Imperfecta. Anteroposterior view of the skull demonstrates a "cracked egg shell" appearance secondary to wormian bones (excess sutural bones). (Photo contributor: John Amodio, MD.)

rib fractures and classic metaphyseal lesions are more specific for physical abuse. Consultation with a radiologist is valuable in a difficult case presenting with multiple fractures and when a diagnosis of child abuse cannot be excluded. Orthopedic consultation in the ED may be required depending on the type and location of the fractures. Goals of therapy include splinting or casting of fractures and maximizing comfort and function. Management of fractures in OI patients with moderate severity is no different from management of fractures in otherwise normal children. Protective orthotics may be needed in children with increased bone fragility. Osteotomies may be needed to straighten bone, and intramedullary rods may be inserted to maintain correct alignment and repair deformities arising both from fractures and from progressive bowing or bending of the skeleton. OI patients need close follow-up by orthopedics and their primary care physicians. Multidisciplinary management with referrals as indicated to a geneticist, an endocrinologist, a dentist, and a social worker for family support may also be needed. In undiagnosed or doubtful cases, diagnosis of OI can be confirmed by DNA sequencing.

Pearls

1. *Osteopenia* is insufficient bone mass resulting from reduced bone production, increased breakdown of bone, or both. *Osteoporosis* is a syndrome resulting from osteopenia that can lead to increased bone fragility and susceptibility to fractures and skeletal deformities.

2. OI or "brittle bone disease" is the most common osteoporosis syndrome in childhood.

3. OI is less common than child abuse. Milder forms of OI may be misdiagnosed as child abuse. Multiple fractures with angular deformities of the long bones, wormian bones, osteopenia, dentinogenesis imperfecta, and a positive family history will help to differentiate the 2 conditions.

4. A history incompatible with injury, the hallmark of abuse, may also be present in OI. When multiple unexplained fractures are present in an infant or toddler, include OI in the differential diagnosis.

5. Spiral or transverse fractures of long bones are more common in OI than metaphyseal fractures; however, metaphyseal fractures resembling abuse are also seen.

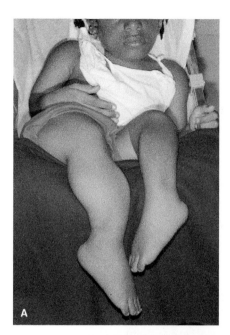
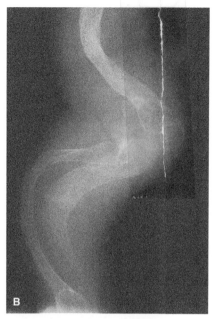
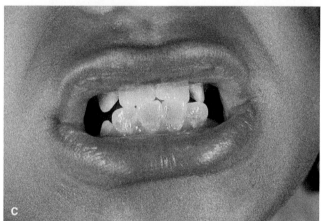

FIGURE 2.49 ■ Osteogenesis Imperfecta (OI). (**A**) Severe bowing and deformities of both upper and lower extremities are seen in this girl with OI, type III. She had normal sclera, triangular facies, and severe bone fragility leading to multiple fractures from early infancy. (**B**) Radiograph of the lower extremity showing generalized osteopenia, thinned cortices, and marked angular deformities of the bones. (**C**) Dentinogenesis imperfecta showing transparent yellow, prematurely eroded teeth. (Photo contributor: Binita R. Shah, MD.)

Clinical Summary

Lichen sclerosus et atrophicus (LSA) is characterized by distinctive white lesions on the genitalia. It is a chronic inflammatory disease of unknown cause predominantly involving girls (female-to-male ration of approximately 8:1). Involvement in boys is called balanitis xerotica obliterans. LSA occurs most commonly between 1 and 13 years of age. Pruritus, burning, constipation, dysuria, dyspareunia, vaginal discharge preceding vulvar lesions (girls), and phimosis and recurrent balanitis (boys) are common presenting symptoms. The skin lesion starts as ivory-colored, shiny, indurated papules that become confluent irregular plaques, which may develop hemorrhagic bullae at their margins. Later lesions atrophy, becoming depressed plaques with a wrinkled surface. The location of lesion in girls is vulvar, perianal, and perineal skin (most common site). Atrophic plaques may lead to shrinkage of the labia and stenosis of the introitus. In boys, the lesion is on the glans and undersurface of prepuce. Extragenital lesions appear as atrophic depigmented patches with cigarette paper–like wrinkling of the surface and sites include neck, axillae,

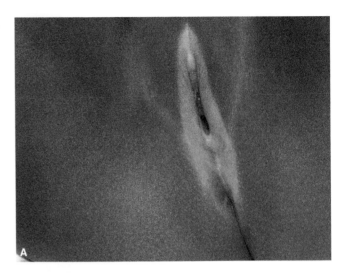

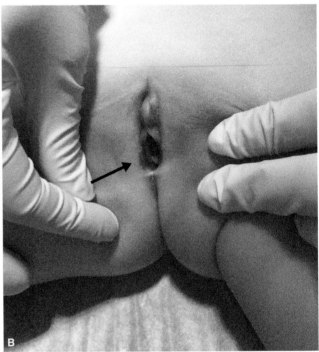

FIGURE 2.51 ■ Lichen Sclerosus et Atrophicus. (**A**) White atrophic plaque with erythema in an hourglass distribution surrounding the vagina and perirectal area is seen in a girl with a complaint of pruritus. (**B**). A hypopigmented atrophic patch surrounding the vaginal opening with a small erosion (arrow) is seen in this 3-year-old girl who presented with vaginal discomfort and constipation. (Photo contributors: Sharon A. Glick, MD [A], and Julie Cantatore-Francis, MD [B].)

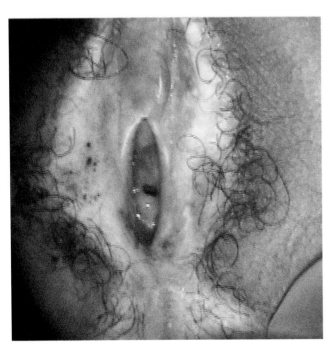

FIGURE 2.50 ■ Lichen Sclerosus et Atrophicus. White atrophic plaque in an hourglass distribution with scattered sites of hemorrhage involving the labia majora, perineum, and perirectal area. This patient presented with a 2-week prior history of dysuria, redness, and vaginal itching followed by spotting. There was no disclosure of sexual abuse. (Photo contributor: Allison M. Jackson, MD, MPH.)

trunk, periumbilical, and flexor surfaces of wrists and around eyes.

Differential diagnosis includes vitiligo, postinflammatory hypopigmentation, sexual abuse, bacterial vulvovaginitis, and intertrigo.

Emergency Department Treatment and Disposition

Topical steroid cream is the initial treatment, and the patient needs to be referred to a dermatologist or a primary care physician for ongoing treatment and follow-ups. Use of barrier protection (eg, petrolatum-based emollients) may help in alleviating symptoms of pruritus and pain with defecation or urination. Advise patient to avoid bubble baths or fragrances containing soaps. Data are conflicting on the spontaneous involution rate of LSA around puberty.

Pearls

1. LSA is one of the most common dermatitides mistaken for sexual abuse, especially when it presents with purpura of the vulva.
2. LSA lesions are atrophic. porcelain-white plaque around the anus and vulva forming a figure-8 or hourglass configuration. This most distinctive pattern is seen in prepubertal females as well as in adults.
3. Nearly all affected boys with LSA present with phimosis in a previously retractable foreskin with an atrophic depigmented plaque at the tip of the penis.

Clinical Summary

Perianal bacterial dermatitis (PBD) is a superficial bacterial infection caused typically by group A β-hemolytic *Streptococcus* (GABHS) or *S aureus* (including methicillin-resistant strains) in the perianal area. PBD is also referred to as perianal bacterial cellulitis. Chronic PBD may present *without* any signs of cellulitis; thus, the preferred term is PBD. It primarily occurs in children between 6 months and 10 years of age. About 70% of cases involve boys. Intrafamily spread can occur (eg, family members bathing together). Siblings may be either asymptomatic with only GABHS-positive cultures, or they may develop similar dermatitis.

Perianal dermatitis and pruritus are the most common presenting symptoms, followed by painful defecation with rectal pain, perianal pain, constipation, blood-streaked stools, and anal discharge. Systemic symptoms are usually absent. During the acute phase (<6 weeks), the perianal area may show bright red erythema (without induration) that is tender and confluent from the anus outward. Size varies from a few to several centimeters. During the chronic phase, patients may present with painful perirectal fissures, dried mucoid discharge leading to irritation and excoriation, proctocolitis, or bleeding with little or no erythema. Psoriasiform plaques with yellow peripheral crust may also be seen. Infection may involve the penis or vulva.

Differential diagnosis includes sexual abuse; candidiasis; contact, atopic, or seborrheic dermatitis; chronic diaper dermatitis; psoriasis; pinworm infestation; inflammatory bowel disease; or local trauma.

PBD is diagnosed by its characteristic distribution and confirmed by a culture obtained from the perianal area. In addition to obtaining a general culture, *a specific request should be made of the laboratory to look for GABHS and S aureus.* Culture the index patient and family members as indicated. A moderate to heavy growth of GABHS or *S aureus* will confirm the diagnosis (children with asymptomatic perianal colonization have light growth of bacteria, eg, GABHS). A throat culture may also be positive when GABHS is the inciting agent.

Emergency Department Treatment and Disposition

PBD should be treated with systemic antibiotic therapy augmented by topical therapy. Drug of choice is penicillin given

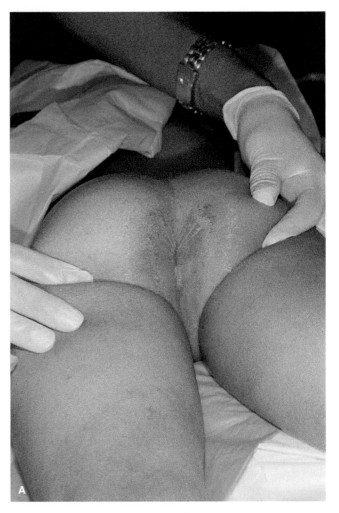

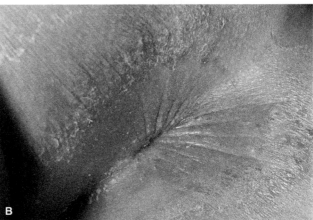

FIGURE 2.52 ■ Perianal Streptococcal Dermatitis. (**A**) This young girl was referred to "rule out" sexual abuse. This rash was present for several weeks, and she received different ointments without response. (**B**) A close-up showing perianal erythema, fissuring, and excoriation with crusting at the periphery. A rectal culture was positive for GABHS. Perianal and vulvar streptococcal infections are not correlated with sexual abuse. Patients, however, may still have a history of sexual abuse. (Photo contributor: Binita R. Shah, MD.)

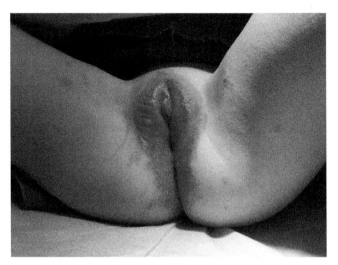

FIGURE 2.53 ■ Perianal Streptococcal Dermatitis. This 7-year-old girl presented with extreme vaginal discomfort. She has vaginal and perianal erythema and edema with open, crusted ulcerations. This is a combination of an irritant contact dermatitis from fragrant flushable wipes and a vaginal/perianal superinfection caused by GABHS. She was treated with antibiotics and a topical steroid and improved within 1 week. (Photo contributor: Julie Cantatore-Francis, MD.)

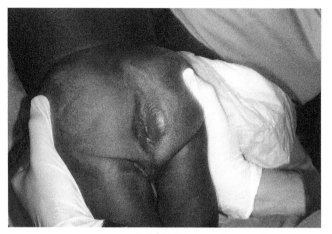

FIGURE 2.54 ■ Perianal Streptococcal Dermatitis. A young male child was referred for evaluation of sexual abuse. He had a history of constipation associated with painful defecation. Intense perianal erythema was seen with fissuring. A rectal culture was positive for GABHS. (Photo contributor: Binita R. Shah, MD.)

Pearls

either orally or parenterally. Amoxicillin may be used instead of penicillin (better-tasting preparation). Erythromycin or clindamycin is used for patients who are allergic to penicillin. These alternative antibiotic treatments may also be helpful for patients who have not responded to a course of penicillin or who are infected with *S aureus*. Topical therapy is with mupirocin ointment. The patient needs to be followed by the primary care physician for monitoring of response to therapy and to document bacteriologic cure after treatment. Recurrences can occur.

1. PBD is a bright-red, sharply demarcated perianal dermatitis caused by GABHS or *S aureus*.
2. PBD often gets mistakenly diagnosed as sexual abuse or contact or atopic dermatitis.
3. Patients with PBD are subjected to treatments for a variety of different diagnoses without success. Failures to respond to prior therapy with topical antifungal or corticosteroids or therapy for pinworms are important clues in suspecting PBD.
4. Undiagnosed and inappropriately treated patients with PBD develop perianal fissures, bleeding, pain during defecation, and constipation.

Clinical Summary

Labial adhesion is fusion of the labia minora, usually extending from an area immediately inferior to the clitoris to the fourchette. The extent of the adhesion is variable and is thickest posteriorly. Labial fusion and labial or vulvar agglutination or synechiae are synonyms commonly used. This is an acquired condition and occurs as a result of labial abrasion that culminates in medial surfaces of labia minor adhering to one another followed by epithelialization. Fusion occurs secondary to local inflammation in the presence of the hypoestrogenic state of a preadolescent child (inflamed/injured epithelium is more likely to fuse in a low-estrogen environment). Nonspecific vulvovaginitis, poor perineal hygiene, diaper rash, and use of harsh soaps are common contributory factors. Other etiologies include lichen sclerosus, atopic or seborrheic dermatitis, herpes or pinworm infection, and sexual abuse.

Labial adhesion occurs most commonly between 3 months and 6 years of age (peak: 13–23 months); however, it can occur at any age. It is rare in newborns (exposure to high levels of maternal estrogens) and in postpubertal premenopausal women. The majority of patients are asymptomatic, and it is usually accidentally noted by a parent or by a physician during examination. Symptoms of UTI such as dysuria and frequency may be present (related to pooling of urine in the vagina leading to recurrent vulvovaginitis [vaginal voider]). Other symptoms include urinary retention or altered urinary stream. Patients with labial adhesions have normal female genitalia; however, the hymen and introitus are obscured because of adhesions. With complete adhesions, the urethra is usually not visualized. Urine may be seen dribbling at the anterior end (just posterior to clitoris). Labial adhesions may also reoccur.

Differential diagnosis includes imperforate hymen, sexual abuse, ambiguous genitalia, congenital absence of vagina, and scarring following female circumcision.

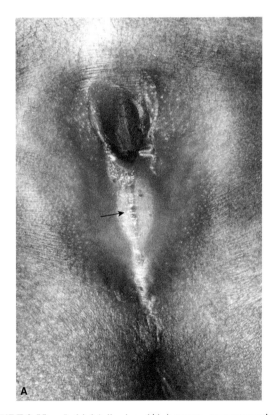
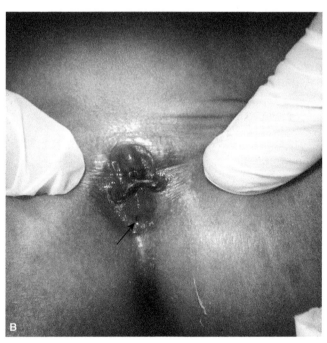

FIGURE 2.55 ■ Labial Adhesion. (**A**) A young, asymptomatic girl was accidentally found by her parents to have "abnormal looking private parts." With complete adhesions, the introitus is not seen, and this is often interpreted by parents as "absence of vagina." It may also appear that there is no urethral opening. A thin line of central raphe (arrow) where the labia are fused is seen. Visualization of a midline raphe excludes the diagnosis of imperforate hymen. (**B**) Almost complete adhesions are seen in this infant, with a very small opening seen near the posterior fourchette (arrow). This patient presented with acute urinary retention. (Photo contributor: Binita R. Shah, MD.)

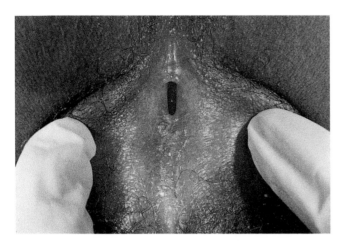

FIGURE 2.56 ■ Female Circumcision (Infibulation). This 10-year-old girl underwent excision of her clitoris and labia minora (as ritual female circumcision) during her early childhood in Africa. Scarred tissue and a narrowed introitus following surgery may mimic labial adhesion or trauma due to sexual abuse. The practice of female circumcision is seen in populations from Africa and the Middle East and in Muslim populations of Indonesia and Malaysia. The type of mutilation ranges from simple excision of the prepuce of the clitoris to complete excision of all elements of the vulvar region, leaving a very small opening for the passage of urine and menstrual fluid. Female circumcision is a form of child abuse and is internationally viewed as a violation of human rights according to the World Health Organization. (Photo contributor: Swati Mehta, MD.)

Emergency Department Treatment and Disposition

Spontaneous resolution (without therapy) occurs in the majority of children. With endogenous estrogen production and the vaginal pH becoming more acidic at puberty, labial adhesions almost always resolve spontaneously. No treatment except reassurance is indicated for patients with asymptomatic adhesions. General measures include reassurance to the family about the presence of normal female genitalia, improving perineal hygiene (eg, regular changing of diapers and thorough wiping after each bowel movement from anterior to posterior), removal of irritants such as caustic soaps, treatment of diaper dermatitis, loose-fitting cotton underwear, and sitz baths. Estrogen cream may be considered for patients with nearly complete adhesions with or without urinary symptoms or for patients with significant parental anxiety. Patients will need to follow up with the primary care physician. A small quantity of estrogen cream is applied topically at bedtime with gentle traction for 2 to 4 weeks. An additional few weeks of application of an inert ointment (eg, petroleum jelly) keeps labia apart while healing is completed. Prolonged use of estrogen cream should be discouraged because of side effects (eg, breast enlargement and/or tenderness, vulvar pigmentation), and the caregiver needs to be educated about this. If the patient presents with acute urinary symptoms, a gentle attempt to separate labia with a Calgiswab can be made (only if adhesions appear to separate easily) after applying 5% lidocaine ointment.

Labial adhesions can result from sexual abuse, but in absence of other evidence, presence of adhesions alone is not diagnostic of sexual abuse. Consider possibility of sexual abuse in girls (especially older) presenting with adhesions many years after the toilet training or without any prior history of adhesions or any predisposing skin condition or presenting with thick adhesions that are difficult to treat.

Pearls

1. A thin vertical raphe (line of adherence) in the midline where labia are fused is pathognomonic for labial adhesions.
2. Labial adhesions should not be separated manually by force; it is painful, and resulting raw surfaces have a greater tendency to reagglutinate.
3. Patients with labial adhesions usually have normal female genitalia; however, hymen and introitus are obscured because of adhesions.

URETHRAL PROLAPSE

Clinical Summary

Urethral prolapse is an eversion of the distal urethral mucosa protruding through the urethral meatus and may be partial or complete. Predisposing factors include increased intra-abdominal pressure (eg, violent coughing, constipation) in a hypoestrogenic state and preceding trauma (eg, straddle injury or sexual abuse). Constriction of the prolapsed mucosa at the urethral meatus may lead to impairment of the venous blood flow with subsequent edema and erythema or purplish appearance of the mucosa. Thrombosis and necrosis of the mucosa may result if the process is not corrected.

Urethral prolapse is seen almost exclusively in premenarcheal girls, with a peak incidence between 4 and 10 years of

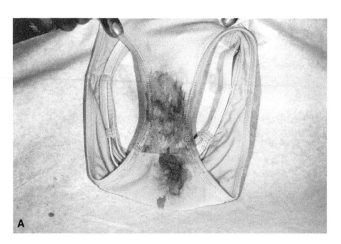

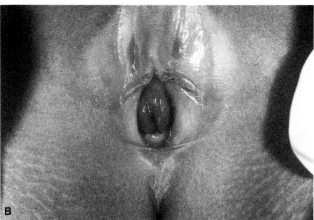

FIGURE 2.57 ■ Urethral Prolapse. (**A**) Blood-stained underwear from an asymptomatic 4-year-old African American girl is shown. Painless bleeding or spotting on underwear, the most common symptom of urethral prolapse, often gets mistaken for vaginal bleeding, hematuria, or rectal bleeding. (**B**) Urethral prolapse is usually a complete circle forming a doughnut-shaped, hyperemic, edematous mass obscuring the vaginal introitus. Center of the "doughnut" is the urethral orifice. (Photo contributor: Binita R. Shah, MD.)

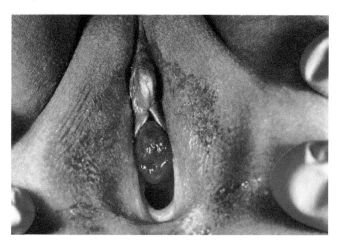

FIGURE 2.58 ■ Urethral Prolapse. The prolapse may be large enough to conceal the introitus. Retraction of the vulva gently in a downward and lateral direction or placing the child in a knee-chest position may help in appreciating the anatomy clearly, with the vaginal introitus seen as a separate structure posterior to the prolapsed urethra. (Photo contributor: Binita R. Shah, MD.)

age, and about 95% of patients are African American. The most common presenting symptom is painless bleeding or spotting on the underwear (90% of patients). Other symptoms may include dysuria and/or urinary frequency (due to urethral inflammation), difficulty voiding or urinary retention (prolapse may occlude urethral meatus), or perineal discomfort. Patient may also be completely asymptomatic and prolapse may be noted on routine examination.

Clinical signs of a prolapsed urethra include cherry-red doughnut or prolapsed cervix-like circular, nontender mass at the introitus. It may appear as a friable rosette of red or

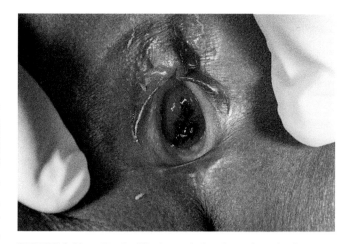

FIGURE 2.59 ■ Urethral Prolapse. A doughnut-shaped, edematous mass with hemorrhagic mucosa obscuring the vaginal introitus is seen. This finding can be mistakenly attributed to trauma caused by sexual abuse. (Photo contributor: Binita R. Shah, MD.)

hemorrhagic tissue and may be ulcerated, gangrenous (necrotic), or infected. A centrally located urethral meatus may not be visible in the presence of severe edema or strangulation. Differential diagnosis of urethral prolapse includes hematoma of hymen from sexual abuse, straddle injury, hematometrocolpos, prolapsed ectopic ureterocele or urethral polyp, urethral cysts, condylomata acuminata, hemangioma, and sarcoma botryoides.

Emergency Department Treatment and Disposition

Urethral prolapse is a clinical diagnosis. Conservative therapy is used for mild cases without necrotic mucosa. This includes warm sitz baths and emollient cream. If indicated, topical antibacterial therapy or topical estrogen therapy (the distal urethra is estrogen dependent) twice a day for 10 to 14 days can be used. It usually resolves spontaneously or with the above therapy in 2 to 3 weeks. Urologic or surgical consultation is required for patients with necrotic mucosa or recurrent prolapse. Indications for surgery (excision and reapproximation of the mucosal edges or carbon dioxide laser therapy) include prolapse with necrotic mucosa at the time of presentation, persistent prolapse with failed medical therapy, recurrent symptomatic prolapse, or urinary retention. Recurrences may be observed weeks to months after the initial resolution following medical therapy. Recurrence is uncommon after surgery.

Pearls

1. Urethral prolapse is the most common cause of apparent vaginal bleeding in premenarcheal girls.
2. Urethral prolapse presents as an interlabial mass and is the only lesion that has a circular mass of tissue surrounding the urethral meatus. If in doubt, catheterization of the bladder through the central dimple of the mass or observation of the child during voiding will aid in the diagnosis.
3. Clinical findings of urethral prolapse can be mistakenly attributed to sexual abuse, especially when prolapsed mucosa has become hemorrhagic and friable.
4. Urethral prolapse cannot be reduced manually.

STRADDLE INJURY

Clinical Summary

Straddle injuries are the most common type of accidental injuries to the genitalia and rarely involve penetration. Soft tissues get crushed between the pubic bone (eg, pubic symphysis, ischiopubic ramus) and a hard object during impact, such as accidentally falling on a furniture arm, bed, bicycle crossbar, balance beam, fence, toilet seat, concrete wall, or playground equipment.

Straddle injuries are usually unilateral and involve the anterior portion of external genitalia in both girls and boys. Injuries to internal genital structures or the anus are rare (protected by soft tissues of the buttocks, bones of the pelvis, and labia in girls). The most common location in girls is the labia majora and labia minora. Other sites may include

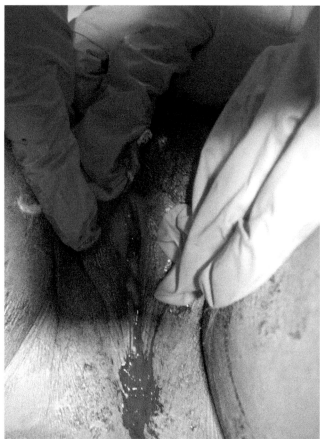

FIGURE 2.61 ■ Straddle Injury. A laceration of the vaginal wall is evident here at 11:00 o'clock after this teenager crashed her bicycle into another rider. Look for other signs of trauma and try to confirm the story with bystanders to make sure it is not fabricated to cover up the abuse. (Photo contributor: Mark Silverberg, MD.)

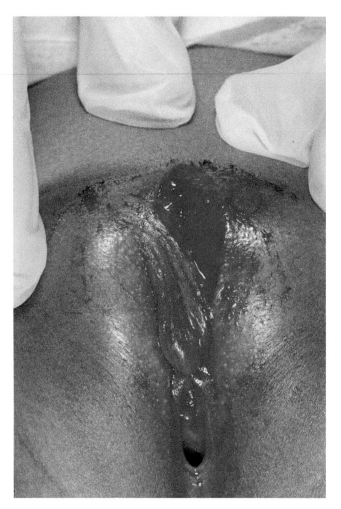

FIGURE 2.60 ■ Straddle Injury. Laceration of the labia majora extending into periurethral tissue secondary to a fall onto the bar of a bicycle is seen in this girl. Her injury was unilateral and did not involve the urethra, hymen, or vagina. (Photo contributor: Binita R. Shah, MD.)

clitoral hood, clitoris, periurethral tissue, or posterior fourchette, but hymen and vagina are usually not involved (unless accidental penetrating injury). Typical injuries are linear abrasions, bruising, or hematoma of labia majora or minora. Small posterior fourchette tears may be seen. Swelling, pain, and bleeding are common symptoms. Findings in boys include ecchymosis or minor laceration of scrotum and/or penis. Scrotal contents may be contused or crushed. Injury to anterior urethra is suggested by blood at the meatus, periurethral or perineal swelling, and difficulty voiding. Injury to the perineum, hymen, penis, and anus have also been reported when a pedestrian's pelvis and torso have been rolled over by a slow-moving vehicle.

Differential diagnosis of straddle injuries includes self-inflicted injuries, which are exceedingly rare in children. Normal masturbation in girls is clitoral or labial and does not cause genital injury. Self-inserted foreign bodies also do

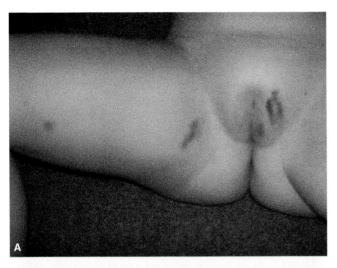

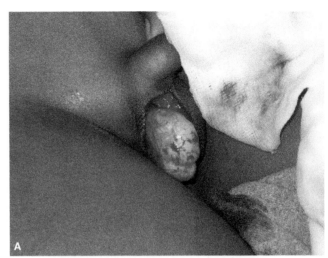

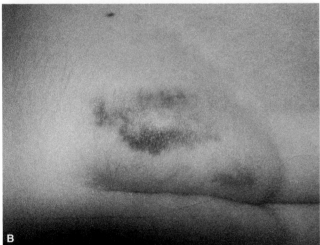

FIGURE 2.62 ▪ Straddle Injury. (**A, B**). The bruises sustained on this child's labia and medial thighs were secondary to her slipping when coming out of the tub while straddling the tub wall. While painful, they healed without event. (Photo contributor: Eve J. Lowenstein, MD, PhD.)

not cause injuries to the hymen. Scrotal ecchymosis can also result from abdominal trauma as blood travels fascial planes settling in the scrotum.

Emergency Department Treatment and Disposition

During the evaluation, other associated injuries, including injury to the urethra, must be excluded. Lacerations may be obscured because of swelling. Examination may be limited as a result of intense pain and fear, and the patient may need procedural sedation. If internal injuries cannot be excluded

FIGURE 2.63 ▪ Straddle Injury Versus Nonaccidental Trauma (NAT). (**A**) Scrotal laceration is seen in this 3-year-old child after an accidental fall on the playground equipment (history substantiated with witnesses at the playground). He underwent exploration in the operating room by the urologist and was found to have no other associated injuries, and the laceration was repaired. (**B**) A 2-year-old child was brought to the ED with a large scrotal laceration that occurred "sometime in the overnight period," which mom and her boyfriend attributed to the child "scratching at his eczema." He was also noted to have bilateral ear bruises (see Figure 1.14 (A, B)) and a prior history of bilateral subgaleal hematomas from a "fall between the bed and a nightstand". Given a lack of history to explain these injuries, Child Protective Services investigation was initiated for NAT. (Photo contributors: Stuart A. Bradin, DO [A], and Earl R. Hartwig, MD [B].)

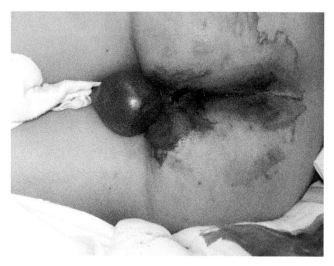

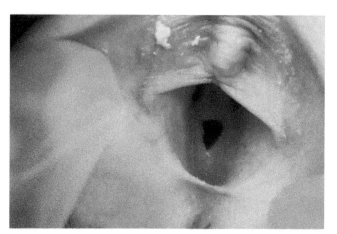

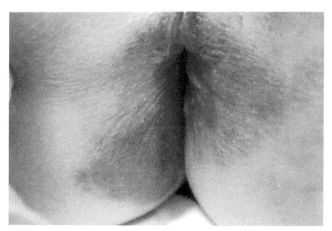

FIGURE 2.64 ■ Straddle Injury. This scrotal hematoma was sustained after consensual rectal intercourse involving a foreign body in a teenager, although abuse needs to be considered. Notice also the laceration of the anterior rectal commissure. (Photo contributor: Mark Silverberg, MD.)

in girls, examination under anesthesia and evaluation by a pediatric surgeon or gynecologist is required. If clinically indicated, a scrotal US to assess testicular injuries and a retrograde urethrogram to assess urethral injuries (extravasation) may be ordered. Boys will need evaluation by a urologist for urethral, testicular (eg, hematoma, rupture), or scrotal injuries (eg, lacerations extending through the dartos). If intra-abdominal injury is suspected, a contrast-enhanced CT scan of the abdomen and pelvis is indicated. Hematomas and superficial lacerations are managed with supportive care, and resolution occurs spontaneously. Patient's ability to void without any difficulty must be confirmed before the discharge. To minimize discomfort, patient can be advised to take sitz baths. Voiding in bath of warm water also may ease the dysuria. Local application of antibiotics may help in promoting healing. Child abuse specialist or Child Protective Services may be consulted prior to discharge if the diagnosis is unclear.

Pearls

1. Straddle injuries are the most common type of accidental injuries involving the genitalia and may be difficult to differentiate from injuries due to sexual abuse. A plausible

FIGURE 2.65 ■ Anogenital Trauma From Motor Vehicular Accident (MVA). An 8-year-old girl presented with fractures of the right tibia and fibula and a degloving injury of the right foot following an MVA while crossing the street. Her anogenital exam was notable for a crescentic hymen with a smooth uninterrupted boarder, erythema at the posterior commissure, few petechiae in the left vestibule, a perineal laceration extending to 12 o'clock perianally without any bleeding, and red and purple perianal bruising extending to her buttocks bilaterally. She made no disclosures of sexual abuse and STI testing was negative. (Photo contributor: Allison M. Jackson, MD, MPH.)

explanation and physical examination that support the history are important in arriving at the correct diagnosis.

2. Suspect sexual abuse if there is a lack of correlation between history and clinical findings, evidence of injuries in other areas, genital injuries in nonambulatory children, extensive injuries, or vaginal, perianal, rectal, or hymenal injuries without a clear history of penetrating trauma.

Chapter 3

INFECTIOUS DISEASES

Michelle W. Parker
Samir S. Shah

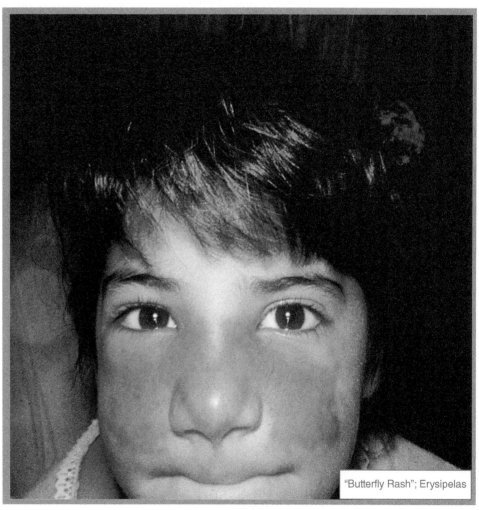

"Butterfly Rash"; Erysipelas

(Photo contributor: Binita R. Shah, MD)

The authors acknowledge the special contributions of Vikas S. Shah, MD, and Binita R. Shah, MD, to prior edition.

STREPTOCOCCAL PHARYNGITIS AND SCARLET FEVER

Clinical Summary

Streptococcal pharyngitis, commonly referred to as "*Strep throat*" is acute tonsillopharyngitis most often caused by *Streptococcus pyogenes* (group A β-hemolytic streptococci [GABHS]), and occasionally by other serogroups, such as C and G. Streptococcal pharyngitis is seen among schoolchildren (5–15 years) with a peak incidence during the first few years of school. The incubation period is 2 to 4 days. Presenting symptoms are abrupt onset with high fever, sore throat, pain on swallowing, malaise, headache, and abdominal pain. The pharynx, palate, and uvula are erythematous and in most instances, the palate and uvula will be edematous and covered with petechiae. The tonsils are enlarged with patches of a gray-white exudate giving a "strawberry" appearance (intensity of exudates ranges from absent in mild cases to a distinct membrane covering the entire pharynx in severe cases). Tender anterior cervical lymphadenopathy at the angles of the mandibles is palpable.

Scarlet fever rash may appear 12 to 24 hours after the onset of fever. The patient's forehead and cheeks are flushed with circumoral pallor. Patients often have a rash characterized by tiny papules that appear like a "sunburn with goose pimples," sandpaper texture, and blanches with pressure. This rash begins in the axilla, groin, and neck and generalizes, sparing the palms, soles, and face, within 24 hours. Other findings include strawberry tongue, exudative tonsillopharyngitis, and

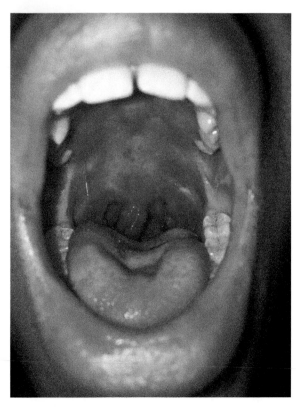

FIGURE 3.2 ■ Acute Uvulitis. Markedly swollen uvula with petechiae on the soft palate and exudative tonsillopharyngitis is seen in this adolescent male presenting with fever, sore throat, and "foreign body" sensation in the throat. His throat culture was positive for GABHS. (Photo contributor: Aditi Jayanth, MD.)

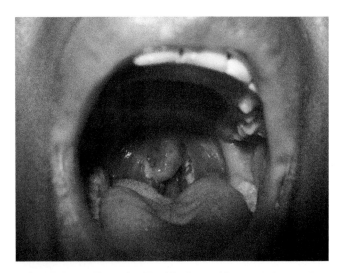

FIGURE 3.1 ■ Exudative Tonsillopharyngitis. Exudative tonsillopharyngitis in an adolescent presenting with high fever, sore throat, and tender anterior cervical adenopathy and a throat culture positive for GABHS. Intensity of exudates can be absent in mild cases to formation of a membrane covering the entire pharynx in severe cases. (Photo contributor: Mark Silverberg, MD.)

Pastia sign (an accentuation of the rash in skin folds with fine line of petechiae). Desquamation may occur after 7 to 10 days and usually continues for 2 to 3 weeks, but can last up to 2 months. When desquamation occurs, it begins as fine flakes on the face, then proceeds over the trunk, hands, and feet. The extent and duration of desquamation are directly related to the intensity of the rash. Scarlet fever rash is caused by 1 or more of several erythrogenic exotoxins produced by GABHS strains and occurs in children who lack immunity to the exotoxin. The portal of entry is the oropharynx in the majority of cases and rarely a surgical wound (*surgical scarlet fever*). Most cases occur in children between 2 and 8 years of age, typically in winter and early spring.

Both streptococcal pharyngitis and scarlet fever are self-limited diseases. Fever abates within 3 to 5 days (in absence of suppurative complications) with resolution of all signs and symptoms within 1 week. Tonsillar hypertrophy and lymph nodes take several weeks to return to their usual size. Suppurative complications include acute cervical lymphadenitis,

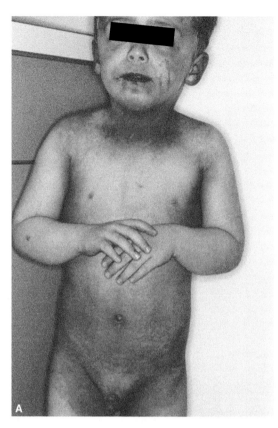
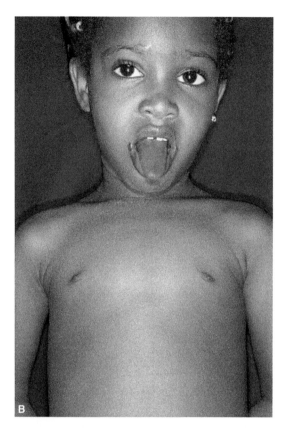

FIGURE 3.3 ■ Scarlet Fever. (**A**) Erythematous scarlatiniform rash with sore throat and fever were seen in this child. Note the prominence of the rash in the neck, axillae, and groin (all pressure sites). (**B**) In dark-skinned patients, the scarlet fever rash may be more easily palpated as "sandpaper texture" than seen. Note the accentuation of the rash in the neck area and absence of conjunctival injection and red lips (characteristic features of Kawasaki disease that also presents with scarlatiniform rash). (Photo contributors: Bipin Patel MD [A] and Binita R. Shah, MD [B].)

peritonsillar cellulitis or peritonsillar abscess, retropharyngeal abscess, acute otitis media, acute sinusitis, mastoiditis, pneumonia, toxic shock syndrome (TSS), intracranial complications (eg, meningitis, brain abscess), and bacteremic spread with metastatic infection (eg, septic arthritis, osteomyelitis). Nonsuppurative complications include acute rheumatic fever (ARF) and acute glomerulonephritis. Acute glomerulonephritis may develop after 1 to 3 weeks despite adequate treatment of streptococcal pharyngitis. Differential diagnosis of exudative tonsillopharyngitis includes viral infections (eg, adenovirus, Epstein-Barr virus [EBV], herpes simplex virus [HSV] [shallow tonsillar ulcers with gray exudates]), other bacterial infections (diphtheria, tularemia), and *Candida* (immunosuppressed patients). Differential diagnosis of scarlet fever includes Kawasaki disease (KD), staphylococcal scarlatina, staphylococcal scalded skin syndrome (SSSS), viral exanthems, *Mycoplasma* infection, TSS, drug hypersensitivity reactions, severe sunburn, and *Arcanobacterium*

haemolyticum infection (tonsillopharyngitis with scarlatiniform rash on the extensor surfaces of the arms and legs; seen in adolescents and young adults).

Emergency Department Treatment and Disposition

Confirm diagnosis by performing either a throat culture (vigorously swab tonsils and posterior pharynx to obtain an adequate sample) or rapid antigen detection test as accurate clinical differentiation of viral and GABHS pharyngitis is not possible. A positive rapid antigen test is diagnostic of GABHS infection; a negative test requires a throat culture. A throat culture is also required to detect non-GABHS streptococcal infection (eg, group C, G, or F streptococcal infection), although these pathogens are not associated with ARF. Consider initiating therapy after a positive rapid antigen detection test; withholding therapy for 24 to 48 hours while

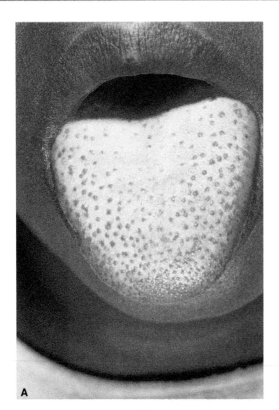
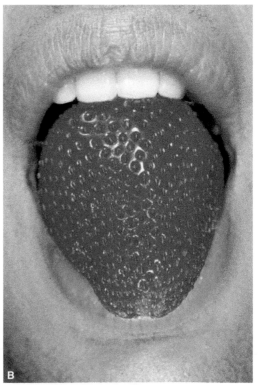
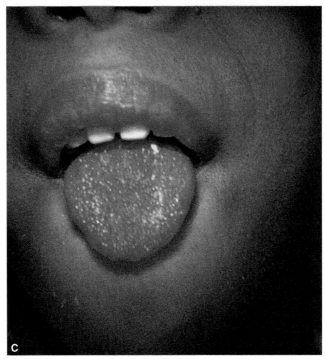

FIGURE 3.4 ■ "Strawberry Tongue" of Scarlet Fever. (**A**) White strawberry tongue (edematous red papillae projecting through white-coated tongue is seen on the second day of illness in a child with scarlet fever). (**B**) The real "red strawberry tongue"? (**C**) Red strawberry tongue (as white coating disappears, red tongue is seen studded with prominent papillae that stand out). Other differential of strawberry tongue includes Kawasaki disease and toxic shock syndrome (TSS; *Staphylococcus aureus*–mediated TSS and streptococcal-mediated TSS). (Photo contributor: Binita R. Shah, MD.)

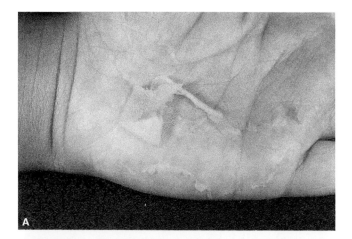

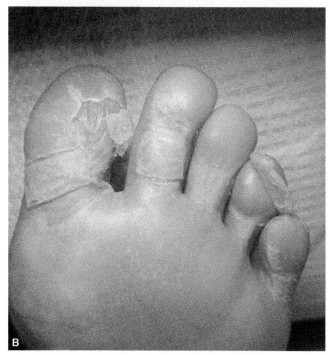

FIGURE 3.5 ▪ Desquamation of the Hand and Foot in Scarlet Fever. (**A, B**) Photographs taken on the eighth day of illness in a child with scarlet fever. (Photo contributor: Binita R. Shah, MD.)

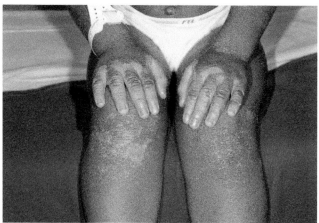

FIGURE 3.6 ▪ Desquamation as Presenting Sign of Scarlet Fever. This child was brought to ED because of this prominent (and frightening to parents) desquamation seen in both hands and lower extremities. He had a sore throat and low-grade fever with "goose bumps" 9 days before this finding. Desquamation may be a presenting sign of scarlet fever (if the initial acute phase is mild and overlooked). Large sheaths of epidermis may be shed from the palms and soles in a glove-like pattern, exposing new and tender epidermis beneath. (Photo contributor: Binita R. Shah, MD.)

awaiting throat culture results does not increase the risk of ARF. Prescribe antibiotics (before throat culture result) for patients with any of the following: prior history of ARF, scarlet fever, suppurative complications (eg, peritonsillar cellulitis or abscess), or patients unavailable for follow-up. Prescribe penicillin V (drug of choice) orally for 10 days (emphasize the importance of completing the *full 10-day course* regardless of clinical improvement to prevent ARF). If compliance is an issue, alternatives include amoxicillin (single daily dose for 10 days) or benzathine penicillin G or mixtures of benzathine

penicillin G with procaine penicillin (to reduce pain) given intramuscularly as a single dose. For patients allergic to penicillin, clarithromycin, azithromycin, and clindamycin are alternatives. Children can return to school after 24 hours of antibiotic therapy. Routine posttreatment follow-up culture is not needed.

Pearls

1. Most common clinical illness produced by GABHS is acute tonsillopharyngitis.
2. Coryza, cough, conjunctivitis, hoarseness, diarrhea, discrete ulcers, or stomatitis in a child with pharyngitis strongly suggests a viral etiology and not GABHS infection.
3. Exudative pharyngitis in children <3 years of age is rarely of streptococcal etiology, and diagnostic studies for GABHS are not recommended routinely.
4. Scarlet fever occurs most commonly in association with pharyngitis and rarely with pyoderma or an infected wound. Tonsillopharyngitis is absent in surgical scarlet fever.
5. Skin tenderness is absent in scarlet fever, as opposed to the prominent skin tenderness of staphylococcal scarlatina.

Clinical Summary

Impetigo is a contagious superficial skin infection occurring in 2 forms: bullous and nonbullous (accounts for >70% of cases). Bullous impetigo is caused by *Staphylococcus aureus,* whereas the nonbullous form is caused by either *S pyogenes* (GABHS), *S aureus,* or both. Nonbullous impetigo is most commonly seen in preschoolers and begins as

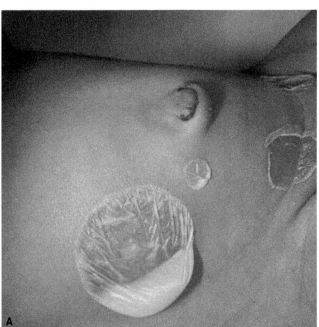

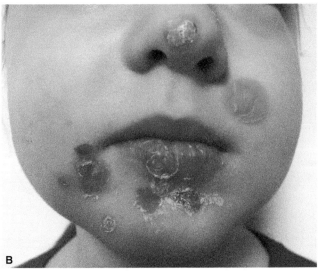

FIGURE 3.8 ■ Bullous Impetigo. (**A**) An intact bullous lesion filled with pus is seen in a 10-day-old neonate. He also had several round, ruptured erosions with a moist, red surface that were surrounded by a narrow ring of scale. Intact or ruptured bullae are round or oval in shape. (**B**) Five-year-old child with multiple superficial bullae in the perioral and perinasal areas, some with classic yellow crusting. (Photo contributors: Binita R. Shah, MD [A], and Jeannette Jakus, MD [B].)

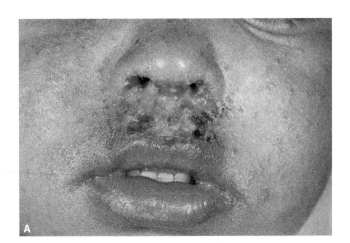

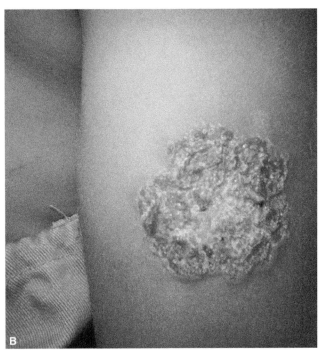

FIGURE 3.7 ■ Nonbullous Impetigo. (**A**) Exposed body surfaces such as the face (around the nose and mouth) are the most common sites. (**B**) Lesion with a honey-colored crust on the upper extremity. Removal of the crust reveals bright red, shiny erosions. (Photo contributor: Binita R. Shah, MD.)

small vesicles progressing to pustules that extend radially with satellite lesions. Vesiculopustular lesions rupture, exposing a red, moist base and purulent discharge, which forms thick, yellow, or honey-colored adherent crusts. Lesions

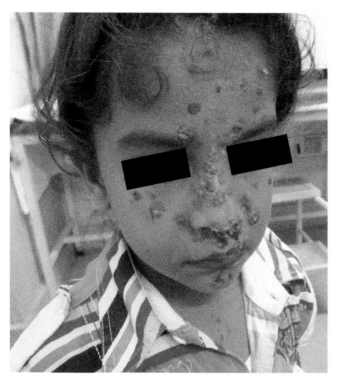

FIGURE 3.9 ■ Bullous Impetigo. Multiple superficial bullae in the perioral and perinasal areas of the face, some with classic yellow crusting, are seen in this girl. (Photo contributor: Raj Pal Singh, MD.)

are usually painless but commonly pruritic, have little surrounding erythema, and tend to occur on traumatized skin (eg, insect bite, abrasion), commonly in hot, muggy summer months. Exposed body surfaces such as the face, nose, mouth,

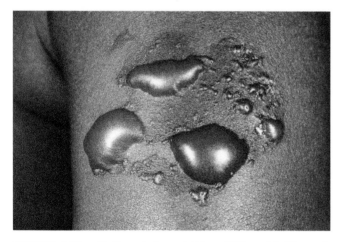

FIGURE 3.10 ■ Bullous Arthropod Bites; Differential Diagnosis of Bullous Impetigo. Close-up of bullous lesions on upper extremity (exposed area) due to arthropod bites. These lesions can be mistaken for either second-degree burns or bullous impetigo. (Photo contributor: Binita R. Shah, MD.)

or extremities are most commonly affected. Skin scratching causes lesions to spread through autoinoculation. Regional lymphadenopathy is common, but constitutional symptoms are absent or minimal.

Bullous impetigo is most commonly seen in newborns, infants, and preschoolers. There is no seasonal predilection. The bacterial reservoir is the upper respiratory tract (eg, nose, conjunctiva) of asymptomatic carriers who spread the pathogen to the child's skin. Lesions result from exfoliative toxin produced by bacteria at the contact site and begin as vesicles that progress to flaccid bullae with little or no surrounding erythema and clear to cloudy contents. Rupture leaves a narrow rim of scale at the edge of shallow, moist, red erosions (scalded skin appearance). Nikolsky sign is absent (unlike staphylococcal scalded skin syndrome [SSSS]). Lesions may be few and localized (usually covered areas) or numerous and widely scattered. Common sites are trunk, perineum, buttocks, and extremities. Lesions heal without scarring.

Complications include acute poststreptococcal glomerulonephritis (impetigo by GABHS) and rarely serious secondary infections (eg, osteomyelitis, septic arthritis). Differential diagnosis of nonbullous impetigo includes ecthyma, HSV infection, varicella, tinea corporis, and localized acute pustular psoriasis. In contrast, differential diagnosis of bullous impetigo includes bullous arthropod bites, poison ivy, child abuse (abusive burn injury), autoimmune blistering disease (eg, linear immunoglobulin A [IgA] dermatosis, pemphigus), and epidermolysis bullosa.

Emergency Department Treatment and Disposition

The diagnosis is clinical, although the aspirate from the lesion may be cultured and Gram stain smear obtained. Although usually self-limited, untreated infection may last for weeks or months. Advise patients and caregivers to wash the affected area with antibacterial soap once or twice a day and remove crusts, which can be softened by soaking the area with a wet cloth compress, before applying topical therapy. Prescribe topical mupirocin ointment for localized impetigo (bullous or nonbullous) to eradicate the infection and prevent person-to-person spread. For generalized impetigo or if there is involvement of multiple family members, prescribe systemic antibiotics covering mixed pathogens (GABHS and

S aureus). First-line oral therapy should account for local methicillin resistance patterns and may include penicillinase-resistant β-lactam drugs (eg, dicloxacillin), a first- or second-generation cephalosporin, clindamycin, doxycycline for children >8 years of age, or trimethoprim-sulfamethoxazole for bullous impetigo. Dicloxacillin may be challenging to administer to young children given its suboptimal palatability and requirement for frequent dosing (4 times each day) and administration on an empty stomach. Refer patients with recurrence for evaluation and treatment of nasal carriage of *S aureus.*

Pearls

1. A pathognomonic finding of bullous impetigo is a ring of scale at the periphery of an eroded lesion with a varnished surface.
2. Impetigo is a highly contagious infection, and spread is facilitated by poor hygiene.
3. Staphylococci can be isolated from bullous impetigo lesions in contrast to culture of SSSS lesions.

Clinical Summary

Ecthyma is a skin infection caused by *S pyogenes* (GABHS) and/or *S aureus*. Unlike impetigo, which is superficial, ecthyma involves deeper layers of the skin (the entire thickness of the epidermis to the upper reaches of the dermis). Ecthyma is seen in children of all ages and more frequently during summer. Predisposing factors include preceding minor skin trauma (eg, abrasions, insect bites), conditions associated with pruritus (eg, scabies, pediculosis), poor hygiene, and malnutrition. Lesions begin as vesicles or vesiculopustules with an erythematous base and rupture to form crusts and erode through the epidermis into the dermis, forming indolent "punched-out" ulcers with elevated margins. Ulcers become elevated and obscured by thick, dark greenish-yellow, tightly adherent crusts that contribute to the persistence of the infection. Lesions are discrete and round, and the most common site is lower legs. Lesions spread by autoinoculation and heal with scarring (unlike impetigo). Complications include cellulitis (untreated ecthyma) and poststreptococcal glomerulonephritis. Differential diagnosis includes cigarette burns (due to child abuse) and ecthyma gangrenosum (EG) (*Pseudomonas aeruginosa* infection in patients who may be immunocompromised).

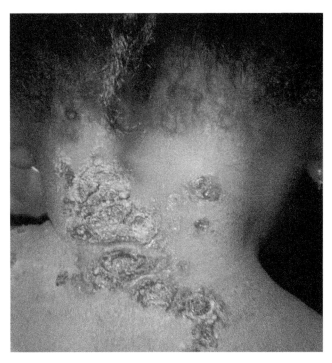

FIGURE 3.12 ■ Ecthyma. Multiple ecthyma lesions on the neck. (Photo contributor: Binita R. Shah, MD.)

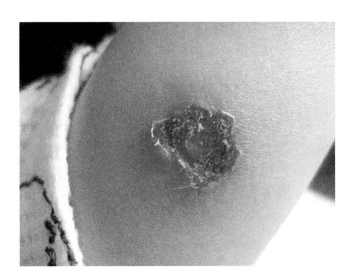

FIGURE 3.11 ■ Ecthyma. An enlarging, slightly painful lesion that started as a "blister" on the forearm (without any prior history of trauma). Culture grew *S pyogenes*. Ecthyma is a discrete, round lesion with a dark crust in the center surrounded by a rim of shallow ulceration. (Photo contributor: Andrea Marmor, MD.)

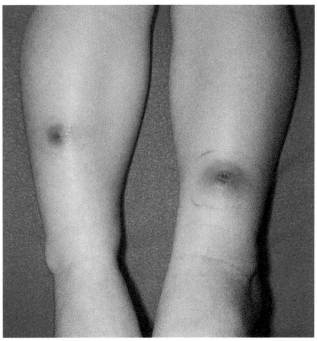

FIGURE 3.13 ■ Ecthyma. Ecthyma in a 2-year-old child. (Photo contributor: Samir S. Shah, MD, MSCE.)

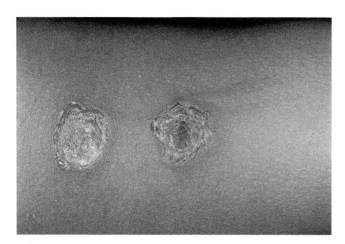

FIGURE 3.14 ■ Ecthyma. Ecthyma may be confused with cigarette burns. Ecthyma lesions are frequently of different sizes and are associated with crusting. Cigarette burns are circular punched-out lesions of uniform size with an average diameter of about 8 to 10 mm and have a smooth well-defined edge. (Photo contributor: Binita R. Shah, MD.)

Emergency Department Treatment and Disposition

Diagnosis is clinical. Culture of the exudate (beneath an unroofed crust) reveals GABHS or *S aureus.* Advise washing the affected area with antibacterial soap and removal of the crust (facilitated by softening the crust by soaking with a wet cloth compress). Prescribe topical mupirocin therapy until all lesions have cleared. Depending on the prevalence of methicillin-resistant or methicillin-sensitive *S aureus* in the community, antibiotic options include oral penicillinase-resistant β-lactam drugs (eg, dicloxacillin) or a first- or second-generation cephalosporin, clindamycin or doxycycline (children >8 years of age).

Pearls

1. Thick crusts and underlying ulcers differentiate ecthyma from nonbullous impetigo.
2. Ecthyma can be mistaken for cigarette burns of child abuse.

Clinical Summary

Erysipelas is a distinct skin infection involving the uppermost layers of the subcutaneous tissue and cutaneous lymphatic vessels. It is caused by *S pyogenes* (GABHS) in the majority of patients and rarely by groups G, C, and B streptococci. It occurs most frequently in infants, young children, older adults, and debilitated patients. The organism gains access to the deeper layers of the skin through breaks (eg, abrasions, lacerations, wounds, chronic ulcers). Predisposing factors include lymphedema, local lymphatic dysfunction, venous stasis, diabetes mellitus, malnutrition, and immunocompromised states. Onset is usually abrupt with

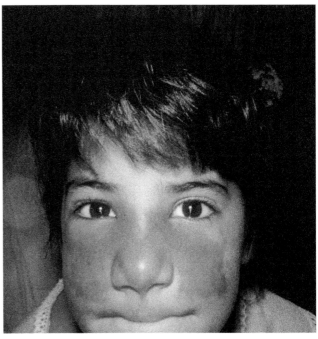

FIGURE 3.16 ■ Butterfly Rash of Erysipelas. A rapidly spreading (<12-hour duration), tender, erythematous, indurated facial rash was seen in this girl with very high fever and leukocytosis. The sharp demarcation between erythema and the normal surrounding skin is evident. Erysipelas may create a "butterfly" appearance (mimicking the rash of systemic lupus erythematosus) on the face. She gave a history of falling off the monkey bar 2 days prior to appearance of this rash. Within 6 months after this infection, she presented again with a second episode of erysipelas at the same site. (Reproduced with permission from Shah BR, Santucci K, Tunnessen W Jr: Erysipelas. *Arch Pediatr Adolesc Med* 1995; Jan;149(1):55-56.)

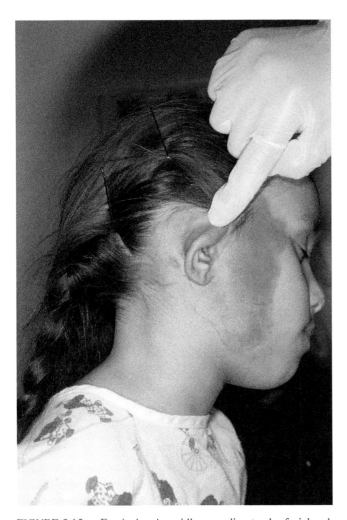

FIGURE 3.15 ■ Erysipelas. A rapidly spreading tender facial rash and high fever were complaints of this girl. She had scratch marks on her cheek (portal of entry). The sharp demarcation between the salmon-red erythema and the normal surrounding skin is evident. Marking the margins of the erythema with ink (as shown) helps in following the clinical course (progression or regression) of the infection. (Photo contributor: Binita R. Shah, MD.)

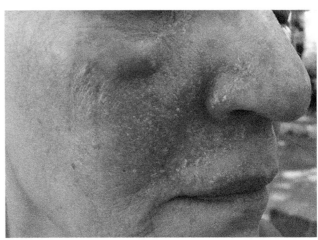

FIGURE 3.17 ■ Erysipelas. Erythematous rash with classic honey-colored crust is seen in this facial erysipelas caused by GABHS. (Photo contributor: Rajni P. Shah, MD.)

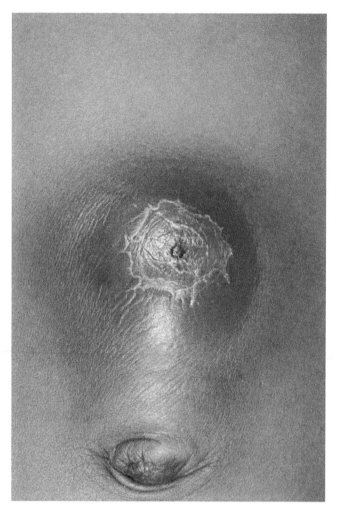

FIGURE 3.18 ■ Cellulitis; Differential Diagnosis of Erysipelas. Cellulitis spreads more slowly and extends more deeply into the subcutaneous tissues; hence, the borders of cellulitis are ill-defined (in contrast to erysipelas). *S pyogenes* and *S aureus* are common pathogens causing cellulitis. *S pneumoniae* and *H influenzae* can cause buccal cellulitis associated with bacteremia in unimmunized young children. (Photo contributor: Binita R. Shah, MD.)

constitutional symptoms (eg, fever, chills, malaise). Common sites are extremities (usually associated with a wound) and face (usually associated with pharyngitis). Initiating lesion is frequently inconspicuous and spreads peripherally with a raised, advancing border. The lesion is a fiery red or salmon colored, warm, tender, tense, indurated well-circumscribed plaque (sometimes with peau d'orange appearance) with a sharp demarcated border distinguishing it from the surrounding normal tissue. Erythematous lymphatic streaks projecting from the margins of the lesion toward regional nodes may be

noted. Intense edema may lead to formation of vesicles or tense bullae that later rupture and crust (bullous erysipelas). A "butterfly" appearance with involvement of both cheeks and nasal bridge may occur with involvement of the face. Regional lymphadenopathy may be present. Desquamation of involved skin may occur 5 to 10 days into the illness. Complications are the same as with any GABHS infection (see pages 94–95). Erysipelas produces lymphatic obstruction, leading to impaired lymphatic drainage causing lymphedema, which predisposes to recurrent episodes of erysipelas frequently at the same site and permanent local swelling. Differential diagnosis includes cellulitis, erysipelas-like presentation due to other bacterial infection (eg, *Streptococcus pneumoniae*, *S aureus*), necrotizing fasciitis, and contact dermatitis.

Emergency Department Treatment and Disposition

The diagnosis is clinical. Hospitalize patients with infection involving the face and those with systemic signs for parenteral antibiotics (eg, ceftriaxone) until improvement is noted or progression is halted (typically 24–48 hours). A CBC is not routinely necessary but, if performed, may reveal leukocytosis with a left shift. Blood cultures are not routinely required but should be considered in ill-appearing and immunocompromised patients. Although not typically necessary, a culture obtained by subcutaneous injection of nonbacteriostatic saline followed by aspiration from the advancing margin of the lesion may yield the organism. If cellulitis due to *S aureus* cannot be excluded by examination, depending on the prevalence of methicillin-resistant or methicillin-sensitive *S aureus* in the community, antibiotic options include penicillinase-resistant β-lactam drugs (eg, oxacillin) or clindamycin. Prescribe oral antibiotics for patients with milder presentations with a close follow-up. Advise rest, immobilization, and elevation of the affected part, and cool, wet dressings as supportive therapy. Extension into deeper soft tissues is rare.

Pearl

1. Erysipelas is commonly referred as St. Anthony's fire because it spreads rapidly like a fire, affecting a very large area of the skin within a short period of time.

Clinical Summary

Necrotizing fasciitis (NF; also known as streptococcal gangrene, flesh-eating bacteria syndrome, hospital gangrene, or necrotizing erysipelas or necrotizing cellulites) is a life-threatening bacterial infection of the fascia and subcutaneous tissues. Patients present with an erythematous, indurated, tender, ill-defined plaque (often mistaken for cellulitis) that manifests disproportionate pain and tenderness. The lesion evolves to a dusky purple color with vesicles/bullae sometimes filled with maroon or violaceous fluid. Subcutaneous emphysema or crepitus may be present, and there may be loss of sensation

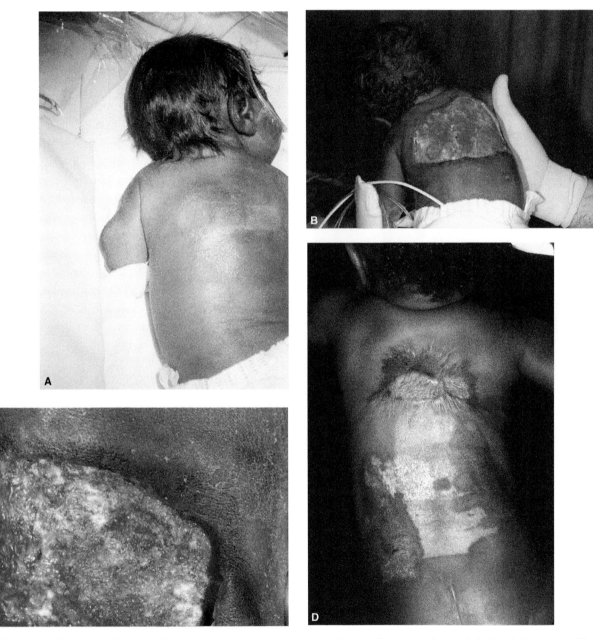

FIGURE 3.19 ■ Necrotizing Fasciitis. (**A**) A 9-day-old neonate presented with high fever, moaning, and slightly indurated swelling with bluish discoloration on the back. (**B, C**) Within 12 hours, there was vesiculation and purplish discoloration. These photographs were taken 8 hours following the first surgical exploration and debridement and shows necrotic borders and pus over the underlying muscle. Both blood and tissue cultures grew *S aureus*. (**D**) Multiple surgical explorations and debridement were performed followed by skin grafting during recovery. (Photo contributor: Binita R. Shah, MD.)

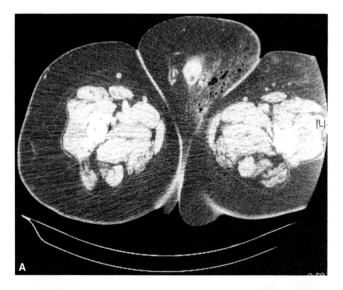

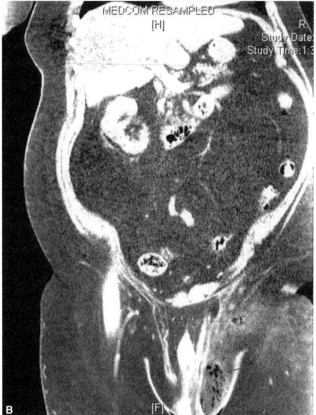

FIGURE 3.20 ■ Necrotizing Fasciitis; Fournier's Gangrene. (A, B) Coronal and axial CT images demonstrate air within the soft tissues of the left perineal region (arrows) compatible with necrotizing fasciitis. (Photo/legend contributors: Nikita Joshi, MD, and John Amodio, MD.)

of the affected area. The lesion expands rapidly with undermining of overlying skin (*important clue for diagnosis*), progressing to necrosis and gangrene. Signs of toxicity include high fever, malaise, altered sensorium, and shock. Fournier gangrene is NF of the perineum, scrotum, and penis. Predisposing factors include infections (eg, varicella), contaminated surgical wounds, IV drug or alcohol abuse, and immunocompromised states. Bacterial myonecrosis, or involvement of the muscle, may be present. Various etiologies include *S pyogenes* (GABHS; most common pathogen); groups B, C, or G streptococci; *S aureus*; *P aeruginosa*; anaerobes (eg, *Bacteroides, Peptostreptococcus, Clostridium* spp); and polymicrobial (gram-negative bacilli [eg, *Escherichia coli, Proteus* spp] and anaerobic bacteria). The majority of cases occur as extensions from localized nearby skin infections that expand along fascial planes, leading to edema, vascular injury, and thrombosis, resulting in widespread necrosis of the superficial fascia, adjoining tissues, and dermis, with associated compression or destruction of nerves innervating skin. Differential diagnosis includes erysipelas, cellulitis, and purpura fulminans. Complications include multiorgan failure with oliguria, acute respiratory distress syndrome, disseminated intravascular coagulation (DIC), myocardial failure, and fluid and electrolyte disturbances (extravasation of intravascular fluid into tissues).

Emergency Department Treatment and Disposition

NF is a medical emergency. Consult surgery emergently for surgical exploration, biopsy (frozen-section biopsy allows rapid evaluation of the pathology to confirm the diagnosis and identification of pathogens underlying the intact skin), debridement of all necrotic tissue, and fasciotomy. Consult an infectious disease specialist and begin empiric broad-spectrum IV antibiotics (eg, ampicillin-sulbactam or ampicillin with either clindamycin or metronidazole and vancomycin). Obtain CBC, comprehensive metabolic panel, and coagulation profile because leukocytosis with immature cells, anemia, hyponatremia, hypocalcemia, hypoproteinemia, evidence of DIC, and elevated values of BUN, creatinine, and liver enzymes may be noted. Perform fine-needle aspiration from the involved area (may show presence of pus and bacteria on Gram stain), and send aspirated material and blood culture for both aerobic and anaerobic pathogens. A radiograph of the affected area may show presence of subcutaneous gas, which mandates rapid surgical exploration; however, absence of soft tissue gas does not exclude diagnosis. Consider CT, US, or MRI of the affected area for the diagnosis in patients with early signs (when diagnosis is unclear); however, these modalities should never delay immediate surgical exploration in patients with obvious signs. Hospitalize all suspected cases of NF to the ICU for ongoing management. Repeat debridement within 24 to 48 hours may be necessary because of continued spread of the infection into surrounding tissues. Other treatment modalities may include hyperbaric oxygen.

Pearls

1. Sine qua non of NF is fascial necrosis with widespread undermining of the skin. The ability to pass a sterile instrument along a plane superficial to the deep fascia without resistance is indicative of NF.
2. Presence of an indurated "wooden" plaque adjacent to infected skin coupled with extreme pain in an area of rapidly advancing edema and inflammation are important clues.
3. Marked systemic toxicity and pain out of proportion to the local findings (in contrast to the usual patient with cellulitis) suggests NF.

Clinical Summary

Ecthyma gangrenosum (EG) is a pathognomonic cutaneous manifestation of *P aeruginosa* septicemia; other skin lesions include subcutaneous nodules, vesicular lesions, gangrenous cellulitis, and petechial rash. EG usually occurs as a result of bloodborne metastatic seeding to the skin from the bacteremia, or rarely as a primary lesion without bacteremia. Predisposing factors for *Pseudomonas* septicemia include immunosuppression (eg, malignancy, diabetes, malnutrition, cystic fibrosis), debilitated preterm newborns, severe thermal burns, disorders leading to severe neutropenia or pancytopenia, hospitalized patients on intensive antibiotic treatment, or those with indwelling urinary, arterial, or venous catheters. Skin lesions begin as hemorrhagic (purpuric) macular, vesicular, pustular, or bullous lesions and evolve into punched-out necrotic ulcers with raised edges with a rim of erythema. Lesions remain localized or more typically extend over several centimeters, ultimately becoming a round, indurated, painless lesion with a characteristic central gray-black eschar. Either a single ulcer or multiple (noncontiguous) ulcers may be seen. Common sites include perineal or gluteal region, extremities, trunk, face, intertriginous areas, and axilla. Lesions take a few weeks to heal. Differential diagnosis includes EG-like lesions in sepsis from other pathogens (eg, *Candida* spp, *S aureus*, *S pyogenes*), thermal burns, pyoderma gangrenosum, purpura fulminans, and brown recluse spider bite.

Emergency Department Treatment and Disposition

Stabilize the patient based on abnormal vital signs (patients with EG are usually septic). Hospitalize to the ICU for parenteral antibiotic therapy and general supportive care including wound care. Begin antibiotic therapy with an aminoglycoside (eg, tobramycin, gentamicin) and an antipseudomonal penicillin (eg, ticarcillin, piperacillin). Obtain CBC (usually neutropenia especially with septicemia), comprehensive metabolic panel, coagulation profile, blood culture, and needle aspiration and culture of the lesion (Gram stain may show presence of bacteria). Consult dermatologist if diagnosis is unclear; a skin biopsy may show numerous bacteria invading the blood vessels (invasion of media and adventitia of vein walls deep in the dermis with very few inflammatory cells).

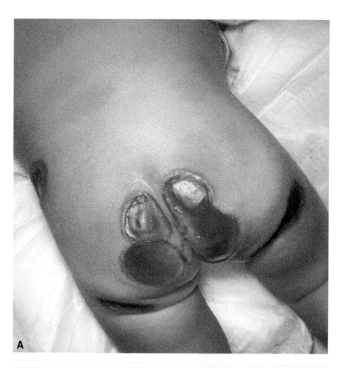

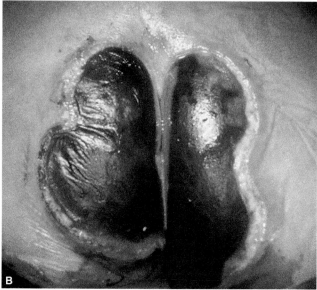

FIGURE 3.21 ■ Ecthyma Gangrenosum. (**A**) Purpuric macular lesions involving the perineum, buttocks, and trunk in a malnourished infant (fed only diluted soy formula) presenting in septic shock. (**B**) Close-up of lesions showing progression to necrotic ulcers with dense black eschars in the center. Note the surrounding erythematous halo with raised edges. Both blood and wound cultures were positive for *Pseudomonas aeruginosa*. (Reproduced with permission from Secord A, Milla C, Shah BR, et al: Picture of the month. Ecthyma gangrenosum. *Am J Dis Child* 1993;Jul;147(7):795-796.)

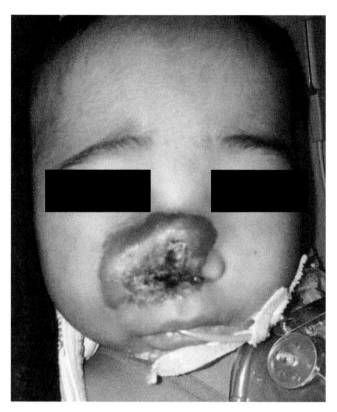

FIGURE 3.22 ▪ Ecthyma Gangrenosum. This infant presented with fever, septic shock, and blackish discoloration of the tip of the nose that rapidly worsened as shown. Her blood culture was positive for *Pseudomonas aeruginosa.* (Photo contributor: Samridhi Goyal, MD.)

Pearl

1. The characteristic findings of EG are punched-out ulcers with a black eschar, surrounded by a rim of erythema.

TOXIC SHOCK SYNDROME

Clinical Summary

Toxic shock syndrome (TSS) is a potentially fatal systemic infection by toxin-producing strains of either *S aureus* (*S aureus*–mediated TSS) or *S pyogenes* (*S pyogenes*–mediated TSS). Diagnosis is made using published criteria. *S pyogenes*–mediated TSS occurs commonly in young children. Predisposing factors include varicella, HIV infection, diabetes mellitus, IV drug use, and invasive infections (eg, bacteremia, pneumonia, osteomyelitis, endocarditis).

S aureus–mediated TSS is seen less commonly in children, and most cases occur in women aged 15 to 34 years (reflecting association with menses). Nonmenstrual cases occur in people of all ages and in both sexes. Predisposing factors include use of tampons during menstruation, foreign body placements (eg, contraceptive sponge, central lines), primary *S aureus* infections (eg, cellulitis, endocarditis), postoperative wound infections, skin or mucous membrane disruptions (eg, burns, insect bites), and vaginal or pharyngeal colonization. Onset may be abrupt or preceded by a prodromal illness of fever, chills, and myalgias. Rash (seen almost always in first 24 hours of illness) may be faint and often mistaken for flush associated with fever. Beefy, red hyperemia of mucous membranes, conjunctival injection, strawberry tongue, erythema, and edema of palms and soles (findings similar to KD) are often seen. Pelvic exam is usually normal except for subtle erythema and edema of the skin of the inner thigh and

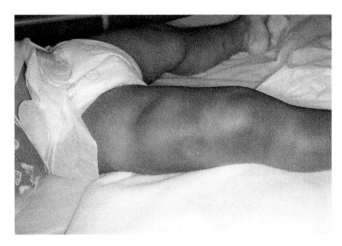

FIGURE 3.24 ■ Cellulitis in Streptococcal Toxic Shock Syndrome (TSS). Cellulitis involving the thigh and lower leg was seen in this child with AIDS. He presented with septic shock and multiorgan failure with a blood culture positive for *S pyogenes*. (Photo contributor: Binita R. Shah, MD.)

perineum in menstrual TSS. The focus of the staphylococcal infection may be inconspicuous, with absent signs of inflammation in skin or wound lesions in nonmenstrual TSS.

Complications of TSS include acute renal failure, acute respiratory distress syndrome, overwhelming sepsis, DIC, and multiorgan failure leading to death. Differential diagnosis includes KD, scarlet fever, septic shock from other etiology (eg, meningococcemia, Rocky Mountain spotted fever

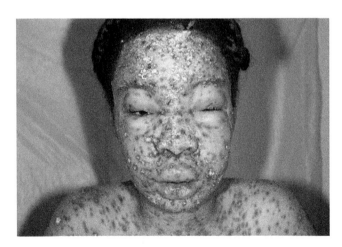

FIGURE 3.23 ■ Streptococcal Toxic Shock Syndrome. An 8-year-old girl presented with fever, hypotension, oliguria, and infected varicella lesions with honey-colored crust. Note also the bilateral periorbital edema. Her blood culture was positive for *S pyogenes*. (Photo contributor: Binita R. Shah, MD.)

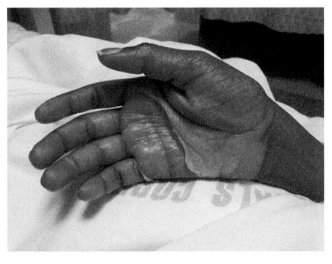

FIGURE 3.25 ■ Desquamation in Streptococcal Toxic Shock Syndrome (TSS). Shown here is desquamation that developed on the seventh day of the illness in an adolescent girl admitted with streptococcal TSS. (Photo contributor: Haamid Chamdawala, MD.)

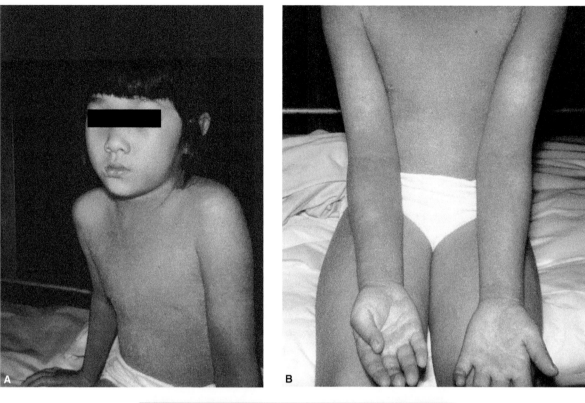

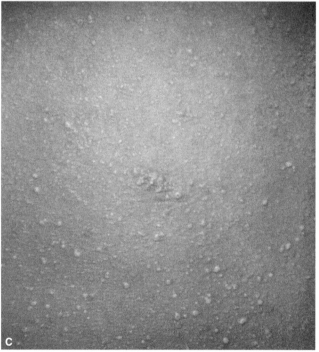

FIGURE 3.26 ■ Staphylococcal Toxic Shock Syndrome (TSS). (**A, B**) Diffuse erythroderma with innumerable pustular lesions, high fever, vomiting, and diarrhea were the presenting complaints of this patient with TSS. Her blood culture was positive for *S aureus*. (**C**) Close-up showing pustular lesions. Culture of these pustules was negative for *S aureus*. (Photo contributor: Binita R. Shah, MD.)

TABLE 3.1 ■ STREPTOCOCCAL TOXIC SHOCK SYNDROME: CLINICAL CASE DEFINITION

Confirmed case	Presence of all laboratory and clinical findings below	
Probable case	Positive culture from nonsterile site and all clinical findings below (and no other cause for illness identified)	
Laboratory findings	Isolation of *S pyogenes*	
	From a normally sterile site (eg, blood, CSF, peritoneal fluid, tissue biopsy specimen)	
	From a nonsterile site (eg, throat, sputum, vagina, surgical wound, or superficial skin lesion)	
Clinical findings		
Hypotension	Systolic BP ≤90 mm Hg in adults or <5th percentile for age in children	
Multisystem involvement (at least two of following)	Renal	Creatinine ≥2 mg/dL for adults or ≥2 times the upper limit of normal for age
	Coagulopathy	Platelets ≤100,000/mm³ and/or DIC
	Hepatic	Serum alanine and aspartate aminotransferases or total bilirubin values ≥2 times the upper limit of normal for age
	Pulmonary	Acute respiratory distress syndrome
	Skin	Erythematous macular rash that may desquamate
	Soft tissue	Necrosis, including necrotizing fasciitis or myositis, or gangrene

TABLE 3.2 ■ STAPHYLOCOCCAL TOXIC SHOCK SYNDROME: CLINICAL CASE DEFINITION

Probable case	Meets laboratory criteria below and has 4–5 of the clinical findings listed below	
Confirmed case	Meets laboratory criteria and all 5 clinical findings below, including desquamation, unless the patient dies before desquamation occurs	
Laboratory criteria	Negative results on following tests (if obtained)	
	Blood, throat, or cerebrospinal fluid cultures (blood culture may be positive for *S aureus*)	
	Serologic tests for Rocky Mountain spotted fever, leptospirosis, or measles	
Clinical findings		
Fever	38.9°C (102.0°F) or greater	
Rash	Diffuse macular erythroderma (nonpruritic)	
Desquamation	1–2 weeks after onset (particularly palms, soles, fingers, toes)	
Hypotension	Systolic BP ≤90 mm Hg for adults	
	<5th percentile for age for children <16 years of age	
	Orthostatic drop in diastolic BP ≥15 mm Hg from lying to sitting	
	Orthostatic syncope or orthostatic dizziness	
Multisystem involvement (3 or more of the following)	Gastrointestinal	Vomiting or diarrhea at onset of illness
	Muscular	Severe myalgia or creatinine phosphokinase >2 times the upper limit of normal
	Mucous membrane	Vaginal, oropharyngeal, or conjunctival hyperemia
	Renal	Blood urea nitrogen or serum creatinine level >2 times upper limit of normal or urinary sediment with ≥5 white blood cells per high-power field in absence of UTI
	Hepatic	Total bilirubin, aspartate, or alanine aminotransferase level >2 times the upper limit of normal
	Hematologic	Platelet count ≤100,000/mm³
	Central nervous system-related	Disorientation or alterations in consciousness without focal neuro- logic signs when fever and hypotension are absent

(RMSF), gram-negative sepsis), measles or atypical measles, ehrlichiosis, leptospirosis, and drug hypersensitivity (eg, Stevens-Johnson syndrome, toxic epidermal necrolysis).

Emergency Department Treatment and Disposition

Assess and stabilize vital signs, including fluid resuscitation and vasopressor agents, as indicated for septic shock. It may be impossible to distinguish clinically both forms of TSS; begin empiric antibiotic therapy that includes antistaphylococcal agents (eg, vancomycin and nafcillin) and a protein synthesis–inhibiting agent (eg, clindamycin). Obtain CBC, blood culture, cultures from the site of infection (skin or soft tissues), vaginal culture (for suspected menstrual TSS), serum electrolytes, BUN, creatinine, liver enzymes, and radiologic studies (as indicated). Consult surgery for exploration, biopsy, and resection of necrotic tissue in NF; drainage of the infected sites; or removal of foreign bodies. Hospitalize patients to the ICU for further management based on clinical severity. The benefit of IV immunoglobulin as an adjunct to antibiotic therapy has not been established.

Pearls

1. Fever, rash, desquamation, hypotension, and multiorgan involvement are the hallmarks of TSS.
2. TSS can be confused with many other causes of fever with mucocutaneous manifestations.
3. Do not use clindamycin alone as an initial empiric therapy, as 1% to 2% of S pyogenes organisms in the United States are resistant to clindamycin.
4. Women with menses-related TSS may experience 1 or more recurrent episodes. Advise against use of tampons and barrier methods of contraception for those with a prior history of TSS.

STAPHYLOCOCCAL SCALDED SKIN SYNDROME

Clinical Summary

Staphylococcal scalded skin syndrome (SSSS), also known as Ritter disease (SSSS of the newborn) and Lyell disease, is a toxin-mediated disease caused by *S aureus* that produces exfoliative toxins (ETA and ETB). *S aureus* colonizes mucous membranes of the nasopharynx, eyes, and other areas (eg, umbilical stump, circumcision site), producing a localized infection. Toxin produced in these areas circulates and acts specifically at the zona granulosa of the epidermis, leading to characteristic exfoliation. SSSS is most commonly seen in infants and young children (90% of cases <6 years; 62% <2 years of age). Infection in older children and adults is related to a decreased renal clearance of the toxin (eg, patients with renal insufficiency) or immunosuppression (eg, HIV infection).

Patients present with a sudden onset of fever and irritability. Prominent crusting around the eyes and mouth occurs early. Pharyngitis, conjunctivitis, or superficial erosions of lips may be noted, but intraoral mucosal surfaces are spared. The rash begins with an exquisite tenderness of the skin (eg, infant cries when held) and a diffuse erythematous scarlatiniform eruption (sandpaper texture, accentuation in perioral and flexural areas). Within 24 to 48 hours, the skin wrinkles and flaccid bullae develop, followed by exfoliation in sheets revealing a moist, red, shiny scalded-looking surface. Borders of exfoliating skin are rolled like wet tissue paper. Nikolsky sign is positive (slight rubbing of normal-looking adjacent skin results in blistering). Exfoliation can spread to the entire body surface area with severe disease. Drying of exfoliated areas occur with flaky desquamation lasting 3 to 5 days, and the rash heals without scarring in 7 to 14 days. An associated staphylococcal infection such as impetigo or purulent conjunctivitis may be present.

Complications include fluid and electrolyte losses (loss of epidermal barrier) leading to hypovolemia, temperature dysregulation, cutaneous infection (cellulitis), pneumonia, and septicemia. Differential diagnosis includes streptococcal scarlet fever, staphylococcal scarlatina or staphylococcal scarlet fever (some cases of SSSS do not progress beyond staphylococcal scarlatina [forme fruste of SSSS]), bullous impetigo, drug eruptions (eg, Stevens-Johnson syndrome or toxic epidermal necrolysis [TEN]), TSS, epidermolysis bullosa, and pemphigus.

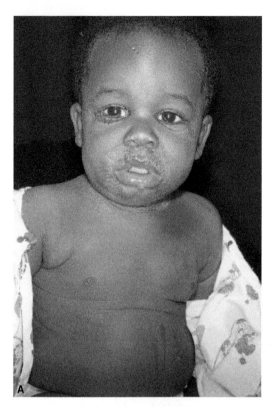

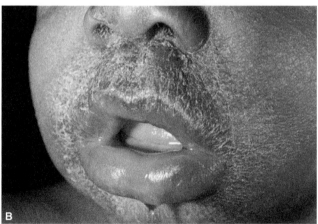

FIGURE 3.27 ■ Staphylococcal Scalded Skin Syndrome (SSSS). (**A, B**) Radial sunburst crusting and fissuring around the orifices (mouth, eyes, nose) are hallmarks of SSSS (first day of rash in this patient). Note the absence of any mucous membrane (MM) involvement of the mouth or eyes (unlike prominent MM involvement of toxic epidermal necrolysis/Stevens-Johnson syndrome). Within 24 hours after these photographs were taken, the skin over the trunk and perineum started wrinkling and flaccid bullae developed, followed by exfoliation in sheets. (Photo contributor: Binita R. Shah, MD.)

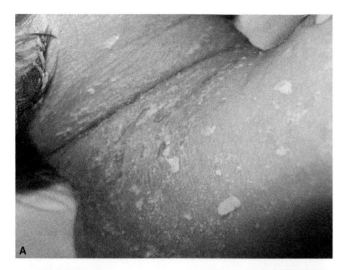

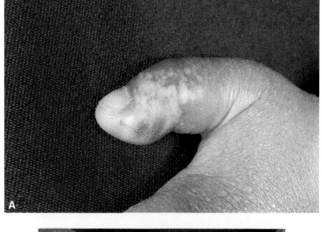

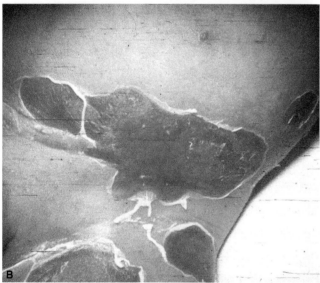

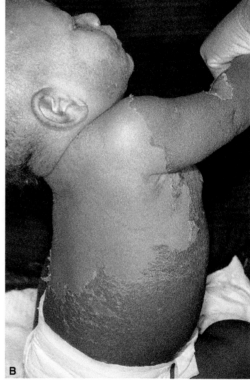

FIGURE 3.28 ■ Staphylococcal Scalded Skin Syndrome. (**A**) Diffuse erythematous rash with flexural accentuation in the neck, widespread exfoliation, and a ruptured bullous lesion is seen in a school-age child. (**B**) Large areas of exfoliation in a different patient revealing a red scalded-looking surface are shown. The borders of the exfoliating skin look like wet tissue paper. (Photo contributor: Samir S. Shah, MD, MSCE [A]; and [B] reproduced with permission from: Shah BR, Laude TL. *Atlas of Pediatric Clinical Diagnosis*. WB Saunders; Philadelphia, PA, 2000.)

FIGURE 3.29 ■ Staphylococcal Scalded Skin Syndrome. (**A**) A 15-month-old infant presented with pustular lesions with cellulitis on the thumb, fever, and generalized scarlatiniform rash associated with skin tenderness. Subsequently, he developed exfoliation in sheets, revealing a scalded-looking surface. (**B**) Photograph taken on the third day after hospitalization shows drying of exfoliated area with flaky desquamation. (Photo contributor: Binita R. Shah, MD.)

Emergency Department Treatment and Disposition

Obtain cultures from the colonized sites such as the mucous membranes of the nasopharynx, conjunctiva, or umbilical stump in neonates (typically blood culture and cultures of the skin and intact bullae are negative for staphylococci). Consult dermatology if the diagnosis is unclear. A skin biopsy specimen (or a frozen section of an induced peel for a rapid diagnosis) will help to distinguish between SSSS and TEN.

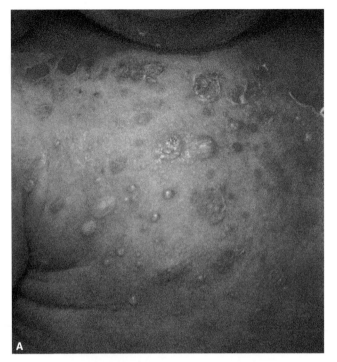

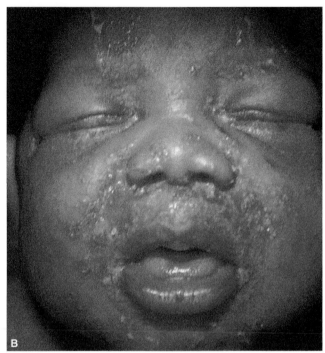

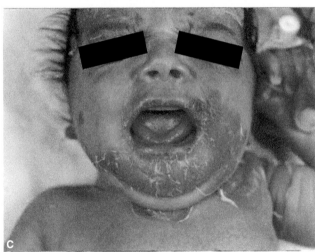

FIGURE 3.30 ■ Staphylococcal Scalded Skin Syndrome in a Neonate (Ritter Disease). (**A, B**) Following circumcision at birth, this 1-week-old neonate presented with extreme irritability, fever, numerous pus-filled intact bullae with some exfoliating lesions, and purulent conjunctivitis. Within 48 hours after these photos, generalized exfoliation over the entire body was seen. (**C**) A different neonate on the fifth day following an exchange transfusion (done for hyperbilirubinemia) developed this rapidly spreading rash with exfoliation that was present on the face and upper trunk. Her blood culture was positive for MRSA. (Photo contributors: Binita R. Shah, MD [A, B], and Prerna Batra, MD [C].)

Admit all patients with widespread erosions and denuded skin for monitoring of fluid and electrolyte deficits, IV antibiotic therapy, and pain control. Depending on the community prevalence of methicillin-resistant *S aureus* (MRSA) and methicillin-sensitive *S aureus*, initial empiric antibiotic options vary. Use a combination of vancomycin and nafcillin for life-threatening illness with sepsis; clindamycin may be added to inhibit bacterial ribosomal exotoxin production. Clindamycin alone may be used for illness without sepsis in areas with substantial community rates of MRSA and low prevalence of clindamycin resistance, or vancomycin alone when rates of MRSA and clindamycin resistance are high. For penicillin-allergic patients, give vancomycin. The usual duration of therapy is 5 to 7 days; bacteremic or immunocompromised patients require a longer duration of therapy. Treat patients with localized SSSS with oral antibiotic therapy (eg, trimethoprim-sulfamethoxazole) with a close follow-up. Topical antibiotic is not required. Advise gently moistening and cleaning the skin with isotonic saline or Burow solution, applying an emollient to provide lubrication and avoiding wet dressings (may cause further drying and cracking).

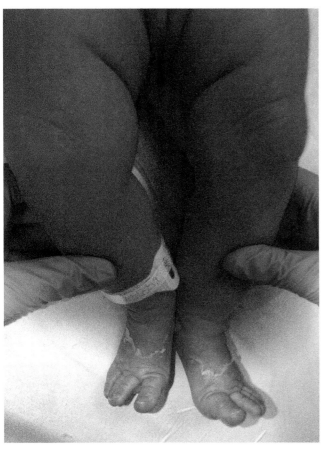

FIGURE 3.31 ■ Staphylococcal Scalded Skin Syndrome. Mild bilateral acral peeling is seen in a 40-day-old, afebrile, and otherwise well-appearing female infant. This was the *only* location where this peeling was seen. Cultures of the nasopharynx, bilateral conjunctivae, and umbilicus were positive for *S aureus*. (Photo contributor: Daniel R. Mazori, MD.)

Pearls

1. Radial sunburst crusting and fissuring around the orifices (mouth, eyes) are hallmarks of SSSS.
2. Nikolsky sign is a hallmark of SSSS, although this is also seen in Stevens-Johnson syndrome, TEN, and pemphigus vulgaris.
3. Early distinction between SSSS and TEN is extremely important. Therapy for SSSS includes antistaphylococcal antibiotics, whereas *discontinuation of the offending drug* is the treatment for TEN.

TABLE 3.3 ■ COMPARISON OF STAPHYLOCOCCAL SCALDED SKIN SYNDROME (SSSS) AND TOXIC EPIDERMAL NECROLYSIS (TEN)

	Age	Cause	Skin Tenderness	Skin Findings	Biopsy Finding Level of Split	Treatment
SSSS	Infants	*S aureus*	Always	Exfoliating skin white No scarring	Granular layer within epidermis	Antibiotics
TEN	Older children	Drugs	Sometimes	Necrosis Frequent scarring	Full-thickness epidermis	Discontinue drug; provide care in burn unit

MENINGOCOCCEMIA

Clinical Summary

Meningococcal infections are caused by *Neisseria meningitidis*. Invasive infection usually results in meningococcemia, meningitis, or both. Strains belonging to groups A, B, C, Y, and W-135 account for most infections. Meningococcal

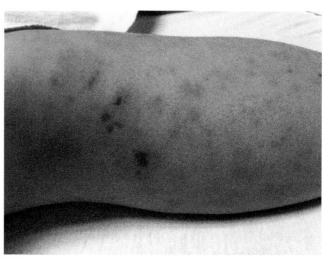

FIGURE 3.33 ■ Meningococcemia. Meningococcemia in a teenager presenting with fever, chills, fatigue, progressive purpuric rash, and hypotension. (Photo contributor: Samir S. Shah, MD, MSCE.)

conjugate vaccination is recommended for preteens and teens at 11-12 years old with a booster dose at 16 years and children and adults at increased risk for meningococcal disease. Centers for Disease Control and Prevention (CDC) recommends routine serogroup B vaccination for 10 years of age

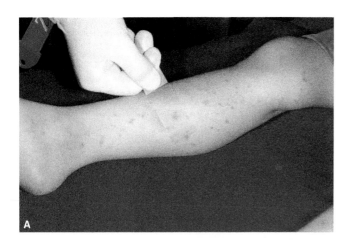

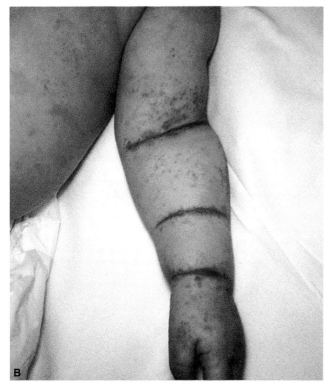

FIGURE 3.32 ■ Meningococcemia. (**A**) Fever and petechial eruption (discrete pinpoint nonblanching lesions measuring 1–2 mm in diameter) associated with septic shock were the presenting signs in this child with meningococcemia. Use of a glass slide (as shown) helps in determining if the rash is blanching or not. (**B**) An infant presenting with petechiae, septic shock, and DIC with meningococcemia. (Photo contributor: Binita R. Shah, MD.)

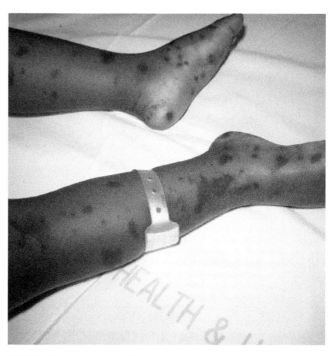

FIGURE 3.34 ■ Purpura Fulminans of Meningococcemia. Purpuric lesions of <10 hours in duration seen on the foot of an 18-month-old infant who presented with septic shock with DIC with meningococcemia. (Photo contributor: Binita R. Shah, MD.)

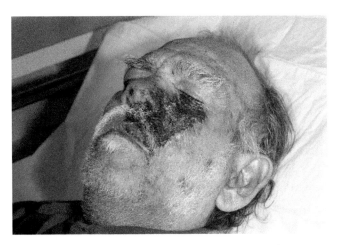

FIGURE 3.35 ▪ Purpura Fulminans. Purpura fulminans is a cutaneous infarction and/or acral gangrene due to DIC. It can be seen in any overwhelming bacterial sepsis. Lesions of purpura fulminans are usually seen at the distal extremities, areas of pressure, and lips, ears, nose, and trunk. (Photo contributor: Binita R. Shah, MD.)

Complications include DIC; purpura fulminans (PF); cardiac (eg, myocarditis, congestive heart failure), pulmonary (eg, pneumonia, lung abscess), and neurologic sequelae from meningitis (eg, subdural effusion or empyema, brain abscess); and Waterhouse-Friderichsen syndrome (bleeding into adrenals, shock, coma, and death). Poor prognostic factors include hypotension, hypothermia, leukopenia, thrombocytopenia, absence of meningitis, PF, petechiae <12 hours before presentation, seizures, or shock on presentation.

Emergency Department Treatment and Disposition

Prompt recognition, stabilization, and immediate initiation of antibiotic therapy are essential in reducing morbidity and mortality. Stabilize vital signs, including fluid resuscitation and

and older at increased risk for meningococcal disease. Risk factors include inherited or acquired terminal complement deficiencies (C5 to C9), properdin deficiency, hypogammaglobulinemia, and asplenia (anatomic or functional). Children 2 years of age or younger (peak attack rate: infants <1 year) are most often affected, with another peak in adolescents (15–18 years of age). Incubation period is 1 to 10 days. Presenting signs and symptoms may be nonspecific, mimicking a viral infection (eg, fever, chills, myalgias/weakness, headache), or may include septic shock, lethargy, coma, convulsion, signs of meningitis (nuchal rigidity, Kernig sign, and/or Brudzinski sign), or signs of multiorgan failure. Initial rash may begin as urticaria, macules or maculopapules, or petechiae that may coalesce to form larger ecchymotic areas with ischemic necrosis. Common sites for the rash are the trunk and extremities (may involve any area), mucous membranes (eg, palpebral conjunctivae), and clusters at pressure points. Differential diagnosis of purpura and petechial lesions includes septicemia with gram-negative or gram-positive organisms, enteroviral infections (eg, echovirus, Coxsackie virus), Rocky Mountain spotted fever, Henoch-Schönlein purpura (HSP), petechiae from intractable coughing or vomiting, trauma (eg, child abuse, accidental), factor deficiency (eg, hemophilia), measles/atypical measles, idiopathic thrombocytopenic purpura, thrombocytopenia from other etiology (eg, leukemia), drug reactions (eg, sulfonamides, penicillins), bacterial endocarditis, gonococcemia, epidemic typhus, *Ehrlichia canis* infection, and Stevens-Johnson syndrome.

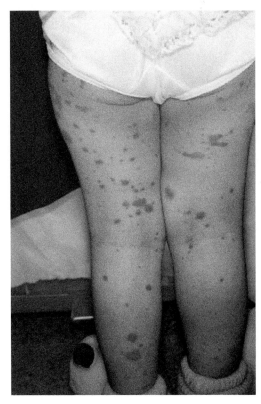

FIGURE 3.36 ▪ Henoch-Schönlein Purpura (HSP); Differential Diagnosis of Meningococcemia. Symmetrically distributed palpable purpuric lesions on both lower extremities and buttocks (usually below the waist) are characteristic features of HSP. Other associated findings (eg, arthralgia/arthritis, abdominal pain, hematuria) also help in differentiating HSP from meningococcemia. Patients with HSP are also usually afebrile and not ill-appearing, and the platelet count is usually elevated or normal. (Photo contributor: Binita R. Shah, MD.)

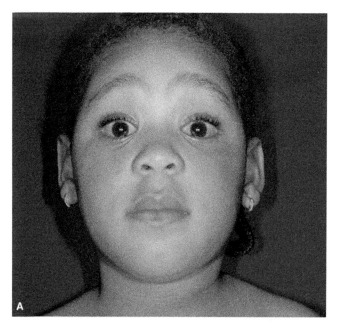

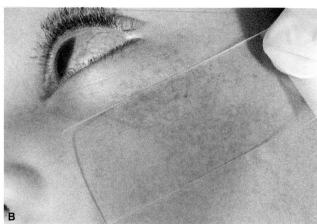

FIGURE 3.37 ■ Petechiae From Other Etiology; Differential Diagnosis of Meningococcemia. (**A, B**) Sudden eruption of petechiae associated with subconjunctival hyperemia appeared only on the face in this afebrile girl following several violent episodes of vomiting due to food poisoning. The remainder of her examination was normal. Petechiae on the face and upper thorax can occur in healthy children following intractable episodes of coughing or vomiting. In contrast, meningococcal infections would cause generalized distribution of petechiae. (Photo contributor: Binita R. Shah, MD.)

pressor agents, as indicated for septic shock. Begin IV antibiotic therapy with cefotaxime *or* ceftriaxone and vancomycin (meningococcemia and meningococcal meningitis are indistinguishable clinically from diseases caused by other bacterial pathogens, including *S pneumoniae*). Do not delay initiation of therapy for completion of diagnostic studies. Obtain a CBC (leukocytosis or leukopenia, thrombocytopenia), coagulation profile (elevated prothrombin time, partial thromboplastin time, D-dimer, fibrin degradation products, and decreased plasma fibrinogen with DIC), serum electrolytes, BUN, creatinine, liver enzymes (multiorgan failure), urinalysis, and blood culture. Gram stain of a petechial skin lesion scraping may also be positive. Perform lumbar puncture only in a stable patient. With meningitis, CSF findings usually will show increased protein and decreased glucose levels, pleocytosis (predominance of polymorphonuclear leukocytes), and a positive culture. Patients with fulminant decompensation may have meningitis in the absence of initial CSF pleocytosis. Hospitalize patient to ICU; droplet precautions in addition to standard precautions are recommended until 24 hours after initiation of therapy.

Advise chemoprophylaxis for close contacts (risk of contracting meningococcal infection among close contacts is 500–800 times the rate for the general population). Throat and nasopharyngeal cultures are of *no* value for deciding who should receive prophylaxis. Antibiotic prophylaxis is given within 24 hours of diagnosis of primary case. Chemoprophylaxis options include rifampin (drug of choice for children) or ceftriaxone, and rifampin, ceftriaxone, or ciprofloxacin for adults. Providers should refer to resources such as American Academy of Pediatrics Red Book or CDC guidelines for definitions of close contacts and post-exposure prophylaxis. Health care workers who did not have direct exposure to the patient's oral secretions *do not* need chemoprophylaxis.

Pearls

1. *N meningitidis* has become the leading cause of bacterial meningitis in children as vaccination for *Haemophilus influenzae* type b and *S pneumoniae* has become available.

2. A transient maculopapular rash mimicking a wide variety of viral exanthems may be a presenting sign of meningococcemia. Conduct a careful examination of skin and mucous membranes for petechiae (a common harbinger of meningococcemia).

3. Classic signs of meningococcal infection (fever with petechiae or purpura) are seen in only 70% of cases. Patients with meningococcal meningitis may also lack CSF abnormalities on initial lumbar puncture (even with a positive CSF culture). Thus, infections by *N meningitidis* must be considered even in the absence of skin lesions or CSF abnormalities.

Clinical Summary

Rocky Mountain spotted fever (RMSF) is an acute febrile exanthematous illness caused by *Rickettsia rickettsii*. RMSF is transmitted by dog tick, wood tick, or Lone Star tick, which are systemically infected and transmit the infection to humans while feeding. RMSF is the second most common (after Lyme disease) tick-borne infection in the United States. RMSF is a misnomer; cases are reported from all parts of the United States. Risk factors include exposure to dogs, residence in wooded areas, and male gender. The tick bite is painless and often goes unrecognized. About 60% of cases are preceded by the removal of an attached and engorged tick. Incidence is highest in children age 5 to 9 years and during the months of April to October. The incubation period ranges from 2 to 14 days, and there may be a prodrome of nonspecific symptoms (mimics viral infection). Classically, patients present with severe headache, myalgia, and bilateral calf pain and may have photophobia, abdominal pain, vomiting, and diarrhea, with abrupt onset of fever and chills. The rash occurs 2 to 4 days after the onset of illness beginning on wrists and ankles and spreading to extremities and trunk within 24 hours; the palms and soles are nearly always affected. Rash begins as erythematous maculopapular lesions that blanch on pressure and becomes petechial and may become confluent with areas of necrosis. An eschar at the site of the bite may be present. The severity of the rash varies from mild evanescent to severe generalized. Involvement of the scrotum and vulva is a diagnostic clue. Desquamation may be seen in severe areas. Conjunctivitis, lymphadenopathy, hepatosplenomegaly, jaundice, and periorbital or peripheral edema may also be present.

Differential diagnosis of RMSF includes meningococcemia, bacterial sepsis from other pathogens (eg, *S pneumoniae*), Henoch-Schönlein purpura, maculopapular rash from viral exanthems (eg, echovirus, Epstein-Barr virus), TSS, idiopathic thrombocytopenic purpura, measles or atypical measles, drug-induced hypersensitivity reactions (eg, sulfonamides, penicillins), secondary syphilis, KD, and other rickettsial diseases, although their presentation is typically less severe.

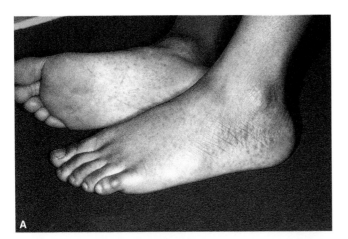

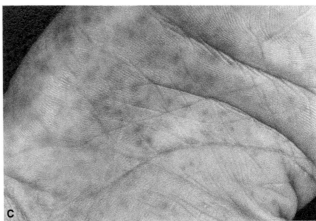

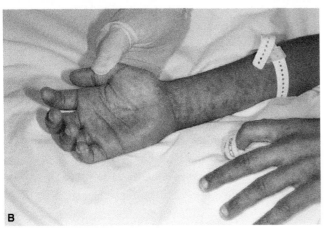

FIGURE 3.38 ■ Rocky Mountain Spotted Fever (RMSF). (**A, B, C**) Erythematous maculopapular eruption that started on the distal extremity and subsequently became petechial and associated fever, severe headache, and myalgia were seen in this adolescent boy. A history of camping during summer vacation in North Carolina 12 days before onset of this rash was obtained. These photographs were taken on the fifth day of the illness. As seen here, the palms and soles are nearly always affected in RMSF. He also had edema of both hands and feet. (Photo contributor: Binita R. Shah, MD.)

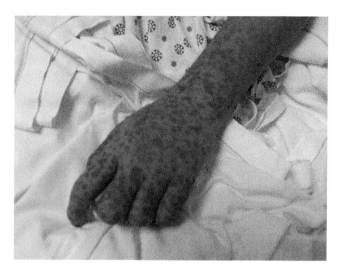

FIGURE 3.39 ■ Meningococcemia; Differential Diagnosis of Rocky Mountain Spotted Fever (RMSF). Purpura with septic shock was the presentation of this adolescent girl. Differentiation between RMSF and meningococcemia is difficult based on clinical presentation alone. (Photo contributor: Vania Kasper, MD.)

Emergency Department Treatment and Disposition

Obtain CBC (a normal or low WBC with bandemia, thrombocytopenia, anemia), comprehensive metabolic panel (hyponatremia, hypoalbuminemia, elevated serum values of creatine

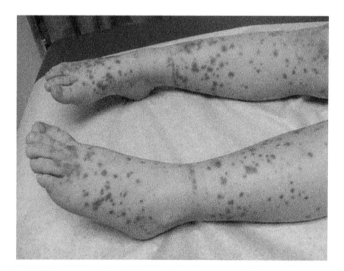

FIGURE 3.40 ■ Henoch-Schönlein Purpura (HSP); Differential Diagnosis of Rocky Mountain Spotted Fever (RMSF). Symmetrically distributed palpable purpuric lesions on both lower extremities and buttocks (usually below the waist) are characteristic features of HSP. Patients with HSP are also usually afebrile, and not ill-appearing like those with RMSF, and the platelet count is usually elevated or normal. (Photo contributor: Anup Singh, MD.)

phosphokinase, and liver enzymes may be seen). If clinically indicated, perform lumbar puncture (CSF exam may be normal or show pleocytosis with an elevated protein and normal glucose values). Obtain specific serologic antibody titers (a 4-fold or greater rise in titer between the acute and convalescent phases is diagnostic; however, it takes 7–10 days into the course of illness to yield results). RMSF is a curable but potentially fatal disease. An important factor in patient survival is early diagnosis and therapy. Admit critically ill patients after ED stabilization including restoration of fluid and electrolyte abnormalities. Begin empiric therapy with IV doxycycline (*drug of choice regardless of age*) and a third-generation cephalosporin to cover for *N meningitidis*. Other alternatives include tetracycline (for patients >8 years of age; tetracycline staining of teeth is dose related; doxycycline is less likely to cause dental staining than other tetracyclines) or chloramphenicol; however, chloramphenicol use is discouraged because of risk of adverse effects, need for monitoring of serum concentrations, and poor coverage of *Ehrlichia* infections. Consult dermatology if diagnosis is unclear. Diagnosis of RMSF can be confirmed rapidly (usually between 4 and 8 days) in patients with a rash. Immunofluorescent staining or PCR of skin biopsy samples demonstrate *R rickettsii*. A 4-fold increase from acute and convalescent serum specimens over a 2- to 3-week period is also diagnostic. Serum PCR assays for *R rickettsii* are available at the CDC in the United States. To remove a tick, grasp the tick with fine tweezers close to the skin and pull gently straight out without twisting. If fingers are used, protect them with tissue and avoid squeezing the body of the tick; thoroughly wash hands after removal.

Pearls

1. Centripetal spread is the hallmark, with rash first appearing on wrists and ankles followed by spreading to trunk within hours.

2. The classic triad of fever, rash, and history of tick bite is present in only 60% to 70% of patients. Neither absence of tick exposure nor absence of rash excludes the diagnosis. A "spotless" form of RMSF occurs in approximately 5% of children infected with *R rickettsii*.

3. The most significant risk factor for death is a delay of appropriate antibiotic therapy; *do not withhold therapy while awaiting confirmation by the serology tests.*

4. Differentiation between RMSF and meningococcemia is difficult based on clinical presentation alone.

TABLE 3.4 ▪ FEATURES OF OTHER RICKETTSIAL INFECTIONS

	Infecting Organism	Host	Vector	Global Distribution	Description
Anaplasmosis	*Anaplasma phagocytophilum*	Mice and other small rodents	Black-legged tick or western black-legged tick	Northeast, mid-Atlantic, upper Midwest and West United States; Europe	Fever, chills, headache, myalgia, malaise, nausea, cough, and confusion 1–2 weeks following bite. Rash rare. Neutropenia, anemia, thrombocytopenia, hyponatremia, and hepatitis may be present.
Ehrlichiosis	*Ehrlichia chaffeensis* and other spp.	White tail deer and other mammals	Lone Star tick primarily	Southeast and South Central United States	Fever, chills, headache, myalgia, malaise, nausea, cough, and confusion 1–2 weeks following bite. Rash may develop 1 week into illness on torso and extremities. Leukopenia, anemia, thrombocytopenia, hyponatremia, and hepatitis may be present.
Epidemic typhus	*Rickettsia prowazekii*	Humans	Body louse	Worldwide but rare in the United States	High fever, chills, headache, myalgia, malaise, nausea, cough, and confusion 1–2 weeks following bite. Rash beginning on the trunk and spreading to extremities appears 4–7 days into the illness and begins as maculopapular, then petechial, then brownish.
Endemic typhus	*Rickettsia typhi*	Cats, rodents, opossums	Fleas	Worldwide but rare in the United States	Similar presentation to epidemic typhus, although less severe. Fever, chills, headache, myalgia, and malaise 1–2 weeks following bite. Macular or maculopapular rash appears 4–7 days into the illness.
Q fever	*Coxiella burnetii* by inhalation or consumption of unpasteurized contaminated milk products	Sheep, cattle, goats		Worldwide	Typically asymptomatic but can cause fever, chills, headache, anorexia, and malaise 2–3 weeks following infection. Cough, chest pain, pneumonia, and hepatitis may occur. Rash rare.

CAT-SCRATCH DISEASE

Clinical Summary

Cat-scratch disease (CSD) is a zoonotic bacterial infection caused by *Bartonella henselae* following a cat scratch (especially kittens or feral cats). Infection is transmitted by cutaneous inoculation. Transmission between cats occurs by the cat flea. Most reported cases occur in people <20 years. A history of a recent contact with a cat is present in >90% of cases. Even though many siblings may play with the same kitten, often, a single family member is usually affected. Occasionally clusters of CSD may be seen in the same family within weeks of one another. The incubation period is 7 to 12 days (from time of scratch to appearance of skin papule) or 5 to 50 days (skin lesion to regional lymphadenopathy). There may be visible signs at the inoculation site, including a scratch or bite with 1 or more small red papules or pustules, although these are often overlooked because of small size. Typically, patients present with regional lymphadenopathy of 1 to 5 cm or more, and this is the most prominent and common symptom, occurring in >90% of cases. Low-grade fever and other constitutional symptoms (eg, malaise, anorexia, fatigue, headache) may be present. Usually, there is involvement of a single lymph node that drains the inoculation site, although occasionally, multiple lymph nodes are involved. The most

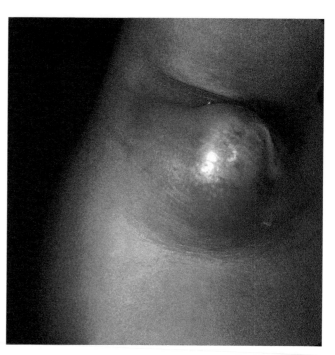

FIGURE 3.42 ■ Bacterial Adenitis/Abscess; Differential Diagnosis of Cat-Scratch Disease. Axillary lymphadenitis (tenderness, erythema, and warmth) and fever of 3 days in duration were the presenting complaints of this child who was prescribed dicloxacillin. An abscess developed requiring incision and drainage, and culture was positive for *S aureus*. (Photo contributor: Binita R. Shah, MD.)

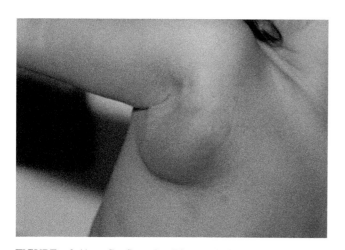

FIGURE 3.41 ■ Cat-Scratch Disease. Axillary lymphadenitis (with tenderness, erythema, and warmth) of 3 weeks in duration is shown in a 4-year-old child who received a kitten as a Christmas gift 2 months before the onset of this swelling. He gave a history of playing roughly and receiving several scratches on his arm by the kitten. A needle aspiration was performed to relieve the symptoms (usually needle aspiration of suppurative nodes is preferred over incision and drainage to avoid prolonged drainage and possible scarring). (Photo contributor: Binita R. Shah, MD.)

commonly involved sites are axilla, cervical, submandibular, preauricular, epitrochlear, femoral, and inguinal lymph nodes. The nodes are tender, warm, erythematous, and indurated, and the lymphadenopathy usually lasts 1 to 2 months, but can last up to 1 year. Spontaneous suppuration is seen in 10% to 40% of cases.

In atypical CSD, there is Parinaud oculoglandular syndrome (involvement of conjunctiva with granuloma but without any discharge or pain, involvement of ipsilateral preauricular lymph node, and possible ipsilateral submandibular or cervical lymphadenopathy).

Rare manifestations of CSD include persistent fever, skin rashes (eg, erythema nodosum, maculopapular rashes), aseptic meningitis, encephalitis, hepatitis, pneumonia, microabscess in liver and spleen, osteolytic lesions, and thrombocytopenic purpura. Differential diagnosis of unilateral lymphadenopathy includes bacterial adenitis, viral infections (eg, infectious mononucleosis [IM]), malignancy (eg, lymphoma), typical or atypical mycobacterial infection, tularemia, brucellosis, histoplasmosis, toxoplasmosis, and lymphogranuloma venereum.

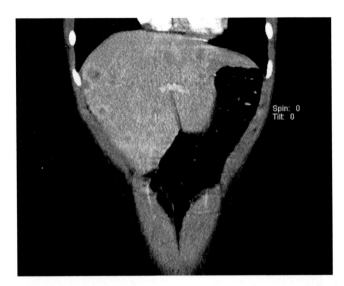

FIGURE 3.43 ■ Hepatosplenic Cat-Scratch Disease. An axial CT image of the abdomen of a teenager with hepatosplenic cat-scratch disease reveals numerous ill-defined, low-attenuation lesions in the hepatic parenchyma, consistent with microabscess formation. (Photo contributor: Samir S. Shah, MD, MSCE.)

Emergency Department Treatment and Disposition

Consult infectious disease specialist for advice on diagnostic tests (eg, indirect fluorescent antibody test for detection of serum antibody to antigens of *Bartonella* species or PCR assay) and management. Consider US for assessing lymph node size and suppuration. CSD is a self-limited infection, and management is primarily symptomatic. Lymphadenopathy may persist for 2 to 4 months, but spontaneous resolution is the rule. Azithromycin treatment can help a more rapid reduction in the size of the lymph node, however, unlikely to change the time to complete resolution of lymphadenopathy. Consider direct needle aspiration of pus to relieve discomfort with suppurative nodes; avoid incision and drainage due to risk of fistula formation. Consider antibiotic therapy for ill patients with systemic symptoms (eg, patients with large painful adenopathy or immunocompromised hosts). Choices include oral (eg, azithromycin, trimethoprim-sulfamethoxazole, ciprofloxacin) and parenteral antibiotics (eg, gentamicin). Educate families that cats require no treatment or quarantine and advice regarding the prevention of CSD (eg, avoid playing roughly with cats/kittens, hand washing after handling the cat, immediately washing sites of cat scratches/bites, and not allowing cats to lick open cuts or wounds).

Pearls

1. Chronic regional lymphadenitis is the hallmark of CSD.
2. Consider CSD in patients with adenopathy, fever, malaise, and history of a feline contact.

Clinical Summary

Lymphadenitis is a localized infection/inflammation of lymph nodes. In children, cervical lymphadenitis is the most common location, but other locations may also occur. Lymphadenitis may be acute, developing over the course of a few days, or subacute or chronic, developing over the course of weeks to months. Bilateral acute cervical lymphadenitis is typically caused by a viral respiratory infection; however, unilateral acute lymphadenitis is more likely to be caused by a bacterial infection. *S aureus* and *S pyogenes* are the most common bacterial causes, but nontuberculous mycobacteria (NTM) and *Bartonella* are also possible and more common in subacute or chronic infections, and may be distinguished by details elicited from history and exam. Important historical details include duration of onset, rate of enlargement, constitutional symptoms, immunization history, travel history, recent soft tissue skin infections in the scalp, throat, or mouth, and animal bites and scratches, especially cats and kittens. Lymphadenitis, in contrast to lymphadenopathy, is characterized by a tender, firm enlargement of the lymph node, often with overlying erythema or cellulitis if secondary to an acute bacterial process, or an overlying violaceous color if secondary to NTM. If a central abscess is present in the lymph node, fluctuance may be felt. Fever and pain are the least common

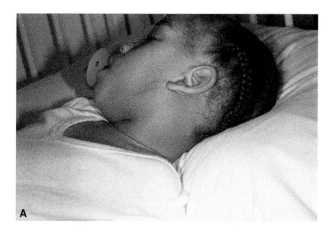

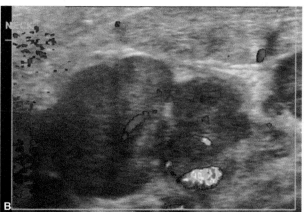

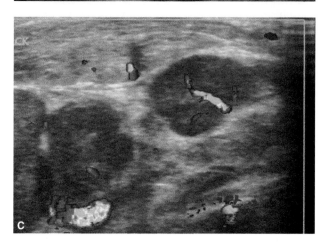

FIGURE 3.45 ■ Acute Suppurative Cervical Lymphadenitis. (**A**) Infected nodes are tender and show warmth and erythema. Fluctuance suggests abscess formation; however, because of induration from the surrounding inflammation, an abscess may be present without fluctuance. *S aureus* adenitis is more likely to suppurate than adenitis from other etiologies. Throat and lymph node aspirate cultures were positive for *S pyogenes* in this patient. (**B, C**) In a different patient, multiple enlarged lymph nodes are demonstrated with increased color flow on color Doppler, compatible with hyperemia from lymphadenitis without evidence of an abscess. (Photo contributors: Binita R. Shah, MD [A], and John Amodio, MD [B, C].)

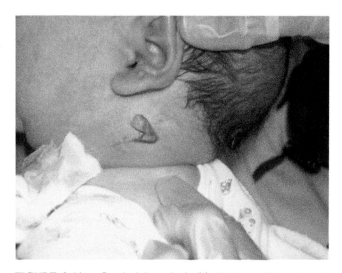

FIGURE 3.44 ■ Cervical Lymphadenitis. Patient with acute unilateral cervical adenitis following incision and drainage with packing material placed. (Reproduced with permission from Shah SS, Kemper AR, Ratner AJ: *Pediatric Infectious Diseases: Essentials for Practice,* 2nd ed. McGraw-Hill Education; New York, NY, 2019.)

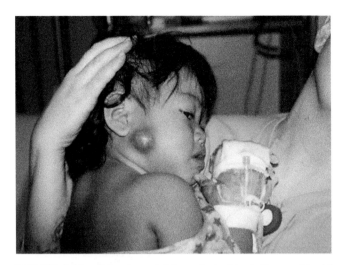

FIGURE 3.46 ▪ Mycobacterial Lymphadenitis. A 2-year-old girl with cervical lymphadenitis caused by nontuberculous mycobacteria. Note the violaceous discoloration of the affected lymph node. (Reproduced with permission from Shah SS, Ludwig S. *Symptom-Based Diagnosis in Pediatrics*. McGraw-Hill Education; New York, NY, 2014.)

in NTM lymphadenitis, and in CSD, the lymphadenitis may be accompanied by prolonged fevers lasting weeks.

Lymphadenitis due to viral causes typically spontaneously resolves, but patients can become secondarily infected with a bacterial pathogen. Acute unilateral lymphadenitis usually resolves with appropriate antibiotic therapy; however, the most common complication despite appropriate treatment is

abscess formation requiring incision and drainage. Less common complications include sepsis, jugular vein thrombosis, carotid artery rupture, septic pulmonary embolus, and mediastinitis. Fistula formation is possible with NTM. Differential diagnosis of lymphadenitis includes leukemia, lymphoma, KD, and collagen vascular diseases. In addition to consideration of the most common causes of lymphadenitis, underlying immunodeficiency such as HIV and other less common bacterial infections such as tuberculosis should be considered.

Emergency Department Treatment and Disposition

The diagnosis of lymphadenitis is clinical. Determination of a drainable fluid collection by identification of fluctuance on exam or by imaging (eg, ultrasound) is important, as drainage will hasten recovery in cases of typical bacterial lymphadenitis. Consult surgery if there is a drainable fluid collection. Incision and drainage should not be performed for suspected NTM or *Bartonella* infections due to risk of fistula formation, so evaluate for suggestive historical or physical exam findings. Hospitalize patients with infection that has failed to respond to outpatient treatment, if there is high risk of requiring surgical intervention, or if the size of the node compromises appropriate oral intake. Prescribe a penicillinase-resistant β-lactam (eg, ampicillin/sulbactam) or clindamycin

TABLE 3.5 ▪ FEATURES OF COMMON CAUSES OF LYMPHADENITIS

	Predisposing Factors	Most Common Location	Associated Symptoms	Distinguishing Features
S aureus and *S pyogenes*	Prior URI or pharyngitis, adjacent soft tissue skin infection or trauma	Cervical	Pain and fever are common	Rapidly progressive with marked tenderness
Nontuberculous *Mycobacterium*, predominantly *M avium*	Oropharyngeal exposure to soil, such as pica and typical developmental hand-to-mouth activities in early childhood	Anterior cervical or submandibular	Systemic signs including fever are rare, as is pain	Enlargement occurs over weeks to months, with development of thinning skin with overlying violaceous discoloration
Bartonella	Contact or known bite or scratch from a cat or kitten	Axillary (common) cervical, submental, inguinal nodes can be affected	Fever and mild systemic symptoms often present; fever may be prolonged	Suspect when lymphadenitis is unresponsive to typical antibiotics and if there is contact with a cat

depending on local *S aureus* susceptibilities for suspected typical bacterial lymphadenitis. Consider CBC (leukocytosis with a left shift) or a blood culture. For suspected NTM infection, *Mycobacterium tuberculosis* should also be considered based on history and risk factors. While surgical excision and antimicrobial therapy may both be successful, excision is typically definitive. *Bartonella* lymphadenitis often spontaneously resolves over the course of 2 to 4 months; however, a 5-day course of azithromycin is preferred. Needle aspiration may be done for symptomatic relief, and surgical excision is typically unnecessary. Prescribe oral antibiotics for patients with milder presentations with a close follow-up. Advise monitoring for worsening swelling or pain, persistent fever, or weight loss, and advise patients to return to ED for compromise in respiratory status or swallowing due to cervical lymphadenitis.

Pearls

1. Unilateral lymphadenitis is most commonly due to *S aureus* and *S pyogenes*.
2. Do not incise and drain suspected NTM or *Bartonella* lymphadenitis due to risk of fistula formation.

Clinical Summary

Chickenpox or varicella is an acute exanthematous illness caused by varicella-zoster virus (VZV), carried only by humans, and spread by person-to-person contact or airborne droplets of infected respiratory tract secretions. Maternal varicella infection can lead to transplacental in utero infection. Incubation period is 10 to 21 days (less in the immunocompromised), and there is usually no prodrome in children. Rash and constitutional symptoms (eg, low-grade fever, headache) occur simultaneously, and the rash lasts 5 to 7 days (longer in immunocompromised hosts and may become hemorrhagic). The rash is vesicular with centripetal distribution, involving the scalp and mucous membranes (eg, conjunctiva, oropharynx). Lesions are round or oval and progress from macule to papule to vesicle to pustule, followed by crusting; *different stages of lesions can be seen together in the same anatomic area* (unlike smallpox). Central umbilication of lesions occurs with healing. Children receiving intermittent courses of corticosteroids (eg, for asthma) may have a more severe course. Differential diagnosis of other papulovesicular eruptions includes herpes zoster, coxsackie virus infections (eg, hand-foot-and-mouth disease), drug eruptions (eg, Stevens-Johnson syndrome), eczema herpeticum, eczema vaccinatum, rickettsialpox, bullous impetigo, impetigo contagiosum, arthropod bites/papular urticaria, dermatitis herpetiformis, and smallpox.

Complications (more common in immunocompromised) include secondary skin infections by *S aureus* and/or *S pyogenes* (eg, cellulitis, impetigo); streptococcal TSS; NF; CNS (eg, meningoencephalitis, cerebellar ataxia), cardiac (eg, myocarditis), hematologic (eg, acute thrombocytopenia, hemorrhagic chickenpox), renal (eg, glomerulonephritis), and bone (eg, reactive arthritis); bronchopneumonia; and hepatitis.

Emergency Department Treatment and Disposition

The diagnosis of chicken pox is clinical. PCR to identify VZV from vesicular fluid is preferred to direct fluorescent antibody testing; Tzanck smear is rarely performed. Chickenpox is typically a benign, self-limiting disease in otherwise healthy children, and oral acyclovir is not recommended for routine use. Acyclovir (given within 24 hours of onset of rash) can be considered in those at increased risk for moderate to severe varicella (eg, patients >12 years of age; patients receiving either long-term salicylates or short, intermittent, or aerosolized courses of corticosteroids; and patients with

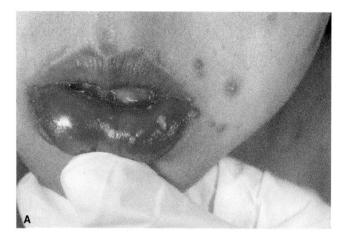

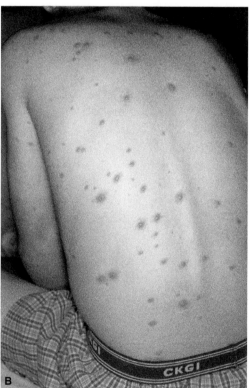

FIGURE 3.47 ■ Chickenpox. (**A, B**). These figures show the presence of lesions in different stages (papule, vesicle, pustule, and crusted lesion) with a centripetal distribution in a child with chickenpox. Lesions are also seen on mucous membranes involving the lips and oropharynx. (Photo contributor: Binita R. Shah, MD.)

chronic cutaneous or pulmonary disorders). Chickenpox is highly contagious (most contagious from 1–2 days before the onset of rash until all the lesions have dried or crusted), with secondary cases occurring in 98% of susceptible persons when exposed. Varicella-zoster immune globulin (VariZIG for passive immunoprophylaxis) is recommended within 96 hours of exposure for contacts at risk of developing severe

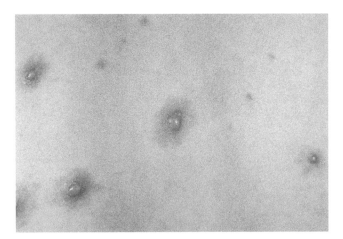

FIGURE 3.48 ■ Chickenpox. Appearance of chickenpox is sometimes described as "dew drops on a rose petal"; the classic vesicles are surrounded by erythema. (Photo contributor: Binita R. Shah, MD.)

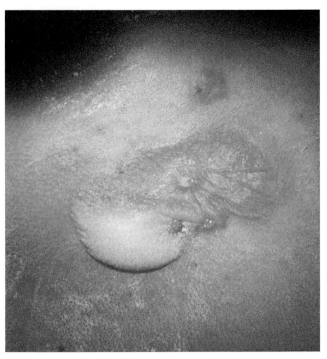

FIGURE 3.49 ■ Bullous Varicella. Close-up of a pus-filled bullous lesion is shown on the trunk of a child with chickenpox resulting from secondary infection with *S aureus*. (Photo contributor: Binita R. Shah, MD.)

varicella, such as immunocompromised patients without evidence of immunity or newborn infants whose mothers have varicella around the time of delivery. If VariZIG cannot be administered, then IV immunoglobulin should be considered. Refer to *American Academy of Pediatrics Red Book* for recommendations on antiviral therapy and VariZIG. Admit immunocompromised patients for IV antiviral therapy. Do not prescribe salicylates (or salicylates-containing products) to children with varicella (association with Reye syndrome). Consider colloidal oatmeal baths and antipruritic lotions such as pramoxine for the pruritus and discomfort. Be careful when prescribing antipruritic medications that cause drowsiness because this side effect may mask lethargy and drowsiness related to complications of chickenpox (eg, meningoencephalitis).

Pearls

1. VZV remains in a latent state in the dorsal root ganglion cells and may get reactivated (as the immunity wanes), resulting in herpes zoster.
2. Chickenpox is more severe in adolescents, adults, and immunocompromised hosts.

Clinical Summary

Herpes zoster or shingles is an acute vesiculopustular eruption occurring in dermatomal distribution caused by VZV and is unusual in children.

A prior clinical or subclinical episode of varicella is a *prerequisite* for the occurrence of herpes zoster. After primary infection has occurred, the virus lies dormant in a sensory ganglion; reactivation of the latent virus results in herpes zoster. Up to 20% of those with history of varicella develop herpes zoster during their lifetime, and multiple attacks can occur (eg, HIV patients). Young infants may develop herpes zoster without prior clinical varicella if in utero exposure occurred. Zoster begins with pain and tingling within the dermatome and progresses to sharp, dull, or burning pain, which precedes the rash by 48 to 72 hours (range, 1–10 days). Pain is minimal when zoster occurs in children, and there is usually a lack of systemic symptoms. The rash begins as erythematous macules and papules that progress to vesicles (12–24 hours), to pustules (3–4 days), and then to crusting (7–10 days). Vesicles are grouped and umbilicated on an erythematous base *in a linear distribution* and erupt along 1 to 3 dermatomes supplied by a spinal or cranial nerve (most common site: thoracic T5–T10 [~75% of cases]). Lesions *do not cross the midline* in immunocompetent hosts.

Ramsay Hunt syndrome is a specific manifestation of zoster that affects geniculate ganglion (facial or auditory nerves) and involves the pinna, auditory canal, tympanic membrane, and anterior two-thirds of the tongue (decreased taste). Patients present with ipsilateral Bell palsy, tinnitus, deafness, vertigo, hearing loss, and otalgia. In herpes zoster ophthalmicus, the ophthalmic branch of the trigeminal nerve is affected and rashes occur on the eyelids; in addition, conjunctivitis, keratitis, iridocyclitis, secondary glaucoma, ocular muscle palsies, ptosis, mydriasis, and panophthalmitis may occur. Hutchinson sign (involvement of nasociliary division of ophthalmic nerve with vesicles on the side and tip of the nose) may be seen. Vesicles occur on the palate, uvula, and tonsillar fossa when the maxillary branch of the trigeminal nerve is involved and on the buccal mucosa, floor of the mouth, and anterior part of the tongue when the mandibular branch is involved. Disseminated zoster (generalized rash with fever) and visceral dissemination (pneumonia, hepatitis, meningoencephalitis) may be seen in patients with persistent depression of cell-mediated immunity. CNS involvement may occur and includes asymptomatic CSF lymphocytic pleocytosis with normal or elevated

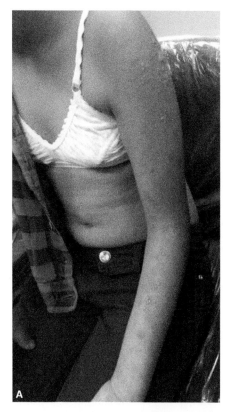

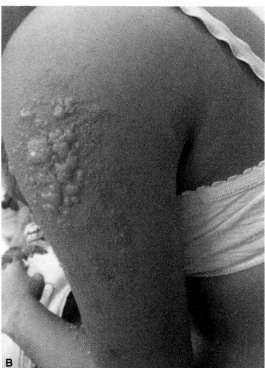

FIGURE 3.50 ■ Herpes Zoster. (**A, B**) Herpes zoster involving dermatomes C7 and C8 is seen in this immunosuppressed 16-year-old girl who had steroid-resistant nephrotic syndrome and was receiving long-term mycophenolate. (Photo contributor: Abhijeet Saha, MD.)

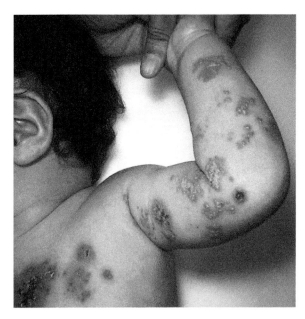

FIGURE 3.51 ▪ Herpes Zoster. An 8-month-old infant with herpes zoster on C5 and C6 dermatomes. This infant never had chickenpox, but his mother had varicella during the last trimester of pregnancy. (Reproduced with permission from Shah BR, Laude TL. *Atlas of Pediatric Clinical Diagnosis*. WB Saunders; Philadelphia, PA, 2000, p. 55.)

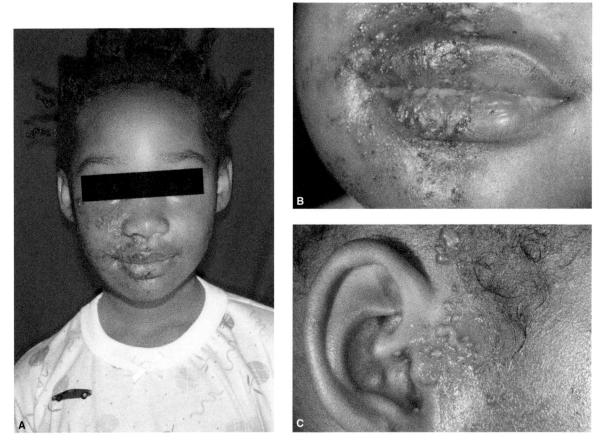

FIGURE 3.52 ▪ Herpes Zoster. (**A, B, C**) Vesicular eruptions were present on the face, lips, anterior two-thirds of the tongue, pinna, auditory canal, and tympanic membrane of this girl. She did not have facial nerve palsy. Note that lesions do not cross the midline in an immunocompetent child. (Photo contributor: Binita R. Shah, MD.)

protein value or symptomatic meningoencephalitis (eg, head-ache, vomiting, photophobia, altered sensorium), transverse myelitis, and zoster paresis (motor weakness and atrophy in associated myotome). Postherpetic neuralgia (pain persisting for >6 weeks after disappearance of the rash) is uncommon in children. Differential diagnosis includes dermatomal herpes simplex infections (eg, anogenital herpes), contact dermatitis, grouped arthropod bites, and localized bacterial or viral skin infections.

Emergency Department Treatment and Disposition

Diagnosis is clinical. PCR to identify VZV from vesicu-lar fluid is preferred to direct fluorescent antibody testing; Tzanck smear is rarely performed. Admit immunocompro-mised patients for IV antiviral therapy, and observe airborne/contact precautions for duration of the illness due to the increased risk of disseminated disease, which is transmissible by droplets. Immunocompetent children usually do not need any treatment and can be discharged with instructions to wash hands after touching lesions and to cover lesions. If lesions cannot be covered, instruct caregivers to keep them home from school or daycare until lesions are crusted. Consult oph-thalmology for patients with zoster ophthalmicus.

Pearl

1. A patient with herpes zoster can transmit varicella, but not herpes zoster, to a susceptible host.

Clinical Summary

Oropharyngeal herpes simplex virus (HSV) infections manifest as acute herpetic gingivostomatitis, herpes labialis, or pharyngitis. HSV-1 infections usually occur above the waist and HSV-2 usually below the waist; however either viral subtype can be isolated from either site, depending on the source of infection. Transmission is by skin-to-skin, mucosa-to-mucosa, or skin-to-mucosa contact. Most primary HSV

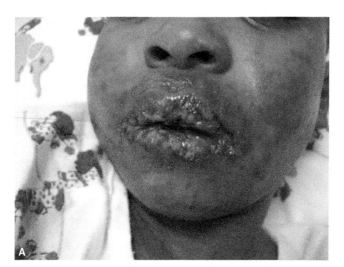

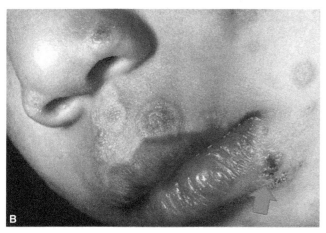

FIGURE 3.53 ■ Recurrent Herpes Labialis and Recurrent Erythema Multiforme (EM). HSV is the most common etiology of EM, and recurrences of EM are common with recurrences of HSV infections as shown in two different patients. (A) Primary HSV infection of the lips in a patient who had target lesions of EM on the face, palms, and soles. (B) Typical erythematosus target lesions with duskiness in the center are seen on the face of this child who had herpes labialis (drying HSV lesions seen around the lower lip [arrow]) 5 days prior to the onset of EM. (Photo contributors: Sharon A. Glick, MD [A], and Binita R. Shah, MD [B].)

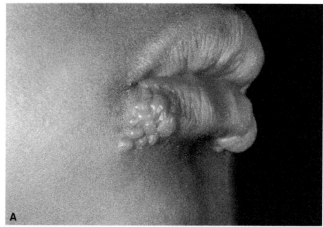

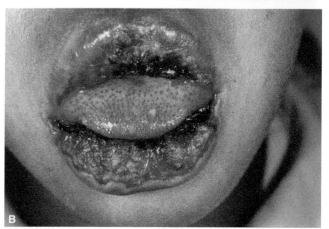

FIGURE 3.54 ■ Herpes Labialis. (A) The hallmark of herpes simplex virus skin infections is grouped vesicles on an erythematous base, as seen here on the mucocutaneous junction of the lip. (B) Recurrent herpetic lesions in a patient with HIV infection. The lesions began with vesicles and healed with crusting. This patient also had lesions on the tongue and buccal mucosa. (Photo contributor: Binita R. Shah, MD.)

infections are asymptomatic, and virus persists for life in a latent form in a sensory ganglion. Reactivation may follow several triggers, including febrile illness, emotional or physical stress, or debilitating activities. In adolescents, primary HSV manifests as pharyngitis (shallow tonsillar ulcers with or without gray exudates).

Gingivostomatitis commonly affects children aged 1 to 3 years, who present with high fever, foul breath, inability to eat or drink, dehydration, drooling, and irritability. Lesions begin as vesicles that rapidly rupture turning into shallow gray ulcers (1–3 mm in size) on an erythematous base. The ulcers are extremely painful, friable, and bleed easily. The gums are swollen, ulcerated, erythematous, friable, and

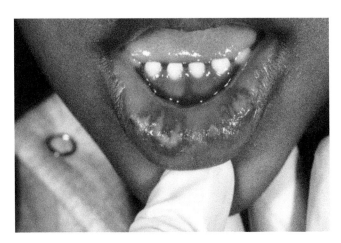

FIGURE 3.55 ■ Herpetic Gingivostomatitis. A child presenting with high fever, refusal to eat, and sores in the mouth. (Photo contributor: Binita R. Shah, MD.)

bleed easily; gingivitis may precede appearance of mucosal vesicles. Lesions are typically located on the anterior tongue, buccal mucosa, gums, and hard and soft palate; lesions may extend to lips, chin, or neck (even in an immunocompetent child). Tender cervical and submandibular/submental lymphadenopathy may be present. Gingivostomatitis is self-limited and usually resolves in 5 to 7 days.

Herpes labialis or fever blisters have a prodrome of pain, burning, tingling, or itching that lasts a few hours; systemic

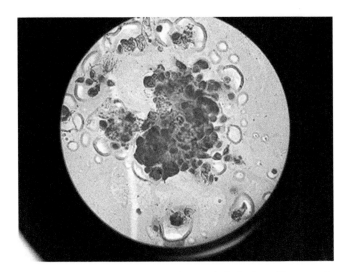

FIGURE 3.56 ■ Tzanck Smear of Herpetic Infection. Giemsa stain of vesicle contents demonstrating multinucleated giant cells (fused virally infected keratinocytes) is indicative of a herpetic infection. (Reproduced with permission from Kane K, Nambudiri VE, Stratigos AJ. *Color Atlas & Synopsis of Pediatric Dermatology*, 3rd ed. McGraw-Hill Education; New York, NY, 2017.)

symptoms are unusual. The lesions begin within 24 to 48 hours after prodrome as the papule progresses to vesicle to ulcer, followed by crusting (within 3–4 days) and healing (within 5–10 days). The lesions are painful, especially at the vesicular stage, and are typically found at the vermilion border of lips, the mucocutaneous junction of the perioral region; lesions are localized in a nondermatomal distribution and recur at the same location or closely adjacent areas.

Differential diagnosis of gingivostomatitis and herpes labialis includes herpangina (posterior pharynx and soft palate lesions usually caused by coxsackieviruses or echovirus), hand-foot-and-mouth disease, aphthous stomatitis (recurrent ulcers with rim of erythema and gray exudates), and zoster ophthalmicus. Differential diagnosis of herpes pharyngitis includes acute exudative tonsillopharyngitis from other etiologies (eg, *S pyogenes*, adenovirus, Epstein-Barr virus).

Emergency Department Treatment and Disposition

Diagnosis is clinical, and tests are usually not performed. Culture of fluid from vesicles or scrapings of the lesion or PCR assay will differentiate between HSV and VZV infections when necessary. Admit immunocompromised patients for IV antiviral therapy (guideline recourses eg, American Academy of Pediatrics, Red Book). For immunocompetent patients, antiviral therapy is not routinely recommended. Advise supportive therapy including antipyretics, hydration, and dietary modifications (eg, cool drinks, popsicles, and soft diet; *avoid citrus juices*). Do not prescribe oral anesthetics (eg, lidocaine viscous) because of the risk of toxicity via absorption through oral mucosa. Exclude children with gingivostomatitis with drooling and active lesions from child care centers.

Pearls

1. In children, the most common manifestation of primary HSV infection is gingivostomatitis, and the most common manifestation of recurrent HSV infection is herpes labialis.

2. Recurrent HSV infections may be associated with recurrent episodes of erythema multiforme.

3. Herpetic gingivostomatitis may be confused with herpangina. Vesicles are usually not seen on the buccal mucosa and anterior portion of the mouth in herpangina.

Clinical Summary

Herpetic whitlow is a cutaneous HSV infection of the terminal phalanx of the fingers or thumb. It is an occupational hazard (eg, dentists) that may also occur in infants and young children; the first episode may accompany herpetic gingivostomatitis. After the primary infection, HSV remains dormant in the sensory ganglia and can recur in the same location. Onset is abrupt with pain or paresthesia at the site. Skin lesion begins as grouped vesicles and/or pustules on an erythematous base, subsequently becoming a painful, erythematous, swollen lesion that usually persists for 7 to 10 days (range, 1–3 weeks). Common sites are terminal phalanx of a finger or thumb. One or more fingertips may be involved. Fever, lymphangitis, and regional lymphadenopathy may accompany the lesion. Differential diagnosis includes contact dermatitis and dyshidrotic eczema.

Emergency Department Treatment and Disposition

Diagnosis is clinical. A needle aspiration of the lesion for HSV PCR or culture will confirm the diagnosis. It usually

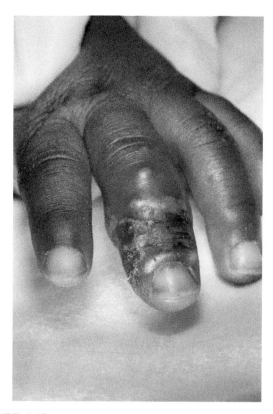

FIGURE 3.58 ■ Herpetic Whitlow. Herpes simplex virus infections like this often get mistaken for paronychia. (Photo contributor: Binita R. Shah, MD.)

resolves without any specific therapy. Supportive therapy includes antipyretics and analgesics for pain as indicated. Topical penciclovir cream may be applied to affected areas every 2 hours. Acyclovir may be used for severe infections.

Pearls

1. Herpetic whitlow is characterized by grouped umbilicated, vesiculopustular lesions on an erythematous base on the distal fingertips or thumb. It is commonly confused with a bacterial paronychia or felon.
2. *Do not* incise or drain herpetic whitlow because surgical debridement may exacerbate the condition.

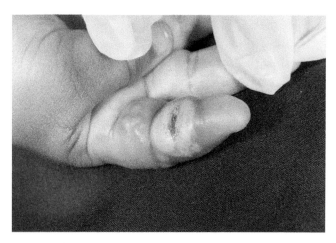

FIGURE 3.57 ■ Herpetic Whitlow. A 4-month-old infant presenting with clusters of vesiculopustular lesions on an erythematous base on the finger. This infant's mother had "cold sores" 7 days prior to developing this rash. Culture of the lesion was positive for HSV-1. (Photo contributor: Binita R. Shah, MD.)

Clinical Summary

Mumps is an acute systemic paramyxovirus infection characterized by swelling of the parotid and other salivary glands. History of exposure to a similar illness is important as humans are the only known natural hosts and the virus is acquired by direct intimate contact with oropharyngeal secretions (droplets). Incubation period ranges from 12 to 25 days after exposure. There is a 1- to 2-day prodrome of fever, headache, malaise, anorexia, and abdominal pain. Bilateral (70% of cases) or unilateral painful, nonerythematous parotid gland swelling follows. This pushes the ear lobe upward and outward, obscuring the mandibular angle. The opening of Stensen duct may be red and edematous. Ingestion of sour liquids may increase pain in the parotid gland. Submaxillary glands may be involved as well. Symptoms occur with (or closely follow) parotitis. Rarely, only submaxillary glands are involved. The opening of Wharton duct may be red and edematous. Sublingual glands are least frequently involved, and bilateral swelling is seen in the submental region and in the floor of the mouth.

Complications include CNS involvement (eg, meningitis or encephalitis), orchitis, or epididymo-orchitis (seen among postpubertal adolescents and young adults). Other rare complications include arthritis, oophoritis, cerebellar ataxia, transverse myelitis, pancreatitis, myocarditis, and deafness. Differential diagnosis of mumps parotitis includes parotitis from other viruses (eg, HIV, parainfluenza, influenza, or coxsackie viruses), bacterial parotitis (eg, *S aureus*), lymphadenitis (eg, anterior cervical or preauricular adenitis), and other causes of parotid swelling (eg, sarcoidosis, parotid duct stone, and long-term wind instrument use). Differential diagnosis of mumps orchitis includes epididymo-orchitis from other etiology (eg, sexually transmitted diseases) and testicular torsion (especially when orchitis precedes parotitis). Differential diagnosis of mumps meningoencephalitis includes meningoencephalitis from other viruses (eg, enterovirus).

Emergency Department Treatment and Disposition

Diagnosis is clinical, and no laboratory tests are usually required. In the first week of illness, PCR testing of buccal secretions may be diagnostic. After the first week, serum IgM is typically positive. Serum amylase is elevated in approximately 70% of cases of parotitis, with peak values during the first week of illness. Treatment is supportive for the majority of cases. Resolution of parotitis takes approximately 10 days. Prescribe support of the testicle, ice packs, and pain management for mumps orchitis with a follow-up. Admit patients with meningitis (or meningoencephalitis) for supportive management. Mumps is contagious; exclude children from school for 5 days from onset of parotid gland swelling. Advise standard and droplet precautions for contagious illness.

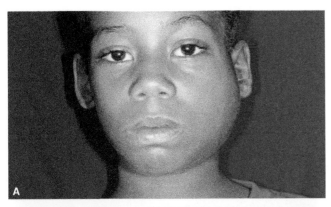
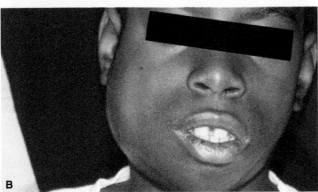

FIGURE 3.59 ■ Parotitis. (**A**) Mumps. Parotid swelling in an unimmunized child who immigrated from Trinidad 14 days before the appearance of this swelling. The parotid gland is normally not palpable. Note swelling extending below the angle of the mandible. (**B**) HIV parotitis. Children with HIV can develop parotitis usually without many symptoms. Typically, the parotid gland is firm, nontender, and chronically enlarged. Involvement can be unilateral or bilateral. (Photo contributor: Binita R. Shah, MD.)

Pearls

1. Mumps presents as either unilateral or bilateral mildly tender parotid gland swellings.
2. Purulent parotitis is unilateral; extreme tenderness and purulent drainage from Stensen duct may be noted and typically children are ill appearing.

ROSEOLA INFANTUM

Clinical Summary

Roseola infantum (also known as exanthem subitum, or roseola or sixth disease) is an acute exanthematous illness caused by human herpesvirus-6 (HHV-6; majority of cases) or HHV-7, for which humans are the only known natural hosts. Infants may have apparent recurrence that is actually sequential infection by the 2 viruses. Roseola cases occur throughout the year without any seasonal predilection. About 95% of cases occur at 6 to 36 months of age (peak: between 6-15 months). The incubation period is 7 to 15 days. There may be a mild prodrome of rhinorrhea, pharyngeal injection, or conjunctival injection; however, absence of a prodrome is most common. Illness begins with an abrupt onset of fever that rises rapidly to 39°C to 41°C and remains elevated consistently or intermittently for 3 to 6 days, after which it defervesces precipitously. Most infants look well during the febrile

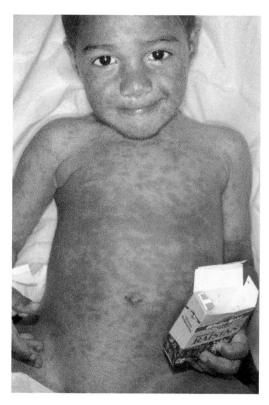

FIGURE 3.61 ■ Roseola Infantum. Diffuse erythematous maculo-papular eruption that developed after 4 days of high fever in this very happy-looking 18-month-old toddler. He was treated for occult bacteremia as an outpatient. He continued to spike fever despite antibiotic therapy, and blood and urine cultures were negative. He was rushed to the ED when this rash appeared on the fifth day (he was afebrile). A diagnosis of roseola infantum was made. (*Important:* A toddler should not be eating raisins due to the risk of choking and foreign body aspiration.) (Photo contributor: Binita R. Shah, MD.)

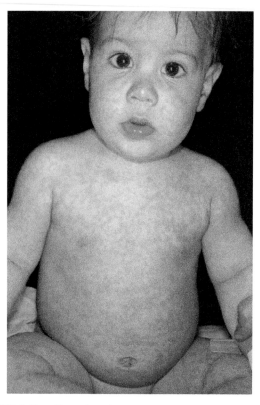

FIGURE 3.60 ■ Roseola Infantum. Diffuse erythematous maculo-papular eruptions that developed after 3 days of intermittently high fever (up to 40°C) in this well-appearing 8-month-old infant who was hospitalized because of bulging fontanelle. All the cultures were negative including CSF. A diagnosis of roseola infantum was made when he developed this rash. Note the absence of conjunctival injection and red lips (characteristic features that are often seen in a highly febrile infant with Kawasaki disease). (Photo contributor: Binita R. Shah, MD.)

period, although there may be a bulging anterior fontanelle and lymphadenopathy (cervical, occipital). After the fever drops (12–24 hours) and, rarely, as it is dropping, a rash of pink- to rose-colored nonpruritic macules or maculopapules occurs on the trunk and then spreads to the face and extremities. Lesions blanch on pressure and do not become vesicular, pustular, or petechial. Lesions usually remain discrete, and the rash is evanescent, lasting from a few hours to 1 to 3 days, after which it clears completely without pigmentation or desquamation. CNS complications include febrile seizures during the febrile prodromal stage (seen in 10%–15% of cases), meningoencephalitis, and encephalitis. Differential diagnosis includes other viral infections (eg, enteroviral infections, infectious mononucleosis and rubella), drug hypersensitivity reactions, and KD.

Emergency Department Treatment and Disposition

Diagnosis of roseola is clinical based on the age, classic history, and clinical findings. During the eruptive phase, no laboratory tests are required as classic roseola is rarely confused with other viral exanthems, and a specific diagnosis of HHV-6 is not usually necessary. During the preeruptive, highly febrile stage of roseola, many infants undergo sepsis workup, receive antibiotic therapy awaiting culture results, and are even hospitalized (especially infants presenting with a bulging anterior fontanelle). CSF examination in infants with HHV-6–associated febrile seizures is usually normal. A diagnosis of roseola is often established in these infants retrospectively when they develop the rash. No therapy is required during this stage except reassuring the family about the benign course of roseola.

Pearls

1. Roseola is the most common exanthem of infants <2 years of age.
2. The sine qua non of roseola is appearance of rash at defervescence; thus, roseola often gets diagnosed retrospectively once the typical febrile course has been observed, followed by appearance of the rash at defervescence.
3. Roseola is frequently misdiagnosed as drug hypersensitivity rash, as these infants are frequently prescribed antibiotics during the febrile preeruptive phase. Detailed history of rash in relation to fever will establish the correct diagnosis.

Clinical Summary

Measles (also known as rubeola or first disease) is a highly contagious exanthematous illness caused by a paramyxovirus. The incubation period is 8 to 12 days, and there is a prominent prodrome of fever, cough, coryza, and conjunctivitis (the 3 C's) with significant photophobia. On the third day of illness, erythematous maculopapular lesions occur along the hairline and spread down the trunk and extremities to the hands and feet, involving palms and soles. On the face and trunk, the rash becomes confluent and initially blanches on pressure; after 3 to 4 days, the rash becomes brownish and does not blanch because of capillary hemorrhages. The rash peaks at the height of fever between the fourth and sixth day of illness and resolves in order of appearance between the seventh and

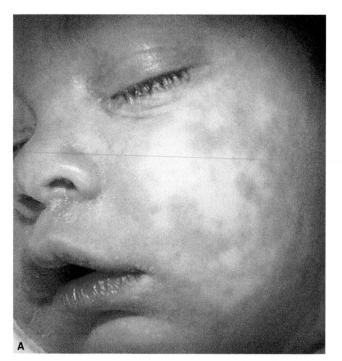

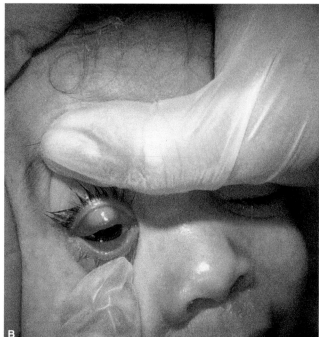

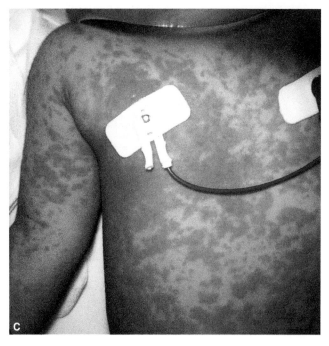

FIGURE 3.62 ■ Measles. (**A, B, C**) An 8-month-old child presented with fever, coryza, and marked conjunctivitis associated with intense photophobia. Confluent, erythematous, and maculopapular rash on the face developed on the fourth day of fever. He developed measles during the measles outbreak seen in New York City in 1993. (Photo contributor: Binita R. Shah, MD [A, B]; [C] reproduced with permission from Shah BR, Laude TL. *Atlas of Pediatric Clinical Diagnosis.* WB Saunders; Philadelphia, PA, 2000.)

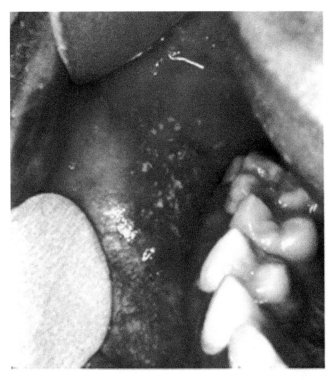

FIGURE 3.63 ■ Koplik's Spots of Measles. Koplik spots present 24 hours before and remain 24 hours after onset of rash. (Reproduced with permission from Tenenbein M, Macias CG, Sharieff GQ, et al. *Strange and Schafermeyer's Pediatric Emergency Medicine*, 5th ed. McGraw-Hill Education; New York, NY, 2019.)

ninth day. Following the rash, a fine, brawny desquamation is seen over sites of most extensive involvement (but not on palms or soles, differentiating it from scarlet fever and KD). Koplik spots are a pathognomonic mucocutaneous exanthem of white papular dots on an erythematous buccal mucosa seen opposite lower molars that may spread to involve entire buccal and labial mucosa. Koplik spots are seen 2 days before and 2 days after the rash and are transient. Absence of Koplik spots does not exclude diagnosis. Modified measles is milder (eg, afebrile course, nonconfluent rash with shorter duration) in infants <9 months old because of a transplacental antibody or administration of immunoglobulin to an exposed individual. Complications include otitis media, pneumonia (interstitial pneumonitis from measles virus or bronchopneumonia from secondary bacterial infection), cervical adenitis, encephalomyelitis, laryngotracheobronchitis, myocarditis, pericarditis, exacerbation of tuberculosis, "black" measles (hemorrhagic

measles, purpura fulminans with DIC), corneal ulceration, and blindness. Subacute sclerosing panencephalitis is a rare but severe late complication of measles infection, leading to neurodegeneration and eventually death. Differential diagnosis includes KD, drug eruptions (eg, Stevens-Johnson syndrome), meningococcemia, rickettsial infections, and other viral exanthems (eg, adenovirus, infectious mononucleosis, and enteroviruses).

Emergency Department Treatment and Disposition

Diagnosis is usually clinical. Report cases immediately to the local health department for assistance in verifying the diagnosis. Serum IgM antibody to measles is one of the simplest methods to confirm diagnosis. Additional tests (eg, measles IgG antibody acute and convalescent titers) may be recommended. Obtain CBC (leukopenia with a relative lymphocytosis seen in uncomplicated measles). CSF examination in suspected encephalitis will show mild pleocytosis with predominance of lymphocytes with increased protein and normal glucose values. Admit infants, malnourished children, or patients with complications (eg, pneumonia, croup, encephalitis). Measles is self-limited, and treatment is supportive. Patients are contagious from 3 to 5 days before to 4 days after the appearance of the rash. Immunocompromised patients are contagious for the duration of the illness (prolonged excretion of the virus in respiratory tract secretions). Vitamin A therapy has been associated with a reduction in morbidity and mortality. Currently, the World Health Organization recommends vitamin A for all children with acute measles, regardless of their country of residence. Follow CDC guidelines for administration of the vaccine and immune globulin in susceptible individuals following exposure to measles.

Pearls

1. Measles is characterized by a prominent prodrome of cough, coryza, and conjunctivitis (the 3 C's) followed by confluent erythematous maculopapular rash.

2. Immunocompromised children may not develop characteristic rash.

RUBELLA

Clinical Summary

Rubella (also known as German measles or 3-day measles) is an exanthematous infection caused by rubella virus. Humans are the only source of infection, which is transmitted through direct or droplet contact from nasopharyngeal secretions. Many cases are subclinical; clinical cases are mild and now seen in susceptible teenagers and young adults. Incubation period varies from 14 to 21 days. Coryza, cough, conjunctivitis (*without photophobia*), and sore throat may occur in adolescents. In children, the prodrome is absent and rash is the first sign of illness. Fever is absent or low grade during rash (*unlike measles*). Palatal enanthem (petechiae or rose spots) may be seen. Rose-pink maculopapular rash starts on the face and neck, becoming generalized within 24 to 48 hours. Lesions are discrete (*unlike striking confluent rash of measles*). By the third day, rash on the face disappears and is present only on the extremities. Eruption usually resolves by the end of the third day, followed by fine brawny desquamation (with intense eruption) or no desquamation. Tender lymphadenopathy involving postauricular and suboccipital

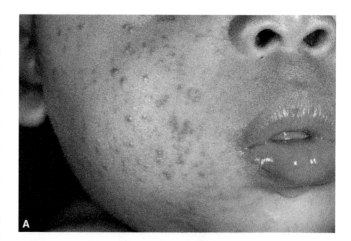

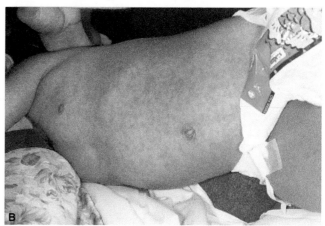

FIGURE 3.65 ■ Rubella. (A, B) Discrete erythematous rose-pink papular rash over the face and subsequently spreading to the trunk in an otherwise well-appearing 16-month-old infant who was not immunized for rubella. The patient also had significant postauricular and suboccipital adenopathy. Adenovirus and enterovirus infections can cause exanthema that mimics rubella. (Photo contributor: Binita R. Shah, MD.)

nodes occurs (most common sites) but can be generalized. Complications include transient polyarthralgia and polyarthritis in adolescent females, purpura (thrombocytopenic or nonthrombocytopenic purpura), and congenital rubella syndrome (CRS). Differential diagnosis includes other viral exanthems (eg, infectious mononucleosis, enteroviral infections) and drug eruptions.

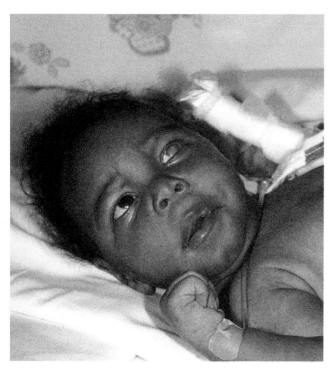

FIGURE 3.64 ■ Congenital Rubella Syndrome (CRS). An infant with glaucoma, microcephaly, and patent ductus arteriosus was born to an unimmunized mother who contracted rubella during the first trimester of pregnancy. Other eye findings of CRS include cataract, anterior uveitis, and micro-ophthalmia. (Photo contributor: Binita R. Shah, MD.)

Emergency Department Treatment and Disposition

Rubella is a difficult clinical diagnosis as most infections are asymptomatic and a similar rash is seen in many other viral infections. Laboratory diagnosis is important when rubella is suspected in pregnant women or newborns; consult an infectious disease specialist (tests may include isolation of virus from nasopharynx or serology such as rubella-specific IgM antibody and a 4-fold rise or seroconversion between acute and convalescent IgG serum titers). Rubella infection requires no therapy, and the majority of patients recover without any sequelae. Patients with arthritis will require therapy directed at pain relief. Children with postnatal rubella should be excluded from schools and child care centers for 7 days after the onset of the rash.

Pearl

1. Rubella causes a 3-day discrete maculopapular rash associated with prominent tender enlargements of postauricular, suboccipital, and cervical lymph nodes.

INFECTIOUS MONONUCLEOSIS

Clinical Summary

Infectious mononucleosis (IM) is caused by Epstein-Barr virus (EBV) in more than 90% of cases. Five to 10% of IM-like illness is caused by cytomegalovirus, *Toxoplasma gondii*, adenovirus, viral hepatitis, and HIV. IM is named for mononuclear lymphocytosis with atypical lymphocytes that accompanies the illness. IM occurs in all age groups with variable clinical expression. In young children, it is often asymptomatic or indistinguishable from other infections. In adolescents and young adults, the presentation is more classic, and the infection is transmitted by oral secretions, by close contact such as kissing (hence called "kissing disease"), or exchange of saliva from child to child (eg, child care centers). The period of communicability is indeterminate. The incubation period is 30 to 50 days. Patients present with fever, myalgias, headache, anorexia, chills, and sore throat with moderate to severe exudative tonsillopharyngitis associated with bilateral anterior and posterior cervical lymphadenopathy (nodes mildly tender to palpation); submandibular, axillary, inguinal, or epitrochlear nodes may also be involved. Other features include hepatic manifestations (transient elevations of liver enzymes [80%–90%]), hepatomegaly (10%–15%), splenomegaly (moderate enlargement in 50%), and skin rash (5%–15% of cases), which can be morbilliform, scarlatiniform, macular, petechial, urticarial, or erythema multiforme–like. Complications include upper airway obstruction, splenic rupture, hematologic (eg, thrombocytopenia, hemolytic anemia),

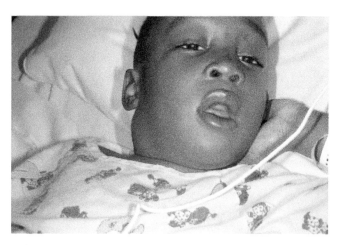

FIGURE 3.67 ■ Infectious Mononucleosis. Cervical lymphadenopathy and mouth breathing were noted in this child who presented with difficulty breathing, fever, and sore throat. His monospot was positive and had 25% atypical lymphocytes on the peripheral smear. (Photo contributor: Binita R. Shah, MD.)

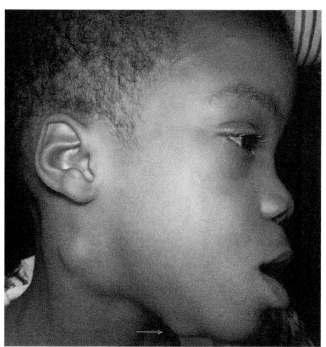

FIGURE 3.68 ■ Infectious Mononucleosis (IM). Cervical and submental lymphadenopathy (arrow) and mouth breathing were seen in this child who presented with "worsening of his snoring," sore throat, and fever. For upper airway obstruction due to IM see also Figure 6.39. (Photo contributor: Binita R. Shah, MD.)

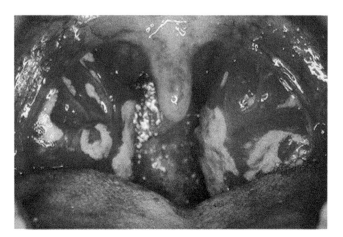

FIGURE 3.66 ■ Exudative Tonsillopharyngitis of Infectious Mononucleosis (IM). Marked white exudates on the tonsils of a child with IM. (Reproduced with permission from Kane K, Nambudiri VE, Stratigos AJ. *Color Atlas & Synopsis of Pediatric Dermatology*, 3rd ed. McGraw-Hill Education; New York, NY, 2017.)

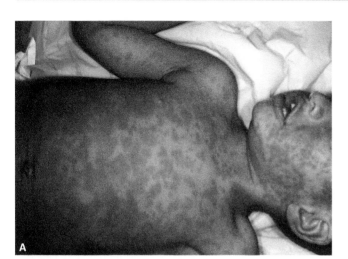
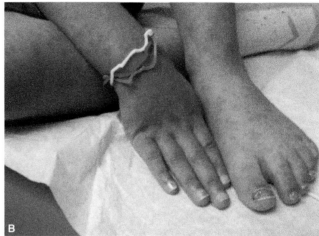

FIGURE 3.69 ■ Rash Related to Ampicillin (or Other Penicillin) in Infectious Mononucleosis (IM). (A) This generalized erythematous papular rash was precipitated by amoxicillin, which was given to this patient 5 days earlier for exudative tonsillopharyngitis (presumed "strep throat"). Fever continued while on amoxicillin. He also had splenomegaly and atypical lymphocytosis. Administration of ampicillin (or other penicillin) produces a rash in up to 90% to 100% of patients with IM. The rash may be pruritic, erythematous, or a copper-colored maculopapular rash that begins 5 to 10 days after the drug is begun and lasts up to 1 week. Involvement can be extensive on trunk, including involvement of palms and soles. (B) Amoxicillin rash in a different patient with IM. This rash is not an allergic reaction to penicillin. True penicillin-allergic skin manifestations include urticaria, erythema multiforme, and Stevens-Johnson syndrome/toxic epidermal necrolysis. (Photo contributors: Binita R. Shah, MD [A], and Andrea Marmor, MD [B].)

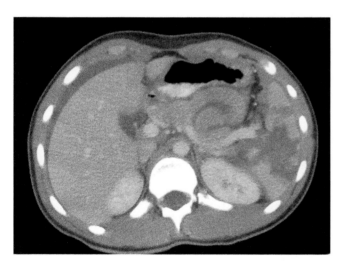

FIGURE 3.70 ■ Splenic Rupture; Infectious Mononucleosis (IM). CT scan of the abdomen demonstrates grade 4 laceration of the spleen, extending to hilum with smaller areas of laceration. Active extravasation was also noted on a different CT image. This 16-year-old adolescent male presented with abdominal pain, left shoulder pain, and feeling dizzy following trauma to his left side of the abdomen while wresting in the school. He had a syncopal episode while in the ED. He had sore throat 2 weeks prior to this. Splenic rupture is a rare but serious complication leading to hemorrhage, shock, and death. Incidence of rupture is highest in the second or third week of illness. Rarely this may a first sign of IM, as seen in this patient. (Photo/legend contributors: Vikas S. Shah, MD, and John Amodio, MD.)

cardiac (eg, myocarditis), disseminated lymphoproliferative disease, and chronic fatigue syndrome. Differential diagnosis includes streptococcal pharyngitis, leukemia, other viral exanthems, viral hepatitis, and diphtheria. *Arcanobacterium haemolyticum* also causes fever, pharyngitis, and cervical lymphadenopathy, typically in adolescents and young adults; one-fourth of affected patients develop a rash on the extensor surfaces of the extremities. Lemierre syndrome (septic thrombophlebitis of the jugular vein caused by *Fusobacterium* spp.) causes pharyngitis and neck pain and may mimic EBV infection.

Emergency Department Treatment and Disposition

Obtain a CBC with peripheral smear, which will show leukocytosis with predominant lymphocytosis and atypical lymphocytes usually >10% (other viral infections usually <10%). Mild thrombocytopenia may also be present. Consider monospot test (usually negative in children <4 years old; heterophil antibody test identifies about 85% of cases of IM in older children during the second week of illness) and, if required, EBV serology tests as mentioned in the table.

TABLE 3.6 ■ INTERPRETATION OF SERUM EPSTEIN-BARR VIRUS ANTIBODIES

	Acute Infection	Recent Infection	Past Infection
Anti-Viral Capsid Antigen IgM	Present	Present/absent	Absent
Anti-Viral Capsid Antigen IgG	Present[a]	Present	Present
Anti-Early Antigen	Absent/present[b]	Present	Present/absent
Anti-Epstein-Barr Nuclear Antigen	Absent	Absent/present[c]	Present

[a]Increases early in illness, always elevated when symptoms are present and persists for life.
[b]Increases weeks to months after symptom onset.
[c]Increases later in illness, typically more than 4 weeks after symptom onset.
Reproduced with permission from Shah SS, Ludwig S. Symptom-Based Diagnosis in Pediatrics. New York: McGraw-Hill Education, 2014.

IM is typically self-limited and patients recover without specific therapy. Admit patients with complications such as upper airway obstruction. Corticosteroid therapy is *not routinely* recommended; however, consider a short course of prednisone given orally for 7 days with subsequent tapering if there is upper airway obstruction and the diagnosis is certain. Advise family/patient to avoid contact sports or heavy lifting until full recovery of splenomegaly (usually 6 weeks), and refer such patients to the primary care physician for monitoring and return-to-play counseling. Educate family about signs of splenic rupture (eg, sudden-onset abdominal pain, especially left-sided; vomiting; pallor; lethargy; or fatigue [signs/symptoms of hemorrhage]).

Pearls

1. Classic IM is an acute illness characterized by a triad of fever, exudative pharyngitis, and cervical adenopathy.

2. IM spectrum varies from asymptomatic infection to fatal infection; most frequent causes of mortality are neurologic complications, splenic rupture, or upper airway obstruction.

3. Streptococcal pharyngitis mimics IM; tender tonsillar and cervical adenopathy and absence of hepatosplenomegaly may help in differentiating between the 2 conditions. Suspect IM when a patient with "strep throat" does not improve within 48 to 72 hours after antibiotics.

4. Ampicillin or amoxicillin given to patients with IM causes nonallergic morbilliform rash that is often mistaken for penicillin allergy.

Clinical Summary

Erythema infectiosum (EI, also known as fifth disease) is an exanthematous illness caused by human parvovirus B19. Sporadic cases are seen throughout the year, while seasonal peaks occur in late winter and spring, most commonly affecting

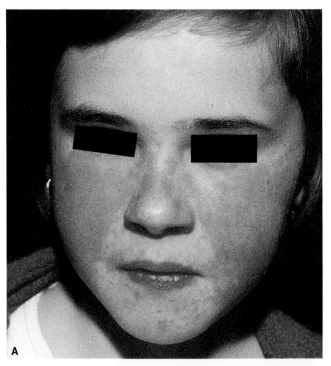

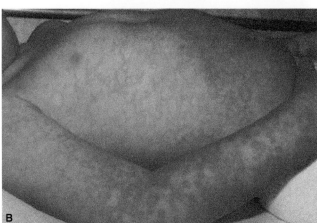

FIGURE 3.71 ■ Erythema Infectiosum (EI). (**A**) Diffuse erythema and edema of the cheeks with "slapped cheek" facies seen in a 10-year-old child with EI. (B) Lacy, reticulated rash on the body of a different child with EI. ([A] Reproduced with permission from Wolff K, Johnson R, Saavedra AP, et al. *Fitzpatrick's Color Atlas and Synopsis of Clinical Dermatology*, 8th ed. McGraw-Hill Education; New York, NY, 2017, and [B] reproduced with permission from Shah BR, Laude TL. *Atlas of Pediatric Clinical Diagnosis*. WB Saunders; Philadelphia, PA, 2000.)

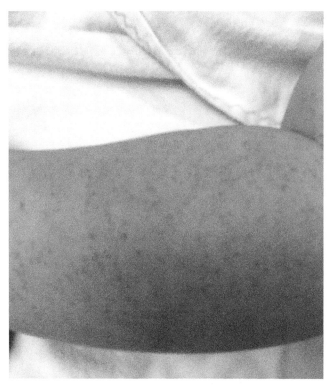

FIGURE 3.72 ■ Erythema Infectiosum. Erythematous, maculopapular rash in an infant with parvovirus B19 infection. (Photo contributor: Samir S. Shah, MD, MSCE.)

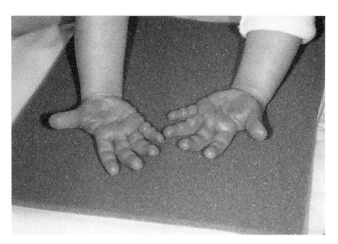

FIGURE 3.73 ■ Papular Purpuric "Gloves-and-Socks" Syndrome in Parvovirus B19 Infection. This syndrome is characterized by petechiae on the hands and feet that appear in a distinct gloves-and-socks distribution (with a clear line of distinction between rash and nonrash areas at wrists and ankles). It is usually seen in older children and adolescents with parvovirus B19 infection. (Photo contributor: Binita R. Shah, MD.)

school-aged children. The incubation period ranges from 4 to 21 days. The prodrome of myalgia and headache may be absent or mild; patients are usually afebrile (or have low-grade fever) and present with a rash. The disease occurs in 3 stages. First is a rash of red flushed cheeks with circumoral pallor (slapped-cheek appearance) lasting 1 to 4 days. This is followed by a symmetric, erythematous maculopapular rash beginning on the trunk and spreading to the arms, buttocks, and thighs. The palms and soles usually are spared, and the rash is more prominent on extensor surfaces. The rash is often pruritic. As the rash clears spontaneously, there is central clearing, making the rash appear reticulated or lace-like. Desquamation does not occur and the rash resolves within 3 weeks. However, in the third stage of the disease, there is recurrent waxing and waning of rash (for weeks or sometimes months) precipitated by a variety of stimuli (eg, sunlight, vigorous exercise, hot shower, stress).

Complications include transient aplastic crisis in patients with hemolytic anemias (eg, sickle cell disease, thalassemia). Adolescent and young adults (more commonly females) may develop symmetrical peripheral polyarthropathy (hands, wrists, knees, ankles) that may last 2 to 4 weeks. Neurologic complications (eg, meningitis, encephalitis), thrombocytopenic purpura, and hydrops fetalis due to intrauterine infection of the fetus are other complications. Differential diagnosis includes other viral exanthems (eg, enteroviral infections), drug eruptions, and collagen vascular diseases (patients presenting with arthralgia/arthritis).

Emergency Department Treatment and Disposition

Diagnosis is clinical based on the exanthema, and no laboratory tests are required for immunocompetent children. For patients with hemolytic anemias, obtain CBC with reticulocyte count. Presence of anti-B19 IgM antibody or parvovirus B19 DNA by PCR on a single serum specimen confirms acute or recent infection. IgG antibodies are detected a few days after IgM antibodies and persist for years. The disease is self-limited, and only supportive therapy is required for immunocompetent patients. Children *do not* need isolation and exclusion from school or day care as they no longer are contagious once the rash appears. Educate family about possible recurrence of the rash. No specific therapy is necessary for arthritis except pain management. Admit patients with hemolytic anemias presenting with aplastic crisis for close monitoring and possible transfusion.

Pearl

1. Slapped-cheek appearance in an otherwise well-appearing child is pathognomonic of EI.

Clinical Summary

Hand-foot-and-mouth disease (HFMD) is a clearly recognizable coxsackie or enterovirus infection commonly seen during late summer and early fall in temperate climates and often occurring in epidemics. HFMD is a highly contagious illness; modes of transmission include fecal–oral, respiratory route, and from fomites. The incubation period ranges from 4 to 7 days. Constitutional symptoms (eg, fever, diarrhea, anorexia) usually precede skin lesions. Locations of lesions include hands/palms (dorsal and palmar surface, sides of

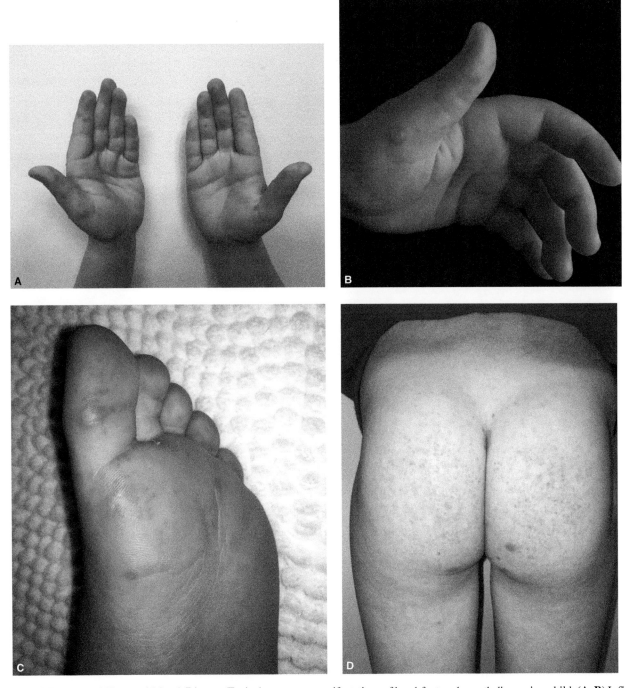

FIGURE 3.74 ■ Hand-Foot-and-Mouth Disease. Typical cutaneous manifestations of hand-foot-and-mouth disease in a child. (**A, B**) Inflammatory vesicles on the hand. (**C**) Inflammatory vesicles on the foot. (**D**) Numerous small erythematous papules and vesicles were also seen on the knees and buttocks. (Photo contributor: Jeannette Jakus, MD.)

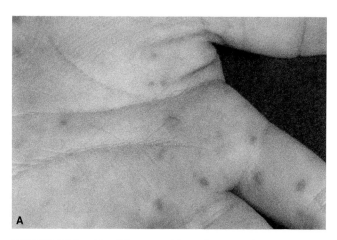

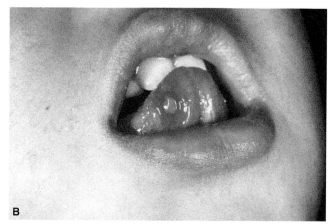

FIGURE 3.75 ■ Hand-Foot-and-Mouth Disease. (**A**) Typical elliptical or oval-shaped papulovesicular lesions with erythematous rims are seen on the hand. (**B**) Ulcers surrounded by a rim of erythema are seen in the mouth. (Photo contributor: Binita R. Shah, MD.)

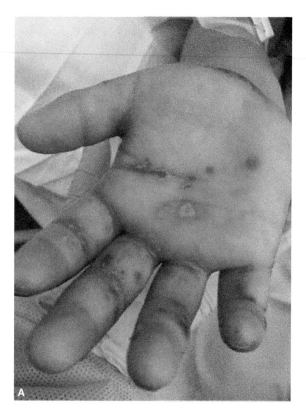

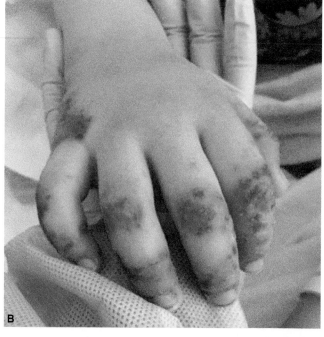

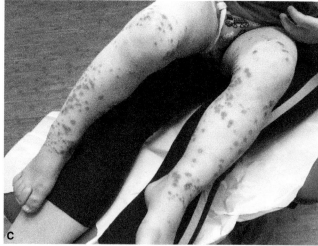

FIGURE 3.76 ■ Eczema Coxsackium. (**A, B**) Atypical presentation of coxsackie virus infection in a 4-year-old child with atopic dermatitis. In addition to the usual manifestations of coxsackie infection, he also developed blisters on palms and soles and exhibited more widespread skin disease, particularly in areas of previous or current eczema. Note the hemorrhagic skin lesions seen, which are also characteristic, on this patient's fingers. Disease in areas of atopic dermatitis may resemble eczema herpeticum, hence the term *eczema coxsackium*. (**C**) This 3-year-old patient had more widespread papules resembling Gianotti-Crosti syndrome, another presentation seen in patients with eczema coxsackium. (Photo contributors: Sharon A. Glick, MD [A, B], and Julie Cantatore-Francis, MD [C].)

fingers), feet (sides of feet and toes, plantar surface of soles), mouth (anterior portion of mouth involving tongue and buccal mucosa, hard palate, gingivae, lips), and buttocks in younger children. Elliptical or oval gray-roofed vesicles with erythematous rims varying in size from 3 to 7 mm (up to 2 cm) and in number from a few to a hundred are seen. Skin lesions are bilateral and symmetric on hands and feet and usually are asymptomatic, whereas mouth lesions are painful. Nonvesicular papular, macular, or petechial lesions may be seen on the buttocks (most common site), upper thighs, and knees. Myocarditis, meningoencephalitis, and aseptic meningitis are rare complications. Differential diagnosis includes other viral exanthems with vesicular lesions (eg, varicella), herpes gingivostomatitis, herpangina, aphthous stomatitis, arthropod bites, and allergic contact dermatitis.

Emergency Department Treatment and Disposition

Diagnosis of HFMD is clinical. Treatment is supportive with antipyretics/analgesics (as indicated) with attention to adequate hydration. Soft diet and cool, non-citrus liquids are often well tolerated in the presence of oral ulcerations. Advise patient and family regarding personal hygiene including hand washing to prevent spread of the infection. HFMD usually is a self-limited disease, with lesions lasting 2 to 7 days and heals *without* scarring.

Pearls

1. HFMD is characterized by vesicular lesions in the mouth, hands, and feet. However, *all 3 anatomic areas need not be affected*. The mouth is most frequently involved, followed by hands and then feet.

2. *Do not* use viscous lidocaine topically for pain relief in the mouth. Systemic toxicity can occur due to absorption of the lidocaine from the buccal mucosa.

Clinical Summary

Herpangina is a characteristic enanthem produced by enteroviruses such as coxsackie A, coxsackie B, and echoviruses, affecting most commonly children between 3 and 10 years old. It is typically seen during summer or early fall in temperate climates. Constitutional symptoms (eg, fever, vomiting, sore throat, dysphagia) may be present. Discrete vesicles and/or ulcers (1–2 mm in diameter) surrounded by an erythematous ring occur on the anterior tonsillar pillars (most frequent site), soft palate, tonsils and uvula, and posterior pharyngeal wall. The number of lesions varies from a few to many, and lesions last for about 1 week. The course is benign in the majority of cases, without any complications. Differential diagnosis includes herpetic gingivostomatitis and HFMD.

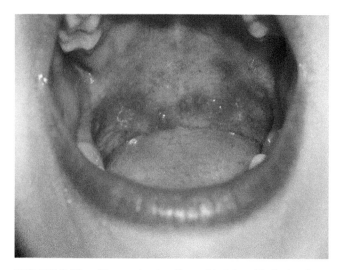

FIGURE 3.77 ■ Herpangina by Coxsackie Virus. Typical yellowish-white ulcers or vesicles that measure usually about 1 to 2 mm in diameter surrounded by an erythematous base are seen. Typically in herpangina, these lesions are seen on the soft palate, tonsils, and uvula. Gingiva, tongue, and buccal mucosa are spared (unlike herpetic gingivostomatitis in which gingiva, tongue, and buccal mucosa are involved). (Photo contributor: Emily Scott, MD. Reproduced with permission from Usatine RP, Sabella C, Smith M, et al. *The Color Atlas of Pediatrics;* McGraw-Hill Education, New York, NY, 2015.)

Emergency Department Treatment and Disposition

Diagnosis is clinical. Treatment is symptomatic, with attention to maintaining good hydration. Soft diet and cool, noncitrus liquids are often well tolerated in the presence of oral ulcerations.

Pearls

1. Herpangina causes tiny vesicles and ulcers on the posterior pharynx. Herpetic gingivostomatitis causes ulcers in the posterior and anterior oropharyngeal mucosa involving tongue, buccal mucosa, and gums, which are swollen and may bleed with minor trauma.
2. HFMD causes oval-shaped vesicles with erythematous rims on hands, feet, and mouth associated with nonvesicular papular, macular, or petechial lesions that may be seen on buttocks, upper thighs, and knees.

Clinical Summary

Cutaneous larvae migrans (CLM; also known as creeping eruption or sandworm disease) is a skin infestation caused most commonly by the larvae of the dog or cat hookworm (eg, *Ancylostoma braziliense*) and rarely by human nematodes (eg,

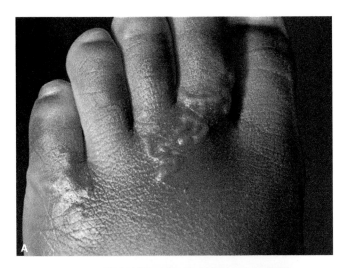

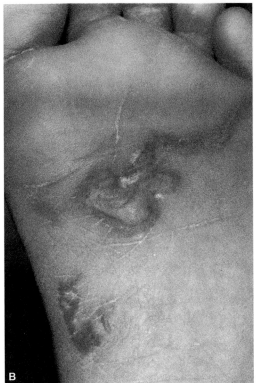

FIGURE 3.78 ■ Cutaneous Larva Migrans. Erythematous, intensely pruritic, tortuous, and serpiginous tracks of migrating larva in a 6-year-old patient with a history of walking barefoot on one of the Caribbean islands. (Photo contributor: Binita R. Shah, MD.)

Ancylostoma duodenale). *A braziliense* larvae infect dogs and cats by burrowing through the skin. Adult hookworms reside in the intestine and shed eggs in feces that are deposited on the ground. The eggs develop into infectious larvae outside the body in places protected from desiccation and temperature extremes, such as sandy, shady areas around beaches or under houses. The larvae penetrate human skin to initiate infection. CLM is commonly seen in people who come into contact with soil contaminated with cat and dog feces (eg, children, gardeners, sunbathers, and those playing in sandboxes, walking barefoot on a beach, and working in tight crawlspaces under houses). Larvae migrate through the skin (at the plane of the epidermal-dermal junction) and advance from several millimeters to a few centimeters a day, producing serpiginous tracks. Larval activity can continue for weeks to months; however, the organisms are unable to penetrate the basement membrane and die within months because they cannot complete their life cycle in the human host. CLM occurs worldwide. Skin lesion begins as a stinging or tingling sensation and reddish papule at the site of larval penetration with an intense localized pruritus. A serpiginous, tortuous, slightly raised track (sometimes with vesicles and bullae) is seen in the upper epidermis; such tracks can grow 1 to 2 cm/day (larva typically located 1–2 cm in front of serpiginous eruption). New areas of involvement may appear every few days. Lesions may be single or numerous (if large areas of the body are exposed, eg, sunbathing). Systemic symptoms are absent. Common sites (any area may be affected) include foot, buttock, hand, and genitalia. Rare presentations include Löffler syndrome (pneumonitis with a large burden of parasites), myositis, and eosinophilic enteritis (larvae reaching the intestine). Peripheral eosinophilia may be present. Skin biopsy is not necessary for the diagnosis (eosinophilic inflammatory infiltrate without migrating parasite seen). Differential diagnosis includes tinea infections, contact dermatitis, granuloma annulare, and cutaneous pili migrans (embedded hair or creeping hair).

Emergency Department Treatment and Disposition

Diagnosis is clinical. When the diagnosis is uncertain, the presence of peripheral eosinophilia should raise suspicion. CLM is usually a self-limited disease. Spontaneous cure occurs usually in several weeks to a few months even without treatment, as the larvae die. However, the intense pruritus often leads to skin excoriation and secondary bacterial infection; therefore, treatment is often prescribed. Oral albendazole or ivermectin are effective. Topical metronidazole has also demonstrated effectiveness.

Pearl

1. An advancing serpiginous growing tunnel in the skin associated with intense pruritus is pathognomonic of CLM.

Clinical Summary

Ascariasis (roundworm) is a nematode infestation by *Ascaris lumbricoides* that occurs at all ages, most commonly in preschool- and early school–aged children. Adult worms live freely in the lumen of the small intestine (commonly in the jejunum and middle ileum) for up to a year, shedding eggs in the stool and leading to fecal–oral transmission. Suboptimal hygiene, poor sanitation, and use of human feces as fertilizer are contributing factors. The majority of patients are asymptomatic. Pulmonary signs and symptoms occur as larvae migrate through the lungs and include fever, shortness of breath/dyspnea, substernal pain, wheezing/asthma, hemoptysis, rales, Löffler syndrome (transient pulmonary infiltrates), and peripheral eosinophilia. Gastrointestinal (GI) signs and symptoms caused by adult worms in the small intestine include abdominal pain (persistent or recurrent) and distension, vomiting (with or without bile), malabsorption, and diarrhea. Worms may be seen in vomitus or stools. Worm migrations at different sites may cause ascending cholangitis, acute pancreatitis, acute appendicitis, diverticulitis, gallstones (dead worms as nidus for stone), perforation, peritonitis, volvulus, intussusception, and acute intestinal obstruction (seen in children with heavy infestation). Stressful conditions (eg, fever, illness) stimulate adult worm migration. Allergic reactions (due to absorption of toxins from products of living or dead worms) include asthma, hay fever, and urticaria. Differential diagnosis of pulmonary ascariasis with eosinophilia includes asthma and Löffler syndrome from other parasites (eg, toxocariasis, strongyloidiasis, hookworm); differential of ascariasis-induced GI diseases includes pancreatitis or appendicitis or cholecystitis from other etiologies.

Emergency Department Treatment and Disposition

Identification of ova on direct smear of a fresh stool specimen or of adult worms in vomitus or feces (often brought to the ED by caretakers) confirms diagnosis. If infestation is uncertain, examine direct smear of stool samples on 3 consecutive mornings. If biliary ascariasis is suspected, obtain US of the biliary tree. Prescribe oral albendazole as a single dose or mebendazole for 3 days. Consult surgery if patient presents with acute

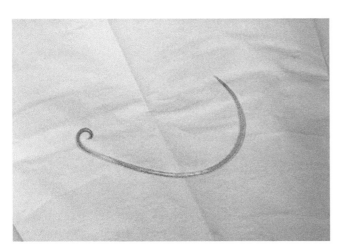

FIGURE 3.79 ■ *Ascaris lumbricoides.* This worm was vomited in the ED by a patient presenting with abdominal pain and several episodes of nonbilious vomiting. Roundworm is the largest intestinal nematode parasite of humans. Sites from which adult worms may be passed include the rectum, the nose (after migration through the nares), and the mouth in vomitus. Characteristic features of roundworms include tapered ends, length between 15 and 40 cm, and white or reddish-yellow in color. (Photo contributor: Binita R. Shah, MD.)

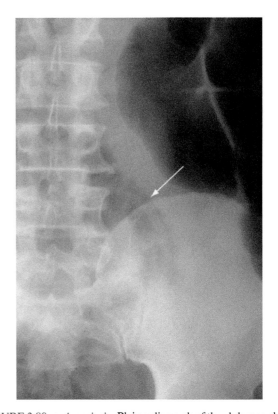

FIGURE 3.80 ■ Ascariasis. Plain radiograph of the abdomen showing a curvilinear radiopaque density in the bowel lumen in the left iliac region (this radiopaque density represents a roundworm, as this patient gave a history of passing roundworms in the stool). He presented with clinical signs of intestinal obstruction. He responded to conservative management and passed several worms after receiving mebendazole therapy. (Photo contributor: Binita R. Shah, MD.)

intestinal obstruction and admit for conservative management (eg, parenteral hydration, nasogastric suctioning), which may resolve symptoms. Surgical intervention may be still needed for obstruction or volvulus. In a patient with a mixed infestation, treat ascariasis first; treatment of other parasites first may stimulate a large worm burden to migrate simultaneously, causing obstruction.

Pearls

1. Ascariasis is the most prevalent human helminthic infestation.
2. Small diameter of the intestinal lumen and propensity to acquire large worm burdens predispose children for acute intestinal obstruction.

Clinical Summary

Malaria is a protozoan infection transmitted to humans by the bite of nocturnal-feeding *Anopheles* mosquitoes. Four species of *Plasmodium* that cause infection include *P falciparum*, *P vivax*, and less commonly *P ovale* and *P malariae*. *P falciparum* tends to cause the most severe infections and *P malariae* the mildest. Less commonly, transmission occurs through transfusion, contaminated needles or syringes, or transplacentally. Malaria affects all ages, and infections can be acute or chronic. Although *Anopheles* mosquitoes are native to the United States, most cases of malaria in the US are imported. Following a 1- to 3-week incubation period in the liver, *Plasmodium* enters a 48- to 72-hour asexual erythrocyte cycle depending on the species. This explains the periodicity of high fever and shaking chills (febrile paroxysms) that are the classic presentation. Sweats, rigors, headache, and muscle aches are also seen. At first, the fever is irregular followed by paroxysms alternating with periods of fatigue in a cyclic pattern (as the infection becomes synchronized). Paroxysms coincide with rupture of schizonts. Nausea, vomiting, diarrhea, abdominal pain, arthralgia, and back pain may be present with paroxysms. Splenomegaly and hepatomegaly may occur and anemia/pallor, thrombocytopenia, leukopenia, leukocytosis, and jaundice may be present. Different species of *Plasmodium* cause specific symptoms.

Emergency Department Treatment and Disposition

Obtain a CBC and comprehensive metabolic panel. Anemia and thrombocytopenia are common, especially with *P falciparum* infection, whereas leukocytosis rarely occurs with malaria. A thick and thin peripheral smear should also be performed (thick smear to detect organisms in erythrocytes and thin smear to determine species). Obtain multiple smears per day and, if possible, at least 1 during or right after a fever spike, which provides the greatest yield. The percentage of erythrocytes harboring parasites and identification of species, both detected from a thin peripheral smear, help determine therapy. Alternatives to blood smear testing are preferred at some hospitals when blood smear expertise is not available. Malaria rapid diagnostic tests, which detect malaria antigens in blood, and PCR tests are both more sensitive and specific than microscopy. Some rapid malaria tests detect only *P falciparum*, whereas others detect multiple species. Neither rapid detection tests nor PCR can quantify parasitemia level. Consult an infectious disease specialist and/or CDC for treatment (https://www.cdc.gov/malaria/about/faqs.html). Patients with severe malaria, which includes signs of CNS or other end-organ involvement, shock, metabolic abnormalities (eg, acidosis, hypoglycemia), or parasitemia >5%, should be admitted to the ICU for monitoring and therapy. Treatment

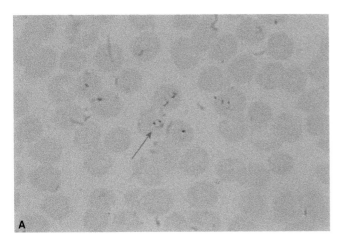
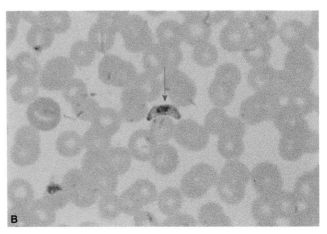

FIGURE 3.81 ■ *Plasmodium falciparum* Malaria: Giemsa-Stained Thin Smear of Peripheral Blood. (**A**) Multiple ring forms of *P falciparum* (arrow). Note that many of the RBCs are infected, and some have 2 ring forms. Some of the rings have double chromatin dots. (**B**) Banana- or crescent-shaped gametocytes (arrow) of *P falciparum*. Note that the RBC membrane has been stretched to enclose the gametocyte. This child immigrated from Africa 2 weeks before his illness. (Photo contributor: Haseeb A. Siddiqi, PhD.)

TABLE 3.7 ■ SPECIFIC SYMPTOMS CAUSED BY DIFFERENT PLASMODIA CAUSING MALARIA

Organism	Incubation Period (days)	Periodicity of Fever	Other Specific Symptoms
P ovale and *P vivax* (benign tertian malaria)	12–18; *P vivax* can be 6–12 months	Schizonts rupture every 48 hours, resulting in daily fever spikes and paroxysms	Hypersplenism (risk for splenic rupture)
			Relapse (up to 3–5 years after primary infection)
P falciparum (malignant tertian malaria)	9–14	Less apparent	Cerebral malaria (fever up to 106°F to 108°F, delirium, coma, seizures, pupillary changes, retinal hemorrhages, hemiplegia, and absent or exaggerated deep tendon reflexes)
			Coagulopathy
			Noncardiogenic pulmonary edema, respiratory failure
			Hypoglycemia, metabolic acidosis, blackwater fever (massive intravascular hemolysis, hemoglobinemia, hemoglobinuria ["black urine"])
			Acute hepatic and renal failure
			Algid malaria (overwhelming infection: hypotension, hypothermia, pallor, vascular collapse, and death)
P malariae (benign quartan malaria)	18–40	Schizonts rupture every 72 hours, resulting in alternate-day or every-third-day fever spikes and paroxysms	Chronic asymptomatic parasitemia (for several years), nephrotic syndrome

regimens for *P vivax* and *P ovale* include primaquine to prevent relapse of infection.

Pearls

1. Presume malaria unless proven otherwise in children with unexplained fever or systemic illness and history of travel or emigration from an endemic area within the previous year.

2. Repeat peripheral smear every 12 to 24 hours over 72 hours if clinical suspicion is strong and an initial smear is negative.

3. Diagnosis of *P falciparum* malaria is a medical emergency.

4. *P vivax* and *P ovale* parasites may cause relapse months to years after initial infection.

5. Malaria is preventable with appropriate chemoprophylaxis and measures to prevent contact with mosquitoes (eg, protective clothing, repellents).

CHAPTER 4

SEXUAL ABUSE, GYNECOLOGY, AND SEXUALLY TRANSMITTED INFECTIONS

Tanya S. Hinds
Angela Lumba-Brown

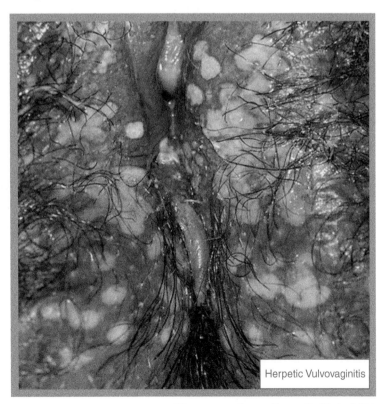

Herpetic Vulvovaginitis

(Photo contributor: Binita R. Shah, MD)

The authors acknowledge the special contributions of Amy Suss, MD, Sarah A. Rawstron, MD, and Konstantinos Agoritsas, MD, to prior edition.

159

Clinical Summary

Sexual assault is sexual activity for which a victim is unable to or cannot give explicit, informed consent. Sexual assault encompasses child sexual abuse (CSA). CSA is completed or attempted any one of the following: (1) contact involving penetration, however slight, between the mouth, vulva, penis, or anus of a child and a perpetrator's hand, penis, or object; (2) intentional touching directly or through clothing of the breast, vulva, penis, anus, groin, buttocks, or inner thigh that is not consistent with child's needs; (3) pornography, voyeurism by an adult, sexual harassment, and commercial sexual exploitation (prostitution, sexual trafficking); (4) confirmed sexually transmitted infections (STIs) in children when perinatal and rare nonsexual transmission has been ruled out. Approximately 1 in 4 females and 1 in 10 males have experienced some form of sexual victimization prior to age 18 years. CSA perpetrators are usually male family members or male acquaintances, not strangers. CSA is most often discovered because of a disclosure by the child weeks to years after event(s). Details are often only incrementally disclosed. Abused children sometimes display explicit or developmentally inappropriate sexual knowledge or behaviors, self-harm, depression, temper tantrums, aggression, phobias, disturbances in sleep and appetite, difficulty in school, abdominal pain, and/or anogenital complaints. The subset of children who have been trafficked (exchanged sexual acts for money, food, shelter, drugs, affection, gifts) often have a history of running away from home, gang involvement, substance use, gender identity concerns, significant nongenital injuries, multiple STIs, and/or current or prior involvement with social services or law enforcement. Adult CSA survivors are at increased risk of sexual dysfunction, depression, and sexual revictimization.

Emergency Department Treatment and Disposition

The diagnosis of suspected CSA is commonly made by careful history taking. History should ideally be obtained from any child older than age 3 years who is willing and able to speak. An open-ended history should begin with an explanation that it is okay for the child to correct the clinician and/or to say the child does not remember or understand. Age-appropriate language and repetition of the child's words followed

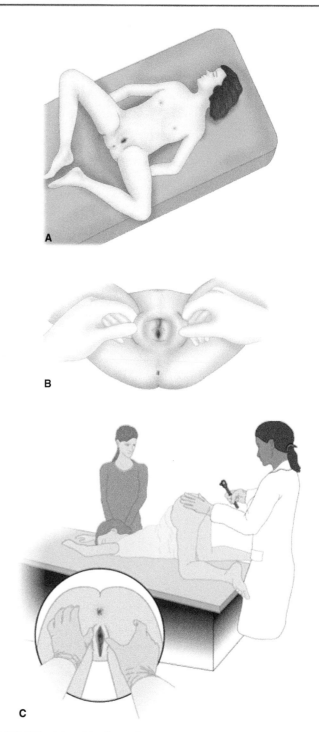

FIGURE 4.1 ■ Physical Examination Positions. (A) Frog-leg position. (B) Labial traction. (C) Girl in knee-chest position with elbows resting on examination table. This position is best for examining the perianal area and the vaginal vault. (Reproduced with permission from Tenenbein M, Macias CG, Sharieff GQ, et al. *Strange and Schafermeyer's Pediatric Emergency Medicine.* 5th ed. McGraw-Hill Education; New York, NY, 2019 [A, B]; and Tintinalli JE, Stapczynski J, Ma O, et al. *Tintinalli's Emergency Medicine: A Comprehensive Study Guide.* 8th ed. McGraw-Hill Education; New York, NY, 2016 [C].)

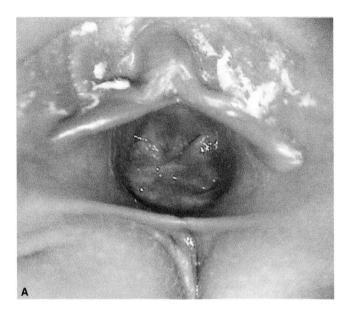

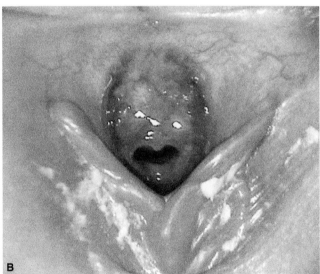

FIGURE 4.2 ▪ Normal Unestrogenized Crescentic Hymen. A 3-year-old girl disclosed that "he [daycare provider] touched me." (**A**) Hymen appeared imperforate due to adherent hymenal edges in a supine frog-leg position with labial traction. (**B**) Unestrogenized cresentic hymen in the same patient in a dorsal knee-chest position. (Photo contributor: Tanya S. Hinds, MD.)

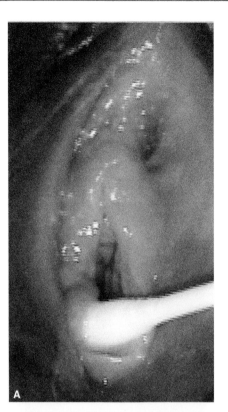

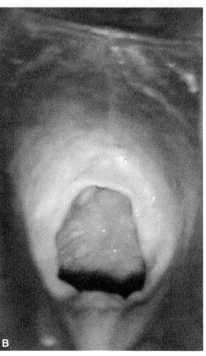

FIGURE 4.3 ▪ Normal Estrogenized Annular Hymen. A 12-year-old girl disclosed "my daddy put his penis in my hole where the blood comes from." (**A**) A possible deep notch at 7 o'clock is seen in a supine lithotomy position. (**B**) Deep notch is not confirmed in a dorsal knee-chest position. A healed injury would remain present in confirmatory dorsal knee-chest position. (Photo contributor: Tanya S. Hinds, MD.)

by "Tell me more" or "And then what happened?" are suggested approaches to obtain relevant details (Table 4.1). The essential elements that should be asked and documented are *who*, put *what, when, where*, and *what happened afterward*.

Acute or healed anogenital injuries are unlikely following CSA, even in cases that involve confessions by perpetrators, STIs, DNA evidence, and/or pregnancy. Nevertheless, a comprehensive medical examination (with attention to demeanor,

TABLE 4.1 ■ ELEMENTS OF A DISCLOSURE[a]

What happened? and what happened afterwards?
Who (name/nickname) did it?
Did it happen one time or more than one time?
When was the last time?
Was lubricant or a condom used?
Was there ejaculation?
Did pain or bleeding occur?
How was urination afterward?
How was defecation afterward?
Did child previously tell?
What are/were reactions to child's disclosure?
Where (location/jurisdiction) did it occur?

[a] Suggested questions. Age-appropriate language must be used. Some questions cannot be asked of young children.

skin, and oral and genital orifices) should be immediate if the child presents acutely (defined as within 72 hours of assault in most jurisdictions within the United States). Forensic sampling (for semen and cellular material) based on local protocols should be obtained during an acute medical examination. The supine frog-leg position is a suggested, initial position to examine the vagina of prepubertal girls and the penis and scrotum of boys of all ages. Manipulation of the prepubertal hymen with a swab or catheter, use of a speculum or proctoscope and/or other invasive techniques should only be performed under sedation. The supine lithotomy position is the initial preferred examination position in pubertal girls. A moistened swab or Foley bladder catheter can also be used to evaluate the thickened, redundant hymenal rim for notches or transections in girls who are Tanner stage III or greater when supine lithotomy is insufficient. The anus can then be examined with children supine holding their knees to their chest or with children on their left side with hips and knees flexed against their chest. The child can be examined in the prone knee-chest position if better anogenital visualization is needed or an ambiguous physical finding is noted that needs to be confirmed or refuted.

If >72 hours have passed since suspected CSA, the child has no acute mental health or medical needs, and presentation for a scheduled examination with a specialist clinician is likely, then an immediate examination in the ED can be deferred. Postponement of the ED examination does not relieve the ED of the responsibility to report suspected CSA based on available historical information. A report to social services and/or law enforcement usually initiates a multidisciplinary investigation in the jurisdiction where the CSA is suspected to have occurred. Social workers, detectives, and specialist clinicians work to ensure the index child and siblings are interviewed, examined, and linked to community-based resources including mental health providers.

Pearls

1. Historical information alone can be the basis for suspicion of CSA and a report to social services and/or law enforcement. Child and caregiver should be spoken with separately if this would likely not be distressing or detrimental to the child.

2. A normal genital exam does not mean sexual assault did not occur. Injury may not occur at the time of CSA, anogenital injury may heal without scarring or sequelae, or injury may be overlooked during examination.

Clinical Summary

Rates of STIs are generally <5% in prepubertal victims of CSA. Teens and victims of sexual trafficking have significantly higher rates. Disclosure of penetrating sexual contact, vaginal discharge, and/or an abnormal genital examination are associated with an increased risk of *Neisseria gonorrhoeae*, *Chlamydia trachomatis*, *Trichomonas vaginalis*, and HIV. Children with pharyngeal and anogenital STIs may also be asymptomatic.

Emergency Department Treatment and Disposition

Screening for STIs is suggested when a child discloses contact that may involve transfer of genital secretions; there is physical evidence of anogenital penetration; the suspected perpetrator is unknown or believed to be at high risk for an STI; a household member has an STI; the prevalence of STIs is high in the community where the child lives; the child has anogenital signs or symptoms of an STI; and/or STI testing is requested by the child or parent. When a prepubescent child has a nucleic acid amplification test (NAAT) that is positive

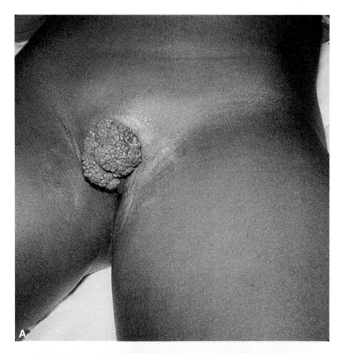

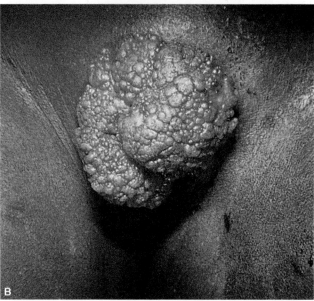

FIGURE 4.5 ■ Condylomata Acuminata (Genital Warts) due to Sexual Abuse. (**A, B**) A cauliflower-like mass present for 1 year on the perineum of this 10-year-old girl is shown. She was repeatedly sexually abused by her stepfather since the age of 8. Condylomata start as pinhead papules that are pink, red, or skin colored. Lesions remain either solitary or develop into grapelike clusters and may coalesce in the rectal or perineal area to form a large cauliflower-like mass. (Photo contributor: Binita R. Shah, MD.)

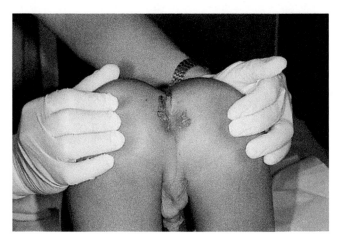

FIGURE 4.4 ■ Condylomata Acuminata (Genital Warts) due to Sexual Abuse. Lesions are seen in the perianal area of this 3-year-old boy who was abused by his maternal uncle. Genital warts are soft, flesh-colored, elongated lesions that develop around mucocutaneous junctions and intertriginous areas (eg, perianally, mucosae of female genitalia). Condylomata acuminata must be differentiated from condylomata lata because both occur in the same areas. (Photo contributor: Binita R. Shah, MD.)

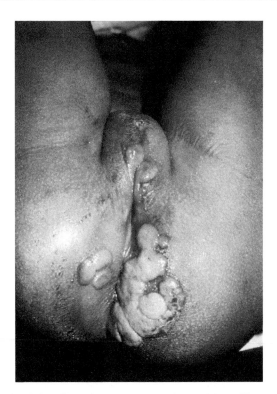

FIGURE 4.6 ■ Condyloma Lata due to Sexual Abuse. Flat-topped, round-oval nodular lesions and plaque (formed by papules that coalesce) with a wide base are seen around the anus and genitalia in a 6-year-old girl who was repeatedly abused by her stepfather. Unlike condylomata acuminata, these lesions are flat and not covered by digitate vegetations. (Reproduced with permission from Shah BR, Laude T. *Atlas of Pediatric Clinical Diagnosis.* WB Saunders; Philadelphia, PA, 2000.)

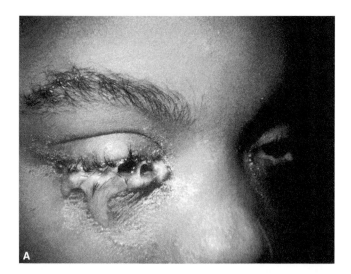

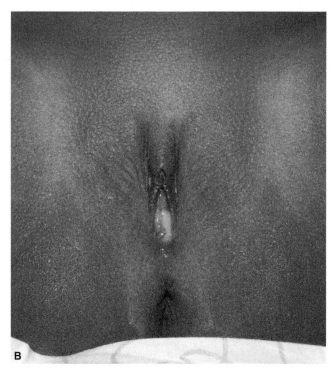

FIGURE 4.8 ■ Gonococcal Infections due to Sexual Abuse. (**A**) Gonococcal conjunctivitis. An 8-year-old girl with profuse mucopurulent discharge. Her eye, pharyngeal, and rectal cultures were positive for *N gonorrhoeae*. Investigation among the family members led to a 21-year-old uncle with gonococcal urethritis, and subsequently, he confessed to sexually abusing this girl. (**B**) Gonococcal vulvovaginitis. A 2-year-old girl presented with purulent vaginal discharge that was positive for *N gonorrhoeae*. The mother was the main caretaker, but this girl was attending a daycare center while the mother was at work. A Child Protective Services investigation found a caretaker at the daycare to be the offender. (Photo contributors: Reproduced with permission from Shah BR, Laude T. *Atlas of Pediatric Clinical Diagnosis.* WB Saunders; Philadelphia, PA, 2000 [A] and Ameer Hassoun, MD [B].)

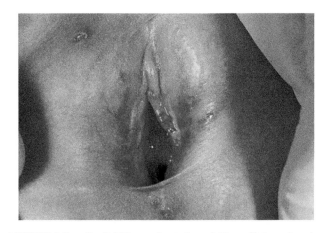

FIGURE 4.7 ■ Genital Herpes due to Sexual Abuse. Extremely painful ulcerative lesions (HSV type 2 culture positive) were seen in an 8-year-old girl who was repeatedly abused by her uncle in the past 2 weeks. Genital herpes is uncommon in children. Lesions usually appear after an incubation period of 2 to 20 days after exposure. Except for perinatal transmission at birth, most HSV-2 genital infections are sexually transmitted. (Photo contributor: Binita R. Shah, MD.)

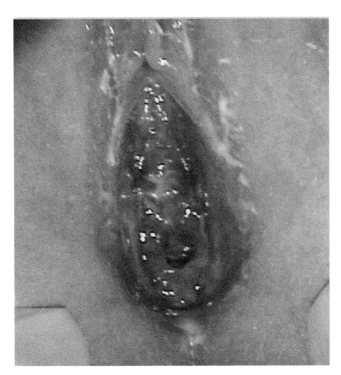

FIGURE 4.9 ■ Chlamydia Vaginitis. A previously healthy 7-year-old girl presented with a 2-week history of vaginal discharge. She did not disclose abuse. Her examination showed a normal, annular hymen without posterior notches. Vaginal culture and NAAT were positive for *Chlamydia trachomatis*. Her discharge resolved after treatment with erythromycin. This is diagnostic of CSA. (Photo contributor: Tanya S. Hinds, MD.)

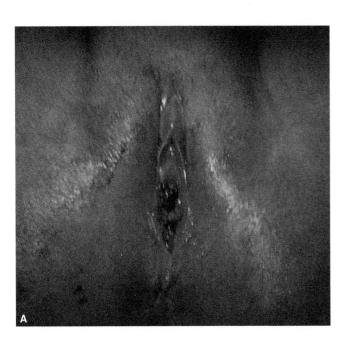

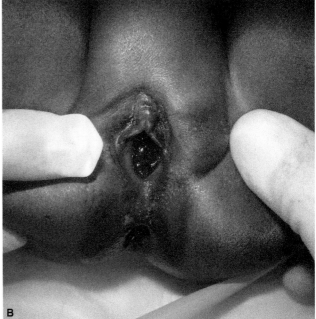

FIGURE 4.10 ■ Sexual Abuse–Related Injuries and Differential Diagnosis. (**A, B**) Sexual abuse. (**A**) Fresh bleeding and blood clots at the introitus and a superficial laceration in the posterior fourchette were seen in this 4-year-old girl who was sexually abused by her uncle. (**B**) A hematoma at the introitus and fresh anal injuries with significant anal dilation were seen in this 4-month-old infant brought to the ED with cardiopulmonary arrest. These injuries occurred while the infant was being cared by the mother's boyfriend. Posterior rib fractures, splenic rupture, and retroperitoneal hematoma were other injuries seen in this infant.

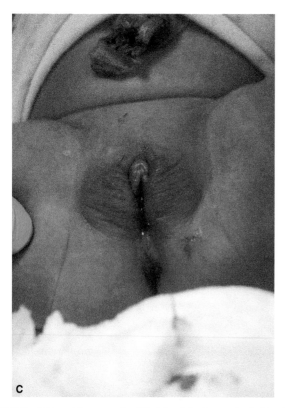

FIGURE 4.10 ▪ (*Continued*) (**C**) Physiologic vaginal bleeding ("neonatal menstruation"). A 3-day-old female neonate, with otherwise unremarkable exam, presented with vaginal bleeding. This is secondary to postnatal sudden withdrawal of maternal hormones resulting in a vaginal discharge that can be blood tinged or frankly bloody. It is seen in some female neonates appearing within a few days after birth. No treatment except reassurance is necessary, and the discharge usually disappears within 10 days. (Photo contributors: Binita R. Shah, MD [A, B], and Ameer Hassoun, MD [C].)

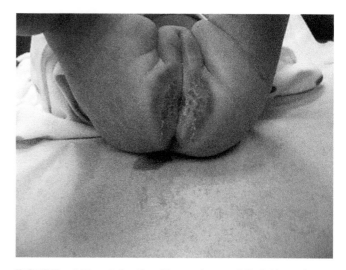

FIGURE 4.11 ▪ Infantile Hemangioma Mimicking Sexual Abuse. A 7-month-old infant with hemangioma with central erosions of the gluteal cleft with extension to the perineum. Evaluation of this midline hemangioma revealed a tethered cord and left-sided duplex ureter, thus fulfilling criteria for PELVIS syndrome (perineal hemangioma, external genitalia malformations, lipomyelomeningocele, vesicorenal abnormalities, imperforate anus, and skin tag). Because of perianal location and erosion, this can be mistakenly attributed to sexual abuse. (Photo contributor: Sharon A. Glick, MD.)

for gonorrhea, *Chlamydia*, or *Trichomonas*, this result must be confirmed with a different NAAT that uses an alternate target or by culture. Confirmation prior to treatment is critical in the prepubertal population where the prevalence of STIs is low and the medicolegal significance of a positive result is high. When perinatal acquisition and/or rare nonsexual transmission are unlikely, confirmation of an STI in a child beyond the neonatal period is diagnostic or suspicious for CSA. There is limited peer-reviewed literature on the age at which perinatal transmission can be excluded for STIs. Specialists should therefore be consulted about likelihood of perinatal transmission, particularly in preverbal children who cannot disclose CSA. Postexposure prophylaxis (PEP) for gonorrhea, *Chlamydia*, and *Trichomonas* is not recommended for prepubertal children who are asymptomatic at time of screening. PEP is recommended for teens, particularly when risk of infection is high and the likelihood of returning for treatment is low. Specialists should be consulted about HIV PEP when children present within 72 hours of an acute sexual assault that presents a substantial risk of HIV transmission.

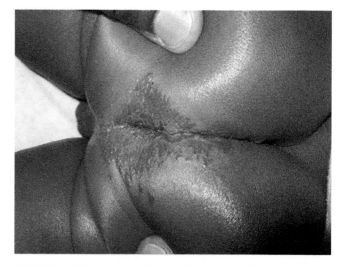

FIGURE 4.12 ▪ Jacquet Diaper Dermatitis Mimicking Sexual Abuse. This severe erythematous erosive eruption is in the differential of diaper dermatitis and can mimic sexual abuse. (Photo contributor: Julie Cantatore-Francis, MD.)

TABLE 4.2 ▪ MANAGEMENT OF SEXUALLY TRANSMITTED INFECTIONS IN YOUNG CHILDREN

Infection	Testing	Prophylaxis and/or Treatment	Sexual Contact	Report Suspected Abuse?
HIV	HIV-1/HIV-2 antigen-antibody immunoassay	Expert consultation	Diagnostic[a]	Yes
Treponema pallidum (syphilis)	VDRL or RPR; if abnormal, FTA-ABS[b]	Penicillin G	Diagnostic[a]	Yes
Neisseria gonorrhea	NAAT[c]; culture preferred for pharynx, anus	Ceftriaxone	Diagnostic[a]	Yes
Chlamydia trachomatis	NAAT[c]; culture preferred for pharynx, anus	Erythromycin, azithromycin, doxycycline	Diagnostic[a]	Yes
Trichomonas vaginalis	NAAT[c], Diamond's media, or InPouch TV culture	Metronidazole, tinidazole	Highly suspicious	Yes
Herpes simplex virus	NAAT[c], or culture	Acyclovir, valacyclovir, famciclovir	HSV-2 highly suspicious HSV-1 suspicious	Yes
Anogenital warts (condyloma acuminata)	Clinical exam: flat, cauliflower or papular warts	Podofilox 0.5% liquid, imiquimod 3.75% or 5% cream, cryotherapy, surgical removal, vaccination	Suspicious[d]	Yes
Bacterial vaginosis	Clue cells, vaginal pH >4.5, positive whiff test	Metronidazole, clindamycin, tinidazole	Unclear	No[e]

[a]When perinatal transmission and rare nonsexual transmission is unlikely.

[b]Venereal Disease Research Laboratory (VDRL) or rapid plasma reagin (RPR); if abnormal, perform a *T pallidum*–specific test (eg, fluorescent treponemal antibody absorption [FTA-ABS]).

[c]Positive nucleic acid amplification test (NAAT) should be confirmed with a different NAAT that uses an alternate target or by culture prior to treatment of a prepubertal child.

[d]First-time anogenital lesions in older children when perinatal transmission, autoinoculation, and diapering are unlikely.

[e]No report if no historical, examination, or other evidence of sexual contact.

Pearls

1. A normal hymen and/or anal examination does not mean sexual abuse did not occur.

2. Sexual contact is the most likely mode of transmission in both young children and teens with *N gonorrhoeae*, *C trachomatis*, and *T vaginalis*.

CONDYLOMATA ACUMINATA

Clinical Summary

Condyloma acuminata (genital warts) are skin-colored, fleshy lesions on mucocutaneous junctions and intertriginous areas that can coalesce into large cauliflower-like lesions. Locations include perianal area, glans penis, scrotum, labia or posterior introitus, vagina, cervix, anus, urethra, mouth, nose, and eyes. Symptoms may include pruritus, burning, bleeding, and pain depending on location and size. Condyloma acuminata is caused by human papillomavirus (HPV), which is prevalent and insidious: >50% of sexually active people are infected, and most infections are asymptomatic, unrecognized, or subclinical and self-limited. Transmission occurs by sexual and nonsexual contact activity. Genital warts in children require careful consideration because approximately 50% are the result of sexual abuse. Serotyping lesions cannot rule out sexual abuse. Nonsexual genital acquisition is usually seen in children younger than 3 years of age occurring via autoinoculation typically from the hands, caregivers with hand warts, genital play among children, and perinatally.

Oncogenic or high-risk HPV types (eg, HPV types 16 and 18) cause cervical cancers and other anogenital cancers. Persistent infection is the strongest risk factor for the development

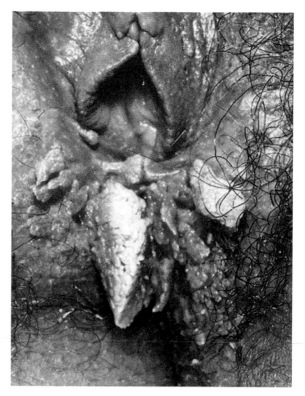

FIGURE 4.14 ■ Condylomata Acuminata due to Sexual Abuse. Venereal warts in a 10-year-old girl who was abused by uncle. (Photo contributor: Binita R. Shah, MD.)

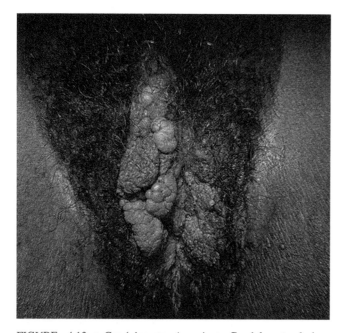

FIGURE 4.13 ■ Condylomata Acuminata. Condylomata lesions grouped into grapelike clusters in a sexually active adolescent girl. These can be pink, red, or skin colored, with a smooth or velvety surface and soft consistency. Lesions may coalesce in the perineal area to form a large cauliflower-like mass. (See also Figure 4.5; Photo contributor: Binita R. Shah, MD.)

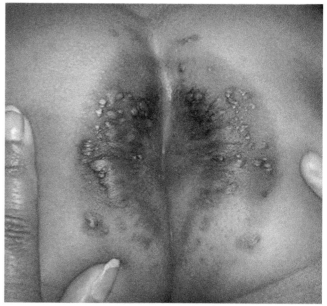

FIGURE 4.15 ■ Condylomata Acuminata. Perianal warts on a young boy evaluated for sexual abuse (treated with topical gentian violet). Infection was most likely due to vertical transmission from mother at birth. (Photo contributor: Sharon A. Glick, MD.)

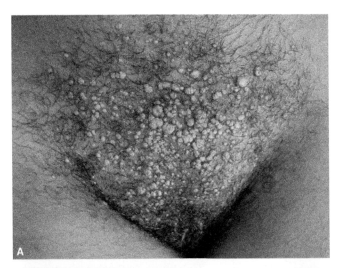

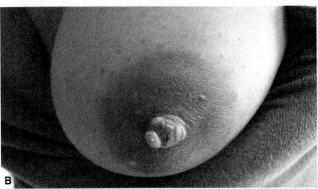

FIGURE 4.16 ■ Condylomata Acuminata. Hundreds of warts on mons pubis (**A**) and a few lesions on breast (**B**) of a teenager with HIV. Warts may occur more frequently and in greater number in the immunocompromised hosts. (Photo contributor: Morgan Rabach, MD.)

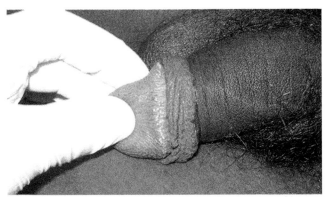

FIGURE 4.17 ■ Pearly Penile Papules; Differential Diagnosis of Condyloma Acuminata. Dome-shaped or hairlike projections on the penile corona are small angiofibromas and represent normal variants that do not require treatment. (Photo contributor: Mark Silverberg, MD.)

of precancerous lesions and cancers. HPV serotypes 6 and 11 account for only 56% of genital warts in children, whereas HPV serotypes 1 to 4, 16, and 18 also contribute. Two HPV vaccines are licensed in the United States: a bivalent vaccine (Cervarix) containing HPV types 16 and 18 and a quadrivalent vaccine (Gardasil) containing HPV types 6, 11, 16, and 18. HPV DNA testing is not recommended because it does not alter clinical management. Differential diagnosis includes condylomata lata, pearly penile papules, and skin tags.

Emergency Department Treatment and Disposition

Untreated, visible warts can resolve on their own, remain unchanged, or increase in size or number. Treatment is aimed at symptom relief, and many factors influence treatment selection including wart size, number, anatomic site, morphology,

patient preference, convenience, adverse effects, and provider experience. The response to therapy is influenced by patient compliance with therapy and the presence of immunosuppression. No treatment has been shown to be superior to any other, and no single treatment is ideal for all patients or all warts. Both patient-applied therapies and provider-administered therapies are available. Patient-applied treatment regimens for external genital warts include podofilox 0.5% solution or gel, imiquimod 5% cream, or sinecatechins 15% ointment. Refer the patient to dermatology if diagnosis is uncertain; the patient is immunocompromised; or warts are fixed, indurated, pigmented, ulcerated, or bleeding. Provider-applied treatment regimens include cryotherapy with liquid nitrogen, surgical removal, curettage, or electrosurgery. When sexual transmission is suspected, screening for other STIs is warranted in addition to history and physical by a child abuse specialist.

Pearls

1. Examination of sexual partners is not required; partners are usually infected at the time a person is diagnosed with HPV infection even in the absence of visible warts.
2. Exclude sexual abuse in children with genital warts.
3. Consult a specialist for management of intra-anal warts because patients may also have warts on the rectal mucosa.
4. Laryngeal papillomatosis has been seen in infants born to mothers with HPV infection delivered vaginally or by cesarean section.

TRICHOMONIASIS

Clinical Summary

T vaginalis infection is almost always sexually transmitted, with peak prevalence rates between the ages of 16 and 35 years. The most common site of infection is the vagina, followed by periurethral glands and urethra. Patients present with pruritus, dysuria, dyspareunia, lower abdominal pain, vaginal discharge, postcoital bleeding, edema and excoriation of the external genitalia, bartholinitis, and urethritis.

Emergency Department Treatment and Disposition

Obtain vaginal secretions for microscopic detection of *Trichomonas* via wet mount (specificity of 60%–70%). NAATs via PCR, such as the Aptima *T vaginalis* assay, performed on vaginal secretions or urine have sensitivity of >95% and specificity >95% and are now considered the gold standard in diagnosis. Culture of *Trichomonas* is warranted when NAATS are unavailable. *T vaginalis* has not been found to infect oral sites, and rectal prevalence appears low; therefore, oral and rectal testing is not recommended.

Treat patients with metronidazole (2 g orally in a single dose *or* 500 mg orally twice a day for 7 days) or tinidazole (2 g orally in a single dose). Both of these regimens have high cure rates of about 95%. Intravaginal or topical metronidazole gel has not been shown to be effective and is not recommended. Certain strains of *T vaginalis* can have diminished susceptibility to metronidazole. If treatment failure occurs with single-dose metronidazole and reinfection is excluded, treat with metronidazole for a 7-day regimen or tinidazole. Treatment of all sex partners is advisable. Because of the high rate of reinfection among patients in whom trichomoniasis is diagnosed, refer the patient to the primary care physician for follow-up.

Pearls

1. Exclude sexual abuse in children with trichomoniasis.
2. Up to 25% to 50% of females may be asymptomatic, whereas up to 75% of males are asymptomatic.
3. Symptomatic females typically have diffuse, malodorous, yellow-green vaginal discharge with vulvar irritation.
4. Cervicitis with hemorrhages, termed "strawberry spots," may be seen in 2% of females.
5. Adverse pregnancy outcomes with trichomoniasis include premature rupture of membranes, preterm delivery, and low birth weight.

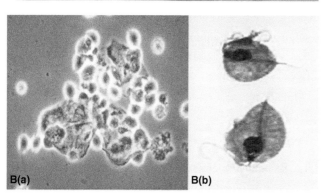

FIGURE 4.18 ■ Trichomoniasis. (**A**) Trichomoniasis caused by *Trichomonas vaginalis*. Note frothy discharge and punctate "strawberry" lesions on cervix. (**B**) *T vaginalis*. Wet mount microscopy [a]. Giemsa stained [b]. (Reproduced with permission from Usatine RP, Smith MA, Mayeaux EJ, et al. *The Color Atlas and Synopsis of Family Medicine*, 3rd ed. McGraw-Hill Education; New York, NY, 2019. [A], and Kline MW. *Rudolph's Pediatrics*. 23rd ed. McGraw-Hill Education; New York, NY, 2018 [B].)

Clinical Summary

Congenital syphilis occurs in babies born to mothers with untreated or inadequately treated syphilis during pregnancy. Transplacental transmission of spirochetes, *Treponema pallidum*, can occur at any stage of pregnancy. Congenital syphilis is divided into early (diagnosed at <2 years of age) and late (diagnosed at >2 years of age). Clinical manifestations are listed in Table 4.3. Infants may present with congenital syphilis after nursery discharge if the mother has early, untreated, asymptomatic primary syphilis with negative serology at delivery (serology is often negative in very early infection) or when the asymptomatic mother's syphilis status was unknown or not reported. Diagnosis relies on clinical findings and reactive syphilis serology (nontreponemal antibody tests such as the Venereal Disease Research Laboratory [VDRL] and rapid plasma reagin [RPR] tests) and is confirmed by a treponemal test (fluorescent treponemal antibody, absorbed [FTA-ABS] and *T pallidum* particle agglutination [TP-PA]). Diagnosis in neonates is difficult, due to lack of clinical signs at birth and because serologic results may reflect maternal antibody status rather than that of the baby. Recommended tests in suspected cases include darkfield microscopy visualization of *T pallidum* or direct fluorescent antibody staining of potentially infected tissues (lesions, umbilical cord, and placenta) or fluids (nasal discharge), CSF or serum PCR for *T pallidum* if available, CBC, serum and CSF examination for VDRL or RPR, cell count and chemistry, liver enzymes, long bone x-rays (usually lower extremities), abdominal US, and an ophthalmologic examination.

Emergency Department Treatment and Disposition

Hospitalize all infants with suspected congenital syphilis for either IV penicillin or IM procaine penicillin therapy for generally 10 days. Therapy is started in the hospital, although IM procaine penicillin can be continued on outpatient basis after diagnostic tests are completed.

Pearl

1. About 60% to 90% of neonates with congenital syphilis are asymptomatic at birth and develop clinical findings within the first 3 months of life.

TABLE 4.3 ■ CLINICAL MANIFESTATIONS OF CONGENITAL SYPHILIS

	Early Congenital Syphilis (presentation <2 years of age)	Late Congenital Syphilis (presentation >2 years of age)
General	Intrauterine growth restriction, lymphadenopathy, pneumonitis, snuffles	Mental retardation, saddle nose, rhagades
Liver	Hepatosplenomegaly, jaundice	
Kidney	Nephrotic syndrome	
Skin	Erythematous maculopapular or papulosquamous or palmoplantar scaling, vesiculobullous hemorrhagic lesions on palms and soles (rare), condyloma lata, and moist patches on lips and mouth	
Bone	Metaphysitis, osteochondritis, periostitis, osteomyelitis, Wimberger sign (bilateral medial tibial metaphyseal osseous destruction)	Hutchinson teeth, frontal bossing, saber shins, and Clutton joints
Blood	Hemolytic anemia, thrombocytopenia, leukopenia, leukocytosis	
Brain	Aseptic meningitis (CSF pleocytosis, elevated CSF protein)	Eighth-nerve deafness, neurosyphilis
Eye	Chorioretinitis, uveitis, glaucoma	Interstitial keratitis

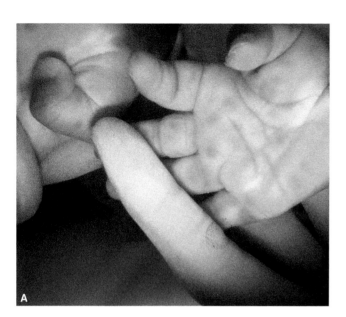
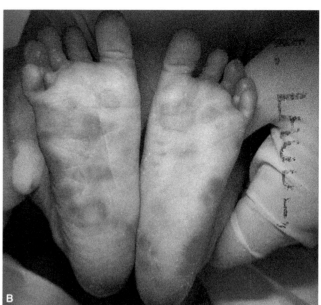

FIGURE 4.19 ▪ Congenital Syphilis. (**A, B**) Erythematous maculopapular round or oval lesions are seen on the hands and feet of a neonate. These lesions fade to coppery brown in color. (Photo contributor: Binita R. Shah, MD.)

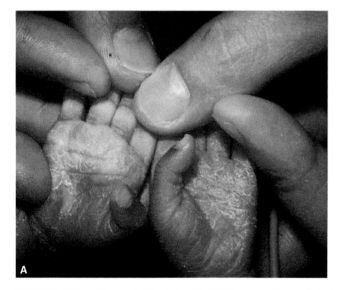
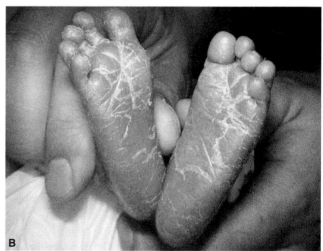

FIGURE 4.20 ▪ Congenital Syphilis. (**A, B**) Desquamation over the hands and feet in a neonate. (Photo contributor: Binita R. Shah, MD.)

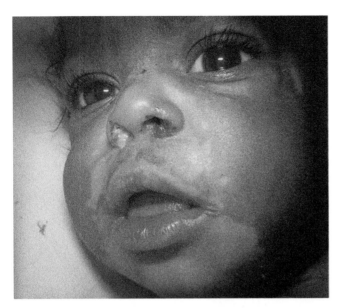

FIGURE 4.21 ■ Snuffles of Congenital Syphilis. Rhinitis of congenital syphilis manifests weeks after birth. Nasal discharge is highly infectious. Postinflammatory hypopigmentation is also seen in this infant due to chronic irritation from nasal discharge. VDRL test was positive with 1:1024 titer. (Photo contributor: Binita R. Shah, MD.)

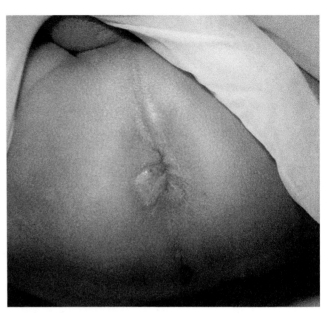

FIGURE 4.22 ■ Condyloma Lata. A single flat-topped, round-oval plaque (formed by papules that coalesce) with a wide base is seen around the anus in this infant. Unlike condylomata acuminata, these lesions are flat and not covered by digitate vegetations. (Photo contributor: Binita R. Shah, MD.)

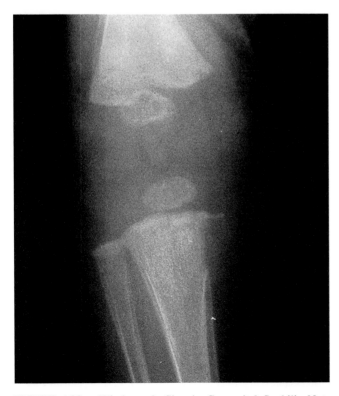

FIGURE 4.23 ■ Wimberger's Sign in Congenital Syphilis. Note metaphyseal lesion along the medial surface of the tibia. These lesions are seen bilaterally and are highly suggestive of congenital syphilis. (Photo contributor: Binita R. Shah, MD.)

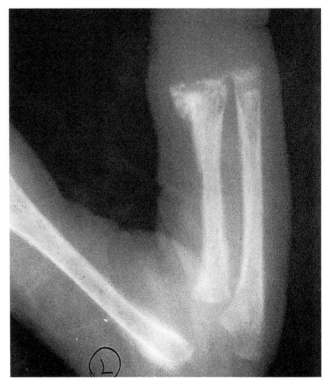

FIGURE 4.24 ■ Bony Lesions in Congenital Syphilis. Metaphysitis, osteochondritis, and periostitis are pathognomonic, and babies with such lesions may present with pseudoparalysis of Parrot (irritability and refusal to move the involved arm or leg due to severe pain). These bone findings are in all extremities (not only in the limb that is painful). (Photo contributor: Binita R. Shah, MD.)

Clinical Summary

Acquired syphilis is contracted through direct sexual contact with ulcerative lesions of skin or mucous membranes of infected people and has 3 stages: primary, secondary, and tertiary. Primary syphilis presents with a round, firm, and painless skin ulcer (chancre) that has a smooth border and a rubbery base. Chancre occurs at the site of contact 10 to 90 days after exposure and heals spontaneously over 3 to 6 weeks. The lesion is usually on the glans penis, cervix, or vagina and less commonly on the lips, nipple, and tongue. Associated painless regional lymphadenopathy may occur 1 to 2 weeks later. Secondary syphilis presents 4 to 10 weeks after the chancre (primary chancre is still present in 10% of patients) usually with a rash that is symmetric and generalized on the trunk, extremities, palms, and soles. Lesions vary and may be polymorphic maculopapular annular, papulopustular, psoriasiform, or follicular; the lesions are often copper colored and nonpruritic. A flu-like syndrome, generalized lymphadenopathy, and splenomegaly may also occur, as may condylomata lata (highly infectious raised white/gray lesions in warm moist areas such as the perineal and anal areas). Some patients have mucous patches in the mouth and alopecia of beard, scalp, or eyebrows. Lesions resolve in 3 to 12 weeks. Tertiary (or late-stage) infection refers to gumma formation (skin, bone, or viscera) and cardiovascular involvement (aortitis). Neurologic infection can occur with any stage of syphilis. Primary and secondary syphilis are sexually transmitted and may be seen in sexually active adolescents or in cases of child abuse. Diagnosis is based on typical skin lesions and confirmed by scraping moist lesions and immediately

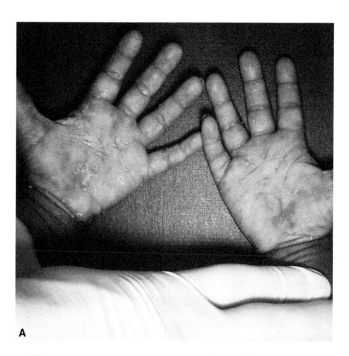

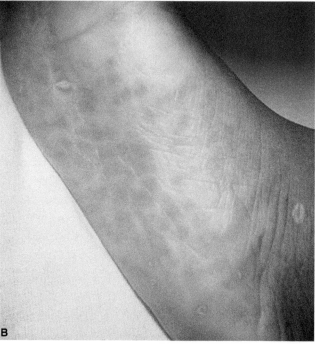

FIGURE 4.26 ■ Secondary Syphilis. (**A, B**) Copper-colored papulosquamous nonpruritic characteristic lesions of secondary syphilis were present on both palms and soles in a 6-year-old girl who was placed in different foster homes since birth and was sexually abused on numerous occasions. (Photo contributor: Binita R. Shah, MD.)

FIGURE 4.25 ■ Primary Syphilis. This teenager showed up in the ED because his girlfriend "made him see a doctor to get the rash on his penis checked out." This totally painless ulcer with raised edges is typical for primary syphilis. (Photo contributor: Mark Silverberg, MD.)

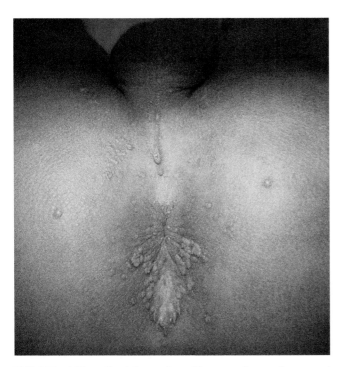

FIGURE 4.27 ■ Condyloma Lata. Flat-topped round to oval plaques (formed by papules that coalesce) with a wide base are seen around the anogenital area in a 5-year-old boy who was repeatedly sexually abused by his stepfather. Unlike condylomata acuminata, these lesions are flat and not covered by digitate vegetations. (Photo contributor: Binita R. Shah, MD.)

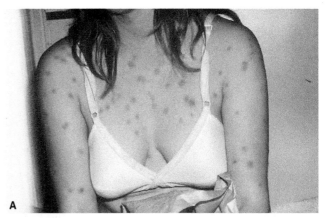

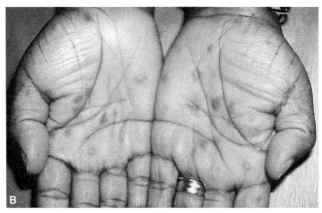

FIGURE 4.28 ■ Secondary Syphilis. (**A, B**) Diffuse papulosquamous lesions with the involvement of palms and soles were seen in this sexually active adolescent patient. (Reproduced with permission from Shah BR, Laude T. *Atlas of Pediatric Clinical Diagnosis.* WB Saunders; Philadelphia, PA, 2000.)

examining the sample with darkfield microscopy. If a darkfield microscope is not available, a slide of the moist material can be made and sent to a laboratory for staining with specific *T pallidum* immunofluorescent antibody. The diagnosis of syphilis (see also page 171) requires both nontreponemal (eg, RPR) and treponemal (eg, FTA-ABS) testing. Generally, standard testing is usually a nontreponemal screening test followed by a confirmatory treponemal test if positive. Nontreponemal antibody titer correlates with disease activity and usually becomes nonreactive after treatment. Most patients with reactive treponemal tests will remain positive for their lifetime regardless of treatment or disease activity. RPR is reactive in only about 80% of patients with primary syphilis at presentation, although darkfield microscopy will be positive. Request test with dilutions of serum in order to prevent a false-negative test due to a prozone phenomenon (most common in secondary syphilis with high titers). False-positive nontreponemal test results may occur due to various medical conditions. All patients who have syphilis should be

tested for HIV infection. Diagnosis of primary or secondary syphilis in a child is evidence of sexual abuse, and the child requires evaluation for other STIs and treatment.

Emergency Department Treatment and Disposition

Treat primary and secondary syphilis with 1 dose of IM benzathine penicillin (50,000 units/kg up to a maximum of 2.4 million units). Nonpregnant patients allergic to penicillin are treated with either doxycycline or tetracycline for 14 days (see the Centers for Disease Control and Prevention's [CDC] STI treatment guidelines). Admit children with suspected primary or secondary syphilis for further evaluation including lumbar puncture and review of the birth mother's medical records to determine if the child has congenital or acquired syphilis. Follow-up requires repeat nontreponemal serologic testing 6 and 12 months after treatment.

Pearls

1. All cutaneous lesions of secondary syphilis are infectious. Relapses can occur up to 1 year after untreated primary infection.

2. Parenteral penicillin is the preferred drug for treatment of all stages of syphilis.

3. Diagnose sexual abuse in any child with postnatally acquired syphilis.

Clinical Summary

Gonorrhea (gonococcal [GC] infections) is one of the most common reportable STIs and is often asymptomatic. Incidence is highest among adolescents. Clinical manifestations are similar to those of *C trachomatis*, and coinfection is frequent. Cervicitis, urethritis, epididymitis, and bartholinitis result from infection. Infection can also spread to cause pelvic inflammatory disease including perihepatitis or pregnancy complications in females. Other susceptible sites of infection include areas of mucosal columnar epithelial cells such as the cervical transition zone, pharynx, rectum, and conjunctiva. Disseminated gonococcal infection (DGI) occurs in up to 3% of infected patients and presents as purulent arthritis or as arthritis-dermatitis syndrome, a triad of tenosynovitis, dermatitis, and polyarthralgias. DGI is more prevalent in females (ratio 4:1), especially those who are pregnant or had menses within the previous 7 days. Other risk factors for DGI include

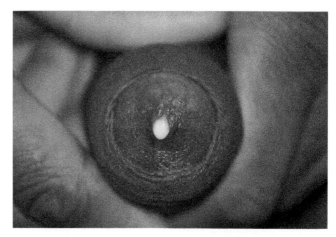

FIGURE 4.30 ■ Gonorrhea. An 18-year-old man with purulent discharge seen at the urethral meatus (discharge expressed by milking the penis). Culture was positive for *N gonorrhoeae*. He was treated for gonorrhea/chlamydia and was advised to inform his sexual partners so that they can receive the treatment. (Photo contributor: Ameer Hassoun, MD.)

pharyngeal gonorrhea, complement deficiency, and immune system diseases such as systemic lupus erythematosus. DGI complications include meningitis, endocarditis, osteomyelitis, pneumonia, and hepatitis. Perinatal GC infection occurs in infants of mothers with GC infection and includes ophthalmia

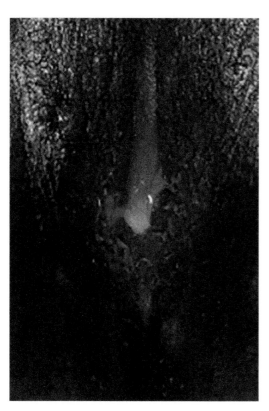

FIGURE 4.29 ■ Gonorrhea. Purulent discharge that grew *N gonorrhoeae* was seen in this sexually active adolescent girl presenting with dysuria and vaginal discharge. (Photo contributor: Binita R. Shah, MD.)

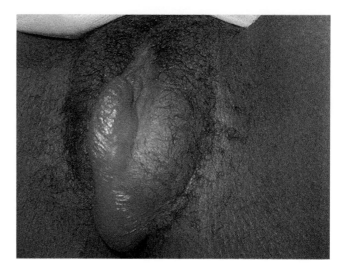

FIGURE 4.31 ■ Bartholin Gland Abscess; Gonococcal Infection. A Bartholin gland abscess (see also Figures 10.44 to 10.45) is a Bartholin glandular or ductal cyst infection usually caused by polymicrobial agents (eg, *N gonorrhoeae*, *Chlamydia trachomatis*, *Escherichia coli*, *Proteus mirabilis*, and anaerobes including *Bacteroides fragilis* and *Peptostreptococcus* spp.). (Photo contributor: Binita R. Shah, MD.)

neonatorum, scalp abscesses at fetal monitor sites, rhinitis, pneumonia, anorectal infections, or disseminated infection.

Emergency Department Treatment and Disposition

Gonorrhea is suspected upon identification of gram-negative intracellular diplococci on Gram stain, with confirmation of diagnosis via culture on Thayer-Martin medium using a type

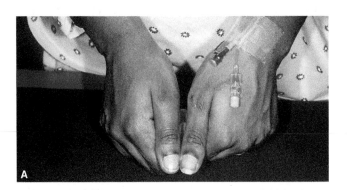

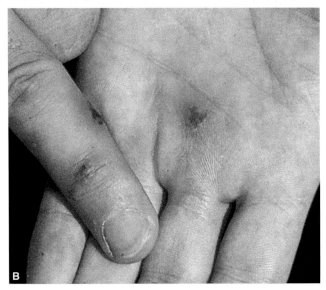

FIGURE 4.32 ▪ Disseminated Gonococcal Infection. (**A**) Swelling of the phalanges of the right thumb and hemorrhagic rash in an adolescent girl. Her blood culture was positive for *N gonorrhoeae*. (**B**) Tender, hemorrhagic, and necrotic pustules on the fingers and palms. (Photo contributor: Binita R. Shah, MD [A], and reproduced with permission from Goldsmith LA, Katz SI, Gilchrest BA, et al. *Fitzpatrick's Dermatology in General Medicine*. 8th ed. McGraw-Hill Education; New York, NY, 2012 [B].)

of chocolate agar, and NAATs (sensitivities and specificities >95%). NAAT testing is the optimal method for diagnosing genital and extragenital GC infections due to its high sensitivity and specificity, rapid results, availability of self-collected vaginal specimens, and identification on urine samples. Culture is useful in failed treatments to determine antimicrobial resistance. In patients with suspected DIG, obtain blood cultures and culture mucosal surfaces.

Treat according to current CDC STI guidelines and with ceftriaxone 250 mg as a single IM dose and azithromycin 1 g as a single oral dose, regardless of chlamydial coinfection status, and with directly observed treatment. Doxycycline 100 mg orally twice daily for 7 days may be administered in cases of intolerance to azithromycin. Do not use quinolone because there are quinolone-resistant *N gonorrhoeae* strains. Admit patients with DGI for IV therapy. Refer to CDC guidelines for the current treatment of complicated GC infections, including extragenital sites, DGI, and infections acquired during pregnancy. Instruct patients to refer their sex partners for evaluation and treatment. Follow-up referrals for counseling and patient education should be provided.

Pearls

1. Diagnose sexual abuse in any child with postnatally acquired gonorrhea.
2. *Treatment failures most often represent reinfection.*
3. Many infections are asymptomatic; thus, screening is important.
4. Symptomatic males infected with genitourinary GC present with dysuria, urinary frequency, and purulent urethral discharge. Symptomatic females infected with genitourinary GC present with abnormal vaginal discharge, intermenstrual bleeding, menorrhagia, or dysuria.
5. DGI is characterized by arthritis/arthralgia, tenosynovitis, and dermatitis (arthritis-dermatitis syndrome).
6. Long-term sequelae in females include tubal scarring, infertility, and ectopic pregnancy.

Clinical Summary

Genital herpes is a lifelong infection with herpes simplex virus (HSV-1 and HSV-2) infection that is sexually transmitted. The majority of genital infections are caused by HSV-2. Most patients infected with HSV-2 have not been diagnosed with genital herpes and have mild or unrecognized infections intermittently shedding virus into the genital tract. Viral shedding is highest during acute eruption of painful vesicular or ulcerative lesions. Recurrences are less symptomatic than primary infections. Incidence of HSV infection increases rapidly after puberty, reaching a peak in the third decade of life.

Emergency Department Treatment and Disposition

A thorough history and physical exam with attention to previous episodes, potentially infected partners, and presence of lesions are critical to diagnosis. Obtain PCR for HSV DNA to

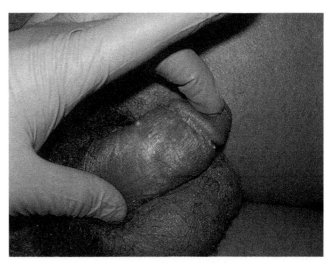

FIGURE 4.34 ■ Genital Herpes. This teenager came to the ED with these very painful sores a few weeks after having sex without a condom. These painful eroded lesions on a red base are quite typical for genital herpes. (Photo contributor: Mark Silverberg, MD.)

diagnose genital herpes. PCR assays have the greatest sensitivity and specificity and are the test of choice for detecting HSV from lesions, in serum, and in spinal fluid. Viral cell culture diagnostic yield is highest early in the course of vesicular eruption, but drops significantly thereafter. Failure to detect HSV does not indicate absence of infection, because viral shedding is intermittent. Treat all patients with a first episode with systemic antiviral drugs such as acyclovir, valacyclovir, or famciclovir. These agents can partially control signs and symptoms of the first clinical episode or recurrent episodes (when given within 1 day of onset of symptoms) or be used as daily suppressive therapy. However, these drugs do not eradicate latent virus and, when stopped, do not affect risk, frequency, or severity of recurrences. Admit patients with severe disease or complications (eg, disseminated infection, pneumonitis, hepatitis, meningitis, or encephalitis) for IV acyclovir therapy. Inform patients with genital herpes that sexual transmission can occur during asymptomatic periods. Advise patients to abstain from sexual activity with uninfected partner(s) when lesions or prodromal symptoms are present and explain the risk of neonatal HSV infection. Pregnant patients should inform their health care providers of HSV infection because delivery via cesarean section is recommended if genital lesions or prodromal symptoms are present during delivery.

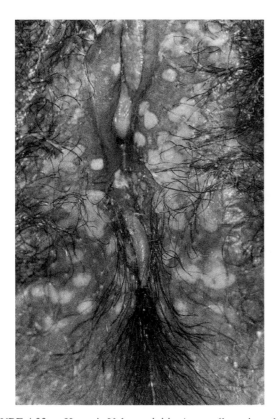

FIGURE 4.33 ■ Herpetic Vulvovaginitis. A sexually active adolescent female patient presented with dysuria, urinary retention, and ulcerated lesions that were surrounded by erythema and edema. Note some of the lesions have coalesced, producing large ulcerated areas and bleeding. This was her first episode of HSV infection. (Photo contributor: Binita R. Shah, MD.)

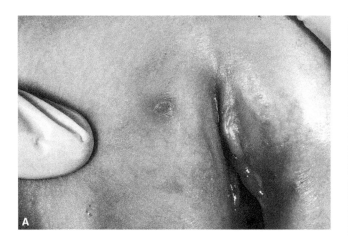

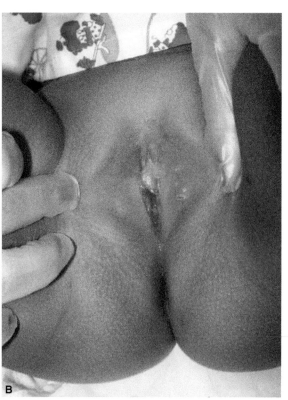

FIGURE 4.35 ■ Herpetic Vulvovaginitis; Sexual Abuse. (**A**) Extremely painful ulcerative lesions (culture-proven HSV type 2) were seen in this girl who was repeatedly abused by her uncle in the past 2 weeks. HSV lesions usually appear after an incubation period of 2 to 20 days after exposure. Genital herpes is uncommon in children. Most HSV-2 genital infections are sexually transmitted in children (except for perinatal transmission at birth). (**B**) These very painful sores on the vulva in this foster child prompted a sexual abuse workup. Foster mother's teenage son was found to be the perpetrator. (Photo contributors: Binita R. Shah, MD [A], and Mark Silverberg, MD [B].)

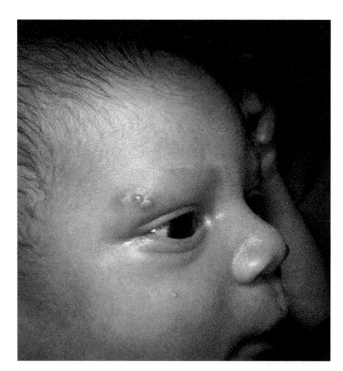

FIGURE 4.36 ■ Herpes Simplex Neonatorum. Infection in the neonate is usually acquired from maternal labial lesions. The risk of transmission to a neonate born to a mother who acquires primary genital HSV infection near the time of delivery is estimated to be 25% to 60%. Localized infection of skin presents with grouped vesicles (seen here) or pustules with varying numbers of lesions seen on the scalp, torso, or extremities usually between the third and sixth days of life; however, lesions may be present at birth (ascending infection) with premature rupture of membranes or with prolonged labor. (Photo contributor: Binita R. Shah, MD.)

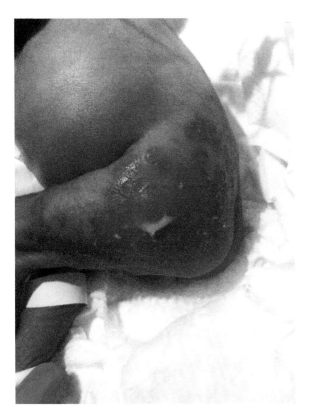

FIGURE 4.37 ■ Herpes Simplex Neonatorum. One-day-old neonate developed this eroded plaque on the left buttock. Birth history was unremarkable except prolonged rupture of membranes leading to cesarean section. He did not respond to systemic antibiotics. On the third day, an eroded plaque expanded with polycyclic borders and satellite erosions and pustules were noted. Diagnosis of cutaneous HSV was confirmed by culture, acyclovir was initiated, and patient responded with resolution of skin findings. (Photo contributor: Deeptej Singh, MD.)

Pearls

1. HSV is the cause of 90% of all vesiculoulcerative lesions of the genitalia.
2. Genital herpes is a recurrent, incurable viral disease.
3. Genital herpes has the ability to become latent and then recur. Latency is lifelong but is interrupted by periods of viral reactivation leading to silent viral shedding.
4. Exclude sexual abuse in any child with acquired HSV.

Clinical Summary

Pelvic inflammatory disease (PID) is an ascending poly-microbial genital tract infection usually found in sexually active females and includes endometritis, parametritis,

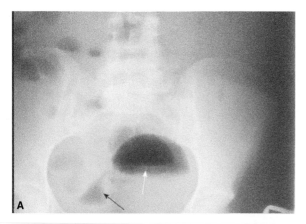

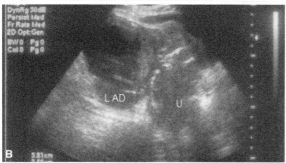

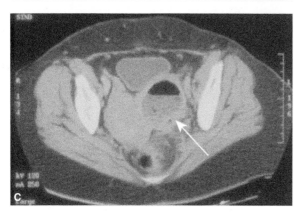

FIGURE 4.38 ■ Tubo-Ovarian Abscess (TOA). (**A**) Plain film of pelvis shows air within uterine cavity (black arrow) and air-fluid level in left adnexa region (white arrow) secondary to left TOA. The abscess contained anaerobic gas-producing organisms, which entered the uterus in a retrograde fashion. (**B**) Corresponding sonographic images show high reflective echoes (air) within the uterus (u) and complex collection, containing highly reflective echoes (air) within the left adnexal region (LAD). (**C**) CT slice of pelvis demonstrates a large left adnexal TOA (arrow). (Photo contributor: Zinn Daniel, MD.)

pelvic peritonitis, salpingitis, oophoritis, tubo-ovarian abscess (TOA), and perihepatitis. Inflammatory disruption of the cervical barrier facilitates movement of microorganisms from the vagina into the normally sterile environment of the uterus. The risk of PID is highest among sexually active females during adolescence (nearly 33% of all cases of PID); females <25 years of age account for 70% of cases. Risk factors for females are younger age, multiple sex partners, unprotected sex, younger age at first intercourse, or previous PID. Menstruation or recent uterine instrumentation (eg, abortion) is believed to facilitate ascension of microorganisms into the upper genital tract. Differential diagnosis of PID includes appendicitis, complications of pregnancy, UTI, reproductive tumors or cysts, adnexal torsion, inflammatory bowel disease, ureteral stones, or calculi.

Emergency Department Treatment and Disposition

Begin empiric treatment with broad-spectrum antibiotics in sexually active females with pelvic or lower abdominal pain, if no cause other than PID can be identified and 1 or more of the following minimum criteria are present on pelvic examination: cervical motion tenderness, uterine tenderness, or adnexal tenderness. Oral temperature >38.3°C (>101°F), abnormal cervical or vaginal mucopurulent discharge, elevated erythrocyte sedimentation rate or elevated C-reactive protein, and

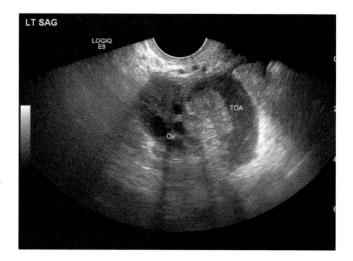

FIGURE 4.39 ■ Tubo-Ovarian Abscess (TOA). An adolescent female with acute pelvic pain. Transvaginal US identifies a normal left ovary (Ov) containing follicles and a distended tubular structure filled with minimally complex material compatible with a TOA. (Photo contributor: Josh Greenstein, MD.)

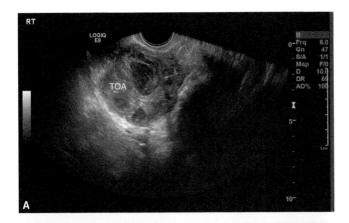

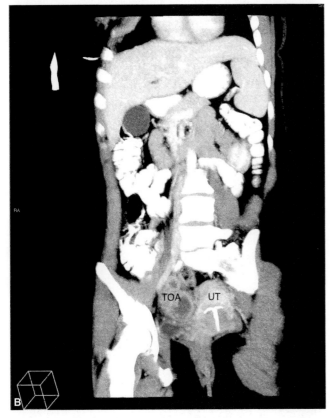

FIGURE 4.40 ■ Tubo-Ovarian Abscess (TOA). A 25-year-old woman with acute right lower quadrant pain. Transvaginal US image [A] demonstrates a complex structure containing hypoechoic tubules and surrounding echogenic inflamed fat. Correlative contrast enhanced oblique maximum intensity projection coronal CT image [B] demonstrates an avidly enhancing tubular structure in the right adnexa compatible with TOA. Adjacent uterus containing an intrauterine device is also seen. (Photo contributor: Josh Greenstein, MD.)

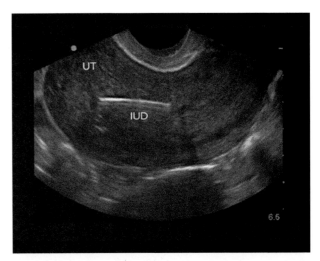

FIGURE 4.41 ■ Intrauterine Device; a Predisposing Factor for Pelvic Inflammatory Disease (PID). A transvaginal image of the uterus (UT) shows a hyperechoic linear foreign body within the endometrial stripe consistent with an intrauterine device (IUD), which increases the risk of PID. (Photo contributor: Michael Secko, MD, RDMS.)

doxycycline. Metronidazole or clindamycin can be added to this regimen with TOA because it provides more effective anaerobic coverage. An outpatient regimen includes a single dose of IM ceftriaxone plus doxycycline given orally with or without metronidazole. Some recommend that all patients be admitted for IV antibiotics. Those with mild or moderate clinical severity may be treated on an outpatient basis. Admit those in whom surgical emergencies (eg, appendicitis) cannot be excluded, those who are pregnant, those who do not respond to or are unable to follow or tolerate an oral regimen, and those with severe illness, nausea, vomiting, or high fever or TOA.

Pearls

1. All females who have PID should also be tested for HIV infection.

2. *N gonorrhoeae* and *C trachomatis* are the most common causative agents of PID, but vaginal and enteric organisms (eg, anaerobes, *Escherichia coli*, genital mycoplasmas, *Gardnerella vaginalis, Streptococcus agalactiae*) also contribute to its pathogenesis.

3. Complications of PID include peritonitis, perihepatitis (Fitz-Hugh–Curtis syndrome), TOA, and adhesions leading to infertility, ectopic pregnancy, and chronic pain.

laboratory documentation of cervical infection with *N gonorrhoeae* or *C trachomatis* also support the diagnosis of PID.

Recommended treatment regimens (refer to CDC STI guidelines) include IV regimen of cefotetan or cefoxitin plus

Clinical Features

Abnormal uterine bleeding (AUB), previously termed *dysfunctional uterine bleeding*, is irregular and/or excessive vaginal bleeding often secondary to excessively thickened endometrial sloughing, frequently in the setting of anovulation, and

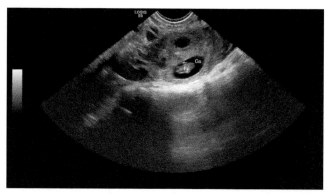

FIGURE 4.43 ■ Ectopic Pregnancy. An adolescent female with a positive pregnancy test and right lower quadrant pain presented with vaginal bleeding. Transvaginal sonogram demonstrates a gestational sac (Gs) with fetal pole (Fp) in the right adnexa compatible with ectopic pregnancy. No intrauterine gestation is present. (Photo contributor: Josh Greenstein, MD.)

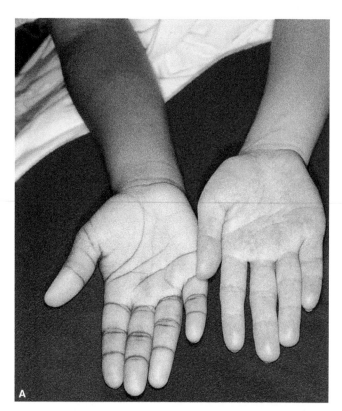

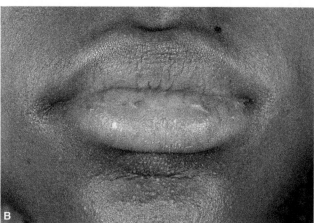

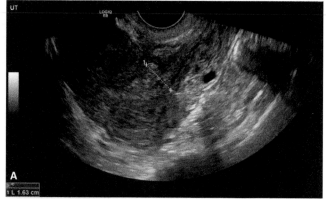

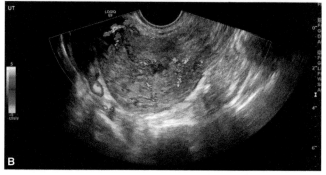

FIGURE 4.42 ■ Extreme Pallor in Abnormal Uterine Bleeding. (**A, B**) A 13-year-old adolescent girl (menarche at 12 years) presented with a history of bleeding for 19 days, feeling tired, weak, pale (hemoglobin/hematocrit: 4.8/15.1), and tachycardic with orthostatic changes. Pallor of her hand (compared with an examiner's hand) and lips is shown. (Photo contributor: Binita R. Shah, MD.)

FIGURE 4.44 ■ Incomplete Abortion. Transvaginal US of a 20-year-old woman presenting to the ED with lower abdominal pain and vaginal bleeding. Pelvic examination showed blood in the vaginal vault with dilated cervical os. (**A**) A thickened endometrial complex measuring 1.6 cm (normal <1.5 cm) containing heterogeneous material is seen. (**B**) Complex material demonstrates color Doppler flow. These findings are consistent with retained products of conception. She underwent dilation and curettage, which confirmed the diagnosis. (Photo contributors: Jonathan Stern, MD, and Ryan Logan Webb, MD.)

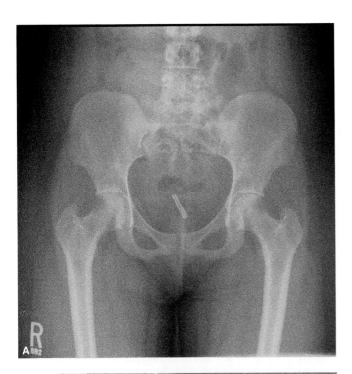

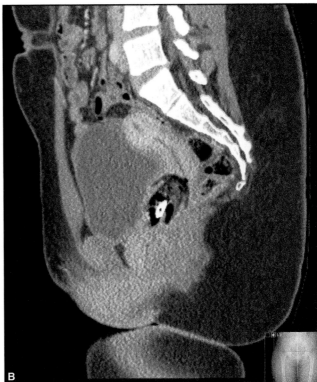

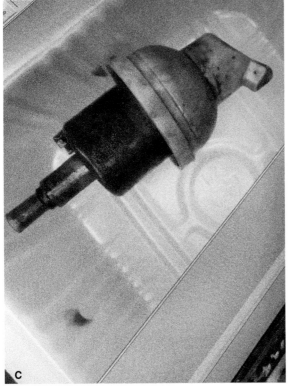

FIGURE 4.45 ■ Intravaginal Foreign Body. An 18-year-old woman with bipolar disorder presented with a history of foul-smelling bloody vaginal discharge for about 6 months. A foreign body (FB) was felt on the pelvic examination but could not be removed. (**A**) Frontal x-ray of the pelvis demonstrates a metallic spring within the lower pelvis region. (**B**) Sagittal CT image with IV contrast shows a metallic FB located inferior to the uterus and between the urinary bladder and rectum. There are surrounding locules of gas and debris. (**C**) Examination and removal of the FB under anesthesia revealed the top of a liquid soap dispenser containing a metal spring in the vagina. The plastic component was not visible on x-ray or CT because plastic is not radiodense. (Photo/legend contributors: Dimpy Mody, MD, Joanne Sheu, MD, and Richard Hong, MD.)

in the absence of structural pathology or anomaly. Up to 50% of menstrual cycles are anovulatory in the first year after menarche and become ovulatory approximately 20 months later. Normal menstrual cycles during adolescence are 21 to 40 days long, with 2 to 7 days of bleeding (20–80 mL of blood loss per cycle). AUB is a common menstrual problem during adolescence, and when severe, it can result in life-threatening anemia. Menorrhagia is prolonged or heavy uterine bleeding that occurs at regular intervals. Metrorrhagia is uterine bleeding that occurs at irregular intervals. Menometrorrhagia is prolonged or heavy bleeding that occurs at irregular intervals. AUB encompasses amenorrhea, menses at irregular intervals or irregular duration, excessive bleeding, or "break-through bleeding." Causes include anovulatory bleeding, polycystic ovarian syndrome, pregnancy and pregnancy-related complications, STIs, bleeding disorders, thyroid disease or other endocrine disorders, life or physical stressors, and medication or drug use.

Emergency Department Treatment and Disposition

Obtain a through history focused on menstrual history, sexual history (including past STIs, pelvic inflammatory disease), history of systemic illness (eg, kidney or liver disease), endocrine history (symptoms of hypothyroidism or hyperthyroidism or hyperandrogenism), use of hormonal contraception or exogenous hormones, other medications, history of other prolonged bleeding or bruising, history of trauma, and family history of polycystic ovarian disease or bleeding diathesis.

Order a pregnancy test, CBC, STI screening if applicable, thyroid function tests, coagulation profile, liver enzymes, BUN, creatinine, type and cross-match (if transfusion is anticipated), and prolactin if a pituitary tumor is suspected. Obtain pelvic US to evaluate for possible structural anomalies or if the pregnancy test is positive. Severe bleeding with hemodynamic instability requires immediate intervention with IV fluids and/or blood transfusions.

If possible, determine whether AUB occurs in the setting of irregular, excessive, or intermenstrual bleeding to narrow differential diagnosis and whether there is a history of amenorrhea. Gynecologic consult may be warranted to guide therapies or further evaluation.

Treatment for AUB including anovulatory bleeding begins with establishing hemodynamic stability with blood transfusion as necessary. If the patient is hemodynamically stable without the concern for significant blood loss in the acute setting, outpatient management may be attempted with close gynecologic follow-up. This may include iron supplementation of 60 mg of elemental iron daily in the setting of anemia and exogenous hormone therapies to return to a pattern of normal menses. Patients should be counseled to keep a menstrual calendar. Hemodynamically unstable patients or patients with severe anemia require stabilization, transfusion, gynecologic consult, and admission.

Pearls

1. The most common reason for AUB during adolescence is anovulatory noncyclic menstrual bleeding secondary to a physiologically immature hypothalamic-pituitary-gonadal axis.

2. While anovulatory bleeding is the most common single cause of AUB in pediatric patients, other causes (eg, pregnancy, endocrinopathies, blood dyscrasias, STIs) should be considered during ED evaluation.

Clinical Summary

Ectopic pregnancy, the implantation of a fertilized egg in the fallopian tube instead of the endometrium (uterus), is the leading cause of maternal morbidity in the first trimester of pregnancy. The most common risk factors are previous tubal infections (eg, PID), previous ectopic pregnancy, prior tubal surgery, and tubal adhesions from a previous appendicitis or abdominal pelvic surgery. Patients may present with mild vaginal bleeding to massive hemorrhage. Acutely ruptured ectopic pregnancy presents with sudden onset of extremely sharp or stabbing unilateral pain, as well as shoulder pain.

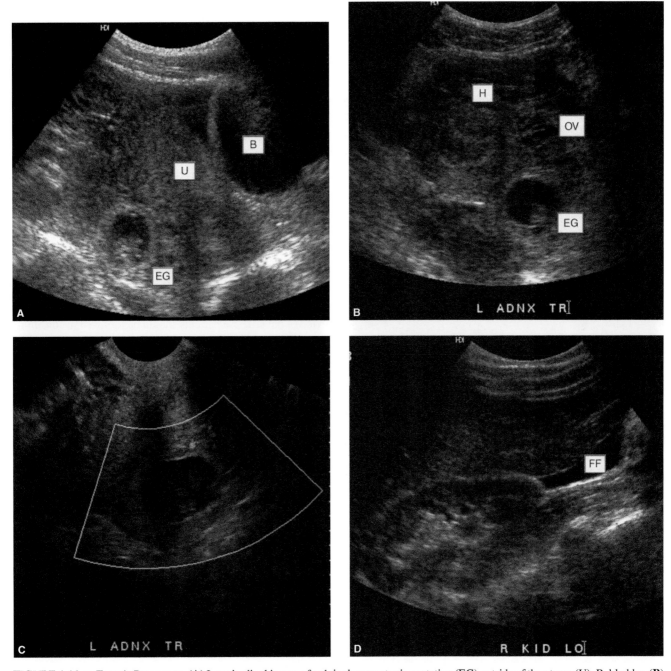

FIGURE 4.46 ■ Ectopic Pregnancy. (**A**) Longitudinal image of pelvis shows ectopic gestation (EG) outside of the uterus (U). B, bladder. (**B**) Longitudinal image of EG in left adnexal region, separate from left ovary (OV) and surrounded by hemorrhage (H). (**C**) Transvaginal image demonstrates fetal pole in EG sac, in left adnexal region. The gestation was live. (**D**) Longitudinal image of right kidney shows free fluid (FF) in Morrison pouch. (Photo contributor: Rachelle Goldfisher, MD.)

Other acute symptoms include dizziness or loss of consciousness from acute intraperitoneal hemorrhage. Differential diagnosis of ectopic pregnancy includes threatened or incomplete abortion, molar pregnancy, ruptured corpus luteum cyst, adnexal torsion, UTI, appendicitis, PID, and ureteral calculi.

Emergency Department Treatment and Disposition

Obtain US to determine if there is intrauterine pregnancy (IUP), which excludes the diagnosis of ectopic pregnancy in singleton pregnancies. The appearance of a gestational sac at

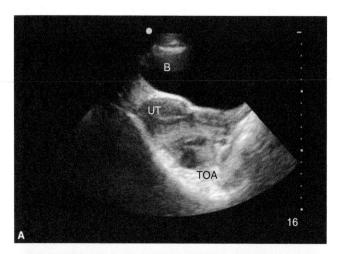

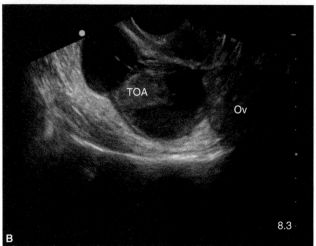

about 5 weeks of pregnancy is the first significant finding on US suggestive of an IUP; however, a definitive diagnosis of IUP should be deferred until a yolk sac is present. Serial measurements of serum β-human chorionic gonadotropin (β-hCG) is useful for trending pregnancy, with increases by at least 66% every 48 hours in a normal pregnancy within the first 30 days after implantation. If β-hCG levels are unchanged or increasing more slowly than normal, the pregnancy is abnormal (it may be an abnormal IUP, or it may be an ectopic pregnancy). Pregnancies that have lower than normal β-hCG levels are more likely to be ectopic. Additional laboratory work includes CBC, type and screen, and coagulation profile.

Ruptured ectopic pregnancy is a surgical emergency. Unstable patients require aggressive resuscitation with fluid and blood followed by surgery. Begin transfusion if clinically indicated, but do not delay surgery for transfusion. Emergency surgery is necessary to stop the bleeding and try to preserve at least a portion of the affected fallopian tube, if it is not completely ruptured. Oophorectomy is not indicated unless the ovary is bleeding uncontrollably or has other pathology. If ectopic pregnancy is probable or possible, management depends on presence of risk factors, serial measurements of serum β-hCG levels, and results of transvaginal US over a period of days. These patients should be followed in consultation with an obstetrician on an outpatient basis.

Pearls

1. Ectopic pregnancies must be considered in pregnant patients with pelvic pain, particularly early in gestation and if associated with abnormal uterine spotting or bleeding.
2. Ectopic pregnancy is suspected if transvaginal US shows no IUP in the setting of positive pregnancy test.

FIGURE 4.47 ■ Tubo-Ovarian Abscess (TOA); Differential Diagnosis of Ectopic Pregnancy. (**A**) A transabdominal sonogram from a phased array probe reveals sagittal view of the uterus (UT) with a cystic adnexal mass posterior to the uterus. B, bladder. (**B**) A transvaginal sonogram reveals complex adnexal structure with an adjacent cystic structure with internal septations. Ov, ovary. (Photo contributor: Michael Secko, MD, RDMS.)

Chapter 5

CARDIOLOGY

Shyam K. Sathanandam
Sushitha Surendran

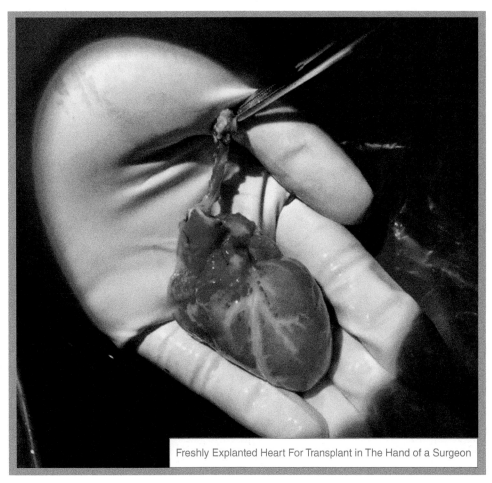

Freshly Explanted Heart For Transplant in The Hand of a Surgeon

(Photo contributor: TK Susheel Kumar, MD)

The authors acknowledge the special contributions of Binita R. Shah, MD, to prior edition.

Clinical Summary

Bradycardia is defined as a heart rate below the normal range for age, and its various etiologies are mentioned in Table 5.1. Clinically significant bradycardia is defined as a heart rate <60 beats per minute (bpm) associated with poor systemic perfusion. Signs of circulatory impairment include poor skin perfusion with pallor; cyanosis; cool mottled extremities; prolonged capillary refill; thready, weak, or absent peripheral pulses; and discrepancy in volume between peripheral and central pulses. Patient is irritable, lethargic, and confused, or has decreased level of consciousness. Respiratory difficulty, decreased pulse pressure of >20 mm Hg, hypotension (decompensated shock), and decreased or no urine output can also be found when severe. The spectrum of bradyarrhythmias includes sinus bradycardia, sinus node dysfunction, sinus node arrest with a slow junctional or ventricular escape rhythm, and atrioventricular (AV) block.

An ECG is necessary to exclude second-degree or complete heart block (CHB). Findings on ECG include a slow heart rate with P waves that may or may not be visible. QRS duration may be normal or prolonged (depending on the location of the intrinsic cardiac pacemaker). Dissociation of P waves and QRS is seen in CHB. P wave with a normal PR interval preceding each QRS complex is seen in sinus bradycardia.

Emergency Department Treatment and Disposition

Patients with bradycardia *not* associated with evidence of poor systemic perfusion need support of ABCs (airway, breathing, and circulation), observation, and reassessment. Hospitalize patient for continued observation, and consult cardiology for asymptomatic bradycardia from drug ingestion, bradycardia resulting from complete AV block or acquired or congenital heart disease (CHD), or patients with refractory bradycardia requiring pacing.

Bradycardia causing cardiorespiratory compromise requires emergent intervention. For symptomatic bradycardia due to hypoxemia (*a sign of cardiopulmonary failure and impending cardiopulmonary arrest*) establish a patent airway. Assist breathing with delivery of 100% oxygen. Perform chest compressions if the patient fails to improve (patient remains unresponsive or flaccid with poor systemic perfusion) or if the heart rate remains <80 bpm in neonates or <60 bpm in infants or children. Pharmacologic interventions are required if there is no response to effective oxygenation and ventilation. Epinephrine is the initial drug of choice. Atropine usually is not effective for hypoxic-ischemic–induced bradycardia. A continuous epinephrine, isoproterenol, or dopamine infusion titrated to effect may be required. For symptomatic

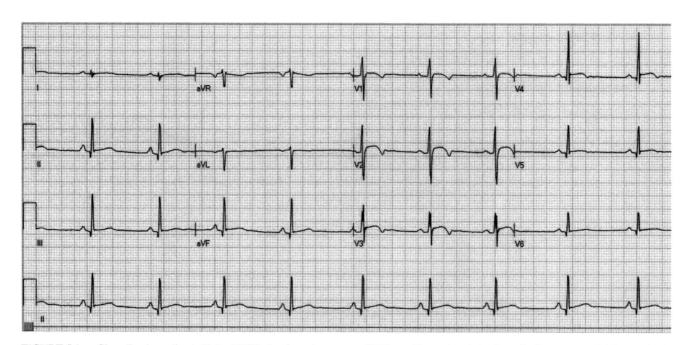

FIGURE 5.1 ■ Sinus Bradycardia. A 12-lead ECG showing a heart rate of 58 bpm. The patient is in sinus rhythm as every QRS complex is preceded by a P wave, a QRS complex follows every P wave, and the P-wave axis is normal. This could be a normal phenomenon in well-trained athletes. (Photo contributor: Shyam K. Sathanandam, MD.)

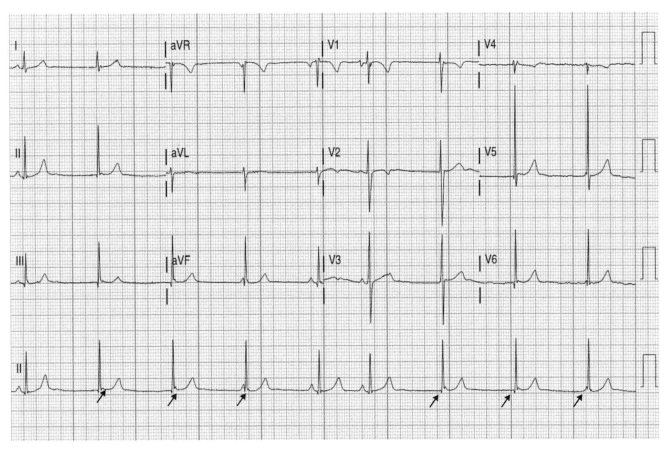

FIGURE 5.2 ■ Sinus Bradycardia with Junctional Escape Rhythm. A 12-lead ECG showing a heart rate of 53 bpm with junctional escape rhythm (arrows) indicated by narrow QRS complex and no relationship between QRS complex and preceding P waves. The P waves and QRS complex are very close to each other, with occasional P waves embedded within the QRS complex. (Photo contributor: Sushitha Surendran, MD.)

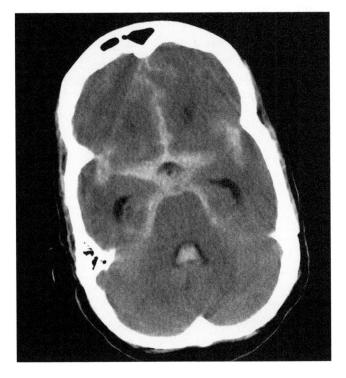

FIGURE 5.3 ■ Differential Diagnosis of Bradycardia. Subarachnoid hemorrhage (SAH) presenting with Cushing triad. A noncontrast head CT scan shows hyperdensity in the basal cisterns in the area of the circle of Willis, with blood in the fourth ventricle (findings typical of SAH) in an adolescent boy presenting to the ED with sudden onset of severe headache, increasing lethargy, and obtundation. Patient had bradycardia, irregular respirations, and hypertension (Cushing triad secondary to increased intracranial pressure). (Photo contributor: Mark Silverberg, MD.)

TABLE 5.1 ■ NORMAL HEART RATE RANGES AND ETIOLOGIES OF BRADYCARDIA

Age	Resting Heart Rate in bpm
Birth–1 week	90–160
1 week–1 year	100–170
1–2 years	80–150
3–7 years	70–135
7–10 years	65–130
11–15 years	60–120

Etiologies of Bradycardia

Respiratory
- During cardiopulmonary resuscitation (CPR; intubated patient): mnemonic *DOPE*

  *D*islodged endotracheal tube (ET) (eg, esophageal intubation or migration to right mainstem bronchus)

  *O*bstructed ET tube (mucus plug)

  *P*neumothorax (inadequate ventilation)

  *E*quipment failure (lack of oxygen leading to hypoxemia)
- Pneumomediastinum

Cardiovascular
- Excessive vagal stimulation (eg, induced by suctioning)
- Cardiomyopathy
- Postoperative atrial cardiac surgery for CHD
- Inflammatory myocarditis

Other
- Increased intracranial pressure (Cushing triad: bradycardia, hypertension, irregular respirations)
- Hypothyroidism

Important contributory causes: H's and T's of CPR:

Hypoxemia	Tension pneumothorax
Hypovolemia	Tamponade
Heart block	Toxins/poisons/drugs (eg,
Hypothermia	organophosphates, cloni-
Head injury	dine, β-blockers, calcium
Hyperkalemia	channel blockers)

TABLE 5.2 ■ COMMON CAUSES OF SINUS BRADYCARDIA

- Conditioned athletes
- Medications
- Hypothyroidism
- Hypothermia
- Anorexia

bradycardia due to vagal stimulation, cholinergic drug toxicity, or primary AV block, atropine is the drug of choice. Vagally induced bradycardia usually resolves once the stimulation is withdrawn. Atropine is very effective if used prophylactically before vagal stimulation in procedures such as endotracheal intubation.

Pacing is not helpful in children with bradycardia secondary to postarrest hypoxic-ischemic myocardial insult. It may be helpful for bradycardia caused by acquired heart disease or CHD causing CHB or sinus node dysfunction. Options include transcutaneous, transvenous, or transesophageal pacing.

Pearls

1. Asymptomatic sinus bradycardia can occur as a normal variant during deep sleep and is also common in highly trained athletes.
2. Most common causes of symptomatic bradycardia are hypoxemia and vagal stimulation, and if not corrected, it may degenerate into full cardiac arrest.
3. Serious causes could include tension pneumothorax and increased intracranial pressure.

Clinical Summary

First-degree AV block is defined as prolongation of the PR interval beyond the norm for age. The PR interval is determined by the point of conduction from the sinus node to the onset of QRS. PR interval is measured from the beginning of P wave to the beginning of QRS complex. The PR interval and QRS duration are age-dependent measures of AV conduction. Impaired conduction is described as first-degree, second-degree, or third-degree heart block (Table 5.3). The normal PR interval changes with both age and heart rate, but it is more age dependent. The AV node is usually the site of conduction delay, although it may occur in the atrium or the infranodal level. ECG findings of first-degree AV block include a regular rhythm that originates in the sinus node with a prolonged PR interval and a normal QRS morphology. First-degree AV block can be a normal finding in approximately 8% of children, and other conditions are mentioned in Table 5.4.

Emergency Department Treatment and Disposition

Consult cardiology, and hospitalize patients with first-degree heart block associated with underlying serious heart disease (eg, acute rheumatic fever, myocarditis) for evaluation and appropriate therapy.

Pearl

1. First-degree AV block alone *does not* lead to hemodynamic compromise and does not need any specific therapy.

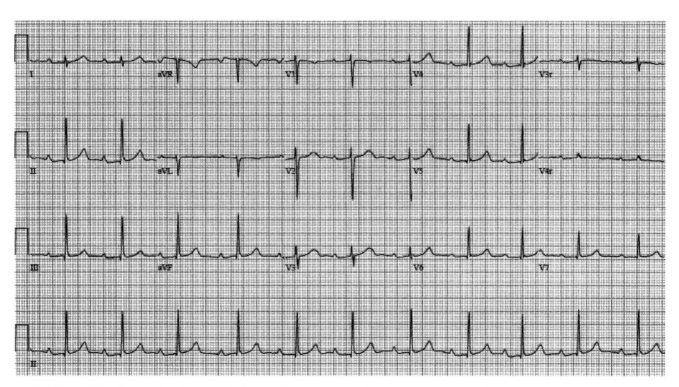

FIGURE 5.4 ■ First-Degree Heart Block. A 12-lead ECG demonstrates a heart rate of 94 bpm and sinus rhythm. The PR interval measures 160 milliseconds, demonstrating first-degree AV block in a patient presenting with acute rheumatic fever (ARF). Prolongation of the PR interval is among the minor modified Jones criteria required for the diagnosis of ARF. The PR interval is measured from the beginning of the P wave to the beginning of the QRS complex. (Photo contributor: Shyam Sathanandam, MD.)

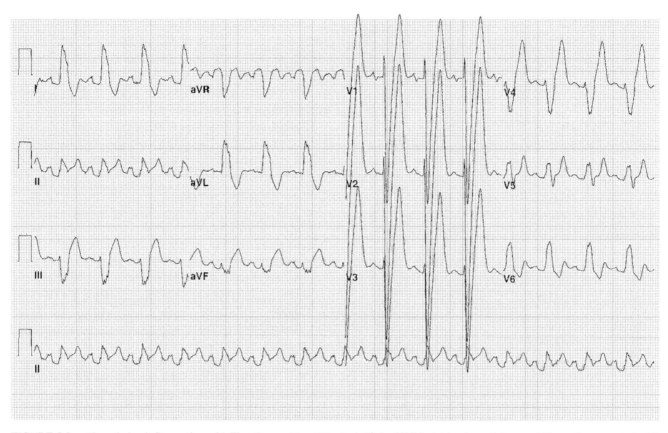

FIGURE 5.5 ■ Hyperkalemia Presenting with First-Degree Heart Block. A 12-lead ECG obtained on a 15-year-old boy who presented with respiratory distress and syncope. The ECG shows sinus rhythm, 92 bpm, first-degree AV block (PR = 0.21 seconds), broad notched P waves, left bundle branch block, diffuse ST abnormalities, and tall tented T waves. His serum potassium level was 7.6 secondary to renal failure. (Photo contributor: Shyam Sathanandam, MD.)

TABLE 5.3 ■ ATRIOVENTRICULAR (AV) BLOCKS

- First-degree AV block: conduction of all atrial impulses into the ventricles, but AV conduction is slower than normal
- Second-degree AV block: intermittent AV conduction (some atrial impulses reach the ventricles and others are blocked)
- Third-degree AV block: complete interruption of AV conduction

TABLE 5.4 ■ FIRST-DEGREE ATRIOVENTRICULAR (AV) BLOCK

- First-degree AV block is present if:
  Infants: PR interval >0.14 second
  Children: PR interval >0.16 second
  Adolescents: PR interval >0.2 second

Conditions Associated with First-Degree AV Block
- Healthy persons (with normal hearts)
- Increased vagal tone (of any etiology)
- Cardiomyopathy
- Untreated congenital heart disease (eg, atrial septal defect, ventricular septal defect)
- Acute rheumatic fever
- Therapy with antiarrhythmic agents (eg, digitalis, β-blockers, calcium channel blockers, amiodarone)
- Postoperative congenital heart disease
- Myocarditis (of any etiology)
- Hyper- or hypokalemia, hyper- or hypocalcemia, hypomagnesemia, hypoglycemia

Clinical Summary

Second-degree AV block is diagnosed when 1 or more (but not all) of the atrial impulses fail to conduct to the ventricles due to impaired conduction. Two distinct types of second-degree AV block are *type I* second-degree AV block (also known as Mobitz I or Wenckebach periodicity) and *type II* second-degree AV block (also known as Mobitz II) (Table 5.5). Mobitz type I heart block can occur as a normal variant (without any symptoms) in children. Patients with Mobitz type II may present with syncope or heart failure. Causes of second-degree AV block include myocarditis, atrial septal defect, acute rheumatic fever, Ebstein anomaly, cardiomyopathy, structural congenital heart disease, drug toxicity (eg, digitalis, β-blockers), increased vagal tone (any etiology), and following surgery near the AV junction. Mobitz type II can also be seen in patients who develop rejection after cardiac transplantation and patients with posttransplantation coronary artery disease. Diagnosis is confirmed by ECG. A CXR may show cardiomegaly, depending on the underlying etiology (eg, myocarditis, cardiomyopathy).

Emergency Department Treatment and Disposition

Evaluate patient and consult cardiology to determine the underlying etiology for the second-degree heart block. Hospitalize patients who are newly diagnosed, those with postcardiac surgery heart block, and symptomatic patients (eg, syncope or dizzy spells) because they may need pacemaker implantation. Mobitz type I AV block by itself does not require any specific therapy. The prognosis of Mobitz type II AV block associated with a wide QRS complex is more ominous, as it may progress to CHB. Emergent treatment is required if signs of hypoperfusion are present with slow ventricular rates. Atropine is the preferred drug. Isoproterenol can be used with caution (eg, in patients with digoxin toxicity); transcutaneous cardiac pacing may be required for patients not responding to atropine. A permanent cardiac pacemaker is required if symptoms of presyncope or syncope occur.

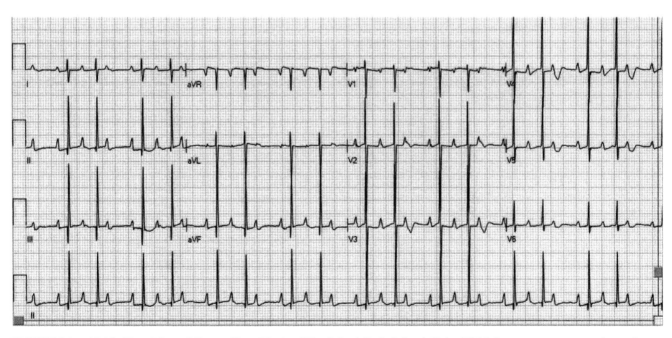

FIGURE 5.6 ■ Mobitz Type I Second-Degree Heart Block or Wenckebach Periodicity. A 12-lead ECG demonstrates a progressive prolongation of the PR interval seen on the ECG on consecutive beats followed by a blocked P wave. This is because of the decremental property of the AV node. After the dropped QRS complex, the PR interval resets, and the cycle repeats giving the impression of paired QRS complexes. (Photo contributor: Shyam Sathanandam, MD.)

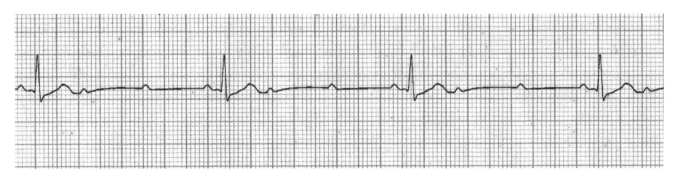

FIGURE 5.7 ■ Mobitz Type II Second-Degree Heart Block. A rhythm strip demonstrating 3:1 AV block. The atrial rate as measured by the P-P interval is 100/min, but only every third P wave is followed by a QRS complex. The PR interval is normal, suggesting the level of block is not at the level of the AV node or above the AV node. This type of second-degree AV block, called Mobitz type II block, is more pathologic because the site of the block is in the more distal conduction system (His-Purkinje system). (Photo contributor: Shyam Sathanandam, MD.)

Pearls

1. Mobitz type I heart block is often transient (eg, seen with myocarditis).
2. Mobitz type II heart block is usually permanent and implies structural damage to the infranodal conducting system.

TABLE 5.5 ■ SECOND-DEGREE ATRIOVENTRICULAR (AV) HEART BLOCK

Mobitz Type I AV Block (Wenckebach Block)

Characteristic features:
- PP interval remains constant.
- Progressive prolongation of the PR interval over several beats until 1 QRS complex drops (usually only a single atrial impulse is blocked).
- After the dropped beat, AV conduction returns to normal.
- Normal QRS morphology.
- Above cycle repeats itself; however, the number of beats in each cycle may not be constant.
- *Some (but not all) atrial impulses fail to conduct to the ventricle.*
- Atrial rate is greater than the ventricular rate.
- Site of the block is almost always at the AV node.
- Normal AV node exposed to very fast atrial rates leads to Wenckebach phenomenon.
- AV block is often due to *reversible depression* of AV nodal conduction.
- No hemodynamic compromise and progression to CHB is unlikely.
- A small percentage may have progressive conduction system disturbance.

Mobitz Type II AV Block

Characteristic features:
- Sudden AV conduction failure.
- QRS drops after a normal P wave.
- One or more beats may be nonconducted at a single time.
- *Absence* of preceding prolongation of the PR interval in normal conducted beats (*thus PR interval remains constant before and after the nonconducted atrial beats*).
- QRS interval may be prolonged (unlike Mobitz type I block).
- Site of block is in the more distal AV conduction system (His-Purkinje system).
- Rhythm may progress to CHB.

Clinical Summary

Third-degree AV block (also known as complete heart block [CHB]; Table 5.6) is a condition in which no impulses from the atria reach the ventricles. Because the impulse is blocked, an accessory pacemaker will typically activate the ventricles (an *escape rhythm*). Third-degree heart block is rare in the pediatric age group. Signs and symptoms in patients with an otherwise normal heart vary. Patients could be bradycardic and asymptomatic. Older children may present with syncope (syncope from a high-degree AV block not related to positional changes or exertion is called a *Stokes-Adams attack*). Older infants may present with night terrors, irritability, or tiredness with frequent naps. Acquired heart block is frequently symptomatic, or present with syncope, congestive heart failure (CHF), shock, or sudden death. Peripheral pulses may be prominent secondary to large compensatory stroke volume. CXR may show cardiomegaly secondary to increased diastolic ventricular filling.

Emergency Department Treatment and Disposition

Hospitalize patients presenting with symptoms (eg, syncope, CHF) or patients newly diagnosed with CHB. Newly diagnosed patients with CHB need an echocardiogram to rule out structural heart disease or myocarditis. Symptomatic newborns (eg, heart failure, evidence of hydrops) with CHB with ventricular rates ≤55 bpm require cardiac pacing. Those with structural heart disease will need a pacemaker if the heart rate is <70 bpm regardless of symptoms. Adrenergic agents (eg, epinephrine or isoproterenol) or a vagolytic agent (eg, atropine) may be tried to increase the heart rate while awaiting placement of the pacemaker. Cardiac pacing (transthoracic, transcutaneous, or transvenous) is also required in symptomatic patients with CHB and CHD. Temporary pacing may be required in postoperative CHB following surgery for CHD.

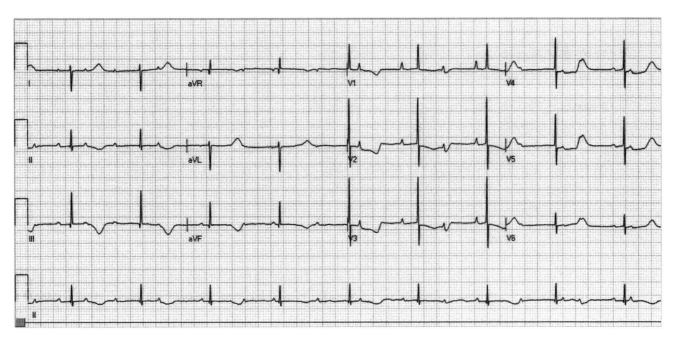

FIGURE 5.8 ■ Complete Heart Block. A 12-lead ECG demonstrates a third-degree AV block with an atrial rate of 92/min and ventricular rate of 42/min. There is no constant relationship between the P waves and the QRS complexes, demonstrating AV dissociation. (Photo contributor: Shyam Sathanandam, MD.)

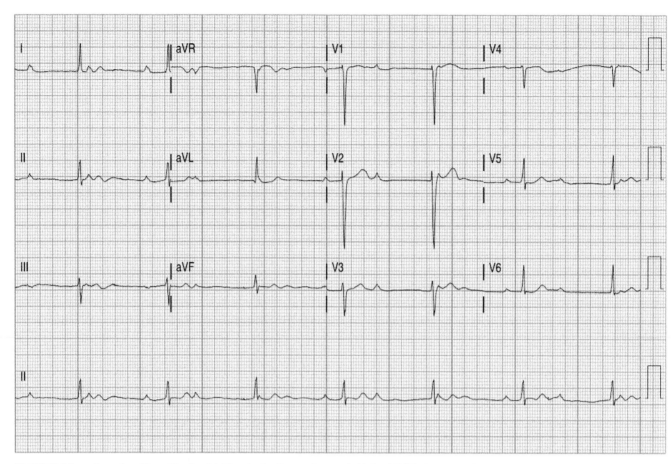

FIGURE 5.9 ■ Complete Heart Block with Ventricular Escape Beats. A 12-lead ECG demonstrating third-degree AV block. The atrial rate is 77 bpm, and the ventricular rate is 43 bpm. There is no constant relationship between the P waves and the QRS complexes, demonstrating atrioventricular dissociation. The QRS complex is wide, showing ventricular escape rhythm. (Photo contributor: Sushitha Surendran, MD.)

Pearls

1. Autoimmune disease accounts for 60% to 70% of all cases of congenital CHB.
2. About 25% to 33% of cases of CHB occur in patients with associated structural heart disease.
3. CHB may not present at birth in infants born to mothers with systemic lupus erythematosus and may develop within the first 3 to 6 months after birth. Unlike other manifestations of neonatal lupus that resolve, CHB is permanent, and patients often require cardiac pacing.
4. An implantable pacemaker is used to prevent sudden death in symptomatic patents with CHB.

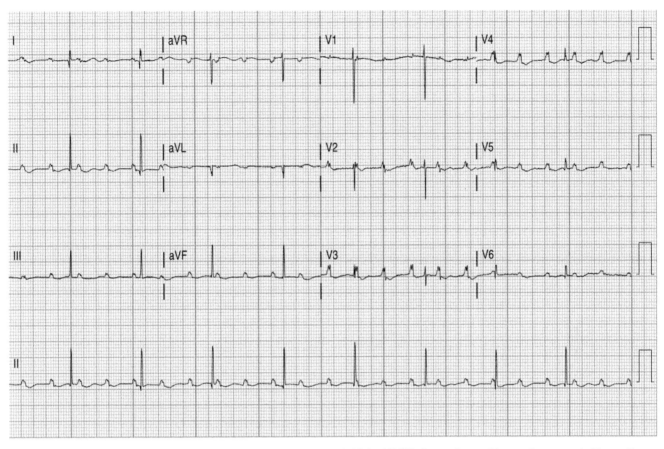

FIGURE 5.10 ■ Complete Heart Block with Junctional Escape Beat. A 12-lead ECG of a newborn with complex congenital heart disease and third-degree AV block. The atrial rate is 138/min, and the ventricular rate is 53/min. There is no constant relationship between the P waves and the QRS complexes demonstrating AV dissociation. The QRS complex is narrow, showing junctional escape rhythm as compared to the previous ECG (see Figure 5.9). (Photo contributor: Sushitha Surendran, MD.)

TABLE 5.6 ■ THIRD-DEGREE ATRIOVENTRICULAR (AV) HEART BLOCK

Characteristic features:
- Failure of conduction of atrial impulses to the ventricles
- AV dissociation (atria and ventricles beat *completely independently,* and P waves and QRS complexes have *no* constant relationship)
- Ventricles are paced by an escape pacemaker at a rate slower than the atrial rate.
- QRS duration may be prolonged or may be normal if the heartbeat is initiated high in the bundle of His (generally, the lower the location of the pacemaker within the ventricular conduction system, the slower the heart rate and wider the QRS complexes).

Some examples of congenital or acquired diseases leading to complete heart block
- Infants born to mothers with systemic lupus erythematosus, rheumatoid arthritis, dermatomyositis, or Sjögren syndrome (autoimmune destruction of AV tracts by maternally derived IgG antibodies)
- Complex congenital heart anomaly (eg, AV septal defects)
- Postsurgical repair of congenital heart disease involving the ventricular septum
- Myocarditis
- Long QT syndrome
- Infections (eg, acute rheumatic fever, Lyme disease, Chagas disease, Rocky Mountain spotted fever)
- Digoxin toxicity

LONG QT SYNDROME

Clinical Summary

Long QT syndrome (LQTS) is characterized by a pathologically prolonged corrected QT interval that is calculated using the formula in Table 5.7. Prolongation of the QTc interval results from a prolongation of the refractory period of the myocardium (during which the atrium is still firing at its regular pace), leading to torsades de pointes (R-on-T phenomenon, a malignant form of ventricular tachycardia [VT]). The condition may be acquired, but more often, it is congenital and inherited (Table 5.8). Common presenting signs and symptoms of LQTS include syncope or presyncope episodes (may be recurrent and often precipitated by exercise, fright, or being startled), seizures, or episodes of paroxysmal VT (often with torsades de pointes morphology that can progress to ventricular fibrillation and sudden death). LQTS may be an incidental ECG finding. About 40% to 50% of patients with genotype-positive LQTS have normal resting QTc. Family history may be positive for occurrence of sudden death in young relatives, syncope with exercise or emotional stress, seizures, arrhythmias, and hearing impairment (congenital LQTS). The QT interval may be very prolonged in neonates and may lead to second-degree or complete heart block.

Emergency Department Treatment and Disposition

Treatment of VT associated with LQTS includes support of airway, breathing, and circulation (ABCs) and providing oxygen and ventilation as needed. Magnesium is the drug of choice in torsades de pointes and helps to terminate the arrhythmia. IV lidocaine, amiodarone, or procainamide can be used. If the above medical therapy fails, synchronized cardioversion is used for stable patients with VT with palpable pulses and defibrillation for patients with pulseless VT, as per Pediatric Advanced Life Support protocols.

Consult cardiology for any patient with LQTS. ECG features of LQTS include low heart rate for age, notched T waves, and T-wave alternans. Stress testing (exertional LQTS) or

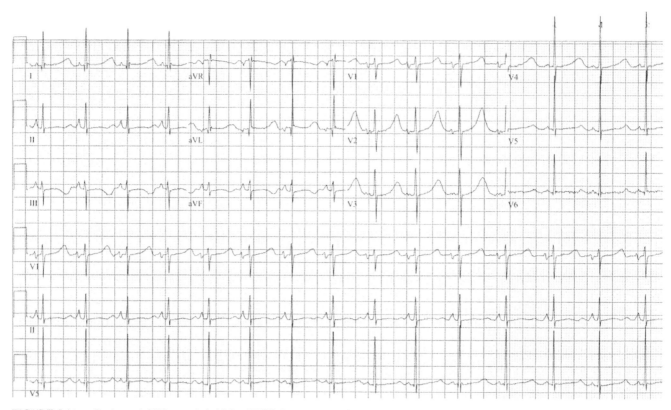

FIGURE 5.11 ■ Prolonged QT interval. A 12-lead ECG demonstrates sinus rhythm with a rate of 95 bpm. There is 1:1 AV conduction. The PR interval and QRS duration are normal. The QT interval is prolonged, and the QTc measures 580 milliseconds. This patient presented with syncope during exercise and was found to have long QT syndrome. (Photo contributor: Shyam Sathanandam, MD.)

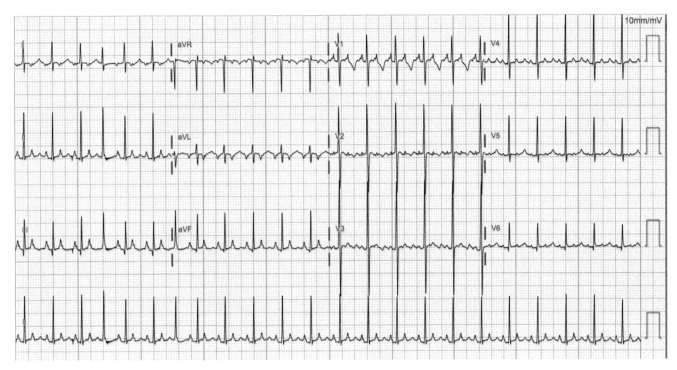

FIGURE 5.12 ■ Long QT Syndrome (LQTS) with 2:1 Block. A 12-lead ECG obtained from a neonate with LQTS. The QTc is 490 milliseconds. There is 2:1 AV block with an atrial rate of 242 bpm and ventricular rate of 132 bpm. LQTS associated with heart block leads to a worse prognosis, and pacemaker insertion is indicated. (Photo contributor: Sushitha Surendran, MD.)

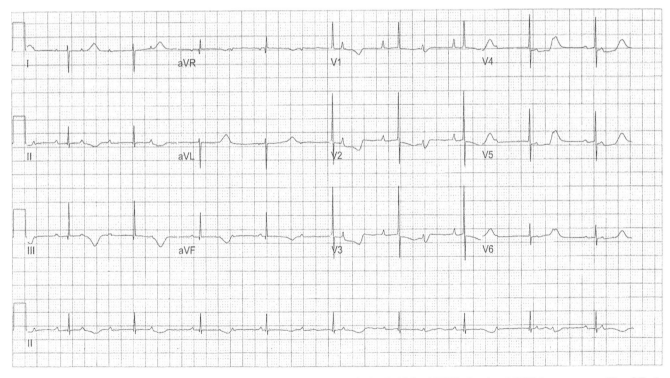

FIGURE 5.13 ■ Long QT Syndrome (LQTS) with Complete Heart Block. A 12-lead ECG showing LQTS in a neonate. The QTc is 600 milliseconds. There is a complete heart block with an atrial rate of 144 bpm and ventricular rate of 40 bpm. There is no constant relationship between the P waves and the QRS complexes. LQTS associated with heart block leads to a worse prognosis, and pacemaker insertion is indicated. (Photo contributor: Shyam Sathanandam, MD.)

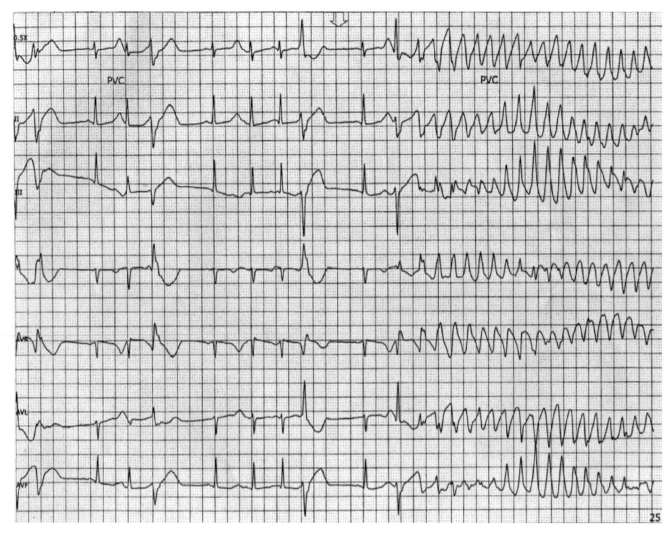

FIGURE 5.14 ■ Long QT Syndrome: Polymorphic Ventricular Tachycardia (VT). A 6-lead ECG obtained on a 12-year-old girl with on and off palpitation and syncope. It demonstrates long QT interval, which leads to polymorphic VT, while the ECG was being recorded. She went in and out of VT, leading to symptoms. An IV infusion of magnesium sulfate or a β-blocker could stop this from progressing to VT. (Photo contributor: Shyam Sathanandam, MD.)

TABLE 5.7 ■ CALCULATION OF QTc

- Should be calculated manually
- Use lead II or V5–V6
- Several successive beats should be measured, with maximum interval taken
- Measure QT interval from the beginning of QRS complex to end of T wave
- The R-R interval preceding the QRS complex should be used for calculation

24-hour Holter monitoring (intermittent LQTS) may help in arriving at the final diagnosis. Long-term goals of therapy for LQTS include β-blockade (eg, propranolol, nadolol) to prevent VT from progressing to ventricular fibrillation and sudden death and to blunt heart rate response to exercise. Therapy should be continued for life. A pacemaker may be required in some patients to overcome profound bradycardia (a common association). Exercise restriction and avoiding drugs that are known to cause prolongation of the QT interval (Table 5.8) are recommended. Advise parents to learn cardiopulmonary

TABLE 5.8 ■ THE QTc INTERVAL

- Formula (Bazett equation) for calculating the corrected QT interval:

$$QTc = \frac{QTm}{\sqrt{R-R}}$$

where QTc = corrected QT interval in seconds; QTm = measured QT interval in seconds; and R-R = interval between previous two consecutive R waves on the ECG in seconds.
- Normally the QT interval is heart rate dependent.
- Above formula corrects measured QT interval to a heart rate of 60 bpm, at which normal R-R interval is 1 second. Since the square root of 1 = 1, the QTc equals the QTm at a heart rate of 60 bpm, with a normal QT interval range of 0.35 to 0.44 seconds.
- Pronged QT interval: QTc >0.45 seconds in adult males and >0.46 seconds in adult females.
- QT interval normally shortens with exercise.
- In patients with LQTS, the QT interval does not shorten appropriately with exercise.
- Useful rule of thumb: normal QT is less than half of preceding R-R interval.

Etiology of Prolonged QT Interval

Congenital (about 50% of cases):
- Two syndromes with LQTS (absence of structural heart disease):
  (1) Romano-Ward syndrome (autosomal dominant inheritance *without* deafness)
  (2) Jervell and Lange-Nielsen syndrome (autosomal recessive inheritance *with* sensorineural deafness)

Acquired:
- Heart disease (eg, myocarditis)
- Electrolyte abnormalities (eg, hypokalemia, hypocalcemia, hypomagnesemia)
- Post cardiac arrest
- Raised intracranial pressure
- Medications (www.qtdrugs.org)
  (1) Cyclic antidepressants (eg, imipramine, amitriptyline)
  (2) Phenothiazines (eg, thioridazine, pimozide)
  (3) Other psychotropic drugs (eg, haloperidol, risperidone, lithium carbonate)
  (4) Gastrointestinal prokinetics (eg, cisapride)
  (5) Antihistamines (eg, diphenhydramine)
  (6) Antiarrhythmics (eg, quinidine, procainamide, amiodarone)
  (7) Antibiotics (eg, trimethoprim, erythromycin, clarithromycin, azithromycin, sulfamethoxazole)
  (8) Antifungals (eg, fluconazole, ketoconazole)
  (9) Epinephrine

resuscitation (because exercise restriction and drug therapy may be ineffective for some children). An implantable cardioverter-defibrillator may be considered in patients with continued episodes of syncope despite therapy and in those with a prior history of cardiac arrest.

Pearls

1. Patients with LQTS may have a normal ECG in the ED.
2. Congenital LQTS results in a mortality rate in excess of 90% if not diagnosed and properly treated.
3. LQTS in association with hypertrophic cardiomyopathy accounts for up to half of the cases of sudden cardiac death.
4. Children with LQTS are predisposed to episodic ventricular arrhythmias, torsades de pointes, syncope, and generalized seizures.
5. Patients with LQTS may develop fatal ventricular arrhythmias, especially if exposed to some medications such as antihistamines, macrolide antibiotics, phenothiazines, or cisapride.
6. All first-degree relatives of a patient with LQTS should undergo a 12-lead ECG (and cardiac evaluation as indicated).
7. Any patient presenting with VT (especially torsades de pointes or a polymorphic type) should have a corrected QT interval determined while in sinus rhythm.

Clinical Summary

Syncope is a sudden and brief loss of consciousness accompanied by a loss of postural tone, from which recovery is spontaneous. All forms of syncope result from a sudden decrease or brief cessation of cerebral blood flow. About 20% of males and 50% of females may have an episode of syncope by the age of 20 resulting in ED visit. Cardiac pathology is found in <5% of children and adolescents with syncope.

Vasovagal syncope (neurocardiogenic syncope, fainting spell) is the most common cause of syncope. Examples include emotional fainting, situational syncope, syncope with panic, and syncope associated with exercise in athletes (without heart disease). Vasovagal syncope is usually seen in adolescents. Most episodes occur after prolonged standing (eg, crowded, warm environment), or with noxious stimuli, strong emotions, hot showers, or fatigue.

Orthostatic syncope occurs while the patient is standing or during a rapid change from a supine or sitting position to standing. Orthostatic BP should be measured 3 minutes after the patient stands up following a supine period of 5 minutes (orthostatic changes present if systolic BP drops by 20 mm Hg and diastolic BP drops by 10 mm Hg). Predisposing events include dehydration, acute blood loss, or use of vasodilator drugs.

Cardiac syncope results from hypoxemia due to cyanotic heart disease or decreased cardiac output secondary to arrhythmia, obstructive lesion, or myocardial dysfunction. Syncope occurs during physical exertion (eg, LQTS). or occurs suddenly without warning.

Breath-holding spells are commonly seen in children between 1 and 5 years of age (peaks around 2 years of age). They resolve spontaneously by school age. There are 2 major types: cyanotic type (about 80%) and pallid type (about 20%). Provoking events include pain, anger, frustration, and vigorous crying followed by forced expiration and apnea (breath-holding spell). Unconsciousness occurs due to decreased cardiac output. Generalized clonic jerks, opisthotonos, and bradycardia and incontinence may occur. Normal physical examination (including cardiac and neurologic examination) is a hallmark.

Emergency Department Treatment and Disposition

Determine the degree of hemodynamic stability, including orthostatic BP and heart rate measurements. Specific treatment of syncope depends on the underlying etiology

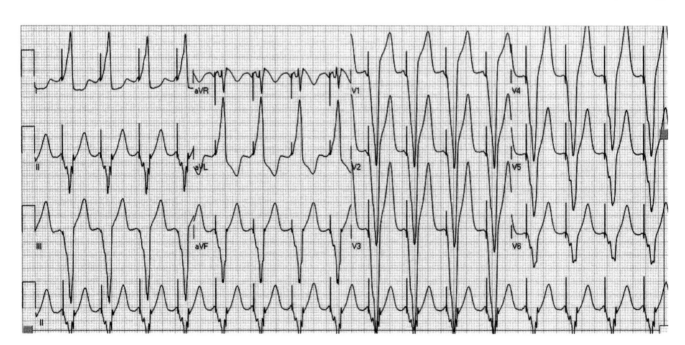

FIGURE 5.15 ■ Ventricular Paced Rhythm. A 12-lead ECG of a 7-year-old child with a history of double outlet right ventricle and complete heart block following surgical repair and subsequent epicardial pacemaker system placement. His ECG shows ventricular pacemaker activity. He is being paced at a rate of 100 bpm. Note the pacing spikes and wide QRS complex. Any patient with a pacemaker presenting with syncope should get a 12-lead ECG and interrogation of the pacemaker to rule out pacemaker malfunction. (Photo contributor: Shyam Sathanandam, MD.)

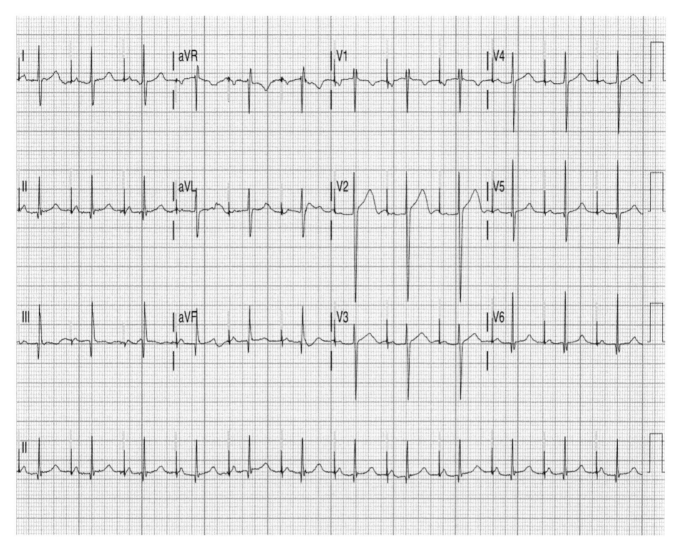

FIGURE 5.16 ■ Atrial Paced Rhythm. A 12-lead ECG of a 21-year-old man with sinus node dysfunction with symptomatic first-degree AV block status post transvenous dual-chamber pacemaker who presented for chest pain. His ECG shows atrial pacemaker activity at a rate of 70 bpm (pacemaker activity represented by green lines). Note the pacing spikes and narrow QRS complex. RSR′ pattern seen in V1 suggests right ventricular conduction delay. (Photo contributor: Sushitha Surendran, MD.)

(eg, LQTS). Routine basic laboratory tests (eg, CBC, electrolytes, glucose) are rarely helpful. Obtain additional tests as guided by the history and examination (eg, toxicology screen, carboxyhemoglobin). Exclude pregnancy in adolescent girls. Obtain a 12-lead ECG (with rhythm strip) in all patients (despite its low yield) because findings can lead to specific therapy (eg, pacemaker for CHB, β-blocker for LQTS). Arrhythmias that lead to syncope may not be present during ED evaluation. Consider 24-hour Holter monitoring or an event monitor, if indicated based on the history or examination. Consult cardiology if cardiac syncope is likely based on history or examination or abnormal ECG findings

or syncope with chest pain, arrhythmias, or palpitations, or a family history of sudden death. Consult neurology if seizures cannot be excluded (Table 5.10) based on the history or with an abnormal neurologic examination.

Reassure and educate patients about the benign nature of syncope for vasovagal syncope, identifying and avoiding precipitating factors (eg, dehydration, excess caffeine), and ensure intake of salty foods during intense physical activity. Educate patients to recognize prodromal symptoms and assume a sitting or supine position with elevation of the feet during such episodes. For orthostatic syncope, provide fluid therapy to patients with volume depletion. Encourage patients

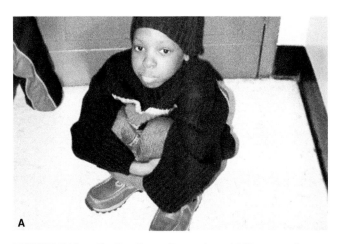
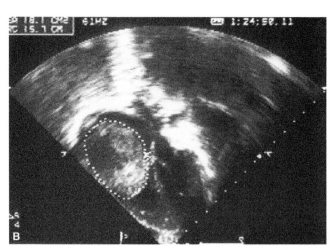

FIGURE 5.17 ■ Cardiac Tumor Presenting with Recurrent Syncope. (**A**) Squatting position assumed by patient while "feeling tired" in the ED. This previously healthy 10-year-old boy presented with recurrent syncope and weakness, increasing tiredness, and shortness of breath of 2 weeks in duration. He had hypotension with blood pressure (BP) of 87/63 mm Hg. (The median systolic BP for children older than 1 year is 90 + [2 × age in years], and the lower limit is 70 + [2 × age in years].) Heart rate was 90 bpm, and he had a normal cardiac examination. Hepatomegaly, right atrial enlargement on ECG, and mild cardiomegaly on CXR were also noted. (**B**) Right atrial mass (arrow) obstructing right ventricular inflow tract on echocardiography. This 6.5 × 5.5 × 4 cm mass was resected and was found to be precursor B lymphoblastic lymphoma/leukemia (intracardiac lymphoblastic lymphoma). (Photo contributors: Barry Hahn, MD, and Sudha Rao, MD.)

to get up slowly after lying or sitting and to discontinue or reduce the dose of any medication that may be responsible for hypotension.

Hospitalize patients presenting with recurrent syncope of undetermined etiology or cardiac syncope (eg, LQTS, tachyarrhythmia, or symptoms suggestive of arrhythmias [eg, syncope associated with palpitations, exertional syncope], AV block, valvular or congenital heart disease, pacemaker malfunction, CHF, cyanotic spells).

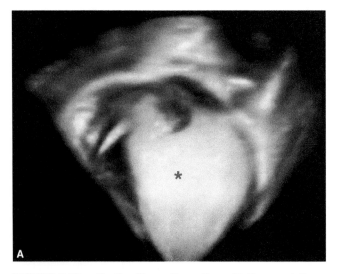
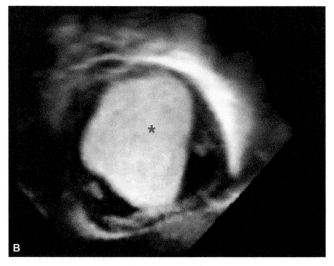

FIGURE 5.18 ■ Cardiac Tumor Presenting with Recurrent Syncope. (**A**) Four-chamber view of a 3-dimensional echocardiography in a young patient with recurrent syncope. There is a large tumor (asterisk) in the interventricular septum that probably caused syncope secondary to obstruction of the left ventricular outflow tract. (**B**) A parasternal short-axis view shows the large tumor in the interventricular septum (asterisk). Primary intracardiac tumor in infants is most likely benign rhabdomyoma that usually regresses, and >50% of these patients have tuberous sclerosis. (Photo contributor: Shyam Sathanandam, MD.)

TABLE 5.9 ■ ETIOLOGY OF SYNCOPE

Cardiac syncope (cardiac lesions causing syncope):
- Tetralogy of Fallot
- Long QT syndrome
- Hypertrophic cardiomyopathy
- Coronary artery anomalies
- Valvular heart disease (critical aortic stenosis, tricuspid stenosis, mitral stenosis)
- Bradydysrhythmia (sick sinus syndrome, heart block [second- and third-degree], pacemaker malfunction)
- Tachydysrhythmia (ventricular tachycardia, supraventricular tachycardia, torsades de pointes)
- Pericardial disease
- Myocardial ischemia/infarction
- Myxoma, adenoma
- Arrhythmogenic right ventricular cardiomyopathy

Noncardiac syncope:
- Autonomic dysfunction (vasovagal, orthostatic, breath-holding spell, situational [cough, micturition, defecation])
- Metabolic (eg, hypoglycemia)
- Hypoxia
- Carbon monoxide poisoning
- Neuropsychiatric syncope (hyperventilation syndrome, atonic seizures (drop attacks), hysterical syncope)

Pearls

1. Syncope is a symptom, not a disease.
2. A thorough history and physical examination are essential for the evaluation of syncope and may lead to or suggest a diagnosis that can be evaluated with directed testing.
3. Vasovagal syncope is the most common cause of fainting in children and adolescents and accounts for >50% of cases of childhood syncope.
4. Dizziness, vertigo, and presyncope do not result in loss of consciousness or postural tone.

TABLE 5.10 ■ DIFFERENTIAL DIAGNOSIS: SYNCOPE VERSUS SEIZURES

	Syncope	Seizures
Precipitants of episodes		
Pain, exercise, stressful event, micturition, defecation	Usually present	Absent
Symptoms before or during episode	Sweating, nausea, feeling of "passing out"	Aura may be present
Disorientation after event	Absent	Present
Slowness in regaining consciousness	Absent	Present
Confusion on awakening	Absent or mild	Marked
Period of unconsciousness	Usually seconds	Minutes or longer
Unconsciousness >5 minutes	Absent	May be present
Rhythmic movements		
Tonic-clonic movements, myoclonic jerks	Occasionally seen	Commonly seen
Incontinence during episode	Absent	May be present
Electroencephalogram	Normal	May be abnormal

SINUS TACHYCARDIA

Clinical Summary

Sinus tachycardia (ST) is defined as a rate of sinus node discharge that is higher than normal for the patient's age (Table 5.1). The usual upper limit of ST in infants and young children (up to 5 years old) is a heart rate up to 200 bpm. The upper limit of ST in older children is a heart rate up to 180 bpm. Tachycardia is a physiologic response to the body's need for increased cardiac output or oxygen delivery (tachycardia is the first sign of hypovolemia: cardiac output = stroke volume × heart rate; thus to maintain cardiac output, a compensatory increase in heart rate occurs, as the child's ability to increase stroke volume is limited). ST is a nonspecific sign of an underlying condition rather than a true arrhythmia (Table 5.11). All P waves are normal in configuration (upright in lead II), and all QRS complexes are preceded by a P wave in ECG. The P-, QRS-, and T-wave morphologies are normal.

Emergency Department Treatment and Disposition

Continuous cardiac and pulse oximetry monitoring helps when monitoring patients presenting with ST that is near the range

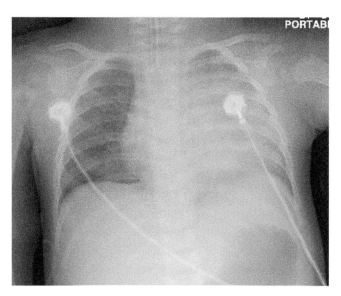

FIGURE 5.20 ■ Differential Diagnosis of Sinus Tachycardia. Myocarditis. A 6-month-old infant presented with a heart rate of 190 bpm, agitation, and cold extremities with poor peripheral pulses (cardiogenic shock) following an upper respiratory tract infection. Myocarditis was clinically suspected. Frontal view of the chest shows very prominent cardiothymic silhouette. Echocardiography showed ejection fraction of 20%. (Photo contributor: John Amodio, MD.)

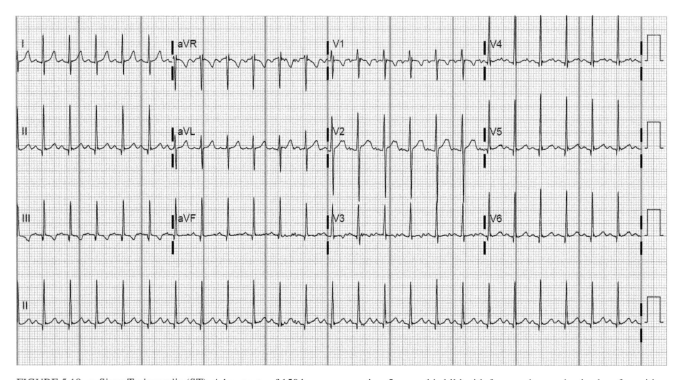

FIGURE 5.19 ■ Sinus Tachycardia (ST). A heart rate of 150 bpm was seen in a 5-year-old child with fever and several episodes of vomiting and diarrhea. In ST, even though there may be some variation in the R-R interval, there is a constant PR interval with a normal P-QRS-T–wave sequence. The P-wave axis is normal (ie, the P waves are normal in configuration), and the QRS duration is normal (<0.08 second). Patient's heart rate improved after resolution of fever and dehydration. (Photo contributor: Shyam Sathanandam, MD.)

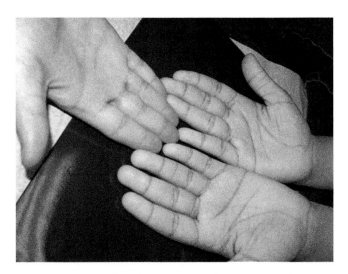

FIGURE 5.21 ■ Differential Diagnosis of Sinus Tachycardia. Severe Anemia. Extreme pallor is seen in this adolescent girl with dysfunctional uterine bleeding presenting to ED with easy fatigability, weakness, and tachycardia (heart rate: 130 bpm) with a hemoglobin value of 3.5 g/dL. (Photo contributor: Binita R. Shah, MD.)

of supraventricular tachycardia (SVT) (eg, HR approaching 200 bpm). Treatment of ST involves treatment of the underlying cause (eg, antipyretics for fever, oxygen therapy for hypoxia, fluid therapy for hypovolemia, pain management).

Do not attempt to decrease the heart rate by pharmacologic or electrical intervention. ST usually resolves once the stressor ceases. The heart rate will return to normal levels with appropriate treatment of the underlying cause.

Pearls

1. ST is the most common rhythm disturbance in children.
2. Treatment of ST involves treatment of the underlying cause.
3. Persistent ST without an apparent inciting cause may be indicative of occult cardiac disease (eg, myocarditis) or an unrecognized noncardiac condition (eg, hypovolemia).

TABLE 5.11 ■ SINUS TACHYCARDIA (ST)

- *Common causes of ST:* Fever, crying, anxiety, exercise, pain
- *Serious causes of ST:*
  (1) Hypovolemia, hypoxia
  (2) Sepsis
  (3) Anemia
  (4) Toxins and drugs (eg, amphetamines, antihistamines, atropine/anticholinergics, cocaine, phencyclidine, cyclic antidepressants, ephedrine/pseudoephedrine, iron, organophosphates, thyroxine, carbon monoxide and cyanide poisoning)
  (5) Myocarditis
  (6) Hyperthyroidism/thyroid storm
  (7) Pericardial tamponade
  (8) Tension pneumothorax

Differential Diagnosis: *ST versus supraventricular tachycardia (SVT)*
- Sometimes difficult to differentiate between ST and SVT
- Beat-to-beat variation is seen in ST, but not in SVT (eg, HR varies with activity in ST, but not in SVT)
- Infants
  (1) Heart rate (HR) >220 bpm = probable SVT
  (2) HR <200 bpm = ST
- Children
  (1) HR >180 bpm = probable SVT
  (2) HR <180 bpm = ST

Clinical Summary

Supraventricular tachycardia (SVT) is defined as heart rate in infants and young children >220 bpm (range: 220–320 bpm) and heart rate in older children >180 bpm (range: 180–250 bpm).

SVT is most commonly caused by a reentry mechanism involving AV nodal tissue, accessory pathways, or increased automaticity. SVT due to accessory pathway conduction (eg, Wolff-Parkinson-White [WPW] syndrome) is the predominant mechanism in the fetus and young infant. AV nodal reentry typically appears in 5- to 10-year-old children and is the predominant mechanism in adults. Primary atrial tachycardia

(eg, AF or fibrillation) accounts for 10% to 15% of SVT at all ages. Associated structural heart disease (eg, Ebstein anomaly, corrected transposition of great arteries) is present in about 20% of cases. Other etiologies include drugs (eg, cold medications containing sympathomimetics), hyperthyroidism, myocarditis, cardiomyopathy, or infections.

Infants usually present with nonspecific symptoms of poor feeding, irritability, or restlessness. If SVT persists for many hours at rapid rates, signs of CHF (eg, tachypnea, tachycardia, hepatomegaly) or cardiogenic shock/cardiovascular collapse (eg, an acutely ill infant with prolonged capillary refill, thready pulses, poor tissue perfusion, ashen color, and metabolic

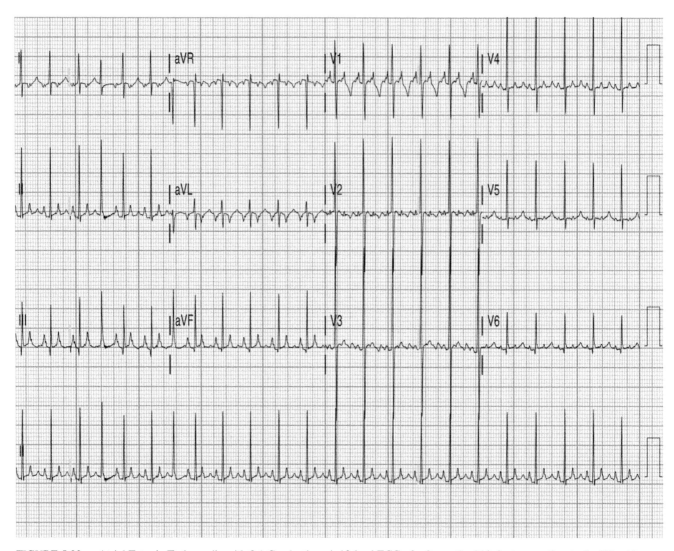

FIGURE 5.22 ■ Atrial Ectopic Tachycardia with 2:1 Conduction. A 12-lead ECG of a 3-month-old infant presenting to the ED with poor feeding and irritability shows atrial ectopic tachycardia at 268 bpm with 2:1 ventricular conduction. Echocardiogram showed severely depressed cardiac function, and multiple attempts at cardioversion were unsuccessful. The patient was placed on extracorporeal membrane oxygenation. (Photo contributor: Sushitha Surendran, MD.)

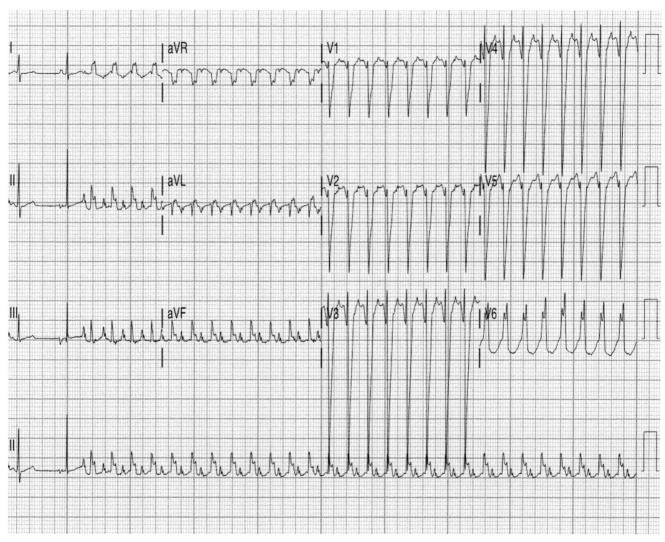

FIGURE 5.23 ■ Atrial Ectopic Tachycardia with Rapid Ventricular Response. A 12-lead ECG of same infant as in Figure 5.22 on extracorporeal membrane oxygenation showing paroxysmal atrial tachycardia with 1:1 ventricular conduction at rate of 194 bpm. Note the abrupt onset of the tachycardia. There is also left bundle branch block (broad or notched "M-shaped" R waves seen in V6). (Photo contributor: Sushitha Surendran, MD.)

acidosis) develop. Infants may be completely asymptomatic, and SVT may be detected during a routine examination. Older children may present with pounding or racing heartbeat, dizziness, diaphoresis, or tiredness. Episodes of SVT are often paroxysmal. Older children may give a history of episodes of a racing heartbeat that starts and stops suddenly. Chest pain is not a usual presenting symptom of SVT. Clinically the heart rate may be too rapid to count.

Most first episodes of childhood SVT occur in the first 2 months of life. About 60% of cases occur in infants <4 months of age and 80% of cases occur in infants <12 months of age. ECG is required to confirm the diagnosis. P waves may not be visible (obscured by the ST segment), which helps distinguish it from ST (Table 5.12); narrow QRS complex is seen in 90% of cases, and wide QRS complex is seen in 10% of cases (aberrant SVT). With persistent tachycardia, ST- and T-wave changes consistent with myocardial ischemia may be seen. Features of WPW syndrome may be seen once the episode of SVT terminates and may include a short PR interval, a delta wave (slow upstroke of QRS complex), and a wide QRS complex. WPW syndrome sometimes closely resembles bundle branch block and must be distinguished. A CXR may show the presence of cardiomegaly suggesting CHF or underlying structural heart disease.

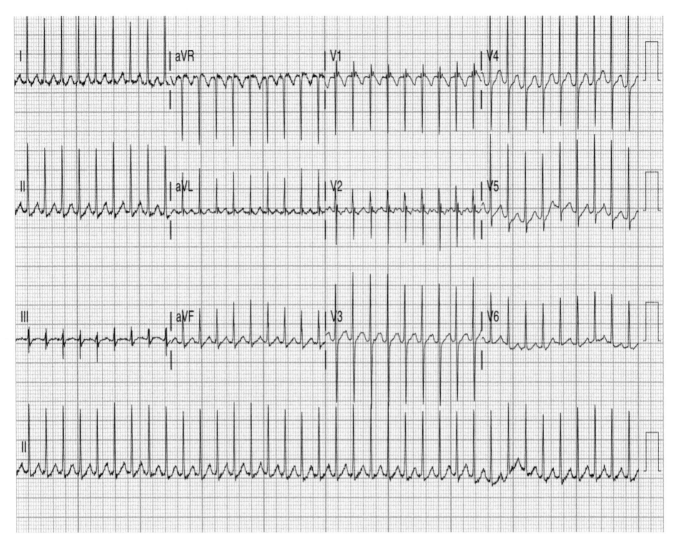

FIGURE 5.24 ■ Supraventricular Tachycardia. A 12-lead ECG of a 6-year-old boy with history of atrioventricular nodal reentry tachycardia who was seen in the ED with symptoms of presyncope. His ECG shows narrow-complex tachycardia with a heart rate of 218 bpm. (Photo contributor: Sushitha Surendran, MD.)

Emergency Department Treatment and Disposition

Evaluate the hemodynamic status and stabilize as indicated, providing high-flow oxygen and continuous cardiac, BP, and pulse oximetry monitoring. Consult cardiology for echocardiography in patients with a first episode of SVT to exclude structural heart disease and to start chronic maintenance therapy (eg, digoxin, propranolol, procainamide, or amiodarone) as indicated with either a first episode or recurrent episodes of SVT. Possible electrophysiology testing and radiofrequency catheter ablation are needed for patients with refractory SVT,

those requiring multiple medications, or those with undesirable side effects from medications.

ED treatment for SVT without circulatory compromise (stable patient) involves vagal maneuvers that heighten the vagal tone to the AV node. Application of an ice bag to the face in infants can be tried first (*Caution: Application of ice to infants should be brief [10 to 20 seconds max], and a cloth or plastic barrier should be used to avoid the occurrence of fat necrosis. Avoid repeated applications of ice to the same location*). Other maneuvers include Valsalva maneuver (asking patient to strain as if straining at stool) and unilateral carotid massage (massage at junction of

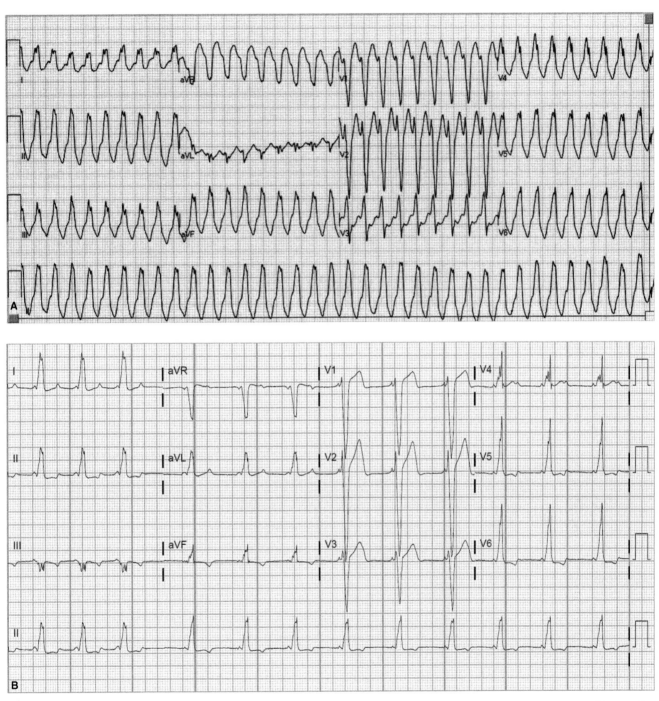

FIGURE 5.25 ■ Supraventricular Tachycardia (SVT) with Aberrancy. (A) A 12-lead ECG demonstrates an apparent wide-complex tachycardia in a 12-year-old adolescent presenting with palpitation. Except for a heart rate of 220 bpm, other vital signs were normal. This is SVT with aberrancy, and it may be difficult to differentiate this from ventricular tachycardia (VT). All wide complex tachycardia should be considered as VT unless proven otherwise, and delay in treatment should be avoided especially if the patient is unstable and awaiting cardiology consult. (B) A 12-lead ECG obtained in the same patient whose tachycardia was terminated without any complication after administration of adenosine. The ECG demonstrates a short PR interval with initial slurring of the QRS complexes, leading to wide QRS complex. (Photo contributor: Shyam Sathanandam, MD.)

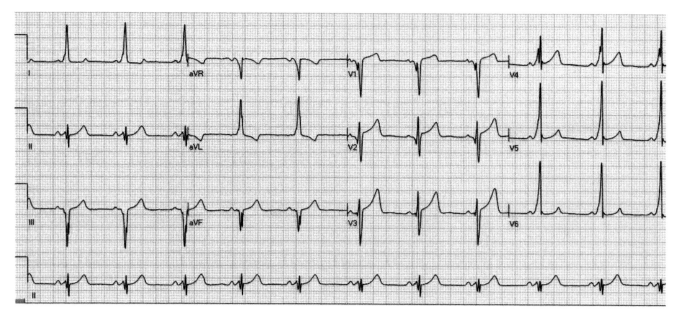

FIGURE 5.26 ■ Wolff-Parkinson-White (WPW) syndrome. A classic ECG of a patient with WPW syndrome showing short PR interval and initial slurring of the QRS complexes, leading to wide QRS complex (pathognomonic for WPW syndrome). This is secondary to conduction via an accessory pathway. Patients with WPW syndrome are at risk for orthodromic-reciprocating tachycardia. (Photo contributor: Shyam Sathanandam, MD.)

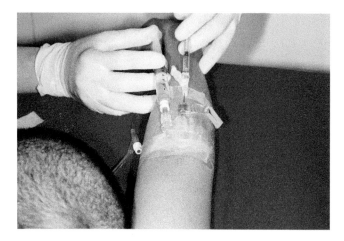

FIGURE 5.27 ■ Two-Hand/Two-Syringe Technique for Administration of Adenosine. Because of its extremely short half-life, adenosine must be given as a rapid IV bolus (inject in 1–3 seconds to maximize the concentration that reaches the heart). While maintaining pressure on the plunger of the syringe containing the adenosine, simultaneously inject a rapid bolus of 3 to 5 mL of normal saline to accelerate delivery to the heart. Injection should be made close to the hub of the catheter, so that it is done closest to the patient. (Photo contributor: Binita R. Shah, MD.)

carotid artery and mandible). Ocular pressure should not be used (risk of retinal detachment).

Medical therapy includes adenosine and verapamil. Do not use verapamil in infants <1 year of age (life-threatening side effects include profound bradycardia, hypotension, cardiac arrest), in children with CHF or myocardial depression, or in those receiving β-blockers. Continuous ECG should be obtained during adenosine push to see the mechanism of termination of tachycardia. This will help the cardiologist in differentiating different types of SVT. For SVT with circulatory compromise or severe CHF (unstable patient with shock or acidosis), adenosine can be tried first if immediate vascular access is available. If not, perform synchronized cardioversion to terminate SVT quickly. Consider sedation in older children (if the patient is conscious and time and clinical condition allow; however, sedation *must not* delay cardioversion). *Reconsider the diagnosis of SVT if conversion to sinus rhythm does not occur; patient may actually have ST.* Admit to the ICU any patient presenting with hemodynamic instability or any patient with a first episode of SVT (for parental and

TABLE 5.12 ▪ DIFFERENTIAL DIAGNOSIS: SINUS TACHYCARDIA VERSUS SUPRAVENTRICULAR TACHYCARDIA

Sinus Tachycardia	Supraventricular Tachycardia
History of volume loss (vomiting, diarrhea, blood loss), fever, hypoxia	History nonspecific (eg, irritability, poor feeding, excessive crying)
Signs of dehydration or hypovolemic shock or sepsis (depending on underlying etiology)	Signs of cardiogenic shock (tachypnea, sweating, pallor, or hypothermia)
Rate > normal for age (usually <220 bpm)	Rate >220 bpm in infants
	Rate >180 bpm in older children
Regular rhythm	Usually regular rhythm (associated AV block extremely rare)
Beat-to-beat variation (some variation in RR interval and heart rate decreases with sleep or when quiet)	*No* beat-to-beat variation; monotonous/fixed rate
Normal P-wave axis	P-wave axis usually abnormal
P wave may not be identifiable (with very high ventricular rate)	P wave may not be identifiable (with very high ventricular rate)
Normal QRS duration	Normal QRS duration in >90% of cases
Heart rate slows gradually with treatment (eg, fluids for dehydration)	Abrupt termination to sinus rhythm (either spontaneously or with treatment)
Normal P-QRS-T–wave sequence	

patient education or beginning maintenance therapy, especially in neonates and infants with possible recurrences of SVT) for further management.

Patients known to have SVT can be discharged home once converted to sinus rhythm with a follow-up appointment with the cardiologist or primary care physician.

TABLE 5.13 ▪ ADENOSINE AND SUPRAVENTRICULAR TACHYCARDIA

- Drug of choice in stable patients or acutely ill patients *with readily available* vascular access
- Relatively safe drug that can be *given to infants and children of all ages,* including full-term and preterm newborn infants
- May also be used in children with WPW syndrome or other AV bypass tracts
- After its administration:
  (1) Transiently depresses sinus and AV nodes, leading to slowed conduction and interruption of the reentry pathway
  (2) *Be prepared to expect brief periods of sinus arrest (asystole).*
  (3) Be prepared to treat cardiac effects such as bradycardia, AV block, atrial fibrillation, atrial flutter, ventricular tachycardia, or ventricular fibrillation.
- Untoward effects are brief (ultra-short half-life [<10 seconds]):
  (1) Dyspnea, flushing, chest pain/discomfort, headache, episodes of apnea
  (2) Bronchospasm (asthma is not a contraindication; be prepared to treat bronchospasm)
- Dose and route of administration:
  (1) Initial dose 0.1–0.3 mg/kg (*maximum first dose: 6 mg*)
  (2) If initial dose is unsuccessful, may double and repeat dose once (*maximum second dose: 12 mg*)
  (3) Maximum single dose: 12 mg
  (4) Use rapid IV bolus followed by normal saline flush (2-hand technique)
  (5) May be given intraosseously
  (6) Adolescents ≥50 kg: 6-mg rapid IV push; if no response after 1–2 min, give 12-mg rapid IV push. May repeat a second 12-mg dose after 1–2 min, if required.

Pearls

1. SVT is the most common dysrhythmia seen in the pediatric age group.
2. Aberrant SVT presents with a wide QRS complex and may resemble VT. If uncertain, all wide-complex tachycardias are assumed to be VT.
3. A diagnosis of sepsis may be mistakenly made in an infant with SVT presenting with poor feeding, irritability, rapid breathing, or shock.
4. Do not delay cardioversion in severely compromised patients while trying to establish vascular access.
5. Do not prescribe sympathomimetics (common in over-the-counter decongestants) for the treatment of URIs in children with SVT, and advise patients also to avoid caffeine.

Clinical Summary

Atrial flutter (AF) is defined as an atrial rate >300 bpm (range: 240–600 bpm) with a ventricular response with varying degrees of block (eg, 2:1, 3:1, 4:1) and normal QRS complexes. It is most commonly caused by an ectopic pacemaker in the atrium, leading to "circus movement" (reentry mechanism) within the atrium. It is most commonly seen in newborns with a structurally normal heart; however, it can happen at any age following heart surgery involving the atria (eg, repair of atrial septal defect). AF in the newborns behaves differently than in older children. The key difference is that, in newborns, AF usually does not recur following conversion, whereas in older children, recurrence is common. AF is characterized by a flutter wave with saw tooth configuration on ECG. The ventricular rate determines eventual cardiac output; a too-rapid ventricular rate may decrease cardiac output. Infants usually present with nonspecific symptoms of poor feeding, irritability, or restlessness. If AF persists for many hours at rapid rates, signs of CHF (eg, tachypnea, tachycardia, hepatomegaly) or cardiogenic shock/cardiovascular collapse (eg, an acutely ill infant with prolonged capillary refill, thready pulses, poor tissue perfusion, ashen color, and metabolic acidosis) develop. Older children may present with pounding or racing heartbeat, dizziness, diaphoresis, or tiredness.

Emergency Department Treatment and Disposition

Evaluate hemodynamic status and stabilize the patient as indicated including high-flow oxygen and continuous cardiac, BP, and pulse oximetry monitoring. Consult cardiology for echocardiography in patients with a first episode of AF to exclude associated structural heart disease or a thrombus in the atrium. If the flutter waves are not clearly seen in the ECG, adenosine can be given to reveal the flutter waves. AF without circulatory compromise requires digitalization provided it is not from digitalis toxicity. Digitalis increases the AV block and thereby slows the ventricular rate. Propranolol may be added to digoxin. Amiodarone is also effective in acute treatment. AF with circulatory compromise or severe CHF may require electrical cardioversion. Patients who are on digoxin cannot undergo cardioversion. Rapid atrial pacing with a catheter in the esophagus or in the right atrium can be effective when cardioversion is contraindicated. Chronic maintenance therapy (eg, digoxin, propranolol, or amiodarone) is usually indicated in patients with either a first episode or recurrent episodes of AF.

Pearls

1. AF is the second most common arrhythmia in the newborn after SVT.
2. Recurrence of AF is less likely in neonates and infants after successful conversion.
3. Suspect a significant cardiac pathology (eg, myocarditis) with AF in an older child with a structurally normal heart.
4. Exclude thrombus in the atrium before cardioversion to prevent embolization especially if it has been going on for couple of days or the duration of AF is unknown.

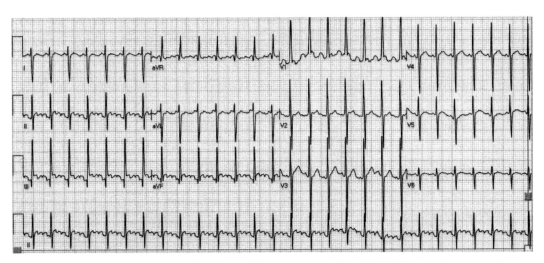

FIGURE 5.28 ■ Atrial Flutter (AF) with Block. A 12-lead ECG demonstrating AF with 2:1 block. The flutter rate is 300 bpm with a ventricular rate of 150 bpm. (Photo contributor: Shyam Sathanandam, MD.)

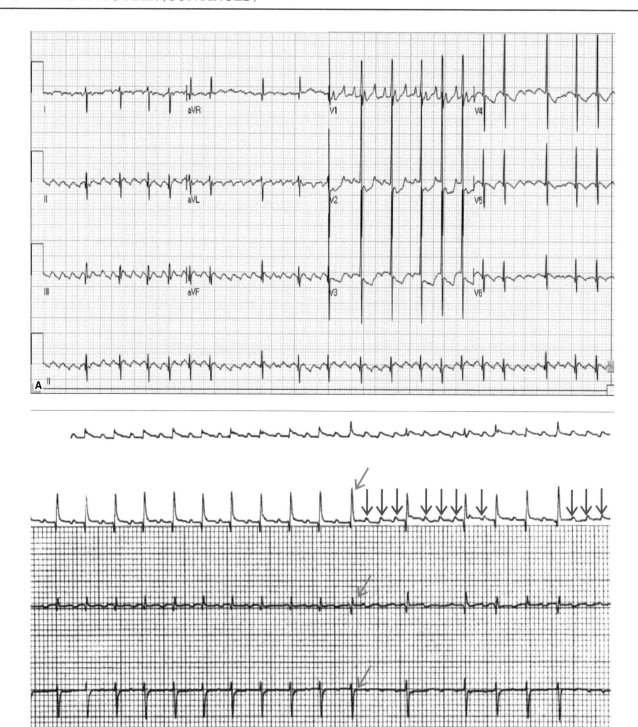

FIGURE 5.29 ▪ Atrial Flutter (AF). (**A**) A 12-lead ECG demonstrating AF with variable conduction in a 10-day-old infant who presented to ED with poor feeding and irritability. AF rate is >300 bpm. (**B**) Simultaneous ECG rhythm strips in different leads showing atrial flutter (AF) and the effect of adenosine. A dose of adenosine is very helpful to differentiate AF from other forms of SVT. Adenosine reversibly blocks the AV node, leading to no AV conduction. As seen here, when adenosine is given (blue arrows), AF waves are not conducted making them more prominent (red arrows), thus confirming the diagnosis. After the effect of adenosine weans off, normal AV node conduction resumes. Adenosine does not terminate the atrial flutter. Adenosine could terminate SVT. (Photo contributor: Shyam Sathanandam, MD.)

Clinical Summary

Premature ventricular contractions (PVCs), also known as ventricular premature contractions and ventricular extrasystoles, are premature, wide, and bizarre-shaped QRS complexes originating from ventricular tissue. PVCs are commonly seen in asymptomatic healthy adolescents but can be seen in any age group including newborns. Presenting signs and symptoms include palpitations or "skipped beats," chest discomfort, chest pain, syncope, dizziness, and difficulty breathing. Sometimes irregular heartbeat is detected during routine examination or as an incidental finding in ECG. Frequent PVCs in the presence of compromised cardiac function may produce signs of CHF. ECG findings include widened, bizarre QRS complexes that are *not* preceded by P waves. P wave may show AV dissociation or retrograde conduction or may be absent. The T-wave polarity usually is opposite to the major QRS deflection. A compensatory pause often follows a PVC. A rhythmic pattern of PVC with a fixed ratio with normal beats is referred to as bigeminy (1:1), trigeminy (2:1), or quadrigeminy (3:1). PVCs could be unifocal or multifocal. If an episode of 3 or more PVCs occur together and lasts for 10 seconds or less, then it is described as nonsustained VT. A 24-hour Holter monitor, exercise stress testing, and echocardiography may be considered per consultation with the cardiologist. About 40% of normal children will have PVCs on a Holter monitor. Exercise stress test will help to determine the response of PVCs to exercise. Usually PVCs decrease with exercise. With an exercise stress test, we can evaluate whether PVCs persist with exercise or increase in number or evaluate for any runs of tachycardia or arrhythmia; this will help the cardiologist in determining further management and medical therapy. Most children with PVC will have a structurally normal heart.

Emergency Department Treatment and Disposition

Patients with "benign" PVCs do not require any treatment. Educate the patient and family about the benign nature and about avoiding stimulants (eg, excess caffeine intake, sympathomimetic agents). Cardiology consultation and hospitalization are necessary for serious PVCs, for patients presenting with cardiac symptoms (eg, syncope, chest pain) with PVCs, and for patients with new onset of PVCs with underlying heart disease. Treatment may include lidocaine, procainamide, propranolol, or amiodarone.

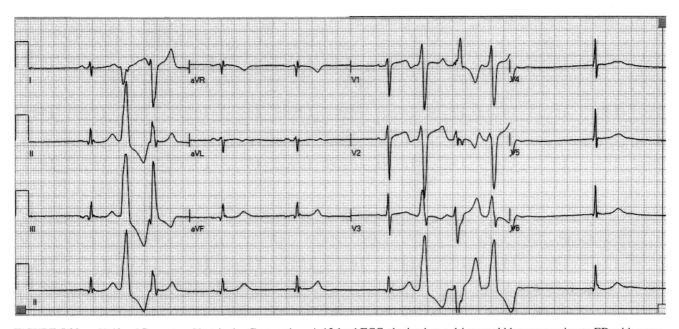

FIGURE 5.30 ■ Unifocal Premature Ventricular Contraction. A 12-lead ECG obtained on a 14-year-old boy presenting to ED with symptoms of "skipped beats." His ECG demonstrates benign monomorphic ventricular ectopics arising from the right ventricular outflow tract. These ectopics were suppressed completely during exercise. (Photo contributor: Shyam Sathanandam, MD.)

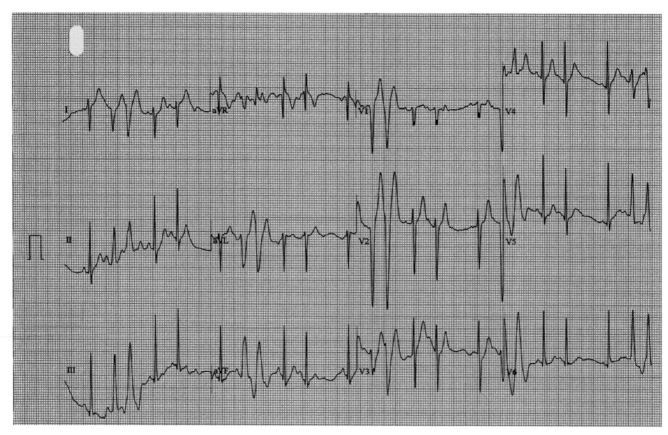

FIGURE 5.31 ■ Multifocal Premature Ventricular Contraction (PVC). Note the multiform morphology of PVCs seen in a child with cardio-myopathy. (Photo contributor: Shyam Sathanandam, MD.)

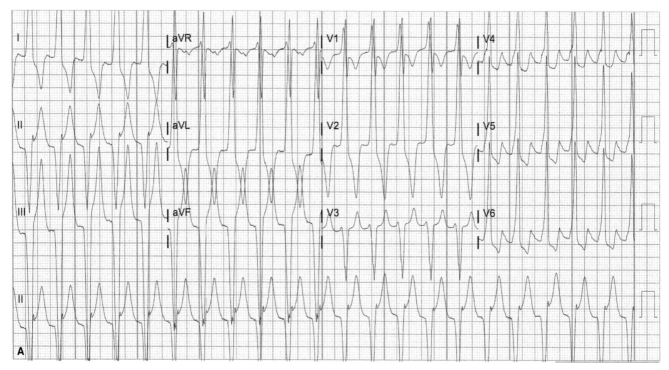

FIGURE 5.32 ■ Monomorphic Ventricular Tachycardia. (A) A 12-lead ECG of a 16-year-old boy with arrhythmogenic right ventricular dysplasia who presented with palpitations and chest pain while playing basketball. The recording shows monomorphic ventricular tachycar-dia (wide-complex tachycardia) at rate of 130 bpm. Patient had an automatic implantable cardioverter-defibrillator placed after this episode.

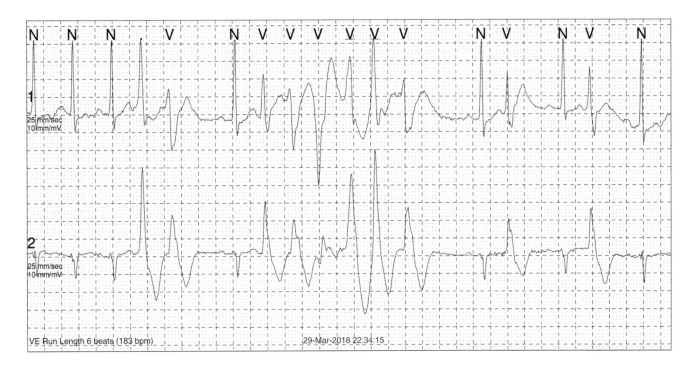

FIGURE 5.32 ■ (*Continued*) (**B**) A Holter monitor recording of the same patient showing ventricular tachycardia with different morphology. (Photo contributor: Sushitha Surendran, MD.)

Pearl

1. If a PVC falls on the T wave of the preceding normal complex (R-on-T phenomenon), it may initiate VT.

TABLE 5.14 ■ PREMATURE VENTRICULAR CONTRACTIONS (PVCs)

Etiology of PVCs
- *Drugs/ingestions:* Sympathomimetics, cyclic antidepressants, digoxin, caffeine, tobacco
- *Electrolyte imbalance:* Hypokalemia, hypocalcemia
- *Underlying heart disease:* Mitral valve prolapse, myocarditis, Lyme myocarditis, cardiomyopathy, coronary artery disease, cardiac tumors, hemochromatosis

Differential of Benign versus Serious PVCs

Benign PVCs:
- Usually asymptomatic adolescents/children
- *Without* underlying heart disease
- Unifocal (uniform morphology)
- Consistent interval from the preceding QRS
- Infrequent; usually single
- *Not* associated with R-on-T phenomenon
- Corrected QT interval normal
- PVCs suppressed by exercise

Serious PVCs:
- Symptomatic
- Associated with underlying heart disease
- Multifocal (different morphology)
- Varying intervals from the preceding QRS
- Pairs of PVCs or runs of PVCs (≥3 PVCs [VT])
- Associated with R-on-T phenomenon
- Associated with prolonged QTc interval
- No effect or increased frequency after exercise

Clinical Summary

Tetralogy of Fallot (TOF) is the most common cyanotic heart disease (Table 5.15). It consists of a spectrum of anatomic abnormalities ("tetrad") that includes a large unrestrictive malaligned ventricular septal defect (VSD), right ventricular (RV) outflow tract obstruction (infundibular pulmonary stenosis [PS]), RV hypertrophy, and overriding of the aorta. The severity of PS ranges from mild to severe PS or to pulmonary atresia. Clinical presentation of TOF depends on the nature and degree of infundibular PS. An ejection systolic murmur is usually heard at the mid-upper left sternal border (murmur of PS) and may radiate toward the back. The loudness of the murmur depends on the volume of blood flowing across the outflow tract. Varying degrees of cyanosis due to right-to-left

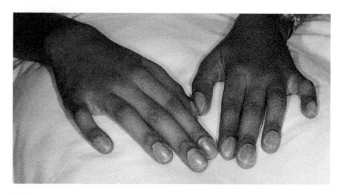

FIGURE 5.34 ■ Clubbing and Cyanotic Nail Beds; Cyanotic Congenital Heart Disease. This 12-year-old patient with tetralogy of Fallot had a hemoglobin value of 22.5 g/dL, a hematocrit of 69.2%, an oxygen saturation of 75%, and a Po_2 of 45 mm Hg on room air. (Photo contributor: Binita R. Shah, MD.)

shunt resulting in an oxygen saturation of 75% to 85% are seen. *Cyanosis shows minimal improvement with oxygen supplementation.* Other findings include increased RV impulse at the lower left sternal border (due to RV hypertrophy), loud single heart sound (pulmonary closure sound very soft), and digital clubbing. Cyanotic spells in infants and children with TOF are referred to as *hypercyanotic spells* (also known as tetralogy spells or tet spells; Table 5.16). Increased RV outflow tract obstruction exaggerates a right-to-left shunt, resulting in

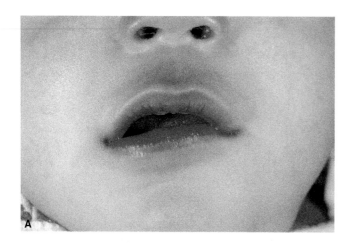

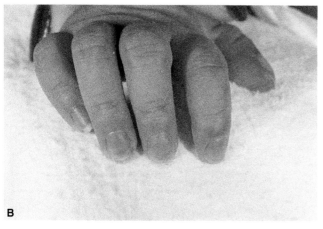

FIGURE 5.33 ■ Cyanotic Congenital Heart Disease. Cyanosis of the lips (**A**) and cyanosis of the nail beds (**B**) are seen in this 4-month-old infant with tetralogy of Fallot presenting with a hypercyanotic spell (lethargy and extreme cyanosis with hyperpnea and notable absence of a heart murmur). These photographs were taken after stabilization. (Photo contributor: Binita R. Shah, MD.)

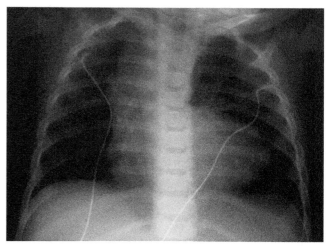

FIGURE 5.35 ■ "Boot-Shaped Heart" in Tetralogy of Fallot (TOF); Cyanotic Congenital Heart Disease. A frontal view of the chest in a 5-month-old infant with unrepaired TOF shows a "boot-shaped heart" (uplifted apex due to the right ventricular enlargement associated with concavity of the upper left heart border due to a small or absent main pulmonary artery segment), diminished pulmonary vascular markings, and a right-sided aortic arch (seen in about 25% of patients with TOF). (Photo contributor: Sushitha Surendran, MD.)

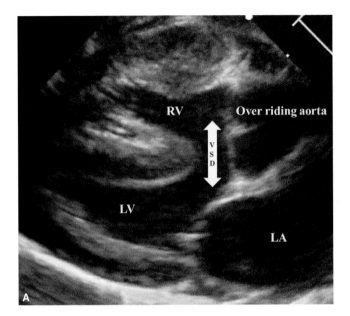

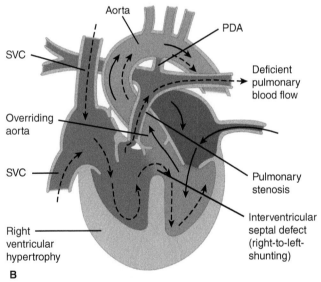

FIGURE 5.36 ■ Tetralogy of Fallot (TOF). **(A)** Parasternal long axis echocardiogram view of a 1-month-old infant presenting to ED with tet spell. His saturations were around 85%. He had severe subpulmonary and pulmonary valve stenosis. LA, left atrium; LV, left ventricle; RV, right ventricle; VSD, ventricular septal defect. **B.** TOF. PDA, patent ductus arteriosus; SVC, superior vena cava. (Photo contributors: Sushitha Surendran, MD [A], and [B] reproduced with permission from Tenenbein M, Macias CG, Sharieff GQ, et al. *Strange and Schafermeyer's Pediatric Emergency Medicine*. 5th ed. McGraw-Hill Education; New York, NY, 2019.)

a decrease in pulmonary blood flow and a hypercyanotic spell (nearly all of the blood in the RV crosses through the VSD and enters the aorta). This leads to decreased Pao_2, increased Pco_2, and decreased pH, resulting in hyperpnea (deep and

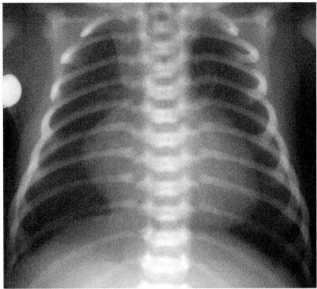

FIGURE 5.37 ■ "Egg on String Appearance" in Transposition of Great Arteries; Cyanotic Congenital Heart Disease. A frontal view of the chest in a 1-week-old baby presenting to the ED with severe cyanosis shows "egg on string appearance" with increased vascularity suggesting a diagnosis of D-transposition of the great arteries. This appearance is secondary to a narrow mediastinum, which is secondary to superimposition of the great vessels. (Photo contributor: Shyam Sathanandam, MD.)

rapid breathing). This can lead to increased venous return to the right heart and increased right-to-left shunt, resulting in a vicious cycle. CBC shows polycythemia (compensatory due to chronic hypoxemia). ECG shows RV hypertrophy with right axis deviation. Radiography in infants may be normal or may show only decreased pulmonary vascular markings. In older children, a boot-shaped heart is seen.

Emergency Department Treatment and Disposition

Hospitalize any patient with a hypercyanotic spell requiring more than oxygen therapy and positional interventions to abate the spell and any patient with complications related to prolonged hypoxemia (eg, seizures). Consult cardiology for further management of the hypercyanotic spell. Maintenance medical therapy may be required to control recurrent hypercyanotic spells (eg, propranolol) while awaiting surgical intervention.

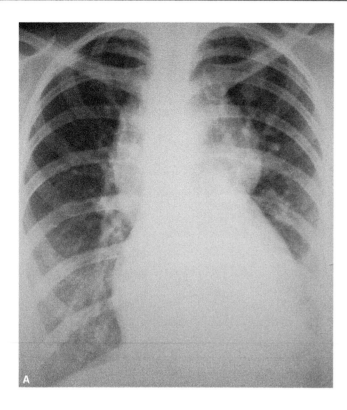

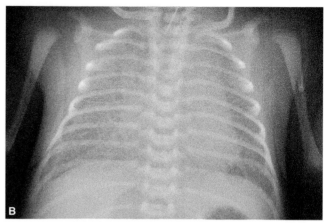

FIGURE 5.38 ■ Total Anomalous Pulmonary Venous Return (TAPVR); Cyanotic Congenital Heart Disease. (**A**) A frontal view of the chest in a 4-week-old infant presenting to the ED with tachypnea shows a "snowman" or a "figure of 8" appearance that is characteristic for supracardiac type of TAPVR. This appearance is secondary to the anomalous pulmonary veins draining into a dilated innominate vein. (**B**) A frontal view of the chest in a 6-day-old neonate presenting to the ED with severe cyanosis, lethargy, and poor feeding shows a ground-glass appearance secondary to obstructed pulmonary veins and a right pleural effusion. Echocardiogram demonstrated an infracardiac type of TAPVR. (Photo contributor: Shyam Sathanandam, MD.)

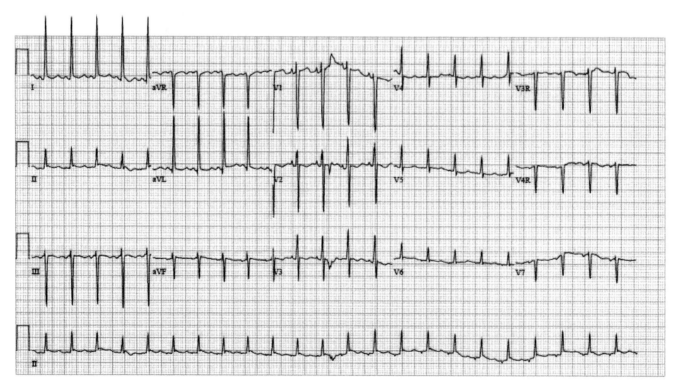

FIGURE 5.39 ■ Tricuspid Atresia; Cyanotic Congenital Heart Disease. A 12-lead ECG obtained on a 3-day-old neonate presenting to the ED with respiratory distress and mild cyanosis shows a left-axis deviation that is virtually pathognomonic for tricuspid atresia. (Photo contributor: Shyam Sathanandam, MD.)

TABLE 5.15 ■ CYANOTIC CONGENITAL HEART DISEASE

5 T's:
- *T*etralogy of Fallot (most common cause of cyanotic *heart disease)*
- *T*runcus arteriosus
- *T*ransposition of the great arteries
- *T*ricuspid atresia
- *T*otal anomalous pulmonary venous connection

Pearls

1. Two hallmarks of TOF are a PS murmur and cyanosis.
2. Hypercyanotic spells of TOF are very dramatic in their presentation. Failure to recognize without immediate intervention may result in hypoxic seizures, profound metabolic acidosis, cerebrovascular accident (due to polycythemia/hyperviscosity), deterioration in cardiac rhythm, and death.
3. Increasing cyanosis in a child with a prior history of heart disease or prior history of squatting with exertion is an important clue indicating a potential hypercyanotic spell.
4. A notable absence or lessening of a previously heard heart murmur in a cyanotic child is the most important clue suggesting a hypercyanotic spell.

TABLE 5.16 ■ HYPERCYANOTIC SPELL OF TETRALOGY OF FALLOT

Presenting features:
- Spells usually occur in the morning shortly after awakening.
- Spells are self-limited and usually last <15–30 minutes.
- Spells may occur spontaneously or be precipitated by events that decrease the systemic vascular resistance such as dehydration, fever, stress, injury, sudden fright, defecation, exertion during feeding, or anything that makes the infant cry.
- Profound cyanosis (or history of increasing cyanosis) in a child with prior history of heart disease.
- Prior history of squatting or knee-chest position with exertion.

During the spell patient, the infant or child may present with any of the following:
(1) Irritability/crying/agitation (signs of hypoxemia)
(2) Lethargy, unconsciousness, or syncope (recurrent or prolonged)
(3) Profound cyanosis
(4) Seizures, cerebrovascular accidents (due to polycythemia)
(5) *Notable absence or decrease in intensity of a previously heard heart murmur* (due to decreased antegrade flow into the pulmonary arteries)
(6) Increased rate and depth of respiration (*hyperpnea, an important feature*)

Management (intervene in the following order, as indicated)

Standard initial therapeutic interventions that result in prompt abatement of the spell:
- Give 100% oxygen via a non-rebreathing facemask.
- Try to calm the child.
- Have the child assume the knee-chest position (knees flexed and drawn up close to the child's chest and pressing on the abdomen); this increases systemic vascular resistance (SVR) in the lower extremities, promoting increased venous return to the heart and increased pulmonary blood flow.
- Morphine sulfate given intramuscularly, subcutaneously, or IV.
- Maintenance rate of IV fluids or correct hypovolemia if present.
- Correct hypoglycemia if present (hypoglycemia may contribute to a spell).

Additional interventions if above measures fail:
- Sodium bicarbonate (corrects metabolic acidosis seen after prolonged hypoxemia)
- Propranolol or esmolol (decreases dynamic contraction of the infundibulum and decreases heart rate)
- Phenylephrine (increases SVR)
- Endotracheal intubation, mechanical ventilation, neuromuscular blockade to reduce oxygen consumption due to increased work of breathing
- *Important: Do not use epinephrine or norepinephrine to abate the spell.*

Clinical Summary

Hypoplastic left heart syndrome (HLHS) refers to a spectrum of CHDs that have in common a very small left ventricle and other associated anatomic abnormalities. There is inadequate antegrade flow to support the systemic circulation because of the hypoplasia of the left heart. Since systemic circulation is supported by the right side of the heart through the ductus arteriosus, these lesions are referred to as ductal-dependent lesions. A few examples of ductal-dependent systemic blood flow lesions include HLHS, critical coarctation of the aorta, and aortic arch interruption. Examples of right-sided ductal-dependent

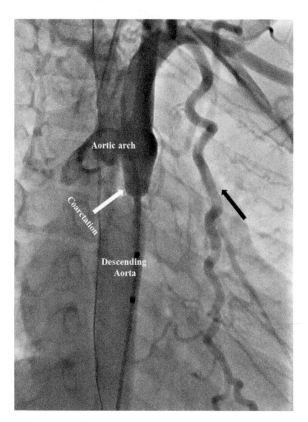

FIGURE 5.41 ■ Coarctation of Aorta. An angiogram of a 10-year-old girl with systemic hypertension shows severe coarctation of aorta (white arrow) with multiple collateral vessels (black arrow). Her lower limb blood pressure was lower than her upper limb pressure, with a 30 mm Hg difference. (Photo contributor: Sushitha Surendran, MD.)

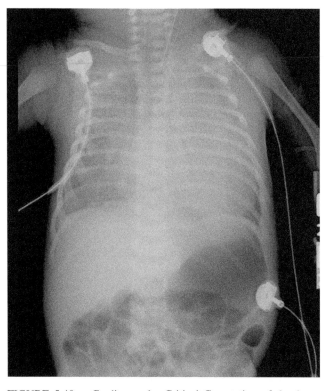

FIGURE 5.40 ■ Cardiomegaly: Critical Coarctation of the Aorta (Left-sided Ductal-Dependent Cardiac Lesion). A frontal view of the chest shows marked cardiomegaly and increased vascularity in a 21-day-old neonate presenting with cyanosis, severe respiratory distress, tachycardia, wheezing, and shock with marked acidosis (arterial pH 6.86, PCO_2 47 mm Hg, PO_2 35.7 mm Hg, and base deficit of –22.4). His wheezing and respiratory distress initially were thought to be due to bronchiolitis, but with findings on the CXR, a possibility of a ductal-dependent cardiac lesion with cardiogenic shock was entertained and prostaglandin E_1 infusion was begun. A diagnosis of critical coarctation of the aorta was confirmed by echocardiography. (Photo contributor: Binita R. Shah, MD.)

lesions (pulmonary circulation dependent on patency of the ductus arteriosus) include pulmonary atresia with intact ventricular septum, tricuspid atresia, and critical pulmonary stenosis. HLHS, a representative of ductal-dependent lesions, is one of the most serious cardiac anomalies presenting in infancy. A neonate born with HLHS appears normal with normal Apgar scores because systemic perfusion and oxygenation are normal in utero. Typically, on day 2 or 3 of life, signs of poor systemic perfusion occur as the ductus arteriosus closes (Table 5.17). All patients with HLHS have a single, loud second heart sound and variable heart murmurs that are usually not diagnostic. ECG may show right atrial enlargement (~30%–40%), right ventricular hypertrophy (~80%–90%), and diminished left ventricular forces (~30%–40%). Radiograph typically shows marked cardiomegaly with normal to increased pulmonary markings.

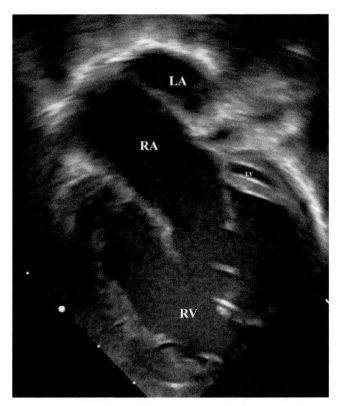

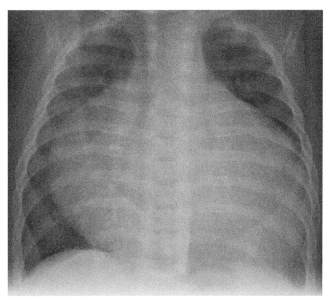

FIGURE 5.43 ■ Ebstein Anomaly: Cyanotic Congenital Heart Disease. A frontal view of the CXR on a 9-month-old baby with Ebstein anomaly shows massive cardiomegaly. This degree of cardiomegaly is seen in only a very few conditions; Ebstein anomaly being one of them. (Photo contributor: Sushitha Surendran, MD.)

FIGURE 5.42 ■ Hypoplastic Left Heart Syndrome. A 4-chamber echocardiogram image of a 2-day-old baby presenting with desaturation, tachypnea, and metabolic acidosis shows hypoplastic left ventricle (LV) and left atrium (LA). The right ventricle (RV) is dilated. RA, right atrium. (Photo contributor: Sushitha Surendran, MD.)

Emergency Department Treatment and Disposition

All ductal-dependent cardiac lesions present in a similar fashion (like HLHS), and the initial medical management is *identical* in all. Support the ABCs and provide continuous cardiac and pulse oximetry. Maintain ductal patency with an infusion of prostaglandin E_1 (PGE$_1$). Treat metabolic acidosis by fluid therapy and sodium bicarbonate (acidosis leads to increased systemic vascular resistance and, in turn, increases pulmonary blood flow). Avoid any maneuver that would decrease pulmonary vascular resistance and pulmonary pressure as this will steal blood flow from the systemic circulation (eg, supplemental oxygen therapy [oxygen acts as pulmonary vasodilator] and hyperventilation [low Pco_2 acts as pulmonary vasodilator]). Aim for the "ideal arterial blood gas with 7.4/40/40" (pH 7.4, Po_2 40 mm Hg, Pco_2 40 mm Hg). This is usually achieved with low (or no) mechanical ventilatory support on room air. After initial stabilization all patients, require admission to the ICU for subsequent management. Consult cardiology (after stabilization) to confirm the diagnosis by 2-dimensional echocardiography and for subsequent referral for surgical management.

Pearls

1. A ductal-dependent cardiac lesion must be considered in any neonate (*up to 28 days old*) with sudden onset of shock, severe hypoxemia, acidosis, or intense cyanosis (systemic circulatory collapse). Hyperoxia test will be helpful in differentiating between a cardiac and a noncardiac cause of cyanosis.

2. Neonates presenting with shock should be treated as having ductal-dependent lesions until proved otherwise; PGE$_1$ infusion, by maintaining patency of the ductus arteriosus, is *lifesaving* in such infants.

TABLE 5.17 ■ DUCTAL-DEPENDENT CARDIAC LESIONS/HYPOPLASTIC LEFT HEART SYNDROME

Characteristic features:
- *Typical age at presentation:* usually within the first few days of life (when the ductus closes; neonates may present as late as 1 or 2 weeks of life and sometimes even older)
- Signs of shock
  - (1) Skin cyanotic or mottled, cool extremities, prolonged capillary refill
  - (2) Peripheral pulses rapid, thready, weak, or absent
  - (3) Discrepancy in volume between peripheral and central pulses
  - (4) Irritability, lethargy, or unresponsiveness
  - (5) Respiratory distress (compensation for severe metabolic acidosis and increased pulmonary blood flow)
  - (6) Hypotension (decompensated shock)
  - (7) Metabolic acidosis due to poor tissue perfusion
  - (8) Decreased or no urine output
- Multisystem organ failure (eg, acute renal failure, seizures)

Treatment of Ductal-Dependent Cardiac Lesions:

PGE_1 infusion
- Vasodilator
- Maintains or reopens the ductus arteriosus
- Given as a continuous infusion (very short half-life)
- Side effects: vasodilator effects (flushing and peripheral edema), fever, jitteriness or convulsions, metabolic (hypoglycemia, hypocalcemia), renal failure, coagulopathies

Life-threatening side effects: apnea, bradycardia, and hypotension
- Load with caffeine to help decrease the apnea due to PGE_1 infusion and start on maintenance dose of caffeine

TABLE 5.18 ■ HYPEROXIA TEST

- Administer 100% oxygen for >10 minutes
- Can be done using an oxyhood or by intubation
- Measure Pao_2 before and after administering 100% oxygen
- If Pao_2 >150 mm Hg = most likely pulmonary in etiology
- If Pao_2 <100 mm Hg or Sao_2 unchanged = most likely cardiac (right-to-left shunt) in etiology

Clinical Summary

Infective endocarditis (IE), a microbial infection of the endocardial/endothelial surface, may be classified as acute or subacute or as native valve endocarditis, prosthetic valve endocarditis, or endocarditis in IV drug abusers. Gram-positive cocci account for 90% of culture-positive endocarditis. Neonates, immunocompromised patients, and injection drug users are at increased risk for gram-negative endocarditis. About 5% to 10% of cases are culture negative. Etiologic agents include *Streptococcus viridans* (most common in all age groups, especially in developing countries where rheumatic heart disease is prevalent) and *Staphylococcus aureus* (second most common and more common in developed countries), followed by coagulase-negative *Staphylococcus epidermidis*, *Enterococcus* species, *Streptococcus pneumoniae*, HACEK group (*Haemophilus* species, *Actinobacillus actinomycetemcomitans*, *Cardiobacterium hominis*, *Eikenella corrodens*, and *Kingella kingae*), and fungi (*Candida* species, *Aspergillus* species). Endocarditis in childhood is seen with preexisting CHD and includes patients with complex cyanotic CHD (eg, TOF), post–cardiac surgery (eg, palliative shunt procedures) patients, and patients with a previous history of endocarditis. Patients with an uncorrected ventricular septal defect, patent ductus arteriosus, atrial septal defect, and bicuspid aortic valve are no longer considered at increased risk for

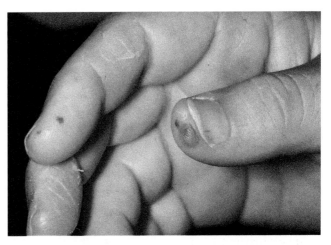

FIGURE 5.45 ■ Osler Nodes. Subcutaneous, purplish, tender nodules in the pulp of fingers known as Osler nodes. (Courtesy of the Armed Forces Institute of Pathology, Bethesda, MD.)

endocarditis, and the American Heart Association (AHA) has exempted these patients from needing prophylaxis.

Endocarditis can also occur without underlying CHD; predisposing factors include infected indwelling central venous catheters. IV drug abuse is not a common predisposing factor in younger children. Bacteremia may occur during severe burns, during any bacterial infection (eg, cellulitis, pneumonia, UTI), following any dental or surgical procedures or any instrumentation of mucosal surfaces, or spontaneously following activities such as brushing teeth. Clinical features of IE are mentioned in Table 5.19. The Modified Duke criteria (refer to AHA website) are a combination of pathologic and

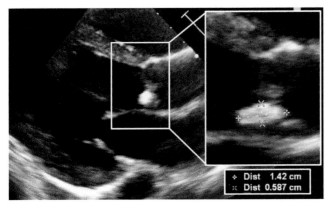

FIGURE 5.44 ■ Infective Endocarditis. Parasternal long axis echocardiogram view of a 15-year-old boy with bicuspid aortic valve showing an echogenic mass attached to the aortic valve cusp. The insert is a zoom-in view of the vegetation on the aortic valve with measurements. He presented with 1-week history of fever, leg pain, and blood culture positive for methicillin-sensitive *Staphylococcus aureus* following a dental procedure. He was treated with 6-week course of cefazolin. (Photo contributor: Sushitha Surendran, MD.)

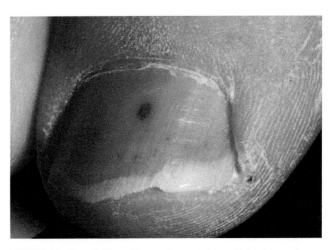

FIGURE 5.46 ■ Splinter Hemorrhages. Note splinter hemorrhages along the distal aspect of the nail plate due to emboli from subacute bacterial endocarditis. (Courtesy of the Armed Forces Institute of Pathology, Bethesda, Maryland.)

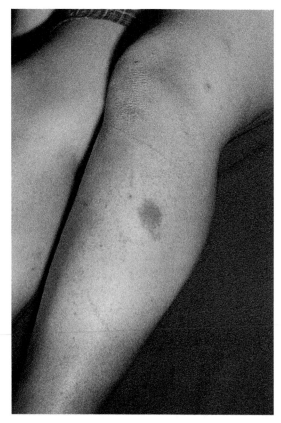

FIGURE 5.47 ■ Petechiae and Purpura. Persistent fever was associated with the petechiae and purpura seen on the lower extremities in this girl with ventricular septal defect. Blood culture was positive for *Streptococcus pneumoniae*. Petechiae and purpura seen in infective endocarditis may mimic a primary vasculitis or primary coagulation disorder. (Photo contributor: Binita R. Shah, MD.)

clinical criteria that help in arriving at the diagnosis of IE. Differential diagnosis of IE includes malignancy, collagen vascular diseases, and other infections affecting the heart (eg, acute rheumatic fever).

Emergency Department Treatment and Disposition

Hospitalize all suspected cases of IE in the ICU, if indicated for acutely ill patients, for confirmation of the diagnosis, IV antibiotic therapy, and continuous cardiac monitoring. Blood cultures are positive in >95% of cases of IE and remain the gold standard for making the diagnosis. Obtain at least 3 sets of blood cultures over a 24-hour period (from separate venipuncture sites and with a large quantity of blood, if possible). Obtain CBC (normocytic normochromic

TABLE 5.19 ■ CLINICAL FEATURES OF INFECTIVE ENDOCARDITIS IN CHILDREN

- Fever (most common symptom), prolonged low-grade fever, rigors, diaphoresis
- Fatigue, nausea, vomiting, abdominal pain, anorexia, weight loss, malaise
- Chest pain
- Arthralgias or arthritis, myalgia
- Splenomegaly (less common than in adults)
- Congestive heart failure (valve destruction, regurgitation)
- Valvulitis (new or changing murmurs)
- Cardiac arrhythmias
- Roth's spots: small, pale, retinal lesions with areas of hemorrhage near the optic disc
- Subungual splinter hemorrhages
- Embolic events (CNS, kidneys, spleen, skin, lungs)
- Cerebral infarction signs/symptoms: seizures, changing mental status, ataxia, aphasia, acute hemiplegia, focal neurologic deficits

Dermatologic Manifestations
- Skin lesions occur in 15%–50% of cases
- Types of skin lesions: petechiae, Osler nodes, and Janeway lesions
  - A. Petechiae or purpura
    - (1) Most common skin manifestation, occur in small crops, usually transient
    - (2) Sites: mucous membranes of the mouth, conjunctiva; upper part of the chest; extremities
  - B. Osler nodes
    - (1) Pea-sized, erythematous, indurated nodules with pale centers; few in number
    - (2) Tender (pain may be elicited by palpating the tips of the digits)
    - (3) Transient; resolves without necrosis or suppuration
    - (4) Sites: pads of fingers and toes (most common), thenar and hypothenar eminences, sides of the fingers, arms
  - C. Janeway lesions (peripheral embolization)
    - (1) Painless; small erythematous macules or small nodular hemorrhages
    - (2) Site: palms or soles

anemia, leukocytosis), erythrocyte sedimentation rate (ESR), C-reactive protein (CRP), and urinalysis (microscopic hematuria, proteinuria). Antibiotic therapy is guided by the identification of the pathogen and sensitivity. It is best not to administer antibiotics in ED while awaiting collection of more blood culture samples and culture results unless patient is very sick. Duration of therapy varies from 2 to 6 weeks.

Pearls

1. Suspect endocarditis in any patient with a heart murmur and persistent unexplained high fever, especially with underlying CHD or condition that increases the risk of bacteremia, or in any febrile IV drug abuser (even in the absence of a heart murmur).

2. Patients with CHD presenting to ED with evidence of soft tissue infections (eg, abscess) must receive appropriate antibiotic coverage prior to debridement or incision and drainage.

Clinical Summary

Acute or chronic pain in the precordial region that may radiate to the neck, arm, or jaw and that is associated with nausea and typically precipitated by exercise is a common presenting symptom in the ED. Relative frequency and causes of chest pain in children are mentioned in the Table 5.20. Initial history should be directed at determining the nature of pain, associated symptoms, and concurrent or precipitating events that may help clarify noncardiac origin of the pain, including focusing on important past and family histories of any unexplained sudden death or drowning, sudden infant death syndrome, and syncope. Associated symptoms such as presyncope, syncope, dizziness, palpitation, dyspnea, cyanosis, sweating, and chest pain with exertion would raise suspicion for a more serious cause of chest pain. Before turning the focus to the chest, perform a thorough physical examination, including observing whether the child is in severe distress from pain, in emotional stress, or hyperventilating. A typical angina pain is located in the precordial or substernal area and radiates to the neck, jaw, arms, back, or abdomen. Patient describes pain as a deep, heavy pressure; the feeling of choking; or a squeezing sensation. Exercise, cold stress, emotional upset, or a large meal typically precipitates angina pain.

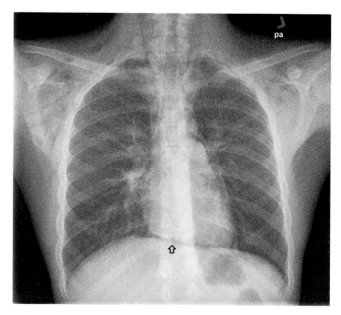

FIGURE 5.49 ■ Differential Diagnosis of Chest Pain. Pneumomediastinum. A frontal view of the chest shows pneumomediastinum and subcutaneous emphysema. Note the continuous diaphragm sign (arrow) diagnostic of pneumomediastinum. This adolescent male presented with flu-like symptoms of cough, rhinorrhea, and several episodes of vomiting followed by chest pain and neck pain. Bilateral crepitus was felt on examination of his neck. (Photo/legend contributors: Caitlin Feeks, DO, and John Amodio, MD.)

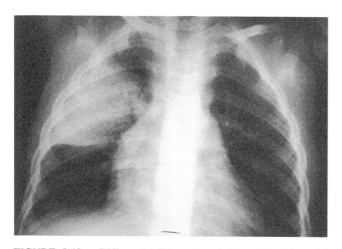

FIGURE 5.48 ■ Differential Diagnosis of Chest Pain. Bacterial Pneumonia. Frontal view of the chest shows right upper lobe consolidation with a slight bulge in the minor fissure in a 7-year-old child presenting to the ED with chest pain and difficulty breathing. Fever, tachypnea, tachycardia, and hypoxemia were additional findings. Her blood culture was positive for *Streptococcus pneumoniae*. (Photo contributor: Binita R. Shah, MD.)

Emergency Department Treatment and Disposition

A 3-step diagnostic approach is recommended. Direct the first step at detecting the 3 most common causes of chest pain: costochondritis, musculoskeletal causes, and respiratory diseases. A through history and physical examination help making the correct diagnosis. The second step is to check for cardiac causes, with cardiac exam, CXR, and ECG, if clinically indicated. If a cardiac cause is not found, the pain is likely due to disease in other systems including psychogenic and idiopathic causes.

Direct the treatment at correcting or improving the cause once a specific cause of chest pain is identified. Consult cardiology when chest pain is anginal in nature; when there are any abnormal findings on CXR or ECG; or when patient has a positive family history of cardiomyopathy, LQTS, or another hereditary disease associated with cardiac abnormalities. Cardiac evaluation requires further studies such as

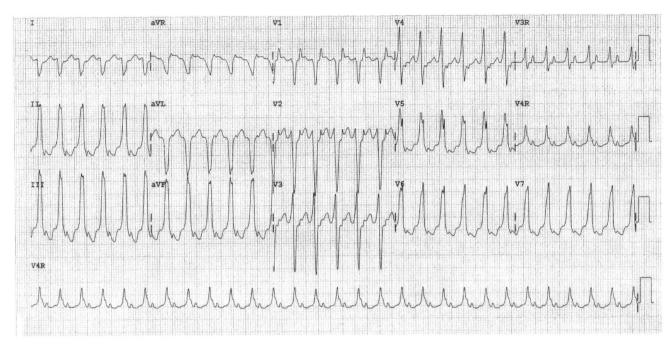

FIGURE 5.50 ■ Differential Diagnosis of Chest Pain. Ventricular Tachycardia (VT). A 16-year-old boy presented with precordial chest pain (dull aching without radiation) lasting for 2 hours following a football practice. He had similar chest pain in the past following football practice and was diagnosed as having exercise-induced asthma and prescribed albuterol before practice. This 12-lead ECG demonstrates a wide-complex tachycardia at a rate of 140 bpm with retrograde P waves best seen in leads V3R and V4R, suggesting that this is VT. There is left bundle branch block and inferior axis (positive QRS in leads II, III, and aVF), suggesting the origin of VT from the right ventricular outflow tract. This is a benign form of VT commonly precipitated by exercise or β-agonists such as albuterol in young men. (Photo contributor: Shyam Sathanandam, MD.)

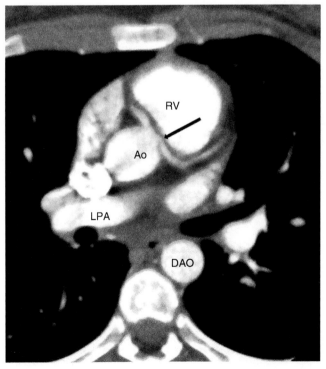

FIGURE 5.51 ■ Anomalous Origin of the Left Main Coronary Artery. A contrast enhanced CT scan axial image of a 13-year-old girl with history of chest pain and syncope shows anomalous origin of the left coronary artery (arrow) from the right sinus of Valsalva with an intramural and interarterial course. The patient underwent unroofing of the anomalous left coronary artery. Ao, aorta; DAO, descending aorta; LPA, left pulmonary artery; RV, right ventricle. (Photo contributor: Sushitha Surendran, MD.)

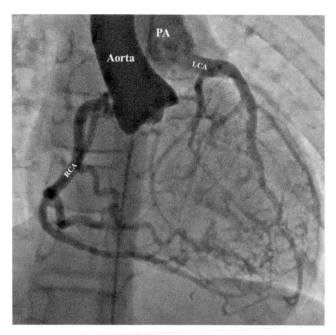

FIGURE 5.52 ■ Anomalous Origin of the Left Coronary Artery from the Pulmonary Artery. A 7-year-old girl with a history of multiple episodes of chest pain while playing was evaluated in the ED after an episode of cardiac arrest and resuscitation. Her angiogram shows anomalous origin of the left coronary artery (LCA), which is filled retrograde by collaterals from the right coronary system, and contrast filling the pulmonary artery (PA) is also seen. RCA, right coronary artery. (Photo contributor: Sushitha Surendran, MD.)

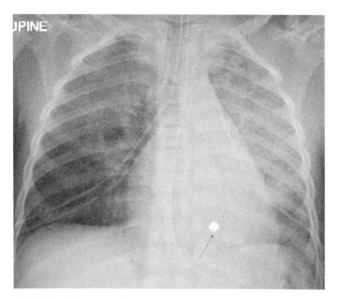

FIGURE 5.53 ■ Gunshot Injury to Heart. CXR of an 8-year-old boy with gunshot injury to left chest with metallic fragment (arrow) left behind in the left ventricle. There is a small left pneumothorax and left chest wall subcutaneous emphysema. Bilateral lung contusions and atelectasis are also seen. (Photo contributor: Sushitha Surendran, MD.)

TABLE 5.20 ■ RELATIVE FREQUENCY OF CAUSES OF CHEST PAIN IN CHILDREN

Idiopathic factors	12%–45%
Costochondritis	9%–22%
Musculoskeletal trauma	21%
Cough, asthma, pneumonia	15%–21%
Psychogenic factors	5%–9%
Gastrointestinal disorders	4%–7%
Cardiac disorders	1%–4%
Sickle cell crisis	2%
Miscellaneous	9%–21%

Noncardiac causes:

A. Thoracic cage:
   (1) Costochondritis (preceded by physical activity, exaggerated by breathing, may be chronic, tenderness on palpation over chondrosternal junction)
   (2) Trauma or muscle strain (history of vigorous exercise or trauma), abnormalities of the ribcage or thoracic spine, and breast tenderness (mastalgia)
B. Respiratory (severe cough or bronchitis, pleural effusion, lobar pneumonia, exercise-induced asthma, spontaneous pneumothorax, pulmonary embolism)
C. Gastrointestinal (esophagitis [burning substernal pain that worsens with reclining posture], peptic ulcer [usually a burning substernal pain that worsens after certain foods], ingestion of foreign body)
D. Psychogenic factors (hyperventilation, anxiety, panic attack, conversion disorder, somatization, and depression)
E. Miscellaneous (Texidor twinge–precordial catch or stitch in the side [lasts for seconds or minutes and associated with bending or slouching], herpes zoster, pleurodynia [devil's grip; coxsackie virus infection, characterized by sudden episodes of sharp chest pain])

Cardiac causes:

A. Structural abnormalities of the heart (eg, severe aortic or pulmonary stenosis, hypertrophic cardiomyopathy, mitral valve prolapse)
B. Coronary artery abnormalities (eg, Kawasaki disease (KD), congenital coronary anomaly, coronary heart disease, hypertension, sickle cell disease), cocaine abuse
C. Aortic dissection and aortic aneurysm (Turner, Marfan, and Noonan syndrome).
D. Inflammatory conditions (pericarditis [viral, bacterial, or rheumatic]), postpericordiotomy syndrome, myocarditis (acute or chronic), KD
E. Arrhythmias (supraventricular tachycardia, frequent premature ventricular contractions, or ventricular tachycardia)

echocardiography, exercise stress test, Holter monitoring, or even cardiac catheterization, and depending on the cause, treatment will be medical or surgical. For teenagers, it is appropriate to perform a urine drug screen also to exclude substance abuse (eg, cocaine), which can cause coronary vasospasm and chest pain. Routine testing for troponin is not recommended unless indicated by history and physical examination or ECG changes. Most musculoskeletal and nonorganic causes of chest pain can be treated with rest, acetaminophen, or nonsteroidal anti-inflammatory agents. If respiratory causes of chest pain are found, treatment is directed at those causes.

Pearls

1. Chest pain is often benign in children. No cause can be found in a majority of patients, even after a moderately extensive investigation.

2. History is the most important information; most cases of chest pain in children originate in organ systems other than the cardiovascular system.

3. Chest pain in children <12 years of age usually has a cardiorespiratory cause; psychogenic causes are more likely in children >12 years of age.

4. ED providers should make every effort to find a specific cause before making a referral to a specialist or reassuring the child and the parents of the benign nature of the complaint.

Clinical Summary

Acute pericarditis, an acute inflammation of the parietal and visceral surfaces of the pericardium, can be infectious or non-infectious in origin and may or may not be associated with pericardial effusion. The most common etiology, particularly in infancy, is viral (eg, coxsackie B virus, adenovirus, enteroviruses, echoviruses, cytomegalovirus, HIV, influenza virus). A few examples of other etiologies include acute rheumatic fever, purulent pericarditis (eg, *S aureus, S pneumoniae, Haemophilus influenzae, Neisseria meningitides,* and streptococci), tuberculosis (constrictive pericarditis), histoplasmosis (endemic areas), heart surgery (postpericardiotomy syndrome), collagen vascular diseases (eg, rheumatoid arthritis, systemic lupus erythematosus), uremia (uremic pericarditis), drug induced (eg, hydralazine, isoniazid, procainamide, phenytoin), and neoplasia (due to metastasis, chemotherapeutic agents, mediastinal irradiation). Pericardial effusion may be serofibrinous, hemorrhagic, chylous, or purulent. Effusion may be completely absorbed or may result in pericardial thickening or chronic constriction (constrictive pericarditis). A rapid accumulation of a large amount of fluid or progressive accumulation of fluid beyond the point of potential pericardial distension can produce cardiac tamponade, which is classically associated with a triad of low arterial BP, jugular venous distention, and distant, muffled heart sounds (Beck triad). Narrowed pulse pressure and pulsus

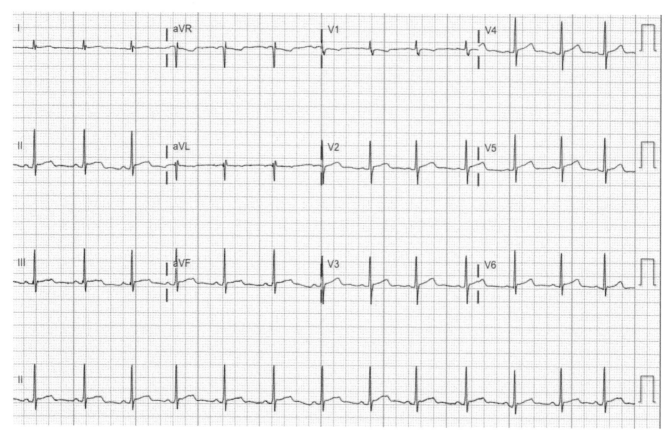

FIGURE 5.54 ■ Acute Pericarditis. A 12-lead ECG obtained in a 15-year-old girl presenting to the ED with chest discomfort and difficulty breathing 1 week after surgical repair of atrial septal defect. This ECG shows mild diffuse ST elevation in anterior and inferior leads. She was found to have pericarditis and a large pericardial effusion. (Photo contributor: Sushitha Surendran, MD.)

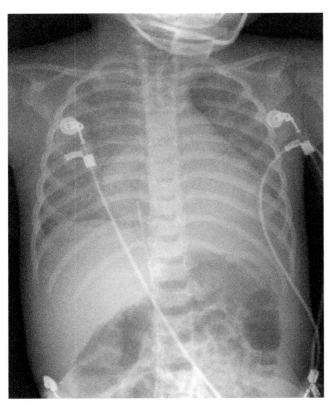

FIGURE 5.55 ■ Acute Pericarditis. Seventeen-month-old toddler presented to ED with difficulty breathing that had progressed over the past 3 days. She had a recent viral upper respiratory tract illness. CXR reveals cardiomegaly and pulmonary edema. This could be viral pericarditis with pericardial effusion or viral myocarditis. Sometimes it is impossible to differentiate the 2 conditions without getting a biopsy. (Photo contributor: Shyam Sathanandam, MD.)

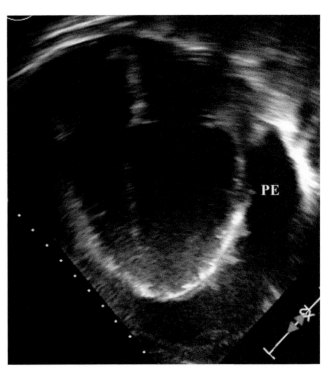

FIGURE 5.56 ■ Pericardial Effusion (PE). A 16-year-old boy presented to the ED with chest pain and difficulty breathing. A 4-chamber echocardiogram view shows a large PE with signs of cardiac tamponade. Pericardiocentesis was performed immediately, and a pericardial drain was placed. A diagnosis of histoplasmosis was confirmed (blood test for *Histoplasma* antigen and antibody panel). Pericardial effusion is an inflammatory response to histoplasmosis rather than an infectious process within the pericardium. CT scan of his chest and abdomen showed multiple granulomatous nodules in his lungs, liver, and spleen and multiple enlarged lymph nodes. (Photo contributor: Sushitha Surendran, MD.)

paradoxus may be observed. Pulsus paradoxus is defined as a decrease in systolic BP >10 mm Hg during inspiration. Cardiac tamponade occurs more commonly with purulent pericarditis.

History may reveal preceding upper respiratory tract infection. Fever and chest pain may be present. Chest pain may be relieved by leaning forward and may be made worse by supine position or deep inspiration. Some patients can present with abdominal pain. Pericardial friction rub (a grating to-and-fro sound in phase with the heart sounds) is the cardinal physical sign. Heart murmur is usually absent. Presence of a cardiac murmur should prompt consideration of acute rheumatic fever or endocarditis.

Emergency Department Treatment and Disposition

Obtain ECG and CXR and consult cardiologist. ECG reveals low-voltage QRS complex (caused by pericardial effusion) and diffuse ST-segment elevation in all precordial and limb leads. CXR will show varying degree of cardiomegaly and increased pulmonary vascular markings (with cardiac tamponade). Echocardiography is the most useful tool to diagnose pericardial effusion. Stabilize patients with hemodynamic compromise. For cardiac tamponade, urgent decompression by surgical drainage or pericardiocentesis is indicated. While getting ready for the procedure, give fluid boluses with plasminate to increase central venous pressure and thereby improve cardiac filling, which can provide temporary emergency stabilization. Medications that decrease the systemic arterial BP (eg, vasodilators, diuretics) should be avoided. Hospitalize patients to ICU who have hemodynamic compromise or are expected to have progressive disease. Salicylates are given for precordial pain and for rheumatic pericarditis. Corticosteroid therapy may be indicated in severe rheumatic carditis or postpericardiotomy syndrome. There is no specific treatment for viral pericarditis. Use of colchicine in addition to nonsteroidal anti-inflammatory agents has been shown to significantly reduce the rate of recurrence in adults. Patients with bacterial pericarditis will need IV antibiotics for 3 to 4 weeks. Pericardiocentesis or surgical drainage to identify the cause of pericarditis is mandatory, especially when purulent or tuberculous pericarditis is suspected. A drainage catheter may be left in place.

Pearls

1. Viral infection is the most common cause of acute pericarditis. A history of upper respiratory tract infection along with the symptom of chest pain that is relieved on leaning forward is helpful in making a diagnosis.

2. The most serious complications of pericarditis are pericardial effusion and cardiac tamponade, the presence of which is an indication for urgent pericardiocentesis.

Clinical Summary

Acute myocarditis is caused by acute inflammation of the myocardium. It can be infectious or noninfectious in origin (Table 5.21). Viral infection is the most common cause. Many viruses that cause acute pericarditis, including parvovirus B19, enteroviruses (coxsackie viruses B and A, echoviruses), adenovirus, cytomegalovirus, HIV, and influenza virus, can also cause acute myocarditis. Older children may have a history of preceding upper respiratory tract or gastrointestinal infection. The illness may have a sudden onset in newborns and infants with anorexia, vomiting, lethargy, respiratory distress, and circulatory shock. Sudden death can also occur. Arrhythmias including SVT or ventricular ectopic beats may be audible. CHB can also occur. The mortality rate is as high as 75% in symptomatic neonates with acute viral myocarditis. The majority of patients with mild disease recover completely. Some patients develop subacute or chronic myocarditis with persistent cardiomegaly and CHF.

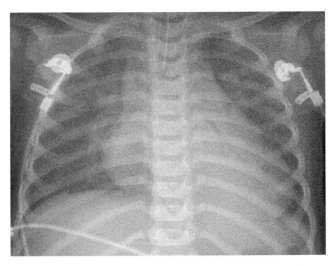

FIGURE 5.57 ■ Acute Myocarditis. Frontal view of the chest shows marked cardiomegaly with pulmonary edema in a 4-year-old child in severe respiratory distress with cyanosis and stupor requiring intubation. Severe metabolic and respiratory acidosis, poor cardiac function noted on echocardiography, and a rapid progression from sinus tachycardia to ventricular tachycardia were seen (see Figure 5.58). Suspect acute fulminant myocarditis in such a scenario. (Photo contributor: Shyam Sathanandam, MD.)

Emergency Department Treatment and Disposition

Obtain ECG and CXR and consult cardiology. Cardiomegaly of varying degrees is seen on CXR. ECG reveals tachycardia with low-voltage QRS complex, ST-T changes, QT prolongation, and arrhythmias, especially PVCs. When there is myocardial damage, wide and notched Q waves may be present. Echocardiography reveals cardiac chamber enlargement, impaired left ventricle function, and pericardial effusion. Occasionally, a thrombus in the left ventricle can be found. Cardiac troponin levels and MB isoenzyme of creatine kinase may be elevated. Serial measurement of brain natriuretic peptide can be useful in evaluating the response to treatment. The best confirmatory test is endomyocardial biopsy, which is not practical in every situation. Cardiac MRI can help to localize areas of inflammation, edema, necrosis, and fibrosis.

Hospitalize patients who are hemodynamically unstable or with aggressive arrhythmias to ICU. Bed rest and limitation of activity are recommended during the acute phase. Arrhythmias should be treated aggressively. When the clinical diagnosis of myocarditis is suspected, it is now recommended to treat with high-dose IV γ-globulin in the hospital. Angiotensin-converting enzyme inhibitors and angiotensin receptor blockers have shown benefits in patients with left ventricular dysfunction and dilation and help in favorable remodeling of the myocardium.

Pearls

1. Myocarditis severe enough to be recognized clinically is rare, but the prevalence of mild and subclinical cases is higher.
2. A high index of suspicion is required to make a clinical diagnosis as it carries a high mortality rate, especially in childhood.
3. Acute myocarditis results in aggressive arrhythmias that may be hard to treat.

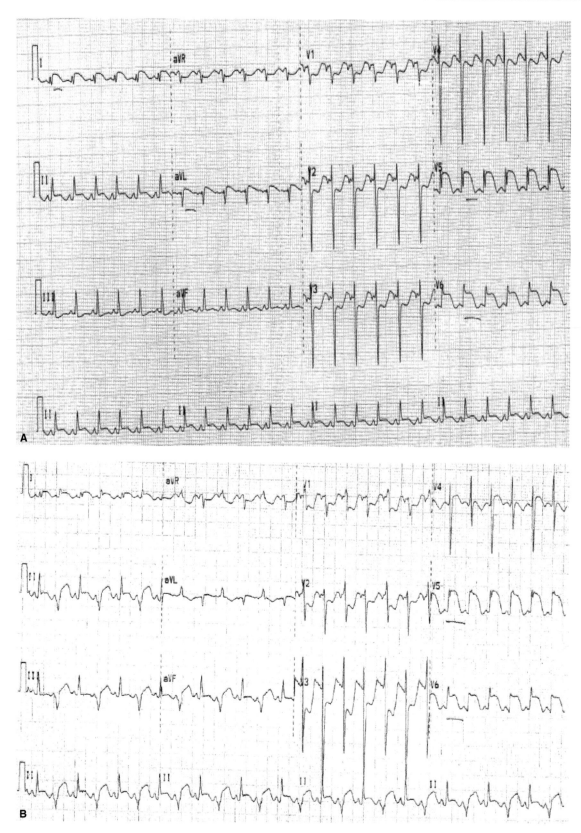

FIGURE 5.58 ■ ECG Changes; Acute Myocarditis. (A–D) Progression of 12-lead ECG obtained from the same patient as described in Figure 5.57 over a 15-minute period. (A) ECG showing sinus tachycardia at a rate of 150 bpm and diffuse ST-T–wave abnormalities. There is hyperacute ST-segment elevation, suggesting myocardial injury or ischemia. (B) ECG obtained 5 minutes later demonstrates sinus tachycardia with ST elevation and ventricular bigeminy.

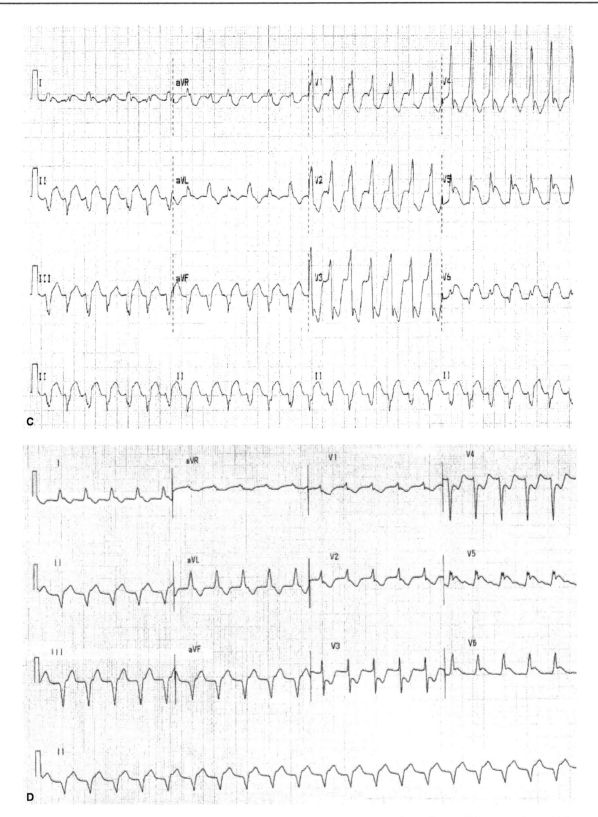

FIGURE 5.58 ■ (*Continued*) (**C**) ECG obtained 5 minutes later shows wide-complex tachycardia, possibly an accelerated idioventricular rhythm with ST elevation. (**D**) ECG showing ventricular tachycardia (15 minutes later from initial presentation) associated with loss of consciousness. Even though the rate of the VT is slow, it is nevertheless an ominous sign. Patients with acute fulminant myocarditis can progress rapidly, and the condition can be fatal if not appropriately managed. (Photo contributor: Shyam Sathanandam, MD.)

TABLE 5.21 ▪ CAUSES OF MYOCARDITIS

Viral causes (a few examples)
- Parvovirus B19
- Human herpesvirus 6
- Enterovirus (coxsackie A and B, echovirus, poliovirus)
- Respiratory syncytial virus
- Adenovirus
- Varicella
- Cytomegalovirus
- Measles
- Herpes
- Mumps
- Influenza
- HIV

Nonviral causes
- Bacterial (eg, *Meningococcus, Klebsiella, Leptospira, Legionella, Mycoplasma*)
- Rickettsiae
- Fungi (eg, actinomycosis, histoplasmosis, *Candida*)
- Protozoal (eg, *Trypanosoma cruzi*, toxoplasmosis, amebiasis)

Noninfectious etiologies
- Hypersensitivity/autoimmune (eg, rheumatoid arthritis, rheumatic fever, systemic lupus erythematosus, scleroderma)
- Drugs (eg, sulfonamides, cyclophosphamide, amphotericin B, acetazolamide)
- Toxic (eg, scorpion, diphtheria)
- Others (eg, sarcoidosis, KD)

Clinical Summary

Congestive heart failure (CHF) is a clinical syndrome in which the heart is unable to pump enough blood to the body to meet its needs. CHF may result from congenital or acquired heart diseases with volume or pressure overload or from myocardial insufficiency. Common defects according to age that lead to CHF are listed in Table 5.22. Volume overload lesions, such as VSD, patent ductus arteriosus (PDA), AV septal defects (AV canal), and systemic arteriovenous fistula, are the most common causes of CHF in the first 6 months of life. Large left-to-right shunts do not cause CHF before 6 to 8 weeks of age because the pulmonary vascular resistance does not fall low enough to cause a large shunt until this age. Atrial septal defect rarely causes CHF, and children with cyanotic heart diseases do not develop CHF unless they have a large systemic to pulmonary artery shunt such as a VSD, PDA, or surgical shunt.

Pulmonary venous congestion in left-sided heart failure leads to tachypnea, dyspnea with exertion, poor feeding, orthopnea in older children, and wheezing and pulmonary crackles. Systemic venous congestion in right-sided heart failure results in hepatomegaly and periorbital edema. Tachycardia, gallop rhythm, and weak, thready pulses are common

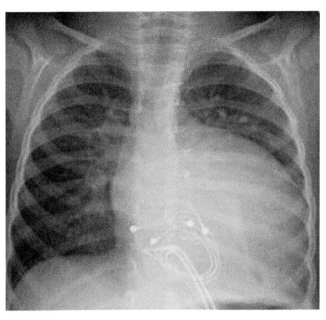

FIGURE 5.60 ■ Dilated Cardiomyopathy. Frontal view of CXR of a 3-year-old child showing cardiomegaly and epicardial pacing leads. He had developed complete heart block after VSD repair and had an epicardial pacemaker system implanted as an infant. He subsequently developed dilated cardiomyopathy (most likely pacemaker-induced cardiomyopathy) (Photo contributor: Sushitha Surendran, MD.)

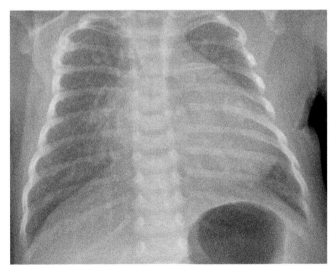

FIGURE 5.59 ■ Ventriculoseptal Defect (VSD) with Congestive Heart Failure (CHF). A 2-month-old infant presented to ED with tachypnea associated with respiratory distress, tachycardia, and decreased feeding. Frontal CXR shows cardiomegaly with pulmonary venous congestion. Echocardiogram confirmed a large VSD. Young infants like this one with CHF often get mistakenly treated as having bronchiolitis especially during respiratory syncytial virus season. (Photo contributor: Sushitha Surendran, MD.)

findings. Distended neck veins and ankle edema may be seen in older children but are not seen in infants. Splenomegaly is not indicative of chronic CHF.

Emergency Department Treatment and Disposition

Obtain ECG and CXR and consult cardiologist. Cardiomegaly is almost always present on CXR, often with increased pulmonary vascular markings. ECG may help determine the type of defect but is not helpful in deciding whether or not CHF is present. Echocardiogram reveals cardiac chamber enlargement and impaired left ventricle function and may help determine the cause of CHF. Hospitalize patients presenting in acute or chronic decompensated heart failure with hemodynamic compromise for inpatient therapy to bring CHF back to a compensated state.

Management of CHF consists of elimination of underlying causes (eg, VSD), elimination of predisposing or contributing causes (eg, anemia, arrhythmia, infection), and control of heart failure. In the ED, heart failure can be controlled using multiple drugs, usually inotropes, diuretics, and afterload-reducing

243

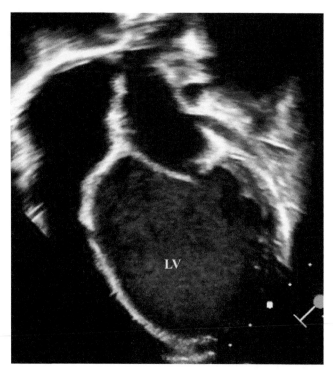

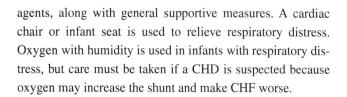

FIGURE 5.61 ■ Dilated Cardiomyopathy. A 4-chamber echocardiogram image of a 3-year-old boy presenting with easy fatigability and shortness of breath with exertion shows severely dilated cardiomyopathy (ejection fraction of 15%). He had developed complete heart block requiring pacemaker implantation following repairs of an atrial and ventricular septal defect in infancy. LV, left ventricle. (Photo contributor: Sushitha Surendran, MD.)

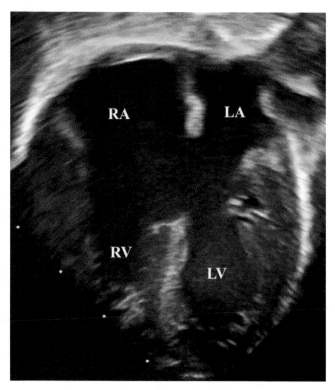

FIGURE 5.62 ■ Complete Atrioventricular Septal Defect. A 4-chamber echocardiogram view of a 6-week-old baby presenting to ED with signs of congestive heart failure and poor weight gain shows a complete balanced atrioventricular septal defect. LA, left atrium; LV, left ventricle; RA, right atrium; RV, right ventricle. (Photo contributor: Sushitha Surendran, MD.)

agents, along with general supportive measures. A cardiac chair or infant seat is used to relieve respiratory distress. Oxygen with humidity is used in infants with respiratory distress, but care must be taken if a CHD is suspected because oxygen may increase the shunt and make CHF worse.

Pearls

1. CHF may result from congenital or acquired heart diseases; knowing the etiologies at various age groups may provide clues for making the proper diagnosis.

2. Signs and symptoms of CHF are different in infants and older children. Infants present with poor feeding of recent onset, tachypnea that worsens during feeding, poor weight gain, and cold sweat on the forehead. Older children may complain of shortness of breath, especially with activity, easy fatigability, puffy eyelids, or swollen feet.

3. Cardiomegaly on CXR is nearly a prerequisite sign of CHF.

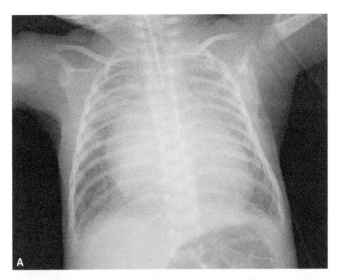

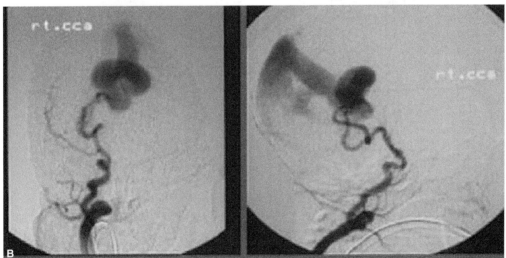

FIGURE 5.63 ■ Vein of Galen Malformation with Congestive Heart Failure. (**A**) Frontal view of CXR demonstrates marked cardiomegaly and vascular congestion (congestive heart failure) in an infant presenting with difficulty breathing. (**B**) Arteriogram demonstrates arteriovenous malformation of the vein of Galen. (Photo contributor: John Amodio, MD.)

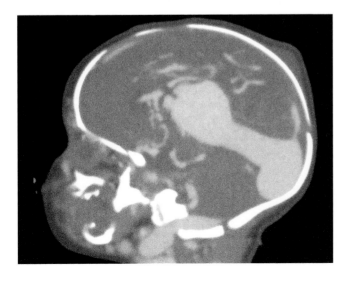

FIGURE 5.64 ■ Vein of Galen Malformation with Congestive Heart Failure (CHF). Head CT with contrast shows a vein of Galen malformation (arteriovenous malformation [AVM]). This 2-month-old presented with respiratory distress and poor feeding. A very active precordium, gallop rhythm, crackles over both lung fields, distended neck veins, and a bruit over the fontanel suggested a cerebral AVM. Systemic AVMs act as left-to-right shunt lesions and lead to CHF in the newborn period. (Photo contributor: Shyam Sathanandam, MD.)

TABLE 5.22 ■ CAUSES OF CONGESTIVE HEART FAILURE

From Congenital Heart Disease

Age of Onset	Cause
At birth	Hypoplastic left heart syndrome
	Large systemic arteriovenous fistula
First week	Transposition of great arteries
	PDA (premature infants)
	Total anomalous pulmonary veins
	Critical aortic or pulmonary stenosis
1–4 weeks	Coarctation of aorta
	Large left-to-right shunts in prematurity
4–6 weeks	AV canal defect
6 weeks–4 months	Large VSD, PDA
	Anomalous left coronary artery from pulmonary artery

Other Etiologies of CHF
- Unrecognized SVT or frequent PVCs (tachycardia-induced cardiomyopathy; at any age)
- Metabolic abnormalities (neonates; eg, severe hypoxia and acidosis, hypoglycemia, hypocalcemia)
- Complete heart block (neonates and early infancy)
- Viral myocarditis (infants)
- Severe anemia (any age)
- Endocardial fibroelastosis (infancy)
- Idiopathic dilated cardiomyopathy (childhood or adolescence)
- Hydrops fetalis (neonates)
- Acute rheumatic carditis (school-age children)
- Rheumatic valvular heart disease
- Acute hypertension (eg, acute postinfectious glomerulonephritis; school-age children)
- Acute cor pulmonale (acute airway obstruction; any age)
- Cardiomyopathy associated with other diseases (eg, muscular dystrophy; adolescents)
- Drug-induced cardiomyopathy (eg, doxorubicin)
- Bronchopulmonary dysplasia (premature infants; right heart failure in early infancy)

Clinical Summary

Acute rheumatic fever (ARF) is an immunogenic multisystem disease that occurs as a delayed sequela of group A streptococcal infection of the pharynx but not the skin. It is relatively uncommon in the United States but is a common cause of heart disease in developing countries. Important predisposing factors include family history of ARF, low socioeconomic status, and age between 6 and 15 years. ARF is diagnosed using the revised Jones criteria (Table 5.23). History of streptococcal pharyngitis is commonly present 1 to 5 weeks before the onset of symptoms, or it may be as long as 2 to 6 months in case of isolated chorea.

Arthritis is the most common manifestation and usually involves large joints either simultaneously or in succession with a characteristic migratory nature. Signs of carditis

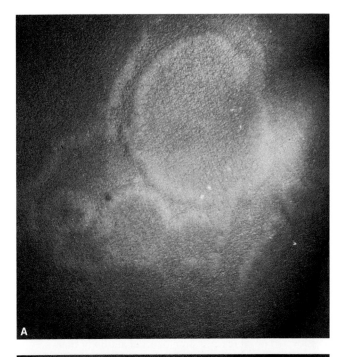

A

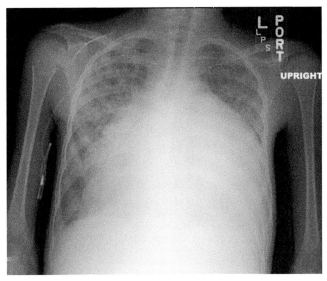

FIGURE 5.65 ■ Rheumatic Carditis. A portable CXR shows severe cardiomegaly and pulmonary edema, suggesting a diagnosis of congestive heart failure in a 16-year-old boy, a recent emigrant from Haiti, presenting with dyspnea, mild cyanosis, tachycardia, and bilateral rales. He had arthritis of the knees. A pansystolic murmur radiating to the axilla was noted. Additional history included fever and a recent sore throat. Echocardiography showed severe mitral regurgitation, pericardial effusion, and poor cardiac function, suggesting the involvement of all layers of the heart. A clinical diagnosis of acute rheumatic fever was made. (Photo contributor: Shyam Sathanandam, MD.)

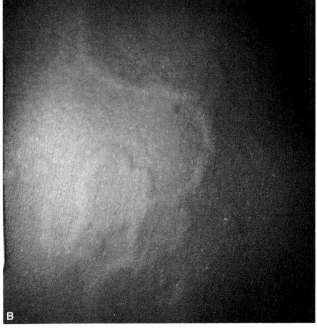

B

FIGURE 5.66 ■ Erythema Marginatum; Acute Rheumatic Fever. (**A**) Annular plaques (complete rings) of varying sizes with flat, pale centers and fairly distinct, raised erythematous margins are seen in an adolescent patient who also had migratory polyarthritis involving knees and elbows. (**B**) Note the serpiginous borders formed by a coalescence of several partial rings. (Reproduced with permission from Shah BR, Laude TL. *Atlas of Pediatric Clinical Diagnosis*. WB Saunders; Philadelphia, PA, 2000.)

TABLE 5.23 ■ GUIDELINES FOR DIAGNOSIS OF RHEUMATIC FEVER

5 Major Manifestations
- Migratory polyarthritis (70%)
- Carditis (50%)
- Sydenham chorea (15%)
- Erythema marginatum (<10%)
- Subcutaneous nodules (10%)

4 Minor Manifestations

Clinical findings:
- Arthralgia
- Fever

Laboratory findings:
- Elevated acute phase reactants (ESR, CRP)
- Prolonged PR interval

Supporting Evidence of Antecedent Group A Streptococcal Pharyngeal Infection
- Positive throat culture or rapid streptococcal antigen test
- Elevated or increasing streptococcal antibody titer

If supported by evidence of preceding group A streptococcal infection, the presence of 2 major manifestations or of 1 major and 2 minor manifestations indicates a high probability of ARF. For chorea, no other criteria or evidence of preceding streptococcal infection is needed.

include (in increasing order of severity) tachycardia out of proportion to the degree of fever, a heart murmur of valvulitis caused by mitral or aortic valve regurgitation, pericarditis (friction rub, pericardial effusion, ECG changes), or signs of CHF (severe carditis). Erythema marginatum is characterized by nonpruritic serpiginous or annular erythematous rashes most prominent on the trunk and the inner proximal portions of the extremities but never on the face. Subcutaneous nodules are hard, painless, nonpruritic, freely mobile swellings of 0.2 to 2 cm in diameter found symmetrically, singly or in clusters, on the extensor surfaces of both large and small joints, over the scalp, or along the spine.

Sydenham chorea (St. Vitus's dance) is more common in prepubertal girls and can be the only manifestation of ARF. It is a neuropsychiatric disorder consisting of both neurologic signs (choreic movement and hypotonia) and psychiatric signs (emotional lability, hyperactivity, separation anxiety, obsessions, and compulsions).

Elevated ESR and CRP levels are objective evidence of an inflammatory process. Positive throat culture or rapid streptococcal antigen tests are less reliable than antibody tests. Antibody tests include ASO titer, anti-DNAase B, and the streptozyme test. Other common but not specific clinical features include abdominal pain, rapid sleeping heart rate, malaise, anemia, epistaxis, and precordial pain. Differential diagnosis includes juvenile rheumatoid arthritis, systemic lupus erythematosus, mixed connective tissue disorder, reactive arthritis, serum sickness, infectious arthritis, and hematologic disorders such as leukemia. Only carditis causes permanent cardiac damage.

Emergency Department Treatment and Disposition

Evaluate hemodynamic status and stabilize as indicated, including high-flow oxygen and continuous cardiac, BP, and pulse oximetry monitoring. Hospitalize any patient when a diagnosis of ARF is made or clinically suspected for further workup and management. Obtain throat culture, ASO and anti-DNase B titers, WBC count, ESR, CRP, ECG, and CXR. ECG may show first-degree heart block, which is 1 of the minor criteria. Consult cardiology for echocardiography in patients with a murmur to diagnose the severity of carditis. Eradication of streptococci (eg, benzathine penicillin G given IM to patients not allergic to penicillin) and anti-inflammatory therapies (eg, salicylates and steroids) are still the mainstay of therapy; however, these therapies must not be started until a definite diagnosis is made. Restriction of activity for 4 to 6 weeks is recommended for carditis.

Pearls

1. The revised Jones criteria are used for the diagnosis of ARF.
2. Maintain a high index of clinical suspicion for ARF because it is uncommon in the United States and must be differentiated from other rheumatologic conditions.

Clinical Summary

Pulmonary hypertension (PH) is defined as the elevation of pulmonary artery pressure due to any cause. It may be idiopathic or heritable with no underlying cause, or it can be due to a specific disease. Pulmonary arterial hypertension is due to pulmonary vascular disease of the precapillary arterioles in the absence of other causes. Persistent pulmonary hypertension of the newborn (PPHN) is the most common cause of PH in the neonatal period.

Clinical presentation can vary from undue shortness of breath, tiredness, fatigue, and chest pain to syncope, seizures, and hemoptysis. Infants can present with poor appetite,

failure to thrive, lethargy, diaphoresis, and tachypnea. On examination, a single and loud P2 without respiratory variation, right ventricular heave, diastolic murmur of pulmonary insufficiency, or holosystolic murmur of tricuspid regurgitation can be appreciated. Signs of right heart failure such as hepatomegaly and peripheral edema can be seen. ECG will show right ventricular hypertrophy with right atrial enlargement and right ventricular strain pattern (ST depression and T-wave inversion in anterior and inferior leads). CXR will show enlargement of the main pulmonary artery and/or right ventricle. Echocardiogram helps to evaluate right ventricular size and function, estimate the pulmonary artery systolic and

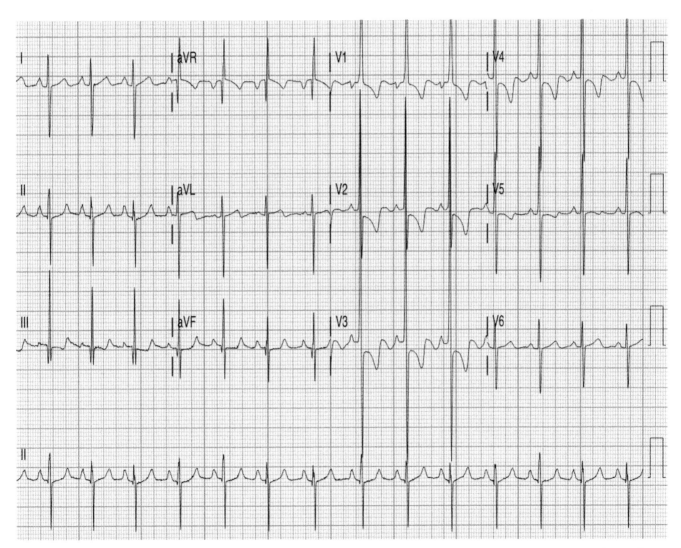

FIGURE 5.67 ■ Right Ventricular Hypertrophy with Strain Pattern. (**A**) A 15-year-old baseball player presented to ED with a history of chest pain for almost a month and shortness of breath. A 12-lead ECG shows right ventricular hypertrophy with right ventricular strain pattern (ST-segment depression in anterior leads and inverted T waves in anterior and lateral leads) and right atrial enlargement with right axis deviation. His echocardiogram showed severe pulmonary hypertension. (Photo contributor: Sushitha Surendran, MD.)

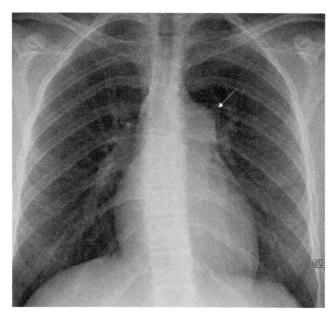

FIGURE 5.68 ■ Pulmonary Hypertension. Frontal CXR of the same patient as shown in Figure 5.69 with pulmonary hypertension shows prominent pulmonary outflow region (arrow). (Photo contributor: Sushitha Surendran, MD.)

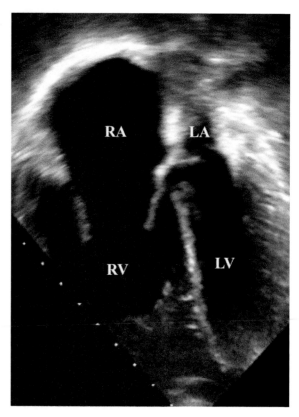

FIGURE 5.69 ■ Pulmonary Hypertension. A15-year-old girl presented to ED with a history of dyspnea and chest pain on exertion for the past 1 year. Her chest x-ray showed cardiomegaly and a dilated pulmonary artery. A 4-chamber echocardiogram view showed a severely dilated right ventricle (RV) and right atrium (RA) with suprasystemic right ventricular systolic pressure. LA, left atrium; LV, left ventricle. (Photo contributor: Sushitha Surendran, MD.)

diastolic pressure, and evaluate for any cardiac cause of PH (Table 5.24) and pericardial effusion. Cardiac catheterization will be helpful to confirm PH and to check pulmonary vasoreactivity before initiation of medication.

Treatment of PH includes pulmonary vasodilators (eg, calcium channel blockers), phosphodiesterase inhibitors (eg, sildenafil, tadalafil), endothelin receptor blockers (eg, bosentan, ambrisentan), and prostacyclin analogs (eg, treprostinil, iloprost). Patient with severe pulmonary hypertension are sometimes on continuous subcutaneous or IV medication via a central line. If PH is due to underlying lung disease, obstructive sleep apnea, thromboembolism, or other etiology, treatment should be directed toward that condition to help decrease the pulmonary artery pressure.

Pulmonary hypertensive crisis refers to an acute rise in pulmonary artery pressure. This causes an acute pressure overload on the right ventricle, leading to decrease in cardiac output and hypoxia. Hypoxia further worsens the pulmonary vascular resistance. This can continue as a vicious cycle and, if untreated, can lead to death. Prompt recognition of pulmonary hypertensive crisis is critical. These patients present with hypoxia, hypotension, tachycardia, and metabolic and respiratory acidosis.

TABLE 5.24 ■ CARDIAC CAUSES OF PULMONARY HYPERTENSION

- **Left-to-right shunt**
  Ventricular septal defect, atrial septal defect, atrioventricular septal defect, patent ductus arteriosus, aortopulmonary window
- **Cyanotic heart disease**
  Transposition of great arteries, truncus arteriosus, tetralogy of Fallot, single ventricle
- **Increased pulmonary venous pressure**
  Mitral stenosis, supravalvar mitral ring, coarctation of aorta, cardiomyopathy, pulmonary vein stenosis, total anomalous pulmonary venous return
- **Pulmonary artery/pulmonary vein anomaly**
  Origin of the pulmonary artery from aorta or ductal origin (Scimitar syndrome)

Emergency Department Treatment and Disposition

Evaluate hemodynamic status and stabilize the patient with endotracheal intubation and continuous cardiac, BP, and pulse oximetry monitoring. Deliver 100% oxygen via the endotracheal tube, and hyperventilate to decrease the carbon dioxide. Maintain PCO_2 around 45 mm Hg. Initiate nitric oxide, which is a pulmonary vasodilator, to help decrease the pulmonary vascular resistance. Maintain lung volume at functional residual capacity to avoid hyperinflation or atelectasis, both of which can worsen the pulmonary vascular resistance. Sedate and paralyze to decrease the metabolic demand, and treat acidosis. Optimize hemoglobin to increase the oxygen-carrying capacity. For patients on subcutaneous or IV therapy, make sure the central line is working properly. Hospitalize all patient to ICU and consult cardiology for further management and for echocardiography to evaluate right ventricular pressure and function. Patient will need inotropic support with epinephrine and/or milrinone to help support the right ventricle. If medical management is unsuccessful, patient may need mechanical support with extracorporeal membrane oxygenation.

Pearls

1. Pulmonary hypertensive crisis is a life-threatening emergency, and prompt recognition is critical.
2. Initiate 100% oxygen and nitric oxide, hyperventilate, and consult cardiology emergently.

Chapter 6

RESPIRATORY DISORDERS

Todd A. Florin
Andrea T. Cruz

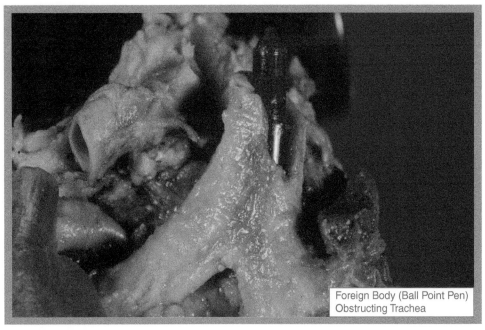

Foreign Body (Ball Point Pen)
Obstructing Trachea

(Photo contributor: David P. Witte, MD)

The authors acknowledge the special contributions of Nooruddin R. Tejani, Diana E. Weaver, Ari J. Goldsmith, Haidy Marzouk, and Jessica Stetz to prior edition.

253

Clinical Features

Foreign body (FB) aspiration, although uncommon, accounts for 7% of deaths in children under 4 years of age. Most aspirated FBs become lodged in the bronchi because their size allows for passage through the larynx and glottis. Large FBs may become impacted in the larynx or trachea, potentially causing complete obstruction, a true emergency. Nuts and seeds are the most commonly aspirated objects, but hot dogs, candy, meat, and grapes are the most implicated objects in choking fatalities. Aspiration of manmade objects is less likely to result in death; balloons, small balls, and beads account for most fatalities. Beans and seeds absorb water and can swell in the airway over time. Organic FBs can cause a surrounding tissue reaction, leading to severe inflammation; nuts and seeds release linoleic acid, which can cause unilateral or bilateral wheezing.

Aspirated FBs can be difficult to diagnose because clinical symptoms may mimic asthma, recurrent pneumonia, bronchiolitis, or URIs. Aspirated FBs should be considered in any young child with new-onset respiratory distress, choking, stridor, cough, or wheezing. Sudden choking and gagging with dyspnea are the first signs of aspiration. However, in up to

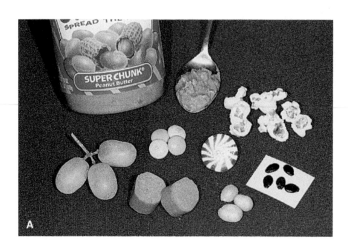

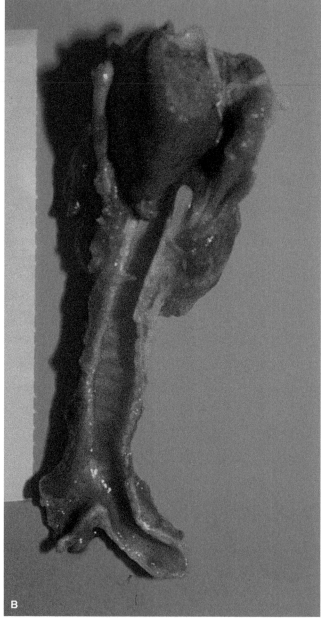

FIGURE 6.1 ■ Aspiration/Asphyxiation by Food Products. (**A**) The most commonly aspirated food products by infants and children include peanuts, chunky peanut butter, hot dogs, popcorn, seeds, grapes, raisins, carrots, meat, and hard candies. Children too young to chew and swallow carefully (usually <5 years of age) should not be given these foods. (**B**) A piece of hot dog is seen lodged in the trachea of a 2.5-year-old child presenting in cardiopulmonary arrest. For children <5 years, hot dogs should be cut longitudinally and not into round pieces. (Photo contributors: Binita R. Shah, MD [A], and Charles Catanese, MD [B].)

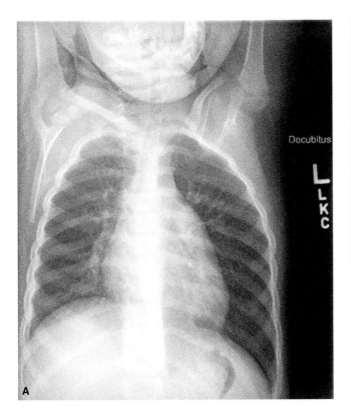

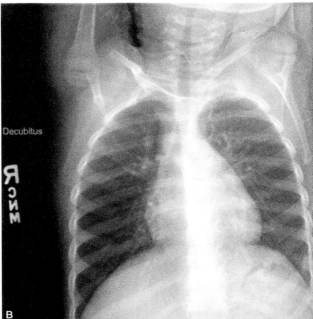

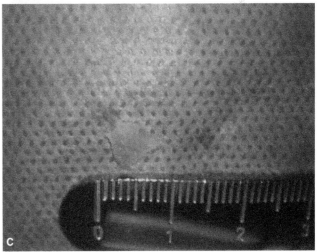

FIGURE 6.2 ■ Carrot Aspiration. A 4-year-old boy had a choking episode while he was running with a carrot in his hand. He presented to the ED with a new onset of bilateral wheezing. (**A, B**) Decubitus views of the chest demonstrate hyperinflation of both lungs, (**C**) Carrot after bronchoscopic removal from the right mainstem bronchus. It is conceivable that initially carrot was in the left mainstem bronchus and subsequently got dislodged during coughing and moved to the right mainstem bronchus. (Photo contributor: Todd A. Florin, MD, MSCE.)

50% of cases, the choking episode is not witnessed. After the initial phase of choking and paroxysms of cough, children often enter into an asymptomatic phase that lasts for hours or even weeks as the FB becomes lodged. In cases of FBs of the larynx or trachea, children may present with hoarseness, stridor, and possibly cyanosis. FBs of the lower respiratory tract occur in younger children, with a slight propensity for the right lung. The classic triad of cough, focal wheezing, and decreased breath sounds is observed in <20% of children with aspiration. When these symptoms are prolonged or atypical, FB should be suspected. Unilateral decreased air entry on chest auscultation is only present in one-third of cases.

Untreated, patients may enter the third phase of the disease course, resulting in complications ranging from atelectasis to pneumonia.

Most FBs are not radiopaque, and small FBs may cause symptoms but no radiologic changes. Frontal view of chest may show air trapping secondary to obstructive emphysema. Bronchial FB results in obstruction during expiration, where air entry is possible during inspiration due to a partial obstruction ("ball-valve") or can result in complete obstruction with poor pneumatization and atelectasis. The sensitivity of plain CXR is increased when inspiratory and expiratory films are taken. Mediastinal shift to the opposite side on the expiratory

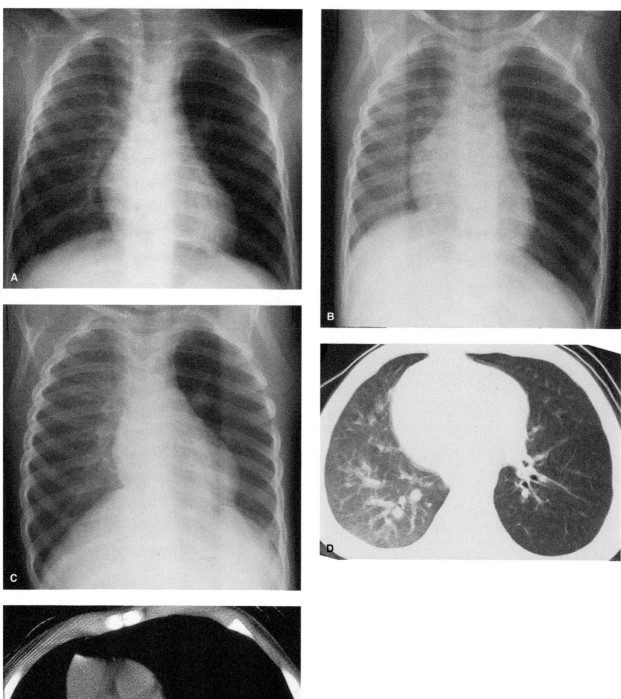

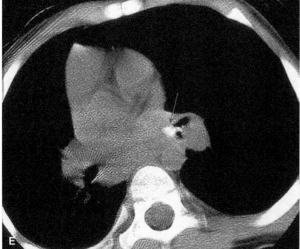

FIGURE 6.3 ■ Foreign Body Aspiration. (**A**) Frontal view of the chest shows hyperinflation of the left lung. (**B, C**) Bilateral decubitus views of the chest show persistent hyperinflation of the left lung with decubitus positioning, consistent with air trapping. (**D**) CT scan shows overinflated left lung with air trapping. (**E**) CT scan showing impacted foreign body in left mainstem bronchus (arrow). (Photo contributor: Rafael Rivera, MD.)

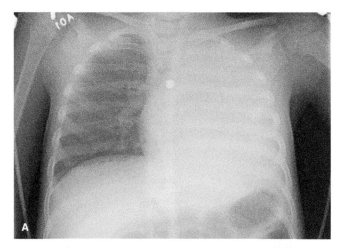

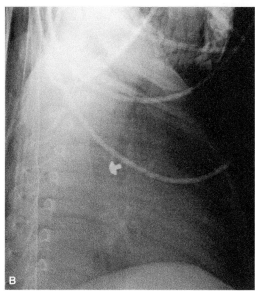

FIGURE 6.4 ■ Radiopaque Foreign Body Aspiration. Frontal and lateral views (**A, B**) of the chest shows a screw in the left mainstem bronchus with atelectasis of the left lung. (Photo contributor: John Amodio, MD.)

phase is diagnostic. Patients who are not old enough to obtain inspiratory and expiratory films should have right and left lateral decubitus radiographs performed. The lung positioned in the dependent position will deflate under the weight of the heart unless it is obstructed. Inspiratory and expiratory CXRs

are normal in 15% of FB aspiration; thus, normal radiographs should not preclude an attempt at FB removal when the clinical history is strongly suggestive. Fluoroscopy, if available, is often useful and may demonstrate air trapping or mediastinal shift. CT scan of the chest, although highly sensitive, is not obtained initially due to increased radiation exposure, unless the patient presents with complications or plain radiographs and fluoroscopy are not diagnostic.

Emergency Department Treatment and Disposition

Bronchoscopy is the most commonly used method for removal of an airway FB. Patients with suspected airway FB must have specialty evaluation by otolaryngology or pulmonary medicine early. Children with laryngotracheal FBs may present in acute and severe airway obstruction. Attempt back blows or chest compressions in infants or the Heimlich maneuver in toddlers and older children first; if unsuccessful in dislodging the FB, attempt laryngoscopy and removal. If the FB cannot be removed by direct laryngoscopy in the ED, use tracheal intubation to advance the FB into a bronchus. Bronchial FBs rarely require emergent intervention. If all of these interventions fail, an emergency airway may be necessary. Give supportive care with oxygen or helium-oxygen (ie, heliox) and monitor closely, including continuous pulse oximetry. Give steroids to reduce airway inflammation as needed.

Pearls

1. Lack of witnessed choking episode and/or normal chest films are the most important factors contributing to delayed diagnosis. Normal radiographs do not preclude the diagnosis of FB aspiration if clinical history is suggestive.
2. The presence of an airway FB should be considered for all patients with new onset of noisy breathing or wheezing (especially in toddlers) or unexplained persistent or recurrent pulmonary findings (eg, pneumonia) regardless of the history of an aspiration event.

Clinical Summary

Pertussis, or whooping cough, is infection of the respiratory tract by *Bordetella pertussis,* a gram-negative pleomorphic bacilli, and is transmitted by respiratory droplets. A related infection, *Bordetella parapertussis* (kennel cough), can be transmitted from dogs and causes a syndrome clinically indistinguishable from pertussis. Mortality due to pertussis is greatest in the first month of life.

The catarrhal stage, consisting of a viral prodrome and mild cough typically lasting 1 to 2 weeks, is followed by a paroxysmal stage of progressive, repetitive, and severe episodes of coughing that lead to a forceful inspiration, producing the characteristic whoop, lasting 2 to 4 weeks. Symptoms take weeks to months to resolve (convalescent stage). Pertussis is most severe in the very young, presenting as gagging, gasping, cyanosis, or apnea without characteristic whoop. Complications among infants include bronchopneumonia (25%), seizures (3%), encephalopathy (1%), cerebral anoxia, and sudden unexpected death. Submucosal bleeding (including subconjunctival hemorrhages and petechiae), diaphragmatic

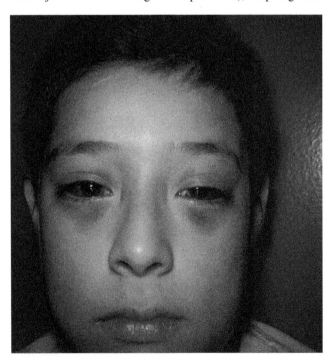

FIGURE 6.5 ■ Bilateral Subconjunctival Hemorrhages and Periorbital Ecchymosis; Pertussis. Violent episodes of coughing leading to hemorrhages (subconjunctival and periorbital) were the presenting complaints of pertussis in this unimmunized adolescent boy from El Salvador. His nasopharyngeal aspirate was positive for *Bordetella pertussis.* (*Important: These findings of subconjunctival hemorrhages and ecchymoses can be mistaken for inflicted injuries from child abuse.*). (Photo contributor: Binita R. Shah, MD.)

rupture, umbilical and inguinal hernias, and rectal prolapse have been reported. Complications among adolescents include syncope, sleep disturbance, incontinence, rib fractures, and pneumonia. A number of other pathogens can cause pertussis-like symptoms (eg, adenoviruses, respiratory syncytial virus [RSV], parainfluenza viruses, influenza viruses, *Mycoplasma, Chlamydia trachomatis*). Leukocytosis with absolute lymphocytosis (total count >50,000 cells/mm^3) may be seen at the beginning of the paroxysmal stage. CXRs may show perihilar, patchy, or diffuse infiltrates, but are often normal. Diagnosis is confirmed by PCR assay using a nasopharyngeal sample.

Emergency Department Treatment and Disposition

Provide supportive care, including suctioning of secretions, humidified oxygen for hypoxia, and maintenance of adequate hydration and nutrition. Treat patients *and their household and close contacts* with macrolide antibiotics (azithromycin, erythromycin, or clarithromycin). Use azithromycin in patients under 1 month old, due to the association between oral erythromycin and infantile hypertrophic pyloric stenosis. Trimethoprim-sulfamethoxazole is an alternative for patients >2 months old who cannot tolerate macrolides. Macrolides given as soon as possible to an exposed person (preferably during the incubation period) will prevent or modify the course of the disease. Of note, antibiotics will not alter the duration of cough or other symptoms but will limit spread of the organism to others. Pertussis vaccine should also be given to unimmunized or incompletely immunized exposed children (DTaP [diphtheria, tetanus, and pertussis] for <7 years of age, Tdap [tetanus, diphtheria, and pertussis] for children 7 years of age and older). Admit patients under 1 year of age and those with apnea or cyanosis during episodes, pneumonia, or respiratory distress. Initiate respiratory droplet precautions for 5 days after initiation of antibiotic therapy or until 3 weeks after the onset of paroxysms without antibiotic therapy.

Pearls

1. Pertussis is a life-threatening infection and is preventable by universal immunization.
2. Neither infection nor immunization provides lifelong immunity to pertussis.
3. Young infants, who are most at risk for severe complications, often do not present with the characteristic whoop of pertussis.

Clinical Summary

Croup is an acute viral inflammation of the larynx and structures inferior to the larynx classically described as acute laryngotracheitis or laryngotracheobronchitis. Spasmodic croup, which is thought to have an allergic component and presents with noninflammatory edema in the subglottic region, is a distinct entity.

Croup affects children aged 6 months to 6 years and occurs in early fall and winter. Patients present with 1 to 3 days of upper respiratory tract symptoms with or without fever, with progression to the characteristic barking cough ("seal-like"), hoarseness, stridor, and respiratory distress. Tachypnea, retractions, hypoxia, and altered mental state are often ominous signs of worsening obstruction. Common etiologies include parainfluenza viruses (most common), RSV, influenza viruses A and B, and adenovirus. The differential diagnosis includes epiglottitis, bacterial tracheitis, foreign body aspiration, retropharyngeal abscess, peritonsillar abscess, angioneurotic edema, congenital anomaly, mediastinal mass (eg, lymphoma), and diphtheria. Routine laboratory studies are not helpful. Plain radiographs of the neck are *not routinely indicated* and should be used only when diagnosis is unclear to exclude other conditions such as retropharyngeal abscess or foreign body aspiration.

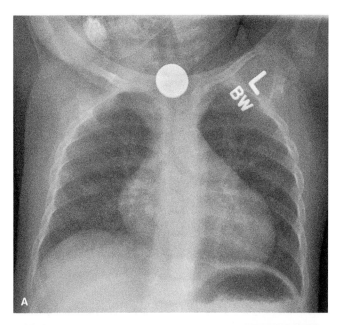

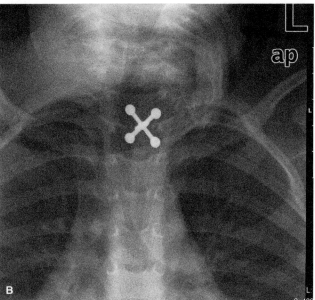

FIGURE 6.7 ■ Foreign Body Ingestions Presenting with Stridor; Differential Diagnosis of Croup. (**A**) Frontal view of the chest shows impacted coin in a child with "noisy breathing" and drooling. (**B**) Frontal view of the neck in a different child shows a jack in the region of the esophagus. This child also presented with a stridor and difficulty swallowing. (Photo contributor: John Amodio, MD.)

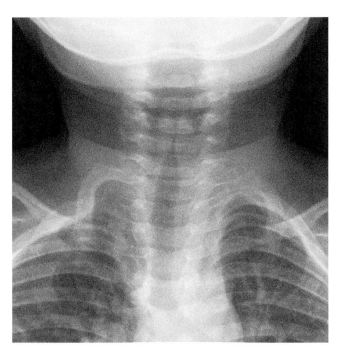

FIGURE 6.6 ■ Croup. Anteroposterior view of the subglottic airway demonstrates narrowing of the airway identified as classic "steeple" sign in a 16-month-old toddler with croup. (Photo contributor: Arnold C. Merrow, Jr., MD.)

Emergency Department Treatment and Disposition

Management of croup depends on the severity of upper airway obstruction. Scales of severity of croup assessment and response to therapy such as the Westley score can be used.

259

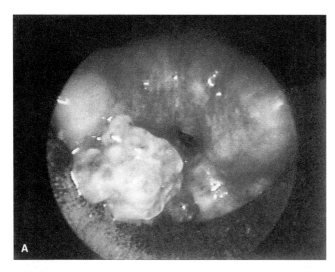 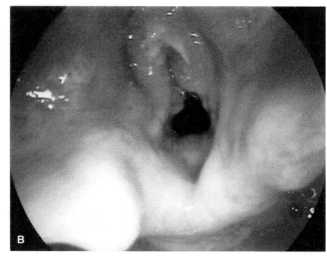

FIGURE 6.8 ■ Laryngeal Papillomatosis Presenting with Stridor; Differential Diagnosis of Croup. (**A**) Respiratory papillomatosis of the left half of the larynx, obstructing the glottic inlet in a patient presenting with hoarseness, stridor, and airway obstruction. (**B**) Papillomatous lesions involving both vocal cords in a different patient with stridor and difficulty breathing. (Photo contributor: Bhuvanesh Singh, MD.)

For mild to moderate croup, the treatment is oral or parenteral steroids, including dexamethasone or prednisolone. For severe croup (eg, stridor at rest, severe respiratory distress), nebulized racemic epinephrine should be given urgently as 2.25% solution diluted in 3 mL of normal saline given over 15 minutes. If racemic epinephrine is not available, then nebulized L-epinephrine 1:1000 can be administered. Improvement of symptoms should occur within 10 to 30 minutes of administration. If after 2 to 4 hours of observation, there is no stridor or chest retractions and the child appears well, he or she may be discharged home. Any child who does not improve after epinephrine administration should be hospitalized. Intubate and admit patients with signs of respiratory failure who do not respond to racemic epinephrine and steroids. Helium-oxygen mixture (heliox) may be useful in the treatment of severe croup as it reduces work of breathing to prevent intubation and allow other medications to reach therapeutic peak. There is no evidence for the use of humidified or cold air, prophylactic antibiotics, or antitussive agents.

Pearls

1. Croup is the most common form of acute upper airway obstruction in infants and children.
2. Regardless of the level of illness acuity, corticosteroid therapy (dexamethasone either orally or intramuscularly) is the standard of care.
3. Drooling, dysphagia, high fever, and toxic appearance are notably absent in viral croup, and thus suggest another diagnosis.

Clinical Summary

Bacterial tracheitis is a potentially fatal, acute infectious upper airway obstruction, occurring in children aged 3 months to 5 years, predominantly in fall and winter. A prodrome of coryza, sore throat, cough, and pyrexia of 1 to 3 days in duration is followed by acute onset of stridor and rapidly worsening respiratory distress, which can lead to airway obstruction and respiratory arrest. Patients with bacterial tracheitis are toxic appearing and show little response to nebulized epinephrine. Visualization of the airways reveals subglottic inflammation, edema of the tracheal mucosa, and copious purulent endotracheal secretions. *Staphylococcus aureus* is the most common bacterial pathogen, followed by *Streptococcus pneumoniae, Streptococcus pyogenes,* nontypable *Haemophilus influenzae, Moraxella catarrhalis,* and *Pseudomonas aeruginosa.* Viral coinfection with influenza A, parainfluenza, RSV, and adenovirus is common. The differential diagnosis includes viral croup, epiglottitis, foreign body aspiration, and retropharyngeal abscess. Complications include cardiorespiratory arrest, acute respiratory distress syndrome, hypotension, toxic shock syndrome, renal failure, pneumothorax, pulmonary edema,

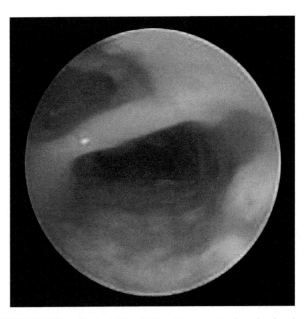

FIGURE 6.10 ■ Bacterial Tracheitis. Photograph of tracheal endoscopy showing pseudomembrane in bacterial tracheitis. (Reproduced with permission from Shah SS. *Pediatric Practice: Infectious Disease.* McGraw-Hill Education; New York, NY, 2009.)

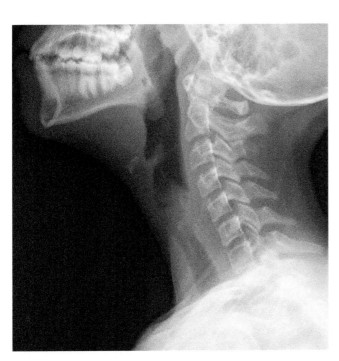

FIGURE 6.9 ■ Bacterial Tracheitis. Lateral view of the neck in a 12-year-old with bacterial tracheitis demonstrates an elongated plaque like filling defect within the upper trachea. The epiglottis is normal. (Photo contributor: Arnold C. Merrow, Jr., MD.)

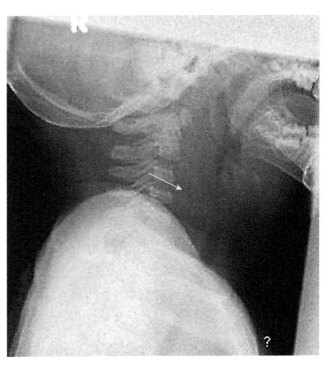

FIGURE 6.11 ■ Retropharyngeal Abscess; Differential Diagnosis of Bacterial Tracheitis. Lateral view of the neck shows collection of air in retropharyngeal soft tissues compatible with abscess. Stridor, drooling, and respiratory distress in a highly febrile child were the presenting signs mimicking bacterial tracheitis. (Photo contributor: John Amodio, MD.)

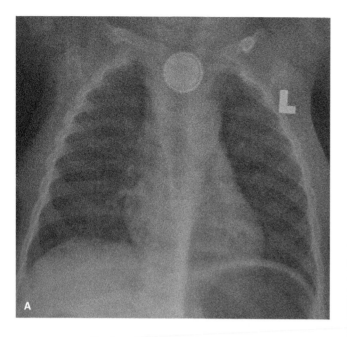

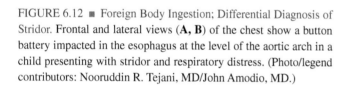

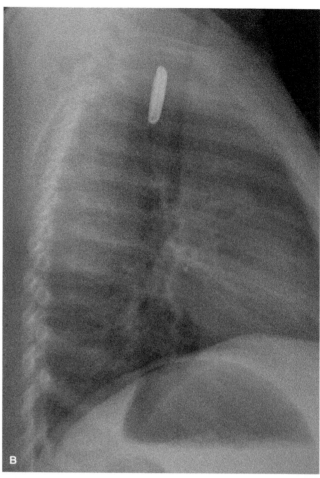

FIGURE 6.12 ■ Foreign Body Ingestion; Differential Diagnosis of Stridor. Frontal and lateral views (**A, B**) of the chest show a button battery impacted in the esophagus at the level of the aortic arch in a child presenting with stridor and respiratory distress. (Photo/legend contributors: Nooruddin R. Tejani, MD/John Amodio, MD.)

and subglottic stenosis. The WBC count is usually elevated or abnormally low. Chest and lateral neck radiographs show subglottic narrowing on posteroanterior view, a hazy tracheal air column and irregular soft tissue densities in trachea (indicating purulent exudate), pneumonia, and pulmonary edema.

Emergency Department Treatment and Disposition

Adequate airway protection with intubation is the single most important therapeutic intervention. Obtain tracheal bacterial cultures at intubation and send secretions for identification of viral agents. Treat hypotension aggressively with isotonic fluid boluses and inotropic support, if necessary. Begin empirical therapy with antistaphylococcal agent (eg,

vancomycin) and a third-generation cephalosporin (eg, ceftriaxone or cefotaxime). Admit all intubated patients to the ICU. With appropriate antimicrobials and aggressive supportive care, rapid improvement and extubation is possible within 72 to 96 hours.

Pearls

1. The clinical hallmark of bacterial tracheitis is toxic appearance and worsening stridor 1 to 3 days after a viral prodrome.
2. In contrast to viral croup, patients with bacterial tracheitis show little response to nebulized epinephrine.
3. Endoscopic visualization of the trachea reveals presence of purulent secretions.

Clinical Summary

Epiglottitis is an acute life-threatening inflammation of the supraglottic structures, including the epiglottis, aryepiglottic folds, arytenoids, and vallecula. It is usually seen in children 2 to 7 years of age and has become rare (0.02 per 100,000 in Western countries) since the introduction of *H influenzae* type b conjugate vaccine. The most common etiologic organisms include *S pyogenes, S aureus, S pneumoniae, Moraxella,* viral agents (parainfluenza, herpes simplex virus type 1, and varicella), and *Candida* species. *H influenzae* type b is still seen in unimmunized children. Noninfectious causes include direct trauma and thermal injuries (eg, scalding burns of face, drinking hot liquids). Symptoms occur with rapid progression and include fever, irritability, toxic appearance, difficulty swallowing, and drooling. *Croupy cough is absent, and stridor is a late finding.* The child usually sits upright with the chin pushed forward (tripod position) to open the airway. Gentle visualization of the oropharynx without the use of a tongue depressor may reveal an erythematous epiglottis protruding at the base of the tongue. In cases of definite epiglottitis, imaging is not necessary. Radiographs should only be used when the diagnosis of epiglottitis is in question to exclude retropharyngeal abscess and foreign bodies. The classic finding of epiglottitis is the "thumbprint sign" on lateral neck radiograph. Contrasted CT scan of the neck may also indicate the presence of epiglottic edema and possibly phlegmon or abscess in the epiglottis or the base of tongue.

Emergency Department Treatment and Disposition

A multidisciplinary team, including pediatric intensive care, anesthesiology, and otolaryngology, is essential to emergent care of epiglottitis. Minimize manipulation of the oropharynx, as this may precipitate sudden airway compromise. The diagnosis should be confirmed emergently by direct visualization in the operating room. Edema with intense erythema of epiglottis ("cherry red") and surrounding structures including arytenoids and aryepiglottic folds and vocal cords is seen. Perform intubation or tracheostomy, as needed. Admit the patient to the ICU for continuous monitoring. Postpone diagnostic tests and placement of IV lines until the airway is secure. Obtain cultures of the blood and epiglottal surface

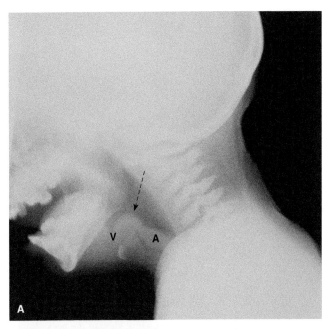

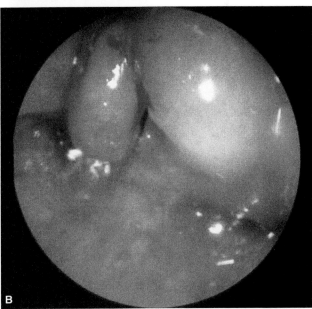

FIGURE 6.13 ■ Epiglottitis. (**A**) Lateral view of the airway shows enlargement of the epiglottis (arrow), thickening of the aryepiglottic folds (A), and amputation of the vallecula (V), leading to the "thumbprint sign." (**B**) Endoscopic view of almost complete airway obstruction secondary to epiglottitis in a different patient. Note the slit-like opening of the airway. (Photo contributor: John Amodio, MD [A], and reproduced with permission from Knoop KJ, Stack LB, Storrow AB, et al. *The Atlas of Emergency Medicine.* 4th ed. McGraw-Hill Education; New York, NY, 2016. Photo contributor: Department of Otolaryngology, Children's Hospital Medical Center, Cincinnati, OH [B].)

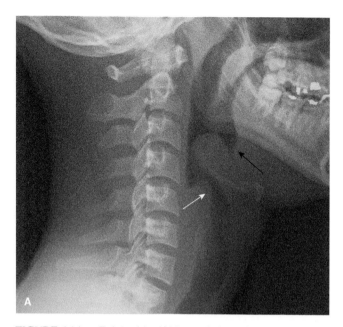
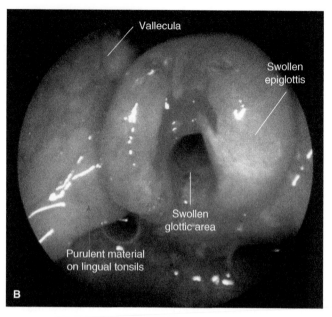

FIGURE 6.14 ■ Epiglottitis. (**A**) Lateral view of the neck shows marked enlargement of the epiglottis, amputation of the vallecula (black arrow), and thickening of the aryepiglottic folds (white arrow) in a 21-year-old patient presenting with history of sore throat, fever, and difficulty handling secretions. His epiglottal culture was positive for *Streptococcus pyogenes*. (**B**) Fiberoptic laryngoscopy showing an edematous epiglottis and glottic area with marked airway compromised in an adult with epiglottitis. ([A] Reproduced with permission from Knoop KJ, Stack LB, Storrow AB et al. *The Atlas of Emergency Medicine,* 4th ed. New York, NY: McGraw-Hill Education; 2016. Photo contributor: Michael Secko, MD. [B] Reproduced with permission from Knoop KJ, Stack LB, Storrow AB et al. *The Atlas of Emergency Medicine,* 4th ed. New York, NY: McGraw-Hill Education; 2016. Photo contributor: Department of Otolaryngology, Children's Hospital Medical Center, Cincinnati, OH.)

for precise microbiologic diagnosis. Treat empirically with a second- or third-generation cephalosporin or ampicillin-sulbactam. Consider addition of an antistaphylococcal agent (eg, vancomycin). Children usually require intubation for 24 to 72 hours, until reduction in airway edema occurs.

Pearls

1. Do not force the patient to lie in a supine position because a gravity-induced change in the position of the epiglottis may lead to total airway obstruction.

2. Do not use a tongue blade to examine the pharynx because it may induce life-threatening laryngospasm.

3. Confirm epiglottitis with direct visualization rather than radiography because patients may develop life-threatening laryngospasm when attempting to hyperextend the neck for the radiograph.

Clinical Summary

Bronchiolitis is clinical syndrome consisting of a viral upper respiratory prodrome followed by increased respiratory effort and wheezing as the infection moves to the lower respiratory tract. It occurs in children under 2 years old, with peak incidence between 3 and 6 months, and is predominantly seen between late fall and spring. Respiratory syncytial virus (RSV) accounts for 40% to 80% of cases; other viral etiologies include parainfluenza virus, rhinovirus, influenza, coronavirus, human bocavirus, adenovirus, and human metapneumovirus. An upper respiratory tract infection prodrome is followed by cough, tachypnea, tachycardia, grunting, flaring, supraclavicular and intercostal retractions, and head bobbing. Infants younger than 2 to 3 months old and premature infants may present with apnea without other clinical symptoms. Nonspecific symptoms include poor feeding and irritability. Examination may reveal work of breathing manifested by retractions, grunting or nasal flaring, and crackles and wheeze on auscultation. A clinical hallmark is minute-to-minute variation in clinical findings, due to respiratory clearance by coughing or changes in a child's behavioral state. Repeated assessments are often necessary to accurately assess disease severity. Fever occurs in one-third of infants, typically early in the disease course, and is usually <39°C (102.2°F). Hypoxemia is primarily due to ventilation/perfusion mismatch, and hypercapnia is a late phenomenon. Progression to respiratory failure may occur. Factors associated with progression to severe disease include age <3 months, gestational age <32 weeks, toxic appearance, respiratory rate >70 breaths per minute, chronic lung disease, congenital cardiac abnormalities, neuromuscular disease, or immune deficiencies. The differential diagnosis includes pneumonia, pertussis, laryngotracheomalacia, foreign body, gastroesophageal reflux, congestive heart failure, vascular ring, cystic fibrosis, mediastinal mass, bronchogenic cyst, and tracheoesophageal fistula.

Emergency Department Treatment and Disposition

The hallmark of management is supportive care; routine imaging or laboratory testing is not recommended for infants with a typical presentation of bronchiolitis. Measure oxygen saturation in all infants with bronchiolitis; oxygen should be initiated only with saturations persistently <90% to 92%. CXR is not recommended routinely, as most radiographs are

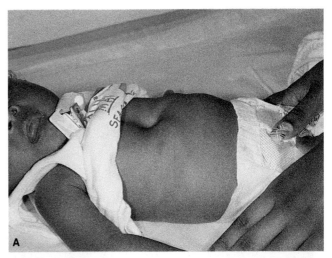

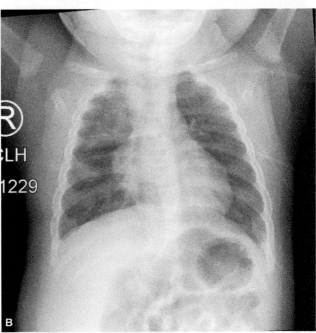

FIGURE 6.15 ■ Bronchiolitis. (**A**) An infant presenting with new onset of wheezing associated with subcostal and intercostal retractions and pulling inward of the sternum with exacerbation of the pectus excavatum deformity. (**B**) A frontal CXR showing hyperinflation, peribronchial thickening, and areas of opacity consistent with atelectasis in the right upper, middle, and left lower lobes. (Photo contributors: Binita R. Shah, MD [A], and Mantosh Rattan, MD [B].)

normal or show findings typical of bronchiolitis that do not change management, including hyperinflation, peribronchial thickening, or atelectasis. CXR should be considered in those with high fever (>39°C), persistently focal crackles, significant hypoxia (oxygen saturation <90%–92%), severe presentations, or lack of resolution of typical symptoms, or those

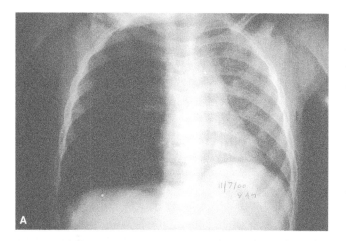

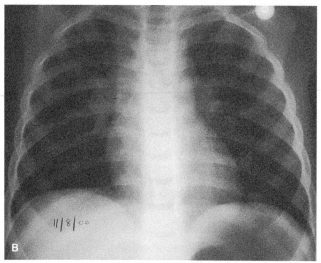

FIGURE 6.16 ■ Foreign Body Aspiration (FBA); Differential Diagnosis of Wheezing. (**A**) Frontal view of chest showing unilateral hyperinflation of the right lung and flattening of the right hemidiaphragm with a slight mediastinal shift to the left. About 20 hours following a choking episode while eating peanuts, this toddler presented with coughing and first episode of wheezing. In bronchiolitis, hyperinflation (a hallmark finding) is present bilaterally, unlike the unilateral hyperinflation seen in FBA. (**B**) Unilateral hyperinflation is no longer seen after extraction of the peanut fragment from the right lower lobe bronchus by rigid bronchoscopy. (Photo contributor: Binita R. Shah, MD.)

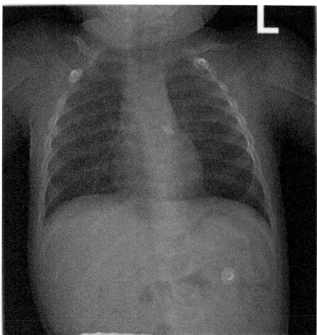

FIGURE 6.17 ■ Foreign Body Aspiration; Differential Diagnosis of Wheezing. Frontal view of chest showing a foreign body (rock) within the left mainstem bronchus. New onset of wheezing and coughing were the presenting complaints of this 9-month-old infant seen in the ED during the RSV season. However, wheezing was unilateral (unlike bronchiolitis), necessitating a radiograph. (Photo contributor: Kanwal Chaudhry, MD.)

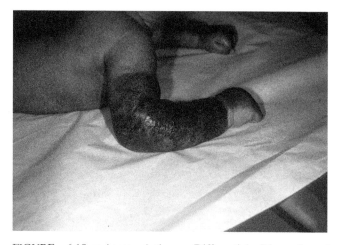

FIGURE 6.18 ■ Acute Asthma; Differential Diagnosis of Wheezing. It is impossible to clinically differentiate bronchiolitis from asthma in a patient with a first episode of wheezing. Reversible bronchospasm, recurrent wheezing, eosinophilia, history of eczema, and family history of asthma or atopy suggest a diagnosis of asthma. This infant presented with a new onset of wheezing and had severe atopic dermatitis with lichenified plaques with exudation over extremities. He responded to bronchodilator therapy. (Photo contributor: Binita R. Shah, MD.)

without the classic clinical presentation for bronchiolitis. Rapid viral antigen tests in outpatients have little impact on management in most cases.

Provide supportive therapy including oxygen therapy and fluid replacement, as necessary. Nasal suctioning may be helpful in improving respiratory distress by clearing nasal secretions, but deep suctioning should be avoided. Provide IV or nasogastric hydration if the infant is having difficulty feeding.

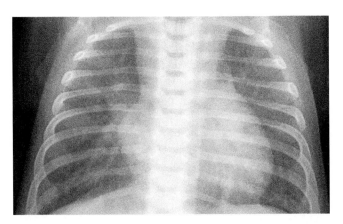

FIGURE 6.19 ■ Congestive Heart Failure (CHF); Differential Diagnosis of Wheezing. Frontal view of the chest shows cardiomegaly and increased markings emanating from the hila, compatible with pulmonary venous congestion (CHF). There are also increased markings extending to the periphery of the lungs, representing pulmonary arterial hypertension secondary to a ventriculoseptal defect. This 3-month-old infant presented with wheezing and tachypnea. Signs and symptoms of CHF (eg, tachypnea, tachycardia, wheezing, rales, respiratory distress, and hepatomegaly) can be easily mistaken for bronchiolitis. (Photo contributor: Shyam Sathanandam, MD.)

Chest physiotherapy should be avoided. There is no proven pharmacologic treatment. Bronchodilators (α- or β-agonists), ipratropium bromide, inhaled or systemic corticosteroids, ribavirin, antileukotriene antagonists, and antibiotics should not be routinely used. A trial of albuterol may be considered *with objective respiratory scoring before and after administration*. Albuterol should be continued only after a documented beneficial response. Nebulized racemic epinephrine may be trialed in severe cases but should not be routinely used. Antibiotics should only be used if there is evidence of a secondary bacterial infection or, in the case of infants younger than 60 days of age, if there is fever and evaluation for a serious bacterial infection. Nebulized hypertonic saline, while potentially associated with decreased hospital length of stay in those with long hospitalizations, has not been shown to be effective in the short-term ED setting. High-flow humidified nasal cannula (at flow rates of 1–2 L/kg/min) may be useful in select infants with severe work of breathing. Admission to the hospital should be considered for those with moderate to severe work of breathing, significant tachypnea, hypoxia (oxygen saturation <90%–92%), dehydration, severe risk factors, or concern for the ability of the infant to follow up.

Pearls

1. Bronchiolitis is the most common wheezing-associated respiratory illness in infants <2 years of age.
2. Apnea may be the presenting manifestation of RSV bronchiolitis in the neonate.
3. Bacterial pneumonia is rare early in the course of viral bronchiolitis. CXRs should not be obtained in routine presentations. Radiographs should be considered in those with high fever, persistently focal crackles, significant hypoxia, severe presentations, or lack of resolution of typical symptoms and those without the classic clinical presentation.
4. Management of bronchiolitis is primarily supportive; routine use of bronchodilators, corticosteroids, and antibiotics should be avoided.

Clinical Summary

Pneumonia, an infection of the lung parenchyma, is one of the most frequent and costly reasons for pediatric hospitalization in the United States. The vast majority of community-acquired pneumonias (CAPs) are caused by viruses, bacteria, or a combination of both. Etiologic determination is challenging due to lack of sensitive and specific noninvasive diagnostic tests and sufficient reference standards; however, a viral etiology is implicated in 60% to 75% of cases, whereas a bacterial etiology is detected in 15% to 30%. Bacterial-viral co-infection is common, accounting for 30% to 50% of cases. Viral pneumonia typically peaks in the late fall and winter months, whereas bacterial pneumonia occurs throughout the year with no seasonal peaks.

Group B *Streptococcus* and gram-negative bacilli are common neonatal bacterial pathogens. *C trachomatis* is seen at about 6 weeks of age, presenting with tachypnea, staccato

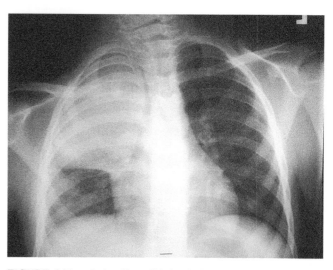

FIGURE 6.21 ■ Lobar Consolidation in Pneumococcal Pneumonia. Frontal CXR shows consolidation of the right upper lobe. Blood culture was positive for *S pneumoniae*. (Photo contributor: Binita R. Shah, MD.)

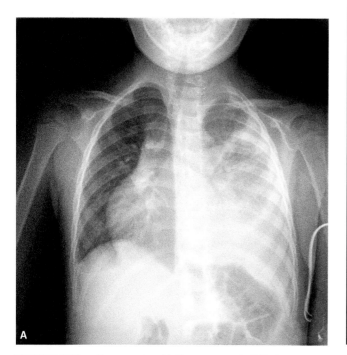

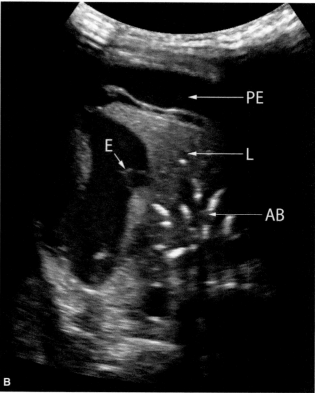

FIGURE 6.20 ■ Pneumonia with Parapneumonic Effusion. (**A**) A frontal radiograph of the chest showing extensive parenchymal consolidation involving the left upper lobe (including lingula) and left lower lobe consistent with pneumonia. There is a concomitant left parapneumonic effusion, resulting in contralateral shift of the heart and mediastinum. (**B**) Transverse US image at the level of the left lower lobe showing consolidated lung (L) with echogenic air bronchograms (AB), marginated by a complex pleural effusion (PE) containing septations/exudate (E). (Photo contributor: Mantosh Rattan, MD.)

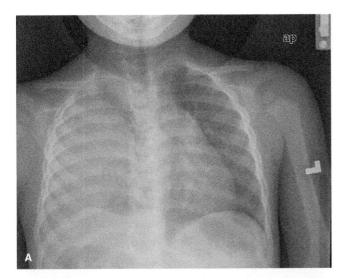

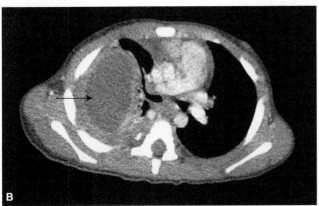

FIGURE 6.22 ■ Pneumococcal Pneumonia with Empyema. (**A**) Frontal CXR shows large soft tissue density in right hemithorax, with mediastinal shift suggesting large pleural collection. (**B**) CT scan shows a large loculated empyema (arrow) with surrounding consolidated lung. Blood and empyema cultures were positive for *S pneumoniae* (serotype A19). (Photo contributor: John Amodio, MD.)

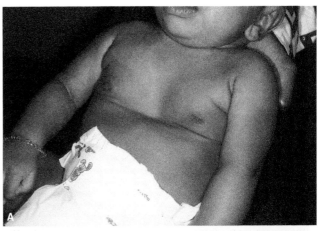

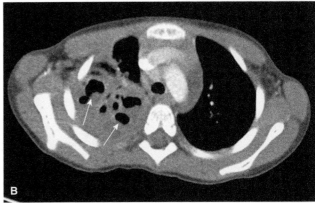

FIGURE 6.23 ■ Staphylococcal Pneumonia. (**A**) A highly febrile infant with respiratory distress. An abrupt onset and rapid progression of pneumonia in very young infants should be considered due to staphylococci until proved otherwise. (**B**) CT slice through upper lobes shows consolidation of the right upper lobe with areas of necrosis (arrows). (Photo contributors: Binita R. Shah, MD [A], and John Amodio, MD [B].)

cough, and absence of fever. From 3 months to 5 years of age, viral etiologies predominate. RSV is the most commonly detected virus. Other viral causes include human metapneumovirus, rhinovirus, influenza, bocavirus, parainfluenza viruses, coronavirus, and adenovirus. *S pneumoniae* is thought to be the most common typical bacterial pathogen, followed by *S aureus* and group A *Streptococcus*. Community-acquired multidrug-resistant *S aureus* resulting in a necrotizing fulminant pneumonia has emerged. Atypical bacterial pathogens are identified in up to 25% of children with CAP. *Chlamydophila pneumoniae* infections occasionally are seen in preschool-age children, whereas in school-aged children, *Mycoplasma pneumoniae* becomes an important pathogen.

Mycobacterium tuberculosis and fungal pneumonia are rarely seen but should be considered in high-risk populations (eg, *M tuberculosis* exposure, immunocompromised).

No single clinical sign or symptom is sufficient to diagnose pneumonia, as there is substantial overlap with other respiratory disorders, such as asthma or bronchiolitis. Symptoms of fever and cough or difficulty breathing are common; tachypnea (respiratory rate >60/min for infants <2 months of age; >50/min for infants 2 months of age up to 1 year; >40/min for children age 1–5 years; >20/min for those >5 years) is the most sensitive sign. Severity is typically assessed based on presence of retractions, grunting, hypoxia, inability to drink, vomiting, or altered mental status. Viral infections are often

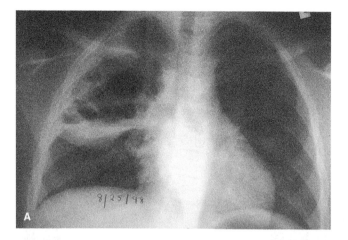

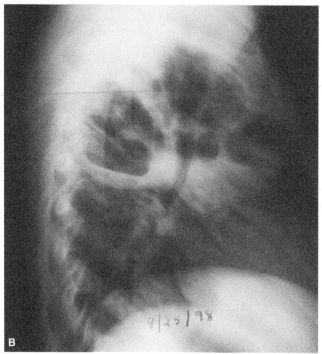

FIGURE 6.24 ■ Staphylococcal Pneumonia. (**A, B**) Frontal and lateral CXRs show involvement of entire right upper lobe with multiple pneumatoceles, some of which have air-fluid levels. The minor fissure is displaced inferiorly ("bulging fissure"). Cystic fibrosis was diagnosed after this pneumonia due to *S aureus*. Clinical deterioration with rapid progression from bronchopneumonia to effusion or pyopneumothorax with or without pneumatoceles is highly suggestive of staphylococcal pneumonia. Other pathogens may also cause empyema or pneumatoceles (eg, *S pneumoniae*, group A streptococci). (Photo contributor: Binita R. Shah, MD.)

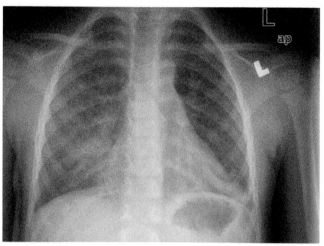

FIGURE 6.25 ■ Viral Pneumonia/Pneumonitis. Frontal view of the chest demonstrates hyperinflation with marked increase in bronchovascular markings emanating from hilum and areas of atelectasis at both bases. (Photo contributor: John Amodio, MD.)

accompanied by symptoms of a URI, such as rhinorrhea, sore throat, and nasal congestion. Lung examination may reveal dullness to percussion, crackles, and decreased breath sounds. Wheezing and chest pain may be present in atypical bacterial infections. Generally, the combination of fever, tachypnea, focal auscultatory findings (decreased breath sounds, crackles), and hypoxia is suggestive of a clinical diagnosis of pneumonia. Pulse oximetry should be performed on every patient with suspected CAP.

Routine CXRs are not necessary if clinical suspicion for CAP is high to confirm pneumonia in children well enough to be treated as outpatients. Two-view (posteroanterior and lateral) CXRs should be obtained in those with hypoxia or significant respiratory distress, those ill enough to warrant hospitalization, those with failure of initial antibiotic therapy, and if complications of pneumonia are suspected. CXRs are limited, however. The intrarater and interrater reliability are modest. In addition, clinical findings may precede radiologic evidence; thus, a negative CXR does not definitively exclude pneumonia in some cases. Follow-up CXRs are not indicated in children with CAP whose symptoms resolve as expected. Chest US, although not yet routinely recommended, often reveals consolidation appearing as hypoechoic areas surrounded by B-lines or air bronchograms appearing as linear and branching echogenic structures. Hepatization of the lung may be seen in lobar involvement. Outpatient management requires no laboratory evaluation. In hospitalized patients with moderate to severe disease, blood cultures should be obtained; the yield will be greatest in those with more severe disease, such as empyema or complicated pneumonia, or underlying medical conditions, such as immunodeficiency.

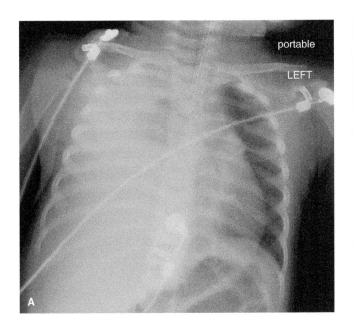

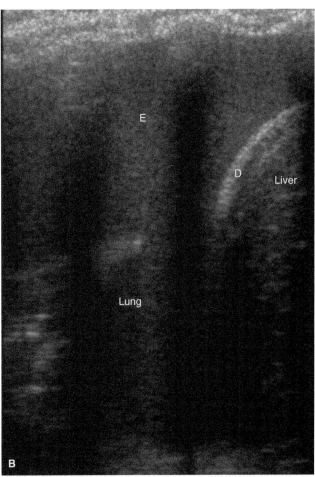

FIGURE 6.26 ■ Influenza A Infection with Secondary Bacterial Infection. (**A**) Frontal view of the chest shows opacification of the right hemithorax with no mediastinal shift, compatible with pleural effusion. This toddler presented with severe respiratory distress associated with fever, cough, and rhinorrhea during flu epidemic. Her nasopharyngeal aspirate was positive for influenza A virus, and blood and empyema cultures were positive for *S pyogenes*. (**B**) Longitudinal sonogram of the right hemithorax shows large complex effusion (E), which was found to be an empyema. (Photo contributor: John Amodio, MD.)

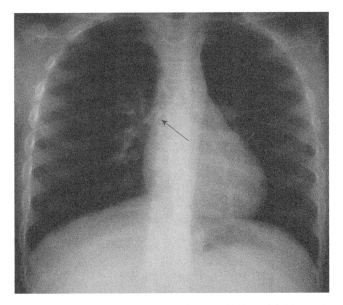

FIGURE 6.27 ■ Foreign Body Aspiration; Differential Diagnosis of Wheezing. Frontal view of the chest shows foreign body (rubber cap) in right mainstem bronchus in a child presenting with coughing and wheezing (which are also common symptoms of viral pneumonia). (Photo contributor: Rafael Rivera, MD.)

Routine measurement of the CBC or acute phase reactants (eg, C-reactive protein) are not warranted in most children with CAP. These tests may be considered in those with severe disease to interpret findings in the context of the clinical examination and other laboratory findings and to look for complications of pneumonia. Electrolytes should be obtained only if significant dehydration or acidosis is expected. Rapid viral testing using sensitive and specific tests may help limit additional testing and treatment. Perform tuberculin skin testing in areas with a high incidence of tuberculosis or if there is high suspicion.

In patients with empyema, pleural fluid should be sent for cell count, Gram stain, and culture. Molecular (eg, PCR) testing of pleural fluid may increase pathogen detection. Generally, other pleural fluid parameters, such as pH, glucose, protein, and lactate dehydrogenase, rarely change management. A chest tube drain or video-assisted thoracoscopic surgery is usually required if pleural fluid is purulent/exudative (empyema) or if the effusion is large, complex, or associated with significant respiratory distress.

Emergency Department Treatment and Disposition

Consider hospitalizing children who are in moderate to severe respiratory distress (eg, dyspnea, retractions, grunting, nasal flaring), have an oxygen saturation <90% on room air, have a toxic appearance or altered mental status, are age <3 months, are immunocompromised, are not able to maintain adequate hydration, have pneumonia with pleural effusion/empyema or a suspected virulent pathogen (eg, S aureus), or if there is concern that home therapy and follow-up will be challenging. Supportive care for pneumonia includes supplemental oxygen if hypoxia is present and IV or nasogastric fluids if there is moderate to severe dehydration.

Generally, children 3 months to 5 years of age well enough to be treated as outpatients do not warrant antibiotics, as the majority of etiologies are viral. When antibiotics are used, age often determines initial empiric therapy. Treat neonates with ampicillin and cefotaxime. A macrolide will cover C trachomatis pneumonitis in neonates (use caution with erythromycin due to increased risk for pyloric stenosis). For older infants and children, amoxicillin is the first-line oral therapy to cover for S pneumoniae. For children who have non–type 1 allergy to amoxicillin, a third-generation cephalosporin (eg, cefdinir) may be used. For those with a history of type 1 reactions, alternatives include macrolides, levofloxacin, or clindamycin. IV ampicillin should be used in hospitalized children. A third-generation cephalosporin (eg, ceftriaxone) should be used as an alternative if the child is incompletely immunized, if local epidemiology demonstrates penicillin-resistant pneumococcus, or in those with life-threatening infections, such as empyema. If Staphylococcus is a concern (including methicillin-resistant S aureus), clindamycin or vancomycin should be added. Give ampicillin-sulbactam or clindamycin to children with aspiration pneumonitis. Macrolides (eg, azithromycin) should be used if atypical pneumonia (C pneumoniae, M pneumoniae) is a concern. A combination of a β-lactam and macrolide should be used in school-aged and adolescent children who are hospitalized when atypical pneumonia is a consideration. If the initial response to IV antibiotics is good, institute oral treatment to complete a 7- to 10-day course in uncomplicated pneumonia and at least a 14- to 21-day course in complicated pneumonia or pneumonia due to S aureus. Use antiviral medications, such as oseltamivir, for treatment of influenza A and B. Respiratory tract secretions are infectious, and good hand hygiene is important. Because viral infections usually are either the direct cause of pneumonia or predispose children to infection with bacterial or atypical pathogens, immunization against influenza is particularly helpful.

Pearls

1. No single clinical finding can be used to diagnosis pneumonia. Hypoxia and work of breathing are more important in the diagnosis than tachypnea and auscultatory findings.

2. Respiratory viruses are the most common etiology of pneumonia in the first few years of life.

3. Most children with cough, runny nose, and fever without the presence of tachypnea or hypoxia do not need antibiotics.

4. Lower lobe pneumonia can present with signs of paralytic ileus and/or referred pain to the right lower quadrant (with right lower lobe pneumonia), mimicking acute abdomen.

5. Children with severe influenza should be evaluated carefully for possible coinfection with bacterial pathogens and may require antimicrobial therapy.

Clinical Summary

Intrathoracic tuberculosis (TB) refers to *Mycobacterium tuberculosis* involvement of the lung parenchyma, pleural space, and intrathoracic lymph nodes. Intrathoracic disease causes approximately 80% to 90% of all TB in children. "Classic" TB symptoms of night sweats are uncommon in children, and in many instances, the only symptoms may be fever and chronic cough. TB should be suspected in any child with a chronic pneumonia unresponsive to therapy for pyogenic infections (eg, pneumococcus), children with weight loss in association with the cough, and immunocompromised children with radiographic abnormalities. Pleural TB is characterized by fever, cough, and pleuritic chest pain. Often, children with TB have a benign examination when compared to the CXRs (ie, the CXR looks "sicker" than the child). The second most common site of TB is in the peripheral lymph nodes, with anterior cervical and supraclavicular nodes being the most commonly involved. The differential diagnosis of intrathoracic TB varies

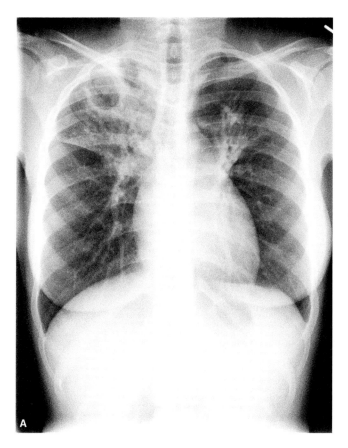

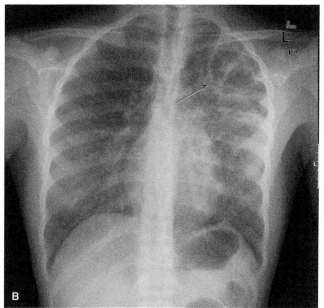

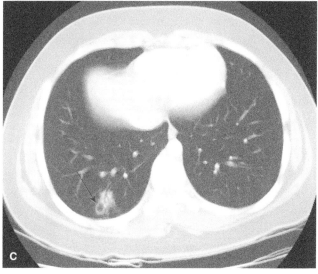

FIGURE 6.28 ■ Cavitary Pulmonary Tuberculosis. (**A**) A cavitary lesion in the right upper lobe with volume loss, reflected in the retraction of the minor fissure upward. There are air bronchograms and the suggestion of >1 cavity. (**B**). Frontal view of chest (different patient) demonstrates a large cavity in the left upper lobe (arrow) with reticulonodular disease (endobronchial spread) of active tuberculosis. (**C**) CT slice of the lower lobe region (different patient) shows air-filled cavity (arrow) compatible with cavitary tuberculosis. (Photo contributors: Andrea T. Cruz, MD, MPH [A], and John Amodio, MD [B, C].)

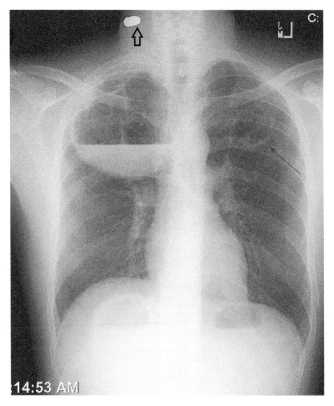

FIGURE 6.29 ■ Reactivation Pulmonary Tuberculosis (TB). Frontal view of chest showing a large cavitary lesion with an air-fluid level in the right upper lobe and a smaller cavitary focus (multiloculated; arrow) in the left upper lobe apical segment in an immunocompromised patient. The air-fluid level on the right represents a secondary infection with development of lung abscess. The most common form of reactivation TB is an infiltrate or cavity in the apex of the upper lobes. This patient's sputum was positive for acid-fast bacillus, and culture was positive for *M tuberculosis*. A radiopaque foreign body (a bullet; patient "accidentally shot" as per history) is also seen in the neck. (Photo contributor: Binita R. Shah, MD.)

based on radiographic findings. For infiltrates, the differential diagnosis includes CAP, fungal pneumonia, and superinfection of congenital lesions (eg, congenital cystic adenomatoid malformations). For pleural effusions, the differential diagnosis includes pyogenic causes of empyema, autoimmune processes, and paraneoplastic phenomena. Intrathoracic adenopathy can be caused by hematologic malignancies (eg, lymphoma), sarcoidosis, and fungal disease.

Emergency Department Treatment and Disposition

CXRs should be obtained in all children with suspected intrathoracic TB. It should be noted that cavitary lesions are more common in adults and there are no radiographic findings that are pathognomonic for TB in children. Radiographs may show focal consolidation, reticulonodular pattern, pleural effusions, adenopathy, or calcifications.

In preschool-aged children, intrathoracic lymph nodes may cause extrinsic compression on bronchi, resulting in distal atelectasis and a ball-valve effect similar to an intrabronchial foreign body. This collapse/consolidation pattern is most common in the right upper lobe in association with enlargement of the azygous node.

Any child with suspected pulmonary TB should have a CBC, liver panel, and HIV testing performed. Because cultures are negative in up to 70% of cases, tests for TB infection should also be obtained; these include the older tuberculin skin test and the newer interferon-γ release assays (QuantiFERON and T-SPOT.TB). The cutoff for skin test induration in children with suspected TB disease is 5 mm.

Providers should consider admitting all children with suspected pulmonary TB for cultures unless (1) the person from whom they acquired TB has known culture results (which can then be used to treat the child) *and* (2) they are well appearing. Otherwise, children should be admitted for gastric

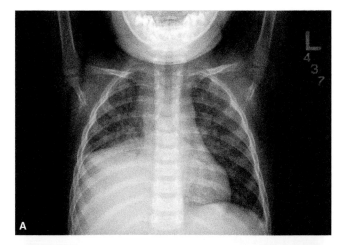

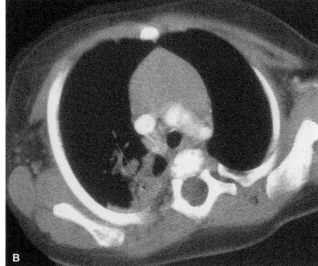

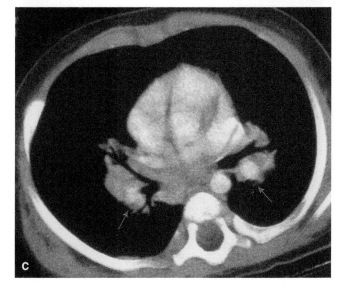

FIGURE 6.30 ▪ Active Pulmonary Tuberculosis (TB). (**A**) Right middle and lower lobe consolidation is seen on a CXR in a toddler presenting with a history of cough for 6 months, exposure to mother with confirmed pulmonary TB, and mild tachypnea on examination. CT scan of the chest in a different patient showing right upper lobe consolidation (**B**, arrow) and bilateral hilar adenopathy (**C**, arrows). Patient also had subcarinal adenopathy. (Photo contributors: Andrea T. Cruz, MD, MPH [A], and John Amodio, MD [B, C].)

aspiration or for collection of expectorated sputa. The former is often needed in young children, who cannot expectorate on command. Several respiratory specimens should be obtained prior to starting therapy. For children with pleural TB and a substantial effusion, pleural fluid should be sent for routine studies, mycobacterial culture, TB PCR, and an adenosine deaminase (ADA) level; ADA levels >40 IU/L are more likely to be seen with TB than with other etiologies. Pleural punch biopsies have a much higher yield than fluid obtained via thoracentesis. Lumbar puncture for routine studies, mycobacterial culture, and TB PCR should be considered for any child <12 months old with suspected pulmonary TB, as the risk of seeding the meningitis is higher for infants than for older

children. The same holds true for suspected pulmonary TB in immunocompromised patients. Any child with suspected TB should be placed in a negative-pressure room pending evaluation. Most children are not contagious with intrathoracic TB; exceptions include children with cavitary lesions, children who are expectorating sputa, patients with suspected laryngeal TB (who can aerosolize the organism just by speaking), and children with draining lesions. However, the noninfectious child may be accompanied by the quite contagious adult from whom they acquired TB. Some hospitals obtain CXRs on caregivers of a child with suspected TB to rapidly identify contagious adults and limit nosocomial spread of the bacterium.

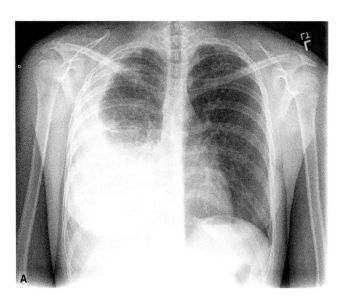
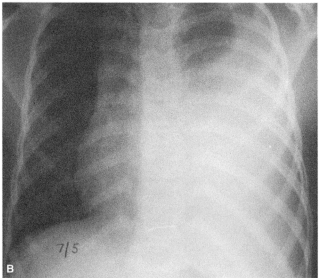

FIGURE 6.31 ■ Pulmonary Tuberculosis with Pleural Effusion. (**A**) Right lower lobe consolidation and a large pleural effusion are seen on a frontal CXR in an adolescent with a history of fever and cough for 3 weeks. Thoracentesis revealed serous, nonpurulent fluid. (**B**) Frontal CXR shows opacification of left middle and lower zones with obliteration of the left cardiac margin, left hemidiaphragm, and costophrenic angle associated with a mediastinal shift to the right in patient with a positive PPD test. The pleural fluid was transudate with a negative AFB smear but positive culture for MTB. (Photo contributors: Andrea T. Cruz, MD, MPH [A], and Binita R. Shah, MD [B].)

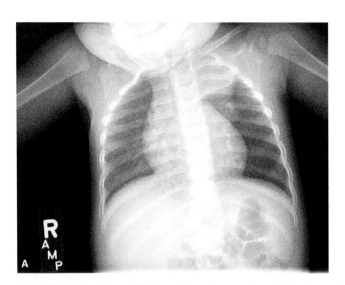
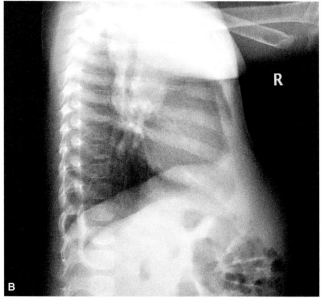

FIGURE 6.32 ■ Lung Collapse Secondary to Bronchial Obstruction From Pulmonary Tuberculosis (TB) Lymphadenopathy. Frontal (**A**) and lateral (**B**) radiographs in an asymptomatic infant with a positive PPD skin test which was placed after her father was diagnosed with pulmonary TB. This child has a left upper lobe atelectatic region caused by compression of the bronchus feeding this part of the lung. The lymphadenopathy is more apparent on the lateral radiograph and appears as the donut-shaped density behind the heart. This region is difficult to see in young children on the frontal view, where it is often obscured by the thymic shadow. (Photo contributor: Andrea T. Cruz, MD, MPH.)

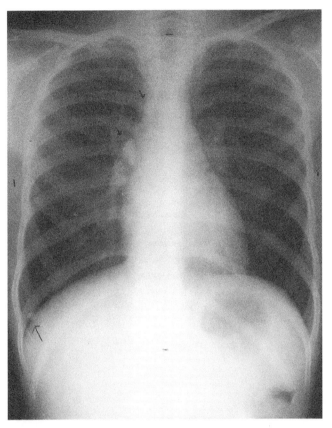

FIGURE 6.33 ▪ Pulmonary Tuberculosis (TB) with Lymph Node Calcifications. The hallmark of childhood pulmonary TB is Ghon primary complex (hilar lymphadenitis and parenchymal focus with or without lymph node calcification). Hilar adenopathy is inevitably present with childhood TB. However, it may not be detected on a plain x-ray in the absence of calcification. A CT scan detects both calcified and noncalcified lymph nodes. (Photo contributor: Binita R. Shah, MD.)

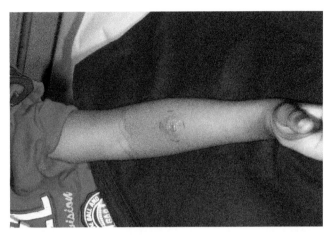

FIGURE 6.34 ▪ Positive Tuberculin Skin Test. A 5-TU (tuberculin unit) purified protein derivative (PPD) skin test result is assessed at 48 to 72 hours after administration. The diameter of induration (*and not erythema*) is measured perpendicularly to the long axis of the forearm. With an intense reaction, a bullous formation may also occur. (Refer to local Department of Health guidelines for interpretation). (Photo contributor: Binita R. Shah, MD.)

Pearls

1. Intrathoracic TB should be suspected in subacute/chronic pneumonia and in patients with certain radiographic features (effusions, intrathoracic nodes, cavities).

2. Many children will not (yet) have a family history of TB, because children are often the first in the family to be diagnosed.

3. Few prepubertal children with intrathoracic TB are contagious, but the same cannot be said of the adults who accompany them; as a consequence, personal protective equipment should be used by all health care workers.

MILIARY TUBERCULOSIS

Clinical Summary

Miliary TB, 1 of the forms of disseminated TB, is named after the "millet seed" appearance on CXR.

This form of TB is most common in young infants and immunocompromised patients. *M tuberculosis* can spread hematogenously through the lung fields and also seed other parts of the body. The most commonly affected sites are the brain and meninges and the reticuloendothelial system, the latter with associated hepatosplenomegaly and, at time, disseminated peripheral lymphadenopathy. Children can present with fever, cough, tachypnea, and failure to thrive. Once seeding of the meninges occurs, children can develop vomiting (due to increased intracranial pressure), cranial nerve palsies (particularly cranial nerves III and VI due to basilar meningitis

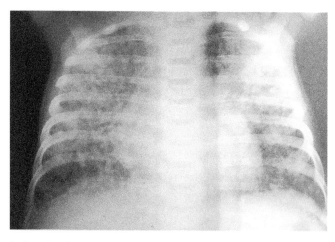

FIGURE 6.36 ■ Miliary Tuberculosis. Frontal CXR showing innumerable bilateral lung parenchymal opacities in an infant who presented with fever, hepatosplenomegaly, and failure to thrive. (Photo contributor: Binita R. Shah, MD.)

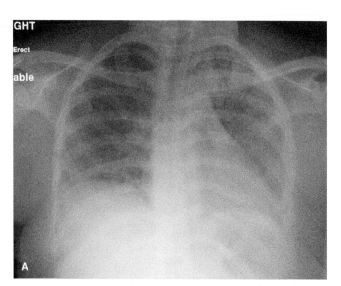

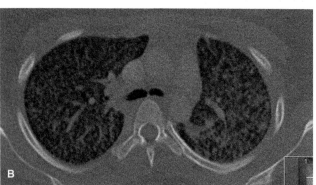

FIGURE 6.35 ■ Miliary Tuberculosis. (**A**) Frontal view of the chest shows multiple tiny nodules bilaterally with more confluent lesions in the left upper lobe. Note the absence of adenopathy. (**B**) CT image through the upper lobes confirms multiple tiny nodules bilaterally. (Photo contributor: John Amodio, MD.)

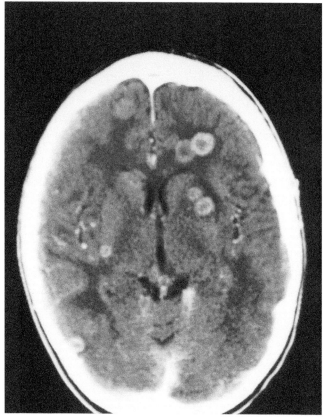

FIGURE 6.37 ■ Tuberculomas. An axial CT image of the brain with contrast shows multiple ring-enhancing lesions bilaterally with surrounding edema in a 5-year-old girl presenting with afebrile seizures. She had a positive PPD with a negative CXR. The most common location of tuberculoma is infratentorial at the base of the brain near the cerebellum, and they can be singular or multiple. (Photo contributor: Binita R. Shah, MD.)

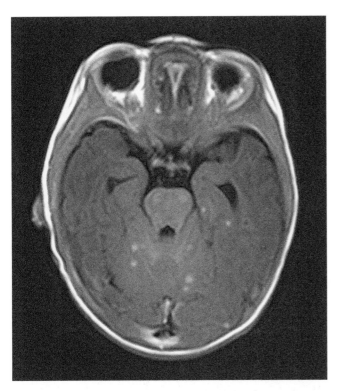

FIGURE 6.38 ■ Tuberculomas. T1-weighted MRI of the brain after gadolinium showing multiple tuberculomas in a 3-month-old infant with miliary tuberculosis. His CSF was normal, showing that tuberculomas can be seen in the absence of meningitis. (Photo contributor: Andrea T. Cruz, MD, MPH.)

causing inflammation where these nerves exit the skull), and altered mental status. The early symptoms of TB meningitis are nonspecific. Children with miliary TB are also at risk for spontaneous pneumothorax caused by expansion of blebs on the surface of the lungs. Few other infections mimic miliary TB on radiography, but disseminated fungal infection, hyaline membrane disease, and lymphocytic interstitial pneumonitis (in HIV-infected patients) can have a similar appearance.

Emergency Department Treatment and Disposition

Please refer to the section on pulmonary TB for other diagnostic tests that should be performed. All children with suspected miliary TB should have a lumbar puncture obtained for routine CSF studies, mycobacterial culture, and *M. tuberculosis* PCR to evaluate for meningitis, as the presence of CNS involvement changes the medications used, the duration of therapy,

and the decision to initiate systemic corticosteroids. Of note, over 90% of all children with TB meningitis also have an abnormal CXR, so TB should be on the differential diagnosis of a child with consistent CSF findings (see below) and an abnormal CXR. Classic CSF findings include a lymphocytic pleocytosis, very high (>200 g/dL) CSF protein, and low CSF glucose; the latter findings are more dramatic the further a child is in the natural history of the infection. Mycobacterial stain of the CSF usually is negative. In addition, children should be admitted for gastric aspiration (daily for 3 days) to be sent for mycobacterial culture. Most children with miliary TB are too young to expectorate sputa, and gastric aspiration is the only way to obtain quality cultures. In the ED, a CT should be obtained if the CSF is concerning for meningitis, as up to 60% of children with TB meningitis will have a noncommunicating hydrocephaly and may require neurosurgical intervention. After admission, consideration should be given to obtaining an MRI scan of the brain in young children with miliary TB, even in the absence of CSF pleocytosis, as tuberculomas can be seen without concomitant meningitis.

As with other forms of TB, children with miliary TB should have a CBC, liver panel, and HIV testing performed prior to the initiation of therapy. In addition, a sodium should be obtained, because both the syndrome of inappropriate secretion of antidiuretic hormone and diabetes insipidus have been described in children with TB meningitis. Children should be admitted to negative-pressure rooms, and health care workers should don N95 masks prior to entering the room to decrease nosocomial spread. Providers performing bronchoscopy or other procedures likely to result in aerosolization of particles should be warned that TB is suspected so that appropriate personal protective equipment can be used.

Pearls

1. Miliary TB is a life-threatening complication of TB predominantly seen in young children.
2. The risk of seeding the meninges is high, and lumbar puncture should be obtained in all children with suspected miliary TB.
3. Children with suspected miliary TB should be admitted, infectious diseases should be consulted, and multidrug therapy for TB should be initiated pending the diagnostic evaluation.

Clinical Summary

Obstructive sleep apnea syndrome (OSAS) is disordered breathing during sleep characterized by intermittent complete airway obstruction and/or prolonged partial obstruction. OSAS disrupts normal ventilation during sleep and normal sleep patterns. Predisposing conditions for OSAS include adenotonsillar hyperplasia (most common cause), obesity, and genetic syndromes with associated craniofacial anomalies such as Pierre-Robin syndrome and Down syndrome. Peak incidence occurs in preschool-aged children between 2 and 6 years old when the tonsils and adenoids are largest in relation to airway size. Nasal polyps (from severe allergic rhinitis or cystic fibrosis), nasal septal deviation, and choanal stenosis are less common causes of OSAS. Once a history of nightly snoring or worsening of snoring with URI is elicited, a more detailed history needs to be obtained. Inquire about repeated URIs and/or recurrent otitis media, labored breathing during sleep, observed apnea episodes described as snoring followed by "choking" or "gasping," restless sleep, enuresis, behavioral issues, school performance, daytime somnolence or fatigue, and morning headaches. Physical examination while awake may be normal or reveal findings related to adenotonsillar hypertrophy such as adenoidal facies, mouth breathing, enlarged tonsils, nasal obstruction during wakefulness, and hyponasal speech. Children may show failure to thrive (inadequate caloric intake during the day and hypermetabolic state at night) or obesity. In longstanding OSAS, pectus excavatum, systemic hypertension, pulmonary hypertension, and cor pulmonale with pulmonary edema (severe cases) may be seen. The main differential diagnosis for OSAS is primary snoring, which is a clinically benign condition (seen in 7%–10% of children) and represents snoring without obstructions, disrupted sleep, or gas exchange abnormalities. Primary snoring is usually exacerbated by URI but does not lead to obstructive apnea.

Emergency Department Treatment and Disposition

Admit any patient presenting with cardiorespiratory failure or worsening of airway obstruction (eg, during URI) to the ICU for continuous cardiac and pulse oximetry monitoring. Use a nasopharyngeal airway to bypass the obstruction or continuous positive airway pressure therapy to establish a temporary airway until a more definitive procedure such as

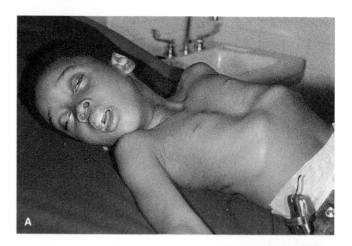

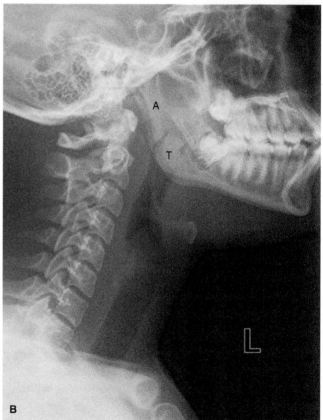

FIGURE 6.39 ■ Obstructive Sleep Apnea (OSA) Syndrome. (**A**) A child presented with worsening of snoring during infection with Epstein-Barr virus (infectious mononucleosis). In ED, he had numerous episodes of OSA during his sleep (cessation of airflow at nose and mouth appreciated by listening with a stethoscope despite apparent, vigorous, inspiratory efforts). His pulse oximetry was 96% while awake and 85% during sleep. Supraclavicular, suprasternal, subcostal, and intercostal retractions are seen. A nasopharyngeal airway was used to relieve his obstruction. (**B**) Lateral view of the neck shows adenoidal enlargement (A) with encroachment on nasopharynx and tonsillar (T) enlargement. (Photo contributor: Binita R. Shah, MD.)

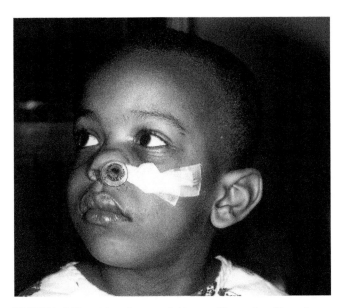

FIGURE 6.40 ▪ Nasopharyngeal Airway; Obstructive Sleep Apnea Syndrome. Obstructive sleep apnea resulting in significant oxygen desaturation occurred in this child who had a long history of snoring. A nasopharyngeal airway (well tolerated in children) was required to acutely relieve the obstruction. (Photo contributor: Binita R. Shah, MD.)

TABLE 6.1 ▪ USEFUL LABORATORY TESTS IN SUSPECTED OBSTRUCTIVE SLEEP APNEA SYNDROME

Hemoglobin/hematocrit:
- May show polycythemia from chronic nocturnal hypoxia

Serum electrolytes:
- Serum CO_2 may be elevated from compensatory metabolic alkalosis (secondary to nocturnal hypoventilation and respiratory acidosis)

CXR:
- Pulmonary edema
- Cardiomegaly
- Aspiration pneumonia

Neck soft tissue radiograph:
- Nasopharyngeal airway narrowing
- Adenotonsillar hypertrophy

ECG and echocardiogram:
- Cardiomegaly, cor pulmonale, pulmonary hypertension

Arterial blood gases:
- Awake: normal Po_2 and Pco_2
- Asleep: elevated Pco_2 and decreased Po_2
- Elevated bicarbonate from compensatory metabolic alkalosis

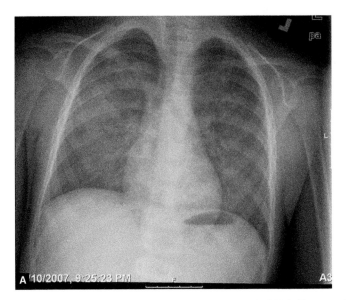
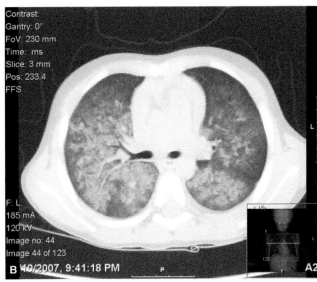

FIGURE 6.41 ▪ Postoperative Pulmonary Edema (POPE). Severe pulmonary edema occurs occasionally within a few hours after extubation in some patients; however, children with OSAS are more likely to experience POPE. (**A**) Fontal radiograph demonstrates normal heart size and pulmonary edema pattern. (**B**) Representative CT slice shows normal heart size and diffuse airspace disease. Follow-up radiograph demonstrated resolution of pulmonary edema pattern in 48 hours. (Photo contributor: John Amodio, MD.)

an adenoidectomy and/or tonsillectomy can be performed. A short course of oral or parenteral corticosteroids can be given to reduce nasopharyngeal lymphoid tissue that may worsen OSAS (eg, in patients with infectious mononucleosis). Refer patients not requiring hospitalization to their primary care physician to arrange for a polysomnogram.

Pearls

1. OSAS is becoming more common in childhood as rates of childhood obesity increase.

2. The 2 most common presenting symptoms of OSAS are snoring and sleep disturbances; however, many children will have behavioral manifestations. Ask parents about sleep-disordered breathing in any child with poor school performance or behavioral problems.

3. A child with suspected OSAS must be examined during sleep, ideally by referral for a formal polysomnogram, including observation of pulse oximetry readings, because physical signs of obstruction may be absent or subtle when the child is awake.

4. Children with OSAS may have an impaired swallowing mechanism or gastroesophageal reflux disease. Both of these entities can lead to aspiration, especially in neurologically impaired children who are also at a higher risk for OSAS.

5. Children with OSAS are also prone to postoperative pulmonary edema syndrome because the upper airway obstruction can predispose to negative-pressure (ie, noncardiogenic) pulmonary edema. This syndrome is manifested by respiratory distress usually immediately after extubation following surgical procedures, but symptoms can be delayed; hence, children with OSAS may require monitoring for 2 to 12 hours after extubation.

Clinical Features

Acute asthma is one of the most common entities treated in the pediatric ED. Asthma exacerbations are acute or subacute episodes of progressively worsening shortness of breath, cough, wheezing, or chest tightness. The hallmark of asthma is reversible airway hyperresponsiveness to external stimuli (eg, viral infections, allergens, tobacco smoke, pollutants, strong odors, emotions, exercise) resulting in bronchial inflammation, edema, excess mucus production, and bronchoconstriction of airway smooth muscle. This leads to airflow limitation, prolonged expiration, air trapping, and hyperinflation. Wheezing (high-pitched, polyphonic "whistling" sounds due to airflow restriction in the lower airways) is the characteristic physical finding during an acute asthma exacerbation. Status asthmaticus occurs when a child continues to have significant respiratory distress and wheezing despite adequate treatment with appropriate bronchodilators. The differential diagnosis for asthma includes any entity that can cause large airway obstruction (eg, foreign body aspiration, tracheomalacia,

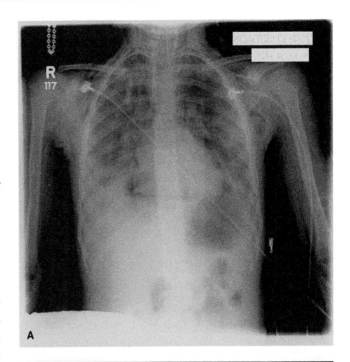

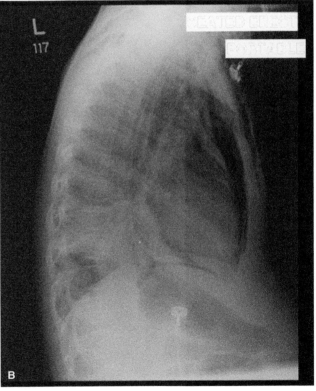

FIGURE 6.43 ■ Acute Asthma with Air-Leak Syndrome. (**A, B**) Frontal and lateral views of chest show extensive subcutaneous emphysema, pneumomediastinum, right pneumothorax, and pneumopericardium. (Photo/legend contributors: Miriam Krinsky, MD/ John Amodio, MD.)

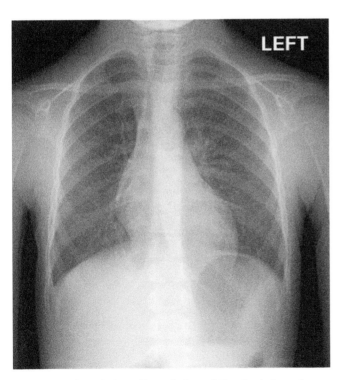

FIGURE 6.42 ■ Asthma. Frontal view of the chest shows hyperinflation, increased bronchovascular markings, and peribronchial cuffing in a child presenting with an acute exacerbation of asthma. (Photo contributor: John Amodio, MD.)

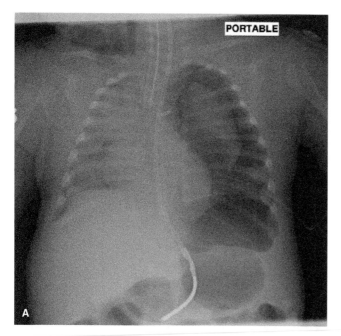

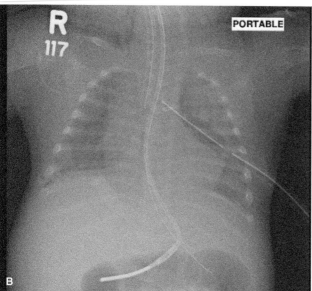

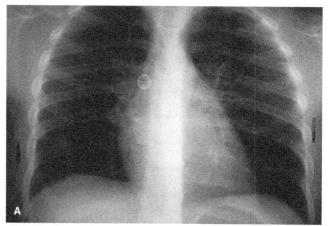

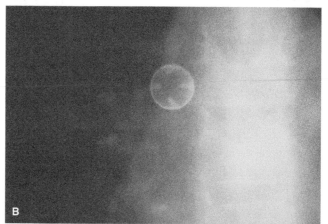

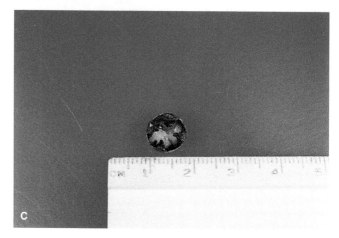

FIGURE 6.44 ■ Tension Pneumothorax; Asthma with Respiratory Failure. (**A**) Frontal view of the chest shows a large tension pneumothorax on the left, a small pneumothorax on the right, and right-sided subcutaneous emphysema in a child with asthma presenting with respiratory failure requiring intubation. (**B**) Frontal view of the chest shows a left chest tube with subsequent diminution of the left tension pneumothorax and persistent right subcutaneous emphysema in the neck. (Photo contributor: Vikas Shah, MD.)

FIGURE 6.45 ■ Foreign Body Aspiration; Differential Diagnosis of Wheezing. (**A**) A round radiopaque density is seen in the area of right mainstem bronchus without a mediastinal shift, air trapping, or distal atelectasis in a 4-year-old patient presenting with worsening cough of 6 days in duration and first episode of wheezing. (**B**) Close-up of the foreign body in anteroposterior view. (**C**) Close-up of brown metal button measuring 1 × 1 × 0.5 cm that was removed from the right bronchus by direct bronchoscopy. (Photo contributor: Binita R. Shah, MD.)

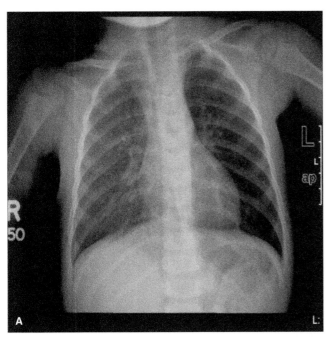
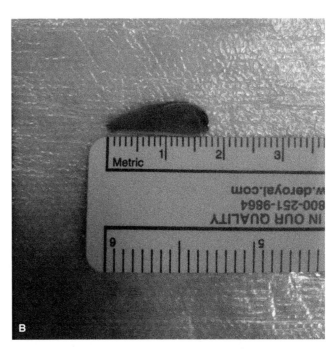

FIGURE 6.46 ■ Foreign Body Aspiration; Differential Diagnosis of Wheezing. (**A**) Single frontal view of the chest shows hyperinflation of the left lung. This 18-month-old toddler presented with persistent wheezing of several days in duration. (**B**) Shell of a sunflower seed that was removed from the right mainstem bronchus. It is conceivable that initially the foreign body was in the left mainstem bronchus and subsequently got dislodged during coughing and moved to the right mainstem bronchus. (Photo contributor: Johnathan Cohen, MD.)

bronchomalacia, endobronchial masses, obstruction from an extrabronchial mass or vascular ring/sling, subglottic stenosis, vocal cord dysfunction) or small airway obstruction (eg, acute viral bronchiolitis, bronchopulmonary dysplasia, chronic aspiration).

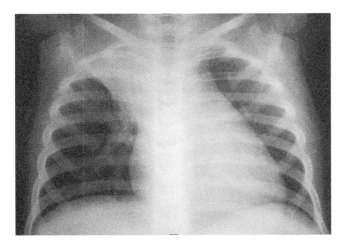

FIGURE 6.47 ■ Endobronchial Tuberculosis; Differential Diagnosis of Wheezing. Frontal CXR shows right upper lobe opacity with an elevation of the right fissure suggesting right upper lobe collapse. This infant presented with unilateral wheezing and coughing. He was cared by a babysitter who had cavitary pulmonary disease. (Photo contributor: Binita R. Shah, MD.)

Emergency Department Treatment and Disposition

The goal of emergent asthma treatment is to reverse bronchospasm and treat airway inflammation. First, quickly assess the severity of the current exacerbation with a physical exam and a brief, focused history including home medications (especially

TABLE 6.2 ■ INDICATIONS FOR INTUBATION IN SEVERE STATUS ASTHMATICUS

Absolute Indications
- Cardiac/respiratory arrest
- Circulatory collapse

Relative Indications
- Respiratory muscle fatigue (paradoxical respirations; rising Pco_2 [>45 mm Hg]; disappearance of pulsus paradoxus)
- Falling pH (<7.25)
- Respiratory rate >40 breaths/min in a child >3 years
- Altered mental status (confused or unresponsive)
- Po_2 <60 mm Hg
- "Silent chest" (obstruction is so severe that there is minimal air exchange)

bronchodilators), past history of hospitalizations, intubation, and known asthma triggers. Validated severity scores for pediatric asthma, such as the Pediatric Asthma Severity Score, should be used to gauge disease severity to direct appropriate therapy. Next determine possible cause(s) of the current exacerbation, and obtain a history of any known allergies. The physical exam should include evaluation of mental status, respiratory rate and effort, heart rate, BP, oxygen saturation, lung auscultation (focusing on severity and location of wheezing), and use of accessory muscles. In children older than 6 years, obtaining peak expiratory flow with a peak flow meter provides an objective measurement of the degree of expiratory flow impairment. Diagnostic tests (eg, arterial blood gas [ABG], CXR, CBC, serum electrolytes) should only be used as indicated; most children presenting with asthma exacerbations require no diagnostic testing.

Inhaled short-acting β-agonists (SABAs) and systemic corticosteroids are the cornerstone of asthma exacerbation management. Inhaled SABAs, such as albuterol, cause bronchodilation through activation of β_2-adrenergic receptors. SABA may be provided by nebulizer or metered-dose inhaler with valved holding chambers (spacers). These devices have been shown to be equivalent with regard to ED length of stay and tachycardia; either may be used for mild to moderate exacerbations. For patients with severe exacerbations, high SABA doses administered by nebulizer are necessary due to the degree of airway obstruction. For moderate to severe exacerbations, administration of 3 doses of albuterol provided 20 minutes apart is first-line therapy. Inhaled ipratropium bromide, an anticholinergic agent, decreases hospitalization rates and improves lung function in severe exacerbations and should be added to albuterol in moderate to severe exacerbations. Systemic corticosteroids, either oral or IV, should also be administered as first-line therapy as early as possible in the ED course to provide maximal effect in decreasing the need for hospitalization. Supplemental oxygen should be provided to maintain oxygen saturation at or above 90% to 92%. In life-threatening attacks, use of adjunct treatments, including IV magnesium sulfate, continuous nebulized albuterol, heliox, IV or subcutaneous terbutaline, or bilevel positive airway pressure should be used early in the ED course to avoid intubation.

Children with mild to moderate attacks who have good response to ED management (ie, no respiratory distress, reassuring physical exam, response to SABA is sustained for ≥60 minutes after last dose, no hypoxia or dehydration) may be discharged with inhaled SABA, a short course of oral corticosteroids (prednisone, prednisolone, or dexamethasone), and close medical follow-up. Consider prescribing inhaled corticosteroids when indicated upon discharge. Patients with residual moderate symptoms despite adequate ED management or requiring SABA more frequently than every 2 to 4 hours should be hospitalized. The National Asthma Education and Prevention Program (NAEPP) guidelines provide additional details on management of asthma.

Pearls

1. Chronic severity classification of asthma (intermittent, mild persistent, moderate persistent, or severe persistent) does not predict the severity of an individual exacerbation.

2. Smaller airways, limited lung elasticity, limited collateral channels of ventilation, softer rib cage, and tendency of respiratory muscles to easily fatigue increase asthma severity risk in infants and young children.

3. Current guidelines do not advocate methylxanthines, aggressive hydration, chest physiotherapy, or mucolytics for status asthmaticus. However, adequate hydration is required when using IV magnesium sulfate because dehydration can potentiate adverse drug effects such as hypotension and hypotonia.

4. Do not forget to consider aspirated foreign bodies, particularly in a child who is not responding to therapy. CXR can be misleading because many children with asthma have atelectasis or asymmetric hyperinflation due to mucous plugging.

Clinical Summary

Pneumothorax is the presence of air or gas between the visceral and parietal pleura and occurs when air enters the pleural space through the chest wall in penetrating trauma or across the lung parenchyma via the visceral pleura. Pneumothoraces may occur in diseased lung (secondary spontaneous pneumothorax), as a result of medical interventions (iatrogenic) or trauma, or without any prior lung pathology or trauma (primary spontaneous pneumothorax [PSP]).

PSP is most commonly seen in adolescent males and is usually caused by rupture of asymptomatic blebs or bullae that were not clinically evident until they resulted in PSP. Although Valsalva maneuvers and increased intrathoracic pressures are described as triggering factors, PSP most commonly occurs at rest. Additional risk factors include a tall, lanky body habitus, smoking, and a prior history of PSP. When air enters the pleural space from a ruptured bleb, the lung will collapse until there is equilibrium or the air leak is sealed; therefore, as the pneumothorax enlarges, the lung volume is diminished. Young, healthy patients can tolerate the resulting reduction in partial pressure of oxygen and vital capacity with minimal to no respiratory distress for several days. Patients generally present with acute onset of chest pain (usually pleuritic), shortness of breath, and sometimes cough. Chest pain will often improve after the first 2 hours even without medical intervention. Tachycardia, tachypnea, and hypoxia may be present. Lung auscultation of the affected side may reveal diminished or absent breath sounds and/or hyperresonance to percussion. Tension pneumothorax is rare in PSP.

Emergency Department Treatment and Disposition

A thorough history should focus on preexisting lung diseases such as asthma, tuberculosis, cystic fibrosis, interstitial lung disease, or congenital pulmonary airway malformation. After initial evaluation, stabilization and supportive care (eg, oxygen), obtain a CXR. Inspiratory and expiratory chest films may be used in subtle cases to better visualize the pneumothorax. CT is not generally indicated in the ED.

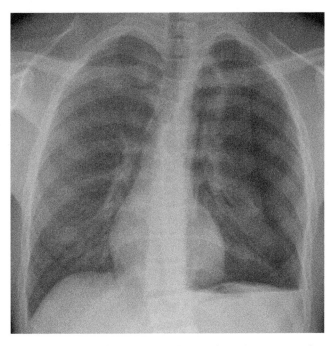

FIGURE 6.48 ■ Primary Spontaneous Pneumothorax. Frontal view of chest shows large pneumothorax on left without mediastinal shift in an adolescent male without any underlying lung pathology. A follow-up study showed resolution of pneumothorax. (Photo contributor: John Amodio, MD.)

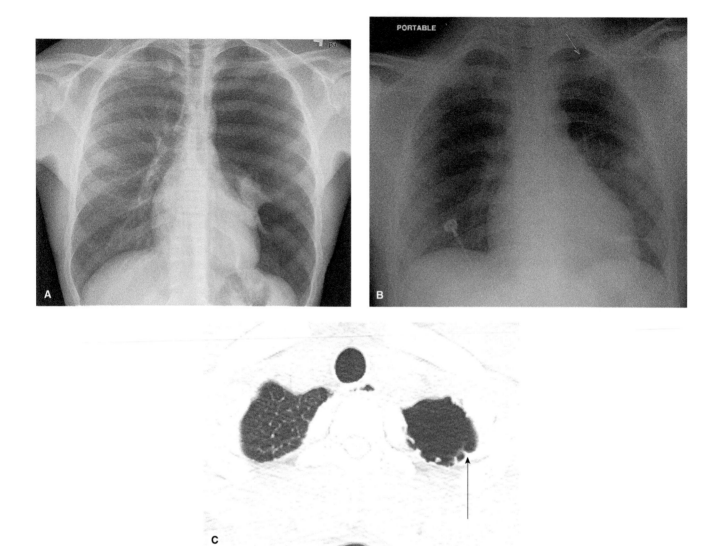

FIGURE 6.49 ■ Primary Spontaneous Pneumothorax. (**A**) Frontal view of the chest shows very large left pneumothorax without evidence of tension in an adolescent male without any underlying lung pathology. (**B**) Frontal view of the chest shows small catheter in left hemithorax with partial reexpansion of the left lung and small residual pneumothorax (arrow). (**C**) CT scan at level of lung apices shows residual pneumothorax on left with small blebs at left lung apex (arrow). (Photo contributor: John Amodio, MD.)

Stable, asymptomatic patients with a small PSP (<3 cm from the apex of the lung to the top margin of the visceral pleura) may be monitored and provided oxygen as needed. Many PSPs resolve with no additional intervention. Consider needle aspiration in those who are symptomatic, but stable, with small (<3 cm) PSP and observe for reaccumulation. Surgical consultation should be considered for larger pneumothoraces. A large

(>3 cm) PSP should be aspirated by pigtail catheter placement to low suction or water seal and patients should be admitted. Treat patients with recurrent PSP (defined as ipsilateral relapse after >1 month) with a chest tube, and consult a surgeon for thoracoscopy (preferably video-assisted thoracoscopic surgery [VATS]) with pleurodesis and possible bullectomy/blebectomy. Consult surgery for the first contralateral PSP.

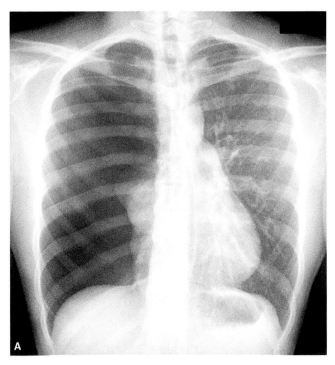 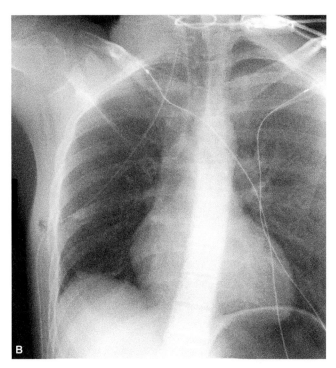

FIGURE 6.50 ■ Tension Pneumothorax From Primary Spontaneous Pneumothorax. (**A**) Frontal radiograph of the chest in a 17-year-old male demonstrates a large right-sided pneumothorax with collapse of the right lung and leftward shift of the cardiomediastinal structures. (**B**) Frontal radiograph of the chest demonstrates placement of a right-sided chest tube with reduced pneumothorax, expansion of the right lung, and decreased cardiomediastinal shift. There is also a small amount of chest wall emphysema at the insertion site of the chest tube. (Photo contributor: Arnold C. Merrow, Jr., MD.)

Pearls

1. All patients with prior PSP must avoid exposure to cigarette smoke. Offer smoking cessation counseling to patients and close family members.
2. Patients with PSP should avoid activities that cause sudden changes in intrathoracic pressure for a minimum of 4 to 6 weeks.
3. Preventive intervention is not required unless patients had a chest tube and thoracoscopy (as part of initial management of PSP), have failure of air leak to resolve after 5 to 7 days, or have a vocation that puts them at high risk for recurrence and puts themselves or others at risk (eg, deep sea diver or airplane pilot).
4. Patients with a second ipsilateral PSP require intervention to prevent recurrence.

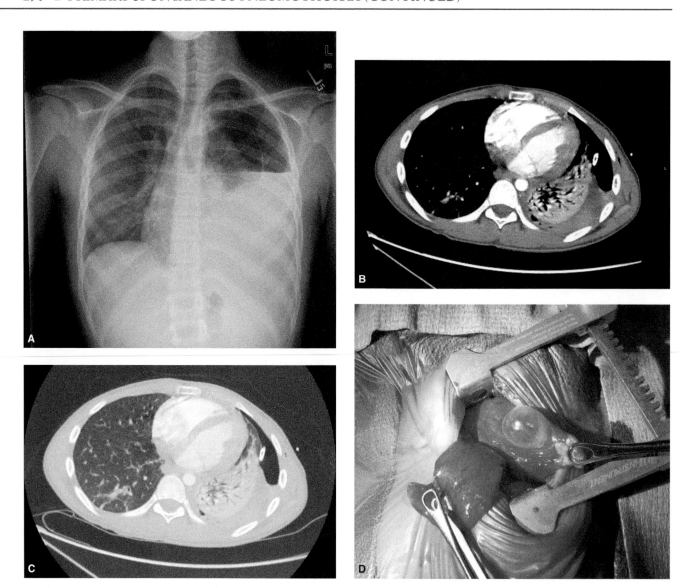

FIGURE 6.51 ▪ Hemopneumothorax and Thoracoscopic Blebectomy. **(A)** Frontal view of the chest demonstrates a large left-sided pleural effusion and pneumothorax. There is also mild rightward shift of the cardiomediastinal structures. Axial contrast-enhanced CT scans of the chest in soft tissue window **(B)** and lung window **(C)** demonstrate a left lung consolidation with air bronchograms. Adjacent pleural effusion and pneumothorax are also depicted. A portion of a chest tube is seen within the pleural space. This was a 14-year-old boy presenting with impending respiratory failure. He denied prior history of trauma or strenuous activity or any known medical problems (raised by foster mother from infancy). A pigtail was placed draining 2 L of serosanguinous fluid. He underwent VATS with blebectomy and decortication with improvement. All investigations for connective tissue disorders and bleeding disorders were negative; however, his HIV tests were positive (tested because of the uncertainty of his birth history, status of biological mother). He was started on antiretroviral therapy. **(D)** A bleb is visualized during VATS in a different patient presenting with recurrent spontaneous pneumothorax. (Photo contributors: Anastasios Drenis, MD, and Richard Hong, MD [A, B, C], and Richard A. Falcone, Jr, MD, MPH [D].)

Clinical Summary

Pulmonary embolism (PE) is difficult to diagnose in children because it is rare and often manifests with an atypical presentation in children with underlying chronic medical conditions. PE is more prevalent in children with sickle cell disease and is precipitated by dehydration and infection. Other predisposing factors include nephrotic syndrome, cancer, chemotherapy, inherited hypercoagulable states (eg, protein C or S deficiency, lupus anticoagulant, factor V Leiden), catheters, surgery, trauma, pregnancy, oral contraceptive use, prolonged immobilization, and cardiomyopathy.

Classic presentations include pleuritic chest pain, shortness of breath, cough, and hemoptysis, although often these are absent in children with PE. Tachypnea is a common physical finding; tachycardia and respiratory distress may also be present. Up to 25% of patients with PE have minimal or no symptoms. Lung auscultation may reveal rales but is often normal. Hypoxia not explained by another disease process should increase suspicion for PE. Signs and symptoms of deep venous thrombosis may or may not be present. The classic Virchow's triad predisposing to thromboembolism consists of any state of relative stasis, prothrombogenic tendency, and injury to the vascular wall. Consideration of disease processes that lead to these factors may aid in diagnosis. Differential diagnosis of PE includes more common diagnoses such as pneumonia, acute chest syndrome in sickle cell disease, pneumothorax, myocarditis, pericarditis, pleural effusion, asthma, and anxiety.

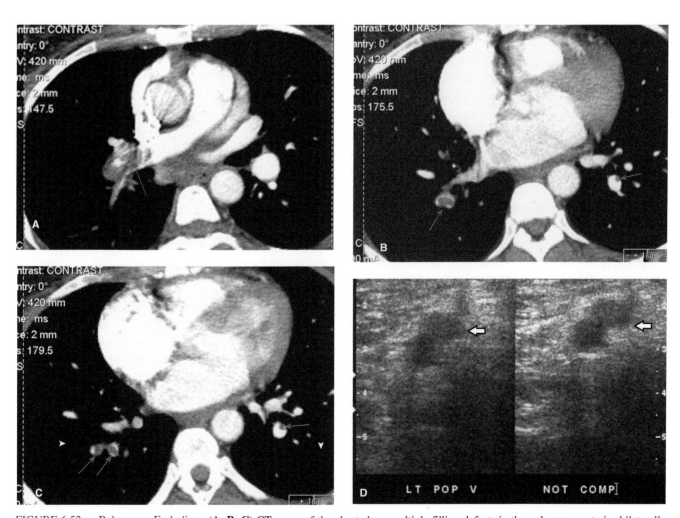

FIGURE 6.52 ■ Pulmonary Embolism. (**A, B, C**) CT scans of the chest show multiple filling defects in the pulmonary arteries bilaterally (arrows). (**D**) Gray scale sonography of the popliteal region demonstrates non-compressibility of the popliteal vein (open black arrow) compatible with thrombosis. Red arrow points to the popliteal artery. (Photo contributor: John Amodio, MD.)

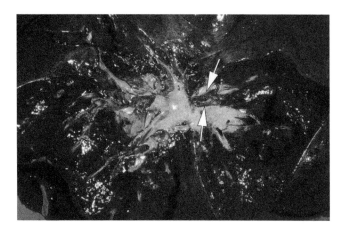

FIGURE 6.53 ■ Pulmonary Embolus (PE). Postmortem pathologic specimen demonstrating pulmonary embolus (arrows) in a 15-year-old boy with paraneoplastic syndrome presenting with PE. (Photo contributor: David P. Witte, MD.)

Emergency Department Treatment and Disposition

Timely detection of PE in children is a significant diagnostic challenge, given its nonspecific presentation and rarity. Laboratory tests are often normal or nonspecific and thus cannot definitively diagnose or exclude PE. ABG may demonstrate an elevated alveolar-arterial gradient; however, the low negative predictive value of a normal Pao_2 may not warrant performing this painful and difficult procedure in children. Respiratory alkalosis may be present, reflecting dyspnea and tachypnea. Conversely, respiratory acidosis may be present, reflecting ventilation/perfusion $(\dot{V}/\dot{Q})$ mismatch. Metabolic acidosis is an ominous sign and reflects poor perfusion. D-dimer enzyme-linked immunosorbent assays have reported sensitivities of 96% to 98% for PE detection but have not been specifically evaluated in children. A positive D-dimer is seen in 90% of adults with PE. A negative result makes PE unlikely; however, a positive result is not specific. It is important to remember that a negative D-dimer in a patient who is *not* considered low risk does not rule out PE, and imaging must be pursued. An ECG should be obtained, although these are often normal or nonspecific. Specific ECG abnormalities include tachycardia, right axis deviation, right heart strain, ST-T–wave changes, or right bundle branch block. The classic S_1-Q_3-T_3 pattern is rarely seen, but suggestive of PE. A CXR should be obtained; it is abnormal in two-thirds of cases, usually with nonspecific findings that are not diagnostic of PE. The most commonly noted abnormal radiographic findings of PE are atelectasis, effusions, and focal infiltrates. Two characteristic radiographic findings of PE are uncommon: a localized area of hypoperfusion (Westermark sign) and a peripheral wedge-shaped density above the diaphragm (Hampton hump). Doppler US should be performed to evaluate for deep vein thrombosis; in the appropriate clinical setting, a positive duplex indirectly corroborates with the presence of a PE. Echocardiography may be used to evaluate signs of right heart strain but is a late finding. Although scan was the historical diagnostic imaging standard, CT angiography (CTA) has become the test of choice and criterion standard for diagnosis of PE because of its relative ease and availability, speed, and ability to evaluate nonvascular structures. Despite relatively strong performance characteristics, CTA is less sensitive for emboli beyond the main, lobar, or segmental pulmonary arteries. Therefore, in a patient at high risk, a negative CTA cannot definitely rule out a PE.

Provide respiratory support, definitive airway management including endotracheal intubation, and ventilation as needed for respiratory compromise. Patients with vital sign instability and hypotension refractory to fluid therapy may require pressor support. In the setting of cardiopulmonary instability, thrombolytic therapy (eg, tissue plasminogen activator) may be considered, although it has not been specifically evaluated in pediatric patients and there is risk of causing life-threatening bleeding. Optimize precipitating factors such as infection, trauma, and heart failure. Admit patients with PE to the ICU for oxygen therapy for hypoxemia and anticoagulation therapy, including unfractionated or low-molecular-weight heparin (LMWH). LMWH is advantageous due to its predictable dosing and minimal need for monitoring.

Pearls

1. Physical exam and laboratory testing are usually nonspecific, and PE diagnosis is usually made by CTA. In high-risk patients with concerning symptoms, a negative CTA cannot definitely rule out a PE due to limitations in imaging the distal arteries.

2. D-dimer is not specific for PE and has not been extensively evaluated in children. A negative D-dimer in a patient who is *not* considered low risk does not rule out PE, and imaging must be pursued.

3. Management of PE in the ED includes supportive respiratory and circulatory care and initiation of anticoagulation to prevent progression of thrombus.

Chapter 7

DERMATOLOGY

Sharon A. Glick
Jeannette Jakus
Julie Cantatore-Francis
Kunal M. Shah

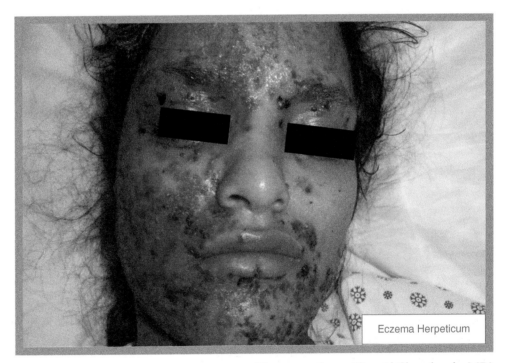

Eczema Herpeticum

(Photo contributor: Haamid Chamdawala, MD)

The authors acknowledge the special contributions of Falguni Asrani, MD, to prior edition.

293

Clinical Features

Urticaria, or hives, are pruritic raised erythematous superficial skin wheals that arise in response to histamine, leukotrienes, prostaglandins, and other substances released by stimulated mast cells. Lesions develop and resolve quickly; individual lesions should resolve in <24 hours. Urticaria is often associated with hypersensitivity reactions, including anaphylaxis. Triggers can include allergic reactions to drugs, foods, insect stings, and rarely aeroallergens. The 2017 guidelines by the National Institute of Allergy and Infectious Diseases recommend introducing all foods including highly allergenic foods such as peanuts, tree nuts, milk, egg, wheat, soy, and shellfish between 5 and 12 months of age, which may result in younger presentations of patient with acute urticaria from

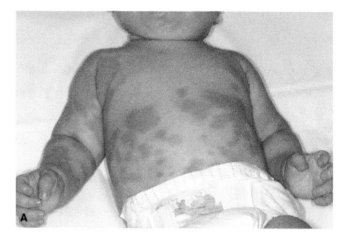

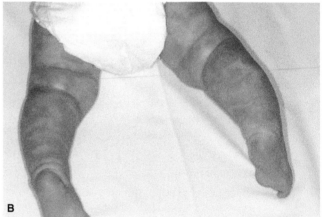

FIGURE 7.2 ■ Acute Urticaria. (**A, B**) An infant with acute urticaria. Etiology of lesions often is undetermined. (Photo contributor: Dawn Davis, MD.)

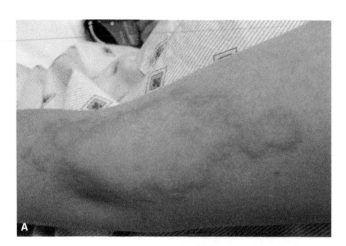

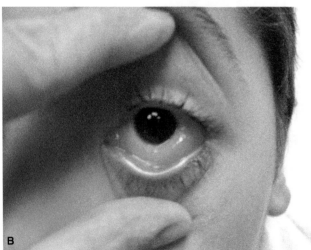

FIGURE 7.1 ■ Acute Urticaria with Chemosis; Anaphylaxis. Erythematous, serpiginous lesions with well-demarcated edges (**A**) and conjunctival edema (**B**) associated with wheezing were seen in this patient. (Photo contributor: Ee Tay, MD.)

food. Infections including hepatitis, Epstein-Barr virus, Lyme disease, *Helicobacter pylori*, helminths, and fungi have been associated with urticaria. In areas where the lone star tick is endemic, there are growing cases of delayed anaphylaxis after ingesting mammalian meat. The reactions can occur up to 48 hours after ingestion from an antibody to alpha-gal, which is a carbohydrate on mammalian meat. Chronic urticaria is when the patient has had symptoms for over 6 weeks. Chronic urticaria can also be caused by physical stimuli including cold, heat, or exercise (cholinergic), pressure, vibration, and sun exposure. Patients with collagen vascular and autoimmune diseases often present with urticaria. Differential diagnosis includes mastocytosis/urticaria pigmentosa (UP), erythema multiforme (EM), bullous skin disorders, or dermatitis herpetiformis. Obtaining a detailed history can help identify an etiology. Urticaria that has been occurring for <6 weeks rarely requires any laboratory workup. Obtaining

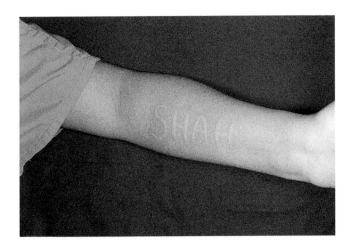

FIGURE 7.3 ■ Dermographism. This "rash" was produced within 3 minutes of stroking the skin with a tongue blade. Dermographism (ability to write on the skin) is an example of physical urticaria. Triggering factors may include contact with clothing, towels, or sheets. It can also occur as an isolated disorder. Linear pruritic wheals appear on skin within 2 to 5 minutes of stroking and usually resolve within 30 minutes to 3 hours. Most patients are without any systemic symptoms. (Photo contributor: Binita R. Shah, MD.)

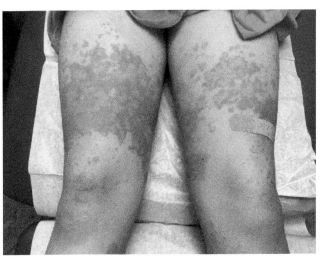

FIGURE 7.4 ■ Urticaria Multiforme. A child with transient, pruritic, polycyclic lesions on the legs (many with dusky centers) after treatment for molluscum contagiosum lesions (pox virus) with cantharidin. Urticaria multiforme is a subtype of annular urticaria and often gets confused with erythema multiforme (see Figures 7.8 to 7.9). (Photo contributor: Julie Cantatore-Francis, MD.)

specific immunoglobulin (Ig) E levels in an acute setting can reflect a falsely negative result. Laboratory tests may be done as indicated for chronic urticaria. Helminth infections and allergies would be associated with eosinophilia.

Emergency Department Treatment and Disposition

Attempt to identify the trigger based on a thorough history. Advise patients to discontinue or avoid the offending agent, if known. Treatment of urticaria includes oral and sometimes parentally administered H$_1$ blockers (eg, diphenhydramine). Second-generation antihistamines (eg, cetirizine) can be used once or twice a day until symptoms resolve. H$_2$ blockers (eg, cimetidine, ranitidine) may be combined with H$_1$ blockers. For patients with severe urticaria, interventions may include epinephrine given subcutaneously, corticosteroids given IV

as hydrocortisone or methylprednisolone, or oral prednisone given first as a bolus followed by a once-daily dose. Suspected anaphylaxis should be treated accordingly (see Figures 18.10 to 18.12). Patients should be educated and sent home with injectable epinephrine. Urticaria can be very frustrating for the patient, and referral to an allergist can often help with management and investigation for the trigger.

Pearls

1. Urticaria is characterized by erythematous, edematous lesions that are pruritic and evanescent.
2. If the lesions last longer than 24 hours or are painful rather than pruritic, refer the patient for skin biopsy to rule out urticarial vasculitis.
3. The underlying cause for chronic urticaria is rarely found.

ANGIOEDEMA

Clinical Features

Angioedema is a swelling of the deeper dermal subcutaneous tissue. Commonly affected areas include the extremities and face, specifically lips and tongue. Airway involvement may occur and is life threatening. It is often painful rather than pruritic. Angioedema occurs secondary to release of various mediators including histamine, leukotrienes, and prostaglandins from stimulated mast cells or abnormalities in the complement or arachidonic acid pathways. Angioedema, like urticaria, is often associated with hypersensitivity reactions, including anaphylaxis. Chronic angioedema is defined by symptoms that last longer than 6 weeks. Acute triggers may include allergic reactions to drugs, foods, and insect stings. Certain medications including angiotensin-converting enzyme (ACE) inhibitors and angiotensin II receptor blockers (ARBs) often cause a non–IgE-mediated reaction manifesting as angioedema even if the patient has been on that medication for many years, and the symptoms may recur 6 to 8 weeks after discontinuation. Some patients who react to ACE inhibitors do not develop symptoms on ARBs, but most patients have modest risk of angioedema recurrence on ARBs. Hereditary angioedema presents as spontaneous recurrent attacks of angioedema often triggered by trauma. There are 3 genetic types, and the most common is inherited in an autosomal dominant fashion; however, many patients have spontaneous mutations. This disorder is characterized by abnormal levels or function of C1 esterase inhibitor. Patients often present with initial attacks around puberty, and many have isolated visceral angioedema that mimics an acute abdomen. Patients often report a prodrome followed by episodes of swelling worsening over a period of 12 to 24 hours, usually with resolution within 3 to 5 days. Edematous lesions are migratory, transient and usually unresponsive to antihistamines. Attacks are usually periodic and are commonly followed by weeks of remission. Laboratory screening is accomplished by obtaining a C4 level that is low during attacks. Further testing with C1 esterase inhibitor level or functional C1 esterase inhibitor assays can be used for confirmatory diagnosis if initial C4 screen is low.

Emergency Department Treatment and Disposition

Anaphylaxis should be treated emergently (see Figures 18.10 to 18.12). For hereditary angioedema, treatment includes supportive care and pain management. Patients presenting with breathing difficulty due to laryngeal swelling may need elective intubation. Epinephrine, corticosteroids, and antihistamines usually do not help patients. Fresh frozen plasma helps in some cases, but exacerbates the condition in others. Refer the patient to an allergist for continuity of care and management. Long-term treatments including synthetic androgen steroids (eg, danazol, stanozolol) may be considered in older children after careful consideration of the risks versus benefits. C1 esterase inhibitor concentrates, plasma kallikrein inhibitors, and bradykinin B2 receptor antagonists are safe and effective.

Pearls

1. Patients with hereditary angioedema usually do not develop urticaria.
2. Family history is important when considering hereditary angioedema.
3. Children with hereditary angioedema may present with severe abdominal pain mimicking acute abdomen and often undergo unnecessary evaluations and sometimes unindicated operative interventions.

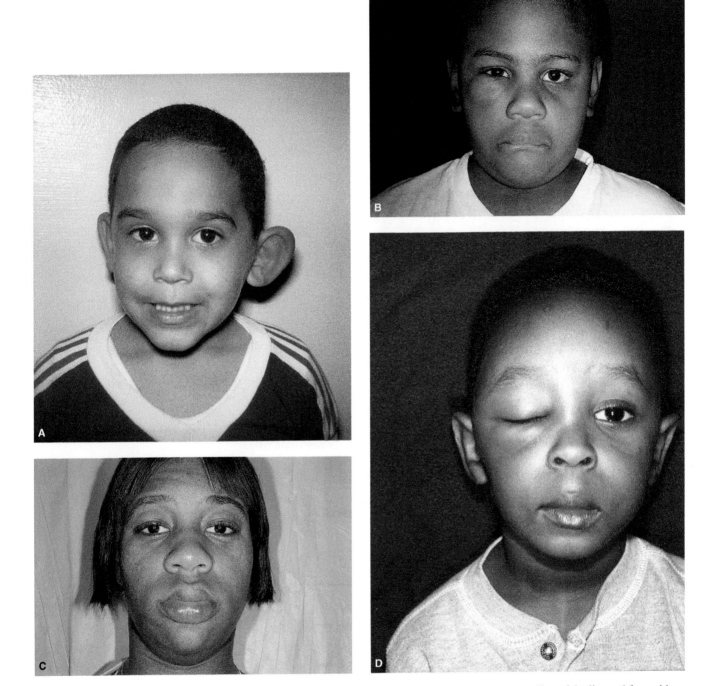

FIGURE 7.5 ■ Angioedema. Swelling of the ear and periorbital area following mosquito bites (**A, B**), swelling of the lips and face with an urticarial rash following ingestion of shellfish (**C**), and swelling of the upper and lower eyelids with facial swelling following ingestion of peanuts (**D**) were the presenting complaints of these children. Angioedema usually involves the loose connective tissues of the ear or the periorbital or perioral areas but may involve the oropharynx or extremities. The edema is nonpitting, well-circumscribed, and usually nonpruritic (unless coexisting with urticaria). (Photo contributor: Binita R. Shah, MD.)

Clinical Summary

Serum sickness is an immune complex–mediated type III hypersensitivity reaction, produced by exposure to a variety of agents. It is characterized by fever, joint involvement, skin rash, lymphadenopathy, splenomegaly, arthralgia, and proteinuria. The classic serum sickness is rarely seen nowadays and can be caused by blood products (eg, human γ-globulin)

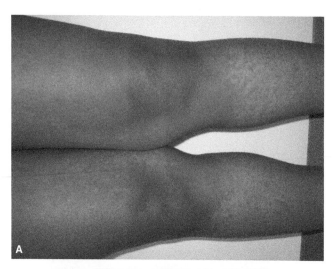

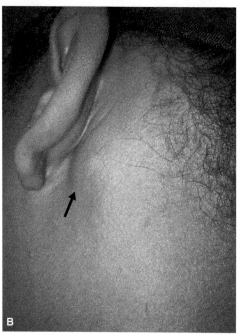

FIGURE 7.6 ■ Serum Sickness–Like Reaction. (A) Erythematous maculopapular and urticarial edematous plaques are seen on the thighs in a patient 2 weeks after receiving Bactrim. (B) Fever, arthralgia, and generalized lymphadenopathy (arrow) were other findings. Patient improved with stoppage of Bactrim and supportive care. (Photo contributor: Erin Gilbert, MD, PhD.)

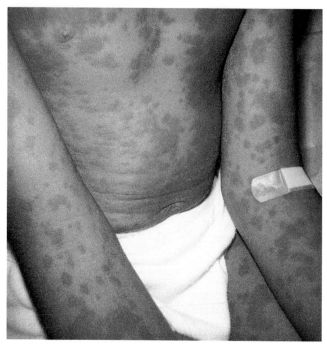

FIGURE 7.7 ■ Serum Sickness–Like Reaction. Morbilliform eruption, swollen, tender knees, elevated ESR, thrombocytopenia, and mild proteinuria were the findings in this patient while receiving cefaclor for 8 days for a sinus infection. Urticarial wheals are the most common type of rash seen with serum sickness–like reaction followed by erythema multiforme–like lesions. (Photo contributor: Binita R. Shah, MD.)

and animal-derived serum (eg, antitoxins for treatment of spider and snake envenomations [eg, Crotalidae antivenin], antitoxins for clostridial intoxication [eg, botulism, gas gangrene], and antirabies serum). Diagnosis is suspected based on history of an exposure to a foreign antigen.

Serum sickness–like reaction (SSLR) is a drug reaction that can be seen 1 to 3 weeks after exposure to the etiologic agent. The mechanism of this reaction is not well understood. The most commonly associated medication in children is cefaclor. Other medications have been implicated, including penicillins, cephalosporins, sulfa drugs, minocycline, propranolol, bupropion, and griseofulvin. Cutaneous morphology can be urticarial, morbilliform, or erythema multiforme–like. Other features are joint swellings, arthralgia, fever, and lymphadenopathy. Unlike classic serum sickness, frank arthritis and hepatic, renal, and CNS involvement are rarely seen. Skin biopsy is not necessary to make the diagnosis. Differential diagnosis includes urticaria, urticarial multiforme (UM), erythema multiforme (EM), vasculitis, and drug reactions. (See Table 7.1 for comparison of UM, EM, and SSLR).

TABLE 7.1 ■ COMPARISON OF FINDINGS FOR URTICARIA MULTIFORME (UM), ERYTHEMA MULTIFORME (EM), AND SERUM SICKNESS–LIKE REACTIONS (SSLR)

Findings	UM	EM	SSLR
Clinical eruption	Transient polycyclic/annular plaques with dusky/clear centers	Fixed target lesions with dusky/violaceous center; may blister	Fixed polycyclic/annular plaques with dusky/clear centers
Mucosal membrane involvement	No	Yes; in EM major	No
Etiology	Infection Antibiotics Immunizations	Herpes virus (most common) Other infections Rarely antibiotics	Antibiotics
Fever	Possible, mild	Possible, mild	Yes, high
Dermatographism	Yes	No	No
Appearance	Well	Well or toxic	Toxic
Facial/acral edema	Yes	No	Yes
Associated symptoms	Pruritus	Pruritis, burning, or skin tenderness	Myalgias, arthralgias, lymphadenopathy

Emergency Department Treatment and Disposition

The majority of SSLRs are self-limited and resolve in 2 to 3 weeks without sequelae in most cases. Patients can be managed by discontinuation of the offending agent (if still receiving it), antihistamines, and NSAIDs as indicated. A short course of systemic corticosteroids may be used in severe cases of arthralgias and myalgias.

Pearls

1. Drugs are the most common cause of SSLR, especially the cephalosporin cefaclor.
2. Typical cutaneous reactions seen in SSLR are urticarial, morbilliform, or erythema multiforme–like eruptions.

URTICARIA MULTIFORME

Clinical Summary

The term *urticaria multiforme* (UM) has been proposed to replace acute annular urticaria (a subtype of acute urticaria) and refers to a benign cutaneous hypersensitivity reaction. UM primarily affects infants and preschool-age children but can be present in young adults and teenagers as well.

Potential triggers include a preceding infection (such as an URI, otitis media, or other viral syndrome), prior antibiotic usage, and recent immunization.

Clinically, UM is characterized by the acute onset of transient, small urticarial macules, papules, or plaques that rapidly expand to large, polycyclic, arcuate and/or annular wheals with central clearing or dusky centers. It can present anywhere on the body including trunk, extremities, and face. Other associated findings include pruritis (very common), facial or acral angioedema, dermatographism, and/or fever.

Diagnosis of UM is usually made clinically. Laboratory testing may show either normal or elevated acute phase reactants. A skin biopsy (not necessary) would show urticaria. UM can frequently be mistaken for other annular skin disorders such as erythema multiforme and SSLRs, but a thorough clinical history and physical examination can differentiate these conditions.

Emergency Department Treatment and Disposition

Reassure patients and their families that this is a self-limited condition which typically resolves within 2 to 12 days. Favorable response occurs to antihistamines within 24 to 48 hours. Treatment includes discontinuation of any antibiotic medication, systemic H_1 (nonsedating in morning such as cetirizine and sedating in evening such as diphenhydramine or hydroxyzine) and H_2 antihistamines, and rarely systemic corticosteroids.

Pearls

1. Duration of individual lesions in UM is <24 hours.
2. Although lesions may have dusky/ecchymotic centers, there is no skin necrosis, blistering, mucous membrane involvement, arthralgias, or arthritis.

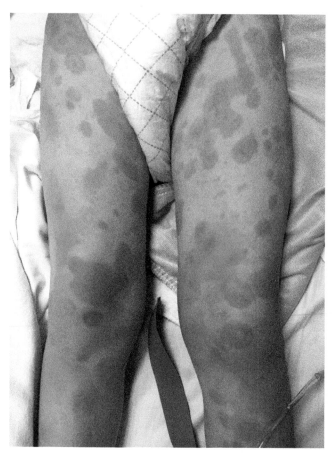

FIGURE 7.8 ■ Urticaria Multiforme. Annular and polycyclic wheals with dusky centers are seen on the lower extremities in this 5-year-old boy who also had periorbital swelling and mild edema of hands and feet. (Photo contributor: Sharon A. Glick, MD.)

3. Systemic symptoms are minimal, and children are non-toxic in appearance.
4. Favorable response to antihistamines should occur within 24 to 48 hours.
5. The patient will often exhibit pruritus and dermatographism.

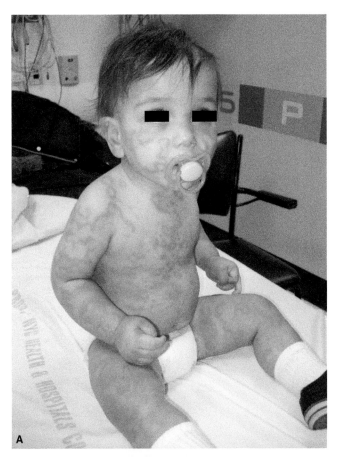

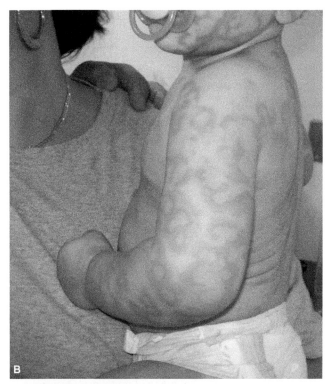

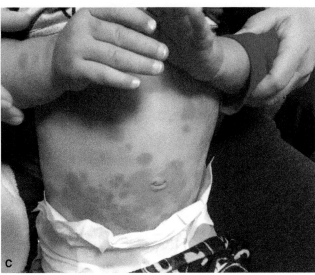

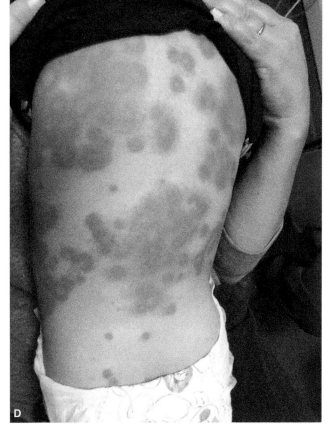

FIGURE 7.9 ▪ Urticaria Multiforme. (**A, B**) Annular and serpiginous urticarial lesions some with dusky centers are seen in this toddler following a viral infection. He also had edema of the hands. This is a subtype of annular urticaria and his rash resolved in <24 hours. (**C, D**) Similar annular and serpiginous urticarial lesions, some with dusky centers, are seen in another toddler associated with edema of the hands. (Photo contributors: Mark Silverberg, MD [A, B], and Yvonne P. Giunta, MD [C, D].)

ERYTHEMA MULTIFORME

Clinical Summary

Erythema multiforme (EM) is an acute hypersensitivity reaction that occurs in response to various etiologic agents such as infections, especially herpes simplex virus (HSV) type 1 and 2, and rarely drugs. It is self-limited but potentially recurring. HSV is the most common cause; others include *Mycoplasma*, *Parapoxvirus*, and *Histoplasma*. Recently, *Mycoplasma pneumoniae*–induced rash and mucositis (MIRM) has been described and is characterized by prominent mucositis involving >1 mucous membrane with sparse to no cutaneous involvement. There is overlap between this entity and EM secondary to *M pneumoniae*. EM is classified into minor and major types, which can be distinguished by the presence or absence of mucosal lesions. EM minor has no or mild mucosal involvement versus EM major, which has severe involvement of 1 mucosal surface. The classic EM lesion is a target "iris" lesion characterized by 3 zones. The innermost zone consists of dusky purpura, hemorrhagic crust, or blistering; the middle zone, the largest, is pale pink and edematous, whereas the outermost zone is composed of a ring of erythema. Occasionally, atypical targetoid (composed of 2 zones only) papular lesions can be present. The classic distribution of EM lesions is symmetric, involving extremities (especially elbow, knees, wrists, and hands), palms, and soles, with few truncal lesions and tends to be fixed for >5 days.

Systemic symptoms are mild or absent. Active HSV lesions or a past history of herpes may be positive. Differential diagnosis of EM includes urticarial multiforme and urticaria (lesions transient), drug eruptions, subacute lupus erythematosus, and vasculitis. If diagnosis is unclear, dermatology consult followed by skin biopsy is indicated.

Emergency Department Treatment and Disposition

No specific therapy is required for EM minor, which is a self-limited disorder. Acyclovir may be given if active HSV lesions are present. Antihistamines, antipyretics, and topical steroids (eg, desonide cream twice a day) can be given for symptomatic relief. Typical patients with EM minor are usually not severely ill and can be managed as outpatients

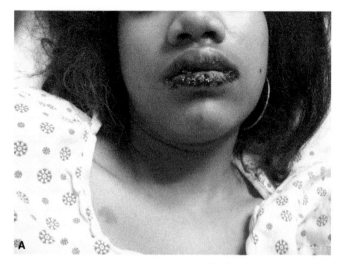

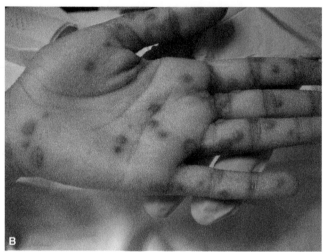

FIGURE 7.10 ■ Herpes Simplex Virus (HSV) Infection and Erythema Multiforme. (**A**) A 15-year-old girl with culture-proven HSV labialis. Her lips have coalescing vesicles with overlying crusts. (**B**) Her palm showing classic iris or target lesions. Note the 3 concentric zones with central necrosis surrounded by a zone of edema and a third surrounding ring of erythema. She also had similar lesions on her soles. (Photo contributor: Sharon A. Glick, MD.)

with follow-up with a primary care provider. Systemic steroids may be considered for severe cases of EM major (eg, prednisone 1–2 mg/kg/day divided once or twice daily for 5–14 days). Prophylactic oral acyclovir can be used for recurrent HSV-induced EM. Prompt treatment of HSV infections in such patients will prevent EM. In cases associated with *M pneumoniae*, the underlying infection should be treated.

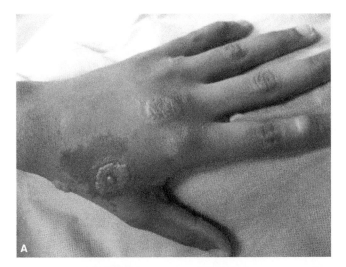

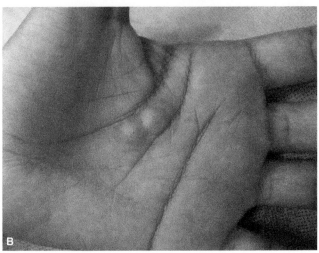

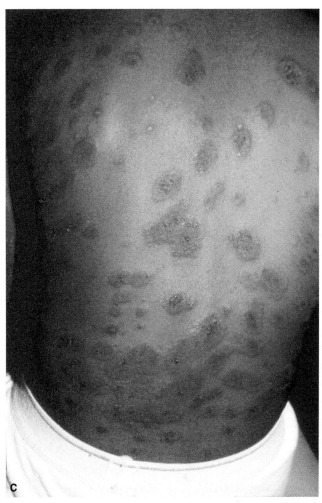

FIGURE 7.11 ■ Erythema Multiforme (EM): Target or "Iris" Lesions. (**A, B**) Bullous EM (a variant of EM) showing "iris" lesions on the hand and palm. (**C**) Classic "iris" lesions of EM in a different patient following herpes simplex virus infection. (Photo contributors: Jeanine Daly, MD [A, B], and [C] reproduced with permission from Shah BR, Laude TL. *Atlas of Pediatric Clinical Diagnosis.* WB Saunders; Philadelphia, PA, 2000.)

Pearls

1. EM is a separate entity from Stevens-Johnson syndrome (SJS) and toxic epidermal necrolysis (TEN). EM does not progress to SJS or TEN.

2. EM is most commonly confused with urticaria multiforme. Skin lesions of urticaria multiforme are transient, lasting <24 hours.

3. EM lesions are fixed, and although lesions may expand, they remain on the same body part for 5 to 7 days.

4. Target or "iris" (with 3 concentric zones) lesions are pathognomonic of EM; however, some of the lesions may be targetoid (with 2 zones) or papular lesions.

5. EM lesions classically are distributed mainly on the extremities including palms and soles, with either none or only 1 mucosal surface involved.

6. Patients with HSV-associated EM may develop target lesions on the lips associated with lip necrosis that can mimic SJS.

7. Patients with MIRM may have multiple mucosal surface involvement.

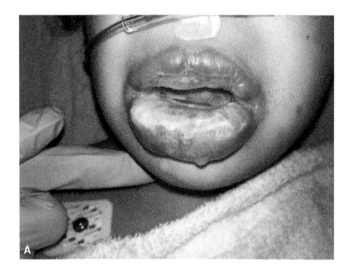

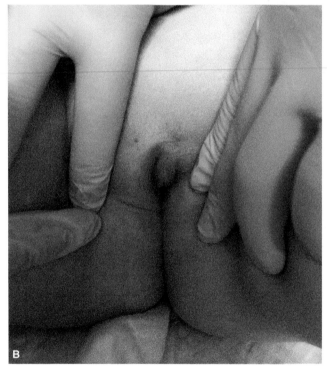

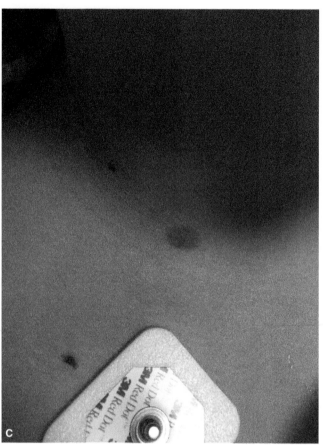

FIGURE 7.12 ■ *Mycoplasma pneumoniae*–Induced Rash and Mucositis (MIRM; see also Figure 7.15). An 8-year-old girl presented to ED with mucositis of lips and oral mucosa (**A**) and erythema of the labia majora and minora (**B**). Note the sparse targetoid eruption on the neck (**C**). She was diagnosed with *M pneumoniae* (positive IgM titers) and treated with azithromycin and supportive care with a full recovery within a week. (Photo contributor: Sharon A. Glick, MD.)

Clinical Summary

Stevens-Johnson syndrome (SJS) and toxic epidermal necrolysis (TEN) are part of a spectrum of hypersensitivity disorders with similar etiologies (most commonly drugs) and can be severe and life threatening. Historically, *M pneumoniae* has been considered an etiology of SJS and typically presents in children and adolescents with mucosal involvement and sparse skin lesions with a less severe prognosis. Recently, this entity has been reclassified as MIRM and is discussed under erythema multiforme (EM). Both SJS and TEN may have severe mucosal involvement as well as epidermal denudation. Depending on area of epidermal denudation, a 3-grade classification has been proposed: SJS (<10% body surface area [BSA]), overlap SJS-TEN (10%–30% BSA), and TEN (>30% BSA). A positive Nikolsky sign is present in both SJS and TEN. Mucosal surfaces of eyes, oral cavity, upper gastrointestinal tract, respiratory tract, and genitals may show blisters, hemorrhagic crusts, painful erosions, and ulcerations.

Most commonly implicated drugs are NSAIDs, antibiotics (penicillins, sulfonamides), and antiepileptics (phenytoin, carbamazepine). The incubation period is usually 7 to 21 days with the initial drug exposure, and prodromal symptoms and mucosal surface involvement may occur before rash and epidermal detachment begins. Clinical features include fever, malaise, upper respiratory tract symptoms, skin pain, and mucocutaneous lesions. The cutaneous lesions may appear targetoid with 2 zones of color characterized by purpura and a tendency to coalesce, with truncal and central distribution. This is distinct from EM, which is characterized by 3 zones and acrofacial distribution. Diagnosis of SJS or TEN is usually made clinically. Leukocytosis, elevated erythrocyte sedimentation rate (ESR), and liver enzyme abnormalities may be present. Frozen section biopsy of skin should be performed for confirmation of diagnosis. Hematoxylin and eosin staining of frozen section of exfoliating skin will show a full-thickness epidermal necrosis.

Complications include secondary bacterial infection, fluid and electrolyte imbalances, and scarring and strictures of the skin and mucosal surfaces. Ocular sequelae include symblepharon, corneal ulceration, and blindness. The course is protracted over 3 to 6 weeks with a mortality rate ranging from 1% to 5% for SJS and 15% to 35% for TEN.

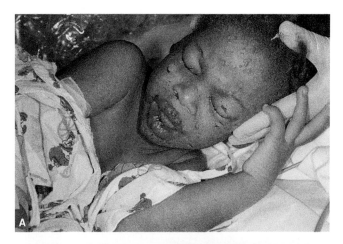

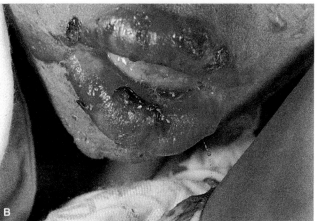

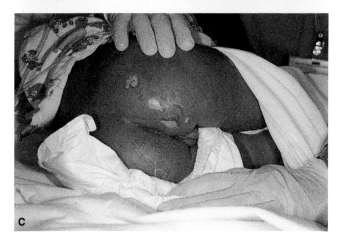

FIGURE 7.13 ■ Stevens-Johnson Syndrome. (**A**) A 7-year-old girl presented with this rash while receiving penicillin (8th day) for pharyngitis. Nikolsky sign was positive with peeling of the epidermis (seen on the face) with minimal pressure. (**B**) Close-up of erosive stomatitis with hemorrhagic-crusted erosions of lips. Erosions were also present on the buccal mucosa, palate, posterior pharynx, and conjunctiva. (**C**) Erythematous and purpuric macules are seen on the back with blistering leading to erosions on the buttocks. Less than 10% of the body surface area was involved. (Photo contributor: Binita R. Shah, MD.)

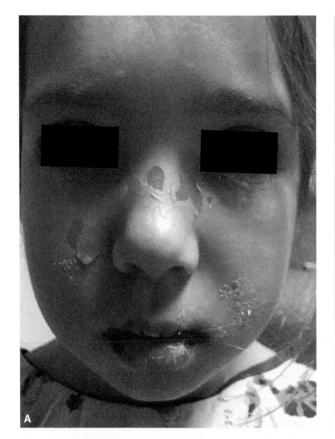

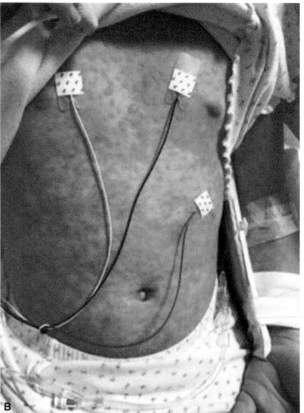

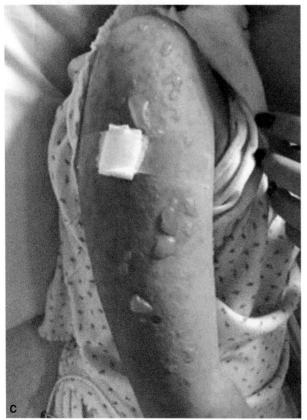

FIGURE 7.14 ■ Stevens-Johnson Syndrome (SJS)/Toxic Epidermal Necrolysis (TEN) Overlap. This 7-year-old girl was started on lamotrigine (Lamictal) 14 days prior to this rash. (**A**) Ruptured bullae are seen on the face with involvement of the oral mucosa. (**B**) Numerous dusky lesions with coalescing flaccid bullae are also seen on the trunk. (**C**) Arm of the same patient with multiple bullae. She had >10% but <30% total body surface involvement, meeting the criteria for SJS/TEN overlap. (Photo contributor: Sharon A. Glick, MD.)

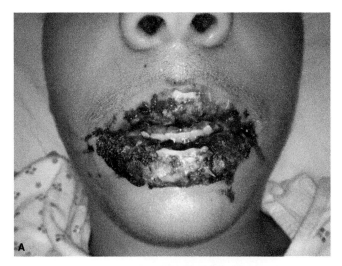

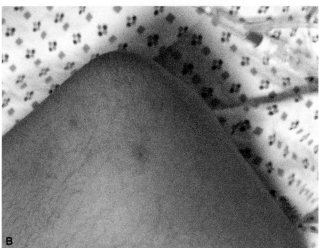

FIGURE 7.15 ■ *Mycoplasma pneumoniae*–Induced Rash and Mucositis (MIRM; see also Figure 7.12). (**A**) Mucous membrane involvement with swelling and severe hemorrhagic and serous crusting of lips. The patient also had conjunctival injection. (**B**) Sparse target lesions on the patient's arm. There were no other cutaneous lesions. Patient was treated with azithromycin and supportive care. (Photo contributor: Sharon A. Glick, MD.)

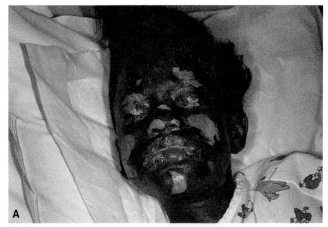

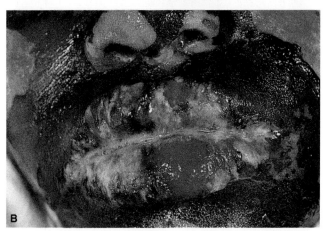

FIGURE 7.16 ■ Toxic Epidermal Necrolysis. Five-year-old girl presented with this rash (100% body surface area involvement) while receiving trimethoprim-sulfamethoxazole (10th day) for a UTI (photographs taken on seventh day of illness). (**A**) Extensive involvement of the face with necrotic skin is seen. (**B**) Close-up of mucosal involvement of the lips showing painful hemorrhagic erosions. (Photo contributor: Binita R. Shah, MD.)

Emergency Department Treatment and Disposition

Hospitalize all patients with suspected diagnosis of SJS or TEN preferably to a burn unit or ICU. Discontinue all drugs introduced within the past month, and do not introduce drugs of a similar class unless the risk of abrupt discontinuation is too high. For example, phenobarbital, carbamazepine, and phenytoin share a common metabolic pathway (cytochrome P450) and may induce a cross-reaction; thus, all 3 drugs are contraindicated after SJS or TEN resulting from any one of them. Obtain urgent dermatology, ophthalmology, urology, and otorhinolaryngology consultations. Supportive care includes management of fluid and electrolytes, pain, thermoregulation, nutritional support, and meticulous skin care (gentle saline soaks and petrolatum gauze to provide barrier over denuded areas). Do not use silver sulfadiazine in patients with sulfonamide-induced SJS or TEN. Provide reverse isolation to prevent secondary bacterial infection. Prophylactic use of systemic antibiotics is not recommended. Systemic corticosteroid use is controversial; there is a risk of increased morbidity and mortality, and hence, routine use is discouraged. Therapy includes IV immunoglobulin (IVIG) given as 1 g/kg/day for 3 days. It helps to reduce development of new

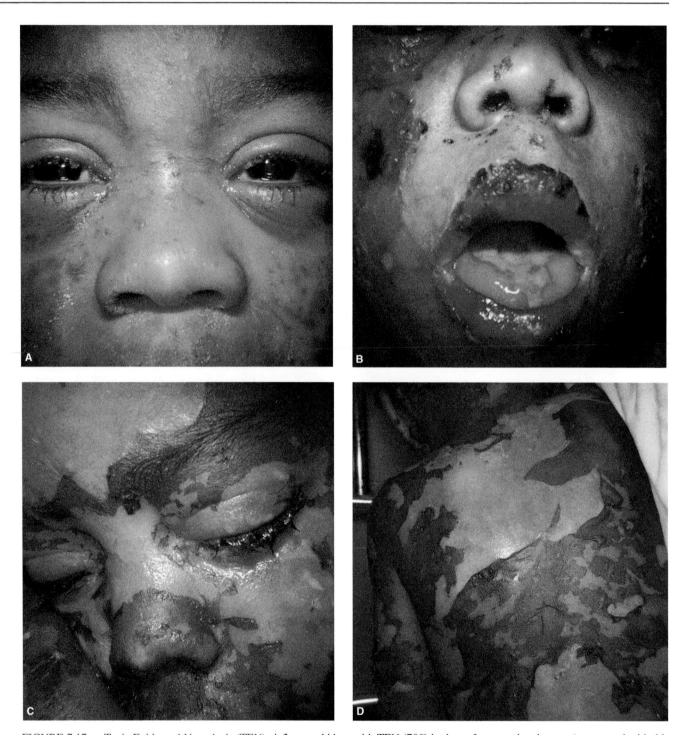

FIGURE 7.17 ■ Toxic Epidermal Necrolysis (TEN). A 3-year-old boy with TEN (70% body surface area involvement) presented with this rash a week after taking phenobarbital for recurrent febrile seizures (photographs taken between second and third day of illness). (**A**) Bilateral eye involvement with mucopurulent discharge. (**B**) Erosive stomatitis and hemorrhagic crusted erosions of the lips. (**C, D**) Abrupt onset and worsening within 24 hours with dark necrotic skin peeling off, leaving a raw dermis were noted. (Photo contributor: Binita R. Shah, MD.)

blisters and helps to arrest disease progression. (IVIG should be free of any IgA to prevent hypersensitivity reaction in IgA-deficient individuals.) Other systemic medications showing efficacy include cyclosporine, infliximab, and etanercept.

Pearls

1. Most common etiology for SJS and TEN are drugs, whereas most common etiology for EM is infectious, with HSV being the most common.
2. In children, SJS is more commonly seen than TEN. Incidence of TEN is more common in HIV patients.
3. Differential diagnosis of SJS or TEN includes staphylococcal scalded skin syndrome (SSSS). TEN is full-thickness epidermal necrosis and denudation, whereas SSSS is a superficial peeling of skin (within the epidermis, below the stratum corneum). Differential diagnosis also includes MIRM, EM, acute generalized exanthematous pustulosis, lupus erythematosus, drug reaction with eosinophils and systemic reaction, and autoimmune blistering disorders.
4. Both SJS and TEN are potentially life-threatening diseases because of multisystem involvement.

Clinical Summary

Adverse drug eruptions generally occur 7 to 21 days after starting a new medication, whereas it takes only a few days for the reaction to occur following second exposure to the same class of medication. The most commonly implicated drugs in exanthematous (maculopapular or morbilliform) eruptions are antibiotics (eg, penicillins, sulfonamides), antiepileptics (eg, phenytoin), NSAIDs, antihypertensives, and anti-HIV medications, although any drug can cause an adverse reaction. Cross-reactivity is common among different drugs of the same class of medications. Drug reactions are more common in HIV-positive individuals. Exanthematous reaction is seen most commonly and has a widespread, bilateral, and symmetric distribution that may involve palms and soles. Fever, malaise, and mild mucosal surface involvement may be presenting symptoms. In a variant known as drug reaction with eosinophilia and systemic symptoms (DRESS), also known as drug-induced hypersensitivity syndrome, the exanthematous drug rash is associated with fever, facial edema, and involvement of at least 1 internal organ with eosinophilia. The incubation period of DRESS is usually 2 to 6 weeks, and it takes weeks to subside, even after drug withdrawal. Another variant is acute generalized exanthematous pustulosis, which is an acute eruption characterized by multiple tiny pustules that heal in 4 to 10 days with desquamation. This is considered an adverse eruption to medications or vaccine administration. Differential diagnosis of drug reactions includes viral exanthems. Eosinophilia is more common in drug eruption than viral exanthems.

Emergency Department Treatment and Disposition

The diagnosis is clinical, and a detailed current and previous drug history with time charting is mandatory to pinpoint the offending drug. If clinical suspicion of an adverse drug reaction is high, discontinue the suspected offending drug. Laboratory tests include CBC, liver enzymes, and urinalysis. Hospitalize children with severe skin findings, evidence of systemic involvement, or inability to maintain hydration (eg, during erythrodermic phase). A dermatology consultation would assist in such decisions. Treatment for morbilliform rashes is mostly supportive and includes skin care (eg, topical steroids to alleviate symptoms) and prevention of infection. Oral or IV steroids are sometimes used in patients with severe systemic involvement and in DRESS to prevent complications.

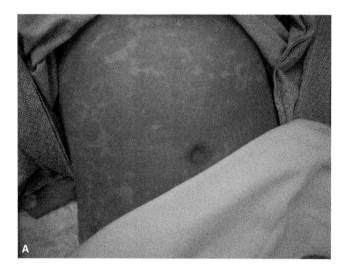 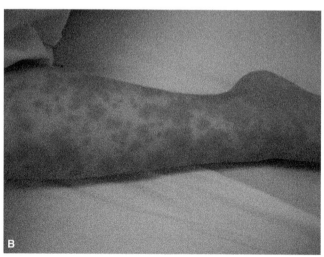

FIGURE 7.18 ■ Drug Rash. (**A, B**) Morbilliform maculopapular drug hypersensitivity reaction seen over the trunk and leg in a child following exposure to azithromycin. The rash improved after stoppage of the drug and supportive management. No mucosa was involved. (Photo contributor: Julie Cantatore-Francis, MD.)

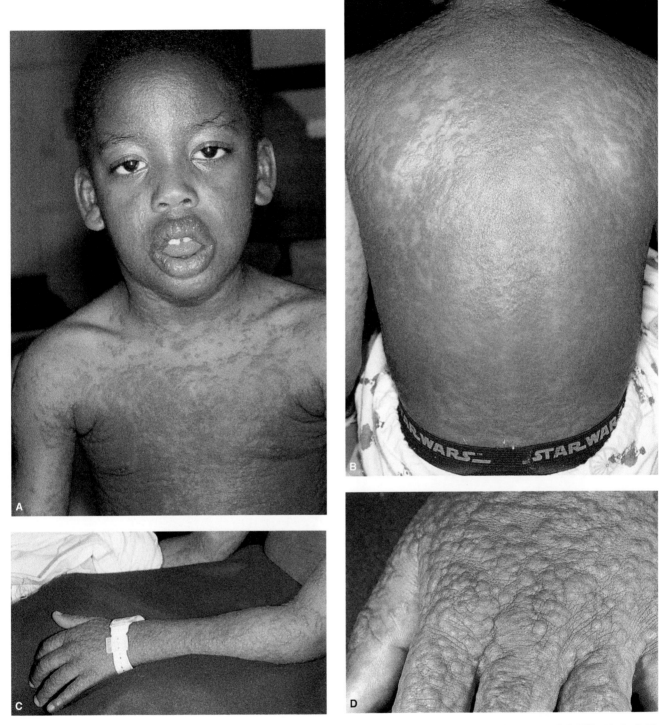

FIGURE 7.19 ■ Drug-Induced Hypersensitivity Syndrome/Drug Reaction with Eosinophilia and Systemic Symptoms (DRESS). (**A, B, C, D**) This child presented with an extensive rash 35 days after starting phenytoin for seizure disorder. He also had fever, facial edema, lymphadenopathy, and elevated liver enzymes requiring hospitalization. He was treated with a slow taper of oral steroids. Monomorphous extensive papular lesions are seen on the face, trunk, both legs, and arms. Mucous membrane involvement in patients with DRESS is either minimal or absent. (**D**) Close-up of his hand shows indurated nature of the rash. (Photo contributor: Binita R. Shah, MD.)

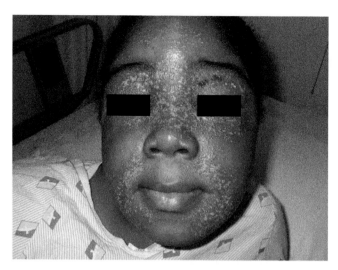

FIGURE 7.20 ■ Acute Generalized Exanthematous Pustulosis. This girl presented with fever and an acute eruption of multiple sterile pustules all over the face, extremities, and trunk following exposure to an antibiotic 2 weeks prior. The lesions healed with desquamation following stoppage of the antibiotic. (Photo contributor: Sharon A. Glick, MD.)

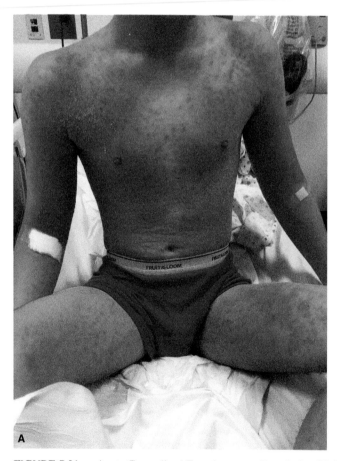

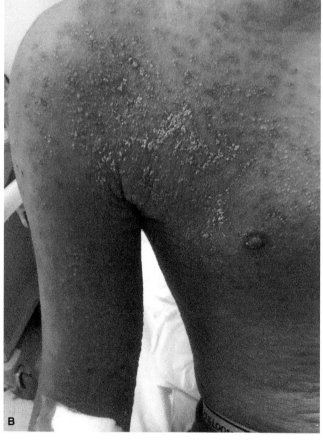

FIGURE 7.21 ■ Acute Generalized Exanthematous Pustulosis. (**A**) An adolescent boy with erythematous papules overlying erythema and coalescing into plaques on chest, abdomen, arms, and thighs. (**B**) Close-up of nonfollicular papulopustules on an erythematous base, some with superficial detachment from epidermis.

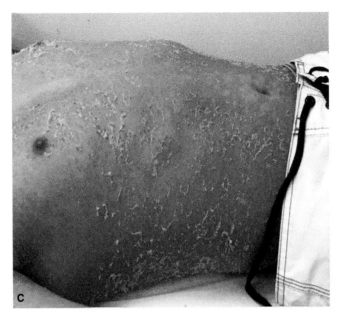

FIGURE 7.21 ■ *(Continued)* (**C**) Several days later, after treatment with topical steroid, patient is healing with desquamation. (Photo contributors: Praneetha Chaganti, MD [A, B], and Sharon A. Glick, MD [C].)

Pearls

1. Exanthematous drug reaction is often misdiagnosed as a viral infection.

2. Prompt recognition and discontinuation of the drug in all types of drug rashes are of the utmost importance in preventing or minimizing the severity and duration of the eruption.

3. Acute generalized exanthematous pustulosis is an acute exanthematous drug eruption, characterized by fever and multiple nonfollicular sterile pustules that subside spontaneously with desquamation. In children, it occurs following a viral infection, vaccine administration, or drugs. The main differential diagnosis is pustular psoriasis.

4. DRESS typically develops 2 to 6 weeks after starting the culprit medication. It is characterized by facial edema and lymphadenopathy.

5. Liver is the most common internal organ involved. Thyroid dysfunction can be delayed, and thyroid function tests should be performed at baseline and 2 to 3 months later.

Clinical Summary

Henoch-Schönlein purpura (HSP) is a small-vessel vasculitis characterized by palpable purpura, arthritis, and gastrointestinal (GI) and renal manifestations and seen in children age 2 to 11 years. About 50% of patients have preceding respiratory infection, mainly group A β-hemolytic streptococcal infection. Other implicated pathogens include hepatitis B virus, adenovirus, *Mycoplasma*, HSV, parvovirus, and HIV. Certain foods, drugs, exposure to cold weather, and insect bites are other predisposing factors. Palpable purpura on lower extremities bilaterally is the presenting sign, and new lesions may develop in crops. This may be associated with fever, joint swelling and arthralgia, abdominal pain, bloody stools, and hematuria.

Complications include bowel obstruction or perforation, intussusceptions, nephrotic syndrome, azotemia, oliguria, chronic glomerulonephritis, hypertensive encephalopathy, CNS manifestations (eg, seizures, coma, paresis), and acute scrotum (mimicking acute testicular torsion).

Emergency Department Treatment and Disposition

Diagnosis of HSP is made clinically. CBC may show leukocytosis, thrombocytosis, and anemia. ESR may be elevated and

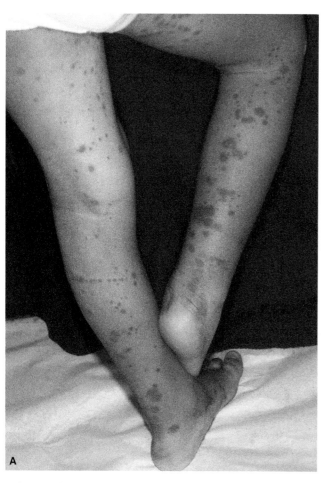
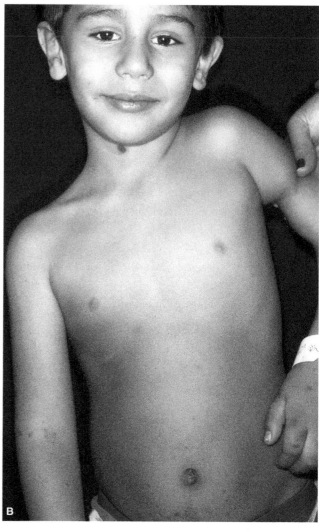

FIGURE 7.22 ■ Henoch-Schönlein Purpura (HSP). (**A**) A 6-year-old boy with crops of palpable purpura on lower extremities and arthritis. (**B**) Shown here is sparing of the trunk and face. Lesions in HSP can also appear on the arms and ears.

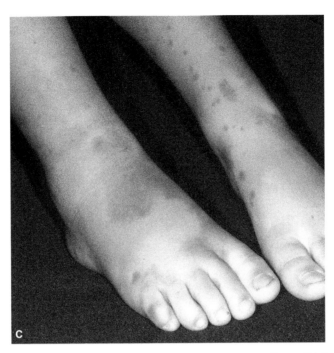

FIGURE 7.22 ■ (*Continued*) (**C**) Close-up of purpura and swollen right ankle. (Photo contributor: Binita R. Shah, MD.)

serum complement levels depressed. Perform urinalysis to screen for renal involvement (may show gross or microscopic hematuria, proteinuria, WBCs, and casts) and stool guaiac to screen for GI involvement. If clinically indicated, use US to evaluate for intussusception and Doppler flow studies to evaluate acute scrotum related to vasculitis. In doubtful cases, skin biopsy helps to confirm leukocytoclastic vasculitis.

There is no specific treatment. The majority of cases are self-limited, and symptoms resolve in a few weeks without permanent residua. Supportive, symptom-directed treatment

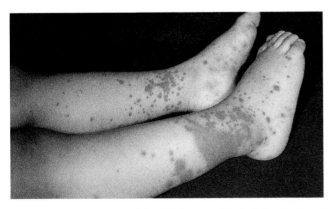

FIGURE 7.23 ■ Henoch-Schönlein Purpura. Typical distribution of palpable purpuric lesions. Angioedema on the right foot is also seen. (Photo contributor: Binita R. Shah, MD.)

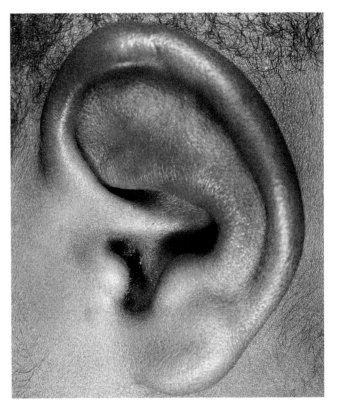

FIGURE 7.24 ■ Henoch-Schönlein Purpura with Vasculitis. Purpuric lesion with edema on ear can be mistaken for child abuse, especially when ear involvement precedes purpura. (Photo contributor: Binita R. Shah, MD.)

includes bed rest, bland diet, and NSAIDs for relief of arthritis and fever. Elevation of the scrotum helps scrotal edema. Hospitalize any patient presenting with complications (eg, hypertension, oliguria, intestinal obstruction, or GI bleeding). Remove the offending antigen, if identified (eg, drugs). Treat the infection if identified (eg, group A β-hemolytic *Streptococcus*). Systemic corticosteroids are indicated for systemic involvement such as severe arthritis, renal involvement, GI complications, and acute scrotum or CNS complications. Corticosteroid therapy does not prevent recurrences, which are usually seen in up to 50% of cases within the first few months (milder and more common in patients with nephritis). Long-term morbidity and mortality are attributed almost exclusively to renal disease. All such patients will need a follow-up by a primary care physician including serial urinalyses and follow-up of renal functions.

Pearls

1. HSP is the most common cause of leukocytoclastic vasculitis in pediatric patients.
2. The classic tetrad associated with HSP is palpable purpura, GI symptoms, renal symptoms, and arthralgias.
3. Arthritis or GI symptoms may precede the appearance of rash by up to 2 weeks.
4. Testicular involvement occurs in up to 35% of patients, and acute scrotal swelling may present prior to purpura and can mimic acute testicular torsion or incarcerated inguinal hernia.
5. Long-term morbidity and mortality are attributed almost exclusively to renal involvement.

Clinical Summary

Acne vulgaris is one of the most common skin problems. Acne is a multifactorial disease caused by interrelated processes, including hyperkeratinization, androgen stimulation, bacterial infection, and inflammation. It is usually not a serious disease, but it can lead to permanent scarring, psychosocial morbidity, and decreased emotional well-being. Acne typically presents with a combination of various lesion types including comedones, papules, pustules, cysts, nodules, scarring, and dyspigmentation. A rare and most severe form of the clinical spectrum of acne vulgaris is *acne fulminans*, occurring most commonly in young males. Patients present with an acute onset of painful, nodular, and occasionally ulcerative pustules concentrated on the chest, shoulders, back, and face. Systemic symptoms such as fever, hepatomegaly, musculoskeletal pain/polyarthralgia, leukocytosis, thrombocytosis, and increased inflammatory markers and transaminases are usually present. Osteolytic bone lesions may be present, especially in the clavicle, sternum, and long bones. The use of isotretinoin is considered a related trigger, which may be dose dependent; the use and cessation of testosterone, bacterial infections, drug-induced disease, and the intake of anabolic androgenic steroids also may be triggers. The skin lesions are usually scarring and leave milia.

Emergency Department Treatment and Disposition

Hospitalization may be required to control the eruption. Systemic steroids are the mainstay of therapy (usually 0.5–1 mg/kg/day for approximately 6 weeks, with dose decreased as the condition improves), with the addition of isotretinoin after the acute inflammatory stage has subsided. Low-dose isotretinoin has been shown to be beneficial in combination with steroids at an initial dose of 0.25 mg/kg/day with a gradual increase to 1 mg/kg/day over 3 to 5 months or longer depending on clinical response. Cyclosporine, dapsone, azathioprine, and infliximab have been used in resistant cases.

Pearls

1. Acne fulminans usually presents in young males with a history of isotretinoin, testosterone, or anabolic steroid use.
2. The presentation is sudden onset of painful and ulcerative pustules on the chest, back, and face in association with systemic symptoms.
3. The recommended treatment is a combination of oral steroids and low-dose isotretinoin once the inflammation has decreased.
4. Acne fulminans usually results in scarring of the affected area.

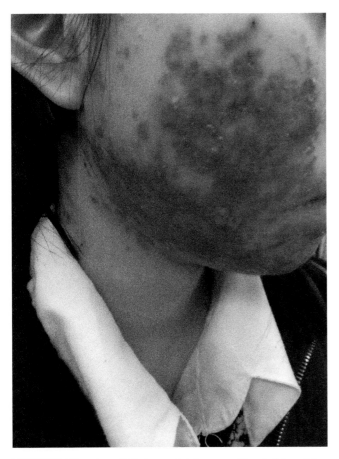

FIGURE 7.25 ■ Acne Fulminans. Adolescent with painful, nodular, and ulcerated pustules on the face. (Photo contributor: Sharon A. Glick, MD.)

SEBORRHEIC DERMATITIS

Clinical Summary

Seborrheic dermatitis is an inflammatory disorder commonly seen in infancy and adolescence. The cause is unknown; however, it has a predilection for areas of high sebaceous gland density and periods of high hormonal levels. In adolescence, seborrheic dermatitis has been linked to *Pityrosporum ovale*, a lipophilic yeast found on the human scalp. Affected areas include the scalp, face, retroauricular areas, mid-chest, axillae, groin, and other intertriginous areas. In infants, it is characterized by an erythematous, greasy, scaly scalp (cradle cap). The lesions may be present in the diaper area including folds

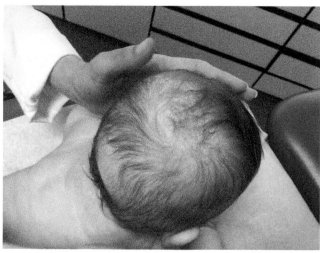

FIGURE 7.27 ■ Seborrheic Dermatitis. Greasy, scaly scalp in a 2-month-old infant. She was treated with a topical corticosteroid oil and ketoconazole shampoo. (Photo contributor: Julie Cantatore-Francis, MD.)

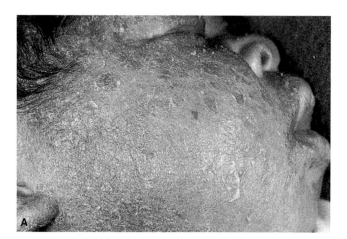

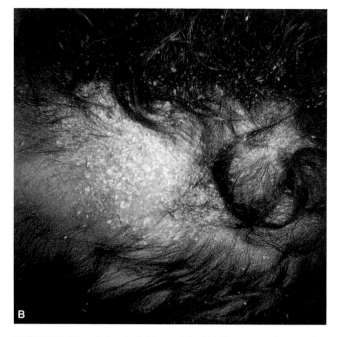

(which are spared in atopic dermatitis). Petaloid, erythematous, noneczematous, scaly, oval plaques may be present on the trunk, back, and flexures. Pruritis is minimal or absent. Secondary monilial infection (due to colonization with *Candida albicans*) and secondary bacterial infections are common, especially in the diaper area. Peak occurrence in infancy is at 3 months of age and usually starts to resolve around 8 to 12 months of age. In adolescence, there may be fine flaky desquamation, with or without erythema, that can

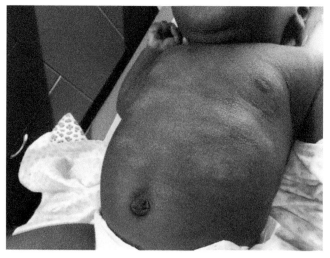

FIGURE 7.26 ■ Seborrheic Dermatitis. (**A**) Greasy papular eruption seen on the face, around the ears, and on the scalp. (**B**) Close-up of scalp showing scaly lesions. (Photo contributor: Binita R. Shah, MD.)

FIGURE 7.28 ■ Seborrheic Dermatitis. Erythematous plaques under the chin, behind the ears, and on the chest area in a 3-month-old infant. (Photo contributor: Julie Cantatore-Francis, MD.)

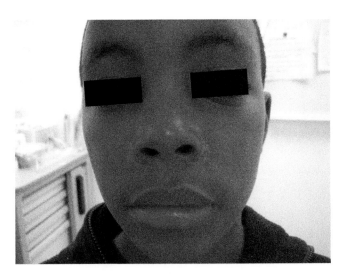

FIGURE 7.29 ■ Seborrheic Dermatitis. Well-defined scaly, greasy plaque seen within the nasolabial folds of a 9-year-old boy. This is an early manifestation of adolescent seborrheic dermatitis. (Photo contributor: Sharon A. Glick, MD.)

spread to the supraorbital area including eyebrows, glabella, nasolabial folds, lips, and aural canal. Hair-bearing areas such as side burns, moustaches, and beards may present with diffuse redness and even pustulation. Blepharitis (inflammation of the eyelid margins) may also occur. The differential diagnosis includes atopic dermatitis, psoriasis, Langerhans cell histiocytosis (in infants), and immunodeficiency disorders. Overlap of atopic dermatitis and seborrheic dermatitis is quite common in infants. Lack of response to topical steroids in suspected atopic dermatitis in an infant should raise the suspicion of seborrheic dermatitis.

Emergency Department Treatment and Disposition

For infants, minor amounts of scale are easily removed by frequent shampooing with products containing sulfur, salicylic acid (eg, Sebulex shampoo), or ketoconazole shampoo. Warm mineral or olive oil compresses followed by washing several hours later and lifting off the scale with a fine-toothed comb may be helpful for scales that are dense, thick, and adherent. For older children and adolescents, antiseborrheic shampoos containing selenium sulfide (eg, Selsun blue), zinc pyrithione (eg, Head & Shoulders), coal tar (eg, Neutrogena T/Gel), or ketoconazole (eg, Nizoral) can be used intermittently (eg, 2–3 times per week). Instruct the patient/parent to lather the shampoo and let it sit on the scalp for 5 to 10 minutes before rinsing. If there is evidence of inflammation, application of a topical low- to mid-potency corticosteroid solution to the scalp and cream to nonhairy inflamed areas is indicated. Caution patients that topical steroids should not be used as maintenance therapy. Topical antifungal agents are also effective.

Pearls

1. Seborrheic dermatitis is the most common rash in the first few months of life.
2. Suspect coexisting atopic dermatitis when lesions are weeping and associated with pruritus.
3. With pronounced localized scaling, seborrheic dermatitis may resemble psoriasis.
4. Seborrheic dermatitis is one of the most common cutaneous manifestations of AIDS in older children and adolescents, and onset usually occurs before AIDS symptoms.
5. Seborrheic dermatitis is a self-limiting disorder and does not cause permanent or scarring alopecia of the scalp.

ALLERGIC CONTACT DERMATITIS

Clinical Summary

Allergic contact dermatitis results from exposure to a topical allergen by a sensitized individual. Percutaneous absorption of an allergen leads to specific T lymphocytes carrying the immune memory to recognize the antigen as a foreign material. Reexposure to the same allergen results in proliferation of sensitized T lymphocytes that release inflammatory mediators, leading to a localized eczematous dermatitis. The most common contact allergens in children include plants (eg, urushiol in poison ivy, poison sumac, poison oak), nickel and cobalt (eg, jewelry, metal wrist band, snap buttons of trouser jeans), shoe materials (eg, rubber and leather [potassium dichromate used for tanning leather]), thimerosal (a preservative in eye drops and vaccines), fragrances, preservatives (in cosmetics, shampoo), hair dye/henna tattoo (paraphenylene diamine), and topical medications (eg, preparations containing neomycin, bacitracin). Allergic contact dermatitis is seen in children, and first exposure to an allergen may occur as early as in infancy.

Diagnosis is based on distribution and morphology of the lesions (eczematous, vesiculation, oozing, and, in chronic lesions, lichenification) and history of exposure. Sharp demarcation between normal and affected skin, with linearity, suggests allergic contact diagnosis. A patch test, done by a dermatologist (if etiology not apparent), can help with a diagnosis. A positive test shows erythema and papules confined to the test site.

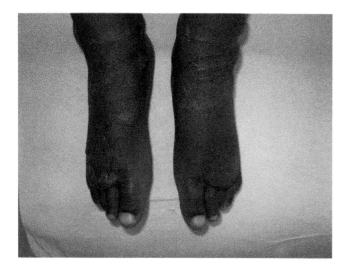

FIGURE 7.30 ■ Allergic Contact Dermatitis. Contact blisters with erythema present on bilateral dorsum of feet, in a patient with allergy to shoe material (most likely rubber). Avoidance of the specific material cures the condition. (Photo contributor: Julie Cantatore-Francis, MD.)

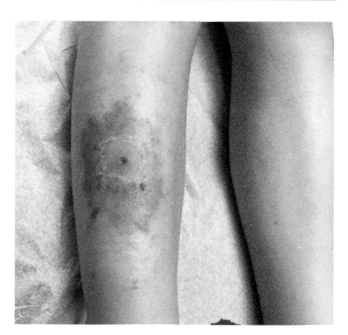

FIGURE 7.31 ■ Allergic Contact Dermatitis. An adolescent male with an erythematous, vesicular, pruritic patch after placing Neosporin on an insect bite. Two days after this rash appeared, he also developed an acute papulovesicular eruption (id eruption) on the arms and hands. (Photo contributor: Julie Cantatore-Francis, MD.)

Emergency Department Treatment and Disposition

Once allergic contact dermatitis has been diagnosed, identification and elimination of the allergen (eg, removal of nickel jewelry) and avoidance of further exposure are necessary. Antihistamines are used (eg, oral diphenhydramine, hydroxyzine) to control the pruritus. Avoid use of topical diphenhydramine because it is a sensitizer (with prolonged use, the patient may develop sensitization). Topical high- or mid-potency corticosteroid cream applied twice a day for 2 to 3 weeks, with avoidance of allergen, treats the condition. Rarely, systemic steroids may be needed (eg, in cases caused by poison ivy, prednisone 1–2 mg/kg/day tapered over 2–3 weeks helps to control the acute inflammation). For poison ivy, if possible, show a picture of the offending plant for patients and family members so they can avoid further exposure. When outdoors, advise using a barrier cream (eg, Ivy Shield), which blocks the resin from touching the skin, and washing the exposed area immediately if accidental exposure occurs. Recurrences are common if the suspected allergen is not eliminated completely; thus, all the ingredients (even in the minutest of proportions) in the suspected allergen should be avoided.

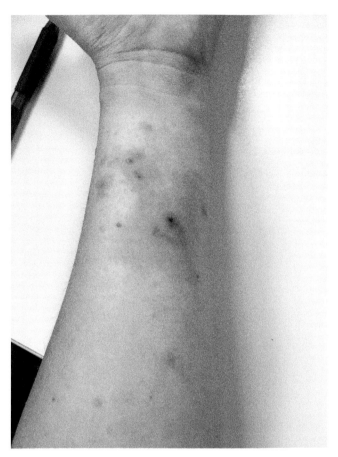

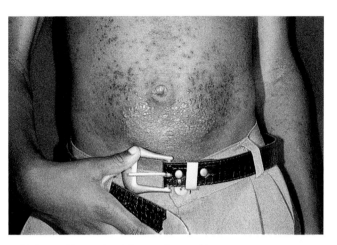

FIGURE 7. 34 ■ Nickel Contact Dermatitis. Nickel sulfate found in a belt buckle was responsible for this rash that was treated with steroid cream without success because patient continued to wear belt. Contact dermatitis from nickel snaps on denim and from belt buckles is often mistaken for eczema (like in this patient). This patient's rash improved only after discontinuation of wearing the belt. (Photo contributor: Binita R. Shah, MD.)

FIGURE 7.32. ■ Poison Ivy Dermatitis. Linear streaks, vesicles, and urticarial wheals seen after exposure to urushiol on the forearm. Super-potent topical corticosteroids were helpful in this case. (Photo contributor: Julie Cantatore-Francis, MD.)

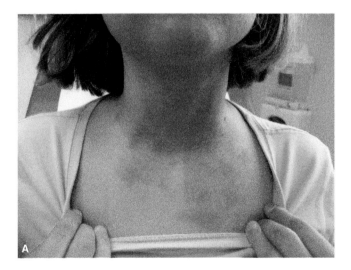

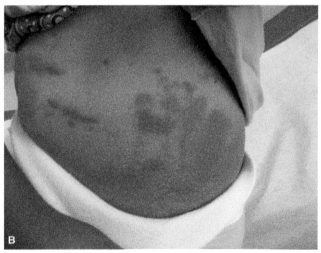

FIGURE 7.33 ■ Allergic Contact Dermatitis. (**A**) Adolescent with recurrence of poison ivy dermatitis seen on neck. Premature termination of oral corticosteroids (patient treated for 3 days only), as occurred in this case, may result in rebound dermatitis. In severe cases, it is important to treat with a steroid taper over 2 to 3 weeks. (**B**) Erythematous linear streaks of urticaria on the abdomen due to spread of urushiol oil. She also had linear array of vesicles on finger. (Photo contributor: Sharon A. Glick, MD.)

Pearls

1. Diagnosis is based on the history of exposure and the pattern of the rash (eg, a symmetrical erythematous rash on both ear lobes in a patient wearing nickel earrings).
2. One of the most common contact allergens in children is urushiol, the sensitizing antigen found in poison ivy.
3. A thorough history is the most important step in management and includes inquiring about animal exposure. Poison ivy dermatitis can result from touching an animal exposed to the plant.
4. Autosensitization dermatitis (id eruption) occurs as acute papulovesicular pruritic symmetric eruptions on the trunk, forearms, extensor surfaces, and rarely on the face and is a hypersensitive reaction to allergic dermatitis and bacterial or fungal infections.
5. Koebner phenomenon (isomorphic phenomenon), in which trauma elicits similar lesions, is also seen in an Id eruption. The diagnosis is clinical, and treatment of the primary dermatitis is crucial. Open wet compresses, antihistamines, and topical steroids may also help.

Clinical Summary

Atopic dermatitis (AD) is a common eczematous dermatitis manifested as a result of persistent inflammation of the skin. It is often associated with allergic diseases such as asthma and allergic rhinitis and manifests as acute, subacute, and chronic dermatitis. AD is thought to be linked to mutations in genes encoding epidermal differentiation (eg, filaggrin), leading to immune dysregulation and epidermal barrier dysfunction, which ultimately result in an abnormal skin reaction to the environment or allergens (eg, dust mite, food, microbes). Diagnosis is based on classic morphology and distribution of dermatitis depending on the age group. The infantile phase is from 2 months to 2 years, characterized by severe pruritus, oozing, vesiculation, eczematous papules, and plaques seen on the face, scalp, extensors of extremities, and trunk. The facial dermatitis is often exacerbated by saliva during feeding and teething, which serves as an irritant. During infancy, the sparing of groin and diaper area (likely due to the increased hydration and protection of triggers by the diaper) helps to differentiate infantile AD from seborrheic dermatitis. The childhood phase lasts from 2 years of age to puberty and is characterized by dry, scaly, lichenified, pruritic plaques seen on the antecubital fossae, popliteal fossae, periorbital and perioral areas, wrists, hands, and feet. Lymphadenopathy may be a prominent feature in affected children. The adult phase begins at puberty and continues into adulthood and is characterized by chronic pruritic lichenified plaques present on the flexors, neck, face, trunk, hands, and feet. Nummular eczema is a variant of AD characterized by discoid, well-circumscribed, annular plaques, commonly seen on the extremities. Associated features of AD include pityriasis alba, periorbital darkening, ichthyosis vulgaris, dermographism, keratosis pilaris, and hyperlinear palms. Elevated serum IgE with peripheral eosinophilia may be seen. Secondary bacterial and viral infections are common including *Staphylococcus aureus* colonization, molluscum contagiosum, and HSV eruptions.

Emergency Department Treatment and Disposition

The majority of patients with AD are treated as outpatients. Management consists of establishing realistic parental expectations that AD is a chronic disorder that involves remissions

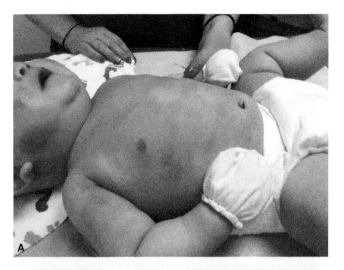

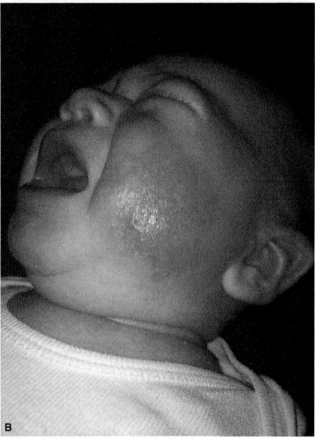

FIGURE 7.35 ■ Infantile Atopic Dermatitis. (**A**) Severe pruritis and erythematous eczematous patches seen on the face, arms, and chest of this 3-month-old boy. Due to severe itching, he has gloves to protect him from excoriations. (**B**) Infants commonly have involvement on the cheeks, as seen in this 3-month-old infant with an oozing plaque. (Photo contributors: Julie Cantatore-Francis, MD [A], and Sharon A. Glick, MD [B].)

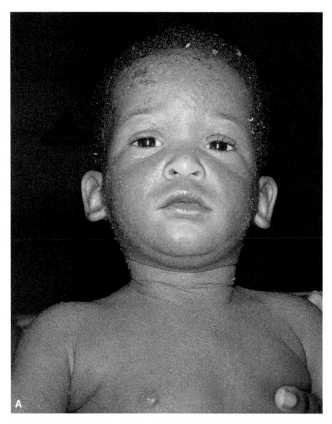
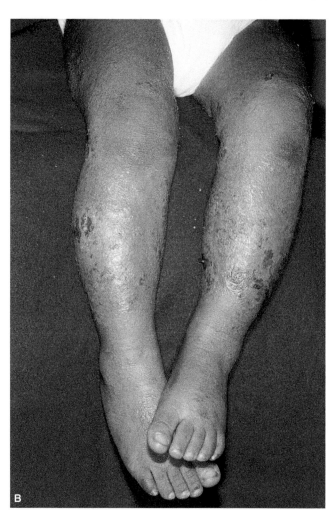

FIGURE 7.36 ◼ Infantile Atopic Dermatitis. Involvement of forehead, scalp, and both cheeks with sparing of the nose ("headlight sign") (**A**), and distribution of lesions in more extensor than flexor surfaces (**B**) are seen. (Photo contributor: Binita R. Shah, MD.)

and exacerbations. Goals of therapy are to control the flare-ups, prevent secondary infections, and keep the skin barrier function intact by constant moisturizing. Advise patient to avoid trigger factors such as hot water; heat; allergens, including dust mites, pollens, molds, and foods such as eggs and peanuts; materials such as wool and fur; exposures to animals (eg, dogs, cats) or items filled with feathers or down (eg, pillows); stress; and infections (eg, *S aureus*, HSV, dermatophytes). Advice on constant and regular care of the dry and xerotic skin includes daily moisturizing, brief baths or showers in lukewarm water lasting not >5 to 10 minutes, use of a mild unscented soap or liquid gentle skin cleanser (eg, Dove fragrance-free soap, Aveeno), and patting (not rubbing) the skin dry, leaving some moisture. Moisturizers (eg, Vaseline,

Aquaphor) are applied all over the skin as soon as the child gets out of the bath or shower to trap moisture in the skin. Moisturizers should be applied to the entire body 2 to 3 times a day. Mid- to high-potency topical steroids are used for body areas (except groin, face, and axillae). Mild topical steroids are used for face, groins, and axillae but not >2 to 3 weeks at a stretch. Topical antibacterial agents (eg, mupirocin) can be used if there is any evidence of excoriations or open wounds. If the infection is severe, oral antibiotics for 7 to 10 days can be used. The addition of dilute sodium hypochlorite (bleach) to a bath or in a shower gel (Puracyn, CLn) can help control dermatitis in children with a history of skin infection. For severe flares, short-term use of wet wraps (using moist pajamas or socks) over diluted topical steroids can be used to increase the

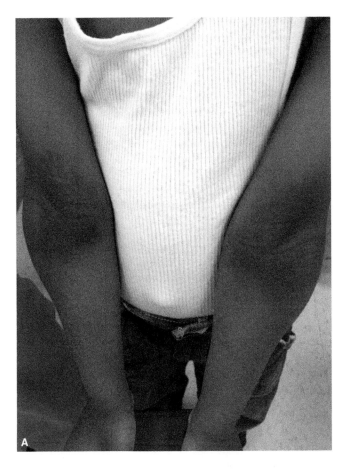

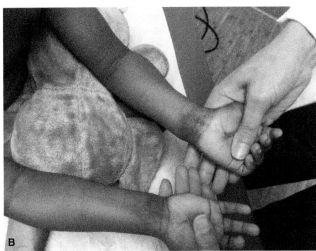

FIGURE 7.37 ■ Atopic Dermatitis. (**A**) Well-defined hyperpigmented, lichenified, pruritic plaques of eczema are seen in the antecubital fossae (a classic site). (**B**) Localized hyperpigmented and thickened plaques on the wrist in a different child. Typical morphology of chronic atopic dermatitis is seen due to constant itching and rubbing on both these children. (Photo contributors: Sharon A. Glick, MD [A], and Julie Cantatore-Francis, MD [B].)

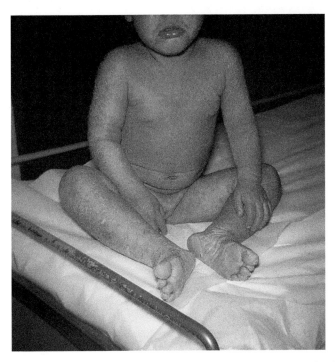

FIGURE 7.38 ■ Generalized Erythroderma. An infant with atopic dermatitis who developed generalized erythroderma. The upper layer of the skin is exfoliating in pieces on a background of generalized erythema. (Photo contributor: Binita R. Shah, MD.)

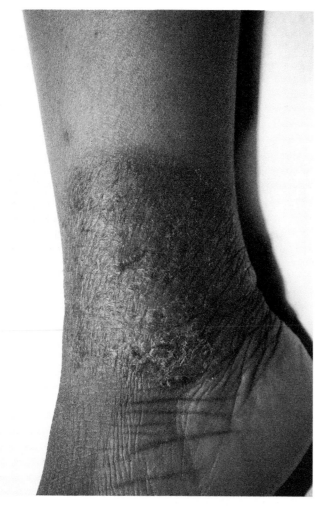

FIGURE 7.39 ■ Atopic Dermatitis with Secondary Bacterial Infection. A lichenified plaque with hyperpigmentation, scaling, and fissuring is seen on the lower extremity. Fissuring and exudation suggest secondary bacterial infection. (Photo contributor: Binita R. Shah, MD.)

steroid absorption over extremities. Topical immunomodulators such as pimecrolimus 1% or tacrolimus 0.03% or 0.1% ointment can be used as steroid-sparing agents. Antihistamine (eg, diphenhydramine, hydroxyzine) is used for control of the severe itch that causes the rash. Systemic immunosuppressive therapy including ultraviolet light treatment should only be considered in chronic, severe AD. Systemic corticosteroid therapy, although acutely effective, has many potential side effects and can result in a rapid rebound effect on atopic patients and thus should be avoided if possible. NSAIDs such as cyclosporine, methotrexate, azathioprine, and mycophenolate mofetil have been used in severe patients, and studies are under way for use of biologics in children with AD. Patients should be referred to a primary care physician or dermatologist for ongoing care.

Pearls

1. AD is the "itch that rashes." Pruritus, xerosis, and eczema are prominent features of AD.
2. Hospitalization is indicated for eczema herpeticum, generalized erythroderma, severe AD with compromised skin barrier causing failure to thrive, or severe flare-ups unresponsive to conventional treatment.
3. Moisturizers form the mainstay of therapy. Topical steroids, antibacterials, and avoidance of trigger factors are the other pillars of the therapy.

Clinical Summary

Eczema herpeticum (EH) is a disseminated cutaneous herpes simplex virus (HSV) infection superimposed on a preexisting active skin condition. A likely cause is the impaired skin barrier in active AD, which allows viral particles to incubate and proliferate quickly, leading to severe dissemination. EH is most commonly caused by HSV-1 and less commonly by HSV-2. Although most commonly seen in patients with AD, it can also occur with other primary dermatologic disorders (eg, seborrheic dermatitis, irritant contact dermatitis, pemphigus, burns, ichthyosis vulgaris, skin grafts). A history of contact with a family member with recurrent oral/facial HSV infection is often found. Clinically, monomorphous vesicles, pustules, and erosions may be seen on a preexisting dermatitis. There may be multiple punctate erosions, some coalescing to form larger polycyclic erosions. EH is more commonly seen on the face, neck, and chest areas and can lead to fatality in infants and young children if not treated promptly.

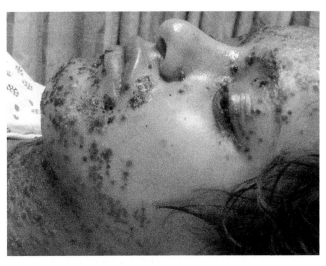

FIGURE 7.41 ■ Eczema Herpeticum. Acute eruption of multiple punctate erosions on the face and neck of an adolescent girl with recalcitrant atopic dermatitis. These punctate erosions also coalesced to form large polycyclic erosions. Viral culture was positive for HSV-1. (Photo contributor: Haamid Chamdawala, MD.)

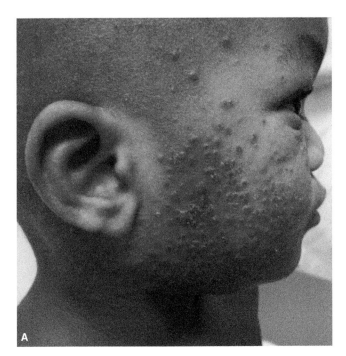

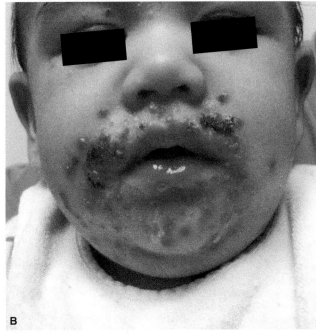

FIGURE 7.40 ■ Eczema Herpeticum. (**A**) Acute eruption of multiple erythematous vesiculopapular lesions with central crusting is seen on the right cheek of a young boy with atopic dermatitis. Because lesions involve the face and are close to the eye, an urgent ophthalmology consult is indicated to exclude corneal involvement. (**B**) Erythematous vesiculopapular lesions around the eyes and mouth with crusting are seen in a different infant. (Photo contributors: Falguni Asrani, MD [A], and Christy Riley, MD [B].)

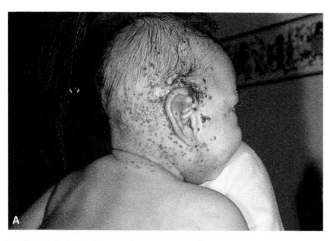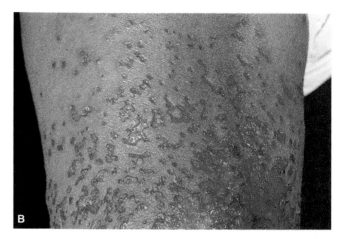

FIGURE 7.42 ■ Eczema Herpeticum. (**A**) Widespread "punched-out" lesions on upper trunk, neck, and extremities in a febrile 4-month-old infant with atopic dermatitis. The mother suffered from recurrent cold sores (herpes simplex labialis) and had cold sores 5 days prior to the appearance of this infant's rash. (**B**) Close-up of the "punched-out" lesions. (Photo contributor: Binita R. Shah, MD.)

Complications include secondary bacterial infection (*Streptococcus pyogenes* and *S aureus*), keratoconjunctivitis, viremia, and scarring.

The major differential diagnosis is eczema coxsackium caused by coxsackie virus type A6, which reemerged in the United States in 2011 as a cause of atypical hand-foot-and-mouth disease. Like EH, eczema coxsackium also favors sites of preexisting dermatitis.

Emergency Department Treatment and Disposition

Diagnosis of EH is usually clinical. A high index of suspicion for EH in patients presenting with a history of "worsening" AD is an important step. Diagnosis can be confirmed by direct fluorescent antibody assays, Tzanck smear, viral culture, and viral DNA polymerase chain reaction for HSV. Dermatology consultation will be valuable in such cases. Ophthalmology consultation is mandatory for periorbital lesions. Hospitalization of infants and young children with EH is indicated in severe cases to prevent complications with prompt administration of IV acyclovir until lesions crust over. Maintaining hydration and skin care are also important. Bland emollients may be applied to the affected areas. Mild cases of EH can be managed as outpatients with acyclovir given orally with a very close follow-up by a primary care physician or a dermatologist. Antistaphylococcal antibiotics should be given along with acyclovir administered either IV (severe EH requiring hospitalization) or orally; topical mupirocin may be used with early, localized, mild cases not requiring hospitalization.

Pearls

1. "Punched out" erosions superimposed on a preexisting active dermatitis such as AD are important clues.
2. Suspect EH when infected-appearing eczema does not respond to appropriate antibiotic therapy; this may indicate HSV infection.
3. Acyclovir and meticulous skin care are key to prompt recovery from EH.

Clinical Summary

Psoriasis is a chronic polygenic skin disorder characterized by well-circumscribed, erythematous plaques with an overlying silvery-white scale affecting about 2% of the general population. The most common clinical variant is plaque psoriasis. Patients often experience a waxing and waning course. Precipitating factors include minor trauma (Koebner phenomenon), infection, stress, and drugs. In the severe form of generalized pustular psoriasis, patients are often ill appearing with fever, generalized erythema, and pustules. Onset is acute, and most patients have an antecedent nonpustular psoriasis or a genetic predisposition. Episodes may be precipitated by

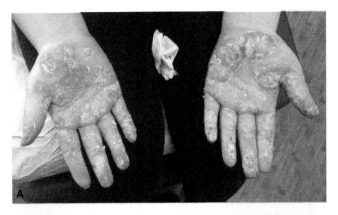

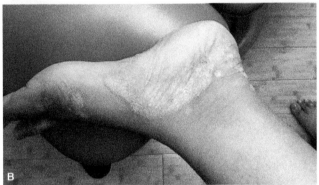

FIGURE 7.44 ■ Palmoplantar Psoriasis. (**A**) An adolescent girl with a history of recurrent pharyngitis presenting with this rash. (**B**) Recalcitrant plantar psoriatic plaques in an adolescent boy who was started on a biologic. (Photo contributor: Julie Cantatore-Francis, MD.)

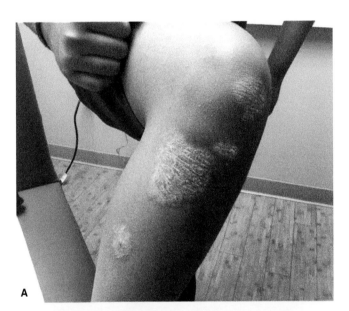

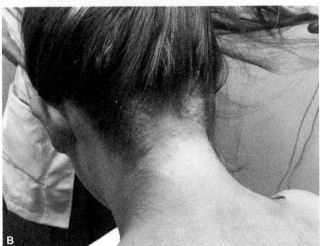

FIGURE 7.43 ■ Psoriasis. Typical well-circumscribed, erythematous plaques with overlying silvery-white scale are seen on the leg (**A**) and scalp (**B**). (Photo contributor: Julie Cantatore-Francis, MD.)

pregnancy, medications (ie, coal tar, lithium), hypocalcemia, or withdrawal of both topical and systemic steroids. Relapses are common.

Diagnosis is usually clinical, and skin biopsy confirms the diagnosis. Complications include generalized exfoliative dermatitis (erythroderma) and psoriatic arthritis. Differential diagnosis includes nummular eczema, tinea corporis, pityriasis rosea, pityriasis rubra pilaris, contact dermatitis, lichen simplex chronicus, Reiter syndrome, psoriasiform drug eruptions, and other conditions of the scalp including seborrheic dermatitis, tinea capitis, and AD.

Emergency Department Treatment and Disposition

Admit patients with severe forms (eg, generalized pustular psoriasis, a serious and, at times, fatal disease). Educate parents about the chronic nature of the condition and relapses

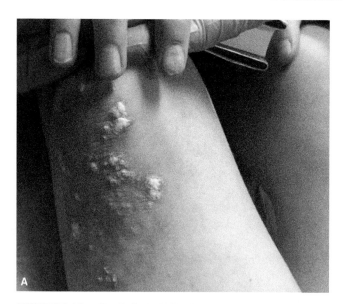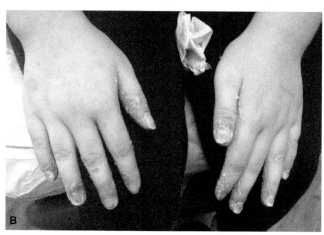

FIGURE 7.45 ■ Psoriasis; Nail Findings. (**A**) Nail pitting in a 14-year-old girl with typical psoriatic plaques. (**B**) Diffuse inflammation of the nail with oil spots, subungual hyperkeratosis, and onycholysis are seen. (Photo contributor: Julie Cantatore-Francis, MD.)

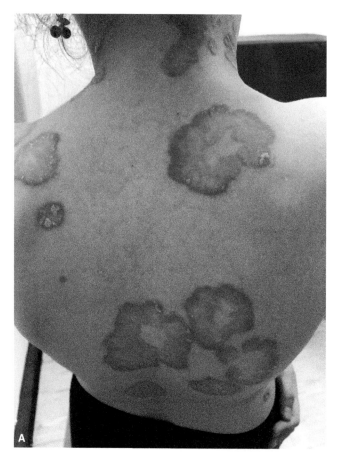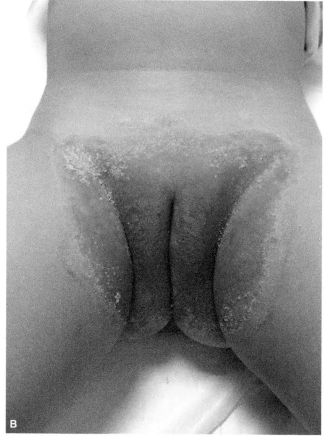

FIGURE 7.46 ■ Psoriasis. (**A**) Annular psoriasis. This 7-year-old girl was misdiagnosed as having tinea corporis. Her fungal culture was negative. She also had nail pitting. She was diagnosed as having annular psoriasis and responded to topical steroids. (**B**) Napkin psoriasis is seen in this infant. Note the overlying scale and sharp demarcation (Photo contributors: Viktoryia Kazlouskaya, MD, PhD [A], and Sharon A. Glick, MD [B].)

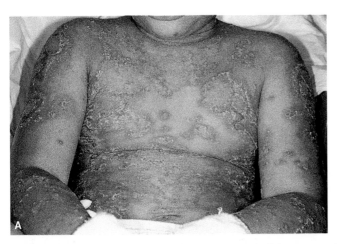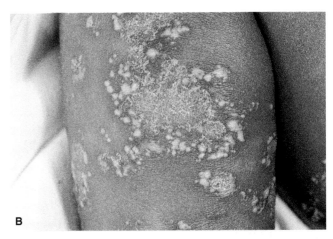

FIGURE 7.47 ■ Generalized Pustular Psoriasis. (**A**) Discrete annular erythematous plaques with a border of pustules. This young girl developed this generalized pustular rash after being treated with oral steroids for presumed atopic dermatitis (steroid withdrawal can trigger pustular psoriasis). The patient was started on methotrexate. (**B**) Close-up of pustular psoriasis. Numerous tiny, sterile pustules evolve from an erythematous base and coalesce into lakes of pus. Pustules are superficial and are easily ruptured. (Photo contributor: Binita R. Shah, MD.)

and remissions. The goal of therapy is to control flare-ups. Advise patients on gentle skin care including lukewarm brief baths (with bath oil or coal tar), gentle soaps, avoiding trauma or scratching the lesions, and use of emollients for skin hydration (eg, Vaseline, petrolatum, mineral oil). For thick scalp lesions, use shampoo 2 or 3 times per week (coal tar, selenium sulfide, or zinc pyrithione). Sunlight exposure helps psoriasis; however, patients should be cautioned to avoid sunburn as this may aggravate their condition. Consider topical corticosteroids creams for management of acute flairs. Low-potency steroid creams may be used on the face and groin (not for >2 weeks) and medium-potency steroid creams on other body parts (not for >2 weeks). High-potency steroid creams (not for >2 weeks) are reserved for older children and adolescents with severely affected areas. Consider antibiotics (eg, penicillin, cephalexin) when a pharyngitis or perianal cellulitis is suspected as precipitating a guttate flare (see Figures 7.50 and 7.51) and obtain cultures for confirmation.

Refer all patients to dermatology. Other therapeutic options in refractory cases include topical vitamin D analog creams or retinoids, phototherapy, or oral therapies including retinoids, methotrexate, or cyclosporine. Biologic agents (eg, etanercept, infliximab) are the newest class of medications being used for treatment.

Pearls

1. Koebner phenomenon (new lesions at the site of trauma) is an important feature of psoriasis.
2. Psoriasis may be seen as early as the first months of life. Diaper area is commonly involved.
3. Pinpoint bleeding where scale is removed (Auspitz sign) is highly characteristic.
4. Involvement of nails is also an important feature and includes nail pitting, oil spots, subungual hyperkeratosis, and onycholysis (detachment of the distal nail plate).

Clinical Summary

Guttate psoriasis is a variant characterized by an abrupt onset of profuse oval or round "guttate" or drop-like lesions, most commonly following group A β-hemolytic streptococcal infections (ie, streptococcal pharyngitis, perianal streptococcal dermatitis, otitis, or sinusitis). Streptococcal pharyngitis or a viral URI precedes the eruption of guttate psoriasis by 1 to 3 weeks.

Emergency Department Treatment and Disposition

Laboratory tests should include a throat culture and serologic titer (eg, antistreptolysin O titer) to confirm streptococcal infection. If infection is confirmed, give antibiotics. The drug of choice is penicillin. Erythromycin or clindamycin is

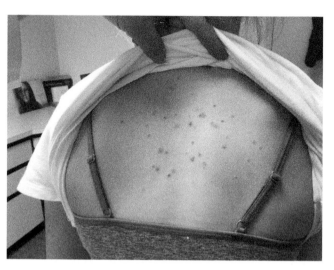

FIGURE 7.49 ■ Guttate Psoriasis. Scattered, drop-like, erythematous papules with silvery scale are seen in a 12-year-old girl who was receiving antibiotics for streptococcal pharyngitis. (Photo contributor: Julie Cantatore-Francis, MD.)

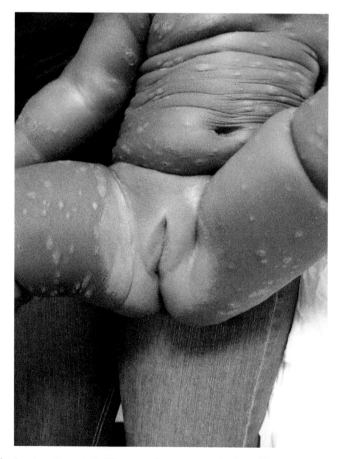

FIGURE 7.48 ■ Guttate Psoriasis. An abrupt onset of diffuse, erythematous, scaly, drop-like plaques in a 15-month-old infant. Note intense erythema of the diaper area. Perianal culture was positive for group A β-hemolytic streptococci. She was treated with penicillin with a complete resolution of the diaper and guttate rash. (Photo contributor: Jeannette Jakus, MD.)

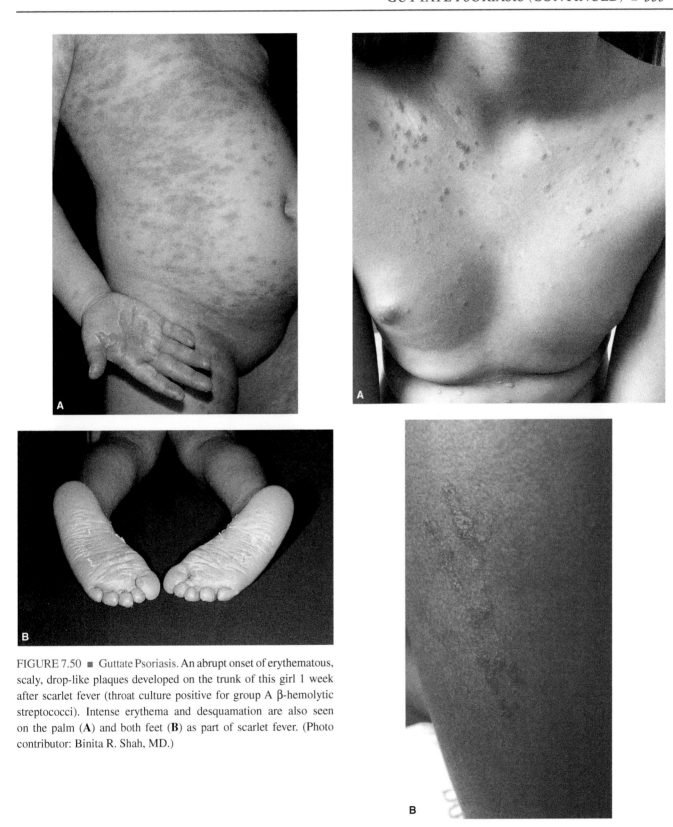

FIGURE 7.50 ■ Guttate Psoriasis. An abrupt onset of erythematous, scaly, drop-like plaques developed on the trunk of this girl 1 week after scarlet fever (throat culture positive for group A β-hemolytic streptococci). Intense erythema and desquamation are also seen on the palm (**A**) and both feet (**B**) as part of scarlet fever. (Photo contributor: Binita R. Shah, MD.)

FIGURE 7.51 ■ Guttate Psoriasis. (**A**) A 9-year-old girl recently treated for strep throat presented with a 1-week history of erythematous scaly thin papules on the face, trunk, and arms. (**B**) The right arm showed evidence of koebnerization. (Photo contributor: Sharon A. Glick, MD.)

a good alternative for patients with penicillin allergy. Refer the patient to a dermatologist for ongoing care. Guttate psoriasis may resolve spontaneously in a few weeks or months, especially with antibiotic therapy. Tonsillectomy or monthly injections of benzathine penicillin may be helpful if flares are precipitated by recurrent streptococcal infections. Exposure to sunlight and broadband or narrowband ultraviolet B phototherapy also help in resolution of lesions. For persistent lesions, the same therapy as that for psoriasis is recommended (see page 329).

Pearls

1. Guttate psoriasis is a variant seen more commonly in children and adolescents and may herald the development of generalized plaque psoriasis.

2. Guttate psoriasis is characterized by an abrupt onset of drop-like lesions, mainly on the trunk, buttocks, hips, and proximal extremities.

Clinical Summary

Pityriasis rosea (PR) is an acute, benign, self-limiting eruption of unknown etiology (presumed viral) with a distinct presentation of a solitary "herald patch" lesion followed by a secondary generalized eruption of smaller papules that appear in crops usually sparing the face, scalp, and distal extremities. About 50% of cases occur before age 20 years, with the highest incidence among adolescents. It is commonly seen during the fall, winter, and spring. About 5% of patients have a prodrome of fever, malaise, arthralgia, and pharyngitis preceding the PR eruption (usually seen with florid PR). Atypical clinical variants of PR are seen in about 25% of cases and include the following:

1. Papular PR (especially in African American children)
2. PR with intensely irritated or inflamed edematous lesions
3. "Inverse form of PR," which includes lesions limited to face, scalp, distal extremities, groin, and axillae

4. PR with vesicular, pustular, urticarial, hemorrhagic (purpuric), or large annular erythema multiforme–like lesions
5. PR with oral lesions

The diagnosis is made clinically, and rarely, a skin biopsy (to exclude other diseases) may be required for atypical cases. Recurrences of PR are rare (about 2% of cases).

Emergency Department Treatment and Disposition

Most patients are asymptomatic and do not need any specific treatment except reassurance about the benign nature and the total duration of the eruption (about 6–8 weeks). Patients are *not* contagious and do not need any isolation. Symptomatic relief from pruritus can be obtained using soothing nonprescription lotions such as calamine, menthol, or pramoxine.

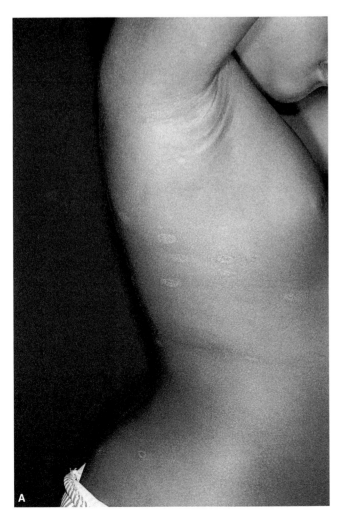

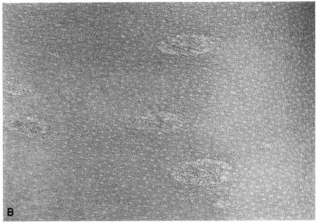

FIGURE 7.52 ■ Pityriasis Rosea (PR). (**A**) Oval-shaped papulosquamous lesions of PR on the trunk. The name PR is derived from Greek (pityriasis = scaly) and Latin (rosea = pink). She had a history of a "round rash" (herald patch) that appeared 10 days prior to this eruption. (**B**) Close-up shows that the long axis of the papulosquamous oval-shaped plaques is oriented along the skin lines. A fine, wrinkled, tissue-like scale remains attached within the border of the plaque, giving the characteristic ring of scale, called collarette scale. (Photo contributor: Binita R. Shah, MD.)

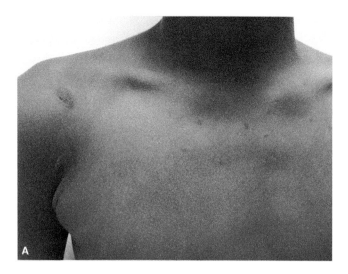

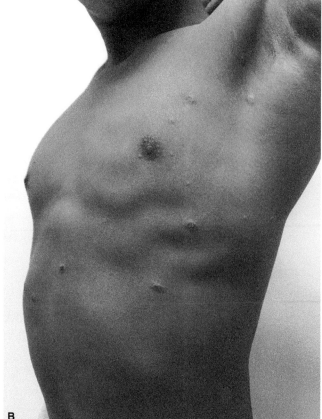

FIGURE 7.53 ▪ Pityriasis Rosea. (**A**) Large, oval, scaly, thin plaque on right shoulder representing a herald patch is seen in a 13-year-old adolescent boy. (**B**) Papules and thin, oval, scaly plaques following skin cleavage lines are also seen. (Photo contributor: Chika Ugorji, MD.)

Lukewarm colloidal oatmeal baths (not hot, as this may intensify itching) may be soothing. Nonfluorinated topical corticosteroids (eg, hydrocortisone 2.5%) and antihistamines may be given for more intense pruritus, especially at night when pruritus is more troublesome. A rare patient with extensive disease with intense itching may respond to a short course of oral prednisone (dose: 0.5–1 mg/kg/day given orally for 7 days). This is rarely indicated in children and is best reserved for patients with intractable pruritus with severe disease. Refer such patients to a dermatologist. Direct sun exposure may hasten the resolution of individual lesions; however, burning should be avoided as this may exacerbate the rash. Alternatively, ultraviolet B administered in 5 consecutive daily erythemogenic exposures results in decreased pruritus and hastens the involution of lesions. Therapy is most beneficial within the first week of eruption and is rarely indicated in children.

Pearls

1. PR is a self-limiting eruption lasting about 6 to 8 weeks and is characterized by pink oval papules or plaques with a collarette of scale affecting the trunk and proximal extremities.

2. Lesions run parallel to the lines of skin cleavage, forming a "Christmas tree" appearance on the back.

3. A herald patch is seen in 70% of cases and heralds the onset of PR; however, its absence does not preclude the diagnosis of PR.

4. Secondary syphilis may be indistinguishable from PR, especially if the herald patch is absent; consider serology for syphilis in all sexually active patients presenting with a rash of PR.

Clinical Summary

Granuloma annulare (GA) is a granulomatous skin disorder of unknown etiology occurring in any age group, especially in school-age children. Multiple associations have been hypothesized including postvaccination (injectables), trauma, insect bites, and sun exposure. A historic association with diabetes has most recently been refuted. The classic and subcutaneous types are common in children. The characteristic morphology is a nonscaly indurated annular or ring-like plaque with a papular border and central clearing. In the classic type, multiple or solitary painless lesions may be seen distributed over the wrists and dorsum of hands and feet but can involve any part of the body. In subcutaneous GA, patients present with multiple or solitary deep nodules (similar distribution as classic form). The differential diagnosis includes tinea corporis and dermal processes such as sarcoidosis. The subcutaneous type may often be confused with rheumatoid nodules or other tumors. The diagnosis is clinical but can be confirmed on biopsy. The histopathology shows palisading granulomas in the dermis with mucin and necrobiotic degenerated collagen.

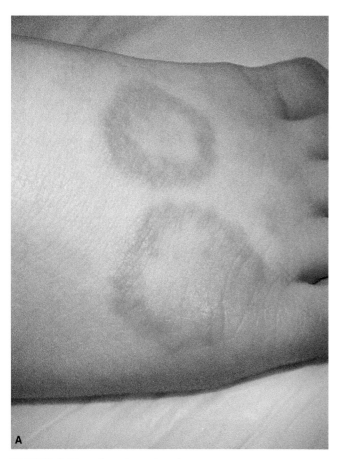

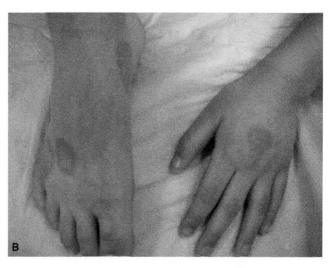

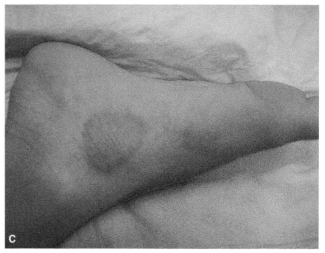

FIGURE 7.54 ■ Granuloma Annulare. (**A**) Well-defined asymptomatic annular plaques with a raised papular indurated border and central clearing, seen on the dorsum of foot, dorsum of hands and feet (**B**), and on the foot (**C**) of a young teenager. (Photo contributor: Jeannette Jakus, MD.)

Emergency Department Treatment and Disposition

GA is a benign chronic condition and is usually followed by a dermatologist and/or primary care physician. It is known to resolve spontaneously in several months to years. Treatment is mainly in the form of topical moderate- to high-potency steroids or injectable steroids (expected to work better).

Pearls

1. GA can be confused with tinea corporis because of its annular configuration and raised papular border. However, unlike tinea corporis, GA lacks superficial scale.

2. GA sometimes resolves spontaneously after a biopsy (not known exactly why this occurs).

Clinical Summary

Scabies is a contagious skin infestation caused by the female mite *Sarcoptes scabiei* subspecies *hominis*. The mite tunnels into the upper layer of the skin, produces a burrow, and deposits 1 to 4 eggs daily for 15 to 30 days. The larvae hatch in a few days, causing intense itching. Only 10% of the eggs develop into adult mites. An infested person has an average of 12 mites on the skin. Signs and symptoms are a result of delayed hypersensitivity cell-mediated immune response to the proteins of the parasite. Nodules are a granulomatous response to the dead mite antigens and feces. The incubation period is 2 to 6 weeks in persons without previous exposure. With a previous infestation, symptoms may develop in 1 to 4 days after reexposure. Scabies affects persons from all socioeconomic levels without regard to age, sex, or standards of personal hygiene; however, it is more common in crowded living quarters and nursing homes. Dogs and cats may be infested by nearly identical organisms (*S scabiei* subspecies *canis*) and sometimes may serve as a source for human infestation.

The diagnosis is clinical based on distribution of lesions, intense pruritus, and a history of affected family members.

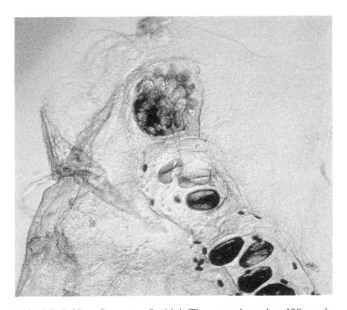

FIGURE 7.55 ■ Sarcoptes Scabiei. The causative mite, 400 μm in size, alongside ova (large black ovals) and feces (scattered smaller black dots). (Reproduced with permission from Kane KS, Bissonette J, Boden HP, et al. *Color Atlas & Synopsis of Pediatric Dermatology.* McGraw-Hill Education; New York, NY, 2002.)

A light microscopic examination of a skin scraping from a burrow or unexcoriated lesion can be done with a no. 15 surgical blade and may demonstrate a mite, egg, or feces. A negative scraping does not rule out scabies. Complications include secondary infection (*S aureus* or *S pyogenes*). Scabies incognito is undiagnosed scabies resulting from the use of topical steroids.

Emergency Department Treatment and Disposition

Untreated scabies can last for months or years. When treating a patient for scabies, it is important to treat all the patient's contacts. The preferred treatment is permethrin 5% cream, which should be applied from the neck down including intertriginous and genital areas, the intergluteal cleft, and under trimmed nails. Because scabies can affect the head, scalp, and neck in infants and young children, treatment of the entire head, neck, and body in this age group is required. The areas around the eyes and mouth should be avoided. The medication should be left on overnight (about 8 hours) and then washed off. Patients should be instructed to change all the clothes and bed sheets the following morning, and the treatment should be repeated 1 week later for optimal results. Side effects include mild, transient burning, stinging, redness, and rash. An alternative treatment for school-aged children, adolescents, and adults includes γ-benzene hexachloride (lindane 1%) cream or lotion. Patients should be cautioned that improper use may lead to a significant systemic absorption, resulting in neurotoxicity. Because of the potential neurotoxicity, lindane should not be used in children younger than age 5 years, premature infants, patients with crusted lesions, children with a prior history of seizure disorders, malnourished children (lindane seeks fat; lack of fat in a malnourished patient may lead to toxicity), children with severe excoriations or inflamed or traumatized skin, children with chronic and preexisting dermatosis, or women who are pregnant or breastfeeding. Other alternative therapies include sulfur (5%–10% precipitated sulfur in petrolatum), crotamiton cream, and oral ivermectin. Advise patients to wash all clothing, towels, and bed linens that have touched the skin (normal washing machine cycle using hot water and a high-heat dryer). Educate patients that itching may continue for days to weeks (3–4 weeks), nodules can persist for weeks to months after effective treatment,

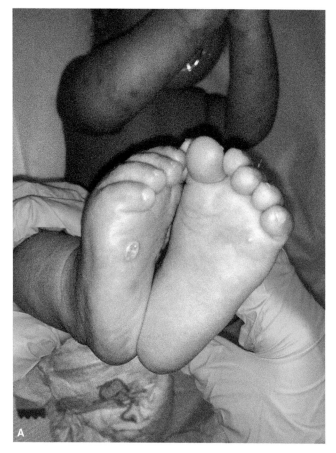

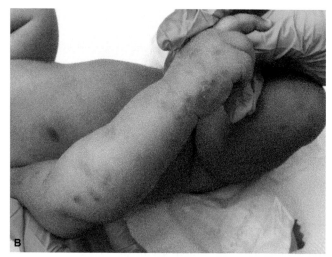

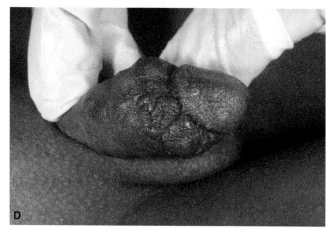

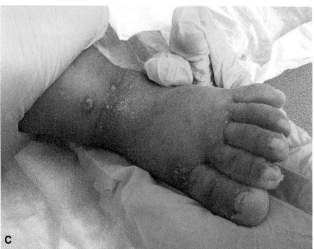

FIGURE 7.56 ▪ Infantile Scabies. Infants commonly have lesions on the palms, soles, and head, and lesions may also involve genitalia. (**A**) Note the vesicular lesions on the sole, which may be seen in babies but are uncommon in older ages. (**B**) Erythematous papules and papulovesicles on the arm extending to the dorsal hand. (**C**) A bullous lesion of the ankle as well as involvement of the dorsal foot and toes. (**D**) Involvement of the penis. (Photo contributors: Sharon A. Glick, MD [A–C], and Binita R. Shah, MD [D].)

and continued application of medication is unnecessary and worsens itching by causing irritation (*overtreatment must be avoided*). Children may return to school or childcare after completing treatment. Consider topical or systemic antibiotic therapy if secondary bacterial infection is suspected. Refer patients to their primary care physician to reexamine for treatment failures in 1 and 4 weeks. Advise isolation of patients with crusted or Norwegian scabies as they carry a high mite load with increased risk of spreading the infection. Several or sequential courses of topical permethrin or γ-benzene hexachloride may be necessary. A single dose of oral ivermectin may also be used.

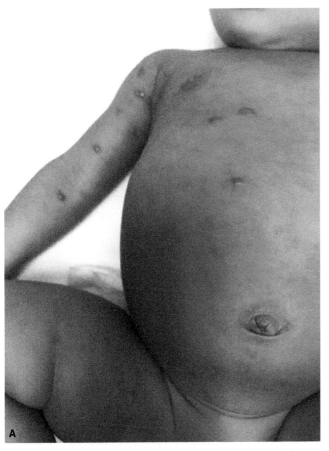
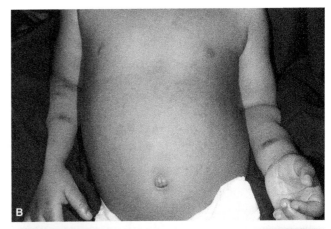
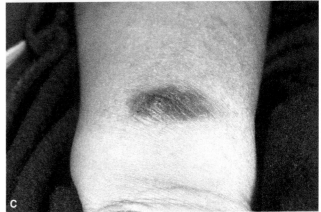

FIGURE 7.57 ■ Scabetic Nodules. (**A**) Scabetic nodules in 2-year-old child previously treated for scabies. (**B**) Scabetic nodule on the wrist of a different infant with scabies and a close-up of the nodule (**C**). (Photo contributors: Sharon A. Glick, MD [A], and Binita R. Shah, MD [B,C].)

Pearls

1. Scabies is an intensely pruritic, erythematous, generalized papular eruption.
2. The presence of a similar rash in other family members is an important clue.
3. Interdigital web lesions are less commonly seen in children.
4. Young infants may have hyperpigmented nodular lesions, especially along the axillary line.
5. Use of bland lubricants or oral antihistamines and topical corticosteroids can help relieve itch.
6. Treatment failures are usually due to failure to treat all the contacts (exposed individuals) simultaneously.

TINEA VERSICOLOR

Clinical Summary

Tinea versicolor is a common superficial skin infection caused by the dimorphic fungus *Malassezia furfur* whose yeast forms are called *Pityrosporum ovale* and *Pityrosporum orbicular*. The organism is part of the normal skin flora and appears in highest numbers in areas with increased sebaceous gland activity. Predisposing factors include malnutrition, burns, immunosuppressive or corticosteroid therapy, Cushing syndrome, and pregnancy. Excess heat and humidity and oily skin or application of oils (eg, cocoa butter, bath oil) on children can lead to yeast overgrowth. The yeast is transmitted by personal contact during periods of scaling. Fungal elements may also be retained in frequently worn garments that are in contact with the skin. Although tinea versicolor is more common in adolescents and young adults (years of higher sebaceous gland activity), it may occur in prepubertal children and infants. The diagnosis is made clinically. It is characterized by multiple small, circular macules of various colors (white, pink, or brown) with scales. Although lesions are typically reddish-brown in light-skinned patients, they can be either hypopigmented (off-white to white) or hyperpigmented (brown) in dark-skinned individuals. Distribution of lesions is highly characteristic, with the upper chest being the most common site of involvement. The back, shoulder, and neck are also often affected. In children, the forehead may be involved. While usually asymptomatic, mild pruritus may be present. Wood's lamp examination may demonstrate yellow-green fluorescence. Scraping the lesions lightly with a surgical blade followed by potassium hydroxide (KOH) examination may show numerous short, rod-shaped hyphae mixed with round spores in grapelike clusters ("chopped spaghetti-and-meatballs" appearance).

Emergency Department Treatment and Disposition

Various topical treatment options include selenium sulfide 2.5% lotion or shampoo. This should to be applied over affected areas and washed off after 10 to 15 minutes daily for 1 week followed by monthly applications for 3 months. Topical antifungal agents (eg, miconazole, clotrimazole, ketoconazole) may also be applied to the affected areas 1 to 2 times a day for 2 to 4 weeks or until clinically inactive. For extensive disease, oral antifungal therapy may be offered. Itraconazole (dose: 200 mg once daily for 5 days) can be used. Alternatively, fluconazole (300 mg) weekly for 2 weeks may be taken. For improved efficacy, patients are instructed to take the medication and then engage in sweat-producing exercise followed by a minimum 12-hour refrain from bathing to allow excretion of the medication onto the skin. The use of oral ketoconazole has fallen out of favor and is now typically avoided due its black-box warning. Recurrence rates of tinea versicolor vary from 15% to 60%. Monthly prophylaxis with 50% propylene glycol in water, selenium shampoo, or azole creams can help prevent recurrences.

Pearls

1. Lesions may be a variety of colors including pink, tan, or white (hypopigmented).
2. The rash begins insidiously and spreads over months to years.
3. Recurrence is high, especially in humid environments, and is considered the rule rather than the exception.
4. Advise patients to exercise one-half hour after taking the oral medication so that the medication may enter the sweat glands for optimal localized treatment.
5. Inform patients that pigmentary changes may take months to resolve even though the treatment was successful.

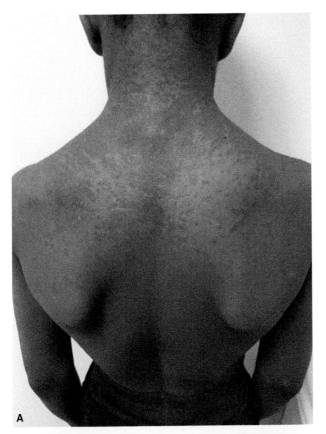

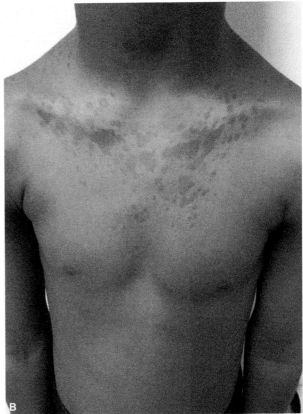

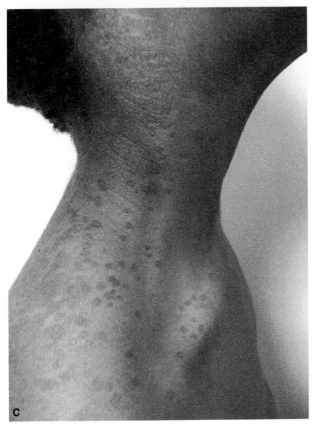

FIGURE 7.58 ■ Tinea Versicolor. Although the back and chest are the most common locations (**A, B**), tinea versicolor can also affect the neck (**C**), face, and arms, as shown here in a teenager. (Photo contributor: Sharon A. Glick, MD.)

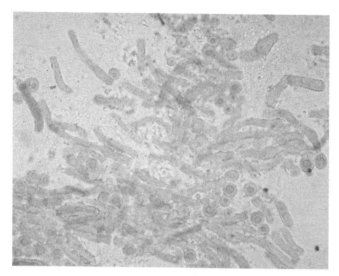

FIGURE 7.59 ■ Tinea Versicolor. KOH preparation demonstrating filamentous hyphae and spores ("spaghetti-and-meatballs") appearance characteristic of tinea versicolor. (Reproduced with permission from Mei Kane KS, Bissonette J, Boden HP, et al. *Color Atlas & Synopsis of Pediatric Dermatology*. McGraw-Hill Education; New York, NY, 2002.)

Clinical Summary

Tinea capitis is a highly contagious fungal scalp infection transmitted by humans and animals. Tinea capitis is more common among African American children than among other racial groups and occurs most commonly in areas of poverty and crowded living conditions. Preschool children (age 3–7 years) are most commonly affected; however, it is increasingly being recognized in adults, infants, and neonates. Infection may be transmitted by sharing personal items such as combs, brushes, blankets, telephones, hats, pillowcases, and barber's shears. Asymptomatic classmates or household members also spread the infection (spores are shed in air in the vicinity of the patient). Thus, tinea of the scalp may be contagious by direct contact or from contaminated fomites. Hair loss occurs because hyphae grow within the shaft, rendering it fragile, so that the hair strands break off 1 to 2 mm above the scalp. Diagnosis is clinical; however, KOH preparation of a diseased hair or fungal culture on dermatophyte test media may aid in diagnosis. When a kerion is present, bacterial culture should be included to exclude superinfection. Complications of tinea capitis include lymphadenitis, bacterial pyoderma, permanent scarring alopecia in severe untreated cases, tinea corporis, and secondary bacterial infection. The presence of an occipital lymph node can aid in diagnosis and is considered by some to be pathognomonic.

Emergency Department Treatment and Disposition

Topical antifungal agents are ineffective, and systemic therapy is required. Griseofulvin is first-line treatment at 20 to 25 mg/kg/day once or twice daily. Advise patients to take the medication with milk or a fatty meal to aid absorption and to continue treatment for 6 weeks or 2 weeks after clinical

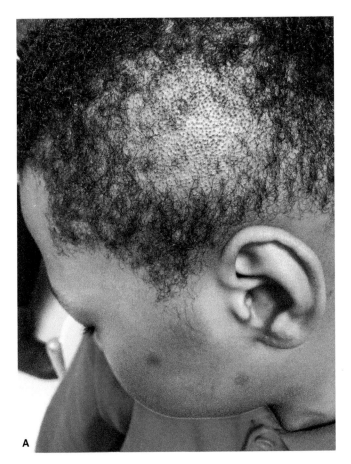

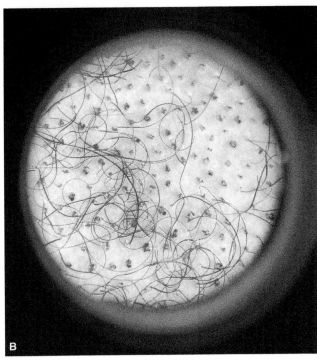

FIGURE 7.60 ■ Tinea Capitis. (**A**) "Black dot" appearance typically seen with infection from *Trichophyton tonsurans*. Arthrospores inside the shafts of infected hairs weaken the hair and causes it to break off at or below the scalp surface, resulting in the "black dot" appearance of the surface. (**B**) Black dot tinea under dermoscopy. (Photo contributor: Sharon A. Glick, MD.)

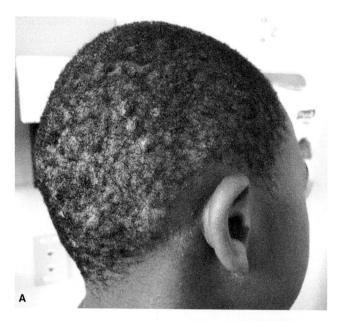

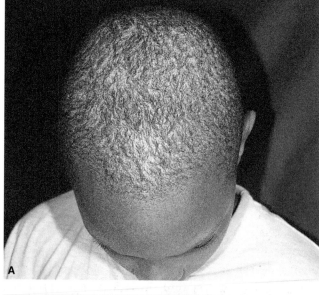

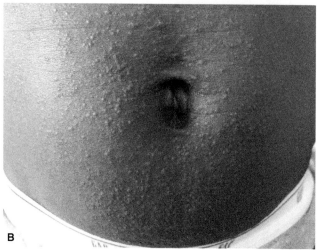

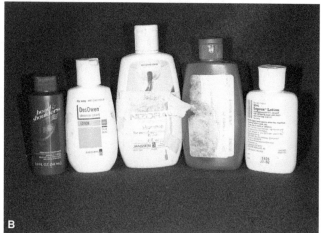

FIGURE 7.61 ■ Tinea Capitis. (**A**) A school-aged boy with tinea capitis resulting in scalp nodules. Occipital lymph node can be appreciated. (**B**) Id reaction. A diffuse monomorphic papulovesicular rash over his trunk, arms, face, and neck consistent with id reaction was also present. (Photo contributor: Jeannette Jakus, MD.)

FIGURE 7.62 ■ Seborrheic Tinea Capitis. (**A**) Diffuse, fine, white adherent scaling on scalp resembling dandruff is seen in this child. Hair loss is minimal with this form of infection. (**B**) Antidandruff medications that were used to treat this child are shown. Patients with this type of tinea are often misdiagnosed and get several antidandruff medications prior to specific antifungal therapy. (Photo contributor: Binita R. Shah, MD.)

resolution of inflammation (overall duration may vary from 6 to 12 weeks). Laboratory monitoring is usually not necessary in a healthy child. Refractory cases may due to drug resistance, poor compliance, or reinfection. Newer antifungals that may be used include itraconazole, fluconazole, or terbinafine. Laboratory monitoring may be necessary when using these medications. Prednisone therapy can dramatically resolve severe inflammation of a kerion. Typical dosing is 1 mg/kg/day for 1 to 2 weeks to calm the inflammation. If bacterial

superinfection in suspected, add oral antibiotics (eg, cephalexin) for the first week of treatment. Antifungal shampoo (eg, selenium sulfide 2.5% or ketoconazole 2%) can be added as adjunct therapy 2 to 3 times per week. Refer patients to their primary care physician for reexamination in 4 weeks. The patient can return to school once treatment is started. Advise patients to use their own towels, hairbrush, comb, and hats and not to share such items with others in order to prevent recurrence or transmission to others. *Trichophyton tonsurans*

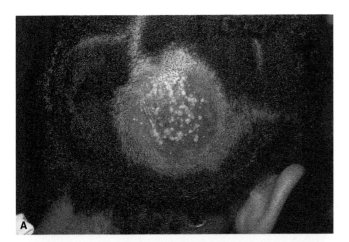

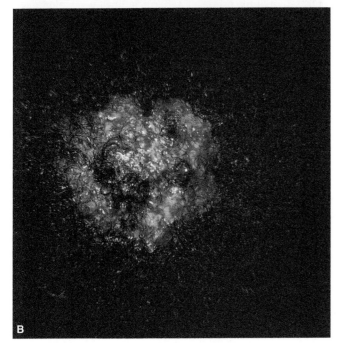

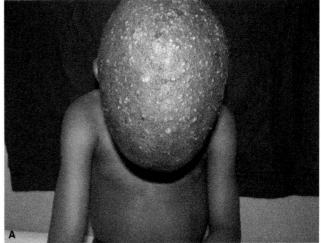

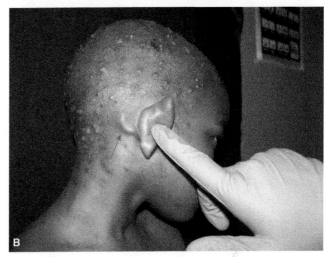

FIGURE 7.64 ■ Pustular Tinea Capitis. Diffuse involvement of the scalp and pustules (**A**) associated with postauricular lymphadenopathy (**B**, arrow) are seen. (Photo contributor: Binita R. Shah, MD.)

FIGURE 7.63 ■ Kerion; Inflammatory Tinea Capitis. (**A**) Indurated, boggy, painful mass with pustules on the scalp. (**B**) Indurated, boggy, painful mass appearing as an abscess on the scalp in a different patient. (Photo contributor: Binita R. Shah, MD.)

lesions may occur outside of the scalp in patients, their families, and their close friends and can serve as a reservoir for reinfection. Evaluation of all siblings or close contacts in the family should be advised.

Pearls

1. Diffuse, patchy, or discrete alopecia; scalp scaling; scalp pruritus; and lymphadenopathy (postauricular or occipital) are characteristic findings.

2. "Black dot" appearance of affected areas represents hairs broken off at surface of scalp.

3. Clinical variants include noninflammatory, inflammatory (kerion), seborrheic, and pustular types.

4. Kerion is characterized by an indurated, boggy, painful scalp and represents the patient's immune response as suggested by a positive skin test to *Trichophyton* antigen.

5. Id reaction, characterized by an acute generalized papulovesicular eruption, may be seen and is commonly misdiagnosed as griseofulvin allergic reaction as the rash frequently coincides with the start of griseofulvin treatment.

Clinical Summary

Tinea corporis is a dermatophyte infection of the body involving the face (excluding the beard area in men), trunk (excluding the groin), or extremities (excluding palms and soles). As the common name "ringworm" implies, it is an annular lesion that spreads peripherally with an active papulovesicular border and central clearing. Tinea corporis is seen in all age groups and may be present concurrently with tinea capitis. It is most commonly seen in warm climates. Infection is transmitted by infected scales from skin lesions of an infected person or from contact with infected scales or hairs deposited on environmental surfaces. *Microsporum canis* infections are usually acquired from infected pets (especially kittens and puppies). The diagnosis of tinea corporis is made clinically, and no tests are required. Direct microscopic examination with KOH preparation or skin scrapings from the scales of the advancing border inoculated on fungal culture (eg, dermatophyte test media) may aid in diagnosis. The differential diagnosis includes other annular plaques, including nummular eczema, pityriasis rosea (herald patch), granuloma annulare, contact dermatitis, psoriasis, seborrhea, tinea versicolor, systemic lupus erythematosus, and erythema chronicum migrans.

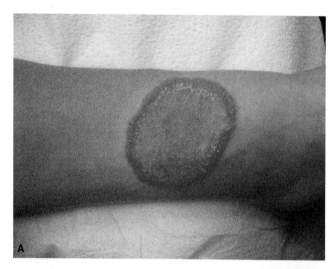

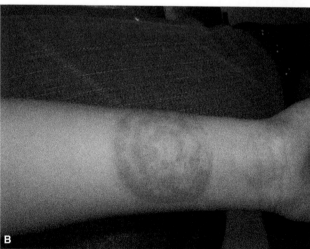

FIGURE 7.65 ■ Tinea Corporis. (**A**) As the name "ringworm" implies, the lesion is an annular lesion that spreads at the periphery with an active, erythematous, scaly, advancing border with a clearing in the center seen in 2 different patients. (**B**) A ring within a ring (1 or 2 rings within a larger ring) may be seen. (Photo contributors: Barry Hahn, MD [A], and Mark Silverberg, MD [B].)

Emergency Department Treatment and Disposition

Topical antifungals are generally effective for treatment. They should be applied twice daily for 10 to 14 days (or until lesions clear) and should be applied at least 2 cm beyond the advancing edge of the skin lesion. Treatment should be continued for 1 more week after clearing to ensure clinical cure. Examples of topical antifungals include the imidazoles (clotrimazole, miconazole, ketoconazole, econazole), allylamines (terbinafine and naftifine), and naphthiomates (tolnaftate). For extensive tinea corporis or if hair-bearing areas are involved, consider griseofulvin given orally with fatty food (dose: 15–20 mg/kg/day for 2–4 weeks).

Pearls

1. Tinea corporis consists of annular plaques with an active, scaly, raised, advancing border and central clearing.
2. Tinea corporis does not fluoresce with Wood's lamp.
3. Tinea incognito is a variant of tinea corporis seen after topical corticosteroid use (when mistaken for nummular eczema). Local immunosuppression causes a loss of characteristic clinical features such as scale and erythema and may make the diagnosis of tinea difficult.
4. Majocchi granuloma, most commonly caused by *Trichophyton rubrum*, is a deep-seeded granulomatous response to dermatophyte infection often due to trauma or use of potent topical steroids.

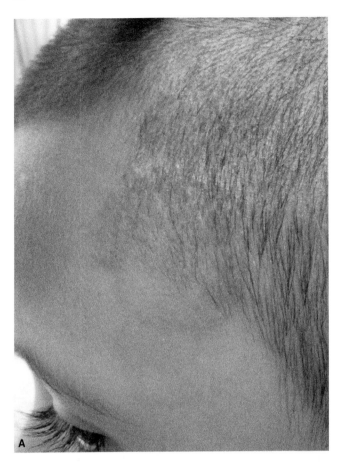

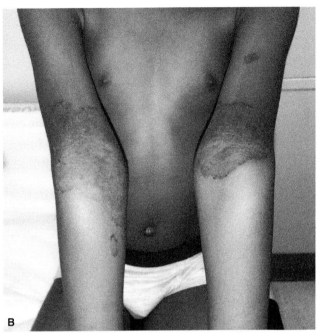

FIGURE 7.66 ■ Tinea Corporis. (**A**) Well-defined annular erythematous scaly plaque with papular border and central clearing on the forehead of a 6-year-old boy (tinea faciei). Because the lesion involved a hair-bearing area, this patient was treated with oral griseofulvin for 6 weeks. (**B**) Extensive tinea corporis involving the antecubital fossae of a boy. Patient was treated with oral antifungals due to extent of his condition with resolution on follow-up. (Photo contributors: Jeannette Jakus, MD [A], and Sharon A. Glick, MD [B].)

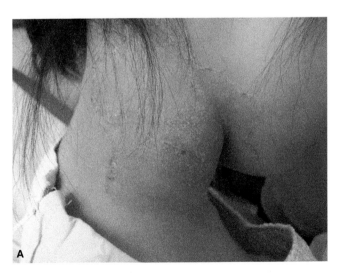

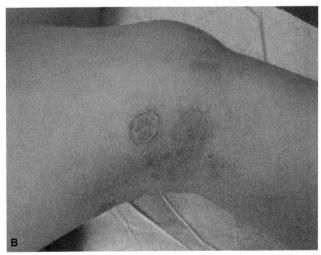

FIGURE 7.67 ■ Tinea Incognito. A 6-year-old girl treated with topical steroids for presumed eczema presented with an expanding lesion of the neck with an erythematous, scaly, raised border extending onto the chest and chin (**A**). Annular, erythematous scaly lesions with central clearing seen in the popliteal fossa (**B**). Cutaneous lesions resolved after 2 weeks of oral griseofulvin therapy. (Photo contributor: Morgan Rabach, MD.)

Clinical Summary

Tinea cruris is a fungal infection of the groin and upper thigh commonly seen in adolescents, young adults, and athletes and is rarely seen in children. Men are affected much more frequently than women. Predisposing factors include concomitant tinea pedis, obesity, a warm humid environment, sweating, and tight (exercise outfits) or wet clothing (bathing suits). The characteristic lesion of tinea cruris is a well-demarcated, erythematous plaque with an active scaly papulovesicular border and central clearing. Infection usually begins in the crural folds and advances to the thigh, forming half-moon–shaped plaques that may extend to the buttock and gluteal cleft. Unlike candidal infection, tinea rarely involves the scrotum or penis. The diagnosis is made clinically. When unsure, diagnosis can be made under direct microscopic examination with KOH preparation from the scales of the advancing border demonstrating hyphae, budding yeasts, or arthrospores. Skin scrapings from the affected area and inoculated on fungal culture (eg, dermatophyte test media) can help identify the specific dermatophyte. The differential diagnosis includes intertrigo, candida, erythrasma, psoriasis, seborrheic dermatitis, or allergic contact dermatitis.

Emergency Department Treatment and Disposition

Topical antifungal therapy with econazole cream twice daily for 2 to 4 weeks is considered first-line treatment of tinea cruris. The use of topical steroids or antifungal preparations combined with high-potency topical steroids should be avoided in the groin as this may quickly lead to skin atrophy or other steroid-related changes. For severe cases, consider use of a short course of griseofulvin. Advise patients to wear loose-fitting underwear. Antifungal powder can be applied daily to help prevent reinfection. If present, tinea pedis should be treated and patients should be instructed to put on socks first before their underwear in order to avoid carrying the fungal elements from the infected feet up to the groin area.

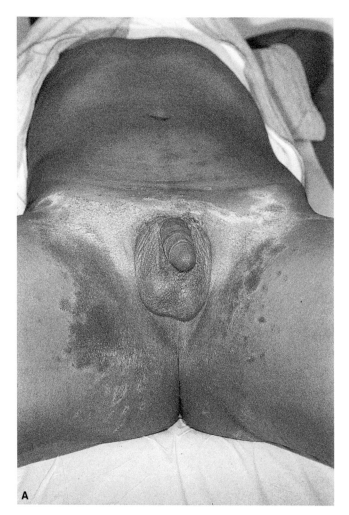

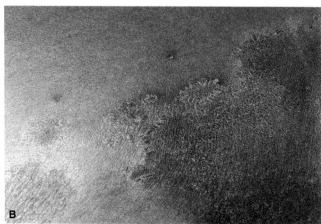

FIGURE 7.68 ■ Tinea Cruris. (**A**) Bilateral, irregular, half-moon–shaped, sharply bordered patches with hyperpigmented, scaly centers are seen. Note the absence of involvement of the scrotum or penis (an important distinction from candidiasis). (**B**) Close-up showing a well-defined advancing border with scaling. KOH preparation of the scale was positive for numerous hyphae. (Photo contributor: Binita R. Shah, MD.)

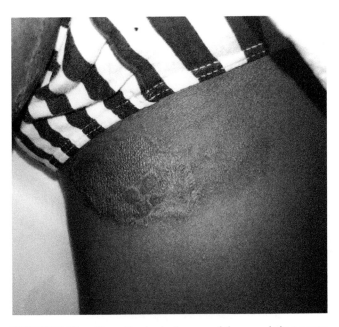

FIGURE 7.69 ■ Tinea Cruris. A close-up of tinea cruris in a young girl is shown. She had bilateral involvement with associated id reaction. (Photo contributor: Jeannette Jakus, MD.)

Pearls

1. Tinea cruris and tinea pedis are commonly seen together in the same patient.
2. Typically, tinea pedis precedes the groin infection (because of spread of infection from the infected feet to the groin).
3. Erythrasma and candidiasis may coexist with tinea cruris.

Clinical Summary

Tinea pedis is a fungal infection of the feet common in adolescents and uncommon in young children. Infection is acquired by contact with skin scales containing fungi or with fungi in damp areas (eg, swimming pools, locker room floors, communal baths, nail salons). Infection in 1 family member tends to spread throughout the household, and communicability persists as long as the infection is present. Once infection is established, the individual becomes a carrier and is more susceptible to recurrences. Predisposing factors include hot, humid weather (summer months) and occlusive footwear. Interdigital infection is almost always present and is characterized by foul odor, pruritus, and dry and fissuring web spaces with white scaling and maceration. Fissuring of the plantar foot surface may be seen. Chronic infection is characterized by diffuse scaling of both soles and occasionally 1 hand. Infection may be associated with a hypersensitivity id reaction (erythematous papulovesicular eruption on legs, trunk, and arms). Secondary infection may occur, as macerated skin serves as portal of entry for bacteria. The diagnosis is made clinically. If unsure, a KOH wet mount may demonstrate fungal elements, which can help differentiate tinea pedis from other conditions. Skin scrapings inoculated on fungal culture (eg, dermatophyte test media) help in confirming the diagnosis. The differential diagnosis includes contact or shoe dermatitis, AD, juvenile plantar dermatosis, dyshidrotic eczema, and candida infection.

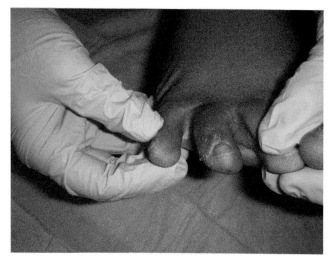

FIGURE 7.70 ■ Tinea Pedis. Maceration and scale in the interdigital web spaces characteristic of tinea pedis. (Photo contributor: Sharon A. Glick, MD.)

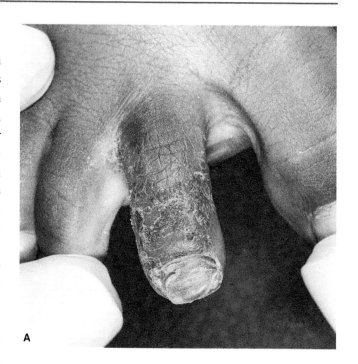

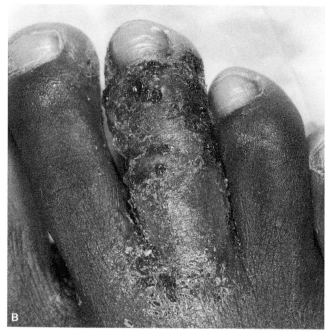

FIGURE 7.71 ■ Tinea Pedis. (**A, B**) The toe web space with macerated scale and inflammation that has extended from the web area onto the dorsum of the foot is seen in 2 different patients. (Photo contributor: Binita R. Shah, MD.)

Emergency Department Treatment and Disposition

Tinea pedis runs a chronic course with frequent exacerbations occurring with hot, humid weather and exercise. General

352

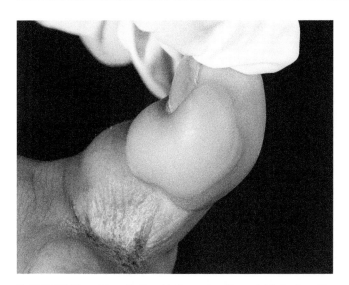

FIGURE 7.72 ■ Tinea Pedis with Secondary Bacterial Infection. The toe web space with macerated scale is seen with a bullous impetigo secondary to *Staphylococcus aureus* infection. (Photo contributor: Binita R. Shah, MD.)

instructions for treatment and to prevent recurrences include good foot hygiene. Advise patients to keep feet cool and dry (especially between the toes), apply absorbent antifungal foot powder daily to help prevent moisture, avoid occlusive footwear (shoes that promote warmth and sweating encouraging fungal growth), use wider shoes (reduces sweating and irritation), use cotton socks instead of nylon or other fabrics (interferes with dissipation of moisture), change wet socks as soon as possible, and dry the groin area before drying feet to avoid inoculating fungal scales into the groin. Topical antifungal preparations are the treatment of choice for tinea pedis. For example, miconazole, clotrimazole, or terbinafine applied twice a day or econazole, ketoconazole, or naftifine applied once a day for 2 to 3 weeks is generally effective. For hyperkeratotic diffuse involvement of the soles, oral treatment may be necessary. Terbinafine given orally for 2 to 6 weeks or griseofulvin given orally for 6 to 8 weeks is

generally well tolerated but should be avoided or used with caution in patients with liver disease. Acute vesicular tinea pedis, a rare acute inflammatory form of tinea pedis, should be treated with griseofulvin given orally for 6 to 8 weeks. Burow's solution–soaked wet compresses applied for 30 minutes several times a day may provide symptomatic relief. Topical antifungal agents can be used once macerated tissue is dried. If secondary bacterial infection is present, antibiotics should be given. Treatment of id reaction includes wet dressings and low-potency topical steroids (rarely, a short course of prednisone therapy). It is important to inquire about other family members with a similar rash and recommend treatment of all infected family members. Advise patients with active infection to avoid swimming pools in order to prevent spread of the infection. Treat tinea cruris simultaneously, if present. Consider and treat toenail involvement when treating tinea pedis because toenail infection can serve as a reservoir for the reinfection of the rest of the foot.

Pearls

1. Tinea pedis is the most common fungal infection in adolescents and adults.
2. Tinea pedis is uncommon in children and should not be confused with eczema or contact dermatitis. Nonetheless, tinea pedis should be considered in the differential diagnosis of foot dermatitis in children, particularly when other household members are affected.
3. Tinea pedis commonly occurs in association with tinea cruris and tinea unguium.
4. Interdigital scaling and fissuring, particularly between the third, fourth, and fifth toes, are clues to diagnosis.
5. "Moccasin-type" or "dry-type" tinea refers to diffuse hyperkeratosis of the soles seen with chronic infection.
6. Look for 2 feet and 1 hand involvement (two feet-one hand syndrome).

TINEA UNGUIUM

Clinical Summary

Fungal infection of the nails is called tinea unguium or onychomycosis. It can be due to *Trichophyton* species, *Epidermophyton floccosum*, or nondermatophyte species such as *C albicans*. Although uncommon, it may be seen in healthy children whose parents have tinea pedis or unguium. Nail infection may occur simultaneously with hand or foot tinea or may occur as an isolated phenomenon. Trauma may predispose to infection. Toenails are more commonly affected than fingernails, and there are 4 patterns of nail infection seen:

1. Distal subungual onychomycosis (infection starting with the free edge of the nail and extending proximally)
2. Proximal subungual onychomycosis (infection starting through the proximal nail fold and extending to the nail plate from below)
3. White superficial onychomycosis (diffuse or speckled white discoloration of nail surface)
4. Candidal onychomycosis (seen in chronic mucocutaneous candidiasis or AIDS)

Fungi are found in the nail plate and in the cornified cells of the nail bed. With clinical suspicion, direct microscopic

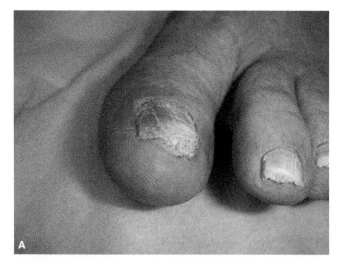

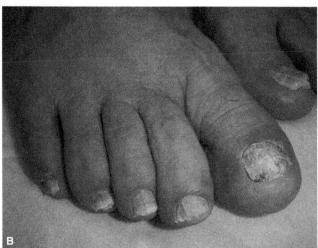

FIGURE 7.74 ■ Tinea Unguium. (**A**) Distal onycholysis, yellow discoloration, and subungual debris are the classic clinical presentation of chronic tinea infection of the nails in an adult patient. (**B**) Extensive involvement of all toenails is best treated with oral antifungals. Patients are also advised to trim and file the nails. (Photo contributor: Heather Schultz, MD.)

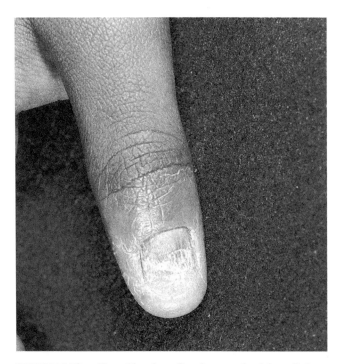

FIGURE 7.73 ■ Tinea Unguium. Onychomycosis of the nail. In an advanced case, infection progresses from the distal end to involve the entire nail plate and the nail plate often separates from the nailbed. (Photo contributor: Binita R. Shah, MD.)

examination of nail clippings or debris in KOH preparation can help in diagnosis. Nail clippings or crumbling debris from under several nails and from different parts of the infected nail can be collected using a curet. Inoculation of these materials on DTM (dermatophyte test media) or Sabouraud media will identify the causative dermatophyte. A periodic acid–Schiff (PAS) stain of an infected nail clipping will show hyphae. The differential diagnosis of tinea unguium includes nail psoriasis, eczema, trauma, leukonychia (white spots or bands on nail), habitual picking of proximal nail fold, and pachyonychia congenita.

Emergency Department Treatment and Disposition

In general, patients will need systemic antifungal therapy; however, newer generation topical solutions claiming good efficacy are now available. Topical antifungal creams and lotions generally do not penetrate the nail plate and are therefore not considered effective except for controlling inflammation at the nail folds. Long-term oral therapy is often followed by reinfection when the oral medication is discontinued. Prolonged use of a topical antifungal agent after clinical response to an oral agent may prevent nail reinfection. Oral antifungal agents that are used for treating onychomycosis include fluconazole, itraconazole, or terbinafine. Given the risk of hepatoxicity with these drugs, it is recommended to obtain a confirmatory (PAS-positive) stain from nail clipping and baseline hepatic function test prior to initiation. The newly approved topicals, efinaconazole and tavaborole, may be effective but must be used for prolonged periods of time (48 weeks or more). These may be a nice option for patients in whom oral antifungals are contraindicated. Other modalities that help in the resolution of infection include mechanical reduction of the infected nail plate with a nail clipper with pliers-type handles (removal of hard, thick debris). Nonsurgical avulsion of symptomatic dystrophic nails with a urea compound may be helpful. Finally, surgical removal of painful or extremely infected nails (eg, great toenail) may be necessary.

Pearls

1. Tinea unguium results in nails that are opaque, thickened, crumbled, and cracked.
2. It typically affects toenails more than fingernails.
3. Infected nails often coexist with normal-appearing nails.

Clinical Summary

Warts are epithelial tumors of the skin and mucous membranes caused by infection with human papillomaviruses (HPVs). HPV strains causing nongenital warts are distinct from those causing anogenital infections. Nongenital warts include the common skin wart (verruca vulgaris), flat warts (verruca plana), plantar warts (verruca plantaris), periungual warts, and threadlike (filiform) warts. Mucous membrane warts include anogenital (condylomata acuminata), oral, nasal, or conjunctival warts and laryngeal papillomatosis. Warts can spread from direct contact or by autoinoculation. The incubation period is estimated to range from 1 month to several years. Warts are commonly seen in school-age children (except condyloma acuminata) and young adults. Laryngeal papillomas occur as the result of aspiration of infectious secretions during passage through an infected birth canal. Special attention should be given to genital warts in children as these may occur after inoculation during birth through an infected birth canal, as a result of sexual abuse, or from incidental spread from cutaneous warts on caregivers. Local trauma promotes infection with the virus; thus, warts are more common on hands, fingers, elbows, and plantar surfaces. Other predisposing underlying conditions for developing warts include infection with HIV, lymphomas, and immunosuppressive therapy.

Diagnosis is clinical; HPV cannot be cultured, and rarely, a biopsy is indicated when a diagnosis is in doubt. Differential diagnosis includes molluscum contagiosum, condyloma lata,

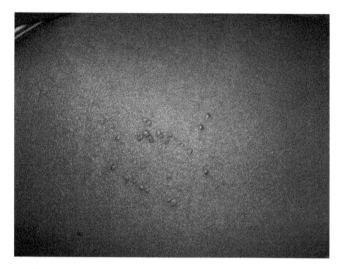

FIGURE 7.76 ■ Flat Warts. Grouped and linear, flat-topped, hyperpigmented papules on the back of a child. The linear pattern may represent koebnerization of warts after scratching. (Photo contributor: Sharon A. Glick, MD.)

skin tags, calluses and corns, lichen planus, lichen nitidus, and squamous cell carcinoma.

Emergency Department Treatment and Disposition

The natural course is highly variable, with about two-thirds of warts resolving spontaneously within 2 years, whereas others may last years or a lifetime. Therapy is decided based on

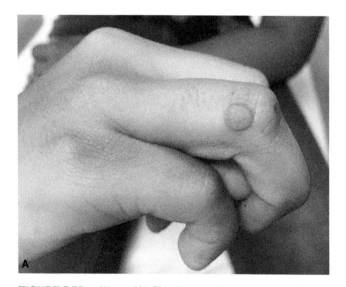

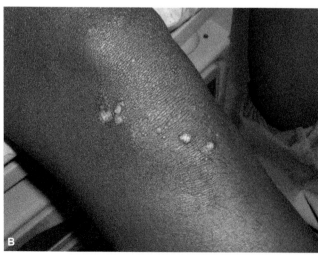

FIGURE 7.75 ■ Warts. (**A**) Classic-appearing common wart on the finger. Common warts tend to favor the fingers and palms. (**B**) Multiple verrucous papules on the knee of a different girl. (Photo contributors: Jeannette Jakus, MD [A], Sharon A. Glick, MD [B].)

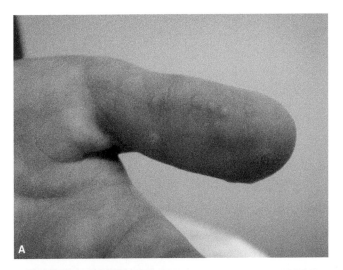

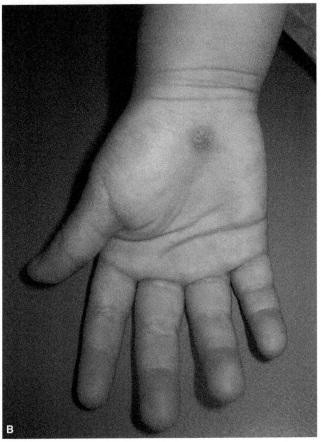

the duration, location, and severity of the warts. Conservative management with watchful waiting may be considered. Educate parents and patients that several treatment sessions are usually required before a cure is achieved. Treatment options for warts that do not resolve spontaneously rely on chemical or physical destruction of the infected epithelium. These treatments include topical application of salicylic acid solution, patches, or plasters (eg, Duofilm, Compound W, Mediplast, Occlusal-HP), tretinoin gel or cream (flat warts), and topical imiquimod. Duct tape, alone or in combination with imiquimod or salicylic acid, can be very effective. Patients should be advised to soak the wart in warm water for 5 minutes before application of medication to remove loose, dry skin and allow the medication to penetrate more effectively. Therapy may be required for up to 12 weeks or more. Patients with warts on the face, periungual warts, large plantar warts, or warts resistant to conservative therapy should be referred to a dermatologist for other therapeutic considerations (eg, cryotherapy, electrodesiccation, laser, or curettage).

Pearls

1. Cutaneous warts are benign infections and self-limiting in a majority of cases.
2. Common warts occur most frequently in children and adolescents. Anogenital warts are most common in young sexually active patients.
3. Genital warts are the most common viral sexually transmitted disease in the United States.
4. Warts will often resolve spontaneously without treatment, and watchful waiting may be done in asymptomatic patients (about two-thirds disappear spontaneously within 2 years); however, failure to treat incurs a risk of spread to other sites.

FIGURE 7.77 ■ Warts. (**A**) Multiple warts on the thumb of a teenager. Black dots seen on the distal lesion represent thrombosed vessels characteristic of common warts. (**B**) Verrucous papule on the palm of a young boy. (Photo contributors: Jeannette Jakus, MD [A], and Sharon A. Glick, MD [B].)

MOLLUSCUM CONTAGIOSUM

Clinical Summary

Molluscum contagiosum is a viral skin infection caused by the poxvirus molluscum contagiosum and characterized by 2- to 5-mm discrete pearly white papules with central umbilication. The face, eyelids, neck, axillae, trunk, and thigh are the most common sites, and occurrence is most common in children between the ages of 3 and 16 years. Swimming pools and communal bathing may be predisposing conditions. Humans are the only known source of the virus, which is spread by direct contact or from autoinoculation via fomites (eg, towels). Predisposing conditions include AD, HIV infection, and other immunodeficiency states including leukemia. Unilateral conjunctivitis may develop with lesions located on or near the eyelids. Rarely, lesions may appear on the conjunctiva or cornea.

Diagnosis is usually made clinically. If in doubt, Wright or Giemsa staining of a crushed papule shows characteristic intracytoplasmic inclusions. Skin biopsy reveals epithelial cells with large intracytoplasmic inclusions (molluscum bodies). A central white core seen on magnification can aid diagnosis. Differential diagnosis includes nevi, acne, milia, warts, or HSV.

Emergency Department Treatment and Disposition

Molluscum contagiosum is a self-limited disease, with an average duration of lesions lasting about 6 to 9 months. However, lesions can persist for years, can spread to distant sites, and may be transmitted to others. In young children and in

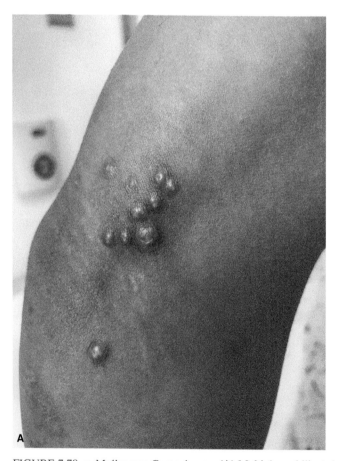
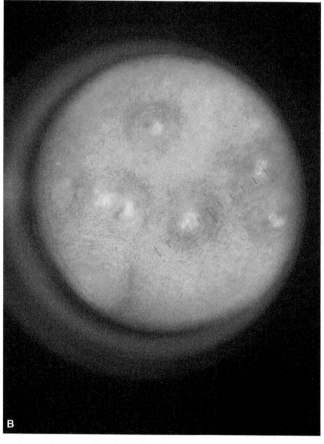

FIGURE 7.78 ■ Molluscum Contagiosum. (**A**) Multiple umbilicated papules on the arm of a child. (**B**) On dermatoscopy magnification, a central white core representing the "molluscum body" can be visualized and may aid in diagnosis. (Photo contributor: Jeannette Jakus, MD.)

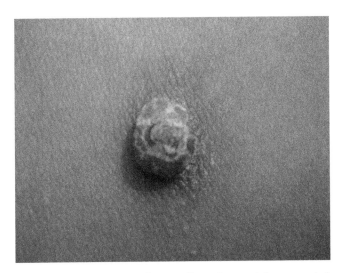

FIGURE 7.79 ▪ Giant Molluscum Contagiosum. A large, crusted, dome-shaped papule with central umbilication on the back of a young boy. Giant molluscum occurs more commonly in immunosuppressed patients, but can occur in any host. It is more difficult to treat and may require surgical excision. This patient also had several typical-appearing molluscum papules on his neck. (Photo contributor: Jeannette Jakus, MD.)

lesions involving sensitive areas (ie, around the eye), a wait-and-see approach should be encouraged. Enlarging or spreading lesions and genital lesions should be definitively treated to prevent spread through sexual contact. Treatment depends on the number and size of lesions, age of the patient, and availability of treatment methods. Mechanical removal of the central core of each lesion with a needle, a sharp curette, or a comedo extractor (lesions involute faster after they are irritated) is often quite effective. Small papules can be removed with a curette with or without local anesthesia (EMLA cream applied 30–60 minutes before treatment effectively prevents pain of curettage). However, this technique should not be used in cosmetically significant areas as scar tissue may form. Topical treatment options include tincture of iodine, salicylic acid (applied each day with or without tape occlusion), tretinoin gel or cream (applied once or twice daily to individual small lesions), or cantharidin (applied in office to each lesion without occlusion and washed off after 2–6 hours). It is important to warn parents that these treatments cause irritation and may lead to blistering. Topical treatments should be applied with a Q-tip to prevent irritation of the surrounding unaffected skin and may require several weeks before results are seen. Patients can alternatively be referred to a dermatologist for other therapeutic modalities that include cantharidin application, manual curettage of large lesions, cryotherapy with liquid nitrogen, electrocautery, or carbon dioxide laser therapy. Finally, patients should be advised to avoid shared baths and towels until the infection is clear.

Pearls

1. Molluscum lesions are benign and self-limited. Lesions can regress spontaneously; treatment may prevent auto-inoculation and spread to other persons.
2. Molluscum lesions may be associated with other venereal diseases.
3. Molluscum lesions are often misdiagnosed as warts or HSV lesions. Visualization of a central white core on magnification may aid in diagnosis. If a dermatoscope is not available, an otoscope may be used.
4. Genital molluscum contagiosum in children may be a manifestation of sexual abuse and should be investigated.
5. Although umbilication of molluscum papules is characteristic, early lesions may not show this feature.

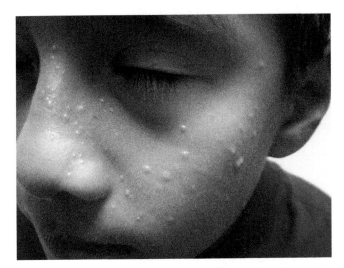

FIGURE 7.80 ▪ Trichoepitheliomas; Differential Diagnosis of Molluscum Contagiosum. Multiple trichoepitheliomas on the face of a 7-year-old boy who was treated for over 4 years for molluscum. This entity should be considered in the differential diagnosis of recalcitrant molluscum. (Photo contributor: Falguni Asrani, MD.)

Clinical Summary

Acropustulosis of infancy is a recurrent, self-limited condition of young children and infants. Most cases begin in infants <10 months old and may recur for weeks to years. It is rarely seen in children older than 3 years of age. Acropustulosis typically affects the acral surfaces—mostly palms and soles and particularly the lateral surfaces of the hands and feet. Pustules may rarely extend to the wrists, ankles, and dorsal surfaces of the hands and feet. Lesions present as erythematous macules and papules and progress to vesicles and pustules over a period of 7 to 10 days. The rash is often intensely pruritic, and children often appear uncomfortable. Most cases resolve after 2 to 3 weeks, but recurrence is common and may occur as frequently as every few weeks to months. The etiology is unknown, although association with preceding scabies has been reported. Diagnosis is clinical. A smear of the vesicle contents reveals neutrophils and may include eosinophils.

Acropustulosis is self-limited and resolves usually by the time the child reaches 2 to 3 years of age. No long-term sequelae associated with this condition are known. Differential diagnosis includes other pustular and papulovesicular eruptions of infancy including pustular psoriasis, cutaneous candidiasis, dyshidrotic eczema, herpes infection, erythema toxicum neonatorum, transient neonatal pustular melanosis, and scabies infection.

Emergency Department Treatment and Disposition

Treatment is symptomatic for relief of itching. High-potency steroids are very effective and can be used safely in limited areas for short periods of time. Oral antihistamines such as diphenhydramine and hydroxyzine may also be helpful. Antibiotics should be considered if bacterial superinfection is suspected.

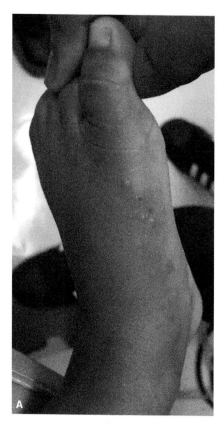
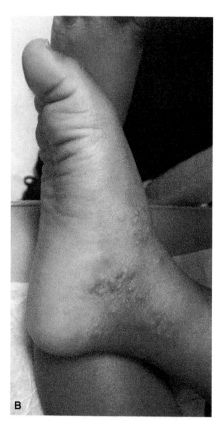

FIGURE 7.81 ■ Acropustulosis of Infancy. (**A, B**) Chronic, recurring, and pruritic eruption on the lateral surfaces of the feet of a young toddler. Lesions of acropustulosis tend to concentrate on the palms and soles and may extend to the ankles and wrists. Pruritus may be intense. (Photo contributor: Jeannette Jakus, MD.)

Pearls

1. Recurrent crops of acral lesions are considered the hallmark of this condition.
2. Patients with acropustulosis of infancy often get misdiagnosis as have scabies. Lack of a family member or contacts with similar rash is an important clue in differentiating the 2 entities.

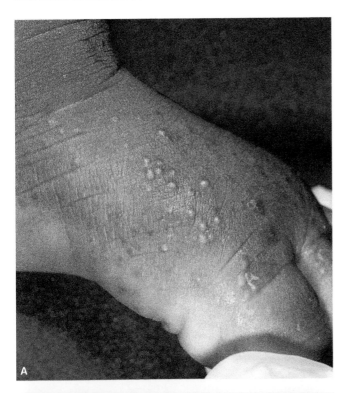

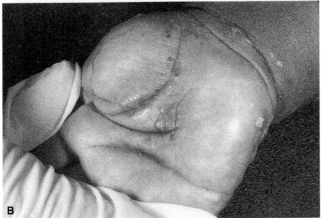

FIGURE 7.82 ▪ Scabies; Differential Diagnosis of Acropustulosis of Infancy. An infant with papulovesicular lesions on the foot (**A**) and palm (**B**). The babysitter had a similar rash involving the wrist and interdigital spaces. Infants with acropustulosis of infancy often get misdiagnosed as having scabies. As seen here, papulovesicular lesions of scabies also typically involve the palms and soles and are intensely pruritic. A history of similar rash in a family member or close contact often is an important clue for scabies. (Photo contributor: Binita R. Shah, MD.)

ERYTHEMA TOXICUM NEONATORUM

Clinical Summary

Erythema toxicum neonatorum (ETN) is a benign skin eruption of unknown etiology seen in the first few days of life in full-term neonates. The characteristic morphology consists of erythematous macules, papules, and pustules that develop between birth and 10 days of life and heal spontaneously within few weeks (about 2 weeks). The face, trunk, back, and extremities are typical sites; it usually spares the palms and soles. There is no mucosal involvement or any systemic complications or internal organ involvement. It often coexists with another benign neonatal skin eruption called transient neonatal pustular melanosis (TNPM; see Figure 7.107). The pustules in TNPM are sterile and need to be differentiated from other pustulosis of neonates, such as impetigo, candidiasis, and herpes infections. The diagnosis of ETN is clinical, and dermatology consultation may be indicated to differentiate this benign disorder from other neonatal pustulosis. Biopsy is rarely indicated; the best diagnostic test is a Wright stain or Tzanck smear from a pustule, which shows presence of multiple eosinophils. Peripheral eosinophilia may be present.

Emergency Department Treatment and Disposition

Recognition and prompt diagnosis of this eruption are the most important steps in the management. No treatment is needed except reassurance to the family because this is a benign, self-limited disorder. Aggressive diagnostic workup including unnecessary use of antibiotics can be avoided. Wright stain or Tzanck smear is the key to diagnosis. Dermatology consultation may be called if the diagnosis is unclear, and if indicated, bacterial, fungal, and viral cultures can be sent to exclude other infectious neonatal pustular conditions.

Pearls

1. ETN does not cause any "toxicity" as the name suggests, and the neonates are otherwise completely asymptomatic.
2. Skin lesions are pale or ivory-colored papules surrounded by blotchy erythema resembling flea bites.
3. It is not seen in premature newborns. It occurs in full-term newborns and is seen more commonly as the gestational age of the neonate increases.

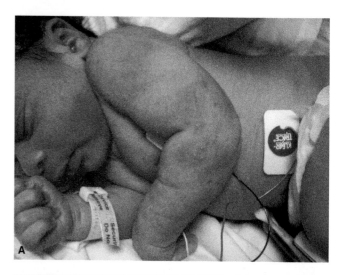

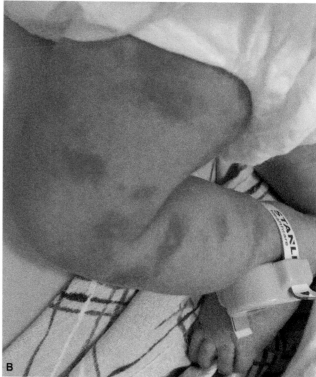

FIGURE 7.83 ■ Erythema Toxicum Neonatorum. (**A**) Erythematous macules topped with yellow-colored papules and pustules seen on the hand of a 3-day-old baby. Tzanck smear of the pustules showed multiple eosinophils. The lesions cleared spontaneously in several days. (**B**) Similar lesions seen on the leg of a different baby. (Photo contributors: Falguni Asrani, MD [A], and Miriam R. Lieberman, MD [B].)

Clinical Summary

Epidermolysis bullosa (EB) is a group of inherited (autosomal dominant or recessive) blistering disorders that occur in 1 in every 50,000 births. Presentation can range from mild to life threatening. Blistering often occurs in areas of trauma or friction. There are 3 major forms of EB: simplex, junctional, and dystrophic (classified based on the level of cleavage in the skin). EB simplex is the most common form. Blisters develop within the epidermis and generally do not lead to scarring. In junctional EB, cleavage occurs at the dermal-epidermal junction. In dystrophic EB, cleavage occurs within the dermis. Both of these forms of EB tend to be more severe and often lead to scarring. Aside from blistering of the skin, patients may experience internal involvement, including the GI and genitourinary tracts as well as ocular involvement. Esophageal, tracheal, and anal strictures may occur, along with retinal neovascularization. Patients may suffer from chronic malabsorption. Pyloric atresia is associated with 1 variant of junctional EB. Internal involvement (ie, strictures, pyloric atresia) should be considered in all patients presenting with dysphagia and/or dyspnea. Diagnosis is made by genetic testing and/or specialized immunofluorescence mapping to determine the level of skin cleavage and the presence of specific antibodies. Prognosis depends on the severity of disease. In patients with the most severe disease, death may occur as early as the first 2 years of life. Secondary infection with sepsis and failure to thrive are the most common causes of death in patients with EB.

Emergency Department Treatment and Disposition

Refer the patient to a dermatologist for ongoing care that is palliative and supportive. Parents should also be referred for

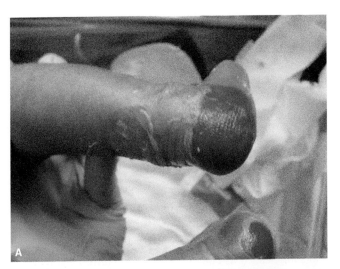

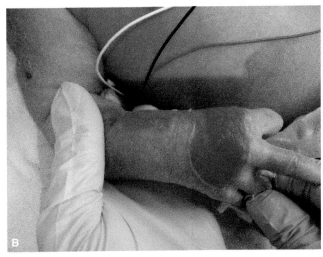

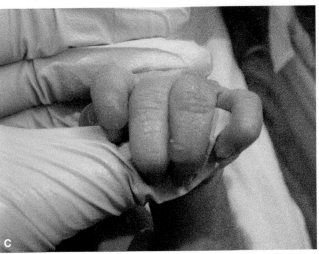

FIGURE 7.84 ■ Epidermolysis Bullosa (EB). (**A**) Blisters in areas of birth trauma in a neonate later diagnosed with dystrophic EB. Blisters in the areas of trauma are characteristic in patients with EB. This neonate also had oral blisters requiring specialized feeding nipples. (**B**) A deep scarring blister on the hand. (**C**) A blister occurring below the nail may cause scarring and permanent loss or damage to the nail matrix. (Photo contributor: Jeannette Jakus, MD.)

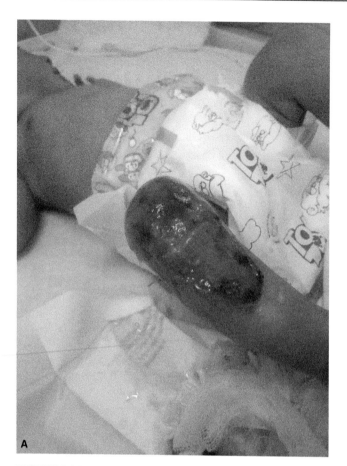

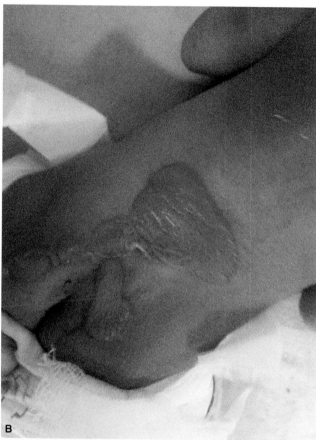

FIGURE 7.85 ■ Epidermolysis Bullosa (EB). (**A, B**) Blisters in the areas of birth trauma in a full-term neonate later diagnosed with dystrophic EB. (Photo contributor: Prerna Batra, MD.)

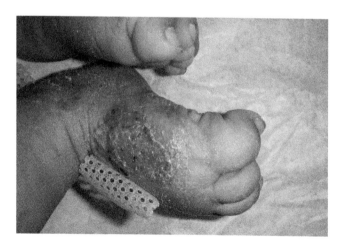

FIGURE 7.86 ■ Epidermolysis Bullosa (EB). A young infant with dystrophic EB. Specialized nonstick dressings are used in wound care. (Photo contributor: Jeannette Jakus, MD.)

genetic counseling and testing to determine the type of EB and risk of recurrence in future pregnancies. Parents should be educated on trauma avoidance. Recommendations include wearing clothing inside out to prevent pressure from seams. Soft fabrics such as cotton are encouraged. Mittens may be helpful, particularly in young babies, to prevent self-inflicted trauma. Young children and toddlers should be encouraged to wear soft, well-fitting shoes. Wound care should include the use of specialized nonstick dressings such as Mepitel (distributed by Mölnlycke Health Care) and Hollister Woundcare. Wounds can be extremely painful, and proper pain management should always be employed. Tense painful bullae may be evacuated using a sterile needle to relieve pressure. Antibiotic ointment should be reserved for cases of suspected infection in order to prevent bacterial resistance. If secondary infection of wounds is suspected, antibiotics should be considered. Patients with failure to thrive will need nutritional supplementation. The Dystrophic Epidermolysis Bullosa Research

Association (DEBRA) is an important and comprehensive resource for both patients and physicians (www.debra.org).

Pearls

1. EB refers to a group of genetic mechanobullous disorders.
2. Blistering of EB can be mistakenly attributed to inflicted burn injuries.
3. Although genetically acquired, bullae, in some milder forms, may not appear until adulthood.
4. Prevention of trauma and infection is the mainstay of treatment.

Clinical Summary

Infantile hemangioma (IH) or its precursor (erythematous, telangiectatic, or hypopigmented patch) is seen in about 5% of infants. Although IHs occur in all races, they are most common in white skin. Risk factors include female sex, prematurity, low birth weight, advanced maternal age, and multiple

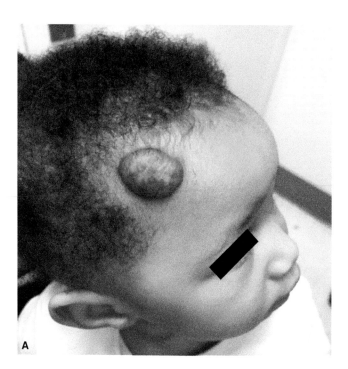

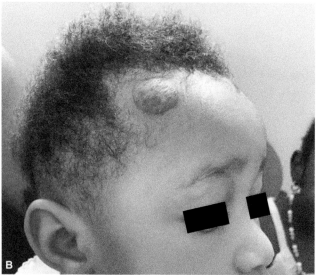

FIGURE 7.87 ■ Infantile Hemangioma. (**A**) Six-month-old infant with superficial hemangioma on the forehead that has started to involute as noted by the dull red color and softening of the lesion. (**B**) Same infant 3 months after treatment with propranolol. (Photo contributor: Sharon A. Glick, MD.)

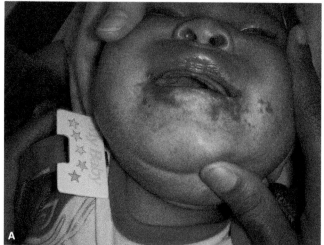

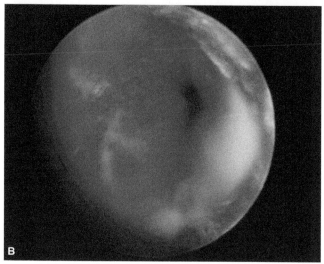

FIGURE 7.88 ■ Infantile Hemangioma (IH). (**A**) This 7-month-old infant with a segmental IH in full beard distribution with lower lip involvement presented with biphasic stridor and respiratory distress. (**B**) Subglottic hemangioma causing airway narrowing was seen during endoscopy. (Photo contributors: Sharon A. Glick, MD [A], and Sydney C. Butts, MD [B].)

gestation pregnancy. Traditionally, IHs have been classified as superficial, deep, or mixed, with the majority located on the head and neck. Most IHs are localized or focal lesions. The less common segmental type are plaque-like and regionally distributed with a higher risk of complications and associated anomalies such as seen in PHACE(S) (posterior fossa malformations, hemangiomas of the face, arterial anomalies, eye abnormalities, and sternal clefting) or LUMBAR syndromes (lower body hemangioma and other cutaneous defects, urogenital anomalies, ulceration, myelopathy, bony deformities,

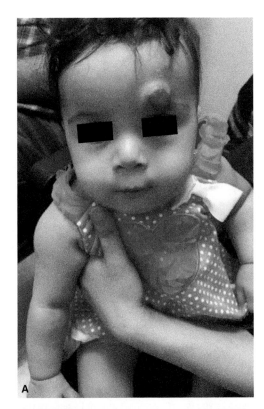

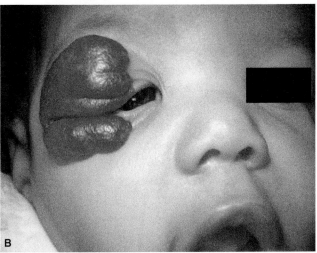

FIGURE 7.89 ■ Infantile Hemangioma. (**A**) A 7-month-old infant with mixed hemangioma showing superficial red overlying the deep component. This infant was started on propranolol therapy. (**B**) This is an example of untreated large periorbital hemangioma of the upper and lower eyelid obstructing the visual axis that may result in amblyopia. (Photo contributors: Sharon A. Glick, MD [A], and Binita R. Shah, MD [B].)

anorectal malformations, arterial anomalies, and renal anomalies). Previously, LUMBAR syndrome was referred to as PELVIS or SACRAL syndrome. The life cycle of IH involves proliferation and involution, with 80% of maximum size

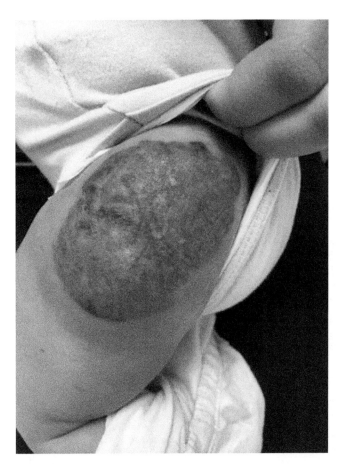

FIGURE 7.90 ■ Infantile Hemangioma. Seven-month-old infant with mixed hemangioma on left thigh. Note the superficial red overlying the deep blue nodular component. (Photo contributor: Sharon A. Glick, MD.)

reached by 3 months of age. The majority of lesions are first noted at 2 to 3 weeks of age. Clinically, involution is indicated by a color change from bright red to pink or gray and softening. The vast majority of IHs can be diagnosed based on history and physical examination. Differential diagnosis includes other vascular lesions such as Kaposiform hemangioendotheliomas and tufted angiomas. Deep hemangiomas may present as nodules with a bluish hue with or without overlying telangiectasias. Their differential includes congenital soft tissue tumors such as fibrosarcoma, rhabdomyosarcoma, and neuroblastoma.

Emergency Department Treatment and Disposition

The majority of IHs do not require any specific intervention other than referral to dermatology for photography

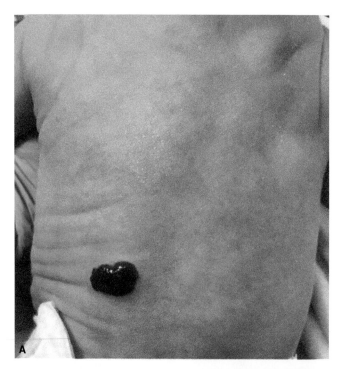

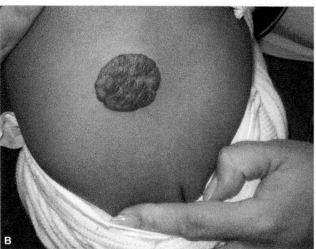

FIGURE 7.91 ■ Infantile Hemangioma. (**A**) Bright red superficial hemangioma on the lower back of a 2-month-old infant. This hemangioma is not in the midline, and patient does not need evaluation to exclude spinal dysmorphism. (**B**) Lumbosacral hemangiomas, like the one shown here, need evaluation to exclude spinal dysmorphism. (Photo contributor: Sharon A. Glick, MD.)

documentation to follow the growth and regression process and to help to reassure parents. The decision to intervene is based on the age of the patient, the location of the lesion, and the likelihood of complications. Treatment indications include life- or function-threatening IH (eg, periorbital lesions causing impairment of vision, beard distribution IH

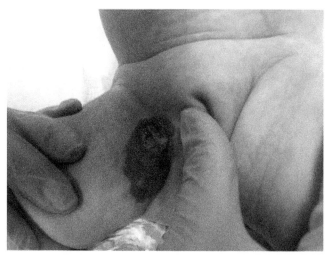

FIGURE 7.92 ■ Infantile Hemangioma with Ulceration. An infant with superficial hemangioma in the diaper area with ulceration. This infant was started on oral propranolol as well as topical petrolatum. Ulceration, the most common complication of hemangiomas, may result in pain, infection, or scarring. Topical occlusive agents such as petrolatum, topical antibiotics, and polyurethane film or hydrocolloid dressings initially treat ulcerations. Pain can be controlled with acetaminophen or, in refractory cases, cautious use of topical lidocaine. Pulsed dye laser treatment is also indicated for ulceration. (Photo contributor: Julie Cantatore-Francis, MD.)

leading to airway compromise, hepatic IH leading to congestive heart failure), locations prone to scarring (eg, nasal tip, perineum or genitalia, lip, or large deep facial lesions), ulceration, or pedunculated IHs that leave fibrofatty residua after involution. Ulceration is the most common complication and a major reason to present to the ED. Besides pain control, initial wound care includes gentle cleansing, barrier ointment such as petrolatum, and nonadherent dressings. Culture malodorous wounds and consider topical empiric treatment with metronidazole or mupirocin. Refer patient to dermatology for further management.

Doppler US, MRI, or CT may help differentiate hemangiomas from other vascular malformations and neoplastic diseases. Patients with large facial hemangiomas also need neuroimaging (MRI/magnetic resonance angiography) to exclude posterior fossa vascular malformations (eg, PHACE syndrome). Patients with midline lumbosacral or perineal hemangiomas need imaging (MRI with contrast and abdominal US) to rule out underlying spinal dysraphism and urogenital anomalies. These techniques also help evaluate for possible visceral involvement. Consult dermatology for complicated hemangiomas requiring intervention.

Pearls

1. Approximately 10% of IHs require treatment during the proliferative phase in order to prevent life- or function-threatening complications or cosmetic disfigurement. It is important to refer early because the period of most rapid proliferation occurs between 5.5 and 7.5 weeks after birth.

2. Refer to a pediatric dermatologist for treatment as well as other subspecialists such as pediatric ophthalmology (eg, periocular hemangiomas and PHACE syndrome), otolaryngology (eg, beard hemangiomas), and cardiology (eg, PHACE syndrome)

3. Segmental hemangiomas are 11 times more likely to be associated with complications, including ulceration and underlying developmental anomalies.

4. Consider referral to a support group such as PHACE Syndrome Community (www.phacesyndromecommunity.org) or Vascular Birthmark Foundation (www.birthmark.org).

5. Propranolol is a US Food and Drug Administration–approved treatment for IH initiated in collaboration with pediatric dermatology. The majority of patients respond within 1 to 2 weeks, with continued improvement over 6 to 12 months of treatment.

Clinical Summary

Mastocytosis is characterized by abnormal proliferation of mast cells in the dermis and viscera; however, in children, the condition is usually confined to the skin. Mastocytosis typically begins before 2 years of age (55% of patients), and overall prognosis is good with spontaneous involution in 50% by puberty. Childhood cutaneous mastocytosis includes a spectrum of single or multiple mastocytomas, urticaria pigmentosa (UP), and diffuse cutaneous mastocytosis (DCM). A positive Darier sign helps in establishing diagnosis in all forms. This sign is highly characteristic and can be elicited in up to 90% of patients by stroking a lesion to induce intense erythema and an urticarial wheal. The most common variant, UP, is characterized by red-brown macules and papules seen most commonly on the trunk and extremities. Mastocytoma may present as a solitary lesion or several skin-toned to yellow-brown plaques or nodules commonly with a peau d'orange surface. These have a tendency to blister and may occur on any cutaneous surface. DCM, the least common variant, is characterized by doughy, thickened skin due to diffuse infiltration with mast cells. These patients may have bullous eruptions as the first sign of disease. Pruritus may be the only symptom with localized cutaneous disease. Patients with extensive disease can experience widespread flushing, intense itching, headaches, bronchospasm, tachycardia, abdominal pain, and anaphylaxis. Triggering factors are described in Table 7.2. Differential diagnosis includes juvenile xanthogranulomas and congenital nevi. Lesions of UP may be mistaken for café-au-lait macules and lentigines.

Emergency Department Treatment and Disposition

Extensive workup in children with mastocytosis is not indicated, except in diffuse disease (widespread UP or DCM) where baseline CBC with peripheral smear, comprehensive metabolic

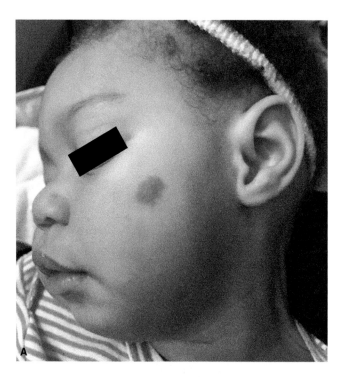

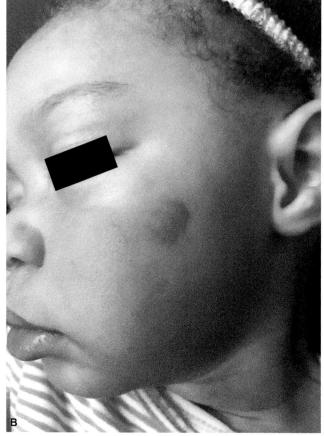

FIGURE 7.93 ■ Solitary Mastocytoma with a Positive Darier Sign. (**A**) An 8- month-old girl with red-brown plaque on left cheek noted by mother since 2 months of age. (**B**) Urtication of lesion with surrounding erythema after rubbing showing a positive Darier sign. (Photo contributor: Sharon A. Glick, MD.)

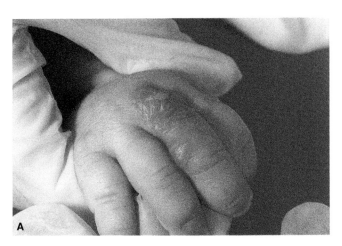 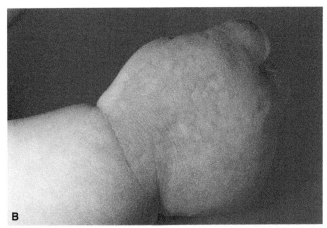

FIGURE 7.94 ■ Solitary Mastocytoma. Erythema and blistering are seen in a 2-month-old infant following rubbing of the finger (**A**). (**B**). Dermographism of intervening normal skin is also common. (Photo contributor: Binita R. Shah, MD.)

panel, and serum tryptase level may be obtained. Further studies should be dictated by symptoms. Direct treatment toward symptomatic relief and avoidance of triggers. Antihistamines are helpful; nonsedating H$_1$ blockers (eg, cetirizine or loratadine) reduce pruritus and flushing, and H$_2$ blockers (eg, cimetidine or ranitidine) may be added for GI symptoms. Topical corticosteroids may be used during acute urtication. Educate patients with widespread UP or DCM to carry an epinephrine pen (EpiPen) because severe allergic reactions can occur. The patient should be given a follow-up appointment with a dermatologist for continuity of care or biopsy when the diagnosis is in doubt. Skin biopsy with Giemsa or methylene blue stain of the tissue will demonstrate infiltration of the dermis with mast cells and their characteristic granules.

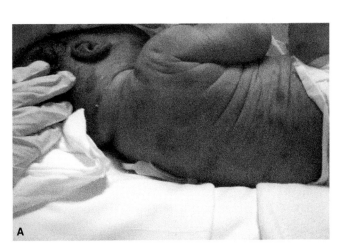 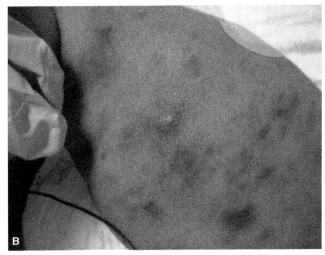

FIGURE 7.95 ■ Urticaria pigmentosa. (**A**) Widespread reddish-brown papules and plaques characteristic of urticaria pigmentosa. (**B**) An example of Darier sign (arrow). (Photo contributor: Sharon A. Glick, MD.)

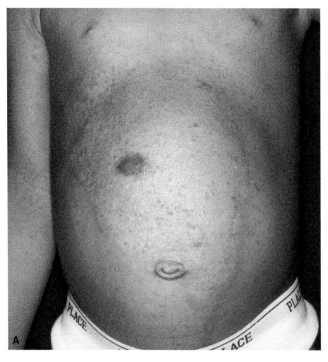 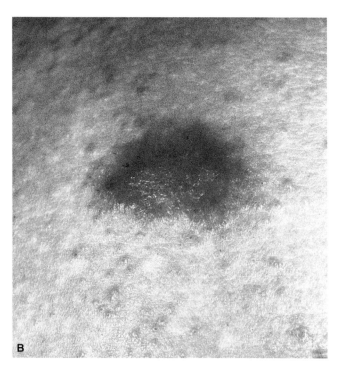

FIGURE 7.96 ■ Diffuse Cutaneous Mastocytosis. Widespread, thickened (**A**), edematous skin is typical of this type of mastocytosis, with a close-up of the lesion (**B**). (Photo contributor: Binita R. Shah, MD.)

Pearls

1. Scabies presenting with red-brown nodules may exhibit a Darier sign and can be confused with mastocytoma.
2. Although overall prognosis is good in childhood-onset mastocytosis, when disease remains into adulthood, patients have the same risks as adult-onset disease.
3. Intense pruritus is a prominent symptom. Systemic signs of histamine release (eg, hypotension, tachycardia, wheezing, syncope, headache, episodic flushing, colic, diarrhea) are seen in more severe types.
4. Dermatographism may be present in up to 50% of patients with UP.

TABLE 7.2 ■ TRIGGERS OF MAST CELL DEGRANULATION

Medications, Oral
Aspirin, alcohol, NSAIDS, codeine, morphine, opiates, vancomycin, dextromethorphan, thiamine, amphotericin B

Medications, Topical
Polymyxin B

Medications in General Anesthesia
D-Tubocurarine, scopolamine, decamethonium, gallamine, pancuronium

Local Anesthetics
Methylparaben, procaine, tetracaine

Physical Stimuli
Hot or cold baths, vigorous toweling, exercise, heat, sunlight, pressure, or friction

Radiation Contrast
Iodinated radiocontrast media

Others
Venoms (honeybee or wasp stings, jellyfish sting), dextran

Clinical Summary

Café-au-lait spots (CALS) are evenly pigmented tan to dark brown macules seen on any cutaneous surface. Solitary CALS are relatively common (prevalence: 3%–36% in general population). In contrast, multiple lesions are an uncommon finding (<1%) at any age, and their presence, particularly in white patients, should encourage further investigation. Multiple CALS is 1 of 7 diagnostic criteria of neurofibromatosis 1 (NF1), which is the most frequent disorder found in patients with CALS. In NF1, patients have at least 6 CALS >5 mm before puberty or >15 mm after puberty. However, not all children with multiple CALS have NF1. Multiple CALS are also seen in Legius syndrome, which also has symptoms of axillary freckling and macrocephaly but, in contradistinction to NF1, no Lisch nodules or neurofibromas. Familial CALS

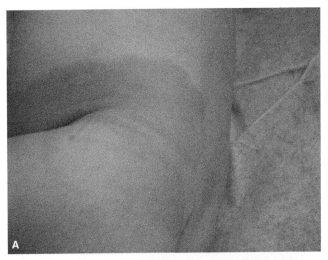

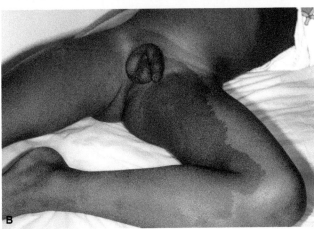

FIGURE 7.98 ■ Segmental Pigmentation Disorder. (**A**) An infant with unilateral block-like hyperpigmentation with a sharp cut-off at the midline of the back. (**B**) A child with unilateral hyperpigmentation of the lower extremity with a sharp cut-off at the midline. (Photo contributors: Sharon A. Glick, MD [A], and Binita R. Shah, MD [B].)

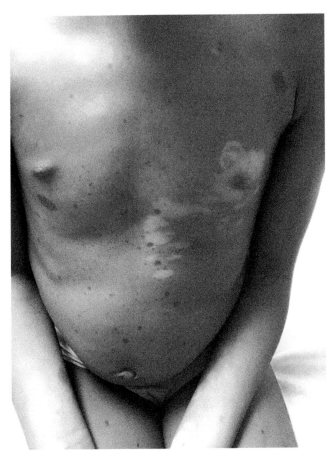

FIGURE 7.97 ■ Café-au-Lait Spots. Multiple café-au-lait macules are noted in this female who meets the criteria for neurofibromatosis. In addition to the café-au-lait macules, she also has axillary freckling and positive genetic testing. Note the segmental vitiligo on the left chest. This is independent of neurofibromatosis. (Photo contributor: Sharon A. Glick, MD.)

segregates as an autosomal dominant disorder but does not appear to confer an increased risk for classic NF1. Segmental NF1 occurs when CALS and/or neurofibromas localize to a specific area of skin without a family history of NF. Other syndromes where CALS can be seen include RASopathies, Legius syndrome, Noonan syndrome, cardiofaciocutaneous syndrome, Costello syndrome, Noonan-like syndrome (formerly Leopard syndrome), piebaldism, familial progressive hyperpigmentation, and familial progressive hyper- and hypopigmentation. Differential diagnosis of a solitary CALS includes speckled lentiginous nevus, lentigo, and congenital melanocytic nevus. Differential diagnosis of large CALS includes McCune-Albright syndrome (triad of large CALS

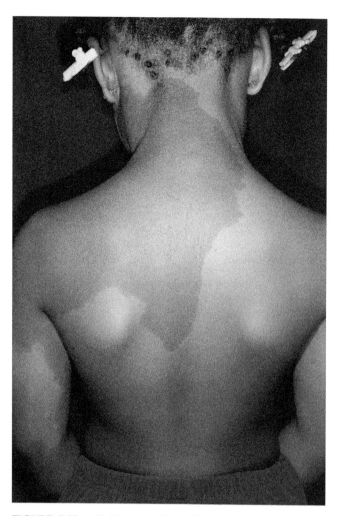

FIGURE 7.99 ■ Café-au-Lait Spots (CALS) in McCune-Albright Syndrome. CALS with irregular, jagged, and shaggy borders are seen on the back of a 4-year-old girl. She also had precocious puberty and polyostotic fibrous dysplasia. (Photo contributor: Binita R. Shah, MD.)

with a jagged border, polyostotic fibrous dysplasia, and endocrine dysfunction), segmental pigmentation disorder, a brown hyperpigmented birthmark seen in a block-like or segmental pattern most commonly on the trunk, and congenital Becker nevus (hamartoma characterized by hyperpigmentation with or without overlying hypertrichosis).

Emergency Department Treatment and Disposition

Treatment of CALS is medically unnecessary. Most patients need only reassurance about the benign nature of these lesions. CALS can be masked by cover-up makeup. Bleaching creams and laser treatment have also been used with variable success for cosmetically significant areas. Patients should be referred to a dermatologist for such interventions. Patients with multiple CALS are at risk of having an underlying disorder. It is important to recognize whether the presence of multiple CALS in a particular patient is normal or indicates an association with a multisystem disorder and refer to the appropriate subspecialty such as dermatology or neurology.

Pearls

1. No investigation is needed for a normal child presenting with a small CALS solitary lesion.
2. Wood lamp examination may accentuate and reveal CALS not apparent in visible light.

Clinical Summary

Erythema nodosum (EN) represents a cell-mediated hypersensitivity reaction to a variety of antigenic stimuli. It occurs in association with several diseases (eg, infections, inflammatory bowel disease, sarcoid) and during drug therapy (eg, sulfonamides, oral contraceptives, phenytoin). EN occurs more commonly in adolescents and young adults (predominant age range: 20–30 years) and is seen more commonly in females (female-to-male ratio of 3:1). The skin lesions are subcutaneous nodules with poorly defined borders that vary in size. They are erythematous, tender, tense, and firm during the first week, but become fluctuant (but do not suppurate) during the second week. The overlying skin changes in color from bright red to violaceous, brownish, yellowish, and green (like resolving hematomas). The most common location is extensor surfaces of shins, and less common locations include the extensor aspects of forearms, thighs, and trunk. The lesions tend to be bilateral and symmetric. The individual lesions disappear in 1 or 2 weeks, but new lesions may appear for 3 to 6 weeks. The lesions are nonulcerating and nonscarring. Low-grade fever, malaise, or arthralgias and arthritis (seen in 50% of patients either during eruptive phase of EN or preceding EN) may be present. Laboratory tests should be done depending on the suspected etiology. Initial evaluation should include throat culture, antistreptolysin O titer, tuberculin skin test, and ESR (usually elevated in patients with EN). CXR may show bilateral hilar adenopathy (seen in EN produced by coccidioidomycosis, histoplasmosis, tuberculosis, streptococcal infections, and as a nonspecific reaction in many cases). The diagnosis is made clinically based on a very characteristic presentation, and in the majority of cases, biopsy is not required.

Emergency Department Treatment and Disposition

In most instances, EN is a self-limited disease and requires only symptomatic treatment, including NSAIDs (eg, indomethacin or naproxen), bed rest, leg elevation, and elastic wraps or support stockings. If possible, it is important to identify the precipitating factor and treat accordingly by specific treatment of the underlying infection or discontinuation of an offending drug.

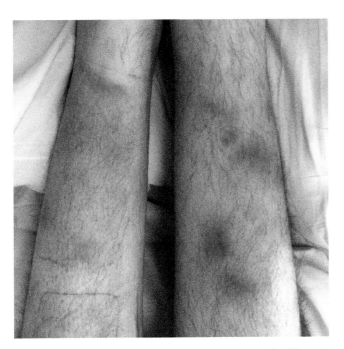

FIGURE 7.100 ■ Erythema Nodosum. Violaceous bruise-like nodules on the extensor aspect of the legs in a 17-year-old boy initially thought to have cellulitis. Further evaluation revealed the underlying diagnosis of inflammatory bowel disease. (Photo contributor: Karen Hammerman, MD.)

Pearls

1. EN lesions are multiple, bilateral, tender nodules that undergo characteristic color changes resulting in temporary bruise-like areas and occur most commonly on the extensor surfaces of the shins.

2. Up to one-half of cases of EN are idiopathic.

3. Most common identified cause of EN is streptococcal infection in children and streptococcal infection and sarcoidosis in adults.

4. EN may recur with recurrent infections (eg, recurrent EN seen in children with recurrent streptococcal infections).

5. The triad of EN, arthritis, and hilar lymphadenopathy is referred to as Löfgren syndrome and is an acute form of sarcoidosis.

ACANTHOSIS NIGRICANS

Clinical Summary

Acanthosis nigricans (AN) is a symmetrically distributed velvety thickening with hyperpigmentation most commonly found within the skin folds of the nape of the neck, axillae, and groin. Other areas of involvement include intramammary, umbilical, knuckles, popliteal, and antecubital fossae. AN can occur at any age and is commonly seen in children. Eight types of AN have been described including benign nevoid, obesity, syndromic, malignancy associated (rarely observed in children), acral, unilateral, medication induced (niacin, oral contraceptives, corticosteroids), and mixed. The most common type in children is related to obesity and insulin resistance. Evidence of abnormal glucose metabolism has been reported in >25% of adolescents with AN. The benign nevoid type may be familial with autosomal dominant inheritance. AN is seen with many syndromes in the categories of obesity-related (Prader-Willi), endocrine dysfunction (polycystic ovarian syndrome, HAIR-AN syndrome [hyperandrogenism, insulin resistance, and AN]), skeletal dysplasias, and autoimmune conditions (lupus erythematosus, dermatomyositis). The diagnosis of AN is made clinically. Laboratory

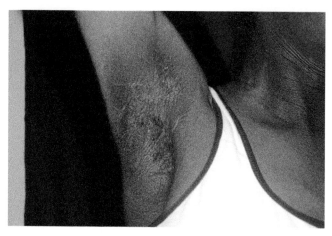

FIGURE 7.102 ■ Acanthosis Nigricans (AN). Velvety hyperpigmentation involving the neck and axilla is seen in this 15-year-old patient. She had HAIR-AN syndrome. This syndrome is usually seen in African American women who present with insulin resistance, hirsutism, polycystic ovaries, elevated testosterone levels, and onset of AN in childhood with subsequent progression during puberty. (Photo contributor: Binita R. Shah, MD.)

tests, as indicated by signs and symptoms, should be performed to exclude any underlying syndromes.

Emergency Department Treatment and Disposition

AN is an important indicator of insulin sensitivity that is independent of body mass index. All children with AN should be classified as to which type they have through history, medication profile, physical examination, and workup, including hemoglobin A1c, fasting serum insulin, glucose, and lipids. Patients can be referred to subspecialty depending on the underlying etiology. Adolescents with AN and hyperandrogenism as evidenced by abnormal menses, acne, or hirsutism should be referred to endocrinology for additional studies. For cosmetic concerns or to promote comfort in areas with thicker lesions, topical retinoids or topical hydroxy acids (eg, lactic acid, 10%–20% urea) may be tried and the patient referred to dermatology for ongoing care.

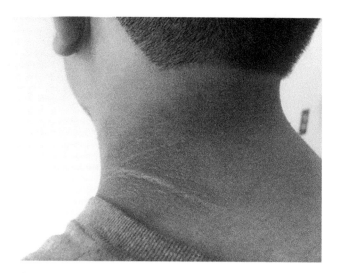

FIGURE 7.101 ■ Acanthosis Nigricans. Mild acanthosis nigricans in an adolescent boy. Screening hemoglobin A1C value was normal. (Photo contributor: Sharon A. Glick, MD.)

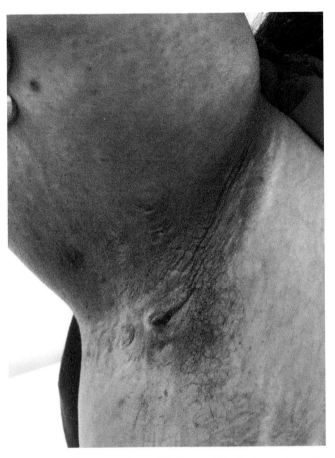

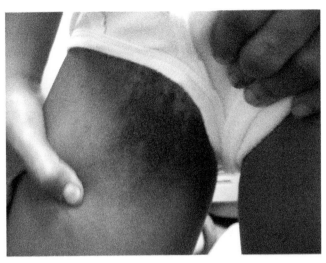

FIGURE 7.104 ■ Acanthosis Nigricans (AN). Benign nevoid AN is seen in the groin of a 7-year-old boy who developed AN at 4 years of age starting on the posterior neck followed by axillae and groin. The major differential diagnosis in this patient is systematized epidermal nevus. (Photo contributor: Sharon A. Glick, MD.)

Pearls

1. The majority of cases of AN are associated with obesity.
2. AN is a cutaneous marker of tissue insulin resistance regardless of its cause.
3. Usually, correction of the underlying disorder improves AN.
4. AN is rarely a sign of malignancy in children; however, a rapidly progressing and widespread AN is caused by malignancy until proven otherwise at any age.

FIGURE 7.103 ■ Acanthosis Nigricans. Velvety hyperpigmentation with a skin tag is seen in this adolescent female with Down syndrome (DS) in the axilla. This condition is seen more frequently in patients with DS. (Photo contributor: Sharon A. Glick, MD.)

HIDRADENITIS SUPPURATIVA

Clinical Summary

Hidradenitis suppurativa (HS) is a chronic, recurrent, inflammatory process due to occlusion of hair follicles of the apocrine gland–bearing areas in the axillary, genital, and perianal regions. HS is characterized by abscesses, deep sinus tracts, and scarring resulting from recurrent rupture and reepithelialization of occluded follicles. Bacteria, although not the primary cause, are thought to play a secondary role in exacerbation of HS. HS is more common in girls, and onset is most often after puberty, in the second to third decade. Although neither smoking nor obesity is implicated as a primary etiology, both have been found to be associated with HS and may exacerbate the condition. The role of hormones and factors such as antiperspirants and deodorants has yet to be defined.

The diagnosis is made clinically. The age of onset and characteristic lesion distribution allow the condition to be readily distinguished from other entities. Most cases occur sporadically, but familial occurrence with autosomal

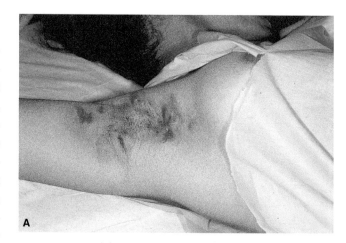

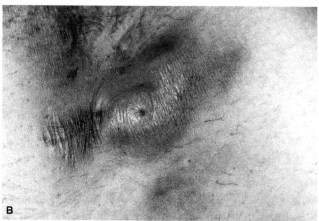

FIGURE 7.106 ■ Hidradenitis Suppurativa. (**A**) Nodules, abscess, and draining sinus tracts involving both axillae were present in this adolescent girl. This was her fourth recurrence. The chronic, malodorous, and unsightly nature of this disease was causing significant social debilitation. Her failure to respond to many courses of antibiotics required surgical extirpation of the apocrine glands. (**B**) Close-up of the cystic nodule with draining sinus. (Photo contributor: Binita R. Shah, MD.)

dominant inheritance has been seen. Complications include anemia, ulceration, and burrowing abscesses that may perforate, forming fistulas and squamous cell carcinoma in areas of long-term scarring. Disease associations with HS include inflammatory bowel disease, autoinflammatory disorders, polycystic ovarian syndrome, and SAPHO (synovitis, acne, pustulosis, hyperostosis, and osteitis) syndrome.

Emergency Department Treatment and Disposition

HS is a difficult condition to treat, and therapy must be individualized based on symptomatology. General measures

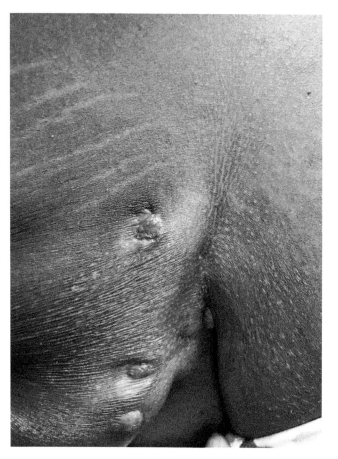

FIGURE 7.105 ■ Hidradenitis Suppurativa. Adolescent female with both intra- and inframammary nodules and friable erosions. (Photo contributor: Sharon A. Glick, MD.)

378

include weight reduction in overweight individuals, wearing loose-fitting clothing, quitting smoking, and decreasing moisture. Dermatology should be consulted for recurrent difficult-to-treat patients and surgery for recalcitrant cases. Initial medical measures include topical antibiotics such as clindamycin, intralesional injection of triamcinolone for early-stage inflammatory lesions, and oral antibiotics guided by bacterial cultures from abscesses. Empirical therapy may be initiated with tetracycline, doxycycline, or minocycline for patients age 8 years or older or combination oral therapy with clindamycin-rifampin. Warm compresses encourage spontaneous rupture of abscesses. Incision and drainage should be used cautiously as there is a high risk of recurrence and the procedure may result in scarring and chronic sinus formation. Recently, adalimumab has been approved by the Food and Drug Administration for the treatment of moderate to severe HS. Second-line therapies include carbon dioxide laser and local excision. In recalcitrant cases, wide excision with primary closure or followed by split-thickness skin grafting may be the only treatment option.

Pearls

1. Apocrinitis (inflammation of apocrine glands) seen with HS is a secondary phenomenon.
2. Characteristic distribution along the axillae, groin, or perineum aids in diagnosis.
3. Severe HS can lead to fistulae, dermal scarring with hypertrophic scars, lymphedema, and even restriction of arm or leg movement.

Clinical Summary

Transient neonatal pustular melanosis (TNPM) is an uncommon benign condition seen predominantly in African American newborns. The cause is unknown. It occurs in full-term infants and manifests with superficial pustules present at birth. The

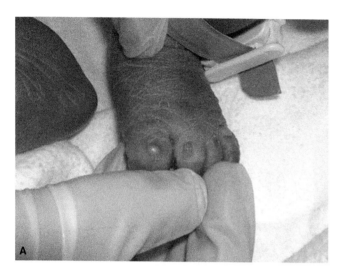

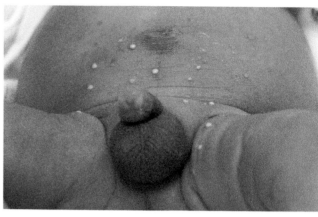

FIGURE 7.108 ■ Transient Neonatal Pustular Melanosis (TNPM) Versus Neonatal *Staphylococcus aureus* Pustulosis. Both TNPM and *S aureus* pustulosis can have similar clinical appearance presenting with pustules and collarettes of scale as seen in this neonate. It is common for neonates to present with multiple pustules in the diaper region with staphylococcal pustulosis. A culture and Gram stain smear will help to determine the etiology. (Photo contributor: Ameer Hassoun, MD.)

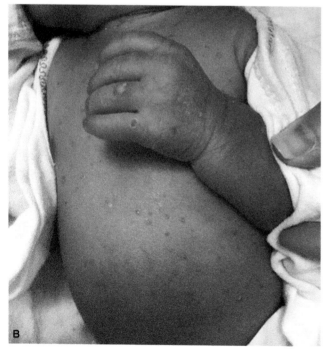

FIGURE 7.107 ■ Transient Neonatal Pustular Melanosis. (**A**) Pustules on the dorsal foot and toes of a newborn. Wright stain revealed numerous neutrophils. (**B**) Note the pustule on the 4th finger of a different newborn. A collarette of scale surrounding a dot of hyperpigmentation is seen on the 5th finger with other dots of hyperpigmentation scattered on the trunk, some with collarettes. (Photo contributor: Sharon A. Glick, MD.)

lesions are typically seen on the underside of the chin, forehead, posterior neck, back, and shins and less commonly on the trunk, dorsal feet, palms, and soles. The pustules easily rupture with residual collarettes of scale and eventually resolve with central brown hyperpigmentation most likely representing postinflammatory hyperpigmentation. These brown macules may last up to several months. The diagnosis is made clinically, so biopsy is rarely indicated. A bedside test helpful for diagnosis is a Giemsa- or Wright-stained smear of a pustule that demonstrates a predominance of neutrophils with few or no eosinophils. The differential diagnosis includes erythema toxicum neonatorum (smear shows a predominance of eosinophils), staphylococcal impetigo (smears shows gram-positive cocci), and neonatal candidiasis (KOH examination positive for pseudohyphae and spores).

Emergency Department Treatment and Disposition

If the clinical diagnosis is in doubt, a Giemsa or Wright stain of a pustule may be performed. No treatment other than parental reassurance is necessary because this is a benign and self-limited condition.

Pearls

1. TNPM and erythema toxicum neonatorum may occur simultaneously in a patient.
2. Newborns brought to the ED after extramural delivery or delivered in the ED may have these pustular lesions, and physicians need to be familiar with this entity.
3. Parents should be told that the hyperpigmented macules take up to several months to resolve.

SUBCUTANEOUS FAT NECROSIS OF THE NEWBORN

Clinical Summary

Subcutaneous fat necrosis (SCFN) is seen in full-term infants during the first weeks of life. Firm, erythematous, well-circumscribed subcutaneous plaques and nodules characterize the condition. The lesions occur over bony prominences on the back, buttocks, thighs, and cheeks and may be solitary or multiple. In general, the condition has a favorable prognosis with spontaneous regression over weeks to months. Several associations that are described in newborns with SCFN include hypothermia, hypoglycemia in infants of mothers with gestational diabetes, hypoxemia due to meconium aspiration, and perinatal asphyxia. It is also seen in healthy infants. Complications of SCFN are uncommon; they include hypercalcemia, thrombocytopenia, and dyslipidemia. Rarely, calcium deposits in persistent lesions may liquefy, drain, and scar. The differential diagnosis of SCFN includes poststeroid panniculitis (distinguished by history of abrupt steroid withdrawal)

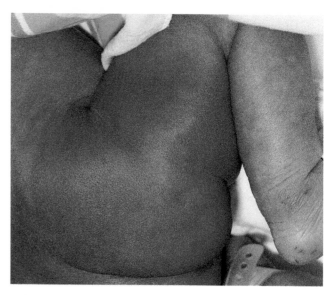

FIGURE 7.110 ■ Subcutaneous Fat Necrosis of the Newborn. Lesions may be present at birth, or they may develop during the first month of life. Most lesions resolve spontaneously over a period of 2 to 4 weeks, but some last significantly longer. There is usually no residual atrophy or scarring. (Reproduced with permission from Prose NS, Kristal L. *Weinberg's Color Atlas of Pediatric Dermatology*, 5th ed. McGraw-Hill Education; New York, NY, 2017.)

and sclerema neonatorum (diffuse cutaneous involvement in a severely ill premature neonate and minimal inflammation seen on histologic examination).

Emergency Department Treatment and Disposition

Refer to dermatology for biopsy confirmation of the diagnosis and follow-up. The biopsy specimen shows a lobular panniculitis with needle-shaped clefts in lipocytes surrounded by lymphocytes, histiocytes, fibroblasts, and giant cells with areas of necrosis or calcification. In the majority of neonates with SCFN, treatment is supportive, with reassurance to caretakers. Hypercalcemia, an uncommon complication, may have a delayed onset requiring monitoring of calcium levels (up to 6 months after birth). Infants found to have asymptomatic hypercalcemia can be managed conservatively through a diet low in calcium and vitamin D or systemically with corticosteroids. Infants with symptomatic hypercalcemia may present with failure to thrive, vomiting, and lethargy and require hospitalization for systemic therapy with calcium metabolism modifiers such as pamidronate.

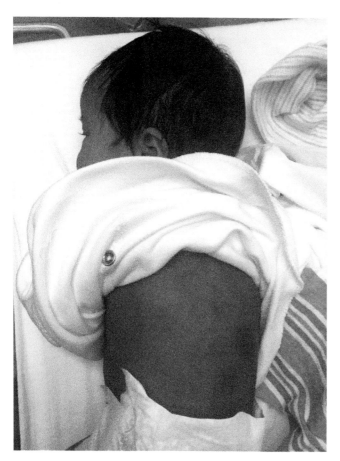

FIGURE 7.109 ■ Subcutaneous Fat Necrosis of the Newborn. Erythematous indurated plaques are seen on mid back of this otherwise healthy 4-day-old full-term infant. (Photo contributor: Amanda Hassler, MD.)

Pearls

1. The etiology of SCFN is unknown but proposed to occur from local injury to neonatal fat, with perinatal asphyxia thought to be the most common association.

2. The lesions can be difficult to appreciate visually and may require palpation for detection of the indurated plaques or nodules.

3. Hypothermia protocols used in newborns with perinatal asphyxia in order to lessen neurologic sequelae may increase the risk for SCFN.

Clinical Summary

Candidal diaper dermatitis is one of the most frequent causes of diaper rash, usually occurring after 2 months of age; other common causes include chafing dermatitis due to chronic friction and irritant dermatitis secondary to contact with topical agents (soaps, detergents, stool, urine, medications). Candidal diaper dermatitis is characterized by beefy-red erythema beginning in the perianal and inguinal folds with

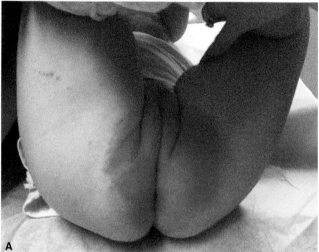

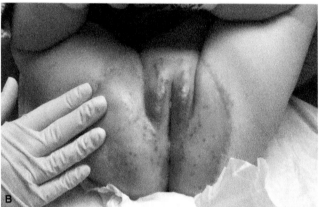

FIGURE 7.112 ■ Candidal Diaper Dermatitis. (**A**) Candidal diaper dermatitis in a 9-month-old infant who developed diarrhea after being treated with antibiotics. (**B**) Dermatitis partially treated with ketoconazole cream. (Photo contributor: Julie Cantatore-Francis, MD.)

satellite papules and pustules. Scale is commonly seen at the peripheral margin of the erythema. In more widespread cases, the condition extends to the buttocks, inner thighs, and lower abdomen. Diagnosis is confirmed by examination of skin scrapings by KOH preparation or fungal culture.

Emergency Department Treatment and Disposition

Candidal diaper dermatitis is treated using imidazole creams (clotrimazole, miconazole, or ketoconazole) with diaper changes. In addition, a barrier cream with zinc oxide and/or petrolatum can be applied with diaper changes in order to prevent contact with irritants such as urine and feces.

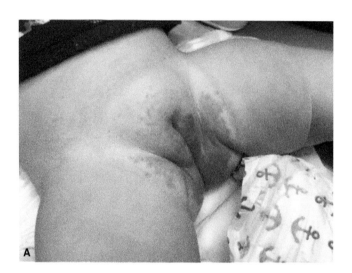

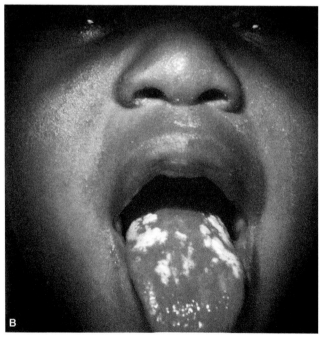

FIGURE 7.111 ■ Candida Infections. (**A**) Candidal diaper rash with satellite papules. (**B**) Candida thrush on the tongue. (Photo contributors: Julie Cantatore-Francis, MD [A], and Binita R. Shah, MD [B].)

Formulations of miconazole, zinc oxide, and petrolatum are available both over the counter (Triple Paste AF) and by prescription (Vusion). In cases of severe inflammation, a low-potency steroid (1% hydrocortisone cream or ointment) may be required for several days. When oral thrush is present with diaper dermatitis, consider adding nystatin solution (100,000 units/mL) to the oral lesions 4 times a day for 1 week. Education regarding the discontinuation of fragranced diaper wipes is helpful, especially in recalcitrant rashes. An inexpensive alternative is the use of a soft cloth moistened with warm water.

Pearls

1. Candidal diaper dermatitis may occur after a course of systemic antibiotics or diarrhea.
2. Check the mouth for white patches of thrush that may occur with candidal diaper dermatitis.
3. Do not use mid- or high-potency steroids or combination creams containing them when treating the diaper area because of increased side effects in this occlusive area.

Clinical Summary

Perioral or periorificial dermatitis (PD) presents as tiny pink to erythematous papules and papulopustules around the mouth, eyes, and nasolabial folds. The etiology is unknown, but a recent retrospective study found that about 70% of patients had a history of topical, inhaled, or systemic steroid use. If untreated, the condition may take months to years to resolve. PD has overlapping features with acne rosacea and is considered to be a juvenile variant by some. However, unlike acne rosacea, PD lacks telangiectasia, a malar component, and ocular inflammation. Granulomatous PD is seen in prepubertal children of African American and Afro-Caribbean descent and represents a less common variant of PD. It is characterized by pink to yellow-brown monomorphous papules in a periorificial distribution. Extrafacial lesions have been rarely reported. Histologic specimens show granulomatous infiltrates of histiocytes and lymphocytes in the dermis. Granulomatous PD usually resolves spontaneously.

Emergency Department Treatment and Disposition

If a history of steroid use is obtained, steroids should be discontinued or tapered. Treatment options include topical metronidazole alone or in combination with oral erythromycin or tetracycline (if the child is older than age 8 years).

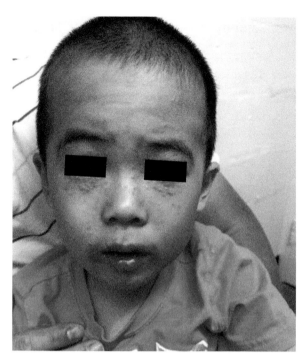

FIGURE 7.114 ■ Periorificial (Perioral) Dermatitis. Periorificial dermatitis is seen in this 3-year-old child secondary to prolonged steroid application on the face. Patient was treated with azithromycin and Protopic (tacrolimus) ointment. (Photo contributor: Alexandra Leonard, MSIV.)

Pearls

1. Parents should be informed that the condition may initially flare with the withdrawal of steroids.
2. In mild cases, topical treatment may be sufficient, and it may take a few weeks to resolve.

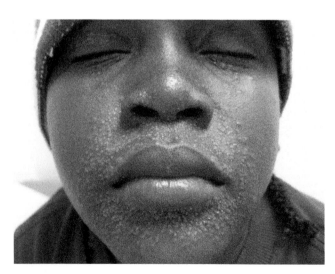

FIGURE 7.113 ■ Perioral Dermatitis. Numerous erythematous papules in a perioral distribution in this adolescent girl. (Photo contributor: Maria Kessides, MD.)

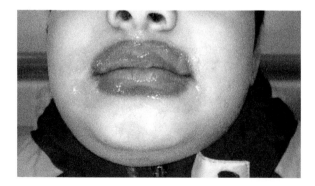

FIGURE 7.115 ■ Contact Irritant Dermatitis in Perioral Distribution. This is an eczematous dermatitis that forms as a result of chronic irritation from continuous licking in a perioral distribution. Management consists of counseling for avoidance of licking habit and use of barrier cream (eg, petrolatum, as seen here). A low- to mid-potency corticosteroid ointment or topical calcineurin inhibitor may also be used. (Photo contributor: Yvonne P. Giunta, MD.)

Clinical Summary

Incontinentia pigmenti (IP) is an inherited X-linked dominant disorder. The majority of cases of IP occur in females. It is considered lethal in the affected males in utero. However, IP has been found in males with Klinefelter syndrome (XXY genotype) or due to somatic mosaicism. This disease can affect the skin, hair, nails, teeth, eyes, skeletal system, CNS, and other organs in varied degrees. Skin findings are often the first observed sign of IP appearing at birth or shortly after and have 4 stages with characteristic lesions in each stage. These lesions tend to follow the lines of Blaschko. These 4 stages may overlap, occur in utero, or be skipped entirely. The 4 stages are vesicular or blistering, verrucous, hyperpigmented, and atrophic or hypopigmented. The vesicular or blistering first stage consists of erythema and superficial yellow or clear vesicles following the lines of Blaschko in a linear distribution on the extremities and a curvilinear or S-shaped configuration on the trunk. Scalp lesions are common. The morphology of lesions may range from papules to vesicles and pustules. This blistering stage is often mistaken for infections such as HSV, varicella, or bullous impetigo. This stage can be differentiated from these entities and other blistering diseases of the newborn based on viral culture, bacterial culture, Gram stain, Tzanck smear, and skin biopsy. In the vesicular or blistering stage, there is marked leukocytosis and eosinophilia. The coexistence of IP and infections has been documented. The verrucous or second stage is characterized by the presence of hyperkeratotic linear plaques or warty papules on 1 or more extremities. The hyperpigmented or third

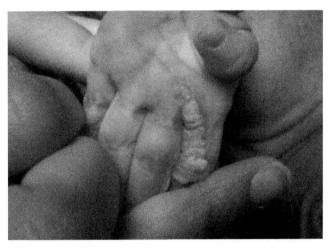

FIGURE 7.117 ■ Incontinentia Pigmenti. Verrucous lesion (stage 2) is shown on the finger of this neonate. (Photo contributor: Sharon A. Glick, MD.)

stage is characterized by linear and whorled grayish brown hyperpigmentation along lines of Blaschko on extremities and trunk. This stage is experienced by almost all individuals with IP. The atrophic or hypopigmented fourth stage consists of pale, hairless atrophic patches or streaks or hypopigmented streaks on extremities. Unlike the other 3 stages, this stage often persists into adulthood.

Additional cutaneous findings include abnormalities of hair (scarring alopecia, coarse hair, hypoplasia of eyebrows and eyelashes), nails (dystrophy/nail ridging, pitting, nail disruption, subungual keratotic tumors associated with bony deformities of the underlying phalanges), and teeth (delayed dentition, missing teeth, pegged and conical teeth). Ocular

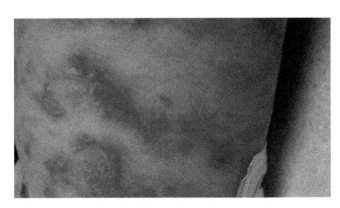

FIGURE 7.116 ■ Incontinentia Pigmenti. Vesicular lesions (stage 1) on the trunk in this newborn are seen. Note the curvilinear distribution following the lines of Blaschko. (Photo contributor: Sharon A. Glick, MD.)

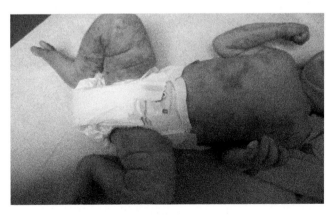

FIGURE 7.118 ■ Incontinentia Pigmenti (IP). Widespread distribution of IP lesions on the trunk and extremities (stages 1 and 2). Often these stages are seen overlapping. (Photo contributor: Sharon A. Glick, MD.)

involvement includes strabismus, nystagmus, optic nerve atrophy, retinal hemorrhages, retinal detachment, and blindness. CNS involvement includes seizures, spasticity, microcephaly, and ataxia, mandating a complete neurologic examination. Neonatal seizures are a poor prognostic sign and may predict developmental delay.

Emergency Department Treatment and Disposition

Patients with IP are usually not acutely ill. No treatment is required for skin lesions of IP. Reassurance should be given to parents. The recognition of the characteristic skin lesions can promote early diagnosis IP as well as presence of associated abnormalities or involvement of other organs. Consult dermatologist if diagnosis is unclear. Refer infants newly diagnosed with IP to ophthalmology and neurology for further evaluation and management as clinically indicated.

Pearls

1. IP is a syndrome with a varied clinical manifestation affecting the skin and other organs.
2. Infants can be born with any stage of skin lesions. Face is usually spared in all stages.
3. Diagnosis of IP does not exclude a coexistent infectious disease. Consider HSV infection and IP in the differential diagnosis of any newborn presenting with vesicular lesions.
4. In addition to clinical appearance, diagnosis of IP is aided by family history, history of miscarriages of male gender, and skin biopsy.

Chapter 8

OPHTHALMOLOGY

Suzanne M. Schmidt
Steven E. Krug

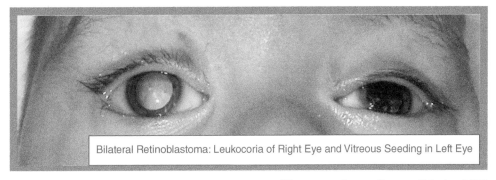

Bilateral Retinoblastoma: Leukocoria of Right Eye and Vitreous Seeding in Left Eye

(Photo contributor: Roman Shinder, MD)

The authors acknowledge the special contributions of Douglas R. Lazzaro, MD, Amy Kulak, MD, and Wayne Scott, MD, to the prior edition.

ORBITAL CELLULITIS

Clinical Summary

Orbital cellulitis is an infection of the soft tissues of the orbit posterior to the orbital septum. Infection may involve any of the orbital structures, including extraocular muscles, sensory and motor nerves, and the optic nerve, and may result in abscess formation (orbital or subperiosteal abscess). Patients present with a moderate to severely inflamed, painful eye, conjunctival injection, swelling of the eyelids, and chemosis (conjunctival swelling). As infection progresses, swelling increases and the eye becomes more chemotic and proptotic. Eye movement is diminished and painful in some areas of gaze, or in severe cases, all areas of gaze (frozen globe). Patients are usually febrile and in significant pain. Orbital cellulitis most often arises as an extension of infection from the paranasal sinuses, although it may also occur as a progression of preseptal cellulitis. Causative pathogens include *Staphylococcus aureus, Streptococcus pneumoniae, Streptococcus pyogenes,* and anaerobes (*Peptostreptococcus, Bacteroides, Fusobacterium*), depending on the source of infection and abscess formation. Differential diagnosis includes preseptal cellulitis, dacryocystitis, dacryoadenitis, intraocular or retrobulbar mass, and retrobulbar hemorrhage from trauma.

Emergency Department Treatment and Disposition

Orbital cellulitis is a true medical emergency, particularly in advanced cases where extension posteriorly to the brain can occur, causing rapid deterioration in the patient's status. Evaluate the orbit and paranasal sinuses with neuroimaging (CT scan with contrast or MRI). Obtain prompt ophthalmology consultation in the ED and otorhinolaryngology (ENT) consultation if sinusitis is present. If a subperiosteal abscess is noted on imaging, surgical drainage may be required. Begin broad-spectrum IV antibiotics while awaiting identification of the source or organism and admit the patient to the hospital. If there is extension posterior to the orbit, the patient may need admission to the ICU.

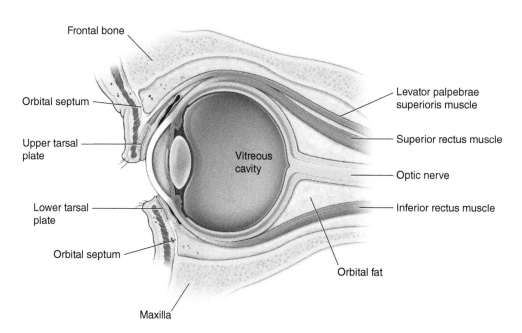

FIGURE 8.1 ■ A Sagittal View of the Orbit. Sagittal view of the orbit illustrating the position of the orbital septum. The orbital septum is an extension of the orbital periosteum to the tarsal plate in both upper and lower eyelids and acts as a physical barrier, preventing spread of a preseptal infection to the orbital contents.

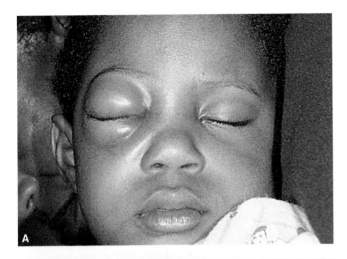

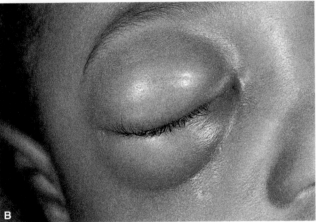

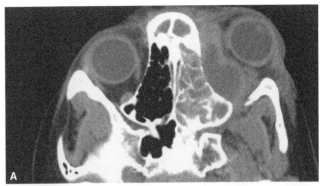

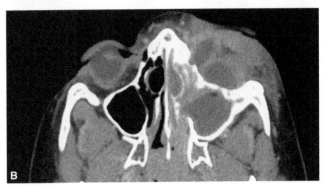

FIGURE 8.4 ■ Orbital Cellulitis. Left orbital cellulitis with subperiosteal abscess and extensive ethmoid and maxillary sinusitis are seen in this postcontrast CT scan. About 75% to 90% of cases of orbital cellulitis are associated with either preceding or concurrent acute paranasal sinusitis (commonly involved sinuses: ethmoid, maxillary, and frontal). (Photo contributor: John Amodio, MD.)

FIGURE 8.2 ■ Orbital Cellulitis. (A, B) Unilateral eye involvement with marked swelling of both upper and lower eyelids, intense erythema, and proptosis in a highly febrile child requiring surgical drainage of a subperiosteal abscess that grew *S aureus*. (Photo contributor: Binita R. Shah, MD.)

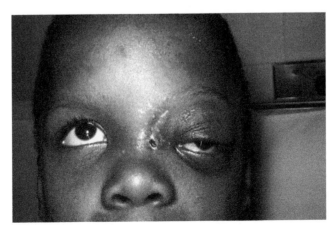

FIGURE 8.3 ■ Orbital Cellulitis. Severe proptosis, malalignment of globe with restriction of eye movements, swelling of eyelids, and unilateral involvement are characteristic findings of orbital cellulitis (photograph taken after drainage of subperiosteal abscess). (Photo contributor: Binita R. Shah, MD.)

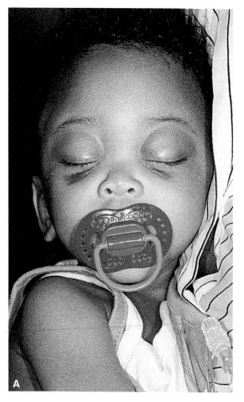
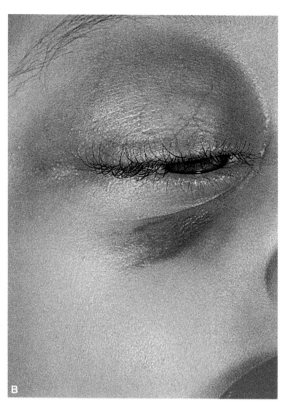
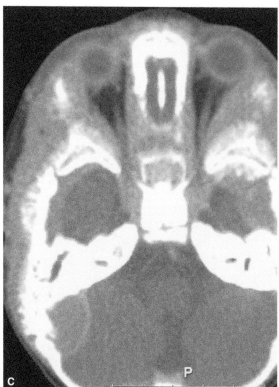

FIGURE 8.5 ■ Metastatic Neuroblastoma: Differential Diagnosis of Proptosis. **(A, B)** An 11-month-old infant with bilateral "raccoon eyes" (periorbital ecchymosis) and orbital proptosis, signs of metastatic neuroblastoma (most common tumor to metastasize to orbit in childhood). **(C)** Aggressive bony erosion and periosteal reaction are seen involving the orbits and temporal bone. Bilateral enhancing soft tissue masses in extraconal spaces with enhancing masses in epidural space and posterior to the right temporal bone. (Photo contributor: Binita R. Shah, MD.)

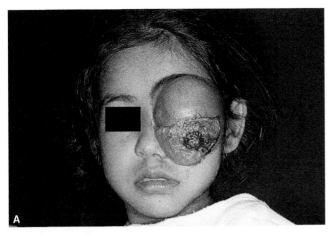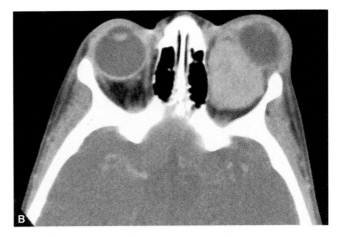

FIGURE 8.6 ■ Rhabdomyosarcoma: Differential Diagnosis of Proptosis. (**A**) A rapidly growing orbital mass in a 7-year-old girl. Rhabdomyosarcoma presents with painless proptosis, globe displacement with edema and erythema of the lids. (**B**) Postcontrast orbital CT scan reveals a large enhancing intraconal soft tissue mass posterior to the left globe causing proptosis. (Photo contributor: Binita R. Shah, MD.)

Pearls

1. Diminished vision can rapidly progress if the orbital infection does not respond to treatment; this is a poor prognostic sign.
2. Orbital cellulitis can be life-threatening if infection spreads intracranially especially to cavernous sinuses.
3. If sinus infection is the source, ENT evaluation with surgical drainage may be indicated.

Clinical Summary

Preseptal cellulitis is infection and inflammation of the eyelids and periorbital soft tissues anterior to the orbital septum. The globe and orbital structures posterior to the septum are not involved; thus, pupillary reaction, visual acuity, and ocular motility should not be affected. Preseptal cellulitis is most often caused by spread of infection from a local skin wound or insect bite. Common pathogens include *S pneumoniae, S aureus,* and *S pyogenes.* Patients present with eyelid erythema, edema, induration, warmth, and tenderness. In severe cases, marked edema may cause eye closure and the patient may be unable to open the eye spontaneously. Low-grade fever is often present. Differential diagnosis includes orbital cellulitis, allergic conjunctivitis, contact dermatitis, chalazion/hordeolum, infectious conjunctivitis with secondary eyelid swelling, dacryoadenitis, dacryocystitis, and trauma.

Emergency Department Treatment and Disposition

Obtain a complete history, including insect bites, trauma, recent dental work, sinus disease, and other infections.

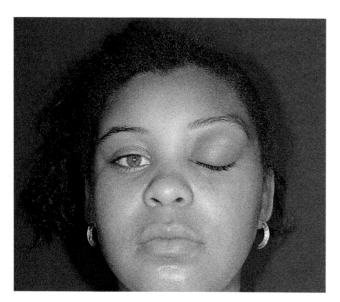

FIGURE 8.7 ■ Preseptal Cellulitis. Intense erythema, edema, and tenderness of the eyelid in an adolescent who had normal vision, full range of eye movements without pain, and absence of proptosis. She also had maxillary sinusitis (clinically swelling and tenderness over the maxillary sinus). (Photo contributor: Binita R. Shah, MD.)

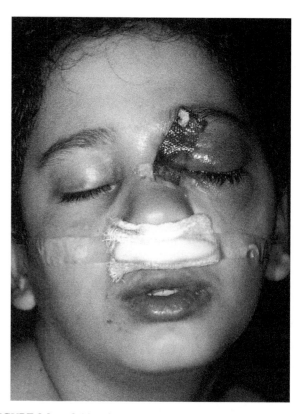

FIGURE 8.8 ■ Orbital Cellulitis: Differential Diagnosis of Preseptal Cellulitis. Orbital cellulitis with proptosis and painful extraocular movements were present in this patient with ethmoid sinusitis and subperiosteal abscess. (Photograph taken after drainage of subperiosteal abscess; reproduced with permission from Shah BR, Laude TL. *Atlas of Pediatric Clinical Diagnosis.* WB Saunders; Philadelphia, PA, 2000.)

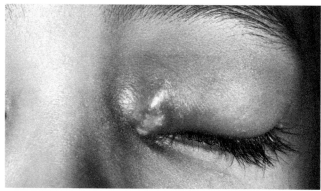

FIGURE 8.9 ■ Hordeolum with Preseptal Cellulitis. Spread from a contiguous infection can lead to preseptal cellulitis. (Photo contributor: Binita R. Shah, MD.)

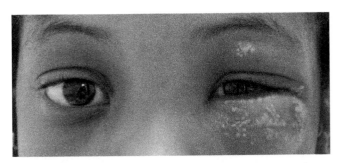

FIGURE 8.10 ■ Herpes Simplex Virus (HSV) Infection: Differential Diagnosis of Preseptal Cellulitis. Multiple grouped vesiculopustular lesions on an erythematous base are seen in HSV infection. Cornea is involved in 10% to 30% of patients with primary ocular HSV infection, and patients need urgent evaluation by an ophthalmologist. (Photo contributor: Douglas R. Lazzaro, MD.)

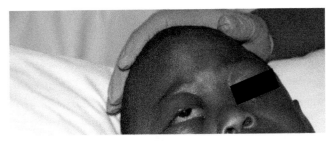

FIGURE 8.12 ■ Rhabdomyosarcoma with Proptosis: Differential Diagnosis of Preseptal Cellulitis. Periorbital edema was misdiagnosed as preseptal cellulitis until it worsened associated with proptosis and chemosis because of a rapidly growing orbital rhabdomyosarcoma in this child. (Photo contributor: Binita R. Shah, MD.)

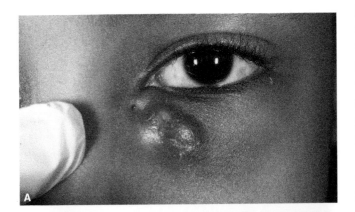

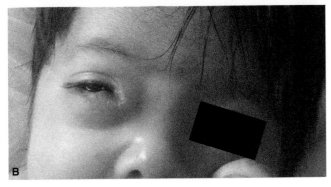

FIGURE 8.11 ■ Dacryocystitis; Differential Diagnosis of Preseptal Cellulitis. (**A, B**) Obstruction of the punctal and nasolacrimal duct can result in fluid accumulation in the nasolacrimal sac (dacryocystocele) and subsequent infection (dacryocystitis). Erythema and swelling are seen in the medial canthal area in both of these patients. Pressure over the lacrimal sac causes pain, and purulent material may be seen at lacrimal puncta. (Photo contributors: Binita R. Shah, MD [A], and Sarah Hilkert, MD [B].)

Perform a thorough eye examination, checking visual acuity, palpating periorbital tissues, assessing pupils and extraocular movements, and looking for conjunctival injection and chemosis. With preseptal cellulitis, the patient should not have any of the following findings: decreased visual acuity, pain with eye movement, chemosis, significant conjunctival injection, abnormal pupillary response or afferent papillary defect, proptosis, or diplopia. Any of the aforementioned findings indicate orbital cellulitis.

Consider obtaining CBC with differential, blood culture, and wound culture, if clinically indicated. If there is concern for sinus disease, orbital extension, or subperiosteal abscess, obtain a CT scan of orbits with thin slices (1- to 2-mm cuts). Patients with mild preseptal cellulitis (not clinically ill, no concern for extension of infection) may be managed as outpatients with oral antibiotics (eg, amoxicillin/clavulanate or clindamycin) for 10 days with close follow-up. If conjunctivitis is present, consider adding topical ophthalmic antibiotics. Children with moderate to severe or rapidly growing preseptal cellulitis, as well as infants younger than 1 year of age, should be admitted for IV antibiotics (eg, ampicillin/sulbactam, ceftriaxone, or vancomycin if methicillin-resistant *S aureus* is a concern).

Pearls

1. Vesicular rash suggests herpetic periorbital infection.
2. Close follow-up is mandatory as preseptal cellulitis may progress to orbital cellulitis, although this is rare.

HORDEOLUM AND CHALAZION

Clinical Summary

A chalazion is a result of obstruction and inflammation of the meibomian glands (oil-secreting glands) of the eyelids. When these glands become obstructed (eg, blepharitis), sebum leaks into surrounding tissue, forming a chalazion filled with lipo-granulomatous material. A hordeolum results from acute infection of the sebaceous glands (stye or external hordeolum) or meibomian glands (internal hordeolum).

Patients present with a visible and palpable circumscribed nodule in the eyelid that is usually solitary but may be bilateral or multiple. With a hordeolum, the localized swelling is tender and erythematous. There may be visible "pointing" of mucopurulent discharge on the external or internal eyelid or drainage/crusting. Patients may complain of chronic itchy eyes associated with blepharitis or have a prior history of a chalazion or hordeolum. Differential diagnosis includes preseptal cellulitis and pyogenic granuloma.

Emergency Department Treatment and Disposition

Perform an ocular exam including visual acuity and an exam of the eyelids and eye, looking for swelling, tenderness, and drainage. Edema is localized to the lesion. The conjunctiva and sclera are usually uninvolved. Consult ophthalmology if

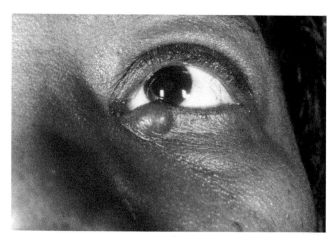

FIGURE 8.14 ■ Chalazion. A pea-sized, mobile, painless, noninflamed nodule is seen within the body of the eyelid. (Photo contributor: Binita R. Shah, MD.)

there is significant conjunctival injection or globe pain. Recommend outpatient treatment with warm compresses to the affected lid for 15 to 20 minutes, 4 times a day with gentle massage of area, or gentle eyelid scrubs with baby shampoo 1 to 2 times daily. If conjunctivitis or purulent eye discharge is present, prescribe topical antibiotics, such as bacitracin or erythromycin ophthalmic ointment. Most chalazions and hordeolums resolve spontaneously with conservative management.

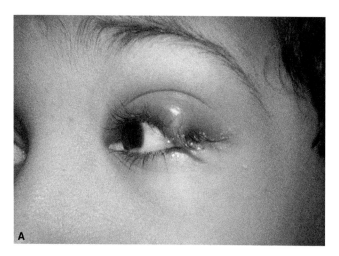

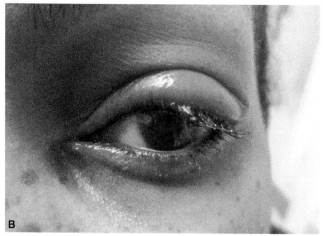

FIGURE 8.13 ■ Hordeolum. (**A**) External hordeolum: erythematous swelling at lid margin with purulent discharge resulting from infection of the sebaceous glands in the eyelash follicles. (**B**) Internal hordeolum: infection of the meibomian glands embedded in the tarsal plate. (Photo contributors: Binita R. Shah, MD [A], and Douglas R. Lazzaro, MD [B].)

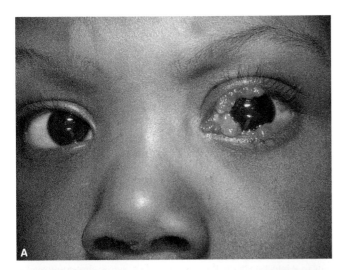

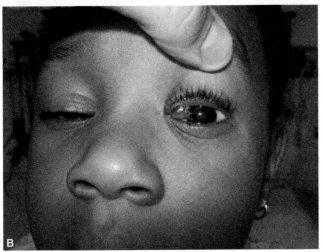

FIGURE 8.15 ■ Differential Diagnosis of Chalazion. (**A**) Conjunctival warts that were present since infancy. He also had warts on his the hand and most likely self-inoculated the virus to the conjunctiva. (**B**) Pyogenic granuloma. (Photo contributors: Binita R. Shah, MD [A], and Mark Silverberg, MD [B].)

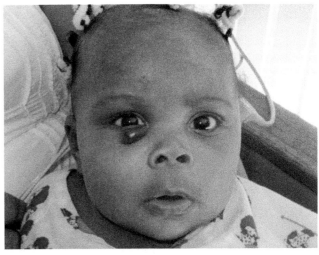

FIGURE 8.16 ■ Infantile Hemangioma: Differential Diagnosis of Chalazion. A rapidly increasing infantile hemangioma in a 4-month-old girl requiring propranolol therapy due to impingement of her vision. (Photo contributor: Haamid Chamdawala, MD.)

Pearls

1. Distinguishing a chalazion from a hordeolum may be difficult; although both have a localized nodule and may have some degree of erythema or discomfort, a hordeolum is usually more tender to palpation.

2. Refer patients with a chalazion lasting >3 weeks for outpatient follow-up with an ophthalmologist.

3. Rarely, a hordeolum may cause preseptal cellulitis or a deeper infection. Treat with systemic antibiotics and consult ophthalmology if edema, erythema, and pain are diffuse or worsen or the patient develops fever.

ACUTE CONJUNCTIVITIS

Clinical Summary

Acute conjunctivitis may be infectious or noninfectious and, by definition, lasts <4 weeks. Patients with infectious conjunctivitis present with conjunctival hyperemia, eye discharge that ranges from watery to purulent, and a history of eyelids sticking together (worse in the morning). Infectious conjunctivitis may present with unilateral or bilateral symptoms, although symptoms often begin in one eye and later progress to involve both eyes.

Bacterial and viral conjunctivitis can be difficult to distinguish from one another, although discharge may be more purulent with a bacterial infection and serous with a viral infection. Numerous bacterial pathogens cause conjunctivitis, including *S aureus*, *S pneumoniae*, *Haemophilus* species, and *Moraxella catarrhalis*. Adenoviral infections are the most common cause of viral conjunctivitis. The presence of pre-auricular lymphadenopathy may help distinguish infectious conjunctivitis from other types.

The severity of symptoms varies from mild injection with scant eye discharge or crusting and little to no lid edema, to severe presentations with moderate to severe mucopurulent discharge with significant scleral injection and lid edema. Copious, hyperacute, mucopurulent discharge may indicate gonococcal conjunctivitis. Consider herpes simplex virus (HSV) infection in unilateral conjunctivitis with a vesicular skin rash or crusted lesions on the eyelid margin.

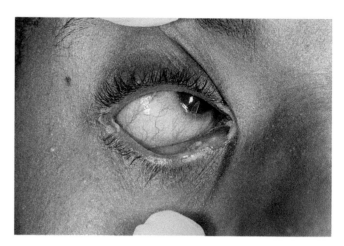

FIGURE 8.18 ■ Bacterial Conjunctivitis. Purulent discharge and conjunctival injection in a patient complaining of eye discharge and matting of lashes on awakening. (Photo contributor: Binita R. Shah, MD.)

Allergic conjunctivitis may present similarly to infectious conjunctivitis but tends to be bilateral with watery discharge, eyelid edema, pruritus, and extensive chemosis.

Differential diagnosis of conjunctivitis includes viral (including HSV), bacterial, and allergic conjunctivitis, vernal conjunctivitis, chemical irritation, foreign body, uveitis, and periorbital cellulitis.

Emergency Department Treatment and Disposition

For viral conjunctivitis, cold compresses and preservative-free artificial tears may provide symptomatic relief, if tolerated. Counsel patients that viral conjunctivitis is self-limited; however, it may get worse in the first 4 to 7 days after onset, but generally resolves in 2 to 3 weeks (longer if there is corneal involvement). Inquire about other contacts with "pink eye." Educate patients on strict hand hygiene, as transmission is through contact and patients may be contagious for up to 12 to 14 days.

If bacterial conjunctivitis is suspected, consider sending eye discharge for culture, and start empiric topical antibiotic therapy (eg, trimethoprim/polymyxin B or erythromycin ointment) for 5 to 7 days. Avoid fluoroquinolone drops in younger children, as systemic side effects are possible. If gonococcal conjunctivitis is suspected, send conjunctival swabs for Gram stain and culture, treat with systemic antibiotics (eg, ceftriaxone), and consult ophthalmology to evaluate for corneal involvement.

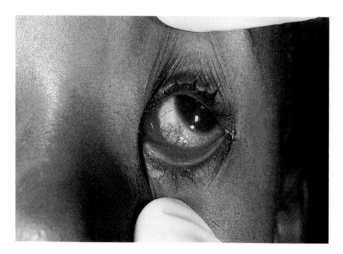

FIGURE 8.17 ■ Adenoviral Conjunctivitis. Severe photophobia, watery discharge, a foreign body sensation, and redness in both eyes (left > right) were seen in this child. Note the intense bulbar and palpebral conjunctival injection and hemorrhages. (Photo contributor: Binita R. Shah, MD.)

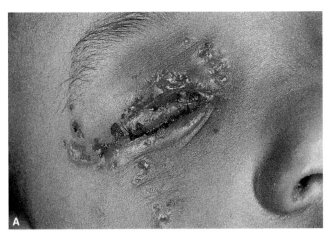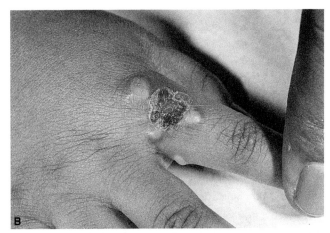

FIGURE 8.19 ■ Herpes Simplex Virus (HSV) Infection. (**A**) Multiple periorbital ulcerated and vesicular lesions in a patient with eczema (predisposing to HSV infection). HSV was cultured from the vesicular fluid. (**B**) Vesicular and ulcerated lesions on the index finger of the same patient (resulting in autoinoculation). (Photo contributor: Binita R. Shah, MD.)

Treatment of allergic conjunctivitis includes avoidance of the offending allergen and symptomatic relief with cool compresses and artificial tears. Oral antihistamines may help with significant pruritis. For moderate cases of allergic conjunctivitis, consider prescribing a topical ophthalmic antihistamine, such as olopatadine 0.1%.

Pearls

1. Check the "ocular vital signs" (red reflex, pupil, visual acuity, and motility) in any child with conjunctivitis.
2. Ocular pain is usually not associated with allergic, viral, or bacterial conjunctivitis and mandates consultation with ophthalmology.

3. Other symptoms that warrant emergent ophthalmology consultation include diminished vision and severe photophobia.
4. Presence of photophobia, pseudomembranes or membranes, marked hyperemia, chemosis, and subconjunctival hemorrhage may indicate epidemic keratoconjunctivitis (EKC), a type of adenoviral conjunctivitis that may involve the cornea. If EKC is suspected, the patient should follow-up with an ophthalmologist.
5. If HSV infection is suspected, consult ophthalmology to evaluate for corneal involvement (risk of corneal involvement is high when lesions are present on eyelid margin).

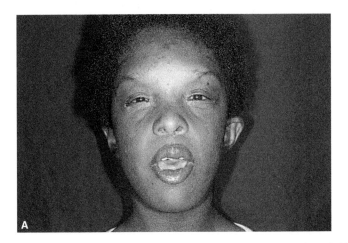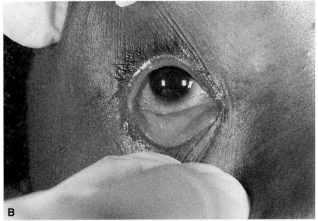

FIGURE 8.20 ■ Allergic Conjunctivitis. (**A**) Intense bilateral eye itching and mucoid discharge in a patient with allergies. Note the crusted discharge at the nostrils and mouth breathing (due to nasal obstruction). (**B**) Conjunctival injection and chemosis (edema of the conjunctiva) are characteristic features of allergic conjunctivitis. (Photo contributor: Binita R. Shah, MD.)

Clinical Summary

Ophthalmia neonatorum is inflammation or infection of the conjunctiva within the first month of life. Neonates present with diffuse conjunctival injection, purulent or mucopurulent discharge, eyelid edema, and chemosis. The time frame of presentation of symptoms is helpful in determining the etiology. Chemical conjunctivitis may be seen within hours of sliver nitrate instillation and last 24 to 36 hours, although this has become rare, as erythromycin ointment has replaced silver nitrate for prophylaxis. In contrast, *Neisseria gonorrhoeae* is usually seen 3 to 4 days after birth and has a variable presentation. Some newborns may present with mild conjunctival hyperemia, whereas others present with hyperacute, copious mucopurulent discharge with severe chemosis, corneal ulceration, or even perforation. Gram stain reveals gram-negative intracellular diplococci. *Chlamydia trachomatis* usually presents 1 to 2 weeks after birth with mild lid swelling, conjunctival injection, tearing, and mucoid discharge. Giemsa stain aids with diagnosis, demonstrating intracellular inclusion bodies in conjunctival epithelial cells or neutrophils. Nongonococcal

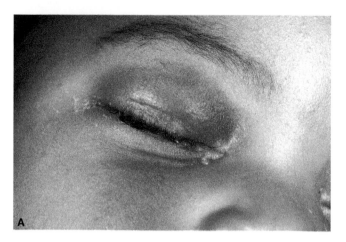

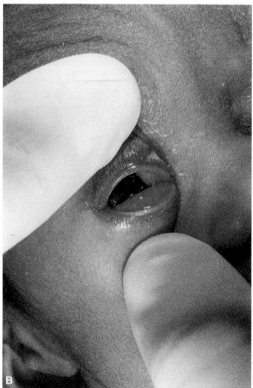

FIGURE 8.22 ■ Chlamydial Ophthalmia. (**A**) This 10-day-old neonate presented with lid swelling, erythema, and mild mucopurulent eye discharge. (**B**) Note the intense hyperemia of the palpebral conjunctiva. Direct fluorescent antibody staining for elementary bodies was positive, and both Gram stain and culture were negative for *N gonorrhoeae*. (Photo contributor: Binita R. Shah, MD.)

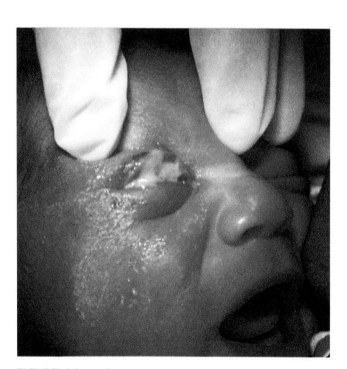

FIGURE 8.21 ■ Gonococcal Ophthalmia. A 5-day-old neonate presented with profuse, mucopurulent eye discharge with bilateral involvement. Note the erythema and swelling of the right lid. Both Gram stain and culture were positive for *N gonorrhoeae*. (Reproduced with permission from Shah BR, Laude TL. *Atlas of Pediatric Clinical Diagnosis*. WB Saunders; Philadelphia, PA, 2000.)

bacterial pathogens, including staphylococci, streptococci, or other gram-negative species, account for 30% to 50% of neonatal conjunctivitis, and these organisms may be seen on Gram stain. Differential diagnosis includes dacryocystitis, nasolacrimal duct obstruction, and congenital glaucoma.

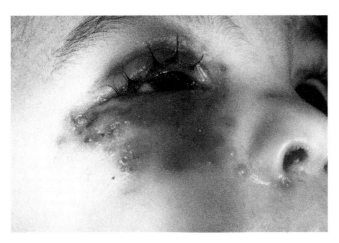

FIGURE 8.23 ■ Herpes Simplex Virus (HSV) Infection. Multiple vesicular lesions on an erythematous base indicate HSV infection. Ocular infections are usually caused by HSV-1, except in newborns, where HSV-2 predominates. (Reproduced with permission from Shah BR, Laude TL. *Atlas of Pediatric Clinical Diagnosis*. WB Saunders; Philadelphia, PA, 2000.)

Emergency Department Treatment and Disposition

Perform a complete eye exam with fluorescein staining to evaluate for corneal involvement. Chemical conjunctivitis does not need treatment, as it is typically self-limited. Arrange follow-up exam in 24 to 48 hours to confirm conjunctivitis is resolving. For neonates with suspected infectious etiology, obtain Gram stain, Giemsa stain, and cultures. Culture of the inferior palpebral conjunctiva will increase the yield. Ophthalmology consultation is recommended to further evaluate and obtain conjunctival scrapings for Gram stain and cultures. Send conjunctival scrapings for chlamydia PCR testing or immunofluorescent antibody testing, as well as for cultures. In neonates with purulent eye discharge concerning for chlamydial or gonococcal infection, evaluate for systemic infection, including blood and CSF studies. Admit the infant to the hospital and treat systemically for both chlamydial (eg, oral erythromycin) and gonococcal (eg, third-generation cephalosporin IV) conjunctivitis. Gram stain and Giemsa stain results may help guide initial therapy. Modify antibacterial treatment based on culture results.

Pearls

1. Suspect chlamydial infection if symptoms persist or worsen despite treatment for gonococcal conjunctivitis; chlamydial conjunctivitis may be accompanied by other systemic manifestations such as pneumonia.
2. Treat the mother and notify her sexual partner(s) for treatment with systemic antibiotics if cultures reveal a sexually transmitted infection.
3. In ophthalmia neonatorum, consider HSV infection, which may require both systemic and topical therapy.

LEUKOCORIA

Clinical Summary

Leukocoria (a white pupillary reflex) can be caused by a number of disease processes including local causes, such as cataract, or a potentially malignant process. Hypopyon with leukocoria in a 1- to 2-year-old child is highly suspicious for malignant retinoblastoma. Leukocoria at birth is suggestive of either a congenital cataract, which may be unilateral or bilateral, or persistent hyperplastic primary vitreous (PHPV). Differential diagnosis includes cataract, retinoblastoma, Coats disease, PHPV, toxocariasis, retinopathy of prematurity, and astrocytic hamartoma. Affected patients present with a white pupil and decreased vision. Physical exam finding of an absent red reflex leads to the diagnosis of leukocoria in many instances.

Emergency Department Treatment and Disposition

Once the diagnosis of leukocoria is made, refer the patient to ophthalmology promptly. Regardless of etiology, a full

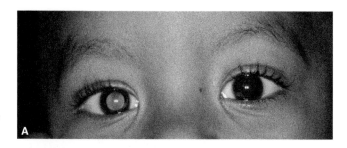
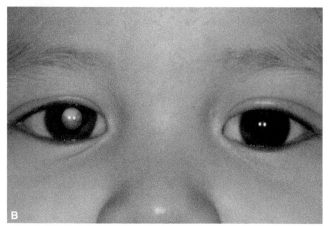
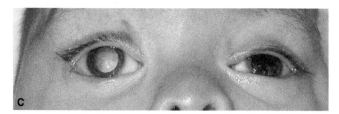

FIGURE 8.25 ■ Leukocoria in Retinoblastoma. (**A, B**) Two different toddlers with unilateral retinoblastoma presenting with leukocoria. (**C**) One-year-old infant with bilateral retinoblastoma presenting with leukocoria of the right eye and vitreous seeding in the left eye. (Photo contributors: Brian P. Marr, MD [A, B], and Roman Shinder, MD [C].)

ophthalmologic exam with imaging is necessary to render a proper diagnosis and exclude life-threatening etiologies. There is no specific treatment in the ED, as the cause of the problem must first be ascertained.

Pearls

1. Absent red reflex (white appearance) and decreased visual acuity are findings of leukocoria.
2. Evaluate for systemic abnormalities. Leukocoria is a marker of underlying pathology.
3. The most common presenting signs of retinoblastoma are leukocoria and strabismus.

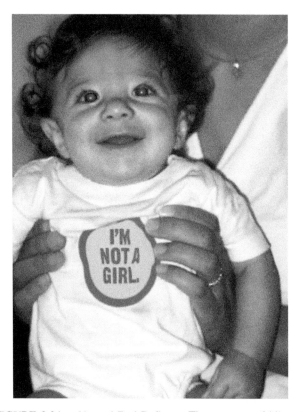

FIGURE 8.24 ■ Normal Red Reflexes. The presence of bilateral red reflexes suggests the absence of cataracts and intraocular pathology. (Photo contributor: Aden Benjamin Spektor and his parents.)

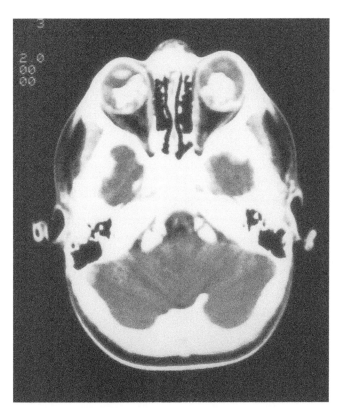

FIGURE 8.26 ■ Bilateral Retinoblastoma. On axial CT scan of the head, soft tissue window demonstrates bilateral large calcified intraorbital masses in a patient with bilateral retinoblastoma. (Reproduced with permission from Shah BR, Laude TL. *Atlas of Pediatric Clinical Diagnosis*. WB Saunders; Philadelphia, PA, 2000.)

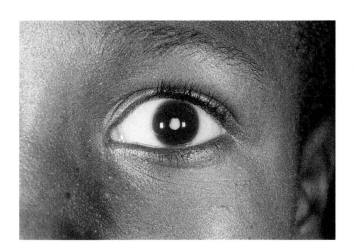

FIGURE 8.27 ■ Cataract: Differential Diagnosis of Leukocoria. (Photo contributor: Binita R. Shah, MD.)

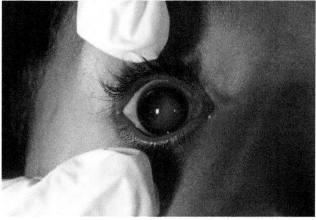

FIGURE 8.28 ■ Coats Disease: Differential Diagnosis of Leukocoria. An opacity is seen in a child presenting with a complaint of decreasing vision. In Coats disease, abnormal retinal blood vessels result in leakage of fluid and exudative retinopathy, seen in this patient on slit lamp examination. (Photo contributor: Binita R. Shah MD.)

Clinical Summary

Infantile glaucoma may be present at birth or diagnosed shortly thereafter; most cases are diagnosed during the first year of life. Sometimes, however, it is not recognized until later in infancy or early childhood. The characteristic signs include the triad of blepharospasm (involuntary blinking/spasm of eyelid), tearing, and photosensitivity. The affected eye of the infant may appear significantly enlarged (buphthalmos) compared to the unaffected eye, with megalocornea, and the cornea may appear cloudy. Infantile glaucoma is bilateral in up to 75% of cases.

Infantile glaucoma may present later in life (up to age 3 years) secondary to a gradual increase in intraocular pressure (IOP). These patients may not present with the typical triad, but with impaired vision and strabismus (crossed eyes). Differential diagnosis includes congenital megalocornea, trauma during delivery with corneal injury, congenital hereditary corneal dystrophy, and congenital infections (eg, congenital rubella, HSV).

Emergency Department Treatment and Disposition

Consult ophthalmology emergently for diagnosis and treatment of glaucoma, which is a vision-threatening disorder. Patients with increased IOP are treated with topical aqueous

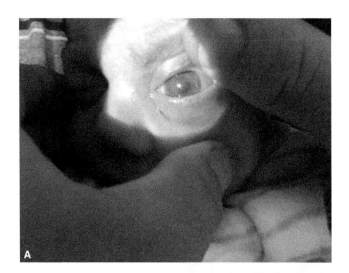
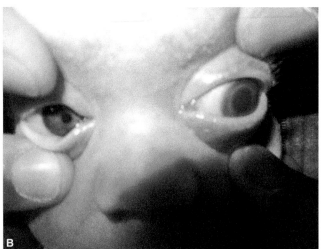
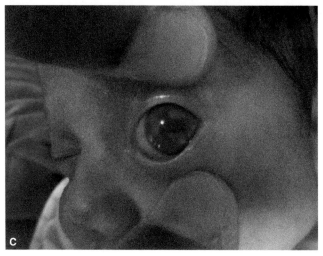

FIGURE 8.29 ■ Infantile Glaucoma. A 33-week preemie at 7 weeks after birth with infantile glaucoma (**A**), with obvious difference in corneal sizes (**B**), and a left buphthalmic eye (**C**) is shown. (Photo contributor: Douglas R. Lazzaro, MD.)

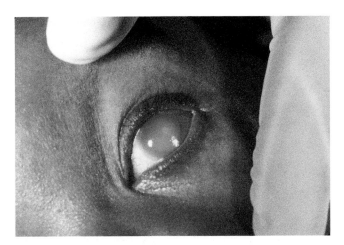

FIGURE 8.30 ▪ Infantile Glaucoma. Corneal clouding in an infant with infantile glaucoma. (Photo contributor: Binita R. Shah, MD.)

suppressants such as β-blockers (eg, timolol), carbonic anhydrase inhibitors (eg, acetazolamide), and prostaglandins (eg, latanoprost). Do not use α-adrenergic aqueous suppressants (eg, brimonidine) in children because they may cause CNS suppression. Surgery is required for definitive treatment. Other causes of excessive tearing and photosensitivity include foreign body, conjunctivitis, and nasolacrimal duct obstruction.

Pearls

1. Infantile glaucoma is a vision-threatening disorder characterized by increased IOP that presents before the age of 3 years.
2. Tearing is the most common sign of infantile glaucoma.
3. The classic triad of blepharospasm, tearing, and photosensitivity is only seen in a third of affected patients at the time of diagnosis.

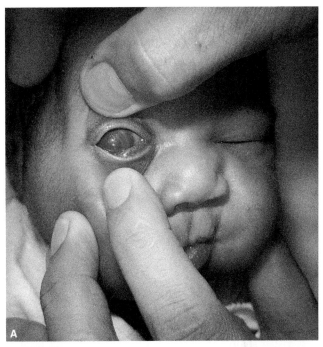

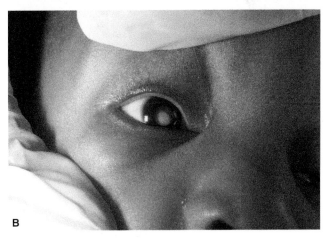

FIGURE 8.31 ▪ Infantile Glaucoma and Cataract with Congenital Rubella Syndrome (CRS). An enlarged, hazy cornea resulting from congenital glaucoma (**A**) and cataract (**B**) are shown in 2 different patients with CRS. Infantile glaucoma is seen in about 10% of patients, and cataract is seen in about 20% of patients with CRS. (Photo contributor: Binita R. Shah, MD.)

CORNEAL FOREIGN BODY

Clinical Summary

Patients with a corneal foreign body (FB) present with eye pain, irritation, and often a sensation of having an FB in the eye. Other symptoms include excessive tearing, photophobia, and redness of the eye. Vision may or may not be affected based on the location of the FB and the amount of inflammation in the surrounding corneal tissue. Historically, many patients will recall the nature and time of the FB occurrence. Rarely, a small FB can cause the aforementioned symptoms without any specific recollection of a causal event. Differential diagnosis includes corneal infection and corneal abrasion.

Emergency Department Treatment and Disposition

Enquire about an FB event. Perform a thorough eye exam, looking for signs of globe injury and presence of FB, and assess visual acuity. The FB can often be found with bright direct illumination if a slit lamp is not available. Evert eyelids to examine for FB. Use fluorescein staining to aid diagnosis and evaluate for associated corneal abrasion. If someone other than an ophthalmologist is attempting removal of the FB, make sure to assess FB depth prior to removal.

A very superficial FB can sometimes be removed by irrigation or with a cotton-tipped applicator if it lies superficially on the corneal or scleral epithelium. Moisten the end of cotton-tipped applicator and softly brush the area where the FB lies. Do not rub firmly because this can further embed the FB into the corneal stroma. Consider instilling topical anesthetic

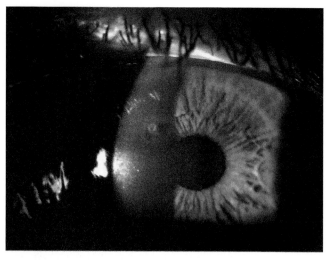

FIGURE 8.32 ■ Corneal Foreign Body. Corneal metallic foreign body. (Photo contributor: Douglas R. Lazzaro, MD.)

drops (eg, tetracaine, proparacaine) prior to removal if the patient is unable to keep the eye open due to pain. Prescribe topical ophthalmic antibiotic ointment for 5 days after removal. For embedded or deeper FBs, consult ophthalmology for removal.

Pearls

1. Pain with a corneal FB is frequently referred to the upper eyelid, and visual acuity is variably affected.
2. Direct visualization or fluorescein staining can reveal the location of the FB.
3. Evert lids when examining for FB.

Clinical Summary

Corneal abrasions occur when the corneal epithelium is damaged. Patients usually present with sharp pain, photophobia, FB sensation (even in the absence of an FB), tearing, and worsening pain with blinking, leading the patient to keep the eye closed. Blurred vision may occur if the abrasion is located in the visual axis. There is often a history of minor trauma, such as being hit in the eye with a toy or a hand, or a history of something flying into the eye or rubbing of the eye. Inquire about use of contact lenses, prior corneal abrasions, and skin lesions. Differential diagnosis includes herpetic keratitis, corneal ulcer, dry eyes, corneal FB, and contact lens overwear.

Emergency Department Treatment and Disposition

Evaluate visual acuity and the anterior portion of the eye and lids for other injury, presence of FB, or visible laceration of the cornea or sclera. Confirm the diagnosis with fluorescein stain of the cornea. If needed, place a drop of topical anesthetic (eg, tetracaine, proparacaine) into the eye and then gently touch a moistened fluorescein strip to the palpebral conjunctiva (not the cornea). Patients with large corneal abrasions, abrasions in the visual axis, or a history of contact lens use should be seen by an ophthalmologist within 12 to 24 hours. Simple corneal abrasions heal rapidly, and routine patching is not necessary. Patching and cycloplegics may be useful with larger epithelial defects. Generally topical ophthalmic antibiotic ointment (eg, erythromycin, polymyxin/trimethoprim) is prescribed to prevent superinfection, although clear evidence to support this is lacking. Ointment may aid with lubrication and healing. Patients should have close outpatient follow-up for repeat evaluation until abrasion is healed.

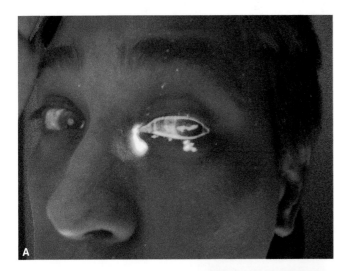

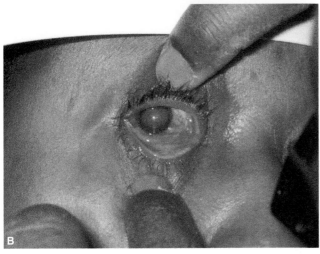

FIGURE 8.33 ■ Corneal Abrasions. (**A**) Sterile, single-use fluorescein strips can be used to help identify abrasions or ulcers. The dye appears green when viewed with a blue cobalt filter light or ultraviolet light source such as a Wood's lamp, as seen in this patient with a linear corneal abrasion. (**B**) This patient experienced severe eye pain after facial trauma from airbag deployment during a motor vehicular collision, resulting in an avulsion of >90% of the cornea. (Photo contributor: Mark Silverberg, MD.)

Pearls

1. Pain and FB sensation are the cardinal symptoms of a corneal abrasion.
2. Vertical linear corneal abrasions suggest the presence of an FB; examine under the eyelids for FB.
3. Never dispense topical anesthetic for continued home use.
4. In a contact lens wearer, select a topical antibiotic with pseudomonal coverage (eg, fluoroquinolone), discontinue contact lens use, and refer urgently to ophthalmology.
5. If the epithelial defect is associated with visible corneal opacities, such as a whitish lesion near fluorescein uptake, suspect a corneal ulcer and consult ophthalmology emergently.

Clinical Summary

Patients with a corneal ulcer present with a painful inflamed eye, sometimes with discharge, complaints of blurred vision, and an FB sensation. Typically, vision is decreased on visual acuity testing and pain may be severe with significant infection. Many patients will have a history of ocular trauma or contact lens use. Photophobia is generally present, and fluorescein staining reveals an epithelial defect. A corneal opacity can sometimes be seen on direct illumination prior to the instillation of fluorescein dye. Bacterial corneal ulcers are rare in children because intact corneal epithelium prevents penetration of bacteria into the corneal stroma. Any condition that leads to a breakdown of the corneal epithelium may lead to a corneal ulcer. Differential diagnosis includes foreign body, herpetic or bacterial infection, and fungal or parasitic keratitis.

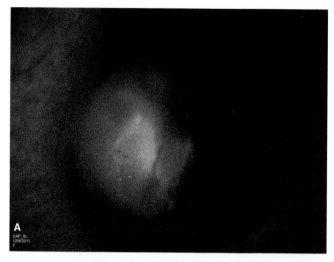

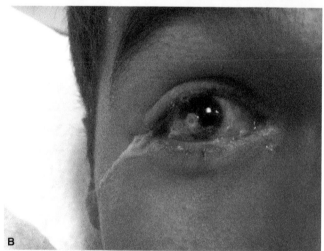

FIGURE 8.35 ■ Corneal Ulcer. (**A, B**) Two patients with corneal ulcers due to *Pseudomonas* associated with contact lens use. (Photo contributors: Douglas R. Lazzaro, MD [A], and Sarah Hilkert, MD [B].)

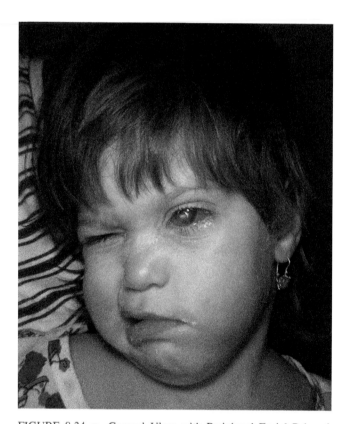

FIGURE 8.34 ■ Corneal Ulcer with Peripheral Facial Palsy. A grayish-white opacity is seen on the cornea with intense erythema. This patient was unable to close her eye due to a facial palsy, resulting in prolonged corneal exposure and a corneal ulcer that grew *Staphylococcus aureus*. Close-up showing hypopyon appears in Figure 8.36. (Photo contributor: Binita R. Shah, MD.)

Emergency Department Treatment and Disposition

Evaluate visual acuity and use bright direct light to identify corneal opacities. Use fluorescein staining to confirm the presence of ulceration. For small ulcers with minimal symptoms and mild decrease in vision, start topical ophthalmic antibiotics and refer the patient for ophthalmologic exam in 12 to 24 hours. For contact lens–associated ulcers, use a topical fourth-generation fluoroquinolone, in addition to a topical antibiotic ointment (eg, polymyxin/trimethoprim). Bacterial culture can be sent from eye discharge or from contact lens case to target therapy. Consult ophthalmology emergently in cases with severely diminished vision, corneal perforation, or an associated hypopyon.

Pearls

1. Suspect herpes simplex keratitis if dendritic ulceration is seen on fluorescein or if corneal ulceration is present with no history of ocular trauma or contact lens use.

2. For contact lens users with possible corneal ulceration, instruct patients to immediately discontinue use of their lenses.

HYPOPYON

Clinical Summary

Hypopyon is the accumulation of leukocytes layered in the anterior chamber of the eye and appears as a white to gray liquid. It is a sign of an infectious or inflammatory process such as endophthalmitis, uveitis, corneal ulcer, or, rarely, retinoblastoma. Patients may present with no history that indicates an etiology (spontaneous) or after significant trauma to the eye. The patient usually has an associated loss of vision, eye pain, and photosensitivity. Differential diagnosis includes corneal ulcer, endophthalmitis, complication of intraocular surgery, posttraumatic inflammation, retained intraocular FB, and retinoblastoma or other tumor in a young child.

Emergency Department Treatment and Disposition

Enquire about contact lens use, trauma, ocular surgery, and family history of ocular problems. Consult ophthalmology

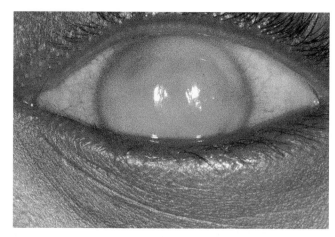

FIGURE 8.37 ■ Hypopyon. A complete anterior chamber hypopyon from retinoblastoma. (Photo contributor: Brian P. Marr, MD.)

emergently. Topical ophthalmic antibiotic or anti-inflammatory medications may be recommended, depending on the ocular and systemic findings, and the suspected underlying etiology.

Pearls

1. A hypopyon is composed of a collection of leukocytes in the anterior chamber.
2. A hypopyon is a medical emergency because it may signal endophthalmitis.

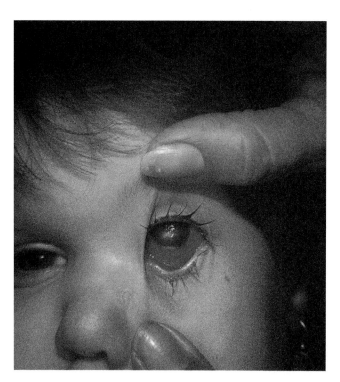

FIGURE 8.36 ■ Hypopyon and Corneal Ulcer in a Patient with Facial Nerve Palsy. Grayish-white opacity on the cornea and accumulation of inflammatory cells in the anterior chamber produce a horizontal layered meniscus (see also Figure 8.34). (Photo contributor: Binita R. Shah, MD.)

Clinical Summary

A hyphema is the accumulation of blood in the anterior chamber of the eye and typically occurs as a result of ocular trauma, but may occur spontaneously in infants with juvenile xanthogranuloma of the iris, retinoblastoma, or a bleeding diathesis. Patients present with eye pain and visible blood in the anterior chamber of the eye and may have a decrease in visual acuity. There is a risk of a spontaneous rebleed within 5 days in cases of trauma, which may lead to further complications such as glaucoma or corneal staining. The amount of blood in the anterior chamber can vary from completely filling the anterior chamber ("8-ball" hyphema) to a microscopic amount seen on slit-lamp evaluation. Risk of complications increases with the size of the hyphema. Patients with sickle cell trait or disease or a bleeding diathesis are at greater risk of severe ocular complications. Differential diagnosis includes neovascularization, trauma, HSV or herpes zoster infection, and intraocular tumor.

Emergency Department Treatment and Disposition

Take a history with attention to bleeding diathesis and sickle cell disease, and test for sickle cell if history is unknown or unreliable. Evaluate for orbital fracture and other traumatic injuries. Consult ophthalmology emergently, place an eye shield that rests on the bony orbit (not an eye patch) over the

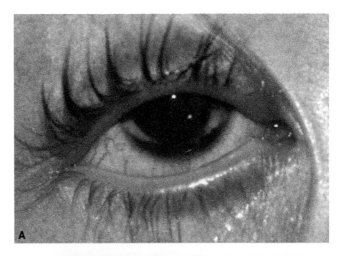
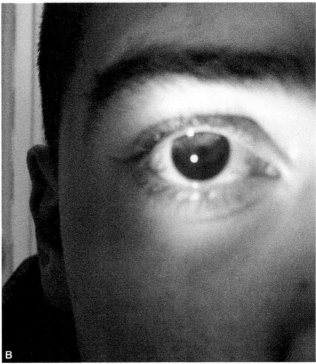

FIGURE 8.39 ■ Hyphema. (**A**) Small hyphema layering in bottom of anterior chamber after blunt trauma. (**B**) Blood filling more than half of anterior chamber after being hit with a snowball. (Photo contributors: Julia K. Lloyd, MD [A], and Barry Hahn, MD [B].)

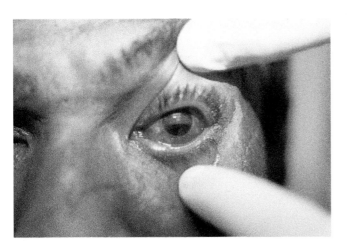

FIGURE 8.38 ■ Hyphema. Blood filling almost one-half of the anterior chamber following blunt trauma. (Photo contributor: Michael Lucchesi, MD.)

injured eye, and avoid any pressure on the eye. Treat pain and nausea to limit an increase in IOP. Bedrest and elevation of the head of the bed are recommended to facilitate layering of the hyphema. Do not give medications with aspirin or NSAIDs. Most patients with a hyphema should be admitted to the hospital for topical ophthalmic medications (cycloplegics and possibly steroids) and frequent reassessment. Low-risk patients with small hyphemas (less than one-third of the anterior chamber) and the ability to comply with restrictions may be managed at home with close ophthalmology follow-up.

Pearls

1. Consult ophthalmology emergently to exclude ruptured globe and to measure IOP.
2. Aspirin and NSAIDs are contraindicated because of the risk of rebleeding.
3. The presence of a hyphema without trauma should prompt an investigation for underlying disease (eg, leukemia, coagulopathy).
4. A small hyphema may be more difficult to discern with a dark-colored iris.

Clinical Summary

Subconjunctival hemorrhage occurs when episcleral and conjunctival blood vessels burst, which may result from direct eye trauma, increased intrathoracic pressure (eg, coughing or vomiting), conjunctivitis, hypertension, bleeding disorders/coagulopathy, or anticoagulant medications. Traumatic subconjunctival hemorrhage may be associated with orbital fracture or other eye injuries. With isolated subconjunctival hemorrhage, vision is normal and there is no associated discharge, tearing, and no pain with eye movements or with palpation over the area of hemorrhage. Presence of these symptoms should prompt consideration of other injuries or disease processes. With recurrent hemorrhages, consider evaluation for thrombocytopenia or other bleeding disorders. Differential diagnosis includes episcleritis, corneal abrasion, and conjunctivitis.

Emergency Department Treatment and Disposition

No treatment is needed for isolated subconjunctival hemorrhage. Reassure the patient of the benign nature of the condition and that it will resolve within 1 to 2 weeks. No workup

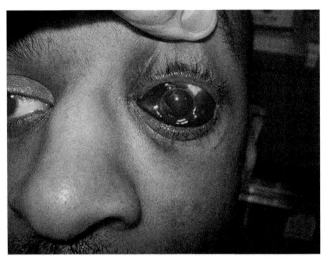

FIGURE 8.41 ■ Subconjunctival Hemorrhage. Severe subconjunctival hemorrhage with bloody chemosis that encircles almost the entire corneal limbus in a patient who was punched in the eye. (Photo contributor: Mark Silverberg, MD.)

is needed unless there are repeated episodes or signs of a systemic bleeding disorder (easy bruising, other bleeding). If there is a history of trauma, exclude associated conditions such as corneal abrasion, globe injury, or orbital fracture.

Pearls

1. Evaluate for injury to the globe if there is severe eye pain, photophobia, decreased visual acuity, or extension of the hemorrhage beyond the limbus.
2. In blunt trauma to the eye with a 360-degree subconjunctival hemorrhage, evaluate for orbital fracture and globe rupture because the hemorrhage may obscure the ruptured globe.

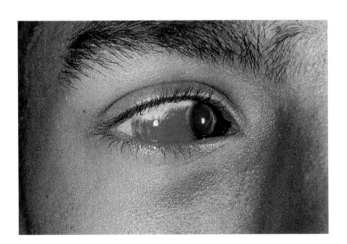

FIGURE 8.40 ■ Subconjunctival Hemorrhage. Subconjunctival hemorrhage following minor trauma is seen in this patient whose ocular examination was otherwise normal. (Photo contributor: Binita R. Shah, MD.)

EYELID LACERATION

Clinical Summary

Eyelid lacerations are classified based on location and involvement of structures: with or without lid margin involvement, medial canthal lacerations, and involvement of the canalicular system or tear-drainage system. Any laceration medial to the punctum is at high risk of canalicular involvement. Patients usually present with a history of trauma and may have other associated ocular injuries, such as scleral, conjunctival, or corneal lacerations, as well as intraocular FB or penetration of the globe.

Emergency Department Treatment and Disposition

Take a careful history to determine the mechanism of injury, and perform a complete examination, including a thorough ocular exam, evaluating for additional injuries. If there is concern for an FB, ruptured globe, or orbital fracture, consider obtaining a CT scan. Consider tetanus and rabies prophylaxis when indicated and administer systemic antibiotics for contaminated wounds, bite wounds, and suspected FB. Consult ophthalmology for evaluation and repair of large or complex lacerations: lacerations with involvement of the lid margin, medial canthus (medial one-third of lower lid), or canalicular system; or if there is concern for additional eye injuries. Prescribe topical ophthalmic antibiotic ointment for the repaired laceration.

Pearls

1. Check "ocular vital signs" (red reflex, pupil, visual acuity, and motility in *both eyes*) in any child presenting with ocular trauma.
2. Lacerations medial to the puncta require probing and irrigation by ophthalmology to determine canalicular involvement.
3. Orbital fat protrusion from the wound represents a deeper laceration in which the orbital septum has been violated. This often requires exploration of the deeper tissues of the eyelid by ophthalmology in the operating room.

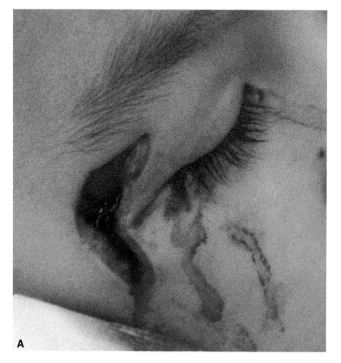

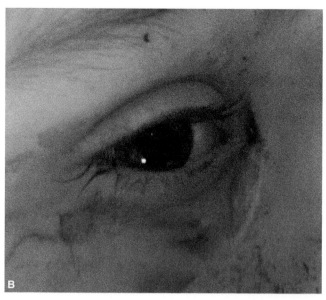

FIGURE 8.42 ■ Eyelid Laceration. (**A**) This laceration lateral to the eye was caused by a flying glass object that penetrated into the orbit, causing associated globe injury. (**B**) This laceration to the medial canthus from a pit bull bite involved the canalicular system and required placement of a stent.

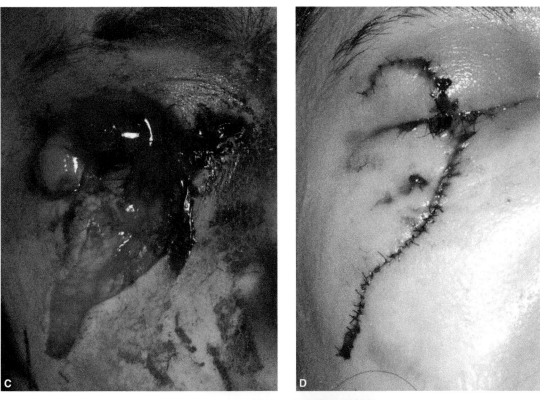

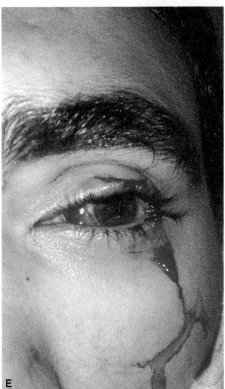

FIGURE 8.42 ■ (*Continued*) (**C, D**) Full-thickness laceration of upper and lower eyelids with associated globe injury from penetrating trauma before and after repair. (**E**) Full-thickness laceration involving left upper eyelid margin with associated subconjunctival hemorrhage following penetrating trauma. (Photo contributors: Sarah Hilkert, MD [A-D], and Douglas R. Lazzaro, MD [E].)

TRAUMATIC GLOBE RUPTURE

Clinical Summary

Patients with globe rupture present with decreased vision and eye pain with a history of direct trauma. Injury may be due to blunt trauma (eg, motor vehicle accidents, projectiles, assault), a fall onto a sharp object, or a penetrating FB. On exam, the eye may have a visible corneal or scleral laceration, choroid or iris prolapse through the injury, a "teardrop" or peaked pupil, or volume loss of the globe. A 360-degree subconjunctival hemorrhage or a hyphema may be present, as well. Pupillary reaction may be abnormal based on the extent of injury. The lens may be in an abnormal location, either in the anterior or posterior chamber or even outside of the eye.

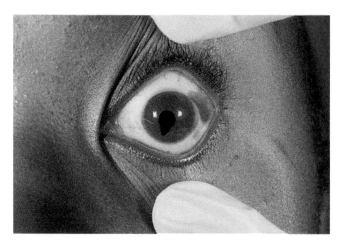

FIGURE 8.44 ■ Teardrop Pupil with Subconjunctival Hemorrhage: Traumatic Ruptured Globe. Immediately after laceration, the iris or choroid may plug the corneal wound. Because of this, the pupil may appear as a teardrop shape with the narrowest segment pointing toward the rupture. (Photo contributor: Binita R. Shah, MD.)

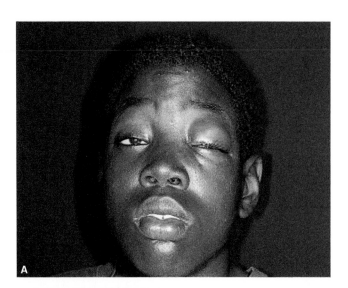

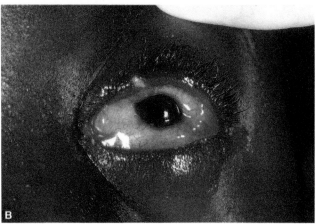

FIGURE 8.43 ■ Traumatic Ruptured Globe. Swelling, redness, eye pain, and blurred vision were the presenting complaints following blunt trauma in this patient (**A**). Severe chemosis is present (**B**). Patients presenting with severe 360-degree subconjunctival chemosis without hemorrhage following trauma should be treated as having a ruptured globe. (Photo contributor: Binita R. Shah, MD.)

Most traumatic globe ruptures occur at the limbal area or at the insertion of the ocular muscles into the globe, and the eye may have limited extraocular movements. Differential diagnosis includes severe eye contusion without rupture, severe infection, and buphthalmic eye (enlarged globe) with possible ruptured cornea.

Emergency Department Treatment and Disposition

Perform a vision assessment, if possible, and evaluate the globe and pupil carefully, without putting pressure on the eye. Place a protective eye shield over the eye, taking care not to put any pressure on the globe, once the diagnosis is made or considered. Imaging with CT may be warranted if there is concern for an intraocular FB (eg, with blast injury) or orbital fracture. Do not use ocular US if globe rupture is suspected because pressure may cause extrusion of intraocular contents. Consult ophthalmology emergently and give broad-spectrum IV antibiotics with activity against gram-positive and gram-negative organisms, including *Bacillus* species if contamination with organic FB. Consider tetanus and rabies prophylaxis, if indicated. Globe rupture requires urgent operative repair; keep patient NPO (nothing by mouth). Minimize patient agitation as much as possible, and provide antiemetics, analgesics, and sedation as needed to prevent increased IOP and expulsion of intraocular contents.

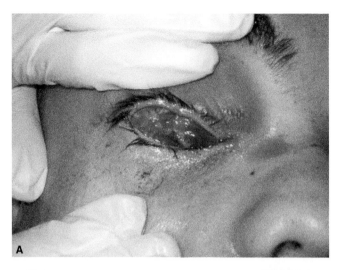

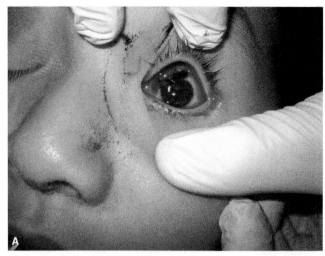

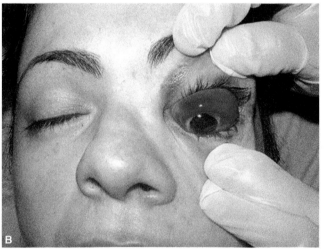

FIGURE 8.45 ■ Traumatic Ruptured Globe. (**A**) Ruptured right globe in a 15-year-old boy from a gunshot wound. (**B**) This adolescent girl was hit in the eye with a softball. Notice the total hyphema ("8-ball" hyphema) filling the entire anterior chamber as well as the bulging sclera overlying the globe rupture site. (Photo contributors: Roman Shinder, MD [A], and Mark Silverberg, MD [B].)

FIGURE 8.46 ■ Traumatic Ruptured Globe. (**A**) Corneal laceration with iris prolapse through the wound is seen in this child due to injury from a broken drinking glass. (**B**) Conjunctival laceration. This can be a sign of a ruptured globe. This patient presented with eye pain and redness following accidental injury from the point of a pencil. (Photo contributors: Bahram Rahmani, MD [A], and Binita R. Shah, MD [B].)

Pearls

1. Traumatic globe rupture represents a true ophthalmic emergency.
2. An abnormally peaked pupil can be a clue to the diagnosis and points in the direction of the injury.
3. Following blunt trauma to the eye, a 360-degree subconjunctival hemorrhage may obscure an underlying ruptured globe.
4. If globe rupture is diagnosed, do not manipulate/examine the eye further. Instead, place a raised protective shield over the eye without putting pressure on the eye.
5. Instruct older patients to avoid Valsalva maneuvers to avoid extrusion of intraocular contents.

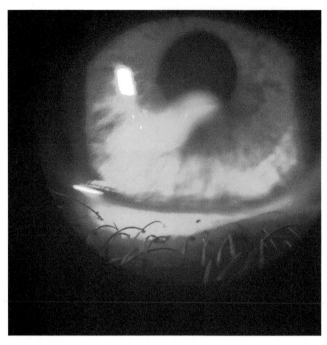

FIGURE 8.47 ■ Positive Seidel Test from Globe Rupture. Fluorescein dye instilled in the superior conjunctiva is diluted by the leak of fluid at the site of the rupture and is noted to stream, helping to identify the presence and location of the injury. (Photo contributor: Sarah Hilkert, MD.)

Clinical Summary

Direct trauma to the face or eye may result in fracture of the bony orbit, in addition to other ocular injuries. The patient presents with eye pain, periorbital bruising, and swelling with tenderness of the bony orbit. Patients may have diplopia with vertical gaze or altered sensation to the cheek, as well as systemic symptoms such as nausea, vomiting, and bradycardia. On examination, limited vertical gaze is highly suspicious for an orbital floor fracture with entrapment of the inferior rectus muscle. Other findings may include decreased vision or a large subconjunctival hemorrhage that extends posteriorly.

Emergency Department Treatment and Disposition

When orbital fracture is suspected, perform a complete eye exam, assessing visual acuity and evaluating for globe rupture, hyphema, and other traumatic injuries. Marked lid swelling may limit your exam. Orbital fractures are diagnosed by CT scan of the orbit. Emergently consult ophthalmology for orbital fractures with muscle entrapment, as urgent surgical repair is necessary. Orbital fractures without muscle entrapment should be seen by an ophthalmologist within 24 hours. Surgery may be required for some patients once the swelling has improved. Consider treatment with prophylactic antibiotics depending on location and extent of fracture.

Pearls

1. With orbital fracture, evaluate carefully for additional eye injuries such as globe injury and retrobulbar hemorrhage (present in 30% to 50% of patients).
2. Periorbital bruising and swelling may not be as apparent in children with orbital fractures ("white-eyed" fracture), so a high index of suspicion must be maintained.
3. Bradycardia, nausea, or syncope in a patient with an orbital fracture suggests muscle entrapment ("oculocardiac reflex"), which requires emergent ophthalmology evaluation and urgent surgical repair.

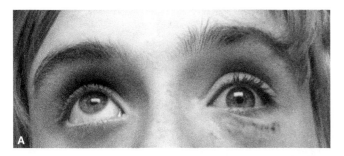
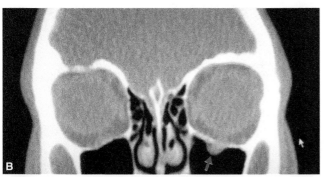
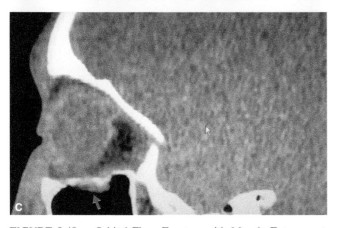

FIGURE 8.48 ■ Orbital Floor Fracture with Muscle Entrapment. (**A**) This patient had limitation of upward gaze on the left from muscle entrapment after being hit in the eye with a baseball. (**B, C**) The patient's CT scan shows an orbital floor fracture and prolapse of the inferior rectus muscle (arrows). (Photo contributor: Sarah Hilkert, MD.)

RETROBULBAR HEMORRHAGE

Clinical Summary

Retrobulbar hemorrhage can occur as a result of direct trauma to the eye or as a complication of orbital surgery or injections and is a true ophthalmologic emergency. Bleeding behind the eye can result in an orbital compartment syndrome with risk of rapid vision loss within 60 to 90 minutes. Patients present with eye pain, proptosis, and vision loss. Other physical exam findings include marked ecchymosis of the eyelids, diffuse subconjunctival hemorrhage, a "hard" eye or eyelid, an abnormal or unreactive pupil, and severely limited extraocular movements.

Emergency Department Treatment and Disposition

Ophthalmology should be emergently consulted for a patient with retrobulbar hemorrhage or ocular compartment syndrome because ischemia and rapid vision loss may occur. Treatment involves decompressing the orbit with a lateral canthotomy and inferior cantholysis, which may be done in the ED setting. There may be associated orbital fracture, and CT scan may be indicated to evaluate for associated injuries but should not delay treatment. Differential diagnosis includes orbital fracture, globe rupture, tumor, and orbital cellulitis.

Pearls

1. Retrobulbar hemorrhage is a vision-threatening emergency requiring immediate intervention to prevent vision loss.
2. The triad of an abnormal or unreactive pupil, severe limitation of extraocular movements, and elevated IOP with the eye itself feeling "hard" is highly concerning for retrobulbar hemorrhage.

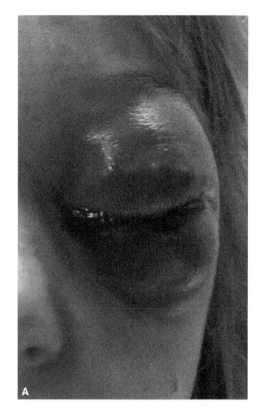

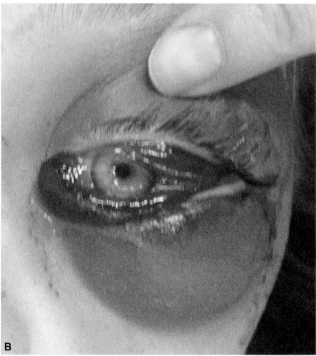

FIGURE 8.49 ■ Retrobulbar Hemorrhage. (**A**) This patient presented with eye pain, marked bruising and swelling of the eyelids, which felt "hard" after blunt trauma. (**B**) Emergent canthotomy and cantholysis were performed with release of the ocular compartment syndrome. (Photo contributor: Sarah Hilkert, MD.)

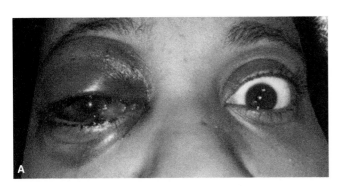 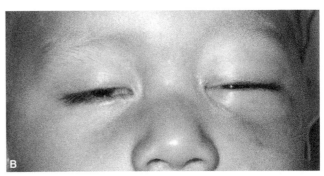

FIGURE 8.50 ■ Retrobulbar Hemorrhage. (**A**) Proptosis, periorbital ecchymosis, and subconjunctival hemorrhage are seen in a 16-year-old after blunt trauma. (**B**) Proptosis, periorbital edema, and ecchymosis are seen in a 3-year-old after blunt trauma. In both these patients, diagnosis of retrobulbar hemorrhage was confirmed by CT scan of the orbit. (Photo contributor: Roman Shinder, MD.)

Clinical Summary

Chemical burns of the eye from acidic or alkaline material are an ophthalmologic emergency. Patients present with eye pain, tearing, and redness after contact with the toxic substance. Swelling of the conjunctiva can be seen, and a corneal epithelial defect will be noted on fluorescein staining. The extent and location of the corneal defect have prognostic significance. In severe injuries, limbal ischemia may occur, causing affected areas to appear pale and result in corneal clouding. Acidic substances tend to precipitate in the eye, which limits penetration and damage to the eye, whereas alkaline substances are more likely to penetrate deeper into the eye,

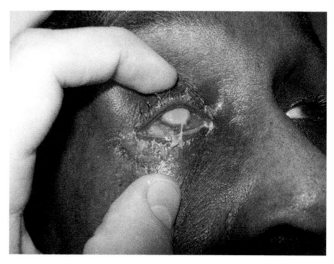

FIGURE 8.52 ■ Chemical Burn. Fluorescein staining demonstrates 100% corneal burn from an acid mist sprayed in this patient's eye while working in a factory. (Photo contributor: Mark Silverberg, MD)

degrading corneal tissue and causing more severe damage to intraocular structures. In severe chemical injury, the cornea may be opacified on presentation, denoting a poor prognosis.

Emergency Department Treatment and Disposition

Chemical eye injury should be treated immediately with copious irrigation. Instilling topical anesthetic drops first can aid in patient tolerance of irrigation. Flush the affected eye

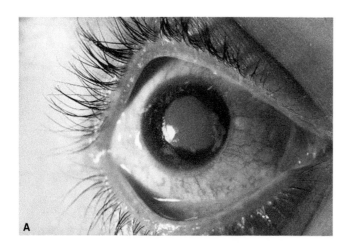

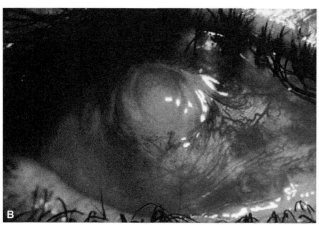

FIGURE 8.51 ■ Chemical Burns. Corneal burns from chemical exposure (**A**) and subacute alkali burn to the conjunctiva and cornea with corneal clouding (**B**). The use of fluorescein confirms injury to the cornea in addition to the conjunctiva. (Reproduced with permission from Hertle RW, Schaffer DB, Foster JA: Pediatric Eye Disease. *Color Atlas and Synopsis.* McGraw-Hill Education; New York, NY, 2002.)

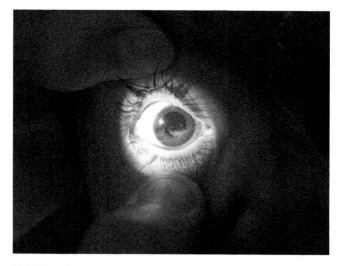

FIGURE 8.53 ■ Chemical Burn. Corneal burn in a child from accidental exposure to calcium hydroxide powder, an alkaline substance used in cooking. (Photo contributor: Bahram Rahmani, MD.)

for a minimum of 20 minutes or with 2 L of normal saline or lactated Ringer's solution using IV tubing and a Morgan Lens, if possible. Particulate matter may accumulate under lids and in fornices. Evert lids and sweep eyelid fornices gently with a moistened cotton-tipped applicator to remove any remaining caustic material. Check ocular pH 10 minutes after irrigation is stopped and continue irrigation until pH of 7.0 to 7.5 is achieved. This may require many liters of fluid or prolonged irrigation. Assess visual acuity and assess corneal damage with fluorescein staining. Consult ophthalmology for all chemical eye injuries. Topical cycloplegics and antibiotic ointment are often indicated, in addition to daily exams by an ophthalmologist. Occasionally admission may be indicated if a child's injuries are bilateral or severe.

Pearls

1. Copious irrigation and restoration of the normal pH are the keys to successful management of ocular chemical injury.
2. Alkali chemical burns tend to be worse than acidic burns and often require more irrigation.

Chapter 9

OTOLARYNGOLOGY

Sydney C. Butts
Nira A. Goldstein
Richard M. Rosenfeld
Aaron L. Thatcher
David J. Brown
Christopher Discolo
Jennifer H. Chao

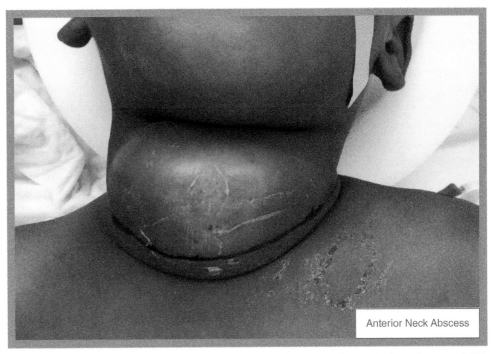

Anterior Neck Abscess

(Photo contributor: Sydney C. Butts, MD)

The authors acknowledge the special contributions of Anita Konka, MD, Matthew Hanson, MD, Miguel Mascaro, MD, Michael C. Singer, MD, Christina DiLoreto, MD, David H. Burstein, MD, Perminder S. Parmar, MD, Marika Fraser, MD, Haidy Marzouk, MD, Jessica W. Lim, MD, and Nur-Ain Nadir, MD, to prior edition.

Clinical Summary

Acute otitis media (AOM) is defined as the rapid onset of signs and symptoms of inflammation in the middle ear. AOM is considered highly likely if *distinct* bulging of the tympanic membrane (TM) or acute purulent otorrhea (not caused by acute otitis externa [AOE]) is seen. AOM is considered possible with *mild* bulging of the TM with recent onset of otalgia plus opacification, distinct erythema, or reduced mobility (on pneumatic otoscopy). AOM is considered unlikely with findings of middle-ear effusion *without* bulging or distinct erythema of the TM (eg, otitis media with effusion). Otalgia or other nonspecific symptoms (eg, fever, irritability) *without* middle-ear effusion or a bulging TM are not consistent with the diagnosis of AOM.

It can be difficult to fully visualize the TM to make the diagnosis; obstructing cerumen can be gently removed with suction or curettage either by ED staff or by the otolaryngology team. AOM should *not* be diagnosed empirically when the TM is poorly visualized.

Emergency Department Treatment and Disposition

Adequate pain relief is an essential part of management, especially in the first 24 hours after AOM diagnosis. Acetaminophen or ibuprofen is recommended; narcotics are rarely

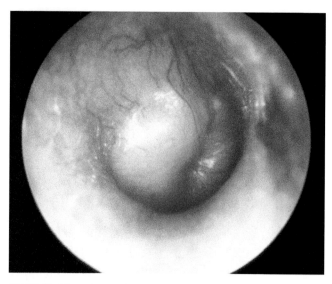

FIGURE 9.2 ■ Acute Otitis Media. Distinct bulging of the tympanic member with purulent middle-ear effusion consistent with acute otitis media. (Photo contributor: Richard Rosenfeld, MD.)

necessary and should be avoided. Antibiotics do not reduce pain associated with AOM in the first 24 to 48 hours and should not be used for this purpose. Topical analgesic drops typically containing benzocaine provide mild pain relief for 20 to 60 minutes after administration and may be useful between administration of oral analgesics and onset of pain relief. Topical analgesic drops should not be used if the TM is perforated or a tympanostomy tube is in place.

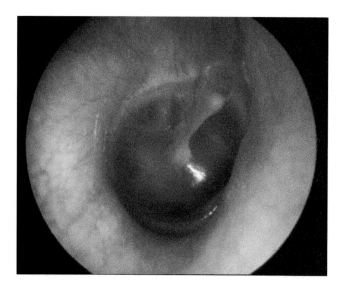

FIGURE 9.1 ■ Normal Tympanic Membrane. Normal tympanic membrane in a neutral position without middle-ear effusion. (Photo contributor: Richard Rosenfeld, MD.)

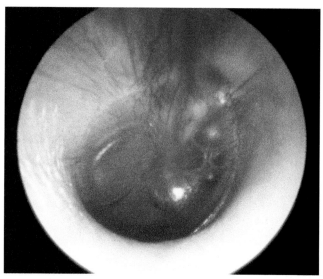

FIGURE 9.3 ■ Otitis Media with Effusion. Nonbulging tympanic membrane with middle-ear effusion consistent with otitis media with effusion. (Photo contributor: Richard Rosenfeld, MD.)

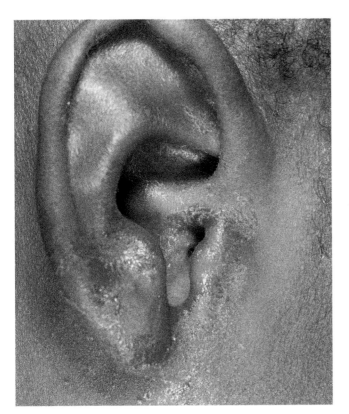

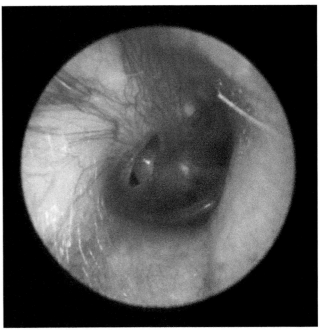

FIGURE 9.5 ■ Tympanic Membrane Perforation; Acute Otitis Media. Perforation of the anterior portion of the right tympanic membrane. (Photo contributor: Sydney C. Butts, MD.)

FIGURE 9.4 ■ Acute Otitis Media Presenting with Otorrhea. Purulent drainage from the external auditory canal (EAC). Various etiologies of otorrhea include AOM with perforation, otitis externa, drainage through tympanostomy tube, foreign body in EAC, cholesteatoma, chronic suppurative otitis media, or basilar skull fracture (bloody otorrhea). (Photo contributor: Binita R. Shah, MD.)

AOM can be managed with watchful waiting, immediate antibiotic prescribing, or delayed antibiotic prescribing. Immediate antibiotic is recommended for infants <6 months of age, in patients with AOM accompanied by otorrhea, or for bilateral AOM in children <2 years of age. If the above criteria are not met, there is a role for delayed antibiotic prescribing in which a *safety-net antibiotic prescription* (SNAP) is given with advice to fill the prescription (and begin therapy) only if the child does not improve within 72 hours of diagnosis or begins to worsen at any time. For many children managed with this strategy, the "delay" becomes indefinite so that the antibiotics are never required.

When an antibiotic is prescribed for AOM, the choice is based on likely pathogens and resistance patterns in the community. Most AOM is caused by *Streptococcus pneumoniae* (20% to 40% penicillin resistant), *Haemophilus influenzae* (30% β-lactamase producing), or *Moraxella catarrhalis*

(100% β-lactamase producing). Recommended first-line antibiotic is amoxicillin with or without clavulanate; children who are allergic to penicillin can be prescribed cefdinir, cefpodoxime, or cefuroxime. For children unable to tolerate cephalosporins, clarithromycin or azithromycin is suitable. Duration of therapy is generally 7 to 10 days, although children aged >2 years may respond to short-course therapy of 5 days. Intramuscular ceftriaxone is appropriate as single-dose treatment for children who cannot tolerate oral antibiotic (eg, severe vomiting) or as a series of 3 consecutive daily injections for children with refractory AOM unresponsive to oral antibiotics.

Drainage of pus from the middle ear by aspiration (tympanocentesis) or incision (myringotomy) is *not* effective for pain relief and should be reserved for (1) complicated infections (eg, mastoiditis, meningitis); (2) severe, refractory AOM that persists despite adequate antibiotic therapy; or (3) when resistant pathogens are suspected and culture is necessary. Management of such children should be with otolaryngology consultation.

Children with recurrent or refractory AOM may benefit from tympanostomy tubes because the tubes (1) ventilate the middle ear, eliminating the pressure gradients that aspirate nasopharyngeal secretions to the middle ear; (2) allow controlled drainage of AOM through the tube, should it recur; and (3) serve as a drug-delivery vehicle for quinolone drops to the middle ear, eliminating the adverse effects of systemic antibiotics and delivering the antibiotic in much higher concentration to the site of infection.

If suppurative complications of AOM are present or suspected (see page 429), obtain diagnostic imaging, and consult otolaryngology for drainage of the middle ear by myringotomy, tympanocentesis, or placement of a tympanostomy tube.

Pearls

1. Counsel caregivers about the importance of prompt and regular pain control in the first 24 to 48 hours; a dose of ibuprofen at bedtime will improve sleep.

2. Topical antibiotic drops are ineffective for AOM with an intact TM and should not be routinely prescribed unless there is a perforated TM or the child has a tympanostomy tube.

3. Children most likely to benefit from immediate antibiotic therapy for AOM are those younger than age 6 months, younger than age 2 years with bilateral AOM, or of any age with AOM accompanied by otorrhea.

4. Delayed antibiotic prescribing (observation option) is best for children aged 6 months or older with unilateral AOM or aged 2 years or older with bilateral AOM; *there is a substantial role for shared decision making with parents when considering this option.*

5. Do not use delayed antibiotic prescribing for children who appear toxic, for children who are severely ill, or if it cannot be ensured that antibiotic will be begun if the child worsens or there is no improvement within 3 days.

Clinical Summary

Although the use of antibiotics has reduced complications of acute and chronic otitis media, those that do develop can be severe. Complications are intratemporal or extratemporal/intracranial and can develop immediately following an episode of AOM. Some develop within several weeks of the initial infection either despite treatment or when treatment was delayed. Complications resulting from chronic middle-ear infections may also develop. Signs of complications include persistent otalgia, postauricular edema and/or erythema, otorrhea, cranial nerve palsies, orbital pain, nystagmus, vertigo, and hearing loss. Presence of focal neurologic deficits, lethargy, altered mental status, or seizure activity raises concern that an intracranial complication has developed.

Intratemporal complications of AOM involves extension of the infection into the bone, often with bony destruction (see Table 9.1). Because the mastoid air cells are continuous

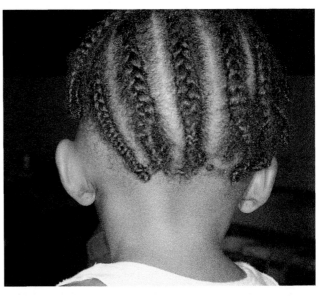

FIGURE 9.7 ■ Acute Mastoiditis. A downward and outward displacement of the auricle associated with erythema and swelling over the mastoid bone in a toddler with purulent otorrhea and tenderness to palpation over the mastoid air cells (postauricular area). (Reproduced with permission from Shah BR, Laude TA. *Atlas of Pediatric Clinical Diagnosis*. WB Saunders; Philadelphia, PA, 2000.)

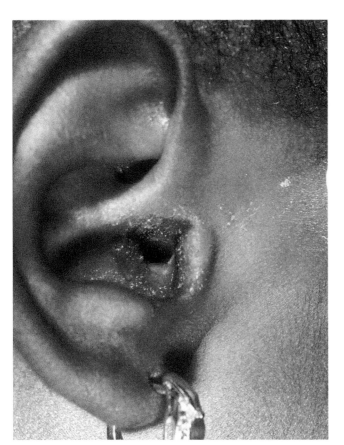

FIGURE 9.6 ■ Acute Otitis Media with Otorrhea. Purulent drainage from the external auditory canal in a patient presenting with fever and earache of 5 days in duration. (Photo contributor: Binita R. Shah, MD.)

with the middle ear, inflammation of the air cells in the mastoid generally accompanies a simple middle-ear infection. In contrast, coalescent mastoiditis is defined as both inflammation and bony necrosis of the mastoid. Patients present with fever, pain, and tenderness over the mastoid process and otorrhea on the order of weeks. Additional hallmarks include postauricular erythema and edema. Mastoiditis is a clinical diagnosis confirmed by CT imaging, where findings of opacification of mastoid air cells and breakdown of the septations of the mastoid cavity will be seen. Fluid in the mastoid cavity alone is not diagnostic of this complication. Progression of the infection can lead to abscess formation, with a purulent collection under the periosteum of the mastoid displacing the auricle anteriorly, which requires drainage mastoidectomy for treatment.

Additional intratemporal complications include extension of an abscess from the mastoid tip and under the sternocleidomastoid muscle into the neck—a Bezold abscess. Abscess collection in the zygomatic process of the temporal bone can also develop and presents as a preauricular collection. Petrositis occurs acutely as an extension of mastoiditis into the petrous apex or from spread of otitis media to the petrous bone via bony erosion, hematogenous spread, or thrombophlebitis. *Gradenigo triad* (abducens nerve palsy, otorrhea,

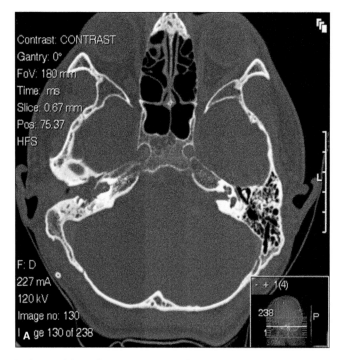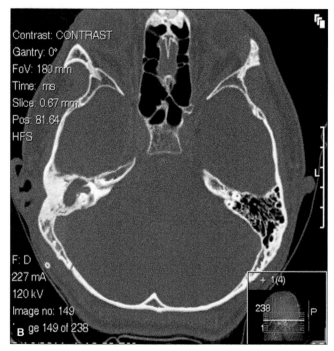

FIGURE 9.8 ■ Chronic Otitis Media with Cholesteatoma and Mastoiditis. (**A**) Axial noncontrast CT of temporal bones shows complete opacification of the right external auditory canal (EAC) and tympanic cavity with nonvisualization of the tympanic membrane and ossicles. This represents a soft tissue mass in the EAC, middle ear, and mastoid with chronic otitis media with cholesteatoma. Opacification and sclerosis of the right mastoid air cells (compared to left) and bony erosion of the tympanic segment seventh nerve canal are also seen. (**B**) Axial CT at a more superior level demonstrates hypoplastic and sclerotic right mastoid air cells, complete opacification of the right tympanic cavity with nonvisualization of the superior semicircular canal (representing cholesteatoma involving and partially eroding the bone of semicircular canal). (Photo/legend contributors: Sydney C. Butts, MD, and Steven Pulitzer, MD.)

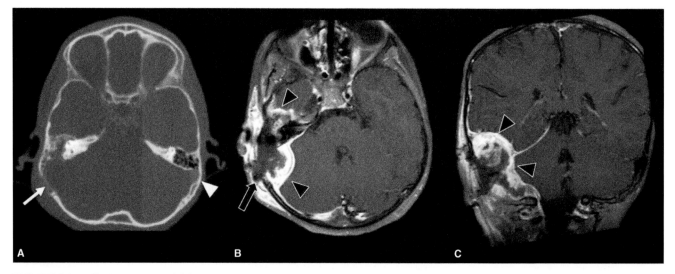

FIGURE 9.9 ■ Coalescent Mastoiditis. A 5-year-old boy with fever, frontal headache, right ear pain, and a "lump" (4 cm × 6 cm) that was hard, tender, and nonerythematous overlying the mastoid area. His right tympanic membrane was erythematous and bulging. (**A**) Note the opacification of the right mastoid air cells with destruction of the normal bony septations. Focal erosion of the bony margin of the right sigmoid sinus (SS) is seen (white arrow), which places the patient at risk for thrombophlebitis. Note normal left SS and preserved surrounding bone (white arrowhead). (**B, C**) Axial and coronal postcontrast T1-weighted MRIs demonstrate a thick-walled rim-enhancing epidural abscess (black arrowheads) extending into the posterior fossa, into the right middle cranial fossa under the temporal lobe, and through a bony defect into the overlying scalp (black arrow, **B**). (Photo/legend contributors: Rabia Malik, MD, and Vinodkumar Velayudhan, DO.)

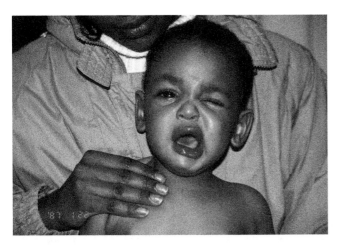

FIGURE 9.10 ■ Facial Palsy; Complication of Acute Otitis Media (AOM). Right-sided peripheral facial palsy associated with right AOM requiring IV antibiotics and myringotomy. Facial palsy results from inflammation directly affecting exposed portions of the facial nerve, which runs through the temporal bone. The facial nerve is usually protected in a bony canal that can either be congenitally absent in portions or eroded by chronic, long-standing otitis media. (Photo contributor: Binita R. Shah, MD.)

and retroorbital pain) indicates infection involving the petrous portion of the temporal bone. Suppurative labyrinthitis occurs when bacterial infection spreads from the middle ear to the inner ear and presents with sudden sensorineural hearing loss, nystagmus, peripheral vertigo, nausea, and vomiting.

Acute and chronic otitis media may also lead to facial nerve paralysis. The facial nerve courses through the mastoid bone and middle ear covered by a bony canal before entering the parotid gland to innervate the facial muscles. In patients with dehiscence of the bone, AOM can result in facial nerve

paralysis. In patients with chronic otitis media, the bone canal is degraded over time resulting in exposure and paresis or paralysis.

Intracranial spread of otitis media may develop when an intratemporal complication develops, but this is not always the case. Meningitis, abscess formation. or intracranial vascular complications will result in symptoms including spiking fevers, neck tenderness, papilledema, and paralysis of the lower cranial nerves.

Emergency Department Treatment and Disposition

Consult otolaryngology for all cases of suspected otitis media complications and neurosurgery for intracranial complications. Order a CT scan with contrast of the temporal bones and brain. Obtain a CBC and blood cultures. Hospitalize such patients for IV antibiotics, and many patients may require operative management.

Pearls

1. Include complications of otitis media in the differential for any patient presenting with facial nerve paralysis. Failing to detect otitis media as the cause of facial paralysis could result in the patient receiving incorrect treatment.

2. Maintain a low threshold for brain imaging in patients who have been on antibiotic therapy, which can mask more obvious manifestations of spread of the infection from otitis media.

TABLE 9.1 ■ COMPLICATIONS OF OTITIS MEDIA

Intratemporal	Extratemporal/Intracranial
Coalescent mastoiditis	Meningitis
Subperiosteal abscess (postauricular)	Otitic hydrocephalus (elevated intracranial pressure in presence of otitis media and absence of bacterial meningitis)
Bezold abscess	Lateral sinus thrombosis
Zygomatic abscess	Epidural abscess
Petrous apicitis	Subdural abscess
Suppurative labyrinthitis	Intraparenchymal abscess (eg, temporal lobe, cerebellum)
Facial nerve paralysis	

Clinical Summary

Acute otitis externa (AOE), commonly referred to as "swimmer's ear," is cellulitis of the external auditory canal (EAC) skin. Diagnosis requires acute onset (within 48 hours) of symptoms *and* signs of EAC inflammation. Symptoms include severe otalgia, EAC pruritus, and ear fullness. Hearing loss and jaw pain may also occur. Signs include hallmark exquisite tenderness of the tragus or pinna, diffuse ear canal edema (which can cause complete obstruction), and erythema. Patients may also have otorrhea, regional lymphadenitis, or cellulitis of the pinna or postauricular skin.

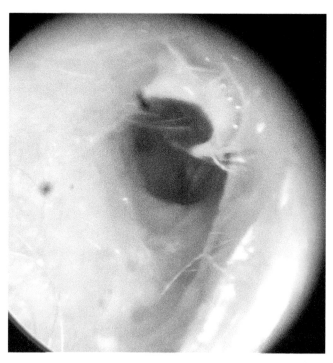

FIGURE 9.12 ■ Acute Otitis Externa. Purulent otorrhea with debris in the external auditory canal with mild to moderate canal edema. Suctioning and removal of this debris along with topic antibiotic therapy are required for prompt resolution of the infection. (Photo contributor: Aaron L. Thatcher, MD.)

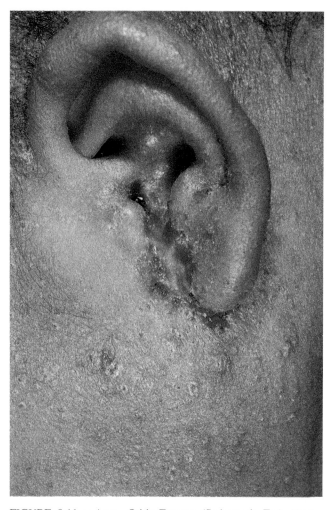

FIGURE 9.11 ■ Acute Otitis Externa (Swimmer's Ear). White-yellow discharge from the external auditory canal (EAC) associated with excoriation of the surrounding skin was seen in this child who was swimming daily during summer camp. His EAC was very edematous and filled with dried debris. Other etiologies of otorrhea from otitis externa (OE) include fungal OE, eczematous OE, and furunculosis (hair follicle infection usually due to *S aureus*). (Photo contributor: Binita R. Shah, MD.)

The majority of AOE is bacterial; the most common pathogens are *Pseudomonas aeruginosa* and *Staphylococcus aureus*. AOE is a clinical diagnosis, and most patients do not require laboratory or radiographic studies. Fungal otitis externa is uncommon in primary AOE but may occur after combination antibiotic/steroid treatment of a previous episode of AOE.

The etiology of AOE is usually multifactorial. Aggressive removal of cerumen removes an important barrier to moisture and infection. Trauma to the EAC predisposes to AOE. Wearing hearing aids, water exposure, and certain dermatologic conditions (eg, eczema, seborrhea, psoriasis) are risk factors for AOE. It is more common in warmer, more humid climates and seasons.

Caution must be taken in patients who are diabetic or immunocompromised. These patients are at risk of developing temporal bone osteomyelitis, also known as malignant otitis externa or necrotizing otitis externa. This disease typically causes the development of granulation tissue in the EAC and chronic mild-to-moderate otalgia. Patients suffering from temporal bone osteomyelitis should be evaluated with temporal bone imaging and inflammatory marker labs, and an otolaryngologist should be consulted.

The differential diagnosis for AOE includes furunculitis, herpes zoster oticus, otitis media with a perforated TM, foreign body with secondary infection, contact dermatitis reaction, and auricular chondritis. Otalgia without signs of inflammation may be referred from nearby structures including the temporomandibular joint or pharynx.

Emergency Department Treatment and Disposition

Definitive treatment for AOE can be provided in the ED. Topical otic antibiotic drops are the first-line treatment for uncomplicated AOE and are highly effective. Systemic antibiotics are not indicated for uncomplicated AOE. They should only be used when the EAC cellulitis has extended to involve the auricle or in patients who are immunocompromised.

Topical therapy can include antibiotics, steroids, acidifying agents, or any combination of the above. Typical treatment courses are 7 to 10 days. Instruction on properly administering drops will improve treatment effect and adherence. The head should be sideways, and the tragus should be pumped after instilling drops.

If the TM is not intact, either because of a perforation or the presence of a tympanostomy tube, ototoxic drops should be avoided. In these patients, fluoroquinolone drops are the safest option.

During treatment, patients should be advised to avoid swimming or head submersion. Water can be kept out of the ear during bathing by applying a petroleum ointment–covered cotton ball to the ear. Patients should be strictly instructed to avoid instrumentation of the EAC, including cotton swabs. In some instances, edema or debris may significantly narrow the EAC, impairing the adequate delivery of topical drops. In these cases, placement of an ear wick in the EAC will enhance penetration of drops to the medial EAC. Ear wicks are compressed, dried sponge material that can be inserted while stiff but expand and become pliable when fluid is absorbed. A wick will stent the edematous canal and convey the medication to the medial EAC. Wick placement can be a painful procedure.

A deep insertion can injure or irritate the TM, but inadequate placement can delay resolution. As canal edema resolves, the wick will often loosen and may fall out spontaneously. Otherwise, wicks are usually changed 2 to 3 days after insertion. Pain control is an important consideration, as the otalgia can be quite intense. Counsel patients on the appropriate use of over-the-counter analgesics. Symptoms of uncomplicated AOE should improve in 48 to 72 hours of appropriate topical antibiotic therapy. Topical anesthetic drops are not approved for treatment of AOE and may mask disease progression.

Immunocompromised patients, including those with diabetes, are at increased risk of complicated AOE. These patients are more likely to have prolonged or recurrent courses, and referral to an otolaryngologist is warranted. Likewise, patients with prolonged or recurrent symptoms despite appropriate first-line treatment may benefit from otolaryngology consultation.

Discharge instructions to the patient should include the following:

1. Patients should maintain dry ear precautions until infection resolution.
2. Instrumentation of the EAC of any kind, including the use of cotton-tipped swabs, should be avoided.
3. Appropriate treatment of uncomplicated AOE should lead to improvement of symptoms within 72 hours and resolution typically in 10 to 14 days.
4. Most patients can follow-up with a primary care physician as needed. Otolaryngology consultation should be sought for case of recurrent, prolonged, or complicated AOE.

Pearls

1. Diagnosis of AOE requires acute-onset otalgia and signs of inflammation in the ear canal.
2. A patient with uncomplicated AOE may be treated as an outpatient with ototopical antibiotic drops.
3. A wick may be required to conduct ear drops through edematous ear canal.
4. Immunocompromised patients are at highest risk for complications such as osteomyelitis or cellulitis.

Clinical Summary

Perichondritis is inflammation of the perichondrium of the external ear, usually caused by a break in the skin barrier, including auricular trauma (blunt or sharp object), piercing of the cartilaginous portions of the external ear, and postoperative wound infections. Progression to chondritis or abscess may follow, and the cartilage may quickly become devitalized and necrotic. Perichondritis is marked by thickening of the perichondrium, making the well-defined shape of the ear less discernible. The skin is often erythematous, and palpation results in marked tenderness. An early auricular abscess may have many of these clinical findings. It is critical to determine if abscess collection has formed so that prompt drainage is done. Edema from a contusion of the ear can usually be distinguished by a history of recent blunt trauma and the appearance of ecchymosis. Other conditions to be excluded include erysipelas, eczema or other dermatitis, otitis externa, and relapsing polychondritis.

Emergency Room Treatment and Disposition

Evaluation including CBC and blood culture should be considered on a case by case basis (eg; patients with high fevers or if an abscess is suspected). Select empiric antibiotic therapy with a quinolone, extended-spectrum penicillin, or cephalosporin, which offers both antipseudomonal and gram-positive bacterial coverage. Quinolones are not approved for use in young children because of concerns about cartilage and bone growth. However, fluoroquinolones offer excellent coverage of gram-negative and -positive bacteria and excellent bioavailability orally. The American Academy of Pediatrics recommends a risk-benefit analysis if quinolones are to be considered and advises that they should be applied only in serious infections caused by multidrug-resistant organisms, where prolonged parenteral therapy represents a downside for the patient, or in patients with allergies to first-line antibiotics. Admit those with severe infections for IV antibiotic therapy to ensure clinical response followed

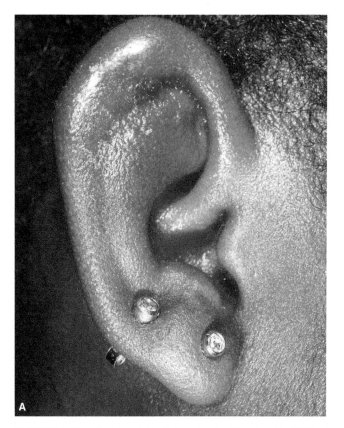 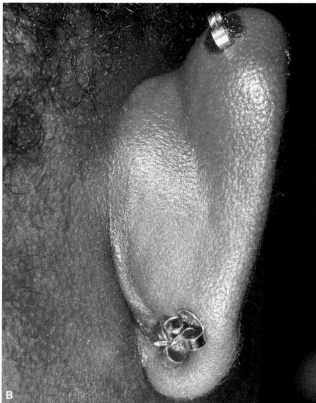

FIGURE 9.13 ■ Perichondritis Following Ear Piercing. (**A, B**) Erythema and swelling of the pinna following the ear piercing (5 days earlier) is seen in an adolescent patient. (Photo contributor: Binita R. Shah, MD.)

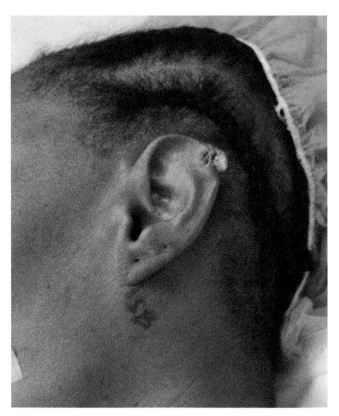

FIGURE 9.14 ■ Perichondritis Leading to Cartilage Necrosis. Cartilage necrosis following an infection from an earring piercing in an adult. (Photo contributor: Sydney C. Butts, MD.)

by oral therapy. Patients with obvious cartilage necrosis or abscess collection require operative management for drainage and/or cartilage debridement. Those who are treated as outpatients need close monitoring by an otolaryngologist. Consult dermatology in complicated cases where an underlying skin condition may have been the source. Appropriate analgesia is also recommended given the significant pain that can be experienced by patients.

Pearls

1. Severity of pain can be a guide to which tissue is involved because perichondritis is often more painful and associated with more tenderness than cellulitis.
2. Treatment failure has significant consequences (eg, chondritis, cartilage necrosis with permanent auricular deformity); thus, obtain an otolaryngology consult in the ED.

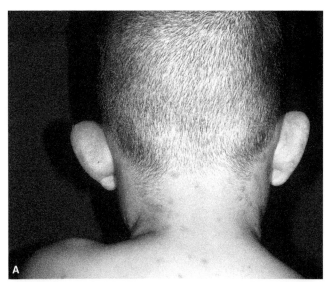

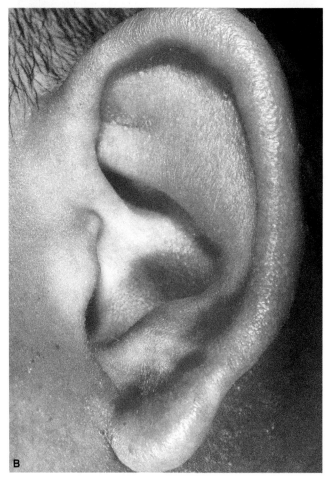

FIGURE 9.15 ■ Swelling of the Ear from Acute Allergic Reaction; Differential Diagnosis of Perichondritis. (**A, B**) Acute-onset swelling of both ears and close-up of swollen, erythematosus pinna in a child with an allergic reaction. (Photo contributor: Binita R. Shah, MD.)

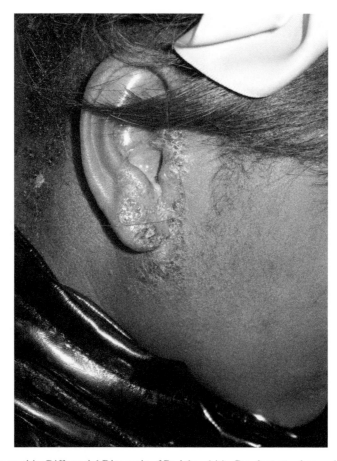

FIGURE 9.16 ■ Eczematous Dermatitis; Differential Diagnosis of Perichondritis. Purulent otorrhea and eczematous dermatitis with excoriations involving the ear are seen in this girl. (Photo contributor: Eve Lowenstein, MD, PhD.)

Clinical Summary

An assortment of foreign bodies (FBs) may be found in the EAC, including plastic beads, cotton swabs, food particles, insects, and button batteries. Patients may be asymptomatic, but more likely, they will report symptoms including otalgia, itching, aural fullness, tinnitus, hearing loss, otorrhea, and bleeding. Even though many auricular FBs have a straightforward presentation and successful outcome, several serious clinical presentations warrant prompt attention. FBs in place for days or weeks can be associated with significant edema of the EAC and frank otitis externa. Sharp FBs can result in injury to the TM or other middle-ear structures.

Emergency Department Treatment and Disposition

Successful removal depends on the type and location of the object and patient cooperation. Take a careful history focused on the type of FB, when and how it entered the ear, and if and how removal was attempted. Carefully inspect the auricle, EAC, and TM, and also look for potential FBs in other orifices (eg, nose). If it appears that the TM has been damaged or if the patient complains of hearing loss, consult otolaryngology before attempting removal.

It is best to use an otoscope with an operating head that will allow adequate visualization. If the FB can be visualized well and is in the proximal EAC, attempt removal with wax curettes, right-angled hooks, alligator forceps, or Frazier

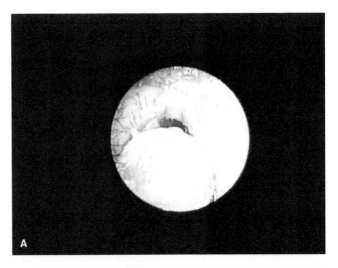

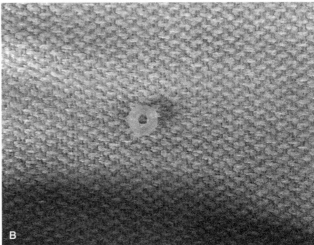

FIGURE 9.18 ■ Auricular Foreign Body. (**A**) A 3-year-old girl presented to the ED after placing a plastic bead in her right ear. The bead is seen filling the external auditory canal. (**B**) Close-up of the plastic bead after removal. (Photo contributor: Sydney C. Butts, MD.)

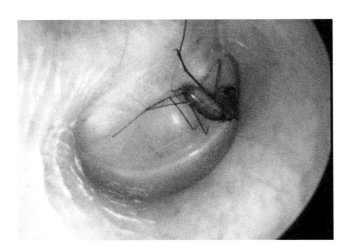

FIGURE 9.17 ■ Auricular Foreign Body (FB). Insects are commonly encountered FBs in the external auditory canal (EAC). Insect in distal EAC sitting directly over the tympanic membrane is seen here. (Photo contributor: Neil Sperling, MD.)

tip suctions (nos. 5 or 7). It is important to avoid iatrogenic trauma, which may cause edema of the EAC, bleeding, distal displacement of the object, or TM perforation; consult otolaryngology if the FB is difficult to remove. Factors associated with unsuccessful ED removal include spherical FBs and an unsuccessful initial attempt at removal. Worsening anxiety of the child and parents results from multiple unsuccessful attempts at removal. When possible, use a microscope that allows adequate lighting and magnification with the patient awake. However, some patients will need to be taken to the operating room for removal.

Assess the patient's hearing before and after FB removal by comparing responses to noise (rubbing fingers together for

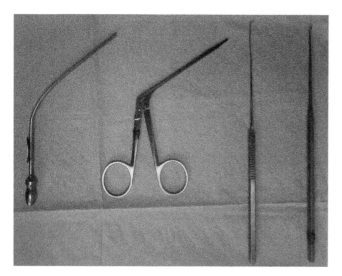

FIGURE 9.19 ■ Otologic Instruments for the Removal of Foreign Bodies (FBs). Multiple otologic instruments are used for safe removal of FBs in the ear canal. From left to right: suction, alligator forceps for grasping, a right-angled hook, and a wax curette are used to deliver round FBs out of the ear canal. The otolaryngologist also uses a microscope that allows use of both hands and a magnified view of the object, which can offer an advantage when FBs are deep within the canal or there is edema or bleeding. (Photo contributor: Sydney C. Butts, MD.)

instance) between the 2 ears or with tuning forks, with 512 Hz being most useful in determining mild to moderate degrees of conductive hearing loss. Perform Rinne and Weber tests to determine whether a conductive or sensorineural hearing loss is present.

Reexamine the EAC and TM after FB removal and check for associated otitis externa (eg, FBs present for days or weeks). Prescribe antibiotic otic drops for infection or with evidence of iatrogenic injury to the canal. Sharp objects can perforate the TM and disrupt the ossicular chain, which results in mild to moderate conductive hearing losses. The most serious injuries involve the round or oval windows with a sensorineural hearing loss and vestibular symptoms (vertigo) that occur because of the leakage of perilymphatic fluid from the inner ear. This is a true emergency requiring immediate evaluation by otolaryngology. In some cases, operative exploration is indicated.

Refer patients with TM perforation for a formal audiogram. All patients should have follow-up with the otolaryngology service within 1 week of discharge from the ED.

Pearls

1. All FBs should be removed to relieve symptoms and to avoid or treat infection.

2. *A battery in the ear canal is an emergency* that can result in severe damage to the surrounding tissues, including TM perforation, ear canal scarring, and eventual stenosis as well as injury to adjacent structures from leakage of the battery. Prompt intervention will prevent significant tissue damage.

3. Do not irrigate the ear canal if absorptive material such as seeds (beans, peas) is suspected because moisture causes them to expand, further occluding EAC.

4. Kill living insects in the EAC before removal by flooding the ear canal with water, alcohol, lidocaine, or mineral oil to drown the insect.

Clinical Summary

Auricular hematoma develops after blunt trauma to the pinna. Frequently, patients describe a blow to the ear with a fist or sports-related activities including boxing and wrestling. The diagnosis is often straightforward because the intricate contours of the anterior surface of the pinna become effaced. The skin and perichondrium covering the auricular cartilage is very adherent anteriorly. Dissection of blood between the adherent soft tissues and the cartilage results in significant pain associated with this injury. Palpation of the affected ear reveals fluctuance. Not all patients will present acutely; in these situations, the hematoma can organize, leading to several possible outcomes. The underlying cartilage may be necrotic from loss of blood supply from the perichondrium, or the hematoma may become infected and progress to an abscess. A persistent hematoma can result in fibrosis of the underlying cartilage. This thickening of the auricular cartilage with obliteration of the auricular contours is often referred to as "cauliflower ear." High-impact blows may also result in fracture of the temporal bone, TM perforation, trauma to the adjacent scalp soft tissues, or injury to the temporomandibular joint.

Emergency Department Treatment and Disposition

Completely evaluate the head and neck and perform a full trauma survey followed by a detailed examination of the ear. It is important to examine the postauricular area down to the mastoid tip as well as the adjacent scalp. Examine the EAC

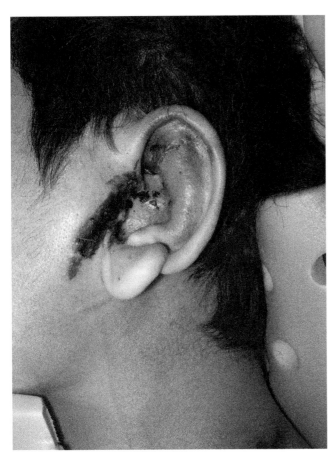

FIGURE 9.20 ■ Auricular Hematoma. This teenager got into an altercation with a classmate and was struck in the ear with the edge of a text book. It is important to make sure blood does not collect beneath the perichondrium to prevent permanent scar formation and the development of a "cauliflower ear." (Photo contributor: Mark Silverberg, MD.)

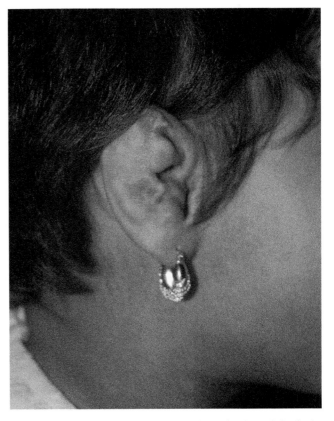

FIGURE 9.21 ■ "Cauliflower Ear"; Complication of Auricular Hematoma. This 5-year-old girl suffered blunt trauma to the right ear due to abuse and was not brought promptly to medical attention. The ear cartilage is thickened and fibrosed with the classic appearance of a "cauliflower ear," which can result when a hematoma develops and is not drained promptly. She was subsequently placed in a foster home. (Photo contributor: Sydney C. Butts, MD.)

and TM. Assess hearing with tuning fork tests, ideally with a 512-Hz tuning fork. Air conduction should be greater than bone conduction when the tuning fork is used.

Consult otolaryngology. Incision and drainage is preferred to simple needle aspiration, which is reported to be associated with higher rates of recurrence. Drain acute hematomas promptly under sterile conditions after infiltration of 1% lidocaine. Use a stab incision in the skin over the area of greatest fluctuance and a curved clamp to open and dissect the cavity, allowing the hematoma to be expressed. Larger hematomas may require multiple incisions for complete drainage. Irrigate the cavity with sterile saline, and suction to ensure clearance of the clot. Reapproximate the perichondrium to the underlying cartilage with bolsters placed anteriorly and posteriorly to provide gentle pressure and prevent reaccumulation of the hematoma. Commonly used bolstering materials include dental rolls, folded petrolatum gauze, or silastic molded to the contour of the ear. Secure the bolsters with nylon or Prolene suture sewn through and through the ear. Instruct the patient and caregiver to keep the bolster in place for 5 to 7 days.

There is not uniform agreement about the need for prophylactic antibiotics, but it is reasonable to give prophylactic antibiotics with gram-positive coverage to immunocompromised patients or those with other systemic illnesses.

Abscess represents a serious complication that should be treated with incision and drainage, copious irrigation of the abscess cavity, and placement of a passive drain in the cavity. This may need to be performed in the operating room if cartilage debridement is required. Admit patients with an auricular abscess for IV antibiotics and close monitoring of the wound.

Pearl

1. Contusions may appear similar to a mild hematoma. The soft tissues are edematous and the overlying skin ecchymotic, making the contours of the ear less distinctive. These patients should be treated conservatively with analgesics and warm compresses. If in doubt, needle aspiration of the area of greatest fullness can be attempted; if negative, no further intervention is required.

Clinical Summary

Most epistaxis in children is caused by digital trauma, nose rubbing, and blunt trauma. Predisposing conditions include upper respiratory tract infections, inhalant allergens, and dry air, especially in the winter months. The peak frequency is in children age 3 to 8 years, and it is uncommon before 2 years. The most common site is the anterior nasal septum at the Kiesselbach plexus or Little's area where the terminal branches of internal and external carotid artery systems merge under a thin, delicate mucosa. Superior epistaxis from terminal branches of anterior or posterior ethmoidal arteries and posterior epistaxis involving terminal branches of the sphenopalatine artery are much less common.

Unilateral epistaxis in a young child warrants evaluation for a nasal FB. Epistaxis from facial trauma usually is caused by injury to the nasal septum. Severe epistaxis after head trauma could be a sign of an internal carotid pseudoaneurysm. Epistaxis after nasal surgery including endoscopic sinus surgery usually occurs within the first 24 hours and resolves with conservative measures. Difficult-to-treat unilateral epistaxis in an adolescent boy may result from a juvenile nasopharyngeal angiofibroma, whereas rhabdomyosarcoma may occur in young children. Unusual causes in children also include hereditary hemorrhagic telangiectasia, primary or acquired coagulopathies, hypertension, and idiopathic thrombocytopenic purpura.

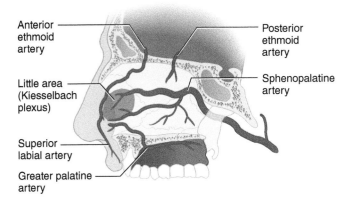

FIGURE 9.22 ■ Arteries That Supply the Nasal Septum. Arterial blood supply to the nasal cavity. The most common site of nasal hemorrhage is at Little's area of the nasal septum. The most common origin of posterior epistaxis is from the sphenopalatine artery. (Reproduced with permission from Tintinalli JE, Stapczynski J, Ma O, et al. *Tintinalli's Emergency Medicine: A Comprehensive Study Guide.* 8th ed. McGraw-Hill Education; New York, NY, 2016.)

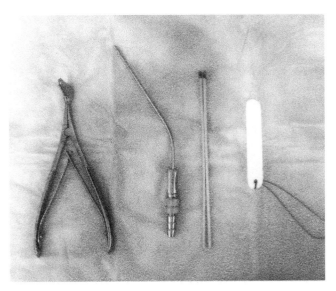

FIGURE 9.23 ■ Epistaxis Tray. Several instruments and packing materials are used to manage patients with epistaxis. The anterior nasal cavity is visualized with the use of a nasal speculum (left), and blood and clots are suctioned using a Frazier suction, which helps to identify the bleeding source. Bleeding can be controlled with cautery using silver nitrate, and for more brisk bleeding, formal nasal packing is applied. Merocel packing (shown here) is one type of intranasal pack that can be used. (Photo contributor: Sydney C. Butts, MD.)

Emergency Department Treatment and Disposition

Assess the child's overall condition and ascertain the degree of blood loss. Take a history with attention to any predisposing factors. Before physical examination, ask the child to blow out all blood and blood clots, if possible. If there is a history of nasal trauma, check for septal hematoma and assess for any fractures (see Figure 20.16). Use topical vasoconstriction and anesthesia by spraying or dripping 0.25% oxymetazoline or phenylephrine and 4% lidocaine into the nose. An otoscope is required for adequate anterior visualization in younger children; a nasal speculum and head light may be used in older children. Remove blood clots with gentle suctioning with a Frazier tip in a cooperative child. Treat active bleeding using local pressure by gently pinching the nasal ala against the bleeding point on the anterior nasal septum for 5 to 10 minutes. If this fails to control the bleeding, limited cautery can be performed by applying a silver nitrate stick to the area around the bleed. Electrocautery, preferably with bipolar forceps, can be performed by an otolaryngologist. Care should be taken to avoid repeated or bilateral cautery because this can lead to avascular cartilage necrosis and perforation. Many hemostatic agents are now available in the form of a biodegradable

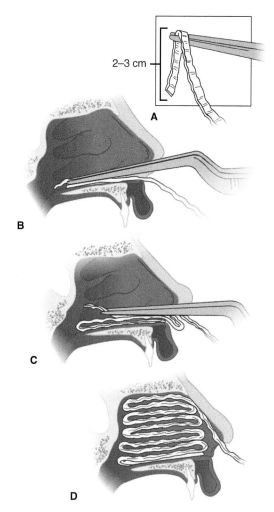

FIGURE 9.24 ▪ Placement of an Anterior Nasal Pack. The key to placement of an anterior nasal pack that will control epistaxis adequately and stay in place is to lay the packing into the nasal cavity in an accordion-like manner so that part of each layer of packing lies anteriorly, preventing the gauze from falling posteriorly into the nasopharynx. (**A**) The first layer of ¼-inch petrolatum-impregnated gauze strip is grasped approximately 2 to 3 cm from its end. (**B**) The first layer is then placed on the floor of the nose through the nasal speculum (not pictured here). The bayonet forceps and nasal speculum are then withdrawn. (**C**) The nasal speculum is reintroduced on top of the first layer of packing, and a second layer is placed in an identical manner. After several layers have been placed, it is often useful to reintroduce the bayonet forceps to push the previously placed packing down onto the floor of the nose, making it tighter and more secure. (**D**) A complete anterior nasal pack can tamponade a bleeding point anywhere in the anterior nasal cavities and will stay in place until removed by the provider or patient. (Reproduced with permission from Tintinalli JE, Stapczynski J, Ma O, et al. *Tintinalli's Emergency Medicine: A Comprehensive Study Guide.* 8th ed. McGraw-Hill Education; New York, NY, 2016.)

matrix hemostatic sealant and may also be directly applied to the area of bleeding.

When anterior epistaxis cannot be controlled with pressure, local cautery, or hemostatic sealants, place an anterior pack. Using a headlight and pediatric nasal speculum, layer packing material impregnated with small amounts of antibiotic ointment from inferior to superior using a Bayonet forceps. Vaseline gauze provides a tight pack, but it needs to be subsequently removed, resulting in further discomfort and the possibility of further injury. Biodegradable oxidized cellulose (Oxycel) or gelatin sponge (Gelfoam) does not need to be removed. A preformed nasal tampon (Merocel) can be inserted along the floor of the nasal cavity where it expands on contact with blood or other liquid. The tampon should be lubricated with gel to facilitate placement. After insertion, it may be wet with a small amount of topical vasoconstrictor or irrigated with saline to help achieve full expansion. After the pack has

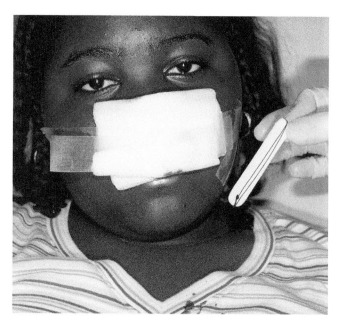

FIGURE 9.25 ▪ Immune Thrombocytopenic Purpura (ITP) Presenting with Epistaxis. Repeated episodes of epistaxis with prolonged bleeding were the presenting complaint of this patient whose platelet count was 5000/mm³ (subsequently diagnosed as chronic ITP). Nasal packing was applied to control her bleeding, and she was hospitalized for close monitoring. A history of prolonged bleeding or a history of easy bruisability in a patient or a family member suggests a systemic disorder, and such patients require a thorough history and physical examination and tests to exclude bleeding disorders. (Photo contributor: Binita R. Shah, MD.)

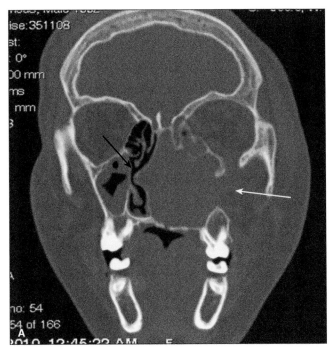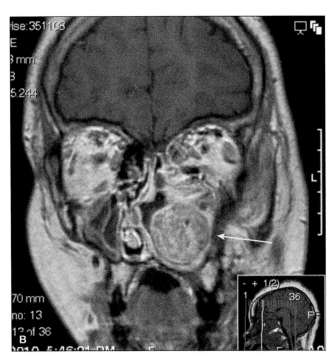

FIGURE 9.26 ▪ Juvenile Nasopharyngeal Angiofibroma Presenting with Epistaxis. (**A**) Coronal noncontrast CT at the level of the nasal cavity demonstrates complete opacification of the left nasal cavity and maxillary sinus with extensive bony remodeling/destruction including destruction of the lateral maxillary sinus wall (white arrow) and deviation of the nasal septum to the right (black arrow). Epistaxis may be caused by sinonasal tumors. This 17-year-old patient had a large left juvenile nasopharyngeal angiofibroma. (**B**) Coronal postcontrast T1-weighted pulse sequence demonstrates a well-circumscribed, heterogenously enhancing mass lesion in the left nasal cavity with extensive bony remodeling and deviation of the nasal septum to the right. There is poor visualization of the lateral left maxillary sinus wall (arrow), and inflammatory changes in the adjacent facial muscles and soft tissues are present. (Photo/legend contributors: Sydney C. Butts, MD, and Steven Pulitzer, MD.)

been inserted, tape a gauze pad over the nose, and instruct the patient and caregiver to change it periodically. Prescribe an antibiotic to prevent toxic shock syndrome. If permanent packing is placed, the patient should be referred to otolaryngology or advised to return to the ED for removal in 2 to 5 days. Consult otolaryngology if anterior nasal examination fails to document a bleeding site or if bleeding cannot be controlled by the above measures. Posterior epistaxis is usually a result of facial fractures, severe coagulopathies, or sinus surgery.

Posterior packing can be performed with urinary catheters, gauze packs, or prefabricated nasal tampons and nasal balloons. Admit children with posterior packs for continuous pulse oximetry as nasal packing can cause iatrogenic sleep apnea syndrome, leading to hypoxia and potentially death. Arterial embolization may be used in patients with severe refractory epistaxis unresponsive to other measures. Risks include those of embolic phenomenon, but the technique is highly successful.

Obtain appropriate imaging studies (CT scan, MRI, angiography) for patients with facial trauma or suspected vascular

tumors. Order CBC, including type and cross-match, in children presenting with signs and symptoms of hypovolemia. Laboratory screening for coagulopathy is mandated for patients with a posterior bleed or with petechiae or easy bruising.

Once epistaxis is controlled, discharge the patient on preventive measures, including humidification with topical nasal saline and/or room humidifiers and application of petroleum- or antibiotic-based ointments. Consult otolaryngology for children with recurrent epistaxis and hematology for children with recurrent epistaxis despite appropriate preventive measures.

Pearls

1. Unilateral epistaxis in a young child, particularly when accompanied by unilateral purulent rhinorrhea and congestion, is highly suspicious for a nasal FB.

2. Vascular tumors such as juvenile nasopharyngeal angiofibroma in adolescent boys and rhabdomyosarcoma in young children can present as difficult-to-treat epistaxis.

Clinical Summary

As with other foreign bodies (FBs) of the upper aerodigestive tract, the clinician is often challenged with piecing together bits of history or may have no history at all in a suspected nasal FB. The key to a successful outcome is including FB in the differential diagnosis once the symptoms have been elicited. Patients with a nasal FB can present with unilateral or bilateral foul-smelling rhinorrhea depending on the number and location of the FBs. Other presenting symptoms include epistaxis and sinusitis. When insertion was not witnessed, as most commonly occurs, the FB could have been in place for days or weeks, and visualization may be hampered by formation of granulation tissue around the FB and the obstruction

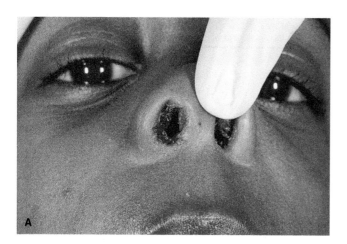

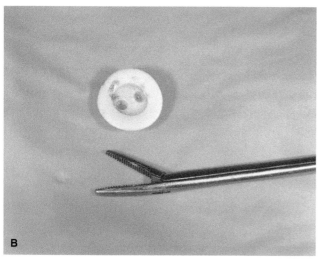

FIGURE 9.27 ■ Nasal Foreign Body. (**A**) A foul-smelling serosanguineous discharge from the right nostril was the presenting complaint in this 6-year-old boy. He confessed to putting a button in his nostril about 1 week prior to this visit. (**B**) Close-up of the button that was removed is shown. (Photo contributor: Binita R. Shah, MD.)

presented by thick secretions. Rhinoliths may also occur in which the FB is a nidus for the crystallization of layers of calcium. The peak age range for nasal FB placement has been reported to be between 2 and 4 years old, with a male predominance.

Emergency Department Treatment and Disposition

Obtain a detailed history from the family about prior medical evaluations, and perform a thorough head and neck exam, with a high suspicion for FBs in other orifices, followed by a non-decongested examination of the anterior nasal cavity. If the object is readily accessible and the patient is able to cooperate, attempt removal in the ED. Have an adult stabilize the child in the examining chair while the physician visualizes the nasal cavity with an appropriately sized nasal speculum and a headlight. Use Frazier tip suctions (no. 5 or 7), a right-angled hook, an angled wax curette, or an alligator forceps for extraction. Having the patient upright minimizes the possibility that the nasal FB could be aspirated during manipulation. If removal is successful, perform a thorough examination of the nasal airway distal to the removed FB to ensure that a second FB is not present. If this is not possible with the nasal speculum, perform an endoscopic examination of the nasal cavity and nasopharynx with either a rigid 0-degree scope or a flexible pediatric fiberoptic scope. Topicalization of the nasal mucosa with decongestant spray and local anesthetic (2% lidocaine spray) is recommended prior to examination with the endoscope. After straightforward removal, the patient is discharged home. Advise the patient to use saline irrigations at home several times a day to help keep any excoriated areas moist. Give oral antibiotics to patients with more extensive inflammatory changes of the mucosa or frank mucopus. Amoxicillin is an appropriate first-line agent to cover the typical organisms that cause sinusitis.

Longstanding FBs will be difficult to visualize, and plain radiographs of the sinuses can be ordered as a screening modality. This is only helpful if the FB is radiopaque. Lateral soft tissue radiograph of the neck may help determine the location of the FB in the anteroposterior dimension. Order CT for radiolucent objects or any unusual presentations such as an infectious process extending beyond the sinonasal cavity. Apply decongestant and local anesthetic sprays prior to examination to decrease local inflammation and prevent bleeding. Consult otolaryngology and obtain a fiberoptic endoscopic

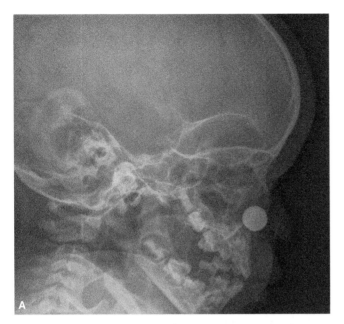

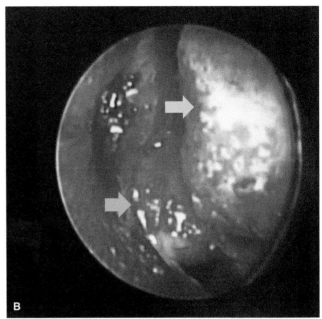

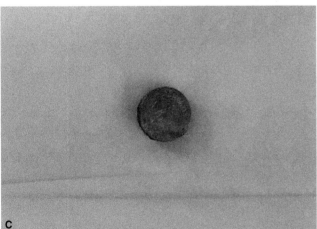

FIGURE 9.28 ■ Nasal Foreign Body; Disc Battery. (**A**) This 2-year-old child presented with a foul-smelling nasal discharged from the left nostril. Lateral radiograph of the face demonstrates a radiopaque foreign body in the left nasal cavity. There is a "halo" or "double ring" appearance well appreciated on this radiograph compatible with a battery. (**B**) Disc battery in the left nasal cavity resulting in a significant inflammation of the surrounding nasal mucosa (blue arrow) is shown. The nasal septum is midline (yellow arrow), and the inferior turbinate is lateral (green arrow). (**C**) Button battery removed from the nasal cavity in a different patient. Injury to mucosal surfaces adjacent to the battery can result in septal perforation, intranasal scarring, and their sequelae. (Photo contributors: Sydney C. Butts, MD [A, C], and Nira Goldstein, MD [B].)

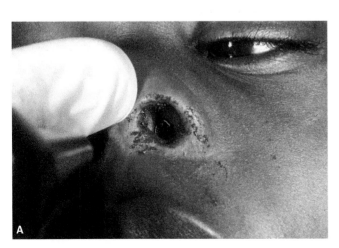

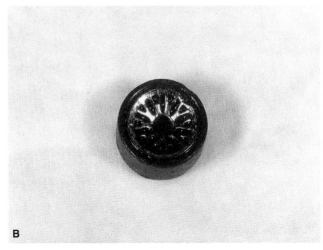

FIGURE 9.29 ■ Nasal Foreign Body. (**A**) A serosanguineous discharge from the left nostril was the presenting complaint in this 5-year-old child. (**B**) Close-up of the wheel of the toy car that was removed is shown. (Photo contributor: Binita R. Shah, MD.)

examination. Patients with longstanding nasal FBs will have a difficult time tolerating manipulation of the object in the ED. Conscious sedation in the ED can be dangerous if the FB is dislodged during manipulation because the patient's protective reflexes are blunted and tracheobronchial aspiration could result. In older children with nasal FBs or children with developmental delays, removal in the operating room may be safer due to difficulty immobilizing the patient. The use of Foley and Fogarty catheters and other similar devices has been described, which involves passage of the catheter distal to the FB with inflation of the balloon posterior to the object and delivery of the FB by removing the catheter. We advise caution in the use of techniques that involve passage with limited visualization and that could change the position of the FB.

Pearl

1. Button/disc batteries cause significant injuries, including septal perforation and saddle nose deformity with extensive septal cartilaginous loss. An intranasal battery is an emergency, and a prompt otolaryngology evaluation and removal are required.

Clinical Summary

Acute sinusitis is an often-misdiagnosed disease because multiple similar conditions have overlapping symptoms and there is no definitive test to distinguish them. Acute bacterial rhinosinusitis (ABRS) is a more accurate term for this condition and must be distinguished from viral upper respiratory illness and allergic rhinitis by history and exam.

The key to distinguishing viral from bacterial rhinosinusitis is in the clinical course of the illness. A viral infection typically has acute-onset symptoms and possibly fever, which generally resolves within 48 hours. ABRS can present in 3 main patterns: (1) as a persistent illness with respiratory symptoms (rhinorrhea, daytime cough with or without fever) for >10 days; (2) as a "double sickening" or recurrence of respiratory symptoms shortly after a viral illness that had been improving; and (3) as persistent fever and severe respiratory symptoms lasting 3 consecutive days. The 4 most specific respiratory symptoms for ABRS are nasal obstruction, facial pressure-type pain, postnasal drip, and purulent rhinorrhea. Detection of purulence from the sinuses may be best detected with nasal endoscopy, which can be performed by the ED or otolaryngology staff. Purulent rhinorrhea alone is not a reliable symptom of ABRS as this symptom commonly occurs during viral illnesses. Sinus palpation is unreliable to diagnose ABRS. Clinical signs and symptoms help to best determine the diagnosis of ABRS. Imaging studies to determine viral versus bacterial sinusitis are not indicated; there are no findings specific to ABRS compared to viral respiratory illnesses. However, imaging should be ordered if a complication of sinusitis is suspected or in the setting of an unusual presentation.

Serious complications of sinusitis fall into 2 main categories: orbital and intracranial. Orbital complications are typically due to direct extension from the ethmoid sinus. Preseptal cellulitis involves the eyelid soft tissues but is not a true intraorbital infection. Four other types of intraorbital infections exist: subperiosteal abscess, orbital cellulitis, orbital abscess, and cavernous sinus thrombosis. Physical findings suggesting orbital complication include periorbital erythema and edema, proptosis, decreased extraocular mobility, and decreased visual acuity.

Intracranial complications often result from direct spread from the sphenoid or frontal sinuses or conduction via venous drainage from the nasal cavity through the cavernous sinus. The complications include epidural abscess, subdural abscess, brain abscess, meningitis, and cavernous sinus thrombosis. Concerning symptoms include severe headache, nuchal rigidity, mental status change, nausea, and vomiting.

Patients with immunocompromised conditions, cystic fibrosis, and ciliary dyskinesia are at increased risk for ABRS and complications. Other complications and sequelae include recurrent ABRS, nasal polyps, chronic sinusitis, and anosmia.

Emergency Department Treatment and Disposition

The initial antibiotic of choice for uncomplicated ABRS is high-dose amoxicillin/clavulanic acid (80 to 90 mg/kg/day). The typical causative pathogens include *S pneumoniae* (30%), nontypeable *H influenzae* (20%), *M catarrhalis* (20%), and *Streptococcus pyogenes* (5%). Impaired susceptibility to penicillins in these organisms has led to the recommendation for amoxicillin/clavulanic acid as the initial treatment over amoxicillin alone. Cephalosporins such as ceftriaxone, cefdinir, cefpodoxime, and cefuroxime are appropriate second-line drugs but *S pneumoniae* may have decreased susceptibility. Trimethoprim-sulfamethoxazole and azithromycin are reported to have less efficacy than previously thought due to resistance by *H influenzae* and *S pneumoniae*.

It is recommended that antibiotics are continued for 7 days after symptom resolution. Therefore, a minimum 10-day course should be prescribed. Patients should be reevaluated

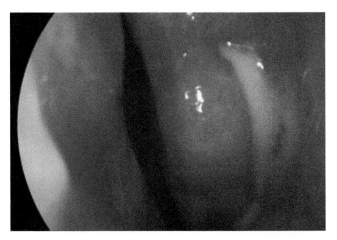

FIGURE 9.30 ■ Acute Bacterial Rhinosinusitis (ABRS). Nasal endoscopy showing purulent rhinorrhea originating from the middle meatus in a case of ABRS. (Photo courtesy of David H. Burstein, MD.)

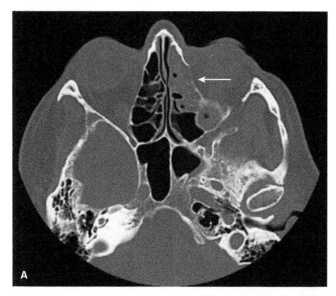

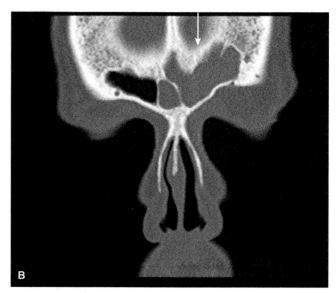

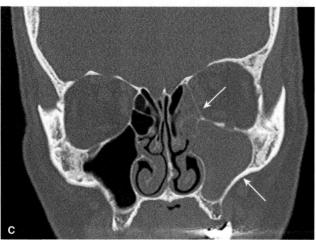

FIGURE 9.31 ■ Acute Bacterial Rhinosinusitis. A classic pattern of unilateral obstruction of the ostiomeatal complex causing infection of the left frontal, anterior ethmoid, and maxillary sinuses. Axial noncontrast CT scan demonstrates opacification of multiple left anterior ethmoid air cells (arrow; **A**). Coronal views demonstrate opacification of the left frontal sinus (arrow; **B**) and a complete opacification of the left maxillary sinus and outflow tract and multiple left ethmoid air cells in an ostiomeatal obstructive pattern (arrows; **C**). (Photo/legend contributors: Sydney C. Butts, MD, and Steven Pulitzer, MD.)

after 72 hours of treatment. Those who fail to improve merit consideration of alternative treatment or alternative diagnosis. Options for alternative antibiotics should be guided by local antibiotic resistance patterns and may include clindamycin and cefixime, linezolid and cefixime, or levofloxacin.

Acute sinusitis in severely immunocompromised patients requires extra consideration. This may be caused by less typical or opportunistic pathogens. Acute invasive fungal sinusitis (AIFS), a rapidly progressive and often lethal condition, should be considered in immunocompromised patients. An otolaryngologist should be consulted to obtain cultures and evaluate for AIFS in this patient group. AIFS diagnosis requires urgent endoscopic evaluation for pale or necrotic nasal tissues and biopsy if there is concern. A diagnosis of AFIS is a surgical emergency. Aggressive systemic antifungal treatment, debridement of involved tissues, and reversal of the immunocompromised state are mainstays of treatment.

Adjuvant medical therapies provide symptomatic relief and treat the underlying etiology impairing mucus clearance. Nasal saline irrigation clears secretions, reduces bacterial load, and improves mucociliary flow. Nasal steroid sprays and antihistamines treat underlying allergic rhinitis or inflammation and reduce mucosal edema. Intranasal decongestant use should be limited to 3 to 4 days to avoid rhinitis medicamentosa. Analgesics should be considered as needed. Mucolytics may be helpful. Management of comorbid conditions should be optimized (eg, asthma, gastroesophageal reflux disease, allergic rhinitis, cystic fibrosis).

Uncomplicated ABRS should be managed on an outpatient basis. Patients should follow-up with their primary care

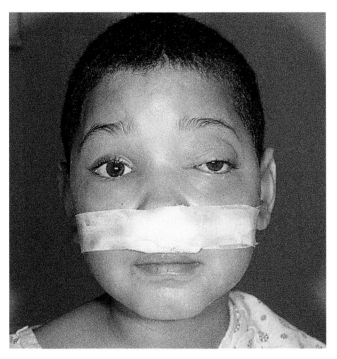

FIGURE 9.32 ■ Orbital Cellulitis Secondary to Acute Bacterial Rhinosinusitis. Unilateral eye involvement with proptosis (outward and inferior displacement of the globe), impaired extraocular movements, and exquisite tenderness over the ethmoid and maxillary sinuses were seen this 8-year-old child. This picture was taken on the second day after surgical drainage. (Photo contributor: Binita R. Shah, MD.)

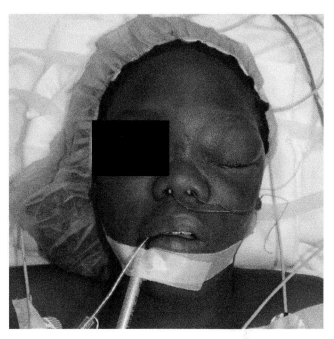

FIGURE 9.33 ■ Acute Ethmoid Sinusitis Complicated by Orbital Abscess. The patient presented with 2 days of worsening left eye swelling and pain. Ethmoid sinus infection broke through the medial orbital wall with abscess formation in the medial orbit. (Photo contributor: Sydney C. Butts, MD.)

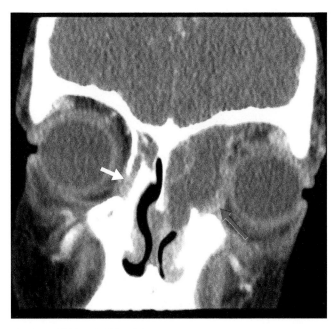

FIGURE 9.34 ■ Intraorbital Complication of Ethmoid Sinusitis. Coronal noncontrast CT scan of 11-year-old boy with bilateral ethmoid sinusitis extending into the left orbit as a subperiosteal abscess (red arrow) causing lateral and inferior displacement of the globe. Note erosion of lamina papyracea inferiorly on the right (white arrow) and completely on the left. (Photo/legend contributors: David J. Brown, MD, and Vinodkumar Velayudhan, DO.)

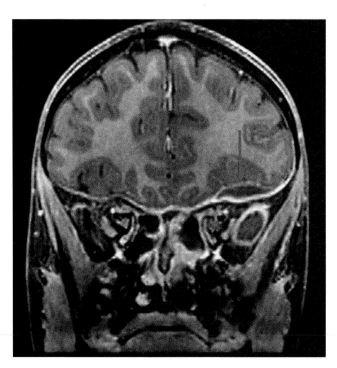

FIGURE 9.35 ■ Intracranial Complication of Acute Sinusitis; Subdural Empyema. Coronal postcontrast T1-weighted MRI of a 12-year-old boy demonstrates a peripherally enhancing fluid collection (arrow) inferior to the left frontal lobe. (Photo/legend contributors: David J. Brown, MD, and Vinodkumar Velayudhan, DO.)

physician during or after completing antibiotic treatment and be instructed to return to the ED if symptoms worsen or persist after 48 hours of antibiotic therapy.

When orbital complications of sinusitis are diagnosed or suspected, urgent ophthalmology and otolaryngology consultations are important to coordinate a comprehensive evaluation and treatment plan. Nearly all patients will require hospitalization and IV antibiotic treatment and possible surgery. With intracranial complications, neurosurgery and otolaryngology consultations are indicated, and patients invariably require hospitalization and IV antibiotics with consideration for surgical intervention.

Pearls

1. Clinical course is the key to distinguish ABRS from a viral rhinosinusitis. Persistent symptoms beyond 10 days, a "second sickening" after initial URI with some recovery, and severe fever and symptoms for 3 consecutive days are the patterns to look for in ABRS.

2. Imaging is not required to make the diagnosis of uncomplicated ABRS. If a complication is suspected, a contrast-enhanced CT of the sinuses is the study of choice with the addition of a dedicated CT scan of the brain if an intracranial complication is suspected.

3. High-dose amoxicillin/clavulanic acid is the preferred initial treatment course and should be continued 7 days beyond symptom resolution.

Clinical Summary

Viral URIs will progress to acute sinusitis in up to 13% of children. Chronic rhinosinusitis (CRS) will develop in a small number of these children and is characterized clinically by 90 continuous days of symptoms that can include nasal obstruction, cough, facial pain or pressure, and purulent rhinorrhea. Ideally, physical exam findings and/or imaging studies support this diagnosis. Persistent inflammation impairs the natural mucociliary clearance of the paranasal sinuses and mucus retention ensues. CRS in children has been shown to exacerbate underlying asthma.

The paranasal sinuses are developing throughout childhood, with the frontal sinuses not reaching full development until the end of the teen years in most individuals. Therefore, pediatric CRS should be thought of as a continuum and not as 1 single disease that affects all pediatric patients similarly. In younger children, the adenoids may play a significant role in the etiology of CRS, but generally, they play less of a role as the child reaches adolescence. Other risk factors for the development of CRS include cystic fibrosis, ciliary dysfunction, environmental allergies, and acquired or congenital immune system dysfunction.

One significant distinction is whether or not polyps are present in the nose. Ongoing research has now clearly shown that CRS with nasal polyps is a different disease entity than CRS without polyps. Therefore, a thorough nasal examination is important in the workup of children with CRS. Anterior rhinoscopy may allow for visualization of polyps, but nasal endoscopy is the gold standard diagnostic tool and should be attempted if possible. Children with nasal polyposis carry an increased risk of having cystic fibrosis, and this diagnosis needs to be considered in this patient population. Other potential comorbid conditions associated with nasal polyps include antrochoanal polyps and allergic fungal sinusitis. There may also be a relationship between allergic rhinitis and the development of nasal polyps.

Emergency Department Treatment and Disposition

Perform a complete head and neck examination including anterior rhinoscopy. Ideally a nasal speculum and head light are used, but in younger children, use of an otoscope can be helpful. Because the most fearsome complications of sinusitis involve spread of infection into the orbit or intracranial space, attention should be paid to these systems. Use of nasal decongestants can improve visualization if needed. It is important to assess for the presence of nasal polyps, which may be easily visualized but are sometimes mistaken for the normal inferior turbinate (especially if the turbinate is hypertrophic). Rigid or flexible endoscopes can be used to perform a more detailed examination of the nose.

If complications are suspected, a CT scan of the sinuses with contrast should be ordered. Imaging should include the orbits and brain. MRI can be a helpful adjunctive test. Otolaryngology consultation should be pursued in addition to neurosurgery and ophthalmology if needed. Patients with impending complications from chronic sinusitis should be admitted to the hospital for IV antibiotics, monitoring, and possibly urgent surgery.

Patients with uncomplicated chronic sinusitis may be discharged home. Consideration should be given to starting saline irrigations and intranasal steroid sprays. Oral steroids and antibiotics may also be prescribed depending on the clinical presentation. Outpatient otolaryngology consultation should be pursued.

Pearls

1. Chronic sinusitis with nasal polyps should raise concern about possible comorbid conditions such as cystic fibrosis or allergic fungal sinusitis.
2. Chronic sinusitis in young children is often related to adenoid hypertrophy or adenoiditis.

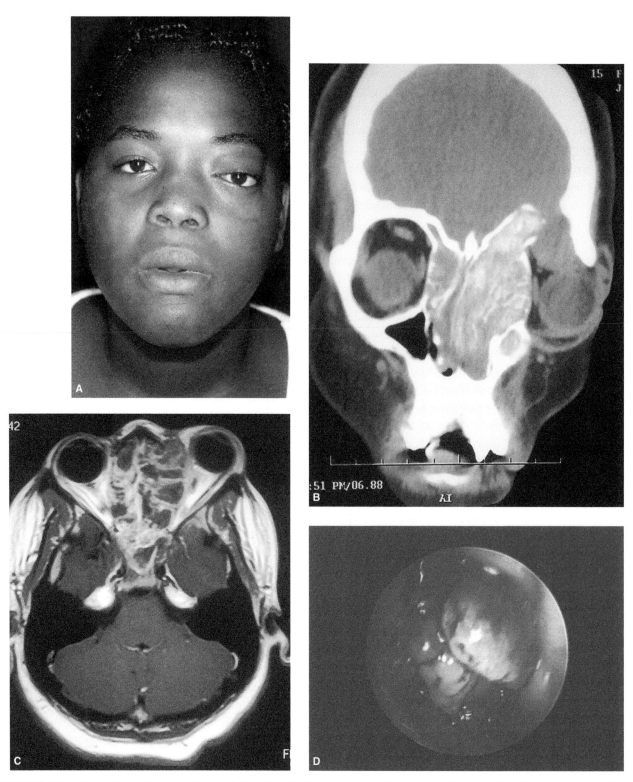

FIGURE 9.36 ■ Proptosis in a Patient with Fungal Sinusitis. (A) An adolescent girl presented with proptosis of her left eye and a history of chronic left nasal obstruction. (B) Coronal noncontrast sinus CT section shows complete opacification of the bilateral ethmoid air cells and frontal sinuses with high-density material compatible with fungal sinusitis. There is suggestion of bony destruction involving the left lateral frontal sinus wall. (C) Axial postcontrast T1-weighted image at the level of the ethmoid sinuses demonstrates opacification and avid enhancement within the mucosal surfaces of the bilateral anterior and posterior ethmoid air cells. (D) Endonasal view of extensive polyps in her left nasal cavity are seen. She underwent bifrontal craniotomy and open sinus surgery. Histopathology of the resected mass confirmed aspergillosis (see Figure 9.37). (Photo/legend contributors: Binita R. Shah, MD, and Steven Pulitzer, MD.)

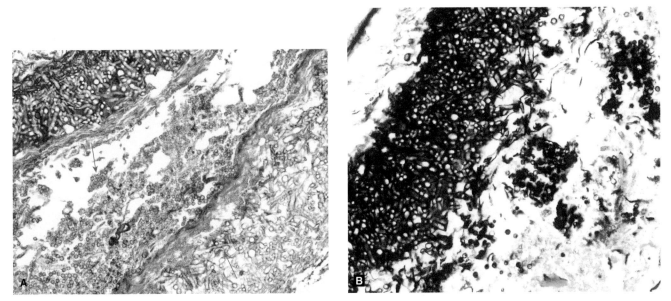

FIGURE 9.37 ■ Nasopharyngeal Aspergillosis. (A) Histologic section of nasopharyngeal mass from the same patient as Figure 9.36 showing hyphae and conidia. These hyphae are branching at acute angles. Nasopharyngeal aspergillosis can be both invasive and noninvasive (aspergilloma; fungus ball). (B) Gomori methenamine-silver stain shows septate hyphae with acute-angle branching, consistent with *Aspergillus*. (Photo/legend contributors: Sydney C. Butts, MD, and Raavi Gupta, MD.)

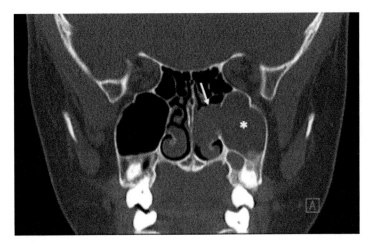

FIGURE 9.38 ■ Antrochoanal Polyp with Chronic Sinusitis. Coronal CT scan without contrast demonstrates an antrochoanal polyp (asterisk) completely opacifying the left maxillary sinus. Note the bowing and expansion of the medial wall of the left maxillary sinus as the polyp spills out of the sinus into the nasal cavity (arrow). Also note the relative lack of any other paranasal sinus disease. (Photo/legend contributors: Christopher Discolo, MD, and Vinodkumar Velayudhan, DO.)

POTT PUFFY TUMOR

Clinical Summary

Pott puffy tumor is an eponym, named for the physician who first described osteomyelitis of the frontal bone associated with subperiosteal abscess. The first description by Pott was in a patient whose finding were secondary to trauma, but most described cases are the result of frontal sinusitis with extension of the infection of the frontal bone (osteomyelitis). Abscess collection between the frontal bone and the periosteum results in the physical examination findings of a soft, fluctuant mass over the frontal bone. The infection can also result in areas of breakdown of the bone of the anterior or posterior table of the frontal sinus with subsequent forehead deformity or intracranial extension of the infection, respectively. Although this complication is not frequently seen in the era of broad-spectrum antibiotics, it can develop in the setting of a neglected or incompletely treated frontal sinusitis. Patients may present with headache, fever, neurologic signs (meningismus, altered mental status), or signs of septicemia.

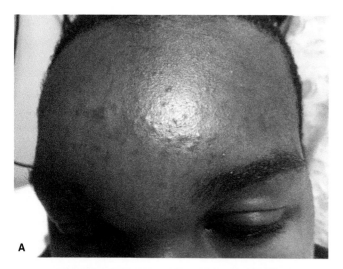

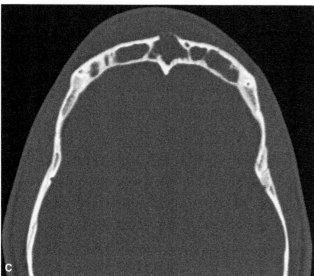

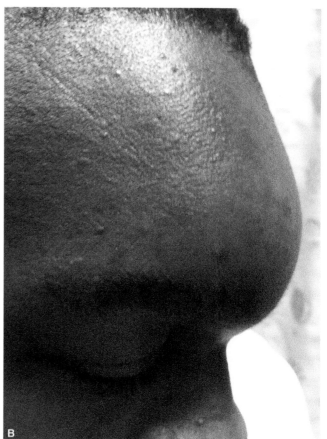

FIGURE 9.39 ■ Pott Puffy Tumor. A 15-year-old adolescent boy presented with severe frontal headache associated with swelling on the forehead as shown (**A, B**). He had symptoms of worsening upper respiratory infection for the past 2 weeks and started developing high fever for 3 days before this presentation. (**C**) His axial noncontrast CT image shows soft tissue within frontal sinuses, with breakthrough of adjacent bone and extension into soft tissues (Photo/legend contributors: Arpan Sinha, MD [A, B], and John Amodio, MD [C].)

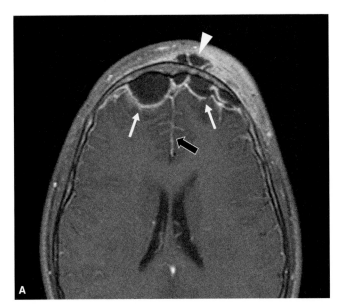 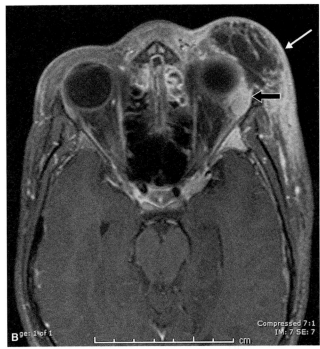

FIGURE 9.40 ■ Pott Puffy Tumor. Axial postcontrast T1-weighted MRIs through the brain (**A**) and orbits (**B**) in a patient with frontal sinusitis (not shown). There are rim-enhancing epidural abscesses exerting mass effect upon the frontal lobes bilaterally (white arrows, **A**). Enhancement in the interhemispheric fissure and adjacent sulci (black arrow) is consistent with meningitis. Abscesses (arrowhead) with surrounding edema and enhancement due to cellulitis are seen in the overlying scalp. The infection spreads to the left orbit (**B**) with an abscess involving the left eyelid (white arrow) and orbital cellulitis resulting in enlargement of the left lacrimal gland (black arrow). Bidirectional spread of infection from the frontal sinuses intracranially and into the overlying scalp is due to the presence of valveless veins that traverse the calvarium. (Photo/legend contributors: Daniel Ostro, MD, and Vinodkumar Velayudhan, DO).

Emergency Department Treatment and Disposition

A history of any prior treatment (antibiotic courses, incision and drainage elsewhere) should be elicited. Some patients may not have high fever or elevated WBC count if they have been on prior antibiotic therapy, but even if some of the typical signs or symptoms of infection are not present, do remember that these patients are potentially critically ill, especially if there is intracranial involvement. In addition to a CBC, blood cultures and culture of any spontaneous purulent drainages from the forehead should be obtained. A CT scan of the brain and sinuses with contrast is mandatory. The patient could also have involvement of other paranasal sinuses or orbital involvement. Patients should be admitted for IV antibiotics in preparation for abscess drainage in the operating room by

an otolaryngologist. If there is any evidence of intracranial involvement, obtain neurology and neurosurgery consultations and have a low threshold for ICU admission for neurologic monitoring.

Pearls

1. Pott puffy tumor is a complication of frontal sinusitis. It is essential to exclude intracranial spread of infection.

2. Surgical drainage (abscess decompression and frontal sinusotomy) is definitive treatment, with prolonged courses of antibiotics in light of osteomyelitis. Early otolaryngology consultation and inpatient admission are initial steps after imaging.

3. Pott puffy tumor often gets mistakenly diagnosed as forehead cellulitis or infected hematoma.

Clinical Summary

Deep neck space infections in children most often include retropharyngeal and parapharyngeal space abscesses. The retropharyngeal space is located between the posterior pharyngeal wall and the prevertebral fascia and extends from the skull base down to the level of the carina. This space

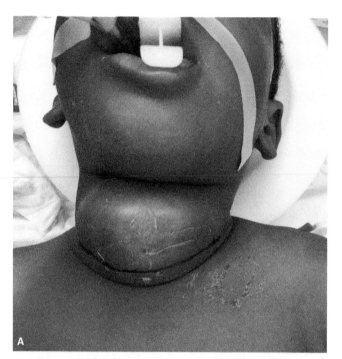

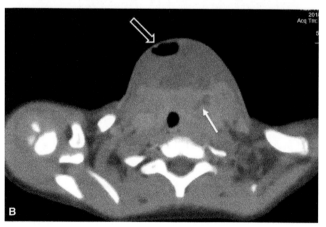

FIGURE 9.41 ■ Anterior Neck Abscess. (**A**) A large anterior neck abscess is seen in this 2-year-old child. (**B**) Contrast-enhanced neck CT scan demonstrates a large multiloculated abscess in the anterior neck containing gas (black arrow). The collection displaces the sternocleidomastoid and strap muscles. It appears to extend into the thyroid gland (white arrow), which raises the possibility of an infected fourth branchial cleft cyst. (Photo/legend contributors: Sydney C. Butts, MD, and Vinodkumar Velayudhan, DO.)

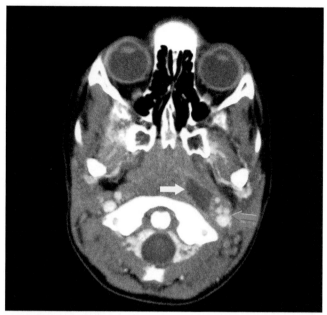

FIGURE 9.42 ■ Parapharyngeal Space Abscess. Axial CT scan with contrast shows a rim-enhancing left parapharyngeal space abscess (yellow arrow). Note how the carotid sheath is lateral to the infection (orange arrow). This allows for transoral incision and drainage to be carried out in a safe manner. Occasionally, these infections are located high in the neck at the base of skull, and this can make drainage more technically challenging. (Photo/legend contributor: Christopher Discolo, MD, and Vinodkumar Velayudhan, DO.)

contains lymph nodes, which can suppurate in the face of infection. These lymph nodes generally regress with age, and this explains why retropharyngeal abscess is less common in older children. The nose, paranasal sinuses, and nasopharynx all drain into the retropharyngeal lymph nodes. Trauma to the posterior pharyngeal wall is a less common route of entry for infection.

The parapharyngeal space resembles an inverted pyramid and extends from the skull base to the level of the hyoid bone. Lymph nodes located in this space do not regress with advancing age. Several anatomic locations within the head and neck can drain into the parapharyngeal space.

Deep neck space infections are often polymicrobial and can contain both aerobic and anaerobic organisms. There is a high incidence of group A β-hemolytic streptococci, but in recent years, *S aureus*, especially methicillin-resistant *S aureus* (MRSA), has become a much more common finding. Less common bacteria that have been implicated in deep neck space infections include *Mycobacterium tuberculosis*, atypical mycobacterium species, *Fusobacterium necrophorum*

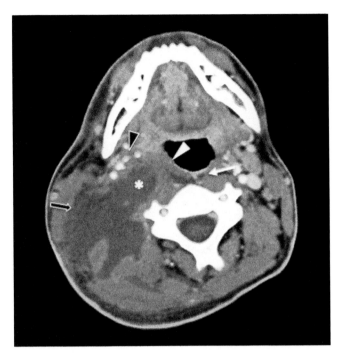

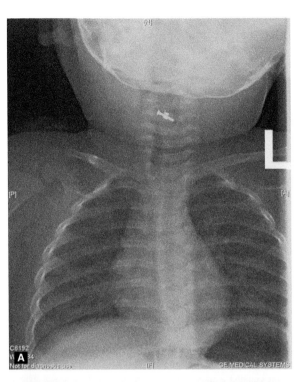

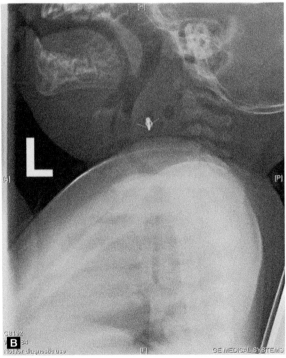

FIGURE 9.43 ■ Deep Neck Abscess Leading to Lemierre Syndrome. Axial contrast-enhanced CT demonstrates a large fluid collection with faint peripheral enhancement extending into multiple deep neck spaces, including the parapharyngeal space (asterisk), retropharyngeal space (white arrow), and posterior cervical space (black arrow). Note how the collection slightly narrows the airway (white arrowhead) and displaces carotid sheath structures (black arrowhead). Large collections in the neck may compromise the airway and affect adjacent neurovascular structures. This patient's cultures revealed *Fusobacterium necrophorum,* confirming the diagnosis of Lemierre syndrome. (Photo/legend contributors: Christopher Discolo, MD, and Vinodkumar Velayudhan, DO.)

(most common etiologic agent of Lemierre syndrome), and *Bartonella henselae* (cat scratch disease).

Deep neck infections generally progress from cellulitis to abscess over the course of 5 to 7 days. Patients often present with odynophagia, dysphagia, trismus, fever, neck pain, and neck stiffness. Drooling and inability to handle secretions can be a sign of impending respiratory compromise. A palpable tender lateral neck mass may be appreciated. Oral examination may reveal lateral pharyngeal wall asymmetry or a bulge in the midline of the pharynx. Complications of deep neck space infections include mediastinitis, sepsis, necrotizing fasciitis, airway collapse, and Lemierre syndrome (internal jugular vein thrombosis; see Figures 9.49 and 9.50). Untreated or advanced abscesses may spontaneously rupture into the pharynx, potentially causing aspiration pneumonia.

FIGURE 9.44 ■ Retropharyngeal Abscess (RPA) Secondary to a Foreign body (FB). (**A, B**) Anteroposterior and lateral views of the neck demonstrate a FB within the region of the esophagus. There is mass effect on the trachea, displacing it anteriorly, and there is extraluminal air noted within the region of the FB. These findings are compatible with an RPA in a 9-month-old infant presenting with persistent drooling. The FB was a hair clip. (Photo/legend contributors: Yvonne Giunta, MD, and John Amodio, MD.)

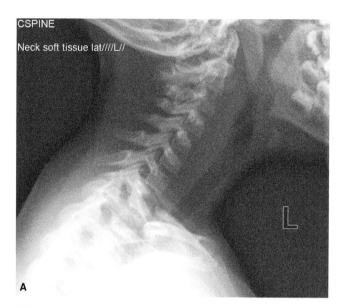

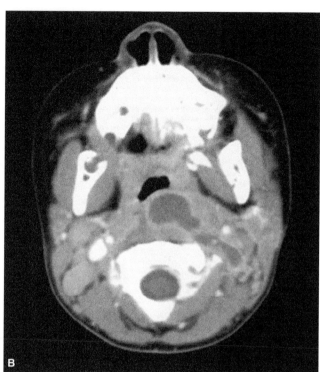

FIGURE 9.45 ■ Retropharyngeal Abscess. (**A**) Lateral view of the neck shows widening of the retropharyngeal space. (**B**) Contrast-enhanced CT scan of the neck reveals a well-defined peripherally enhancing and centrally low-density lesion in the nasopharyngeal region causing a mass effect on the adjacent airspace. These findings are consistent with a retropharyngeal abscess. (Photo/legend contributors: Mark Silverberg, MD, and John Amodio, MD.)

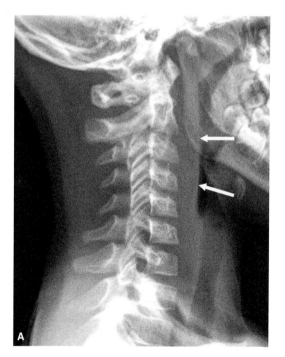

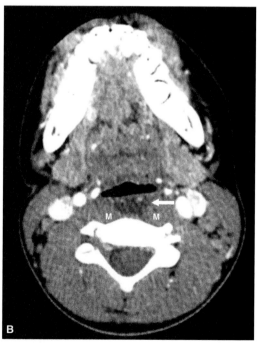

FIGURE 9.46 ■ Retropharyngeal Cellulitis. A 9-year-old boy presented with fever, sore throat, and neck pain for 1 day. He had tenderness to palpation on the left side of his neck with a limited neck rotation to the left. Because of lack of improvement after ibuprofen and dexamethasone, a lateral neck radiograph (**A**) was obtained. It demonstrates soft tissue swelling that may be prevertebral or retropharyngeal (white arrows). (**B**) Axial contrast-enhanced CT scan demonstrates fluid without rim enhancement consistent with edema (white arrow); no abscess is visualized. The position of the fluid anterior to the longus coli muscles (M) confirms its retropharyngeal location. When no rim enhancement is present, as in this case, attempts at drainage will often yield no fluid. (Photo/legend contributors: Tian Liang, MD, and Vinodkumar Velayudhan, DO.)

Emergency Department Treatment and Disposition

Assessment and stabilization (if necessary) of the airway are of paramount importance when children present with deep neck space infections. Signs of potential respiratory embarrassment include worsening stridor, inability to lie supine, inability to handle secretions, and use of accessory respiratory muscles. All patients should be closely monitored with continuous pulse oximetry and frequent vital sign surveys. Otolaryngology should be consulted early if airway symptoms are present.

Lab studies including CBC with differential, blood cultures, and possibly a throat culture should be obtained prior to starting antibiotics.

Imaging is often necessary to differentiate cellulitis from abscess. A contrast-enhanced CT scan of the neck is the current gold standard imaging modality. Young children may require sedation for this test, further demonstrating the importance of an accurate airway assessment. A lateral neck x-ray may have some utility for disorders of the retropharyngeal space but generally cannot differentiate abscess from cellulitis or phlegmon. Transcervical or transoral US has gained popularity in some centers. Benefits of US include avoidance of exposure to ionizing radiation and less need for sedation in younger patients. The main limitation of US is that it is more dependent on the skill of the technician or clinician both performing the exam and interpreting the findings.

Infection in the tissues surrounding the pharynx can lead to edema of the pharynx and airway. Otolaryngology personnel can perform bedside flexible fiberoptic laryngoscopy to assess the patency of the airway. If possible, impending airway collapse should be managed in the operating room, but intubation in the ED setting is sometimes needed. All patients should be made NPO (nothing by mouth) upon arrival to the ED until a definitive diagnosis is made and a treatment plan is formulated.

Empiric antibiotic therapy should be started in the ED setting until further information is available. Antibiotic coverage should include both anaerobic and aerobic organisms as well as those that produce β-lactamase. If MRSA is suspected, vancomycin should be initiated.

Often patients may go directly to the operating room from the ED setting based on clinical presentation and results of lab work and imaging. Inpatient monitoring should be in a high-acuity bed such as the ICU or step-down unit until clinical improvement is documented.

Pearls

1. Deep neck space infections are potentially life threatening, with potential for rapid clinical decline in children.
2. Retropharyngeal abscess is much more common in younger children, whereas parapharyngeal space infections can occur throughout childhood.
3. Contrast-enhanced CT scan remains the imaging modality of choice.

PERITONSILLAR ABSCESS

Clinical Summary

Peritonsillar abscess (PTA) is the most common suppurative infection of the head and neck; cases are more common in children age >10 years, although cases have been described in children <1 year old. Typically, the abscess lies at the superior pole of the potential space between the tonsillar capsule and the surrounding muscle bed. PTA frequently occurs in patients with a history of recurrent tonsillar infection. The infection is often polymicrobial, with group A *Streptococcus* isolated in up to 40% of cultures and anaerobic bacteria isolated in 40% to 75% of cultures. Patients present with throat pain, usually unilateral, for 5 to 7 days. Some may have progression of symptoms despite initiation of antibiotics. The history is also notable for odynophagia, poor oral intake, and inability to tolerate secretions with drooling. A characteristic muffled or "hot potato" voice, neck pain, trismus, and unilateral otalgia may be present. Constitutional symptoms include fever, malaise, and irritability.

Physical examination reveals asymmetric peritonsillar fullness, bulging soft palate, and deviation of the uvula away from the side of infection. Mouth opening may be limited secondary to local pain. The affected tonsil may be erythematous or covered with a purulent exudate. Palpable, tender cervical lymphadenopathy may be present. Complications include spontaneous rupture; extension to the parapharyngeal,

submandibular, and sublingual spaces; aspiration pneumonia; mediastinitis; sepsis; and recurrent PTA.

Emergency Department Treatment and Disposition

Diagnosis is clinical, and CBC is not required. Obtain a throat culture or culture of the aspirate for identification of the pathogens to direct antibiotic therapy. If the patient is uncooperative or the diagnosis is questionable, obtain a transcervical US. A CT scan with contrast is only needed if there is suspected involvement outside the peritonsillar space.

Children with a physical examination suggestive of a PTA or an US positive for a large abscess (>15 mm) require needle aspiration or incision and drainage. Children with smaller abscesses or peritonsillar cellulitis often respond to medical therapy alone. Give IV antibiotics (ampicillin and sulbactam or clindamycin) and a dose of dexamethasone (0.5 mg/kg) and adequate IV fluid hydration before beginning the procedure. Controversy exists over needle aspiration versus formal incision and drainage because little difference in symptom resolution has been found in several studies. Steps involved in incision and drainage of the PTA in the ED include:

1. Ensure needed equipment is available: benzocaine, aminobenzoate, and tetracaine (Cetacaine) spray; tongue depressors; 1% lidocaine with epinephrine; 10-mL syringes; 18-, 21-, and 25-gauge needles; Yankauer suction; emesis basin; headlight; no. 11 blade; curved clamp; and a culture swab.
2. Provide anesthesia: topical Cetacaine spray and local infiltration of 1% lidocaine with epinephrine with the 25-gauge needle may be used for local anesthesia.
3. Aspirate the area of maximal fluctuance with an 18- or 21-gauge needle. Remember that the internal carotid artery is 2 to 2.5 cm posterolateral to the tonsillar fossa.
4. If >3 to 4 mL of pus are aspirated, proceed to incision and drainage. Incise the area of greatest fluctuance with a no. 11 blade and then spread open with clamp. The aspirate may be sent for culture and sensitivity.

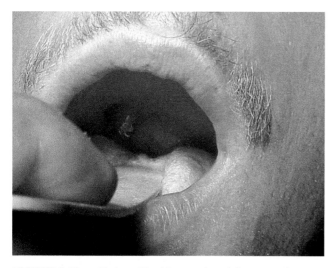

FIGURE 9.47 ■ Peritonsillar Abscess. An adolescent patient presented with a severe sore throat, fever, and difficulty swallowing. He had trismus, fullness, and bulging of the left tonsil, with deviation of the uvula toward the contralateral side. A diffuse white coating on the tongue is also seen. (Photo contributor: Ronak R. Shah, MD.)

Admit patients who are uncooperative, have severe trismus, or remain symptomatic after needle aspirate/incision and drainage. Some children may require incision and drainage in the operating room or quinsy tonsillectomy (tonsillectomy in presence of acute infection). Admit patients who

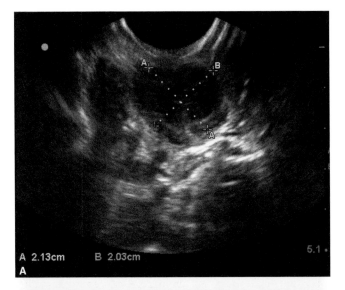

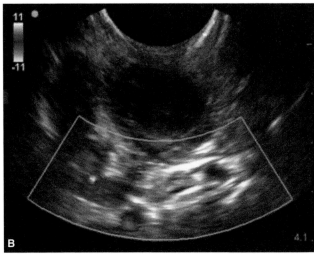

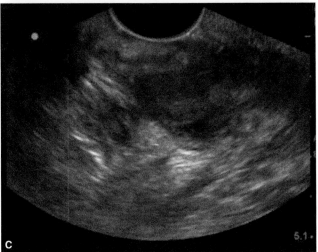

FIGURE 9.48 ■ Peritonsillar Abscess: US Images. (**A**) US image of a 2 × 2 cm peritonsillar abscess. The image is obtained by touching the tip of a covered endocavitary transducer on the patient's swollen tonsil. This technique not only confirms the presence of the abscess, but also the size, depth, and position of the carotid artery posterior to the abscess (note the hypoechoic circle just posterior to and to the left of the abscess cavity [**B**]). (**B**) Doppler mode can be activated and the window placed posterior to the abscess in order to locate and note the depth of the carotid artery behind the tonsil. This allows greater safety and anatomic awareness for drainage of the abscess. (**C**) After drainage of the peritonsillar abscess, the anechoic fluid pocket is collapsed, indicating successful drainage of the abscess (Photo contributor: John P. Gullett, MD.)

cannot tolerate oral intake, appear toxic, or have suspected complications for hydration and IV antibiotics.

Discharge those who can tolerate oral intake after needle aspiration or incision and drainage, providing oral antibiotics (clindamycin or amoxicillin/clavulanate), analgesics, and half-strength hydrogen peroxide oral rinses. Refer to otolaryngology for follow-up in 5 days. Children with recurrent PTAs or 1 episode of PTA but recurrent tonsillitis are candidates for elective tonsillectomy.

Pearls

1. Diagnosis is clinical with the classic triad of trismus, fullness or frank bulging of the superior aspect of the peritonsillar space, and deviation of the uvula toward the contralateral tonsil.
2. Treatment involves needle aspiration with or without formal incision and drainage and antibiotics. Children who are uncooperative or too young to cooperate may require incision and drainage in the operating room or quinsy tonsillectomy.

Clinical Summary

Lemierre syndrome is an acute oropharyngeal infection with secondary septic thrombophlebitis of the internal jugular (IJ) vein. It is generally seen in adolescents and frequently complicated by metastatic infections. The most common pathogen is *F necrophorum* (gram-negative obligate anaerobe normally found in the oral cavity and gastrointestinal and genital tracts). The diagnosis of Lemierre syndrome is mainly clinical. Patients have a history of recent pharyngitis and present with high fevers and rigors, neck pain, or stiffness. The oropharynx can appear normal with exudative tonsillitis or peritonsillar abscess. There may be anterior and posterior cervical lymphadenopathy and/or a tender swelling at the angle of the mandible (site of IJ thrombosis). Patients may also present with pneumonia as pulmonary involvement is frequent. Depending on where the septic emboli have lodged, additional symptoms may include those associated with brain abscess or cavernous sinus thrombosis, skin/soft tissue abscess, osteomyelitis, septic joint, or abdominal abscess. Lemierre syndrome is a great masquerader. The differential includes viral pharyngitis, infectious mononucleosis, atypical and bacterial pneumonia, endocarditis and intra-abdominal sepsis. Morbidity

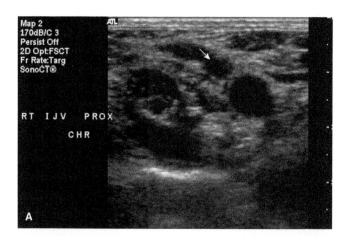

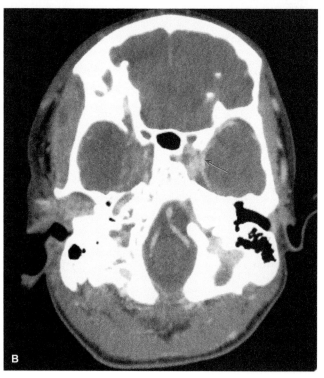

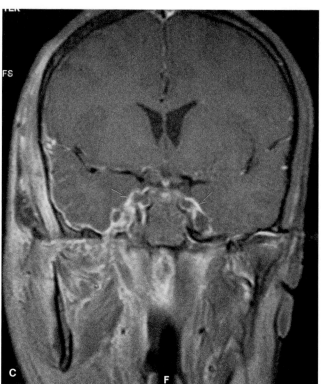

FIGURE 9.49 ■ Lemierre Syndrome. (**A**) A transverse sonographic image of the right internal jugular (IJ) vein shows nonocclusive thrombus within the right IJ in a highly febrile adolescent patient presenting with swelling around the angle of the jaw with altered sensorium. (**B**) Axial CT scan shows inhomogeneous enhancement of the cavernous sinus bilaterally (arrow) compatible with cavernous sinus thrombosis. (**C**) Magnetic resonance coronal postgadolinium image shows right leptomeningeal enhancement and diffuse enhancement of the masticator muscles and right temporalis muscle, compatible with diffuse inflammatory changes. Also note the inhomogeneous enhancement of the cavernous sinuses (arrows) compatible with cavernous sinus thrombosis. (Photo contributor: John Amodio, MD.)

and mortality are related to the extent of septic embolization and sepsis.

Emergency Department Treatment and Disposition

Order a CBC, comprehensive metabolic panel, blood cultures, and a CXR. The CXR will frequently exhibit multiple infiltrates (nodular lesions representing septic thrombi). Order other tests (eg, coagulation studies, lactate, venous blood gas) for evaluation and treatment of septic shock as needed. Radiologic imaging should be guided by the clinical presentation of the individual patient. Order ultrasonography to determine if IJ thrombus is present and CT and/or MRI as indicated to detect metastatic infections. Treat the infection with parenteral metronidazole or clindamycin and either a third-generation cephalosporin or β-lactam with β-lactamase inhibitor because some infections are polymicrobial. Drain any abscesses. Consider anticoagulation if a cavernous sinus thrombosis is present and consult infectious disease, surgery, neurosurgery, and orthopedics as needed for specific abscesses. Admit patients to ICU for ongoing care of sepsis.

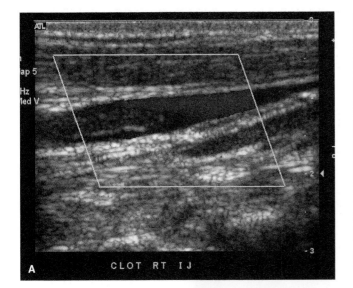

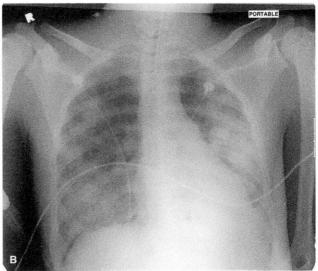

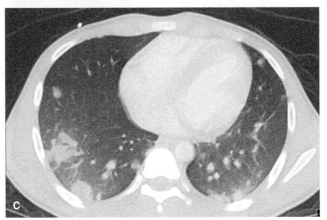

FIGURE 9.50 ■ Lemierre Syndrome. (**A**) A color Doppler scan of the right internal jugular vein demonstrating nonobstructive thrombus in an adolescent patient presenting with pansinusitis and parapharyngeal abscess. (**B**) Portable anteroposterior view of the chest demonstrating multiple infiltrates. (**C**) CT scan through the lower lobe regions demonstrates multiple pulmonary nodules with ill-defined borders consistent with septic emboli.

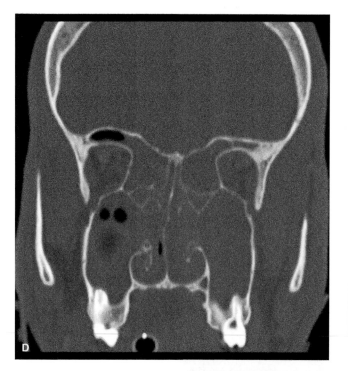
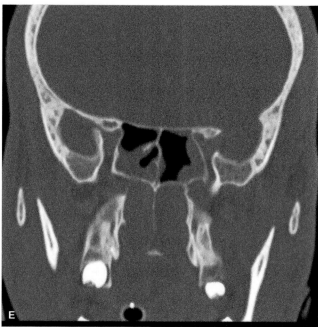
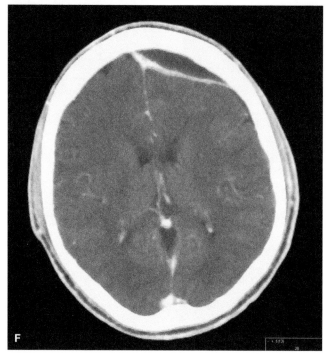

FIGURE 9.50 ■ (*Continued*) (**D, E**) Coronal reconstructions of the paranasal sinuses demonstrate pansinusitis. (**F**) Contrast-enhanced CT image of the brain demonstrates a left epidural abscess. (Photo contributor: John Amodio, MD.)

Pearls

1. High clinical suspicion is the key to diagnosing Lemierre syndrome.

2. Multiorgan dysfunction secondary to septic embolization can be a manifestation of Lemierre syndrome.

3. Drainage of abscesses is integral to treatment.

Chapter 10

SURGICAL AND GENITOURINARY

Neil G. Uspal
Vincent J. Wang

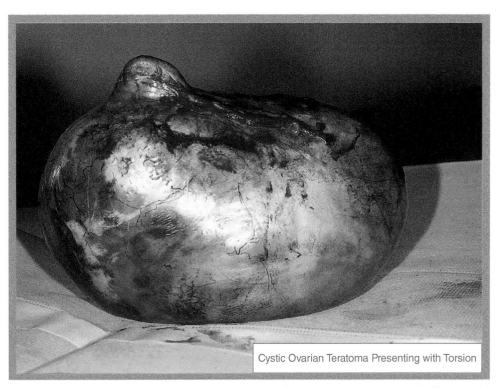

Cystic Ovarian Teratoma Presenting with Torsion

(Photo contributor: Binita R. Shah, MD)

The authors acknowledge the special contributions of Jennifer H. Chao, MD, and Andrea Marmor, MD, to the prior edition.

Clinical Summary

Intussusception occurs when the proximal portion of the intestine invaginates into the distal portion, causing abdominal pain, bowel injury, and eventually bowel obstruction. Early in the process, lymphatic return is impeded; then, as the edema and pressure increase, venous followed by arterial flow becomes compromised, leading to infarction of the entrapped bowel segment. Intussusception usually occurs

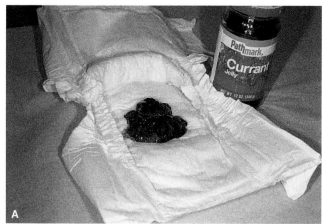

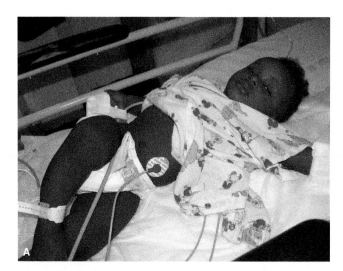

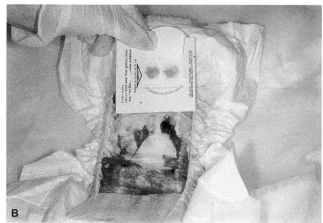

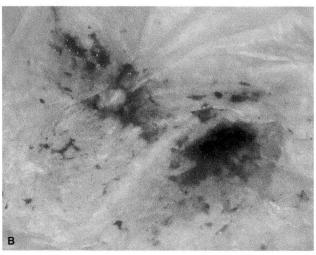

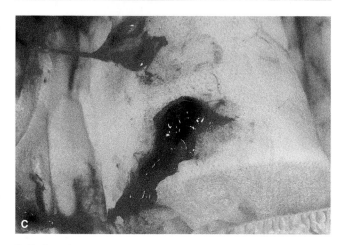

FIGURE 10.1 ■ Intussusception. (**A**) Extreme lethargy was the presenting complaint of this 10-month-old infant. (**B**) While in the ED, he passed this stool mixed with blood and mucus. Other neurologic signs of intussusception include coma or shock-like state (out of proportion to abdominal signs), seizures, hypotonia, or opisthotonic posturing. (Photo contributor: Binita R. Shah, MD.)

FIGURE 10.2 ■ Currant-Jelly Stool in Intussusception. (**A**) Commercially available currant jelly. (**B, C**) Diarrhea containing mucus and blood constitutes the classic currant-jelly stool (seen in about 60% of cases). This Hemoccult-positive stool was passed by an 8-month-old infant presenting with inconsolable crying episodes and bilious vomiting. (Photo contributor: Binita R. Shah, MD.)

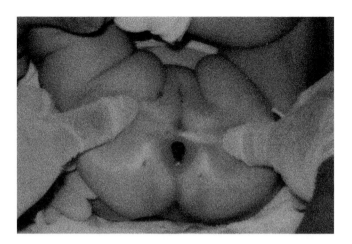

FIGURE 10.3 ■ Intussusception. The apex of the intussusception may extend into the transverse, descending, or sigmoid colon—even to and through the anus, mimicking rectal prolapse. This type of intussusception can be distinguished from rectal prolapse by the separation between the protruding intestine and the rectal wall, which does not exist in rectal prolapse. (Photo contributor: Binita R. Shah, MD.)

between the ages of 3 months to 3 years, with a peak in infants <1 year old. In children <3 years old, it is generally idiopathic and possibly due to prominent lymphoid tissue in the intestine serving as a lead point. The majority of intussusceptions are ileocolic, although they may present anywhere along the lower gastrointestinal (GI) tract. In older patients, lead points include Meckel diverticula, polyps, tumors (lymphomas or hemangiomas) or intramural edema, and hematomas from Henoch-Schönlein purpura. Sites other than ileocolic are also associated with underlying pathology.

Patients typically present with a sudden onset of severe, colicky abdominal pain at regular intervals, vomiting (initially nonbilious, but may progress to bilious), and bloody stool ("currant jelly"—with mucus and gross or occult blood). Patients often curl up to guard the abdomen. The abdominal pain may also increase in intensity over the course of its presentation. Patients may present variably and may not have all of these symptoms. They may also appear well between

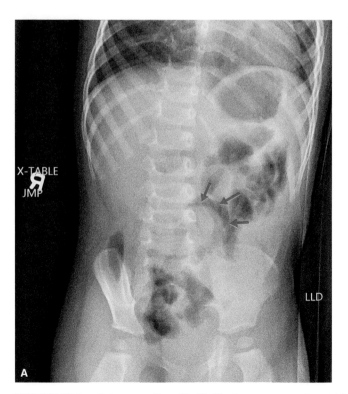

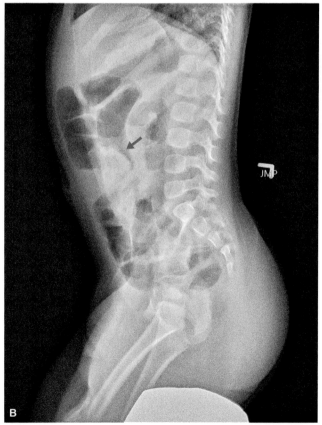

FIGURE 10.4 ■ Intussusception. (**A, B**) Single anteroposterior and lateral view of the abdomen demonstrates the crescent sign of intussusception (arrows) in an 18-month-old infant who presented with 2 days of vomiting, fussiness, and blood in stool. Intussusception was successfully reduced via air enema. (Photo contributor: Neil G. Uspal, MD.)

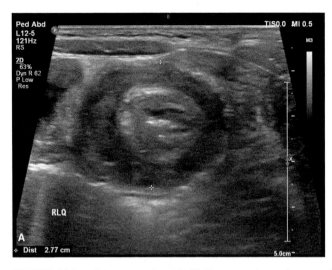
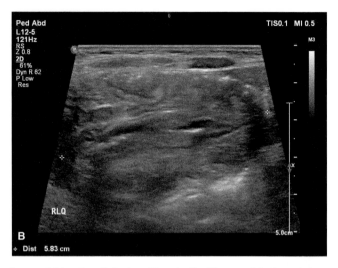

FIGURE 10.5 ■ Intussusception. (**A, B**) Transverse image (concentric rings and "doughnut" sign) and longitudinal image of the bowel show intussusception in a 10-month-old infant presenting with intermittent abdominal pain, vomiting, and bloody stools beginning 24 hours prior to this presentation. (Photo contributor: Neil G. Uspal, MD.)

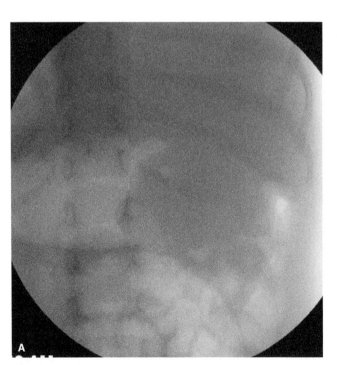
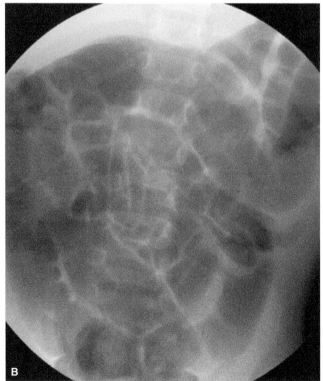

FIGURE 10.6 ■ Intussusception. (**A**) Fluoroscopic image taken in the prone position during an air reduction procedure shows a soft tissue mass, which represents intussusception. (**B**) Fluoroscopic image taken after successful reduction demonstrates air diffusely throughout the colon and small bowel. (Photo contributor: John Amodio, MD.)

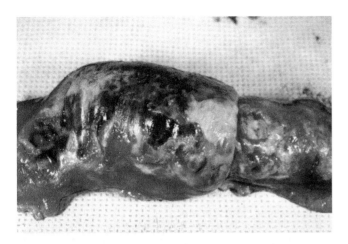

FIGURE 10.7 ■ Intussusception in Henoch-Schönlein Purpura (HSP). A magnified view of ileoileal colic intussusception after bowel resection in a patient with HSP in whom the intussusception could not be reduced by barium enema. The proximal portion of the ileum (intussusceptum) telescopes into the more distal ileum and cecum (intussuscipiens). This image also illustrates necrosis of both the intussusceptum and intussuscipiens. (Photo contributor: Binita R. Shah, MD.)

episodes. Lethargy and irritability may also be prominent. A subset of children, particularly infants, may present with lethargy as the sole clinical manifestation of intussusception. A "sausage-like" abdominal mass may be palpable on physical examination, and the feces frequently test positive for blood.

The differential diagnosis includes gastroenteritis, colitis, constipation, volvulus, toxin ingestion, encephalopathy, and any other condition that produces GI obstruction or lethargy.

Emergency Department Treatment and Disposition

Abdominal radiographs are not sensitive for intussusception but may be used as an initial screening test in certain clinical settings. Supine, prone, and left lateral decubitus views should be obtained if screening radiographs are performed. Radiographs should also be obtained to exclude free air in the abdomen once the diagnosis of intussusception is

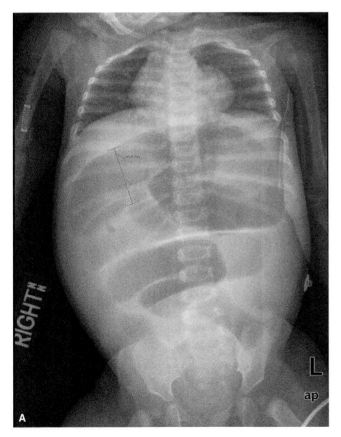

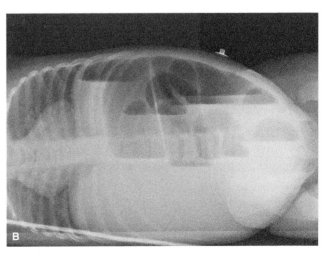

FIGURE 10.8 ■ Intussusception. The 6-month-old infant was brought to the ED a second time with vomiting and lethargy. Her initial ED diagnosis (seen 24 hours earlier) was acute gastroenteritis. She was ill-appearing with tachycardia and distended abdomen. Frontal (**A**) and right side down decubitus (**B**) images show multiple dilated small bowel loops with differential air fluid levels diagnostic of small bowel obstruction.

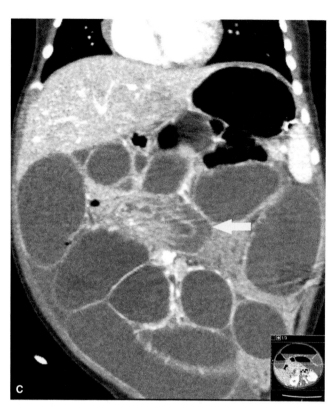

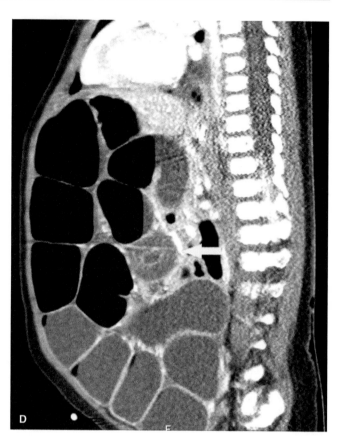

FIGURE 10.8 ▪ (*Continued*) (**C, D**) Coronal and sagittal CT reconstructive images show intussusception (arrow). (Photo/legend contributors: Tian Liang, MD, and John Amodio, MD.)

established. Obtain US for a definitive diagnosis. Surgery should be consulted in confirmed cases. Provide IV hydration and keep patients NPO (nothing by mouth). If abdominal perforation is not present, reduction of intussusceptions involving the colon with hydrostatic enema (air, barium, or water) should be attempted under radiology guidance in the presence of surgeons. Reduction may be guided by ultrasonography or fluoroscopy. If reduction is not achieved after 3 attempts, consider repeated delayed reduction or consult surgery for operative reduction. Ileoileal intussusceptions reduce spontaneously and rarely require operative reduction. Free air on the radiograph or clinical signs of peritonitis are indications for immediate operative intervention. Observation after successful reduction is prudent because of the potential for early recurrence. Protocols vary from the ED observation to hospitalization. It is important to emphasize strict return precautions.

Pearls

1. Intussusception is often misdiagnosed as gastroenteritis.
2. Profound lethargy may be the only symptom of intussusception, and patients may be misdiagnosed with sepsis or other conditions causing lethargy, which may result in a delay in diagnosis.
3. The classic triad (vomiting, pain, and blood in stool) of intussusception is not present in most cases.
4. Gross hematochezia ("currant jelly" stools) is a late finding, and its presence should not be relied upon to make the diagnosis of intussusception.

Clinical Summary

Pyloric stenosis is an idiopathic hypertrophy of the pylorus muscles, which creates a gastric outlet obstruction. Pyloric stenosis occurs in infants between the second week and second month of life (or later in preterm infants). It occurs more frequently in first-born boys, with a male-to-female ratio of about 4:1.

Infants typically present with increasing nonbilious, projectile vomiting soon after feeding, but otherwise may be well appearing. The infant is typically hungry right after vomiting.

The history often includes constipation or a decrease in the number of stools. After several days of vomiting, dehydration and weight loss may occur. Vigorous vomiting may cause a Mallory-Weiss tear that presents with coffee-ground emesis.

Physical exam may reveal a firm, ballotable mass with the size and shape of an olive in the mid epigastrium, as well as a visible peristaltic wave. With delayed presentation, cachexia may be present. However due to easier access to US, it is not common to see infants late in the course of illness. Thus, having a high index of suspicion is prudent in any infant with

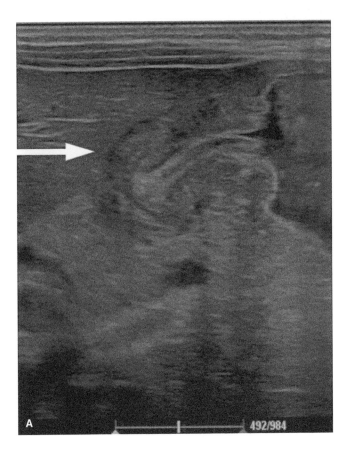

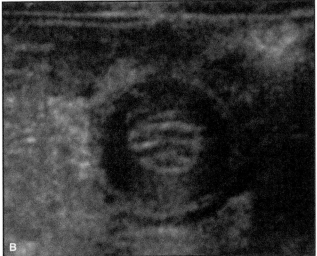

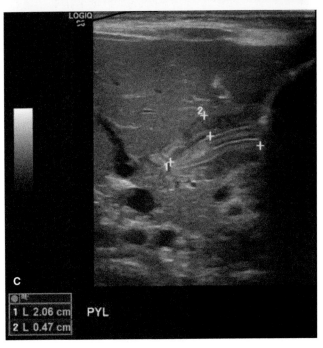

FIGURE 10.9 ■ Hypertrophic Pyloric Stenosis. (**A**) Longitudinal US image (arrow) of the hypertrophied pylorus in a 35-day-old infant with a 2-day history of projectile vomiting. There is thickening of the pyloric wall and hypertrophy of the mucosa, with prolapse into the antrum producing the "nipple sign." (**B**) Transverse image through the pylorus producing the "doughnut sign." (**C**). Hypertrophic pyloric stenosis. The normal pylorus measures <14 mm in length and muscle thickness up to 3 mm in width. (Photo contributors: Sathyaseelan Subramaniam, MD [A], and John Amodio, MD [B, C].)

projectile, nonbilious emesis and failure to thrive or with inadequate weight gain. The differential diagnosis includes gastroesophageal reflux, overfeeding, gastroenteritis, inborn errors of metabolism, adrenal insufficiency, and milk protein allergy. The presence of bilious emesis necessitates emergent evaluation for postpyloric obstruction, such as midgut volvulus.

Emergency Department Treatment and Disposition

Although palpation of an enlarged pylorus ("olive") may be considered diagnostic for pyloric stenosis, US is typically used to confirm the diagnosis. An upper GI study may be performed if the US is inconclusive or if US is not available. Serum electrolytes may reveal a hypochloremic, hypokalemic metabolic alkalosis. Other findings include acidic urine pH (paradoxical aciduria in the face of metabolic alkalosis) and mild hyperbilirubinemia. Dehydration and electrolyte abnormalities should be corrected prior to pyloromyotomy to prevent anesthesia-related perioperative morbidity. A nasogastric tube may be helpful for continued vomiting, although once patients are made NPO, vomiting is usually infrequent. Consult surgery and admit the patient for IV hydration and pyloromyotomy. Most patients will tolerate feeds and be discharged home within 48 hours of surgery.

Pearls

1. Pyloric stenosis is the most common cause of hypochloremic metabolic alkalosis in infancy.
2. The best time to examine for an "olive" is soon after the infant has vomited or while feeding to see the peristaltic wave from left to right.
3. Pyloric stenosis is not a surgical emergency but may be a medical emergency because of electrolyte disturbances and dehydration. Most patients will require rehydration prior to surgery.

Clinical Summary

In the pediatric age spectrum, acute nonperforated appendicitis is most commonly seen in school-aged and teenaged children. Patients classically present with periumbilical pain migrating to the right lower quadrant, fever, anorexia, vomiting, localized peritonitis, and/or guarding. Localization of pain and accompanying complaints vary with the length and position of the appendix, which is highly variable. For example, a retrocecal appendix is likely to cause rectal irritation and diarrhea, whereas an appendix abutting the bladder may cause dysuria, and one that abuts the liver may cause pain in the right upper quadrant. Younger children manifest more nonspecific symptoms such as generalized abdominal pain, irritability, and refusal to ambulate. In this population, the diagnosis is often not made until after appendiceal perforation.

Various signs are used to describe the classic findings of appendicitis. Their presence is variable depending on the position of the appendix. Commonly described signs include McBurney's point tenderness (tenderness one-third the distance from the right anterior superior iliac spine to the umbilicus), Rovsing sign (pain appreciated in the right lower quadrant with palpation of the left lower quadrant), psoas sign (pain with extension of the right hip due to an inflamed appendix adjacent to the psoas muscle), and obturator sign (pain with passive internal rotation of the flexed right hip). The differential diagnoses include constipation, pneumonia, genitourinary pathologies (eg, testicular torsion, pyelonephritis), ovarian pathologies (eg, ovarian torsion, mittelschmerz), ectopic pregnancy, pelvic inflammatory disease, mesenteric adenitis, UTI, and other surgical pathologies (eg, intussusception, midgut volvulus, incarcerated hernia).

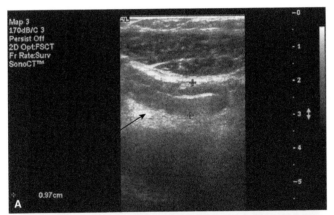

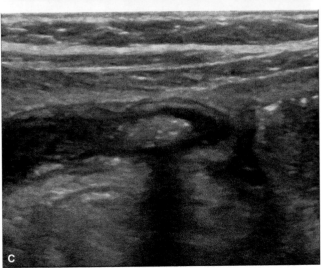

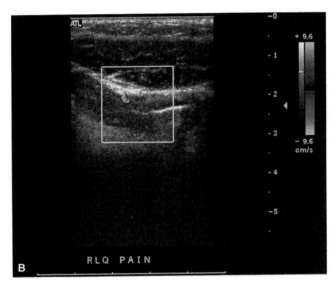

FIGURE 10.10 ■ Acute Nonperforated Appendicitis. (**A**) Longitudinal sonographic image of the right lower quadrant reveals an enlarged (diameter > 6 mm), noncompressible appendix. Note increased echogenicity of the surrounding periappendiceal fat compatible with surrounding inflammation (arrow). (**B**) Same image as above with color flow imaging demonstrating increased flow compatible with hyperemia. (**C**) Longitudinal image of an enlarged appendix with an echogenic focus with acoustical shadowing compatible with an appendicolith. (Photo contributor: John Amodio, MD.)

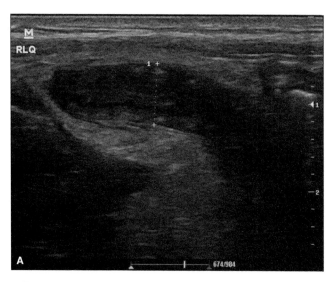
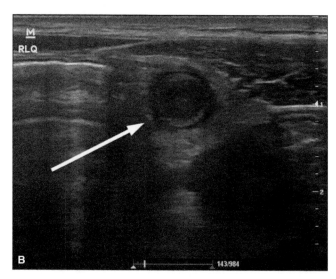

FIGURE 10.11 ■ Acute Nonperforated Appendicitis. (**A, B**) Arrow points to a target sign of an acutely inflamed appendix on a US image seen in an 8-year-old boy presenting with acute-onset right lower quadrant pain, fever, and vomiting for 1 day. (Photo contributor: Sathyaseelan Subramaniam, MD.)

Emergency Department Treatment and Disposition

The diagnosis of appendicitis relies on clinical evaluation and usually the selective use of imaging studies. Clinical prediction rules, such the Pediatric Appendicitis Score (PAS), may be used to risk stratify patients. High-suspicion patients warrant surgical consultation. When uncertain, US is the preferred modality for imaging of the appendix, although CT scan may be used when US is not available or the results are indeterminate. Laboratory tests, including CBC with differential, C-reactive protein, pregnancy test (adolescent females),

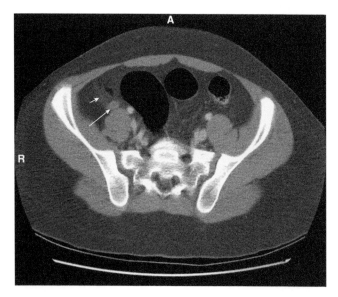

FIGURE 10.12 ■ Acute Nonperforated Appendicitis. CT scan of right lower quadrant shows enlarged, contrast-enhanced appendix (long arrow) with surrounding increased "stranding" of periappendiceal fat (short arrow), compatible with acute appendicitis. (Photo contributor: John Amodio, MD.)

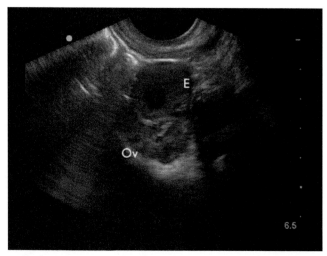

FIGURE 10.13 ■ Ectopic Pregnancy; Differential Diagnosis of Acute Abdomen. A transvaginal coronal image of an ectopic gestational sac (E) adjacent to the ovary (Ov) is seen in an adolescent girl presenting with cramping right lower quadrant abdominal pain. (Photo contributor: Trushar Naik, MD.)

and urinalysis, may facilitate the diagnosis or identify other causes of symptoms. Provide IV hydration and keep patients NPO. Provide adequate analgesia, including morphine as needed, as studies have shown that analgesia does not affect diagnostic accuracy. Consult surgery and consider admission for serial abdominal exams if the diagnosis is unclear. Provide antibiotics (coverage for gram-negative and anaerobic bacteria) after the diagnosis is made and in consultation with surgery.

Pearls

1. Missed appendicitis is one of the most common diagnoses resulting in malpractice claims.
2. An inability to hop up and down on the right leg without pain is often helpful to identify peritonitis.
3. Early in the course of appendicitis, patients may have a normal WBC and normal C-reactive protein; these findings do not exclude the diagnosis.
4. Diarrhea, although more often associated with gastroenteritis, may also be present in appendicitis, and its presence does not exclude the diagnosis.

Clinical Summary

Perforation of appendicitis generally occurs after 48 to 72 hours of symptoms of appendicitis. Clinical symptoms differentiating perforated appendicitis or appendicitis with abscess from simple acute appendicitis include the presence of higher fever, systemic toxicity, diffuse abdominal tenderness and guarding (potentially a rigid abdomen), and elevated markers of inflammation, including WBC count, absolute neutrophil count, and C-reactive protein.

Patients with perforated appendicitis do not like to move and feel most comfortable lying on their sides with the hips and knees flexed. They walk very slowly in a bent-over position with a shuffling gait while holding the right side of the abdomen and will refuse to hop or jump because of extreme pain. Although these symptoms may also be present in patients with nonperforated appendicitis, they may be more pronounced after perforation. When initial perforation occurs, there may be some initial relief of pain, but until abscess formation is complete, generalized peritoneal irritation is typically present.

Emergency Department Treatment and Disposition

When appendiceal perforation is suspected, make all patients NPO. Provide IV fluid resuscitation with crystalloids. Useful adjunctive testing may include a CBC with differential, urinalysis, pregnancy test (as appropriate), and C-reactive

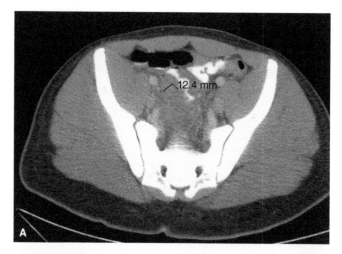

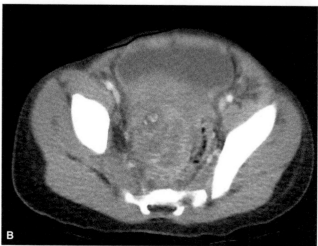

FIGURE 10.15 ■ Perforated Appendicitis. (**A**) CT image through right lower quadrant demonstrate an enlarged, poorly defined appendix with increased density throughout the surrounding periappendiceal fat, compatible with perforation and phlegmon. (**B**) CT scan of the pelvis shows dilated appendix with appendicolith on top of pelvic abscess, compatible with ruptured appendicitis. (Photo contributor: John Amodio, MD.)

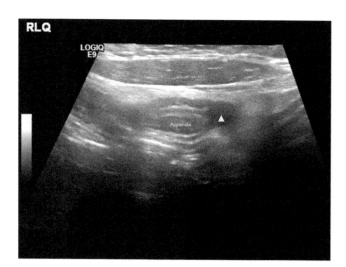

FIGURE 10.14 ■ Perforated Appendicitis. US image demonstrates a dilated appendix with a discontinuous wall and small surrounding collection (triangle) in 4-year-old child presenting with right lower quadrant pain. (Photo contributor: Gregory N. Emmanuel, MD.)

protein. Provide adequate analgesia as needed with morphine or other opiates. Consult surgery emergently. Consider CT for those with delayed presentation of perforated appendicitis to evaluate for abscess. Once the diagnosis is confirmed, start broad-spectrum antibiotics with coverage for gram-negative and anaerobic bacteria.

Definitive management of perforated appendicitis varies based on patient illness severity, presence of abscess, and surgeon preference, although increasing evidence supports appendectomy at presentation. Stable patients with appendiceal abscesses may be candidates for delayed appendectomy. This decision should be made by the surgical service.

Pearls

1. Preschool-age children are often difficult to evaluate for appendicitis and often present with perforated appendicitis.

2. Adequate fluid resuscitation and stabilization prior to surgical intervention is imperative.

3. Patients with peritonitis, as in perforated appendicitis, are often quiet and avoid movement, unlike patients with intestinal obstruction who are restless and often doubled over in pain.

Clinical Summary

Inguinal hernias are more common in boys, especially boys with a history of prematurity, and are caused by failure of the processus vaginalis to fuse after testicular descent. In females, the ovary may be associated with the incarcerated hernia. Patients most often present with a history of an inguinal or scrotal bulge that becomes more prominent with increased abdominal pressure (crying, straining, coughing, laughing). Although most hernias are manually reducible, patients may present with incarcerated hernias that cannot be reduced manually. These patients will present with inguinal swelling alone or in conjunction with pain, vomiting, irritability, poor feeding, lack of bowel movements, or abdominal distension. Palpation reveals a firm, immobile, and often tender and erythematous scrotal or inguinal swelling. Incarceration is more common in patients <2 years old.

Emergency Department Treatment and Disposition

If the diagnosis is unclear, order a US to differentiate hernia from hydrocele, testicular torsion, or other inguinal or testicular pathology. In females, a US should be obtained to assess for ovarian involvement. Incarcerated hernias require emergent reduction. Provide analgesia and sedation as needed, and

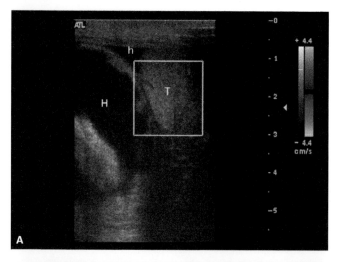

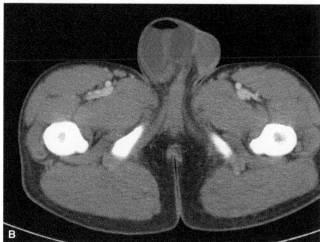

FIGURE 10.17 ■ Incarcerated Inguinal Hernia. (**A**) A sonographic image of the right scrotum showing a normal-appearing testicle (T) with normal color flow. Adjacent to the testicle is a fluid-filled loop of bowel, compatible with a hernia (H). There is a small reactive hydrocele (h). (**B**) CT image of the same patient through the right scrotum showing incarcerated loop of bowel containing air and fluid. (Photo contributor: John Amodio, MD.)

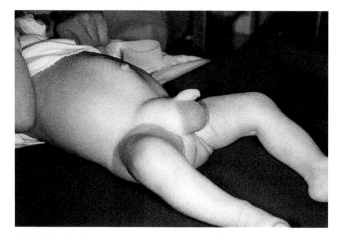

FIGURE 10.16 ■ Incarcerated Inguinal Hernia. This infant presented with inconsolable crying associated with vomiting. His hernia could not be reduced into the abdominal cavity, mandating a surgical repair. Other entities that cause inconsolable crying in infants include testicular torsion, paraphimosis, fracture (child abuse), and hair-tourniquet syndrome. (Photo contributor: Binita R. Shah, MD.)

apply gentle constant manual pressure along the axis of the inguinal canal to decompress the sac and push it in. If the hernia is not reducible or if there is any concern for intestinal perforation or gangrenous bowel, consult surgery emergently for operative management. If there is concern for perforation, order upright or cross-table lateral plain radiographs to assess for free air. Admit patients for observation and surgical repair (usually after 24 hours to allow for resolution of edema), or discharge for delayed repair (after surgical consultation) with clear follow-up plans and very specific instructions to return for recurrence.

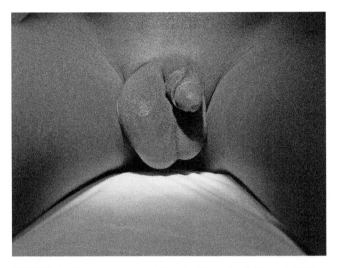

FIGURE 10.18 ■ Incarcerated Inguinal Hernia; Differential Diagnosis of Testicular Torsion. Inguinal hernia can be seen as a distinct bulge separate from the testicle in this image. Both incarcerated inguinal hernia and testicular torsion present with acute onset of painful and swollen scrotum. (Photo contributor: Jennifer H. Chao, MD.)

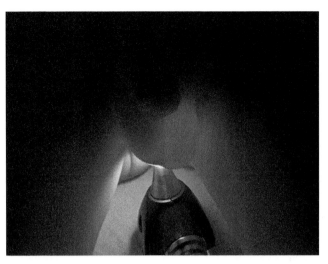

FIGURE 10.20 ■ Hydrocele; Nonpainful Scrotal Swelling; Differential Diagnosis of Acute Scrotum. A positive hydrocele transillumination is seen in this 4-year-old child presenting with nontender left-sided scrotal swelling. (Photo contributor: Ameer Hassoun, MD.)

Pearls

1. Always consider incarcerated hernia as a differential diagnosis in inconsolable infants.
2. Do not attempt to reduce the hernia if there is evidence of peritonitis or the patient is ill appearing.
3. The hernia may cause pressure on the spermatic cord, causing venous congestion and infarction of the testicle.
4. Placing the child in Trendelenburg and maximizing relaxation will aid in successful reduction.

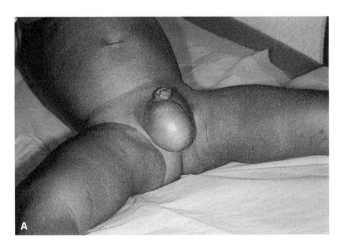

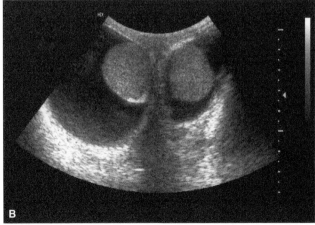

FIGURE 10.19 ■ Hydrocele; Nonpainful Scrotal Swelling; Differential Diagnosis of Acute Scrotum. (A) A swelling of the right hemiscrotum due to a hydrocele is seen in this infant. A hydrocele may be confused with hernia, cannot be reduced, lacks a mass at the inguinal ring, and occurs more often bilaterally. (B) Bilateral hydroceles seen in a sonographic image of scrotum in a different infant. (Photo contributors: Binita R. Shah, MD [A], and Mark Silverberg, MD [B].)

Clinical Summary

Testicular torsion is most common in the newborn and the early adolescent. In adolescents, it occurs most commonly when there is a "bell-clapper" deformity: the testis is inadequately fixed to the tunica vaginalis, allowing twisting of the testicle on the spermatic cord, which obstructs blood flow. Patients typically present with acute onset of severe pain in the groin (sometimes with radiation to the abdomen) and vomiting. Patients may also solely present with lower abdominal pain. Physical exam reveals a swollen, tender testicle, often in a transverse lie, sitting higher than usual. There may also be erythema of the overlying skin, absence of the cremasteric reflex, and lack of relief with elevation of the testicle (a negative Prehn sign). There may be a history of similar episodes as the testes can twist and untwist spontaneously. With delayed diagnosis, the pain may subside, and there is thickening of the scrotal skin. Torsion occurs more often on the left side, likely from the increased length of the spermatic cord.

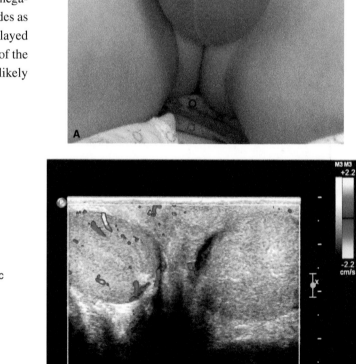

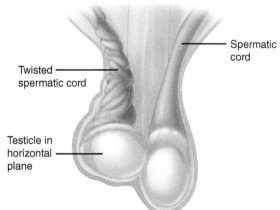

FIGURE 10.21 ■ Bell-Clapper Deformity; Testicular Torsion. Bell-clapper deformity leading to the twisting of the spermatic cord and testicular torsion. This causes the testis to be elevated, with a horizontal lie. The lack of fixation of the tunica vaginalis to the posterior scrotum predisposes the freely movable testis to rotation and subsequent torsion. An elevated testis with a horizontal lie may be seen in asymptomatic patients at risk for torsion. (Reproduced with permission from Tenenbein M, Macias CG, Sharieff GQ, et al. *Strange and Schafermeyer's Pediatric Emergency Medicine*. 5th ed. McGraw-Hill Education; New York, NY, 2019.)

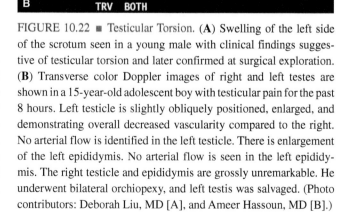

FIGURE 10.22 ■ Testicular Torsion. (A) Swelling of the left side of the scrotum seen in a young male with clinical findings suggestive of testicular torsion and later confirmed at surgical exploration. (B) Transverse color Doppler images of right and left testes are shown in a 15-year-old adolescent boy with testicular pain for the past 8 hours. Left testicle is slightly obliquely positioned, enlarged, and demonstrating overall decreased vascularity compared to the right. No arterial flow is identified in the left testicle. There is enlargement of the left epididymis. No arterial flow is seen in the left epididymis. The right testicle and epididymis are grossly unremarkable. He underwent bilateral orchiopexy, and left testis was salvaged. (Photo contributors: Deborah Liu, MD [A], and Ameer Hassoun, MD [B].)

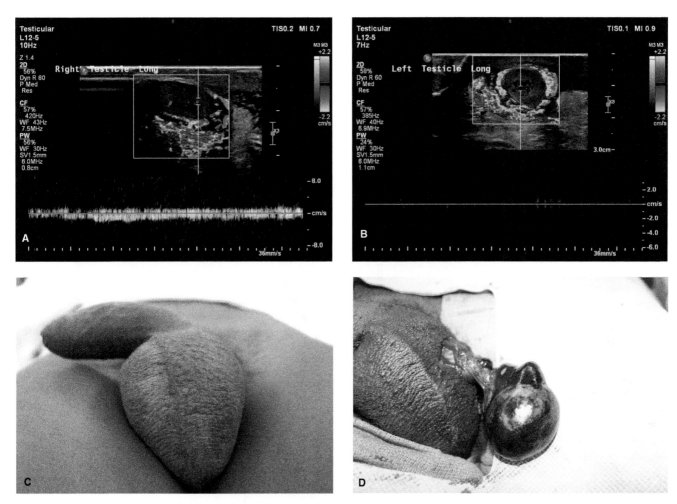

FIGURE 10.23 ■ Testicular Torsion. (**A**) Longitudinal color Doppler sonogram of right testis shows normal peripheral and central vascularity. (**B**) Longitudinal color Doppler sonogram of left testis demonstrates peripheral vascularity but no central vascularity, compatible with missed testicular torsion. This 5-year-old boy presented with one day history of left scrotal swelling and left-sided lower abdominal pain for 3 days. His testicle was successfully de-torsed in the operating room. (**C**) Left-sided scrotal enlargement is seen in this adolescent boy whose symptoms began 18 hours before presenting to the ED. (**D**) An intraoperative picture of the torsed necrotic testicle and epididymis. His testicle was found to be twisted 360 degrees. (Photo contributors: Neil G. Uspal, MD [A, B], and Mark Horowitz, MD [C, D].)

Emergency Department Treatment and Disposition

Consult urology or surgery emergently. Testicular viability is dependent on duration of testicular ischemia. If the diagnosis is unclear, obtain color Doppler sonography. Findings may include diminished to absent blood flow to the testicle, visualization of twisting in the spermatic cord, and changes in the size and echotexture of the testis. In situations in which operative repair is not rapidly available, manual detorsion to improve blood flow to the testicle may be attempted pending surgery. The affected testicle is externally rotated ("opening the book") 1 or 2 360-degree turns. If successful, this will improve pain, the position of the testicle, and blood flow. If unsuccessful, rotation in the opposite direction may be necessary, because up to one-third of torsed testicles will be laterally rotated. Whether torsion is resolved manually or spontaneously, surgical exploration and fixation within the scrotum are required to prevent further episodes.

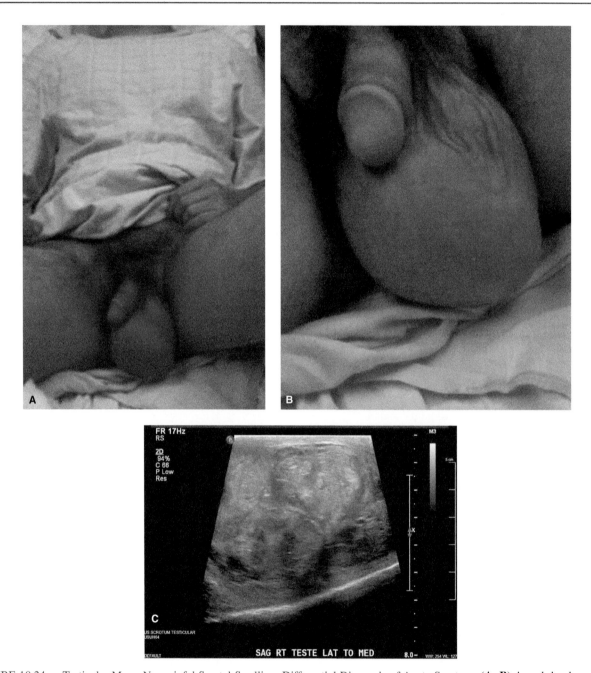

FIGURE 10.24 ■ Testicular Mass; Nonpainful Scrotal Swelling; Differential Diagnosis of Acute Scrotum. (**A, B**) A rock-hard nontender scrotal mass was felt in this 15-year-old adolescent boy who went to primary care physician for sports physical. He had this swelling for more than a year, but he was "too embarrassed and afraid" to tell anyone until recently when he told his dad about "cup being painful." However, he was not examined by anyone prior to this visit. He denied any history of pain or urinary symptoms. (**C**) Sagittal US image shows large mass replacing entire right testicle. Histopathology confirmed germ cell testicular cancer. (Photo contributor: Stuart A. Bradin, DO.)

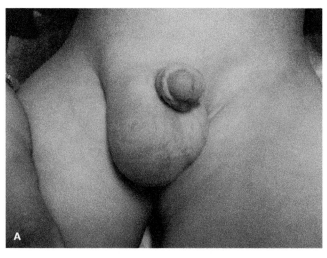
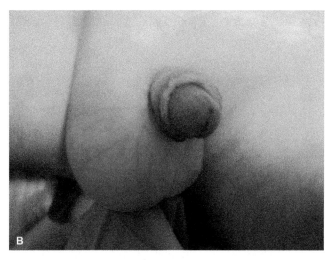

FIGURE 10.25 ■ Hydrocele; Nonpainful Scrotal Swelling; Differential Diagnosis of Acute Scrotum. (**A, B**) Hydrocele without and with transillumination. A hydrocele or hernia will transilluminate, whereas a torsed testicle or other solid scrotal mass will not. (Photo contributor: Ee Tay, MD.)

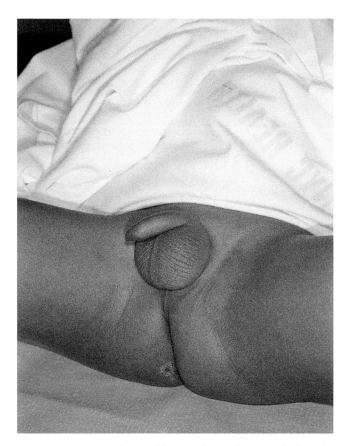

FIGURE 10.26 ■ Cellulitis with Acute Scrotal Swelling; Differential Diagnosis of Acute Scrotum. Acute onset of scrotal swelling, extreme pain, and fever were the presenting complaints of this child. He had impetigo over the perineum with subsequent spread of the infection. (Photo contributor: Binita R. Shah, MD.)

TABLE 10.1 ■ DIFFERENTIAL DIAGNOSIS OF ACUTE PEDIATRIC SCROTUM

Painful and Swollen	Nonpainful and Swollen

• Testicular torsion
• Acute epididymitis (or epididymo-orchitis)
• Orchitis (eg, mumps)
• Torsion of appendix testis
• Torsion of appendix epididymis
• Trauma
  1. Testicular hematoma
  2. Fracture or rupture of testis
• Testicular tumor (hemorrhage within tumor)
• Incarcerated inguinal hernia
• Testicular venous congestion
• Acute hydrocele
• Vasculitis
  1. Henoch-Schönlein purpura
  2. Kawasaki disease
	• Acute idiopathic scrotal edema
	• Hydrocele
	• Reducible inguinal hernia
	• Varicocele
	• Spermatocele
	• Testicular tumor

*Differential Diagnosis of Acute Painful Scrotum
A Diagnostic Dilemma*

• 3 most common etiologies (about 90% of cases)
1. Testicular torsion
2. Acute epididymitis (or epididymo-orchitis)
3. Torsion of appendix testis

TABLE 10.2 ■ DIFFERENTIAL DIAGNOSIS: TESTICULAR TORSION VERSUS ACUTE EPIDIDYMITIS

	Testicular Torsion	Acute Epididymitis
Average age	12–15 years	25 years
Pain	Usually sudden	Gradual
Severity	Peaks in hours	Peaks in days
Fever	Uncommon	Common
Vomiting	Common	Uncommon
Dysuria	Rare	Common
Discharge	Rare	Common
Laterality	Unilateral	Usually unilateral (~10% bilateral)
Testis	Riding high in scrotum	Normal position
Long axis of testis	Horizontal lie	Normal vertical lie
Cremasteric reflex (affected side)	Absent (usually)	Present
Prehn sign	Negative	Positive
Pyuria or bacteriuria	Rare	~50%
Color Doppler flow	Decreased	Increased

• An enlarged epididymis can be felt distinctly on the testis early in the course of acute epididymitis. With time, as edema spreads to the testis as well as to the scrotal wall, it may become difficult to differentiate torsion from epididymo-orchitis.

Pearls

1. Presume testicular torsion until proven otherwise in any boy with acute scrotal pain.
2. Perform a testicular exam to exclude torsion in all boys with abdominal pain.
3. A recent history of trauma may accompany torsion and is often misleading.
4. If there is very high suspicion for torsion, emergent urologic or surgical evaluation or operation takes priority over diagnostic studies.
5. Patients with symptoms for <6 to 12 hours are more likely to have a salvageable testicle. Even if symptoms are present for >12 hours, patients must be explored emergently as salvage is still often possible.

Clinical Summary

Blunt scrotal trauma can result in testicular dislocation, fracture, or rupture, hematoma, and/or hematocele. Patients present with pain (often accompanied by nausea and vomiting), swelling, and ecchymosis. In testicular dislocation, the testicle is out of the scrotum and found in the inguinal, abdominal, penile, or perineal area. Testicular fracture or rupture involves a break in the tunica albuginea, which can be indirectly seen on US as an irregular contour. A testicular hematoma is blood within the testicle, whereas a hematocele is an extratesticular collection of blood.

Emergency Department Treatment and Disposition

Examine the testes in all boys with pelvic or perineal trauma. A thorough exam of the scrotum is also necessary. If there is an empty scrotum, search for a possible dislocated testis, which must be relocated via closed or open reduction. Order a US and consult urology or surgery. Provide adequate analgesia.

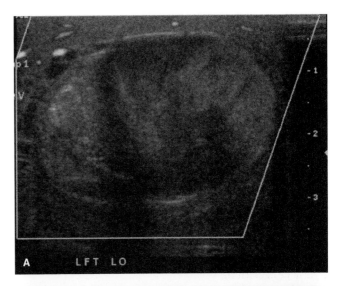

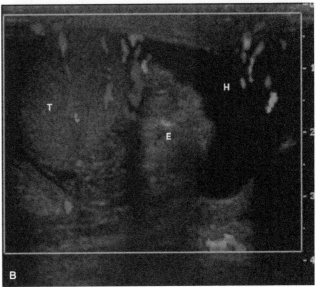

FIGURE 10.28 ■ Testicular Trauma. (**A**) Sagittal sonogram of the left testicle demonstrates a heterogeneous architecture and diffuse skin thickening. (**B**) Transverse sonogram shows poor margination of the lateral aspect of the testicle (T) with the epididymis (E), compatible with rupture. Note reactive hydrocele (H). Vascular supply to the testicle is within normal limits. (Photo contributor: John Amodio, MD.)

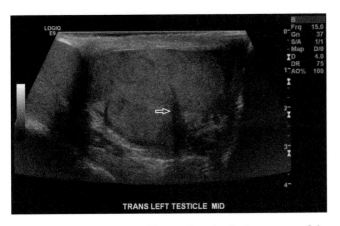

FIGURE 10.27 ■ Testicular Trauma. Longitudinal sonogram of the testicle shows fracture line (arrow), in the setting of trauma. (Photo contributor: John Amodio, MD.)

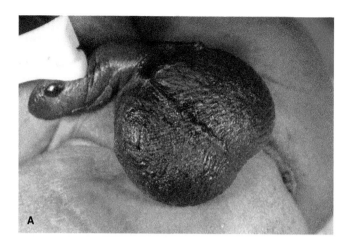

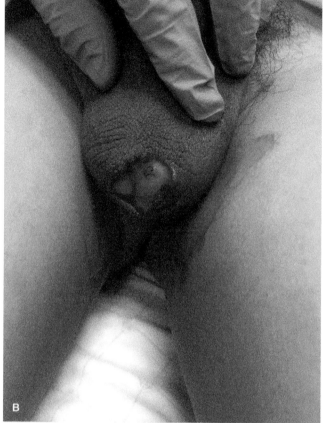

FIGURE 10.29 ■ Scrotal Trauma. (**A**) Birth trauma. Scrotal edema with ecchymosis and a hemorrhagic blister on the penis are seen in a neonate born after breech presentation in a difficult delivery in the ED. Scrotal US showed a hematoma without any testicular trauma. (**B**) Scrotal laceration. Laceration to the inferior scrotum exposing the tunica vaginalis. Such wounds require surgical exploration to evaluate testicular health. (Photo contributors: Binita R. Shah, MD [A], and Karen Kwan, MD [B].)

Testicular fracture or rupture is a surgical emergency, because salvage is more likely within 24 hours. Manage small hematomas and hematoceles conservatively with pain management. Consult urology or surgery for drainage of large hematomas because testicular pressure may cause ischemia and atrophy.

Pearls

1. Consult urology or surgery early because testicular injuries are time sensitive.

2. Administer adequate pain medication to optimize testicular examination.

3. Testicular torsion may present with a history of trauma.

4. Traumatic epididymitis presents in a delayed manner as a recurrence of pain.

5. Painless scrotal swelling in the setting of polytrauma should prompt evaluation for intra-abdominal injury.

Clinical Summary

Epididymo-orchitis is inflammation of the epididymis and the testes, either of which may be found in isolation (either epididymitis or orchitis) or together (epididymo-orchitis). In sexually active patients, *Chlamydia trachomatis, Neisseria gonorrhoeae, Mycoplasma, Ureaplasma,* and *Escherichia coli* (more likely with anal sex) are the most common pathogens. In younger patients, common organisms include *E coli* or other gram-negative uropathogens, usually in conjunction with a UTI, and viruses such as adenovirus, enterovirus, and mumps. Isolated epididymitis is often caused by physical exertion or blunt or repetitive trauma. Patients present with a relatively gradual onset of pain, swelling, and redness (as compared to torsion). Prehn sign (pain relief with elevation of the testis) is often positive, unlike in testicular torsion, in which there is no relief with testicular elevation. However, *this is not a 100% reliable sign to differentiate the 2 diagnoses.* In epididymo-orchitis, the testis is typically in a normal vertical position and the cremasteric reflex is usually present. Patients may also complain of penile discharge, dysuria, urinary urgency, or increased urinary frequency. If inflammation is limited to the epididymis, the pain will be limited to the upper posterior pole of the testis.

Emergency Department Treatment and Disposition

Obtain a urinalysis and urine culture in all patients and test for *N gonorrhoeae* and *C trachomatis* in sexually active adolescents. Consult urology and obtain scrotal US when the diagnosis is unclear. In epididymo-orchitis, US will show increased blood flow and edema to the affected area, often with a reactive hydrocele. Treat sexually active patients with ceftriaxone and either doxycycline or azithromycin for gonorrhea and chlamydia. UTI should be suspected based on abnormal urinalysis, positive urine culture, or a history of anatomic abnormality. Treat with appropriate antibiotics. Patients with no evidence of bacterial infection should be treated solely with supportive care, including scrotal support and NSAIDs for pain.

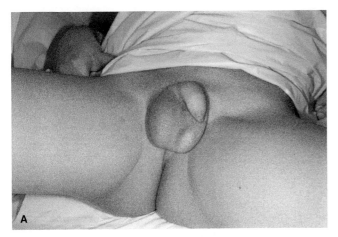

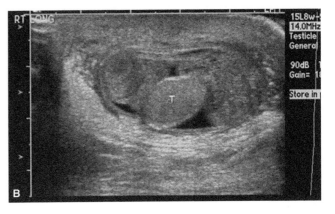

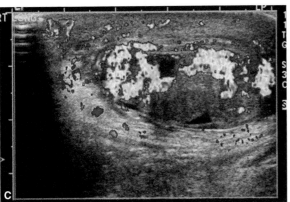

FIGURE 10.30 ■ Acute Epididymitis. (**A**) An erythematous right-sided scrotal swelling of 3 days in duration is seen in this 6-year-old boy. The orientation of the testis was normal, with its long axis parallel to the long axis of the body. (**B, C**) Longitudinal sonographic image demonstrates markedly enlarged epididymis surrounding the testicle (T). There is also marked thickening of the scrotal skin secondary to the inflammatory process. Color Doppler image of epididymitis showing marked increased hyperemia within the epididymis. (Photo contributors: Binita R. Shah, MD [A], and John Amodio, MD [B, C].)

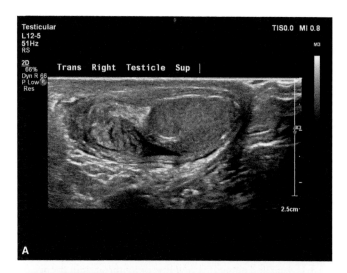

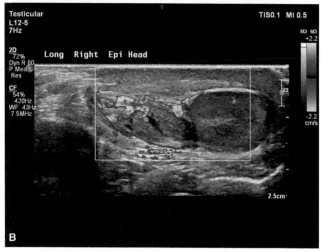

FIGURE 10.31 ▪ Acute Epididymitis. (**A, B**) Sagittal sonograms of the scrotum show an enlarged hyperemic epididymis in an 11-year-old boy with 5 days of right testicular pain. The patient was discharged with analgesics and recommendations for supportive care. (Photo contributor: Neil G. Uspal, MD.)

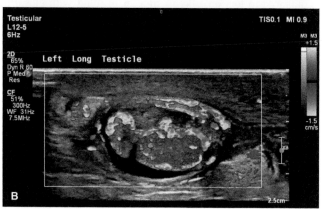

FIGURE 10.32 ▪ Acute Epididymo-orchitis. (**A, B**) Transverse and sagittal color Doppler sonograms of the left testis shows enlarged epididymis and hyperemic epididymis and testis, compatible with epididymo-orchitis in a 9-year-old boy with 24 hours of left scrotal pain and redness. Patient was discharged with recommendations for supportive care. (Photo contributor: Neil G. Uspal, MD.)

Pearls

1. Refer patients with epididymitis or orchitis caused by a UTI for urologic evaluation.
2. Acute epididymitis is the most common alternative diagnosis for patients with suspected testicular torsion. Torsion must be ruled out in an expeditious manner if the diagnosis is unclear.
3. Counsel adolescents with epididymitis or orchitis on safe sex practices and perform comprehensive sexually transmitted disease testing.
4. Epididymitis in prepubertal males with no evidence of UTI may be treated with supportive care alone.

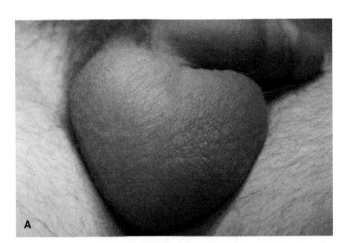
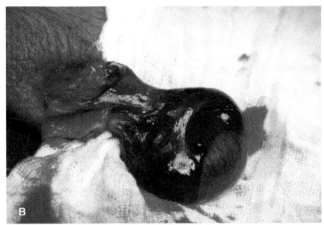

FIGURE 10.33 ■ Testicular Torsion; Differential Diagnosis of Epididymo-orchitis. Right scrotal enlargement and high-riding testicle with some loss of the rugae (compared to the left side) are seen in this image (**A**) taken prior to scrotal exploration. Intraoperative image of a necrotic testis (**B**). This adolescent patient who presented with scrotal pain and swelling was diagnosed as having epididymo-orchitis. He returned to the ED with worsening scrotal pain, and testicular torsion was diagnosed. Acute epididymitis (or epididymo-orchitis) is the most common entity confused with testicular torsion and often indistinguishable from testicular torsion on examination. In addition, no radiologic tests are 100% sensitive or specific. An absent venous flow followed by absent arterial flow is seen in torsion. It is very unusual to see any venous or arterial flow with torsion; you may see flow to the periphery (scrotum), but typically no flow is seen. With infection, there is increased flow to whichever structure is infected. (Photo contributor: Mark Horowitz, MD.)

Clinical Summary

The appendix testis is a vestigial appendage on the upper pole of the testicle that may twist on its stalk, becoming necrotic and painful. This occurs more often before puberty but may occur at any age. It is the most common cause of acute scrotal pain in children. Patients present with pain and swelling of more gradual onset and less severity than seen with testicular torsion. Tenderness and swelling are localized to the superior lateral aspect of the testis distinct from the epididymis. The testis typically has a normal vertical lie, and the cremasteric reflex is usually present.

Torsion of the appendix testis resolves without intervention in 2 to 10 days as the appendage is resorbed. The differential diagnosis includes testicular torsion, acute epididymoorchitis, and other causes of acute scrotum (see Table 10.1).

Emergency Department Treatment and Disposition

Although torsion of the appendix testis is a clinical diagnosis, testicular torsion must be ruled out. Order US if the diagnosis is uncertain and/or consult urology. If testicular torsion cannot

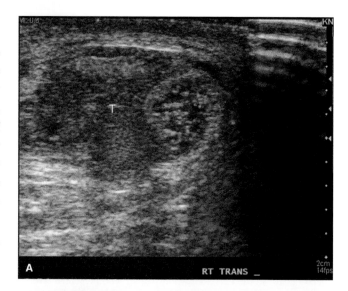

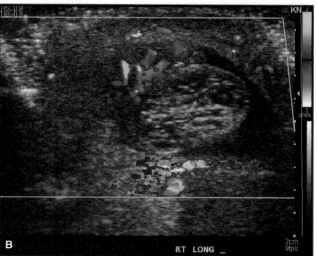

FIGURE 10.35 ■ Torsion of the Appendix Testes. (**A**) Transverse image demonstrates heterogeneous mass medial to testicle (T). Note the characteristic "Swiss cheese" appearance of the torsed appendix testis. (**B**) Absent color flow within mass compatible with torsed appendix testis. (Photo contributor: John Amodio, MD.)

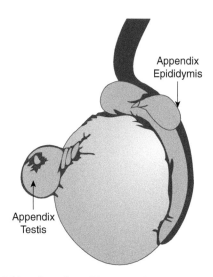

FIGURE 10.34 ■ Location of Intrascrotal Appendages. The appendix testis and appendix epididymis are vestigial remnants of the Müllerian and Wolffian ducts, respectively. These small pedunculated structures are at risk for torsion. The appendix testis is a far more common vestigial structure than the appendix epididymis and thus composes the majority of appendiceal torsions. (Reproduced with permission from Kline MW. *Rudolph's Pediatrics*. 23rd ed. McGraw-Hill Education; New York, NY, 2018.)

be excluded, surgical exploration is warranted. If the diagnosis is clear, treat with rest, scrotal support, and analgesia.

Pearl

1. The classic sign of torsion of the appendix testis is the "blue dot" of the ischemic appendage, although this may not be seen secondary to surrounding edema and skin thickening of the scrotal wall.

Clinical Summary

Foul and/or bloody vaginal discharge in the prepubertal child is often associated with the presence of an occult vaginal foreign body (FB). Other possible diagnoses include nonspecific vaginitis, vaginitis from respiratory or enteric organisms, and sexual abuse. The duration of symptoms may vary from days to years. Toilet tissue is the most common vaginal FB, although other objects may be inserted into the vagina as part of exploratory behavior. A thorough social history must also be taken to rule out abuse.

Emergency Department Treatment and Disposition

Examine patient in either the frog-leg (supine) or knee-chest (prone) position. Consider US if clinical suspicion for an FB is high but an FB is not visualized on exam; however, US will not identify all FBs. Alternatively, an exam under procedural sedation may be necessary to adequately visualize the vaginal vault. Irrigate with lukewarm water through a small catheter or angiocatheter to remove small pieces of toilet paper.

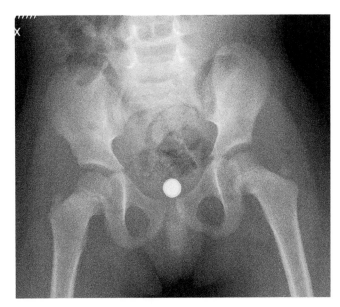

FIGURE 10.37 ■ Vaginal Foreign Body. Anteroposterior radiograph in a 4-year-old girl (with a "history of putting something in her butt") shows a battery in the lower midline portion of the pelvis. A 2.5-cm-diameter button battery from the vagina was retrieved under general anesthesia (GA). She presented again 2 weeks later to the ED with bloody vaginal discharge. Examination under GA revealed multiple ulcers on both anterior and posterior vaginal wall. (Photo contributor: Shyam Sathanandam, MD.)

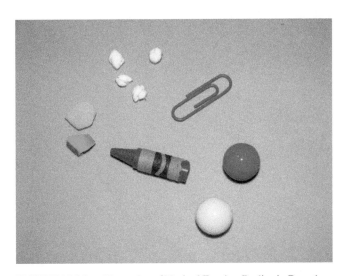

FIGURE 10.36 ■ Examples of Vaginal Foreign Bodies in Prepubertal Children. Examples of objects found in the vagina of prepubertal children by accident or intention are shown and include wads of toilet paper, crayon, pieces of rubber or clay, paper clip, and marbles. Other items include food items, bottle caps, or toys. Foreign objects in a child's vagina may also indicate child sexual abuse. (Photo contributor: Binita R. Shah, MD.)

Provide analgesia and/or sedation prior to removal of any FB, as surrounding tissues are sensitive and friable, and the procedure can cause significant psychological stress. Consult surgery for FB removal in the operating room for large FBs, for potential FB erosion into surrounding structures, or if the FB is not easily visualized on external exam.

Pearls

1. If clinical suspicion for a vaginal FB is high, consider imaging and examination in the operating room even if an FB is not visualized on external exam. Procedural sedation in the ED may also be helpful.

2. Vaginitis secondary to an FB will not resolve until the FB is removed.

3. If a vaginal FB is identified, examine other easily accessible orifices, such as the ears and nose, for additional FBs.

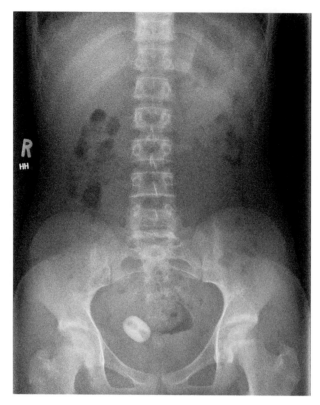

FIGURE 10.38 ■ Vaginal Foreign Body. A foreign body is shown in a 10-year-old girl with a history of autism. She self-reported inserting a 3 × 1 × 1 cm plastic bead into her vagina. The bead was removed in the operating room. (Photo contributor: Photo contributor: Neil G. Uspal, MD; see also Figure 4.45.)

Clinical Summary

An imperforate hymen is usually an isolated anomaly. Hematocolpos (vaginal distension with menstrual products) or hematometrocolpos (distention of the uterus and vagina with menstrual products) may cause abdominal pain and a mass in a pubertal adolescent with primary amenorrhea. There may

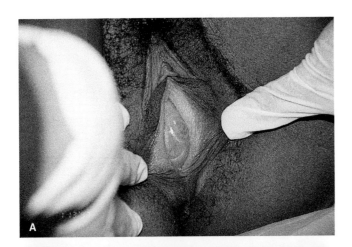

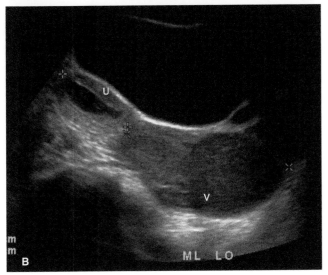

FIGURE 10.39 ■ Congenital Imperforate Hymen with Hematometrocolpos. (**A**) An imperforate hymen with a bulging mass at the introitus is seen in this 12-year-old girl who presented with intermittent crampy abdominal pain of 24 hours in duration. She had similar abdominal pain about 4 weeks prior and was prescribed antacids by her physician. Because of recurrence of pain, she came to ED. She denied any prior menstruation. (**B**) Sagittal sonographic image of the pelvis demonstrates enlarged vagina (V) containing fluid and echogenic material (blood) and fluid-filled uterus (U) in a patient with imperforate hymen. (Photo contributors: Binita R. Shah, MD [A], and John Amodio, MD [B].)

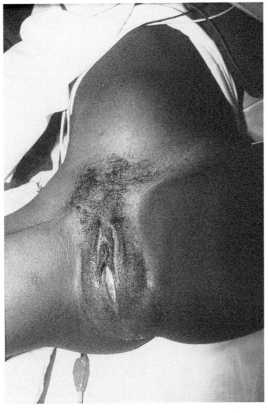

FIGURE 10.40 ■ Congenital Imperforate Hymen with Hematometrocolpos. An imperforate hymen with a bulging mass was visualized at the introitus in this 13-year-old girl presenting with severe abdominal pain and difficulty voiding. She had similar pain about 5 weeks prior to this episode. Her sexual development level was Tanner IV, but she denied having prior menstruation. An abdominal mass (distended uterus) was palpable in the midabdomen. Hymenectomy was performed, leading to drainage of about 1.0 L of blood, fluid, and menstrual debris. (Photo contributor: Binita R. Shah, MD.)

be a history of cyclic abdominal pain or symptoms associated with an abdominal mass, including constipation, urinary retention, or back pain.

Neonates with imperforate hymen may develop a mucocele from distention of the vaginal introitus with mucous secretions produced by intrauterine stimulation of an infant's cervical mucus glands by maternal estrogens. Mucoceles resolve spontaneously, and children remain asymptomatic until puberty. A bluish or purplish bulge in the vaginal vault is noted in the adolescent. The differential diagnosis includes labial adhesion, congenital absence of the vagina, and "acquired imperforate hymen" from genital trauma of sexual abuse (scarring leading to imperforate hymen).

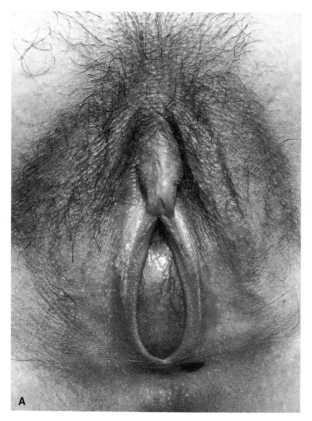

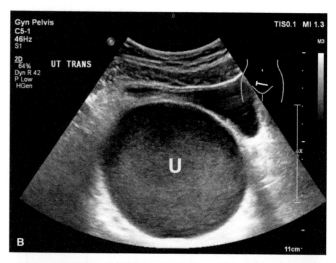

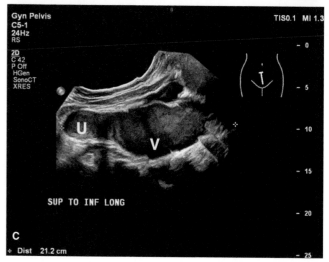

FIGURE 10.41 ■ Imperforate Hymen with Hematometrocolpos. (**A**) A 11-year-old girl presented with a 1-week history of lower crampy abdominal pain and fullness. Her history revealed lack of menses. Her examination revealed a bluish bulging mass at the introitus (hemato-metrocolpos), which was managed by performing a hymenectomy in the operating room. (**B, C**) Transverse and longitudinal sonograms of the uterus (U) and vagina (V) show uterus and vagina to be enlarged and filled with low-level echoes compatible with hematometrocolpos. (Photo contributors: Ameer Hassoun, MD [A], and Neil G. Uspal, MD [B, C].)

Emergency Department Treatment and Disposition

Obtain a pelvic US to delineate local anatomy for patients with an unclear diagnosis or concern for other genitourinary abnormalities. Consult gynecology or surgery for urgent resection of the hymen in the adolescent and drainage of menstrual blood and debris. Reassure patients about the normality of their genitalia.

Pearls

1. Do not puncture the membrane to relieve pressure because this may cause ascending infection.
2. Always perform a genitourinary exam in pubescent girls with abdominal pain.

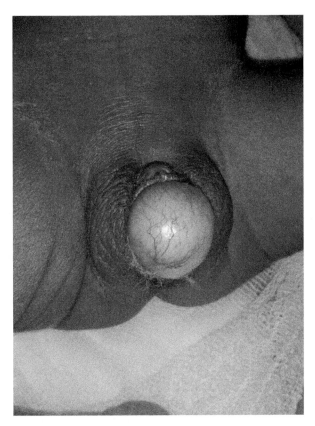

FIGURE 10.42 ■ Imperforate Hymen with Hydrocolpos. This neonate had an intralabial swelling coming from the introitus noted at birth. A cruciate incision was planned but it ruptured spontaneously, draining all the secretions. (Photo contributor: Prerna Batra, MD.)

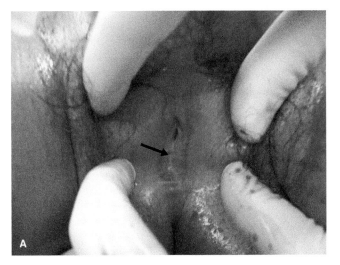
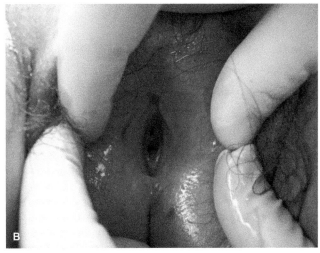

FIGURE 10.43 ■ Labial Fusion; Differential Diagnosis of Imperforate Hymen. (**A**) Labial fusion (adhesions or agglutination) is shown in an adolescent girl. A thin vertical raphe (arrow) in the midline over the site of introitus (where labia are fused) is pathognomonic of labial fusion. Usually with imperforate hymen, a bulge is seen in the vaginal introitus that is not seen with labial fusion. The extent of fusion is variable among patients. A small opening is seen here right below the clitoris. (**B**) Same patient following manual lysis (with anesthesia) of the fusion showing normal female genitalia. Patients can be also treated with Premarin cream. (Photo contributor: Mark Horowitz, MD.)

Clinical Summary

Bartholin glands are situated in the vulva, in the posterior aspect of the vaginal vault, and secrete mucus to lubricate the vagina and vulva. Obstruction of the ducts may lead to a Bartholin gland cyst or abscess that can present in adolescent females. A Bartholin gland cyst is a fluid collection within the gland secondary to an obstruction of the Bartholin duct. It is generally asymptomatic. Cysts can become infected and become Bartholin gland abscesses. Symptoms of a Bartholin gland abscess include unilateral vulvar swelling accompanied by severe pain in the area. Fever may be present as well. Physical examination reveals unilateral swelling in the posterior aspect of the vaginal vault, at approximately the 4 o'clock or 8 o'clock positions, with swelling protruding outward.

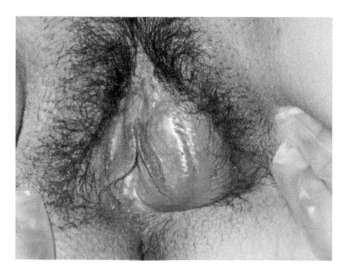

FIGURE 10.45 ■ Bartholin Gland Abscess. This patient presented with a tender area of swelling that was medial to the left labia majora. Incision and drainage of Bartholin gland abscess may require marsupialization to prevent recurrence. (Photo contributor: Janet Semple-Hess, MD.)

The differential diagnosis includes Bartholin gland cyst, other abscesses or cysts in the area, hematoma, FB, hematometrocolpos, condyloma, folliculitis, lipoma, and other soft tissue tumors. Bartholin gland cysts will present as swelling in the same location but should be painless.

Emergency Department Treatment and Disposition

Diagnosis is clinical, and further testing is generally not necessary. Culture of the abscess contents is optional but may help identify the causative organism of infection. Unlike other abscesses, simple incision and drainage frequently leads to recurrence. Definitive treatment of a Bartholin gland abscess involves incising, draining, and placing a Word catheter in the abscess, or incising and draining the abscess and surgically creating a marsupial pouch. Marsupialization generally requires that the procedure be done in the operating room. Follow-up with a gynecologist or a pediatric surgeon is also indicated.

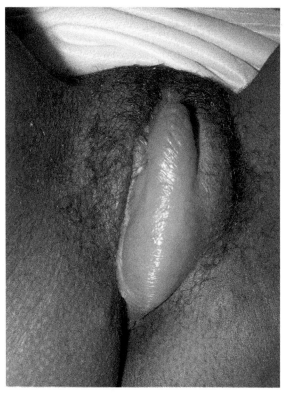

FIGURE 10.44 ■ Bartholin Gland Abscess; Gonococcal Infection. Dysuria and difficulty sitting and walking were the complaints of this sexually active adolescent female. An extremely tender, fluctuant mass with surrounding edema and erythema of the labia majora was seen secondary to Bartholin gland abscess requiring incision and drainage. The culture grew *N gonorrhoeae*. Bartholin's glands are located bilaterally at the posterior introitus and drain through ducts that empty into the vestibule at approximately the 4 o'clock and 8 o'clock positions. These glands are normally pea sized and are neither palpable nor visible unless infected or inflamed. (Photo contributor: Binita R. Shah, MD.)

Pearls

1. Do not perform routine incision and drainage of Bartholin gland abscesses alone. Definitive treatment involves incision and drainage, followed by placing a Word catheter or marsupializing the abscess.

2. Additional diagnostic testing is not necessary.

Clinical Summary

Paraphimosis refers to when the penile foreskin is retracted behind the coronal sulcus and cannot be returned to its normal position. This creates a tourniquet effect on the distal penis and the glans, leading to venous congestion and reduced blood flow. As edema of the distal structures increases, it becomes increasingly difficult to replace the foreskin to the normal position. Patients present with severe pain and swelling of the glans penis. They may have difficulty voiding and urinary retention secondary to urethral obstruction due to edema. If untreated, paraphimosis may lead to local necrosis.

Emergency Department Treatment and Disposition

Diagnosis is made visually; however, it is essential to take a careful history to verify that the patient is uncircumcised, as severe balanoposthitis in the circumcised male or a hair tourniquet may appear similarly. Provide adequate analgesia with topical lidocaine jelly, oral or parenteral anesthesia, or dorsal penile nerve block. Promptly reduce the paraphimosis by first decreasing the edema with constant manual pressure and cold compresses for several minutes, then rolling the foreskin back over the glans with concurrent inward pressure on the glans. If this is not successful, consider puncturing the foreskin with

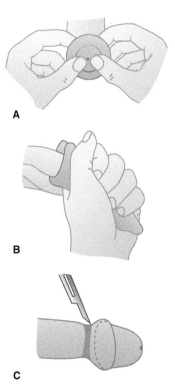

FIGURE 10.47 ■ Acute Paraphimosis. (**A**) Manual reduction. The thumbs are placed on the distal glans penis with the fingers behind the phimotic ring. The thumbs push inward on the penis while the fingers pull the phimotic ring distally over the glans. (**B**) Squeezing with swab. Edematous part of the glans is held in the fist of one hand and squeezed firmly. A gauze swab or warm towelette will help to achieve a firm grip. Continuous pressure is exerted until the edema passes under the constricting collar to the shaft of the penis. The foreskin can then usually be pulled over the glans. (**C**) Dorsal slit incision (if manual reduction methods fails) should be made in the constricting collar of skin proximal to the glans under local or light general anesthesia. The incision allows the foreskin to be advanced and reduces the swelling. Follow-up circumcision should be performed. (Redrawn and modified from Murtagh J. *Murtagh's Practice Tips.* 7th ed. McGraw-Hill Education; New York, NY, 2017.)

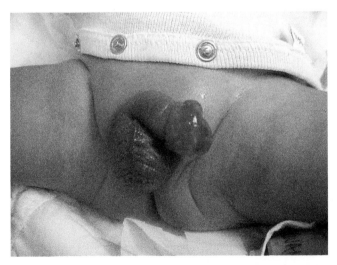

FIGURE 10.46 ■ Paraphimosis. Edema and swelling of foreskin retracted behind glans penis is seen in a 12-month-old uncircumcised male infant presenting to ED with inconsolable crying. (Photo contributor: Mark Silverberg, MD.)

either a 23- or 25-gauge needle (multiple punctures may be required) and manually expressing the fluid before rolling the foreskin back into place. Further measures include dorsal slit of the foreskin or emergency circumcision, which should be performed by urology or surgery. After reduction, instruct the caregiver and/or patient not to retract the foreskin for several days and to follow up with urology or surgery for consideration of circumcision.

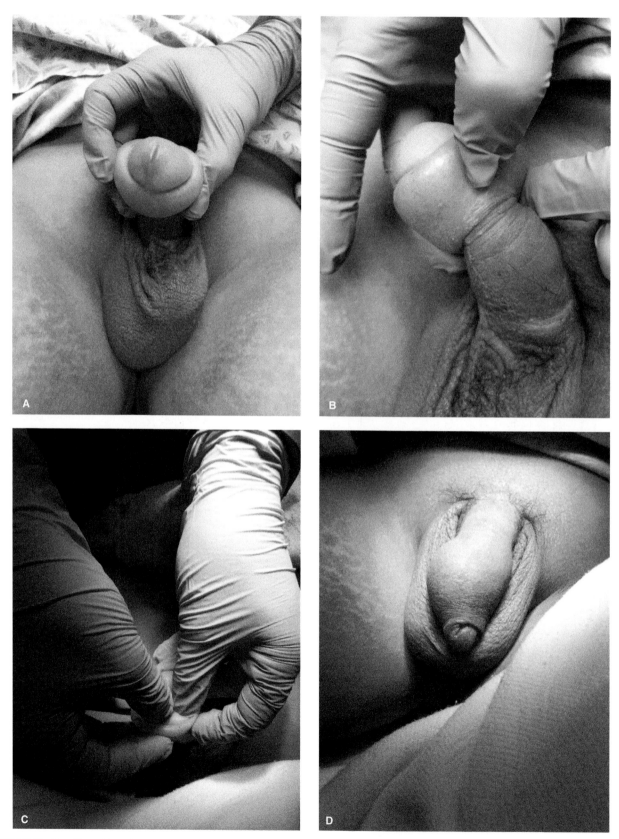

FIGURE 10.48 ■ Paraphimosis and Manual Reduction. Patient with paraphimosis (**A, B**). Images demonstrate the reduction of a paraphimosis, which requires compression of the foreskin and glans of the penis followed by reduction of the foreskin over the glans (**C**), restoring the penis and foreskin to their normal appearance (**D**). (Photo contributor: Deborah R. Liu, MD.)

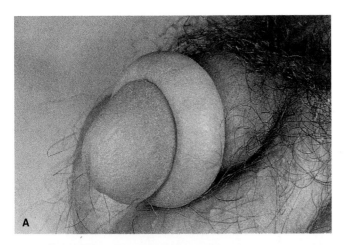

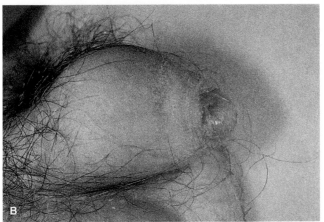

FIGURE 10.49 ■ Paraphimosis. (**A**) An adolescent patient with autism presented with paraphimosis of 3 days in duration. A manual reduction of paraphimosis was performed. (**B**) Postreduction residual penile edema may take hours to days to fully resolve. (Photo contributor: Binita R. Shah, MD.)

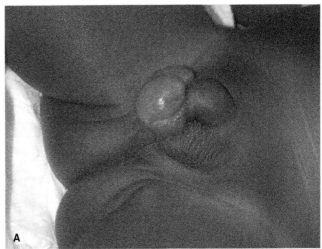

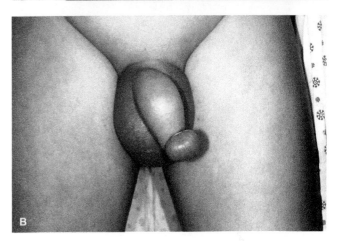

FIGURE 10.50 ■ Paraphimosis-Like Presentations. (**A**) The hair-tourniquet syndrome. This is an emergency similar to paraphimosis. Penile constriction may result in swelling and ischemic injury distal to the constrictive process. Careful examination is required to identify the tourniquet (eg, hair), which is mobilized gently, divided, and removed (see also Figure 2.40). (**B**) Penile edema due to nephrotic syndrome. Severe edema of the glans penis and shaft is seen in a child presenting with anasarca from nephrotic syndrome (see also Figure 16.11). (Photo contributors: Michael Stracher, MD [A], and Binita R. Shah, MD [B].)

Pearls

1. Infants with paraphimosis may present with inconsolable crying (because of pain).
2. Advise families to avoid aggressive retraction of the foreskin with cleaning, as this may lead to paraphimosis.
3. Paraphimosis may be iatrogenic because of retraction of the foreskin for catheterization or medical examination. Always remember to return the foreskin to the proper position after manipulation.

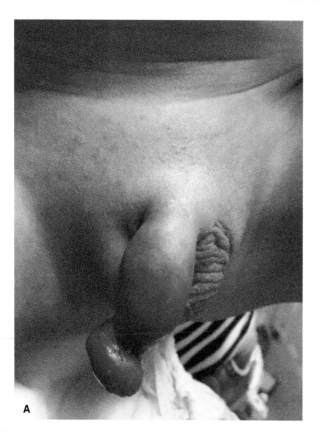
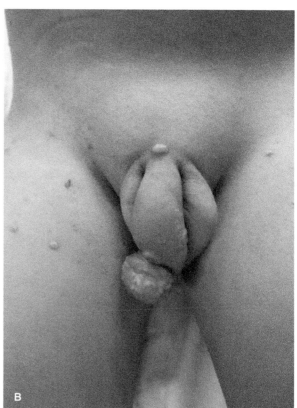

FIGURE 10.51 ■ Balanoposthitis. (**A**) A 23-month-old, febrile, uncircumcised male child presented to the ED with a 1-day history of swelling and redness of the penis. (**B**) Balanoposthitis secondary to infection from chickenpox in a 7-year-old boy with steroid-resistant nephrotic syndrome receiving tacrolimus therapy. (Photo contributors: Maria Chitty Lopez, MD [A], and Abhijeet Saha, MD [B].)

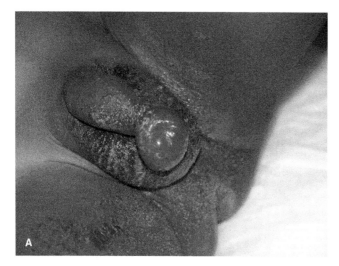
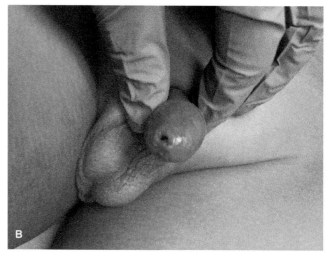

FIGURE 10.52 ■ Balanoposthitis with Phimosis. (**A**) Balanoposthitis in an uncircumcised toddler showing erythema; severe edema and constricted preputial orifice are also shown. Balanoposthitis may look very similar to paraphimosis. (**B**) Recurrent inflammation to the foreskin of the penis can lead to pathologic phimosis. (Photo contributors: Binita R. Shah, MD [A], and Deborah R. Liu, MD [B].)

Clinical Summary

Ovarian torsion occurs most often in late childhood and early adolescence in pediatric patients. A large ovarian cyst or mass of at least 5 cm in diameter is most often the precipitating factor for torsion; however, torsion does occur in normal ovaries, especially before adolescence. Patients present with acute-onset pelvic pain, generally one sided, which may be accompanied by nausea and vomiting. A tender mass may be palpable. Patients may have a prior history of intermittent pain during previous episodes of ovarian torsion and detorsion. Similar to the testes, the viability of the ovary is dependent on the duration of compromised blood supply. Although the likelihood of ovarian nonviability increases with time, viability may be preserved even after 24 hours of symptoms.

Emergency Department Treatment and Disposition

Provide adequate pain management and fluid resuscitation. Order color Doppler sonography. Signs of ovarian torsion on US can include ovarian enlargement, heterogenous ovarian appearance, diminished/absent blood flow on color Doppler, multiple small peripheral follicles (secondary to edema), abnormal ovarian location, or the presence of a "whirlpool sign" (twisting of the vascular pedicle). If there is high clinical suspicion and/or radiographic findings consistent with torsion, consult gynecology and/or pediatric surgery for exploratory laparotomy.

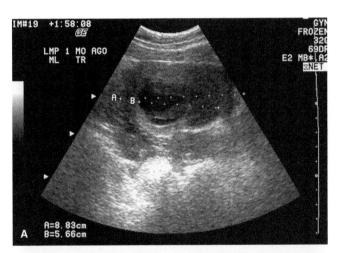
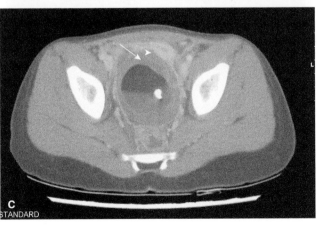
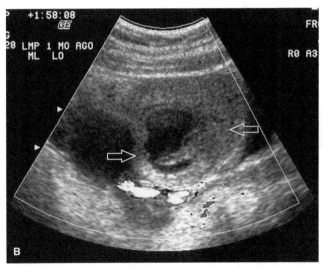

FIGURE 10.53 ■ Ovarian Torsion. (**A**) Longitudinal scan of left ovary shows enlargement of the ovary containing a complex cyst. (**B**) Color Doppler image shows absent color flow within the ovarian tissue (arrows) compatible with torsion. (**C**) CT scan shows a mass with calcification, fluid, and fat within the left ovary compatible with a dermoid (white arrow). There is marked thickening of the ovarian wall (arrowhead) suggestive of torsion of the ovary. (Photo contributor: John Amodio, MD.)

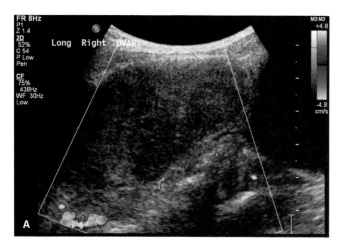
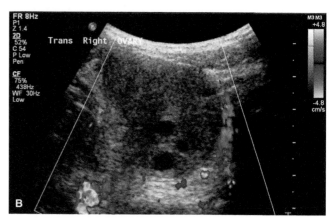

FIGURE 10.54 ▪ Ovarian Torsion. (**A, B**) Sagittal and transverse color Doppler sonograms of the right ovary demonstrate ovarian enlargement and absent flow, compatible with torsion in a 7-year-old girl who presented with a 5-day history of right lower quadrant abdominal pain. The ovary was detorsed in the operating room but appeared to be necrotic on follow-up imaging. (Photo contributor: Neil G. Uspal, MD.)

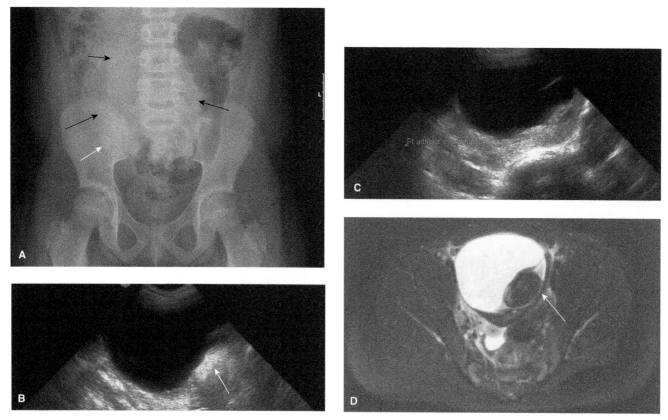

FIGURE 10.55 ▪ Ovarian Teratoma Presenting with Torsion. (**A**) Plain film of abdomen in an 8-year-old girl with abdominal pain shows large midabdominal mass (black arrows) containing a calcification (white arrow). (**B, C**) A cystic mass arising from the right ovary on sonography. Notice fat plug (white arrow). (**D**) MRI showing cystic mass above uterus with a fat plug (white arrow). The ovary was noted to be torsed at surgery. (Photo contributor: John Amodio, MD.)

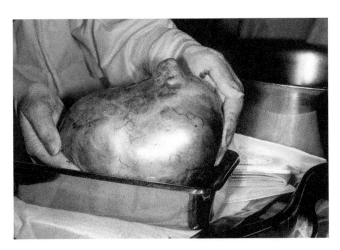

FIGURE 10.56 ■ Ovarian Teratoma Presenting with Torsion. Cystic ovarian teratoma was removed from an adolescent patient presenting with severe abdominal pain from the ovarian torsion. (Photo contributor: Binita R. Shah, MD.)

Pearls

1. Ovarian torsion must be treated as an emergent condition, equal to testicular torsion.
2. The difficulty of diagnosis often delays surgical intervention. A high degree of suspicion is imperative.
3. The presence of blood flow to the ovary on Doppler US does not rule out the presence of ovarian torsion.

Clinical Summary

Intestinal malrotation occurs during fetal development when the intestine does not fully rotate and thus does not allow attachment of the cecum to the right lower quadrant. The cecum instead ends up in the mid-upper abdomen fixed to the abdominal wall by Ladd bands of peritoneum, which override and can obstruct the duodenum. The narrowed mesenteric base of the intestine allows for twisting of the duodenum on the cecum, leading to volvulus. Most patients present in the first year, and many in the first month of life, typically with bilious emesis and signs of intestinal obstruction. Stools may demonstrate occult or frank blood. Patients may present in septic or hypovolemic shock. The younger the infant, the more likely obstruction will be severe with necrosis.

Emergency Department Treatment and Disposition

Stabilize the patient as needed including aggressive resuscitation in cases of shock. Consult surgery emergently. Place a nasogastric tube for gastric decompression. Obtain CBC, electrolytes and glucose, lactate, and type and cross for evaluation and management of shock and preparation for surgery. Give broad-spectrum antibiotics for possible bowel necrosis

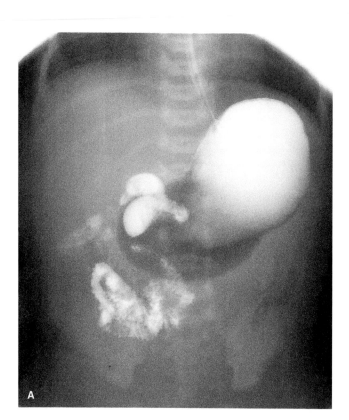
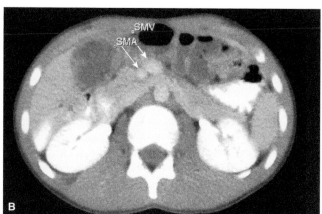
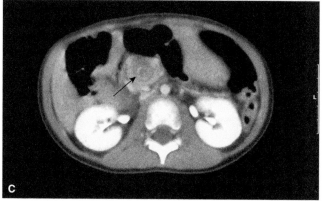

FIGURE 10.57 ■ Malrotation and Volvulus. (**A**) Supine image from upper GI study demonstrates small bowel loops to the right of the left pedicles of the spine, compatible with malrotation. In addition, the upper small bowel loops have a "twisted" configuration suggestive of volvulus. (**B**) CT image of a child with malrotation demonstrating reversal of the normal relationship of the superior mesenteric artery (SMA) and superior mesenteric vein (SMV). Normally, the SMV is to the right of the SMA. (**C**) CT image of a child with volvulus of the duodenum. Note the "swirl" appearance (arrow) of the mesentery and vessels. This 2-year-old child presented with a history of intermittent abdominal pain associated with bilious vomiting. Patient had 1 prior admission at 3 months of age for inconsolable crying with vomiting and bloody stool that resolved spontaneously. (Photo contributor: John Amodio, MD.)

and perforation. If patients are hemodynamically unstable and have symptoms consistent with volvulus, they should be taken to the operating room for emergent exploratory laparotomy without further imaging in the ED. For patients who are hemodynamically stable, order an upper GI series. With malrotation, the upper GI series will show abnormal positioning of the duodenojejunal flexure (ligament of Treitz). With volvulus, upper GI will show a corkscrew sign (spiraled appearance of the duodenum and jejunum).

Pearls

1. Infants with bilious vomiting must be presumed to have malrotation or volvulus until proven otherwise.
2. Infants may present with septic shock.
3. Older children may present with a history of multiple episodes of intermittent emesis and abdominal pain.
4. Patients found to have a malrotation of any type, even without current signs of obstruction, must be evaluated by surgery to prevent future volvulus.

Clinical Summary

Umbilical granulomas consist of granulation tissue persisting at the base of the umbilicus after cord separation. Granulomas are 3 to 10 mm, typically pedunculated, moist, and mucosal in appearance, and may be friable. No purulent discharge or redness of the skin is seen around the umbilicus, which are signs of omphalitis. The differential diagnosis includes umbilical polyps and other remnants of the urachus or omphalomesenteric duct. Umbilical polyps are firm masses of intestinal epithelium or uroepithelium, usually red, and generally larger than an umbilical granuloma, but otherwise similar in appearance. Polyps are distinguished from granulomas in that they do not respond to silver nitrate cauterization and require surgical excision. Rarely, a complete connection remains between the umbilicus and bladder or intestine secondary to failure of the urachus or omphalomesenteric duct to close. This is identified clinically by a patent fistula in the umbilical mass draining urine or stool. The diagnosis is supported by US. With any of these anomalies, further evaluation for associated GI or genitourinary anomalies is recommended.

Emergency Department Treatment and Disposition

Treat umbilical granulomas with application of topical silver nitrate. Blot the area dry, and then roll the silver nitrate

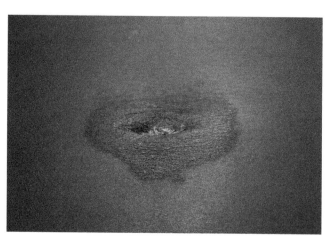

FIGURE 10.59 ■ Silver Nitrate Burn. Burn is seen in this 1-month-old infant 1 day after the application of topical silver nitrate application for umbilical granuloma. This complication can be avoided with a topical application of bland emollient (eg, petrolatum) on the skin around the umbilicus. Such application acts as a physical barrier and prevents burns that occur after accidental touching of the skin during silver nitrate application. (Photo contributor: Ameer Hassoun, MD.)

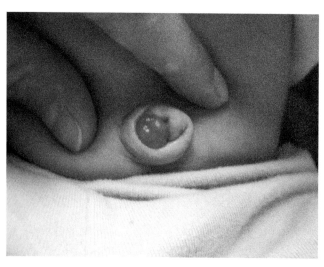

FIGURE 10.58 ■ Umbilical Granuloma. A 6-week-old infant, otherwise well, with a growing, moist mass in his belly button is shown. This granuloma was noted about 1 to 2 weeks after cord separation and regressed promptly after cauterization. (Photo contributor: Andrea Marmor, MD.)

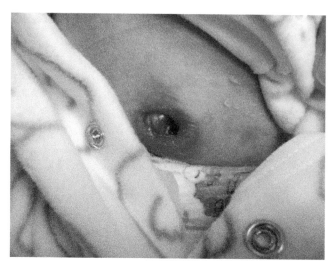

FIGURE 10.60 ■ Omphalitis; Differential Diagnosis of Umbilical Granuloma. Although exudate and odor from the umbilical stump or cord remnant are common benign findings, erythema or induration *around* the umbilical stump or cord remnant may herald a severe, life-threatening infection. Omphalitis, usually a polymicrobial bacterial infection of the umbilical stump, occurs in neonates who may appear well or systemically ill. Hospitalization and treatment with systemic broad-spectrum antibiotics are required. Risk factors for omphalitis include preterm delivery, maternal infection, and umbilical catheterization. (Photo contributor: Andrea Marmor, MD.)

stick tip over the moist, pink tissue, leaving a grayish residue. Repeat treatments may be needed 1 to 2 times per week for several weeks, until the granuloma epithelializes.

Pearls

1. Moist, pedunculated umbilical masses can be safely cauterized using silver nitrate in the ED.

2. An umbilical mass with a draining fistula requires further evaluation with US and referral to a pediatric surgeon.

3. Use care in applying silver nitrate to umbilical granulomas, because silver nitrate can cause chemical burns and skin staining when it comes in contact with skin.

Clinical Summary

Fascial openings through the umbilical area allow passage of umbilical vessels from mother to fetus antenatally. The umbilical ring usually closes spontaneously after birth, but in some children, the opening persists and is apparent clinically as an umbilical hernia. An umbilical hernia presents at birth or shortly after as a protruding umbilicus. The mass is typically noted by parents to appear or enlarge when the infant is crying or straining and may be firm during these activities but should be soft and reducible when the infant is calm. Air content in the bowel can be felt in the mass, and the borders of the fascial opening can often be palpated. The vast majority of umbilical hernias decrease in size and eventually close. The best predictor of failure to close is the size of the fascial opening (>1.5 cm).

Emergency Department Management and Disposition

An umbilical hernia that is reducible (when the infant is calm) is a benign condition, and only reassurance is recommended. Although extremely rare, if signs of incarceration are present, surgery should be consulted to prevent progression to strangulation. Recommend surgical referral for hernias that are symptomatic or large (fascial opening >1.5 cm) and that fail to decrease in size after 3 to 5 years of age.

Pearls

1. Umbilical hernias are a very common, usually self-resolving condition, and surgical intervention is rarely needed.
2. Signs of incarceration include a hard, nonreducible mass, with or without persistent vomiting or signs of intestinal obstruction.

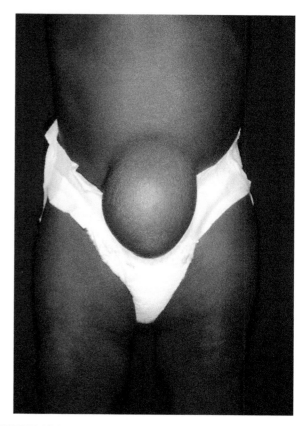

FIGURE 10.61 ■ Umbilical Hernia. Umbilical hernia can be quite impressive as seen in this toddler, and even though incarceration is uncommon, the family needs to be educated regarding symptoms of incarceration. (Photo contributor: Binita R. Shah, MD.)

Chapter 11

HEMATOLOGY AND ONCOLOGY

Scott T. Miller
Kusum Viswanathan

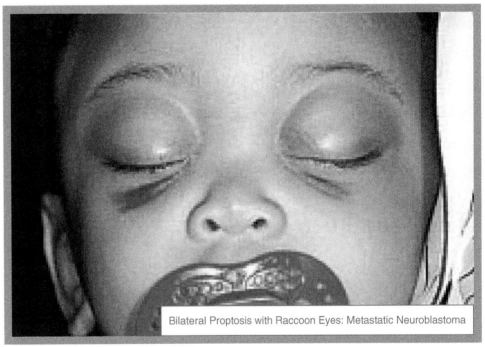

Bilateral Proptosis with Raccoon Eyes: Metastatic Neuroblastoma

(Photo contributor: Binita R. Shah, MD)

The authors acknowledge the special contributions of Sreedhar P. Rao, MD, and Shahina Qureshi, MD, to prior edition.

509

Clinical Summary

Fever in a child with sickle cell disease (SCD) is a medical emergency because of the possibility of overwhelming *Streptococcus pneumoniae* sepsis. By age 1 year, 30% to 50% of infants with homozygous sickle cell anemia (HbSS) have diminished or absent spleen function, with this rate being >90% by age 4 years. The prevalence of splenic dysfunction is likely similar in children with sickle β^0-thalassemia, and although splenic hypofunction occurs less commonly and at a later age in children with hemoglobin SC (HbSC) and sickle β^+-thalassemia, they should also be considered at risk. Although availability of conjugated pneumococcal vaccines (most recently Prevnar 13) has reduced the prevalence of invasive pneumococcal disease, prompt empiric therapy with an appropriate antibiotic remains critically important. To some extent, use of Prevnar 7 resulted in emergence of nonvaccine, penicillin-sensitive serotypes as causes of invasive disease, and children age <5 years should be receiving prophylaxis with penicillin. Patients with pneumococcal bacteremia are often well looking for a period of several hours prior to sudden circulatory collapse and death; the presence of otitis media or other localized infection does not exclude the possibility of bacteremia. Children with high fever (temperature > 40°C) and/or headache may require lumbar puncture. Although children with acute chest syndrome (ACS) may present with obvious respiratory distress, presentation may be subtle, and careful clinical and radiographic assessment is required. Parents are advised to bring febrile children with SCD for evaluation of sepsis because of their increased risk despite the fact that majority of such febrile episodes may not be bacterial in origin.

Emergency Department Treatment and Disposition

Children presenting with fever should be urgently triaged and immediately seen by an ED provider. After brief examination, blood should be obtained for a CBC with a reticulocyte count, blood culture, and any other indicated tests, and if there is no known allergy, a dose of a long-acting cephalosporin (eg, ceftriaxone) should be administered IV. If penicillin resistance is common in the community, and especially if meningitis is present, treatment with vancomycin is recommended. Patients should then be observed carefully as laboratory results are retrieved and any additional evaluation completed.

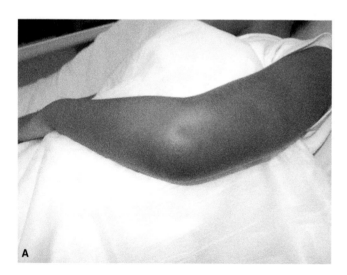

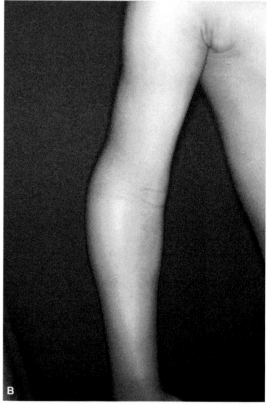

FIGURE 11.1 ■ Sickle Cell Anemia. Fever, pain, and swelling with erythema can be seen in both osteomyelitis and vaso-occlusive crisis (VOC) usually due to bone marrow infarction; clinical differentiation between the 2 may be difficult. (**A**) Osteomyelitis of the humerus with erythema, swelling, and fever were seen in this child with SCD. (**B**) Swelling of the elbow and forearm with pain, fever, and similar signs of inflammation were seen in a different child with VOC. (Photo contributor: Binita R. Shah, MD.)

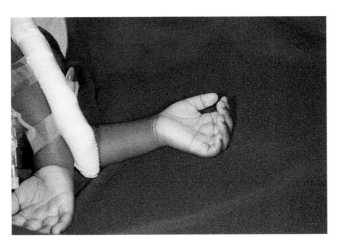

FIGURE 11.2 ■ Sickle Cell Anemia with Transient Aplastic Crisis. Fever and rhinorrhea for 3 days followed by irritability were the presenting complaints of this infant whose Hg value was 3 g/dL with reticulocytopenia. Aplastic crisis is caused by parvovirus B19 infection, and patients may present with weakness, listlessness, dizziness, and extreme pallor. (Photo contributor: Binita R. Shah, MD.)

All patients should have a CXR as part of their assessment. Even immunized children taking penicillin should be managed urgently and receive empiric therapy. Children with high fever, pain, and/or ACS should be admitted to the hospital. However, the majority of children with fever can be managed on an ambulatory basis; clinical criteria published in 1993 were highly effective in identifying a higher risk group of children best hospitalized and should still be used by ED physicians for appropriate disposition of febrile children. Children with any of the following characteristics should be hospitalized to continue antibiotics pending culture results:

1. Toxic appearance
2. Temperature ≥40°C
3. Infiltrate on CXR, abnormal oxygen saturation, tachypnea in excess of that attributable to fever, or clinical signs of consolidation (see ACS; Figure 11.5)

4. WBC count >30,000/mm^3 or <5000/mm^3
5. Platelet count <100,000/mm^3
6. Hemoglobin <5 g/dL or >2 g/dL below baseline
7. History of sepsis due to *S pneumoniae*
8. Poor oral intake or signs of dehydration
9. Concurrent pain episode

Others who require admission include any child without a reliable caretaker, source of primary care, and/or hematology follow-up; children with no telephone or poor access to the hospital; and unimmunized, noncompliant children. Others generally can be sent home. A hematologist should be called to ensure adequate follow-up and to obtain any further critical information that may be available. If discharged, the child must be reevaluated in the ED or at the hematology clinic 24 hours after administration of parental antibiotics. Depending on culture results and other factors, a second dose of cephalosporin, an oral course of antibiotics, or discontinuation of antibiotic therapy might be recommended. This decision should be made in conjunction with the hematologist.

Pearls

1. Fever in a child with SCD is a medical emergency that needs prompt evaluation and empiric antibiotic therapy to prevent death/morbidity from pneumococcal sepsis.
2. Prompt empiric therapy is required even if the child has been immunized, is taking prophylactic penicillin, and/or has a "source" for the fever.
3. Criteria are available that permit most children to be discharged and managed on an ambulatory basis.

SICKLE CELL ANEMIA WITH ACUTE PAIN

Clinical Summary

Pain is one of the most common manifestations of sickle cell anemia and can occur in any part of the body. It is often associated with bone marrow infarction and may be accompanied by prominent inflammatory changes (warmth, tenderness, and erythema) over the painful area, or there may be minimal or no physical findings. Pain may be due to "sludging" of sickle cells in the capillary bed with vascular obstruction and tissue ischemia or infarction; sickle cell vasculopathy and inflammatory mediators may contribute to tissue injury. However, the subjective complaint of pain is often unaccompanied by objective physical findings, and the patient must be relied upon to assess analgesic response. There are no clinical, radiographic, or laboratory parameters proven to confirm or refute pain. Radiographs are generally not useful in assessment of acute pain; even with acute infarction, bone films will be normal for 7 to 10 days after onset. Nuclear medicine scans (gallium, indium, and bone or bone marrow) have been used to attempt to differentiate acute bone infarction from osteomyelitis but are also often not definitive and should not be ordered in the ED. Other potential causes of pain should be assessed. Patients with chest pain should be examined carefully for rib tenderness and/or clinical findings of consolidation. If hospitalized, they also must be continuously monitored for splinting/hypoventilation as a potential precipitant of ACS. Careful performance of the physical examination with auscultation for rales or diminished breath sounds is critical; clinical findings often precede radiographic findings. Tachypnea may be subtle, with shallow but rapid respiratory rate. Sickle cell patients with concurrent asthma may be at increased risk for ACS. Abdominal pain and/or distension may be a presenting symptom of ACS or sometimes a complication. Any patient with abdominal pain requires careful monitoring of pulmonary status and oxygen saturation. Other potential causes of abdominal pain need to be considered, both sickle cell related (ie, cholecystitis, gallstone pancreatitis) and those occurring in the general pediatric population. If appendicitis is suspected, hematology consultation must be obtained before surgery. Although acute infarction of cranial bones can occur, severe or persistent headache should prompt a careful neurologic assessment for meningitis or acute cerebral hemorrhage; cerebral infarction is not usually associated with pain. Low-grade (or sometimes high) fever can complicate pain episodes, especially in patients with local inflammatory findings. A workup for possible infection should be

done, and empiric antibiotic therapy may be required. Prior to antibiotic administration, it may be appropriate to consult orthopedics regarding aspiration of an inflamed bone or joint to attempt to obtain material for culture.

Emergency Department Treatment and Disposition

The patient's assessment is the only tool available for adequate pain management, and they should be asked to quantitate their pain using an assessment scale (eg, a numerical pain intensity scale [visual analog scale] or the Wong-Baker FACES scale for younger children). A numerical goal should be agreed upon, and patients should be reassessed and retreated at intervals until adequate control is achieved. Patients receiving opioid analgesia should also be assessed with a sedation scale and have the dosage modified as required. Patients should be monitored, most commonly with a pulse oximeter. Patients will often suggest what medications and dosages have provided relief on previous episodes; this information should be used in designing a treatment regimen. IV fluids are often administered at a maintenance rate. Although most children with pain are somewhat dehydrated, aggressive hydration may risk pulmonary edema and ACS; patients with concurrent ACS generally should receive only maintenance fluids or less. If the patient is drinking liquids, decrease the IV fluid accordingly. Most patients receive IV ketorolac (see below) and generally require a "rescue" dose of IV morphine sulfate. A patient should be reassessed in 30 minutes, and if pain is poorly relieved and sedation acceptable, additional morphine should be given. Once relief is achieved, morphine should be given at 2- to 3-hour intervals to maintain adequate analgesia. An alternative to morphine is hydromorphone, which has a slightly longer duration of action and is given every 3 to 4 hours. There is also some experience with nalbuphine, an agonist/antagonist agent that may be less of a respiratory depressant and perhaps less associated with development of nosocomial ACS. Both morphine and hydromorphone may be used via patient-controlled analgesia (PCA), allowing the patient to titrate medication to achieve pain control. The optimal dosing for PCA (generally a continuous infusion supplemented by demand doses by the patient) has not been established for children with SCD, and use should be restricted to physicians or pain teams with experience. Ketorolac, a nonopioid NSAID that is not a respiratory depressant,

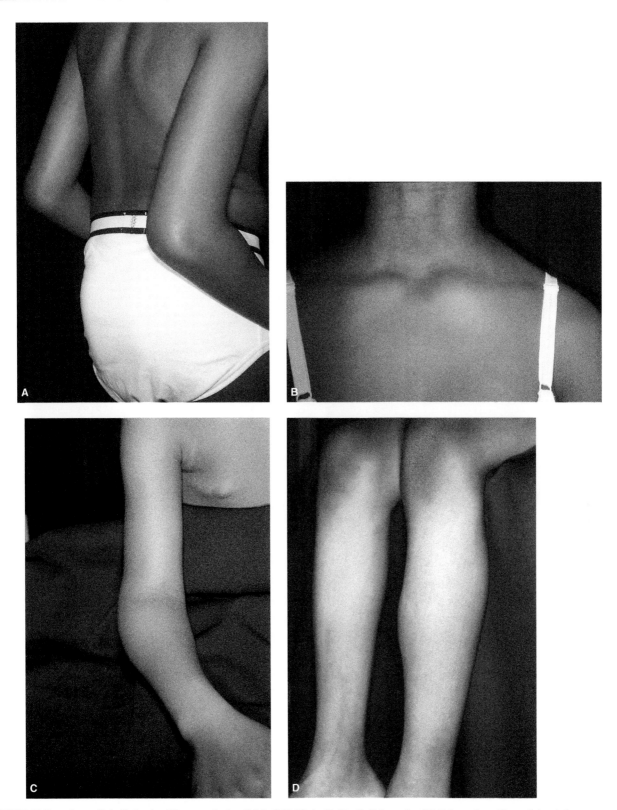

FIGURE 11.3 ▪ Acute Pain Episodes (Vaso-occlusive Crisis [VOC]) in Sickle Cell Anemia. (**A**) Pain and swelling of the right upper arm as a manifestation of VOC. (**B**) Pain and swelling over the left medial clavicle as a manifestation of VOC. (**C**) Pain and swelling around elbow as a manifestation of VOC. (Photo contributor: Binita R. Shah, MD [A–C].) (**D**) Pain and swelling of lower extremity as a manifestation of VOC. (Reproduced with permission from Shah BR, Laude TL. *Atlas of Pediatric Clinical Diagnosis*. WB Saunders; Philadelphia, PA, 2000.)

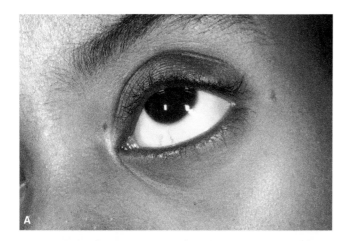

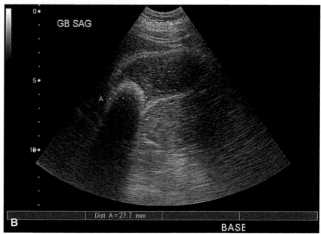

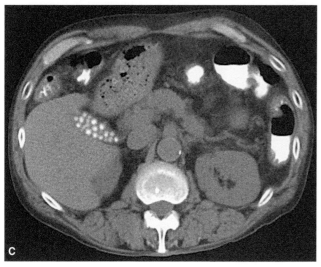

FIGURE 11.4 ■ Right Upper Quadrant (RUQ) Syndrome in Sickle Cell Anemia. (**A**) Worsening jaundice and right-sided abdominal pain were the presenting complaints in this adolescent girl with sickle cell disease. Sickle cell–related causes of RUQ syndrome include cholecystitis, gallstone, pancreatitis, and sickle cell hepatopathy. (**B**) US shows a large stone within the gallbladder with acoustical shadowing. There is also sludge within the gallbladder lumen. (**C**) CT scan shows multiple calcified calculi within the gallbladder in a different patient presenting with right-sided pain. (Photo contributors: Binita R. Shah, MD [A], and Mark Silverberg, MD [B, C].)

may thus be especially useful in patients with chest or back pain. However, it is not approved by the US Food and Drug Administration for repetitive dosing in children and may be associated with nephrotoxicity. It should not be used with ibuprofen or by patients with impaired renal function. If pain is poorly controlled on usual doses of opioids and/or the need for parenteral analgesia continues, the patient should be hospitalized. If pain is, in the assessment of the patient, under control, it may be appropriate to substitute an oral analgesic prior to discharge to ensure continued adequacy of analgesia on discharge. The dose of morphine when changed from parenteral to oral administration needs to be increased 3-fold and hydromorphone 4-fold to achieve comparable analgesia. Oxycodone is an alternative. Use of codeine in children under 12 years of age has recently been discouraged due to variability in metabolism; a substantial minority of patients may not metabolically activate codeine, and it may be ineffective.

Codeine and oxycodone are often dispensed in combination with acetaminophen; if combinations are prescribed (we generally discourage), parents should be reminded not to supplement with additional acetaminophen. Ibuprofen and/or acetaminophen should generally be continued with the oral opioid preparation. Patients should be provided with sufficient analgesia to last up to 5 days and be encouraged to follow up with the hematologist or primary care physician, who will determine whether additional duration of opioid treatment may be required. Fortunately, chronic pain is unusual in children with SCD; the unusual child who requires chronic pain treatment clearly needs careful and ongoing physician follow-up. Those who use the ED primarily and do not show evidence of an ongoing relationship with a health care provider should be referred for psychosocial assessment. Nonpharmacologic interventions should be encouraged, including psychosocial strategies (distraction or psychotherapy), behavioral strategies (deep breathing, relaxation, self-hypnosis), and physical strategies (heat, massage). Regular (10 puffs every 2 hours while awake) use of incentive spirometry is proven to reduce the incidence of nosocomial ACS and, especially if a prolonged stay in the ED is anticipated, should be prescribed. Patients with recurrent episodes of pain and/or ACS are candidates for hydroxyurea therapy (preferably after consultation with a hematologist). Hydroxyurea is safe and effective in reducing the frequency of pain and ACS in children as young as age 9 months and convincingly improves life expectancy in adults.

Pearls

1. The patient is the only person who can assess his or her pain and may have a useful opinion as to the most effective analgesic regimen. Listen to the patient!

2. *Do not administer placebo*; response to placebo does not prove that the patient is not in pain.

3. Meperidine is a less effective pain reliever and has a higher potential for toxicity (neurotoxic); its use is discouraged except perhaps in patients who are truly allergic to morphine (and thus hydromorphone and codeine as well).

4. Patients who received opioids for pain relief in the recent past or for more than a few days may develop pharmacologic tolerance to the drug and require higher doses for pain relief. Rapid cessation of opioid therapy after several days of treatment may result in withdrawal symptoms, sometimes manifested as recurrent pain. Opioid dosage should be tapered over several days in such cases.

5. Use of NSAIDs offers the advantage of lack of respiratory depression and habituation, and NSAIDs are frequently used as initial and supplemental therapy but are potentially nephrotoxic.

6. Causes of pain other than those attributable to acute vaso-occlusion must be excluded.

Clinical Summary

ACS is defined as acute pulmonary findings and a new infiltrate on chest radiograph in a child with SCD. These findings may include tachypnea, which is sometimes subtle; retractions; diminished (often asymmetrical) breath sounds; and rales, vesicular sounds, or other signs of consolidation. Hypoxemia is often present, and new pulmonary findings may be seen on CXR. However, many patients present with clinical findings of ACS that precede abnormal radiographic findings by 24 to 48 hours. Because of multiple and sometimes overlapping etiologies, all children with ACS should be treated for both infectious and sickle cell–related etiologies. The most common identifiable infectious pathogens are atypical bacteria (*Mycoplasma pneumoniae* and *Chlamydia pneumoniae*); bacterial infection (including *S pneumoniae*) may occur in approximately 5% of cases. The most common identifiable noninfectious cause of ACS is pulmonary fat embolization from infarcted bone marrow; marrow infarction is a frequent cause of an acute pain episode. Transfusion therapy may be important in preventing multiorgan failure and death

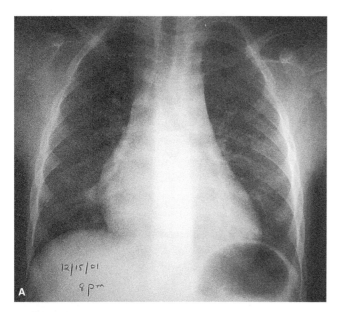

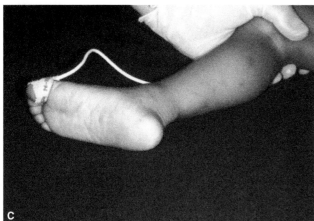

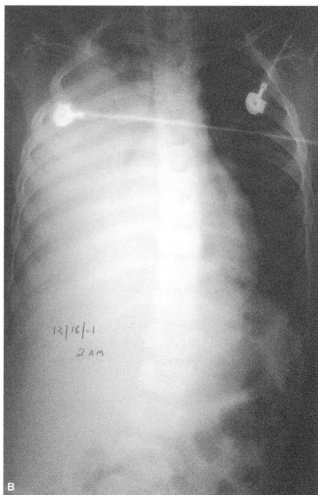

FIGURE 11.5 ■ Acute Chest Syndrome (ACS). (**A**) Frontal radiograph showing cardiomegaly with a minimal ill-defined parenchymal infiltrate in the right lower lobe in a patient presenting with chest pain, cough, and fever. (**B**) A repeat radiograph taken 6 hours later shows near complete opacification of the right hemithorax, with a mediastinal shift to the contralateral side resulting in severe respiratory distress and hypoxemia. These findings may represent a large consolidation with or without pleural effusion. There is also levoscoliosis most likely secondary to splinting from the right-sided process. (**C**) Pallor. A significant drop in hemoglobin value from baseline often occurs during ACS. (Photo contributor: Binita R. Shah, MD.)

due to severe fat embolization syndrome (approximately 70% of children are ultimately transfused during a course of ACS). Abdominal pain and/or distension may be a presenting symptom of ACS or sometimes a complication. Any patient with abdominal pain requires careful monitoring of pulmonary status and oxygen saturation. Neurologic problems may occur because of embolization of bone marrow fat from the lungs to the brain or ischemia/infarction due to systemic hypoxemia and underlying cerebrovascular disease. There is a temporal association of ACS with stroke.

Emergency Department Treatment and Disposition

Examine patients carefully, especially those with fever, chest or back pain, and abdominal pain or distension; an accurate respiratory rate is simple and critical. A CBC with reticulocyte count is required. It often shows a significant drop in hemoglobin (Hb) value from baseline, a decrease in platelet count, and an elevated number of nucleated RBCs. Chest radiograph may initially be normal or involve 1 or several lobes and rapidly progress to "white-out" of 1 or both lungs. Pleural effusions may be present. Because radiologic findings may lag behind clinical findings, treatment should precede confirmatory radiograph in children with symptoms and signs of ACS. A specimen for type and screening should be sent to the blood bank with the alert that the patient has SCD. Many blood banks will have a complete RBC phenotype on file to extend the compatibility profile; at a minimum, patients who require transfusion should receive RBCs compatible with types C, E, and Kell (historically the most antigenic in sickle cell populations). Because most Rh (D)–negative Caucasian donors are C and E negative as well, if the need for blood is urgent, Rh- and Kell-negative units can generally be released promptly and safely. Hydration should be cautious (maintenance fluids or less) with close monitoring of intake and output to avoid pulmonary edema–induced worsening of ACS. Careful choice and dosing of analgesic therapy is needed to prevent hypoventilation secondary to splinting and/or sedation/respiratory depression (hypoventilation may lead to atelectasis and hypoxemia); ketorolac use may be desirable

in older patients. Incentive spirometry, as prescribed for pain, should be offered, especially if a prolonged stay in the ED is anticipated. All patients with ACS should receive macrolide therapy to cover possible atypical bacteria. Although bacteria, including *S pneumoniae*, are uncommon pathogens, younger patients (especially nonimmunized) with high fever, high WBC count, or a toxic appearance may also be given antipneumococcal therapy pending culture results. Simple transfusion with packed RBCs is often given for a moderate to severe episode, especially when associated with a drop in Hb concentration. Unless a prolonged stay in the ED is required and a patient is clinically distressed, transfusion is best administered in the inpatient area. Simple transfusion rather than exchange should be the front-line therapy unless a patient is less anemic than average (ie, Hb >9 g/dL) and thus cannot safely be given a simple transfusion because of viscosity concerns (posttransfusion Hb should never exceed 11 g/dL in an acutely ill, urgently transfused patient). Activation of various cytokines and upregulation of adhesion molecules are manifestations of an often robust and sometimes deleterious inflammatory response. Use of dexamethasone (given every 12 hours for 4 doses) attenuates the course of ACS but appears to be associated with a high readmission rate for pain shortly after recovery from ACS. An "asthma regimen" of prednisone for 5 to 7 days may be less associated with readmission and perhaps efficacious in reducing the need for transfusion; however, this regimen has not been assessed prospectively and should *not* be initiated in the ED. Children with a concurrent diagnosis of asthma may be at increased risk for ACS and increased severity; while bronchodilator therapy is not uniformly given to treat ACS, in those with wheezing and/or a history of asthma, administration of bronchodilator treatment is appropriate. Because of its variable and often severe clinical course, all patients with ACS should be hospitalized, preferably in an ICU or well-observed bed with oxygen therapy and continuous cardiac and pulse oximetry monitoring. A pediatric hematologist should be consulted for management of a patient with ACS and in decisions about antibiotic coverage, transfusion, and steroid therapy. All patients who experience even a single episode of ACS should be made aware of the role of hydroxyurea therapy in potentially reducing the risk of recurrent ACS and other sickle cell complications.

Pearls

1. A careful physical examination, with particular attention to respiratory rate and effort, is critical in diagnosis of ACS.

2. Fever may be the only early manifestation of ACS; all febrile sickle cell patients should have a chest radiograph as part of their evaluation, even if respiratory signs and symptoms are not identified.

3. Clinical or radiologic diagnosis of ACS mandates hospitalization. Radiographic findings may lag and need not be present to make a clinical diagnosis of ACS.

4. All patients with ACS and hypoxia and/or tachypnea should receive supplemental oxygen.

5. The blood bank should always be aware of a sickle cell diagnosis, so extended antigen matching, at least to include C, E, and Kell antigens, is done.

6. Children with wheezing and/or a history of asthma may benefit from bronchodilator therapy.

Clinical Features

Stroke affects 5% to 10% of children with SCD. The majority of ischemic strokes are due to watershed infarcts resulting from sickle cell vasculopathy of major cerebral vessels.

It is speculated that abnormal adherence of sickled RBCs and WBCs to the vascular endothelium and perhaps nitric oxide depletion result in vessel injury and intimal hyperplasia. Hyperplasia leads to gradual stenosis and ultimately occlusion of the large- and middle-caliber cerebral arteries,

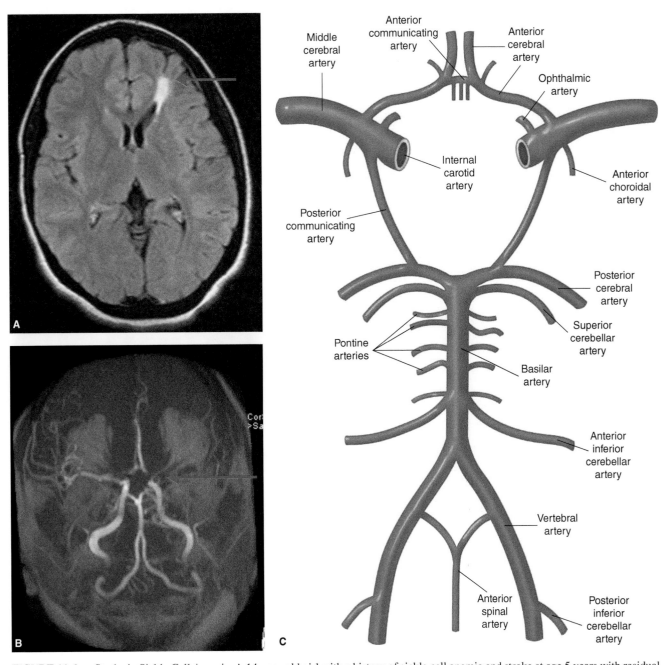

FIGURE 11.6 ■ Stroke in Sickle Cell Anemia. A 14-year-old girl with a history of sickle cell anemia and stroke at age 5 years with residual right lower limb weakness presented to the ED with history of headaches. (**A**) Axial FLAIR MRI shows an old ischemic lesion in the left frontal region (arrow). (**B**) MRA of the circle of Willis shows lack of flow in the left middle cerebral artery (arrow). (**C**) Circle of Willis. Two internal carotid arteries and 2 vertebral arteries come together at the base of the skull to form the circle of Willis. (Photo contributor: Geetha Chari, MD [A, B], and [C] reproduced with permission from Samady H, Fearon WF, Yeung AC, et al. *Interventional Cardiology*. 2nd ed. McGraw-Hill Education; New York, NY, 2017.)

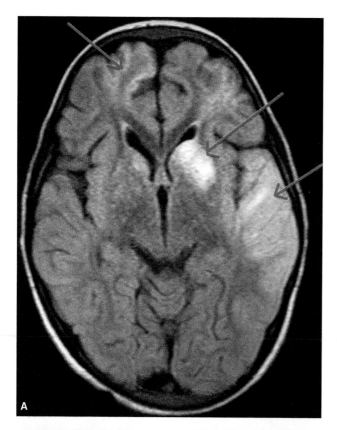

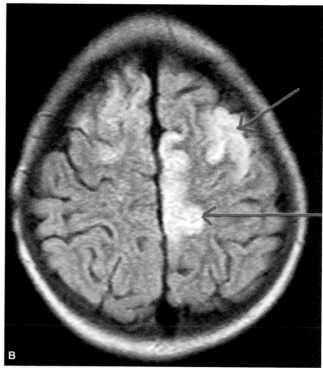

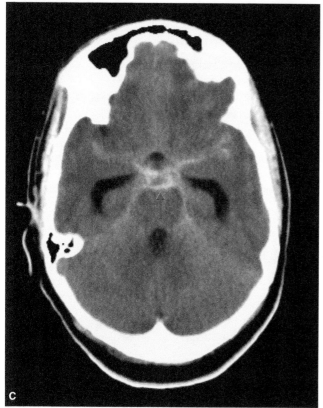

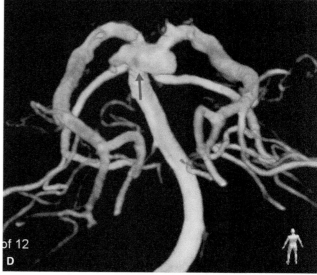

FIGURE 11.7 ■ Stroke in Sickle Cell Anemia. (**A, B**) A 6-year-old girl presented to the ED with history of sudden onset of right hemiplegia. MRI FLAIR axial images reveal new ischemic stroke (red arrows) with high signal in the left caudate nucleus and frontal/parietal white matter, involving both middle and anterior cerebral artery distribution. Evidence of old stroke (blue arrow) can be seen in the right frontal region (hyperintense signal following the gyri). (**C, D**) A 17-year-old girl presented with syncope and headache. CT scan of head (**C**) reveals subarachnoid hemorrhage (hyperdensity in the basal cisterns, arrow), with enlargement of the temporal horns of the lateral ventricles. Angiogram (with 3-dimensional reconstruction; **D**) revealed a large aneurysm at the top of the basilar artery (arrow). (Photo contributor: Geetha Chari, MD.)

particularly the middle cerebral artery; often multiple vessels are involved. Approximately 70% to 90% of children with SCD who have strokes due to infarction have cerebrovascular disease of major vessels. An additional 10% to 30% may have microvascular disease; typically, these lesions are in deep periventricular white matter. Hemorrhagic stroke (subarachnoid and/or intracerebral hemorrhage) occurs less commonly during childhood but becomes progressively more common with increasing age. A sudden onset of hemiparesis is the most common presentation in children. Weakness or numbness of an extremity or a painless limp may be patient or parent complaints. Cranial neuropathies are sometimes seen, but infarction in the brainstem and areas fed by the posterior circulation (cerebellum) are uncommon. Patients may have bilateral findings at the time of initial diagnosis because of previously unrecognized infarcts. Intracranial hemorrhage can present with headache, although headache is not often seen in infarctive strokes. Patients with transient ischemic attacks (TIAs) may have similar symptoms that resolve spontaneously within 24 hours of onset. TIAs are associated with an increased risk of subsequent stroke, and patients with TIA should be investigated carefully for underlying cerebrovascular disease. Transcranial Doppler (TCD) ultrasonography is a screening method to identify children at increased risk for stroke, who, once identified, can receive preventive chronic transfusion therapy. Screening appears to substantially reduce stroke incidence and is recommended at least annually for all children with HbSS or sickle β^0-thalassemia from age 2 through 16 years. Prompt TCD screening may be useful in an individual patient with TIA or equivocal neurologic findings to establish stroke risk but must be performed by an examiner familiar with the screening protocol and interpretation required for children with SCD.

Emergency Department Treatment and Disposition

A pediatric hematologist and a pediatric neurologist should be consulted emergently regarding a patient with suspected stroke to confirm the neurologic findings and initiate therapy. Patients should be given oxygen, and specimens should be sent for CBC, coagulation screen, and alloantibody screening. A specimen should also be sent for complete RBC phenotyping to facilitate extended antigen matching of blood and ultimately chronic transfusion therapy. A CT scan of the brain is generally done urgently to rule out intracranial hemorrhage. CT scans are relatively insensitive for infarction,

although sensitivity improves after 3 to 4 days. Patients who are found to have intracranial bleeding on CT scan should have urgent neurosurgical consultation. If conventional angiography is needed, it is best done after exchange transfusion (see below) and using low ionic strength contrast medium. A diffusion-weighted MRI scan should be done to confirm cerebral ischemia or infarction, with magnetic resonance angiography (MRA) done concurrently to establish the extent of cerebrovascular disease. It is convention that patients with newly diagnosed stroke be treated with exchange transfusion; recovery is often substantial after the procedure. Although no prospective trials have compared exchange transfusion to simple transfusion repeated at weekly intervals to achieve the traditional goal of <30% HbS, a retrospective review suggested that patients exchanged promptly had a lower risk of stroke recurrence. A simple transfusion may be given to patients with Hb <9 g/dL while preparing for exchange. An exchange transfusion requires admission to the hospital, most appropriately to an ICU, and can be done manually or by erythrocytapheresis. TIA patients should be transfused while awaiting complete evaluation for cerebrovascular disease and the decision as to whether to continue a chronic transfusion program. Most patients who are found to have a new acute cerebral infarction, or TIA with significant vascular disease, are placed on a chronic transfusion program for at least several years. Although anticoagulation and thrombolytic therapy are increasingly used in adults with acute stroke, appropriate use of these therapies has not been established in patients with SCD; standard therapy is exchange transfusion.

Pearls

1. The most common cause of stroke in children with SCD is cerebral infarction due to vasculopathy of the major cerebral vessels.
2. A painless limp or weakness (hemiparesis) is the most common presentation of stroke. In younger children, a limp or unwillingness to walk may occasionally be mistakenly diagnosed as a pain episode. A lack of complaint of pain, local tenderness, or inflammatory findings in the extremities should prompt neurologic assessment.
3. All patients with SCD presenting with a seizure or neurologic symptoms and signs must be assessed for possible stroke.
4. Stroke in patients with SCD usually develops as an isolated event; however, it may occur during other types of crisis (eg, aplastic crisis, ACS, or splenic sequestration).

Clinical Summary

Priapism is defined as an unwanted painful penile erection. Clinically, it can be a single prolonged (24 hours to several days) episode or shorter, often recurrent, "stuttering" episodes. Prolonged episodes are generally low flow and ischemic, presumably because of sludging and stasis of blood in the cavernosal spaces. Ischemia and infarction will injure cavernosal smooth muscle and ultimately result in fibrosis and impotence. The pathophysiology of high-flow priapism is not clear. It may be related to vascular disease and autonomic dysfunction and/or nitric oxide depletion with derangement of normal regulatory pathways. Stuttering episodes are more commonly seen in prepubertal males, and the prognosis is probably better than in older patients with low-flow episodes; however, in a large series from Jamaica, all patients with stuttering ultimately did have a prolonged episode lasting longer than 24 hours. Noninvasive methods used to assess penile perfusion include radionuclide penile scan and Doppler ultrasonography. The glans and corpus spongiosum are generally spared in sickle cell–related priapism, providing a rationale for surgical shunting. Tricorporal priapism is associated with a more prolonged, difficult course and more severe systemic disease.

Emergency Department Treatment and Disposition

Emergent consultation with urology and pediatric hematology is needed for patients who have a priapism episode lasting >2 hours; many of these episodes will extend to 24 hours and beyond without intervention. Episodes lasting >48 hours are associated with a high incidence of subsequent impotence; intervention should begin as early as possible after a patient appears in the ED. Patients should be treated with fluids at 1.5 times maintenance and given adequate analgesia (ie, morphine sulfate). Aspiration of the corpora cavernosum and irrigation with approximately 10 mL of a 1:1,000,000 dilution of epinephrine should be performed by an experienced urologist within a few hours of presentation as it nearly always achieves at least temporary detumescence. Depending on the patient, it is performed with local or regional anesthesia and/or moderate sedation; younger children may require admission to the hospital for deep sedation or general anesthesia. The first blood aspirated may be sent for analysis of pH, Pco_2, and Po_2 to establish cavernosal flow status. If aspiration fails or priapism recurs after brief detumescence, the patient should be hospitalized. Although there is no proven benefit from blood

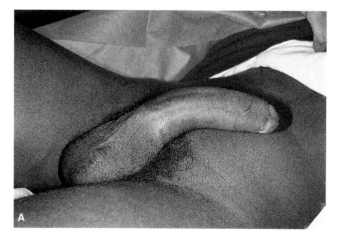 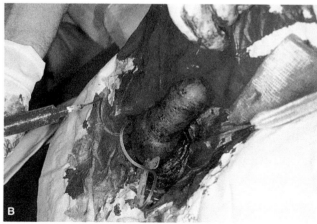

FIGURE 11.8 ■ Priapism in Sickle Cell Anemia. (**A**) An adolescent patient presented with a swollen, edematous, and very tender penile erection of 5 hours in duration. The diagnosis of priapism is usually made by clinical examination. Both corporal bodies are turgid and tender, whereas the glans penis and spongiosum are usually spared. (**B**) A 21-gauge butterfly needle was placed in the corpora cavernosum after lidocaine injection; aspiration and irrigation with saline and phenylephrine were performed, with subsequent resolution of the priapism. (Photo contributor: Binita R. Shah, MD.)

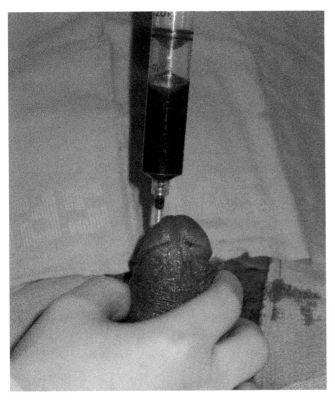

FIGURE 11.9 ■ Priapism in Sickle Cell Anemia. When medical therapy fails, priapism becomes a surgical emergency. Notice how dark the blood is when drained from this patient's corpora due to stasis. (Photo contributor: Mark Silverberg, MD.)

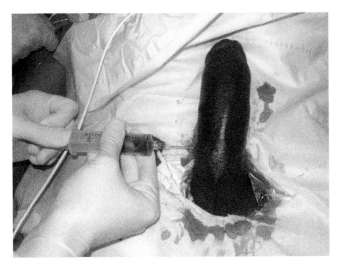

FIGURE 11.10 ■ Priapism in Sickle Cell Anemia. Intracorporeal irrigation with phenylephrine was carried out to reduce the priapism in this patient using the lateral approach. (Photo contributor: Mark Silverberg, MD.)

transfusion in the acute management of priapism, it may be useful to transfuse (simple transfusion in most cases) after an unsuccessful aspiration and prior to a repeat; subsequent aspiration will then allow "normal" transfused blood to enter the cavernosal spaces. Blood transfused to a patient during a low-flow episode will not enter the cavernosae and is unlikely to be effective. If detumescence occurs after initial aspiration, the patient may be discharged from the ED. Pseudoephedrine 30 to 60 mg each night may reduce risk of recurrent stuttering episodes, and a dose at onset of an episode may also be helpful. Recurrent priapism episodes that resolve spontaneously or with aspiration should be referred to a hematologist and/or urologist familiar with the disorder. Additional preventive treatment for recurrent priapism may include chronic transfusion therapy to maintain HbS <30% for 6 to 12 months, hydroxyurea therapy, stilbestrol therapy (unacceptable side effects), injections of leuprolide (suppresses production of testosterone), or oral finasteride. Ketoconazole will lower testosterone levels and may reduce stuttering, but requires corticosteroid replacement dosing. Paradoxically, sildenafil, a cyclic guanosine monophosphate–specific phosphodiesterase type 5 inhibitor commonly prescribed for erectile dysfunction, has been shown to be beneficial in some sickle cell patients with recurrent priapism, presumably by restoring nitric oxide homeostasis disrupted by hemolysis-related nitric oxide depletion.

Pearls

1. Priapism is a persistent, painful erection associated or unassociated with sexual stimulation.
2. Penile aspiration/irrigation with epinephrine should be done within a few hours of presentation and is usually effective in achieving detumescence.
3. A common complication of priapism is impotence. The risk of impotence increases with the number of recurrent episodes and increased duration of episodes. Patients who have persistent priapism for >48 hours prior to intervention often are left impotent.
4. Males with recurrent episodes should be referred for consideration of chronic preventive therapy.

Clinical Features

The combination of jaundice and right upper quadrant pain, tenderness, and sometimes hepatic enlargement is termed *right upper quadrant syndrome* (RUQ syndrome). Although children with SCD have normal susceptibility to viral or immune hepatitis, generally the differential diagnosis of concern in children presenting with RUQ syndrome is obstructive choledocholithiasis versus sickle cell hepatopathy. Gallstones are extremely common in children with SCD, with estimates that 30% of children age 2 to 10, 50% of adolescents, and 80% of adults with SCD likely have gallstones. These are often bilirubinate stones and not calcified; 90% are not radiopaque. Although stones are most commonly asymptomatic, stones will occasionally occlude the common bile duct and cause obstructive jaundice; pancreatitis can sometimes accompany common bile duct obstruction. Despite this risk, most do not recommend routine cholecystectomy for asymptomatic stones. Sickle cell hepatopathy is due to intrahepatic sickling and cholestasis. In children, this most often is an extreme benign hyperbilirubinemia; children generally look fairly well, with or without liver enlargement or tenderness, despite sometimes markedly elevated levels of total and direct bilirubin and mild elevation of hepatic transaminases. Symptoms generally resolve in a few days, although jaundice may persist for weeks. Adults and (usually) older children may be at risk for a more dangerous form of hepatopathy in which hyperbilirubinemia is accompanied by signs of hepatic dysfunction (coagulation abnormalities, hyperammonemia, CNS changes). Children who have hepatic dysfunction at presentation may have a severe or life-threatening course and require transfusion (perhaps exchange transfusion) to avoid a mortal outcome. Of note, children with the more fulminant direct hyperbilirubinemia often have serum bilirubin levels of 30 to 80 mg/dL, whereas those with the more benign hyperbilirubinemia generally have levels from 10 to 30 mg/dL. It is important to note that children with sickle cell anemia frequently have mild unconjugated hyperbilirubinemia due to hemolysis. In addition, a significant subgroup of children have a total serum bilirubin level >4 mg/dL, which cannot be attributed to hemolysis alone. Nearly all such children have Gilbert syndrome and are homozygous for mutations in the glucuronosyl transferase gene (*UGT1A*). The incidence of

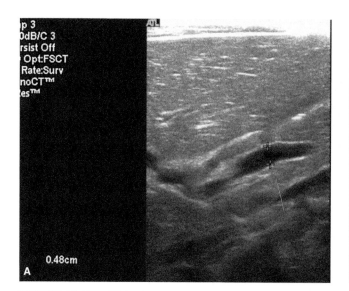
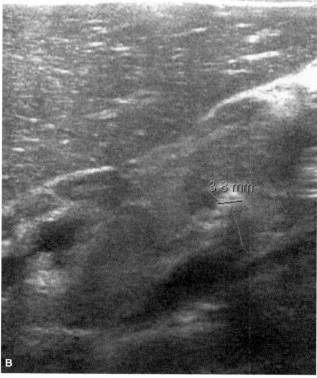

FIGURE 11.11 ■ Right Upper Quadrant Syndrome; Acute Cholecystitis. (**A**) Longitudinal image of a dilated common duct, measuring 0.48 cm in anteroposterior diameter (arrow). (**B**) Transverse image at level of the head of the pancreas demonstrating calculi impacted in the distal common duct (arrow).

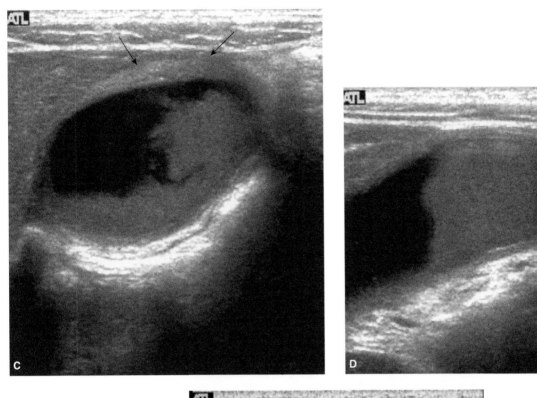

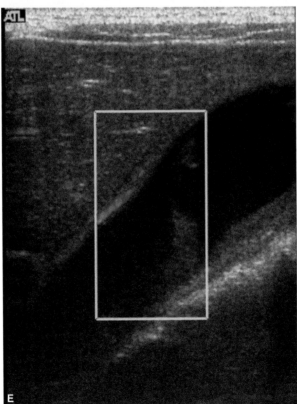

FIGURE 11.11 ▪ (*Continued*) (**C, D**) Longitudinal images of the gallbladder, which appears distended with sludge and stones. Notice the thickened gallbladder wall (arrows). (**E**) Longitudinal color Doppler image of the gallbladder showing hyperemia of the wall. (Photo contributor: John Amodio, MD.)

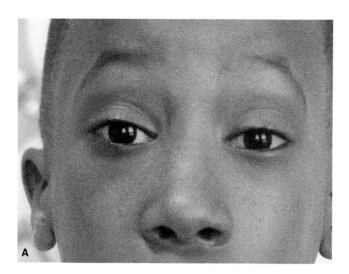
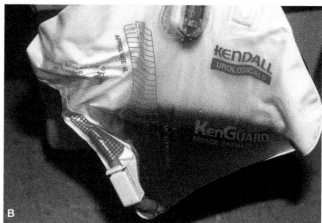

FIGURE 11.12 ■ Right Upper Quadrant Syndrome; Sickle Cell Hepatopathy. (**A**) Right upper quadrant pain associated with progressive worsening of scleral icterus was the presenting complaint of this 10-year-old child with SCD. He had mild elevations of liver enzymes with a total bilirubin of 56 mg/dL and direct bilirubin of 18 mg/dL. (**B**) It is useful to examine the urine. Conjugated bilirubin is water soluble and may result in tea-colored urine; bilirubinuria implies an elevated serum level of conjugated bilirubin. Urinary urobilinogen is increased in hemolysis and is colorless, although oxidation of urobilinogen may produce urobilins, which are yellow-brown in color. The presence of bilirubinuria without urobilinogen suggests biliary obstruction. (Photo contributors: Haamid Chamdawala, MD [A], and Binita R. Shah, MD [B].)

Gilbert syndrome in sickle cell populations is 12% to 25%; an additional 50% may be heterozygous with somewhat higher bilirubin levels than individuals with the normal genotype. Higher indirect bilirubin levels are associated with increased risk for gallstones.

Emergency Department Treatment and Disposition

Patients should be examined with attention to hepatic enlargement and/or tenderness, mental status, and presence or absence of asterixis. Blood work should include CBC and reticulocyte count, coagulation profile, liver enzymes with total and direct bilirubin, and serum amylase, lipase, and ammonia. Patients found to have only indirect hyperbilirubinemia, even with levels >4 mg/dL, require no further evaluation and can be informed they likely have inherited Gilbert syndrome, which contributes to their jaundice. All patients with direct hyperbilirubinemia should be hospitalized for diagnostic imaging and IV hydration. Abdominal US is generally the initial imaging but can miss common bile duct stones (up to 30%). Sensitivity is improved by magnetic resonance cholangiopancreatography or endoscopic ultrasonography. Children found

to have obstructive choledocholithiasis (dilated common bile duct or hepatic ducts) may spontaneously pass obstructing stones but are candidates for endoscopic retrograde cholangiopancreatography (ERCP) for confirmation of the diagnosis and therapeutic commissurotomy. Elective laparoscopic cholecystectomy is usually done 4 to 6 weeks after the acute episode (timing is somewhat dependent on the institution). Patients found to have no evidence of obstruction on imaging and who do not have hepatitis have sickle cell hepatopathy and can generally be managed conservatively. However, those with hepatic dysfunction should be transfused promptly, perhaps with exchange transfusion to lower the HbS to <30% of the total.

Pearls

1. All children with direct hyperbilirubinemia should be hospitalized for evaluation and at least conservative management.

2. For patients with common bile duct obstruction, ERCP should be offered if available for relief of obstruction to be followed by elective laparoscopic cholecystectomy.

Clinical Summary

There are 3 causes of acute exacerbations of anemia in children with SCD: acute splenic sequestration (see page 529), transient aplastic crisis (TAC), and hyperhemolysis. Hyperhemolysis is relatively unusual and is often seen in association with viral illness. It may be due to activation of the reticuloendothelial macrophage system by an infectious agent, with enhanced removal of sickle cells and generally appropriate response by the bone marrow. It is not apparently related to concurrent glucose-6-phosphate dehydrogenase deficiency (as previously thought). In 70% to 100% of cases, TAC is due to infection by parvovirus B19. This virus is the cause of erythema infectiosum (fifth disease) in the general population. Infection results in transient, profound inhibition of erythropoiesis because of viral incorporation into RBC precursors after entry via the P blood antigen receptor (also known as globoside). In individuals with normal Hb, this results in reticulocytopenia for 7 to 10 days but no clinically significant drop in Hb concentration due to normal RBC survival of 120 days. Patients with SCD may a have much shorter RBC life span and thus become profoundly anemic and reticulocytopenic (reticulocyte count <1% and often <0.1%). Children receiving hydroxyurea therapy may become less anemic and less frequently require transfusion than those who are not treated; hydroxyurea does not appear to impede the immune response to parvovirus B19 infection. Usually patients with

TAC compensate well because of the gradual progression of anemia and often complain of nonspecific symptoms of tiredness, headache, or malaise at presentation. The prodromal symptoms and rash associated with parvovirus infection in the general population are often not observed in children with SCD. Leukoerythroblastosis, sometimes extreme, is often seen during the recovery phase of TAC; such patients are sometimes misdiagnosed as having hyperhemolysis and generally will not require transfusion (or even hospitalization).

Emergency Department Treatment and Disposition

Infants and children presenting with pallor and/or tachycardia should be seen immediately by a physician with assessment for cardiovascular compromise. Blood should be drawn for CBC, reticulocyte count, and type and screen. Patients who have severe anemia and profound reticulocytopenia due to clinically suspected parvovirus P19 infection should be provided oxygen and hospitalized for cautious transfusion to achieve near-baseline Hb levels (7–9 g/dL) and to relieve symptoms. These patients often show minimal cardiovascular compromise but are at risk for high-output congestive heart failure if transfused too rapidly. Transfusions should ideally be phenotype compatible for at least C, E, and Kell antigens. Hematology consultation would assist

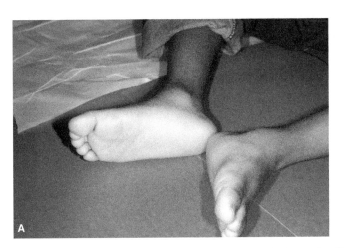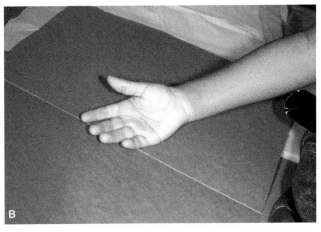

FIGURE 11.13 ■ Transient Aplastic Crisis in Sickle Cell Anemia. (**A, B**) Pallor and tiredness were the presenting complaint of this child whose Hb was 4.0 g/dL and reticulocyte count was 2%. Parvovirus B19 IgM serology was positive. Even the modest reticulocytosis with the presence of B19 IgM suggest early recovery. (Photo contributor: Binita R. Shah, MD.)

in such decisions. During hospitalization, patients should be isolated from other sickle cell children, immunocompromised patients (may acquire chronic parvoviremia), and pregnant women (increased fetal loss, hydrops fetalis) until reticulocytes recover, indicating resolution of parvoviremia and infectivity. Diagnosis can be confirmed by detection of parvovirus DNA during the reticulocytopenic phase or by detection of anti-B19 IgM with recovery. Families should be advised to bring siblings with SCD to be checked for reticulocytopenia.

Pearls

1. Infants and children with acute splenic sequestration crisis are generally hypovolemic and require fluid resuscitation and urgent, rapid transfusion, whereas those with TAC are generally well compensated and require very cautious transfusion therapy.

2. Diagnosis of aplastic crisis with B19 infection can be confirmed by B19 IgM serology *only* after reticulocyte production has resumed. Diagnosis during the aplastic episode requires detection of viral DNA.

Clinical Summary

Acute splenic sequestration crisis (ASSC) is a life-threatening complication seen most commonly in infants with SCD under age 4 years. It can occur in any of the common genotypes, but in older children, it becomes more common in those with HbSC, sickle β-thalassemia, or HbSS with α-thalassemia. In many patients today, SCD is diagnosed by newborn screening programs, allowing early instruction of parents in splenic palpation; studies have shown that this intervention increases the frequency of diagnosis of ASSC but reduces mortality. ED personnel must be aware that parents often become proficient at splenic palpation and should take their observation seriously. Patients who present with severe ASSC often have massive splenomegaly, tachycardia, and hypovolemia; Hb levels below baseline; reticulocytosis; and often thrombocytopenia. Subacute presentations with mild to moderate exacerbation of anemia and newly discovered splenomegaly also occur. The differential diagnosis of acute exacerbations of anemia in children with SCD includes ASSC, TAC (see page 527), and hyperhemolysis.

Emergency Department Treatment and Disposition

Infants and children who present with pallor, tachycardia, or parental complaint of splenic enlargement should be seen immediately by a physician with assessment for cardiovascular compromise and splenic enlargement. Blood should be

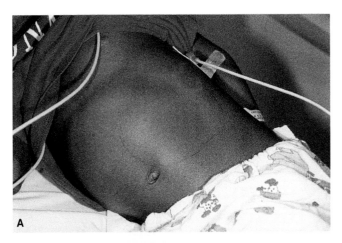

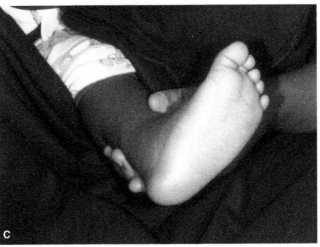

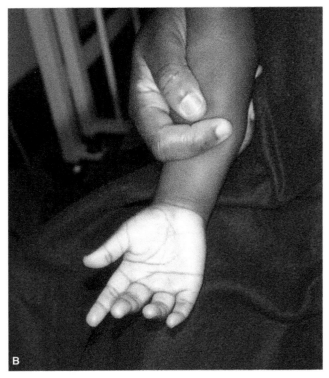

FIGURE 11.14 ■ Acute Splenic Sequestration. (**A**) Abdominal fullness with massive splenomegaly were seen in this child who presented with lethargy, weakness, extreme pallor, and tachycardia. (**B, C**) Severe pallor. Sudden, rapid enlargement of the spleen due to acute trapping of the blood occurs in acute sequestration crisis resulting in a fall in Hb level (despite a persistently elevated reticulocyte count). (Photo contributor: Binita R. Shah, MD.)

drawn for CBC, reticulocyte count, and type and screen. After stabilization of vital signs, often requiring fluid resuscitation, and provision of oxygen therapy, patients should be hospitalized to the pediatric ICU or to a monitored bed. These patients usually need urgent transfusion to achieve approximate baseline Hb levels. Patients should not be overtransfused, because cells trapped in the spleen surprisingly often recirculate after transfusion and the Hb level may increase to levels above that predicted based on volume transfused. Transfusions should ideally be phenotype compatible for at least C, E, and Kell antigens. A hematology consultation would assist in such decisions. Patients presenting with subacute presentations may also require hospitalization for careful monitoring of splenic size, vital signs, and Hb for 24 hours. After a first episode of ASSC, parents are reeducated regarding splenic palpation and warned that recurrences are common (50%–90%). After a second episode, splenectomy may be recommended by the hematologist, especially since the risk of pneumococcal sepsis has diminished because of availability of conjugated pneumococcal vaccines; however, postsplenectomy thrombocytosis may exacerbate underlying thrombophilia. Some may recommend splenectomy after a first episode if there are concerns about adequate parental monitoring of spleen size or lack of proximity to a hospital.

Pearls

1. Patients with ASSC may rapidly progress to cardiovascular collapse and death.
2. Infants and children with ASSC are generally hypovolemic and require fluid resuscitation and urgent, rapid transfusion, whereas those with TAC are generally well compensated and require very cautious transfusion therapy.
3. Parents may be quite proficient at splenic palpation. Their complaint of a newly palpable or enlarged spleen should be taken seriously.
4. Children with less common genotypes of SCD (HbSC, sickle thalassemias) may be at risk for ASSC throughout childhood.

Clinical Summary

Newly diagnosed immune thrombocytopenia (ITP) is characterized by sudden onset of skin and/or mucosal bleeding in otherwise healthy children. Bleeding may include petechiae, ecchymosis, oral mucosal bleeding, epistaxis, and hematuria. Menorrhagia may be seen in adolescent females. CNS bleeding is seen in 0.1% to 0.5% of children with ITP. Peak age at presentation is from 2 to 6 years with equal gender prevalence, in contrast to female preponderance in adolescents and adults with ITP. Often, there is history of a viral illness in the weeks prior to onset of the illness. Physical examination is unremarkable except for skin and mucosal bleeding. Lymphadenopathy and hepatosplenomegaly are not seen except when ITP is associated with infectious mononucleosis. The platelet count is generally <20,000/mm³ in nearly 80% of children, although the severity of thrombocytopenia is variable. Blood smear shows some large platelets indicative of increased platelet turnover. Hb level may be low due to bleeding; WBC count and differential are usually normal. Prothrombin time (PT), partial thromboplastin time (PTT), fibrinogen, and fibrin split products, although generally not done, are normal. Antinuclear antibody and tests for HIV infection are done mostly in adolescents or as indicated. Bone marrow aspiration shows normal erythroid and granulocytic series with normal to increased numbers of megakaryocytes. A bone marrow is not needed for diagnosis in most patients, but it is recommended in patients with features that suggest malignancy, such as lymph node enlargement, splenomegaly, joint pains, leukocytosis, and atypical lymphocytes, or if there is neutropenia and anemia and bone marrow failure is suspected. It is also indicated in children who respond poorly to initial therapy.

Newly diagnosed ITP is a clinical diagnosis reached by exclusion of other causes of thrombocytopenia such as leukemia or aplastic anemia. Acute leukemia almost never presents with isolated thrombocytopenia. ITP can be a presenting manifestation of systemic lupus erythematosus, Evans syndrome, or AIDS, particularly in adolescents.

Emergency Department Treatment and Disposition

In the absence of significant mucosal hemorrhages, patients with platelet counts between 20,000/mm³ and 50,000/mm³ can be observed without specific therapy and followed as outpatients with once- or twice-weekly evaluation and blood count. Hospitalization and hematology consultation are recommended for patients with severe mucosal bleeding and platelet count <20,000/mm³. These patients may receive IV immunoglobulin (IVIG), IVIG against D-antigen (anti-D), or glucocorticoid. Advantages of IVIG given at a dose of 1 g/kg/day for 1 to 3 days include rapid onset of action and increase in platelet count in 80% to 90% of recipients. IVIG can be given *without* a bone marrow examination. The administration may not be suitable for ED administration since IV infusion takes 6 to 8 hours. Other treatment options are IV methylprednisolone (30 mg/kg/day up to 1 g for 3–4 days) or oral prednisone (4 mg/kg for 7 days followed by 2 mg/kg

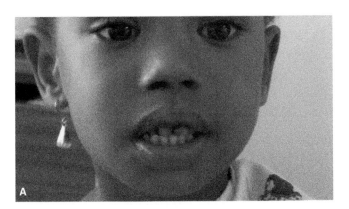
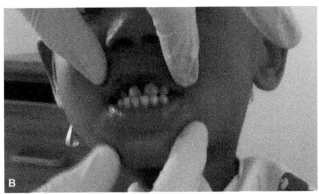

FIGURE 11.15 ■ Newly Diagnosed Immune Thrombocytopenia. (**A, B**) Spontaneous nose and gum bleeding developed in this healthy 3-year-old girl with a preceding history of upper respiratory tract infection. Her CBC was normal except platelet count of 23,000/mm³. After a dose of anti-D immunoglobulin, her platelet count rose to 148,000/mm³. (Photo contributor: Haamid Chamdawala, MD.)

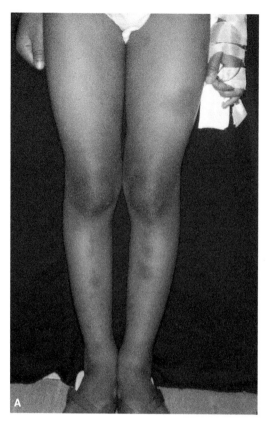
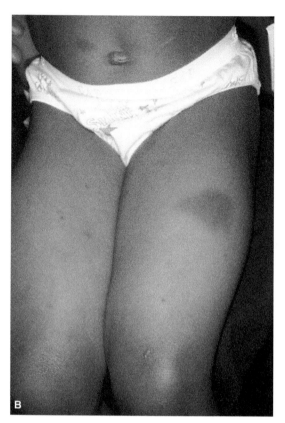

FIGURE 11.16 ■ ■ Newly Diagnosed Immune Thrombocytopenia (ITP). (**A**) Sudden onset of petechiae and ecchymoses over the hands and lower extremities (seen here on shins of tibia and thigh) developed in this otherwise healthy girl. Her WBC count, differential, and Hb values were normal, and platelet count was 15,000/mm³. Purpura is typically asymmetrical in ITP. (**B**) Close-up of ecchymotic lesion on the thigh. (Photo contributor: Binita R. Shah, MD.)

with tapering over next 2 weeks or 4 mg/kg/day for 4 days without tapering). Advantages of prednisone therapy include inexpensive therapy, oral administration, and effectiveness in 75% to 80% of patients. A bone marrow examination is recommended by some pediatric hematologists before starting corticosteroids. Anti-D of Rh blood group system, when given to Rh-positive children with ITP, produces a rapid rise in platelet count. The advantage is that it can be given by IV infusion over 3 minutes at a dose of 75 μg/kg (375 IU/kg) to patients who are Rh positive and have a negative direct antiglobulin test. Patients who are Rh negative cannot receive anti-D. The patient should be observed for 6 to 8 hours after anti-D administration for evidence of intravascular hemolysis. Premedication with prednisone and acetaminophen prior to anti-D is known to result in higher platelet count with fewer side effects. The most common adverse effect is a decrease in Hb concentration by 1 to 2 g/dL. For life-threatening hemorrhages (eg, intracranial bleeding or retroperitoneal bleeding), the patient needs to be hospitalized and managed in an ICU setting. Treatment that may be started in the ED prior to

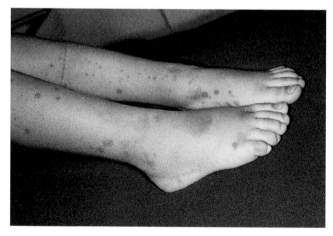

FIGURE 11.17 ■ Henoch-Schönlein Purpura (HSP): Differential Diagnosis of Newly Diagnosed Immune Thrombocytopenia (ITP). Palpable purpuric lesions are symmetrically distributed over the lower extremities in HSP. Angioedema of both feet is also seen in this child. Other systemic involvement, such as of the joints (eg, arthritis), renal system (eg, hematuria), and gastrointestinal system (eg, abdominal pain), and normal or elevated platelet count in HSP help to differentiate HSP from ITP. (Photo contributor: Binita R. Shah, MD.)

admission in such patients includes IV methylprednisolone, initiation of IVIG infusion, and a slow IV push of anti-D (if the patient is D positive). The dosing will be recommended by a hematologist. Platelet transfusions are given every 6 to 8 hours. Although platelet survival following platelet transfusion is poor, it is better when combined with corticosteroids and IVIG or anti-D immunoglobulin.

Pearls

1. Newly diagnosed ITP typically presents with sudden onset of petechiae and ecchymoses in an otherwise healthy child.

2. Newly diagnosed ITP is a diagnosis of exclusion. Bone marrow aspiration is not required for diagnosis if patients are observed without specific therapy or receive IVIG or anti-D therapy.

3. Newly diagnosed ITP is a self-limiting disease (~90% of patients recover by 6 months from the diagnosis).

Clinical Summary

Hemophilia is an X-linked recessive disorder due to deficiency of factor VIII (hemophilia A) or factor IX (hemophilia B). Hemophilia A affects 1 in 5000 to 10,000 males, and hemophilia B affects 1 in 30,000 males. Bleeding manifestations are identical in patients with factor VIII or IX deficiency. Patients with mild (factor level 6%–30%) and moderate hemophilia (factor level 1%–5%) usually bleed after trauma. Those with severe hemophilia (factor level <1%) bleed either spontaneously or after minor injury. Hemarthrosis and bleeding into the muscle are characteristic of bleeding in patients with hemophilia. Other manifestations include oral bleeding, hematuria, gastrointestinal bleeding, or CNS bleeding. One to 2% of patients with hemophilia may experience intracranial bleeding. Only a third of hemophilia patients bleed after circumcision. In most patients, diagnosis is made at birth because of family history; in nearly a third of the patients, hemophilia is due to a new mutation. When the diagnosis of hemophilia is suspected, the following laboratory studies should be done: PT, PTT, and mixing studies when either of these is prolonged to determine if the prolongation is due to deficiency or antibody. Confirmation includes assays for factors VIII, IX, XI and studies to exclude von Willebrand disease (von Willebrand panel that includes von Willebrand factor [VWF] antigen, VWF activity [ristocetin cofactor activity, VWF collagen binding, and factor VIII clotting activity]).

Emergency Department Treatment and Disposition

Urgent hematology consultation is recommended for all children with hemophilia who present with bleeding. Patients presenting with severe or life-threatening bleeding (CNS, gastrointestinal, or airway) need stabilization of vital signs. For patients with hemophilia A, factor VIII 50 units/kg IV (to achieve 100% factor VIII level) is started in the ED followed by 3 to 6 units/kg/h by continuous IV infusion for 24 hours, and the patient is admitted to the ICU for ongoing monitoring and additional therapy. For patients with hemophilia B, 80 to 100 units/kg of factor IX is given IV followed by 20 to 40 units/kg every 12 hours. Additional therapy is continued in the ICU. A history of head injury should be taken seriously. Even in the absence of external bleeding, the patient should be given appropriate clotting factor in a dose of 50 units/kg (factor VIII) or 80 units/kg (factor IX) prior to any imaging studies. Obtain a head CT scan soon after factor infusion. Any patient with significant head injury (eg, loss of memory, hematoma, or laceration) should be hospitalized after factor replacement in the ED and receive factor replacement for 3 to 5 days even if head CT scan is negative. Monitoring the levels of coagulation factor is mandatory in patients receiving factor replacement for serious and life-threatening bleeding.

In patients with hemophilia A and hemarthrosis or muscle or large subcutaneous hematoma, give factor VIII concentrate

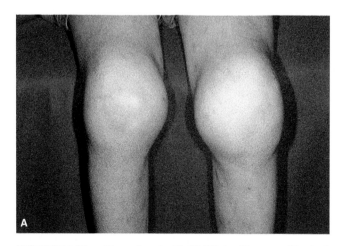
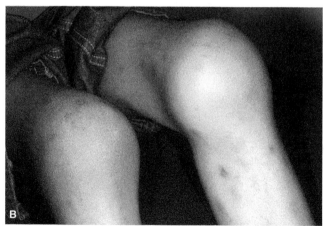

FIGURE 11.18 ■ Hemarthrosis. (**A, B**) Bilateral knee swelling is shown in 2 different patients with hemophilia A presenting with significant pain and limitation of movement. Markedly swollen knees seen here represent an acute bleeding with hemophilic arthropathy or synovitis. (Photo contributor: Binita R. Shah, MD.)

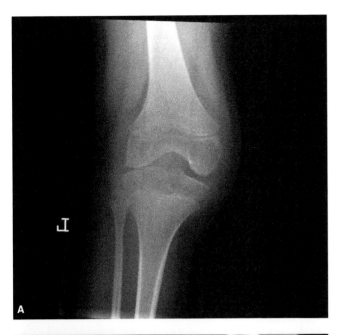

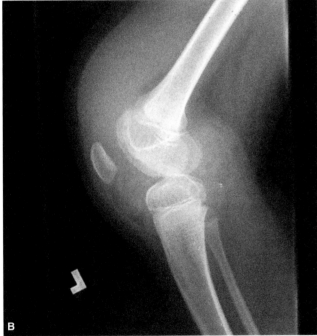

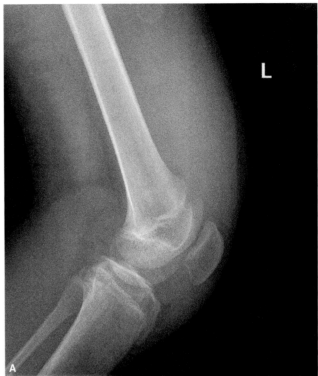

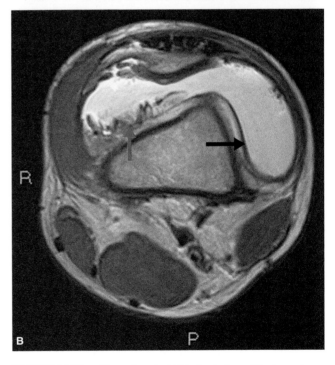

FIGURE 11.19 ■ Hemarthrosis. Posteroanterior (**A**) and lateral (**B**) views of the knee demonstrate swelling with a large joint effusion and widening of the intercondylar notch, compatible with bleeding into the joint space in a child with hemophilia. (Photo contributor: John Amodio, MD.)

FIGURE 11.20 ■ Hemarthrosis. (**A**) Lateral view of the knee shows large joint effusion in an adolescent with hemophilia. (**B**). Axial T2-weighted image demonstrates large joint effusion (black arrow) with frond like projections (red arrow), which are of decreased signal on T2-weighted image compatible with hemorrhagic synovium. (Photo contributor: John Amodio, MD.)

(preferably recombinant factor VIII) 50 units/kg via slow IV push initially and then 20 units/kg on the next day; additional doses are given if clinically indicated. For hemophilia B patients, infuse factor IX (concentrate or recombinant factor IX) in a dose of 80 units/kg followed by 40 units/kg the next day. Sometimes, hemarthrosis may not be clinically evident, but a history of injury and/or a complaint of stiffness and a warm sensation even before there is pain and swelling in the joint are indications to treat with factor.

For oral bleeding or dental extraction in patients with hemophilia A, administer factor VIII 20 units/kg or factor IX 40 units/kg for molar extraction and antifibrinolytic therapy (ε-amino caproic acid or Amicar) by mouth before extraction and 4 to 5 days after extraction. For patients with hemophilia B, administer factor IX 40 units/kg (80 units/kg if molar extraction) along with antifibrinolytic therapy as in hemophilia A.

IV desmopressin (DDAVP) or nasal desmopressin (Stimate) can be used to treat bleeding in mild hemophilia A. An IV infusion of DDAVP is given over 30 minutes. The patient should have had previous documentation of a good response to DDAVP with a 2- to 4-fold increase in factor VIII activity. The dose may be repeated at 24-hour intervals for 2 or 3 days only because further doses will be ineffective (tachyphylaxis). Stimate nasal spray requires 1 spray in 1 nostril (150 µg) for patients weighing <50 kg or 1 spray in each nostril (total dose 300 µg) for patients who weigh >50 kg. During the acute phase, immobilization is recommended as required by bed rest, ice, compression, and elevation.

Pearls

1. Accurate diagnosis of the type of hemophilia (factor VIII or IX deficiency) is essential for the proper management of the patient.

2. If patients with hemophilia are on home therapy and bring in their factor to the ED, it may be used for treating the patients if the same product is not readily available in the ED.

3. It is also important to know if the patient has history of inhibitors to factor VIII or IX. Patients with inhibitors are treated with either prothrombin complex concentrates (eg, FEIBA [factor VIII inhibitor bypassing activity]) or recombinant factor VIIa.

4. DDAVP is an option for treatment of some patients with mild hemophilia A if its efficacy has been previously documented.

5. Do not prescribe DDAVP nasal spray that is used to treat patients with diabetes insipidus because it only delivers 10 µg per spray; instead, prescribe Stimate nasal spray, which delivers 150 µg per spray.

6. Aminocaproic acid or tranexamic acid is an important medication when treating oral bleeding in patients with hemophilia.

7. CT scan of the head must be done if there is a history of head trauma—even if symptoms are minimal. All head injuries should be treated aggressively with factor infusion, even if there are no signs of intracranial bleeding.

Clinical Summary

Lymphadenopathy is defined as painless enlargement of the lymph nodes measuring >1 cm in diameter in the neck and axillary region and 1.5 cm for inguinal nodes. In the supraclavicular or epitrochlear region, nodes >0.5 cm can be considered lymphadenopathy. Regional lymphadenopathy involves 1 or 2 contiguous regions; generalized lymphadenopathy involves more than 2 noncontiguous regions and is usually due to systemic disease. The etiology is determined by whether adenopathy is regional or generalized, presence or absence of signs of local inflammation, and whether there are systemic symptoms (eg, fever, weight loss). Clinical features depend on the cause of lymphadenopathy. During evaluation, location, size, consistency, and signs of inflammation (warmth, tenderness, erythema, fluctuance) of lymph nodes are noted. Erythema of skin over the node and tenderness indicate acute infection. Matted or fixed nodes to the skin or underlying structures may be seen in tuberculosis or malignancy. Cervical lymphadenopathy may be seen in oropharyngeal infections, cat-scratch disease, leukemia, lymphoma, metastatic neuroblastoma, infectious mononucleosis, tuberculosis, histiocytic disorders, and autoimmune lymphoproliferative disease. An enlarged thyroid gland with cervical adenopathy suggests thyroid carcinoma. Right supraclavicular adenopathy is usually due to an intrathoracic malignancy or infection in the mediastinum; left supraclavicular adenopathy is usually

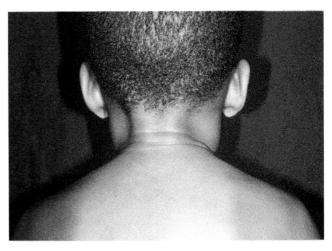

FIGURE 11.22 ■ Bilateral Cervical Lymphadenopathy; Infectious Mononucleosis. Splenomegaly, exudative tonsillopharyngitis, and atypical lymphocytosis were other findings. This patient's lymphadenopathy completely resolved in 3 weeks. (Photo contributor: Binita R. Shah, MD.)

due to an intra-abdominal malignancy. Lymph node biopsy is indicated if there is no decrease in size of lymph nodes in 4 to 6 weeks or no regression to normal size in 8 to 12 weeks. Lymph node biopsy in the majority of patients reveals nonspecific lymphoid hyperplasia. In such cases, close follow-up for persistent signs and symptoms is essential, and a repeat lymph node biopsy may be needed to make the diagnosis if the problem is not resolved. Lymph node biopsy should be considered in patients whose adenopathy persists or increases in size. Consider doing a biopsy if there are associated signs and symptoms of persistent or unexplained fever; weight loss; night sweats; lymph nodes that are hard, rubbery in consistency, matted together, or fixed to the surrounding structures or to the overlying skin; or mediastinal adenopathy.

Emergency Department Treatment and Disposition

Hematology/oncology consultations are recommended for suspected malignancy. Tests, as clinically indicated, include CBC (screening for anemia, thrombocytopenia, abnormal WBCs); peripheral blood smear to look for atypical lymphocytes or any abnormal morphology (eg, lymphoblasts); throat culture for *Streptococcus pyogenes*; intradermal tuberculin (5 tuberculin unit purified protein derivative) test; serology tests for Epstein-Barr virus, cytomegalovirus, HIV, and toxoplasmosis; erythrocyte sedimentation rate (ESR);

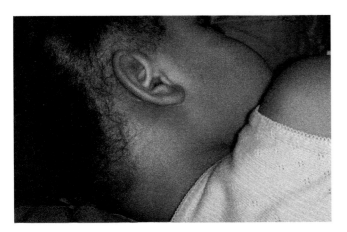

FIGURE 11.21 ■ Acute Suppurative Cervical Lymphadenitis. Infected nodes are tender and show warmth and erythema. Fluctuance suggests abscess formation; however, because of induration from the surrounding inflammation, an abscess may be present without fluctuance. *Staphylococcus aureus* adenitis is more likely to suppurate than adenitis from other etiologies. (Photo contributor: Barry Hahn, MD.)

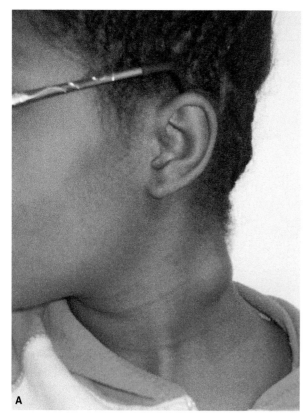

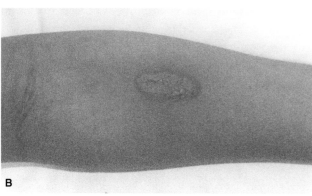

FIGURE 11.23 ■ Mycobacterial Cervical Lymphadenitis. (**A**) A 6-year-old girl presented with a 3-month history of a slowly growing left neck mass. She denied any history of fever, cough, weight loss, night sweats, or any exposure to pets or any family member with tuberculosis. She had traveled to Guyana 1 year ago. About a month prior to this presentation, she was seen by her primary physician and prescribed antibiotics without any response. Her CBC and CXR were negative. Her purified protein derivative test was positive, as shown (**B**). A fine-needle aspiration biopsy confirmed diagnosis of tuberculosis, and she was started on therapy. (Photo contributor: Haamid Chamdawala, MD.)

comprehensive metabolic panel including serum lactate dehydrogenase (LDH) and uric acid; and a CXR (hilar or mediastinal adenopathy). Needle aspiration of the affected node, if clinically indicated, may be done and aspirate sent for Gram stain and acid-fast stains and aerobic and anaerobic cultures. Patients with suppurative adenitis (painful, enlarged, tender nodes) require antibiotics after appropriate laboratory evaluation (CBC with differential, blood culture). If the patient is febrile and looks ill, he or she may be admitted for IV antibiotic therapy and for possible incision and drainage. Patients with significant leukocytosis, an abnormal differential, hyperuricemia, high serum LDH, or mediastinal or hilar adenopathy should be admitted with urgent consultation from the hematology/oncology service. A diagnosis of leukemia can be made by bone marrow aspiration/biopsy, thus avoiding the need for lymph node biopsy. Do not give steroids for treating enlarged lymph nodes as this may result in partial treatment of leukemia or lymphoma, will confuse the clinical picture, will delay the diagnosis, and may worsen the prognosis for the patient.

Pearls

1. The majority of patients with lymphadenopathy have benign, self-limited disease that resolves without specific therapy.
2. Enlarged nodes anterior to the sternocleidomastoid muscle are usually benign (exception: thyroid cancer).
3. Approximately 50% of masses in the posterior triangle or multiple masses extending across both the anterior and posterior triangles represent malignancies, the majority of which are of lymphoid in origin.
4. Suspect malignancy in case of large, painless, firm, and rubbery lymph nodes in the posterior triangle.
5. Supraclavicular lymphadenopathy strongly suggests malignancy.
6. Bacterial lymphadenitis commonly presents with fever and painful, enlarged, tender lymph nodes with local signs of inflammation.

Clinical Summary

Acute leukemia is the most common malignancy in childhood. Of the approximately 2900 cases diagnosed in the United States every year, 75% are acute lymphoblastic leukemia (ALL) and the remaining are acute nonlymphoblastic leukemia. Childhood ALL has a peak between 2 and 6 years of age and occurs more commonly in boys. It may be T or B cell in origin. There are a variety of predisposing or contributing factors such as environmental carcinogens, viral infections, genetic syndromes, Bloom syndrome, Fanconi anemia, immunodeficiency states such as Wiskott-Aldrich syndrome, ataxia telangiectasia, and ionizing radiation. The presenting signs and symptoms reflect the degree of bone marrow

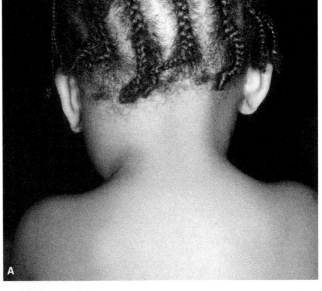

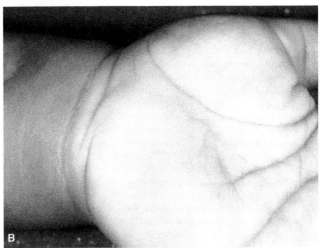

FIGURE 11.25 ■ Acute Lymphoblastic Leukemia (ALL). (**A**) Lymphadenopathy in a child with ALL. Lymph nodes are nontender, firm, and may be matted or fixed to the skin or underlying structures. (**B**) Severe pallor with a Hg value of 4.8 g/dL in the same child. His WBC count was 260,000/mm³ and platelet count was 16,000/mm³. (Photo contributor: Binita R. Shah, MD.)

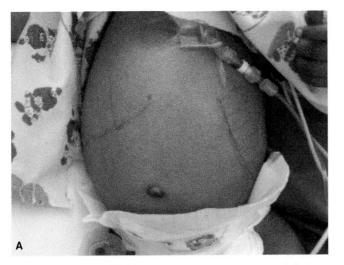

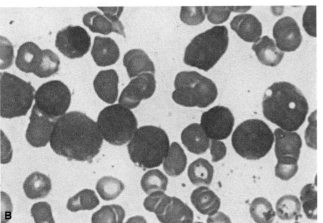

FIGURE 11.24 ■ Acute Lymphoblastic Leukemia. (**A**) A child with massive hepatosplenomegaly and generalized adenopathy. (**B**) Lymphoblasts (L1 subtype: small uniform cells with scanty cytoplasm and rounded nuclei) in a peripheral smear. (Photo contributors: Haamid Chamdawala [A], and Shahina Quereshi, MD [B].)

infiltration with lymphoblasts and the extent of extramedullary spread. Low-grade unexplained fever is present in 80% of patients. Pallor and fatigue due to anemia and epistaxis, petechiae, and purpura due to thrombocytopenia may be seen. Anorexia is common, but significant weight loss is uncommon. The duration of symptoms varies from days to weeks. There is multiorgan involvement due to leukemic infiltration with differing signs and symptoms. Bone pain is present in 25% of patients. Long bones are affected with involvement

539

of the periosteum. Patients present with limping and tenderness, and the condition may be misdiagnosed as rheumatoid arthritis or osteomyelitis. Extramedullary spread leads to lymphadenopathy and hepatosplenomegaly. Hepatic dysfunction from liver infiltration is mild with LDH elevation. T-cell ALL usually presents with a high WBC count and a mediastinal mass. Compression of the trachea or superior vena cava causes dyspnea, plethora, and facial edema (superior vena cava syndrome [SVCS]). Infiltration of the kidneys causes renal enlargement. CNS involvement is rare at presentation. Males may have testicular infiltration, and the testes should be examined for painless enlargement clinically and by US if suspected. The testes serve as a sanctuary site and need specific therapy. Hyperuricemia, hyperkalemia, hyperphosphatemia, and hypocalcemia due to tumor lysis may lead to uric acid nephropathy and subsequent renal failure. Differential diagnosis of ALL includes ITP, aplastic anemia, infectious mononucleosis, and other malignancies such as neuroblastoma and lymphoma.

Emergency Department Treatment and Disposition

All clinically suspected patients with ALL require hematology consultation and hospitalization for confirmation of the diagnosis by a bone marrow examination and further management. Laboratory tests include CBC with a differential and peripheral smear, blood culture, renal and liver function tests, uric acid, LDH, PT, PTT, type and cross match, and urine analysis. CXR is obtained to look for hilar lymphadenopathy and/or mediastinal mass. IV hydration is initiated with the anticipation of tumor lysis syndrome (TLS). Although leukemic blasts may be identified in the peripheral smear in some patients, bone marrow examination is mandatory for establishing a definitive diagnosis, to establish that >25% of the marrow has blasts, to identify the immunologic subtypes (T-cell ALL and B-cell ALL), and for cytogenetic evaluation. These are all necessary for risk stratification and treatment. Lumbar puncture is done after admission to look for blasts in CSF and for administration of intrathecal chemotherapy. A traumatic tap will confuse the cytologic assessment and potentially seed the CNS with lymphoblasts. Supportive care includes packed RBC and platelet transfusions (especially for bleeding and prior to lumbar puncture), prevention and treatment of infections, and treatment of TLS. Blood products should be irradiated and cytomegalovirus negative. After the initial 4-week induction therapy, the presence of measurable residual disease is an important prognostic factor for long-term relapse-free survival. Multiagent chemotherapy is given for 2 to 3 years after risk stratification. Four-year event-free survival is >95% for low-risk ALL, 90% to 95% for standard-risk ALL, and 88% for high-risk ALL. Patients deemed to be very high risk with unfavorable chromosomes and failure to achieve remission are treated with aggressive chemotherapy and hematopoietic stem cell transplantation.

Pearls

1. TLS and SVCS are medical emergencies and require immediate intervention. It is important to perform a bone marrow aspirate before treatment is given.
2. Unexplained fever, weight loss, lymphadenopathy, hepatosplenomegaly, and bone pain require investigations for malignancy.
3. Patients with ALL may have leukopenia or leukocytosis at presentation.

Clinical Summary

Hodgkin lymphoma (HL) accounts for 7% of pediatric cancers. It is most common in adolescents between 15 and 19 years of age. The overall incidence is higher in adolescent females than males; however, in the younger age group, males have a higher incidence. Risk factors include a family history of HL (3- to 5-fold increase in close relatives) and history of Epstein-Barr virus infection, immunosuppression, and autoimmune disorders. The clinical presentation includes the presence of painless, firm or hard lymph nodes that may be immobile, bulky, and attached to each other and the underlying structures. They are in the cervical, axillary, supraclavicular, and inguinal regions. Patients can have nonspecific fatigue and anorexia. Fever, weight loss >10% in the previous 6 months, and night sweats are considered "B" symptoms and are important for staging and prognosis. It is important to look for hepatosplenomegaly. Most patients have a mediastinal mass on CXR, and if this is bulky, it can lead to dyspnea, cough, or stridor (SVCS). The differential diagnosis includes leukemia, non-Hodgkin lymphoma, infections, systemic lupus erythematosus, and reactive hyperplasia.

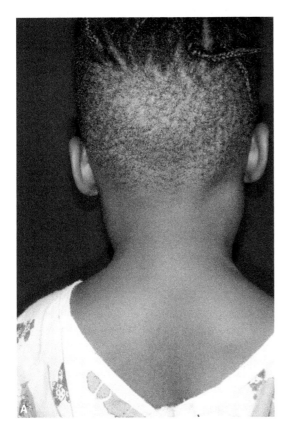

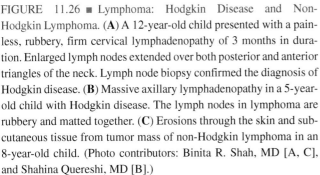

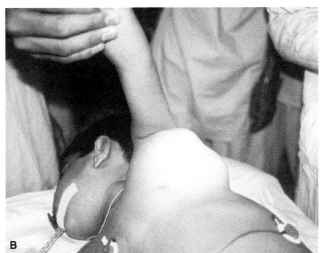

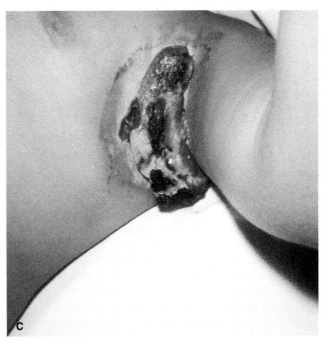

FIGURE 11.26 ■ Lymphoma: Hodgkin Disease and Non-Hodgkin Lymphoma. (**A**) A 12-year-old child presented with a painless, rubbery, firm cervical lymphadenopathy of 3 months in duration. Enlarged lymph nodes extended over both posterior and anterior triangles of the neck. Lymph node biopsy confirmed the diagnosis of Hodgkin disease. (**B**) Massive axillary lymphadenopathy in a 5-year-old child with Hodgkin disease. The lymph nodes in lymphoma are rubbery and matted together. (**C**) Erosions through the skin and subcutaneous tissue from tumor mass of non-Hodgkin lymphoma in an 8-year-old child. (Photo contributors: Binita R. Shah, MD [A, C], and Shahina Quereshi, MD [B].)

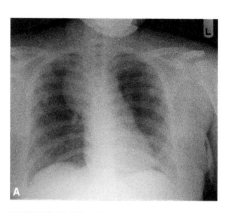 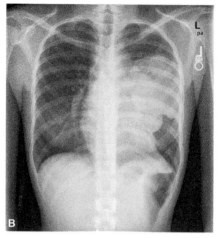 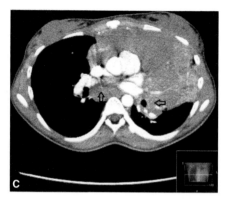

FIGURE 11.27 ■ Hodgkin Lymphoma Presenting as Anterior Mediastinal Mass. (**A**) A 14-year-old girl with a history of fever, dyspnea, fatigue, and weight loss of 30 lb was noted to have autoimmune hemolytic anemia (Hg 3.7 g/dL, reticulocyte count of 26% with positive direct Coombs) and a mediastinal mass, as seen here on anteroposterior view of the chest. A postcontrast axial CT image confirmed a large homogeneous soft tissue density mass in the anterior and middle mediastinum later confirmed as Hodgkin lymphoma. (**B**) A 17-year-old very emaciated adolescent girl presented with a recent history of pneumonia, worsening chest pain, productive sputum, joint pains, and weight loss. Examination revealed decreased air entry on the left side with wrist and knee swelling. Posteroanterior view of the chest shows large anterior mediastinal mass. (**C**) Axial CT scan confirms anterior mediastinal mass with adenopathy also seen in left hilum and middle mediastinum (arrows). Diagnosis of Hodgkin lymphoma was confirmed. (Photo/legend contributors: Mario Peichev, MD, and Eric Minkin, MD [A]; Majo Joseph, MD, and John Amodio, MD [B, C].)

Emergency Department Treatment and Disposition

All patients with suspected HL should be evaluated by the pediatric oncologist. Laboratory tests include CBC, ESR, liver and renal function tests, LDH and uric acid, PT, PTT, type and cross match, and urinalysis. A CXR should be done because it often shows a mediastinal mass. Additional tests include a CT scan of the neck, chest, abdomen, and pelvis with and without contrast and a PET/CT scan. The diagnosis is made by an excisional biopsy by the surgeon working in conjunction with pediatric oncology. Patients with a large mediastinal mass need to be evaluated with care, and a biopsy should be done under local anesthesia. Classical HL accounts for 90% to 95% of cases. Therapy and prognosis depend on the stage. In stage I and II, there is involvement of lymph nodes or extralymphatic organs on the same side of the diaphragm. Involvement of lymph nodes on both sides of the

diaphragm indicates stage III disease, and distant metastases indicate stage IV disease. The presence of "B" symptoms is recorded for staging and is important for decisions regarding therapy. Treatment is a combination of chemotherapy and radiation therapy and is stratified based on risk; risk is defined as low, intermediate, or high based on the stage. This is particularly important because the cure rate is high and the aim is to reduce side effects of therapy. The overall survival rate is >95%.

Pearls

1. Painless firm or hard lymphadenopathy is the most common presentation of HL.
2. It is important to ask about the presence of fever, night sweats, and weight loss.
3. Early-stage disease requires less intense chemotherapy and has a better prognosis.

Clinical Summary

Any abdominal mass in a child requires urgent medical attention because it may be a presenting manifestation of a malignant tumor. These masses tend to be retroperitoneal in origin. In infants, most abdominal masses tend to be due to benign conditions. Any mass detected during a routine well-child visit may increase the chance of early diagnosis and treatment of a malignant tumor and a favorable outcome. It is essential to obtain a detailed history including the duration of the mass and rapidity of increase in the size of the mass, pain, constipation (suggests either a tumor compressing the bowel or that the mass is stool), diarrhea, urinary symptoms, fever, and weight loss and to perform a thorough physical exam in each

patient. An irritable or cachectic child may have a malignancy; high blood pressure suggests Wilms tumor, neuroblastoma, hydronephrosis, or multicystic kidney. Proptosis and periorbital ecchymosis suggest metastatic neuroblastoma. Sporadic

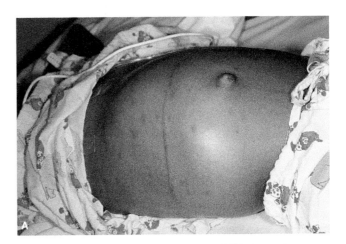

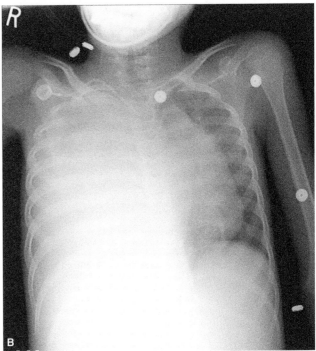

FIGURE 11.29 ■ Wilms Tumor. (**A**) A 7-year-old child presented with a huge abdominal mass and respiratory distress. Wilms tumor diagnosis was confirmed by biopsy. Wilms tumor most often presents as an asymptomatic mass in the flank. Because of the retroperitoneal location of the kidney, these tumors can be quite large at diagnosis. (**B**) Almost complete opacification of the right hemithorax with mediastinal shift to the left is seen. Approximately 10% to 15% of patients with Wilms tumor will have hematogenous metastatic disease at presentation; the most common site is lungs (80%–85%) followed by liver (15%). (Photo contributor: Binita R. Shah, MD.)

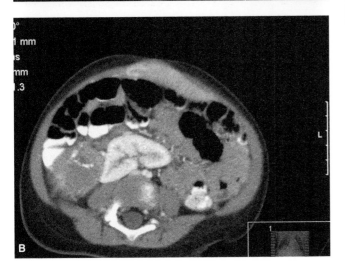

FIGURE 11.28 ■ Hepatoblastoma. (**A, B**) Very large, heavily calcified mass occupying the right lobe of the liver. Note displacement of the right kidney, which is rotated 90 degrees on its axis. (Photo contributor: John Amodio, MD.)

543

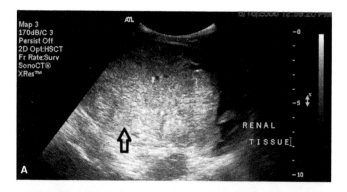

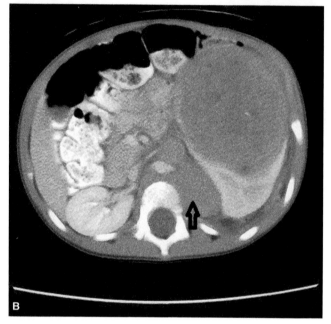

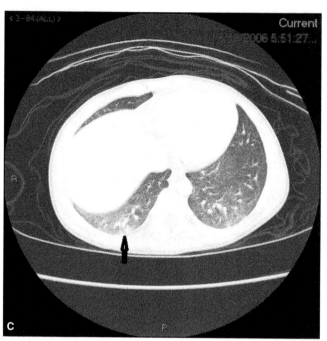

FIGURE 11.30 ■ Wilms Tumor. (**A**) Longitudinal sonogram of the left kidney demonstrates a large mass (arrow) within the left kidney. (**B**) CT scan demonstrates large mass arising from left kidney and para-aortic lymphadenopathy (arrow). (**C**) CT scan of the chest demonstrates metastatic nodule (arrow) within the right lower lobe of the lung. (Photo contributor: John Amodio, MD.)

aniridia or hemihypertrophy may be associated with Wilms tumor. Marked pallor and petechiae suggest marrow infiltration by the tumor, typically neuroblastoma. Fecal masses are usually mobile, multiple, and palpable in the left lower quadrant or on the entire left side corresponding to the course of the descending colon. Rectal examination confirming that the rectum is filled with stool suggests that the abdominal mass may be a stool mass. Fecal masses usually disappear after a cleansing enema. Less common abdominal masses include intussusception (mass in right lower or upper quadrant) or incarcerated hernia; imperforate hymen with an abdominal mass suggests hydrocolpos, hydrometrocolpos, hematocolpos, or hematometrocolpos (see Figure 10.40).

In the differential diagnosis of abdominal masses in children, the age of the child is an important consideration. Greater than 50% of masses in neonates are of renal origin, and of these, most are caused by multicystic kidney disease or congenital

hydronephrosis. Abdominal masses in infants and children are either retroperitoneal tumors (eg, Wilms tumor or neuroblastoma) or enlarged liver and spleen (often from diseases such as leukemia or lymphoma). Laboratory evaluation includes CBC, comprehensive metabolic panel, serum LDH, uric acid, calcium, phosphate, urinalysis, and pregnancy test, particularly when dealing with a midline abdominal mass in an adolescent female. Severe anemia or pancytopenia suggests bleeding into tumor or extensive marrow infiltration, respectively. Anemia with thrombocytosis is a frequent finding in neuroblastoma. LDH is elevated most often in lymphoma, neuroblastoma, and germ cell tumors. High uric acid, potassium, and phosphate (evidence of tumor lysis syndrome) prior to therapy is seen typically in Burkitt lymphoma. Hypercalcemia is seen in some patients with lymphoblastic leukemia, mesoblastic nephroma, and rhabdoid kidney tumor. Hematuria may be seen in patients with Wilms tumor or renal cell carcinoma.

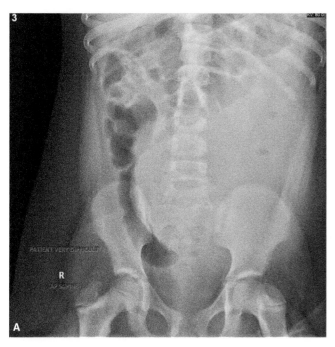

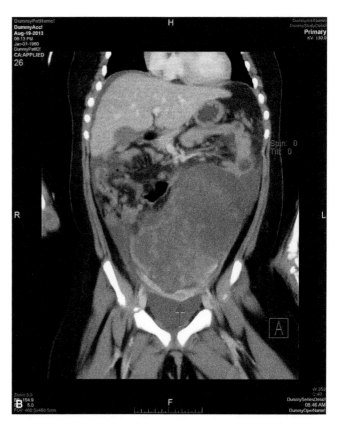

FIGURE 11.31 ▪ Rhabdomyosarcoma. An 8-year-old girl presented with a history of limping, abdominal pain, and constipation. (**A**) Supine abdominal x-ray showing a soft tissue mass in the left side of the abdomen displacing the bowel loops superiorly and to the right. (**B**) Coronal postcontrast CT image showing a large heterogeneously enhancing soft tissue mass just superior to the uterus (arrow) and displacing the bowel superiorly and to the right. (Photo/legend contributors: Kusum Viswanathan, MD, and Eric Minkin, MD.)

Emergency Department Treatment and Disposition

Plain CXR is done for evidence of mediastinal adenopathy (eg, lymphoma), posterior mediastinal mass (eg, neuroblastoma), or pulmonary metastasis (eg, Wilms tumor, rhabdomyosarcoma, or hepatoblastoma). Plain radiograph of the abdomen is obtained for evidence of intestinal obstruction (eg, intussusception presenting with an abdominal mass) or calcification in a solid mass (eg, neuroblastoma, Wilms tumor, hepatoblastoma, or ovarian teratoma). Abdominal US will determine the structure of origin and whether the mass is solid or cystic. A CT scan with contrast will provide details of the extent of the mass, invasion of adjacent structures, and presence or absence of enlarged nodes. MRI is superior in evaluating paraspinal masses such as neuroblastoma that may invade the spinal canal. If a mass is thought to be secondary to constipation, an enema may resolve the problem. Pediatric hematology/oncology, pediatric surgery, and pediatric nephrology service consultations are obtained depending on the probable clinical diagnosis. Management of abdominal mass usually depends on the underlying etiology. Most patients with abdominal mass due to clinically suspected malignancy need hospitalization for prompt evaluation and treatment by the pediatric oncologist. Hymenotomy is performed for abdominal mass due to imperforate hymen with hydrometrocolpos (abdominal mass will disappear as the secretions/menstrual products are drained). Air contrast enema may reduce (or if indicated, surgical reduction) an intussusception and result in disappearance of the mass.

Pearls

1. Any abdominal mass in a child requires urgent medical attention because it may be a presenting sign of malignancy.

2. A history of fever, bone pain, and weight loss suggests metastatic neuroblastoma or lymphoma.

Clinical Features

Neuroblastoma is the third most common childhood cancer, after leukemia and brain tumors. It is the most common cancer in the first year of age, and approximately 75% of patients present between birth and 2 years of age. The tumor arises from the sympathetic chain and is seen often in the adrenal gland and the abdomen. Signs and symptoms include an abdominal mass (retroperitoneal or hepatic), abdominal pain, proptosis, "raccoon eyes" (periorbital ecchymosis caused by orbital metastases), Horner syndrome, localized back pain and weakness (spinal cord compression), constipation, and skin nodules. Some patients can present with opsoclonus-myoclonus syndrome (OMS) with rapid, spontaneous, irregular dancing eye movements and rhythmic jerking of the limbs. Neuroblastoma is the most common malignancy with OMS in children. Metastases to the bones and bone marrow can cause bone pain and changes in blood count, and skin metastases can be seen as firm, nontender nodules. Metastases can also occur to lymph nodes and liver.

Tumors can undergo spontaneous regression, mature to a benign ganglioneuroma, or be aggressive with metastatic dissemination. Age, tumor stage, histology, cytogenetics, and molecular genetics play a role in prognosis and therapy. Infants <18 months old who have stage IVS neuroblastoma with a resectable primary tumor and metastases limited to the liver, skin, and bone marrow can have spontaneous regression. Differential diagnosis includes other tumors presenting with abdominal mass (eg, Wilms tumor), other catecholamine-secreting tumors, and other cancers with metastatic bone marrow involvement (eg, leukemia).

Emergency Department Treatment and Disposition

Patients presenting with an abdominal mass need a US followed by an MRI of the chest, abdomen, and pelvis. A CBC, comprehensive metabolic panel, LDH, ferritin, and urine collection for vanillylmandelic acid and homovanillic acid are important. Further evaluation with an ^{123}I-metaiodobenzylguanidine (MIBG) scan is done to look for metastatic disease. Treatment is guided by staging of the tumor and could involve initial surgery or biopsy, chemotherapy, and radiation therapy based on tumor characteristics. Amplification of the *n-myc* oncogene is associated with poor prognosis. Patients will need to be admitted for further evaluation by a multidisciplinary

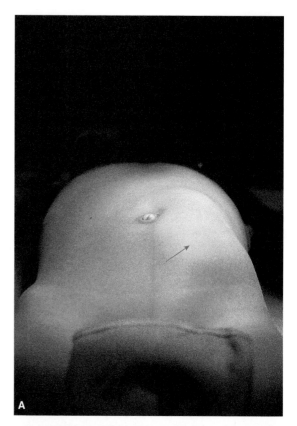

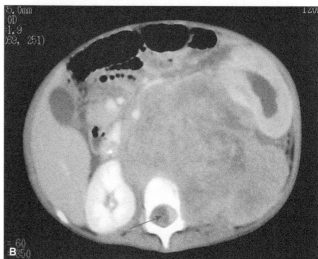

FIGURE 11.32 ■ Neuroblastoma. (**A**) An abdominal mass (arrow) and weight loss were seen this 3-year-old girl. Excessive catecholamine secretion by neuroblastoma may result in tachycardia, hypertension, diarrhea, and skin flushing. Other findings include exophthalmos, periorbital ecchymoses ("raccoon eyes"; see chapter opener figure), abdominal pain, localized back pain, and weakness. (**B**) Complex predominantly left-sided heterogenous mass with necrotic areas and calcifications arising from the retroperitoneum is seen on CT scan. Left kidney is displaced anteriorly with hydronephrosis. Invasion of spinal canal is seen (arrow). Histology confirmed the diagnosis of neuroblastoma. (Photo contributor: Binita R. Shah, MD.)

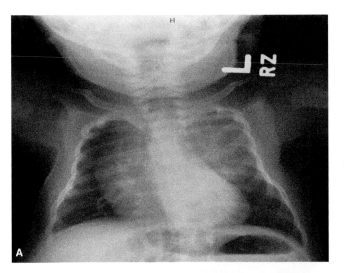

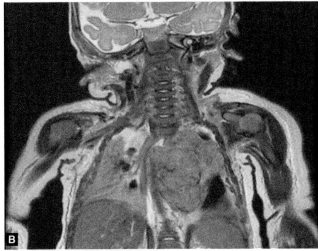

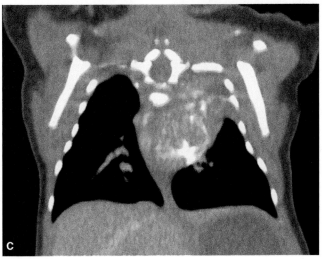

FIGURE 11.33 ■ Congenital Neuroblastoma. **(A)** A 7-week-old infant presented with decreased activity and flaccid paralysis of bilateral lower extremities. Frontal view of the chest demonstrates a large left-sided posterior mediastinal mass with calcifications. There is thinning and splaying of the ribs by the mass. **(B, C)** Coronal MRI and coronal CT reconstruction show calcified posterior mediastinal mass. Surgical debulking was done, and pathology confirmed neuroblastoma. (Photo/legend contributors: Yagnaram Ravichandran, MD, and John Amodio, MD.)

team including pediatric hematologist/oncologist, pediatric radiologist, and surgeon. Some tumors near the spine can grow through the neural foramina and invade the spinal canal (dumbbell shaped), causing neurologic symptoms, and may need immediate intervention.

Pearls

1. Neuroblastoma is the most common cancer in the first year of life.

2. Neuroblastoma is the most common metastatic tumor of the orbit. The presence of "raccoon eyes" without a history of trauma is an important red flag.

3. Prognosis and treatment are guided by age, stage, histology, cytogenetics, and molecular features of the tumor.

4. Some infants with stage IVS can have spontaneous regression.

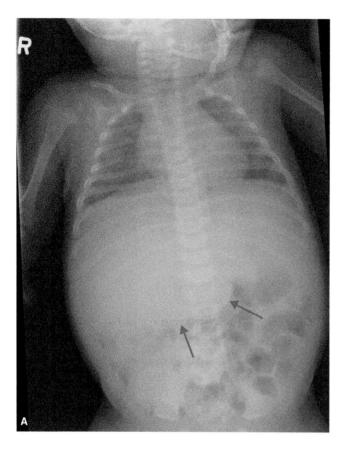

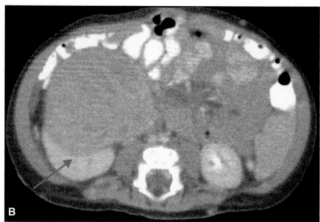

FIGURE 11.34 ■ Congenital Neuroblastoma. (**A**) A supine view of the abdomen shows a soft tissue mass in the right upper quadrant (arrows) displacing the bowel inferiorly and to the left in this 3-month-old infant who presented with skin lesions and an abdominal mass. (**B**) Axial postcontrast CT image shows a heterogeneous soft tissue density mass in the right side of the abdomen compressing and posteriorly displacing the right kidney (arrow). He had neuroblastoma stage IVS, which spontaneously resolved. (Photo/legend contributors: Kusum Viswanathan, MD, and Eric Minkin, MD.)

Clinical Summary

Ovarian tumors and rhabdomyosarcoma are the 2 common pelvic tumors in girls. Ovarian tumors are rare, accounting for 1% of childhood malignancies, and are of different pathologic subtypes. Most ovarian tumors are benign; however, 10% to 20% may be malignant. Malignant ovarian tumors are uncommon in childhood and are seen in adolescence with a peak incidence at 19 years of age. Two-thirds of pediatric ovarian tumors are of germ cell origin. The most common malignant ovarian tumor is dysgerminoma, which is rapidly growing but curable with surgery and chemotherapy. Next are teratomas, the majority of which present in the premenarchal age. These arise from the 3 germ cell layers and can be solid or cystic with or without calcifications. The immature teratomas contain fetal immature tissue, which is neuroectodermal in origin and can be malignant. Mature teratomas are histologically benign but can present with ovarian torsion and can rupture spontaneously, leading to peritonitis in 1% to 3% of cases. Endodermal sinus or yolk sac tumors are associated with an increase in serum α-fetoprotein (AFP) level and can present with metastases to the lung, liver, or lymph nodes. In embryonal carcinoma, human chorionic gonadotrophin (HCG) level is increased, and precocious puberty, amenorrhea, or hirsutism may be seen. Choriocarcinoma is rare in children and may present with an increase in serum HCG level and metastases to the lung and liver. Other rare tumors are mixed germ cell tumors and gonadoblastomas that are associated with dysgenetic gonads and sexual maldevelopment. The most common signs and symptoms of ovarian tumors are abdominal mass, abdominal distention, and abdominal or back pain. Pain can be chronic but may mimic an acute abdomen, especially if presenting with torsion. Fever, constipation, amenorrhea, vaginal bleeding, urinary frequency, or dysuria may be present. Differential diagnosis includes appendicitis, ovarian cyst, ovarian torsion, tubo-ovarian abscess with pelvic inflammatory disease, UTI, and ectopic pregnancy.

Emergency Department Treatment and Disposition

Any patient presenting with an abdominal or pelvic mass needs an immediate sonogram because most ovarian tumors can be identified by US. A solid mass is considered malignant and needs further evaluation. A CBC may show decreased Hb

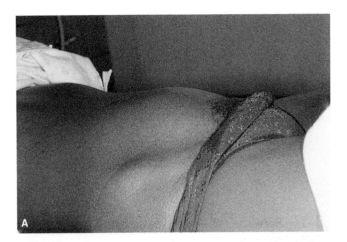
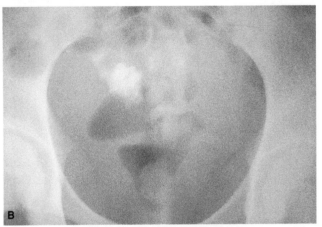
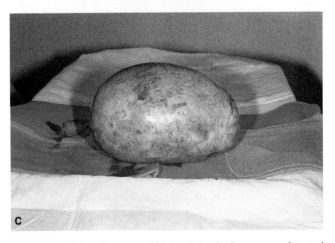

FIGURE 11.35 ■ Teratoma. (**A**) An abdominal mass was detected on a routine examination from a completely asymptomatic 13-year-old adolescent girl. (**B**) Supine kidney-ureter-bladder (KUB) film of the abdomen shows clusters of calcifications in the pelvis on the right side. A pelvic US confirmed a cystic mass arising from the right ovary. (**C**) Mature cystic teratoma that was removed. Teratomas may be unilateral (85%–90%) or bilateral (10%–15%). The most common presentation is a suprapubic mass, and the majority of patients are asymptomatic. (Photo contributor: Binita R. Shah, MD.)

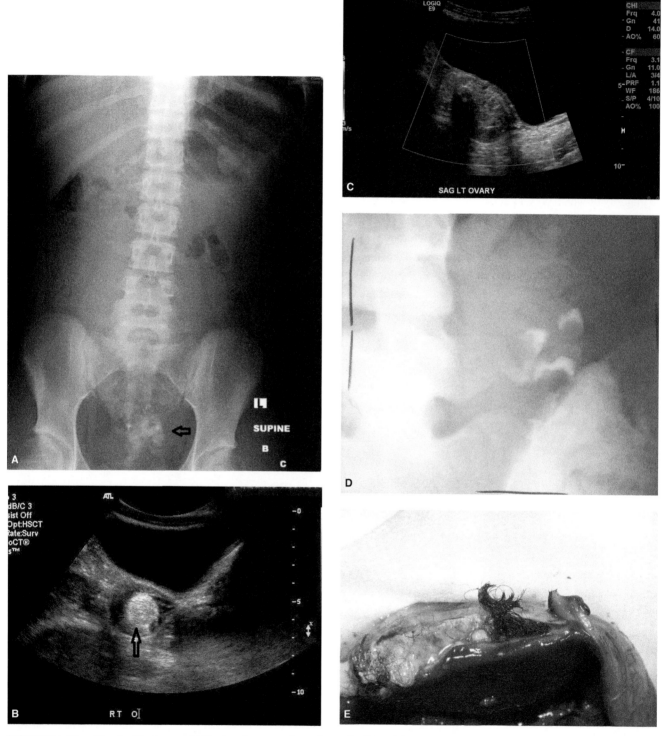

FIGURE 11.36 ■ Ovarian Teratoma. (**A**) Single anteroposterior radiograph of the abdomen demonstrates a calcified mass (arrow) in the pelvis, compatible with an ovarian teratoma in an adolescent female. (**B**) Sonogram of the right ovary in a different patient demonstrates echogenic focus (arrow) representing fat within right ovarian cyst, compatible with ovarian teratoma. (**C**) Sagittal image of the left ovary shows calcified mass with strong acoustical shadowing compatible with ovarian teratoma. (**D**) Close-up of plain film of the abdomen showing clusters of teeth within a mass (teratoma) in a 17-year-old girl. Presence of calcification is a hallmark of a benign teratoma. (**E**) Opened mature cystic teratoma of ovary showing hair, calcium, and a mixture of tissues. (Photo contributors: John Amodio, MD [A, B, C], and Binita R. Shah, MD [E], and [D] reproduced with permission from Shah BR, Laude TL. *Atlas of Pediatric Clinical Diagnosis*. WB Saunders; Philadelphia, PA, 2000.)

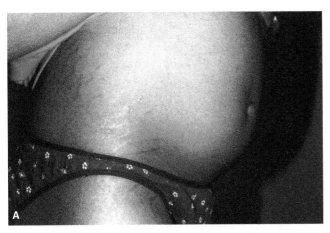
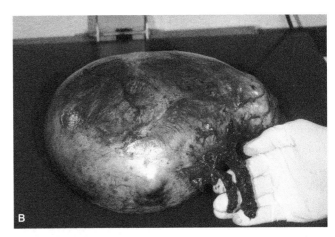

FIGURE 11.37 ■ Teratoma Mimicking Pregnancy! (**A, B**) A steadily increasing abdominal girth was thought to be a possible pregnancy in this 12-year-old adolescent girl. She was seen on several occasions by her primary care physician who had performed several pregnancy tests. The "pregnancy" turned out to be a cystic ovarian teratoma weighing 10 pounds! (Photo contributor: Binita R. Shah, MD.)

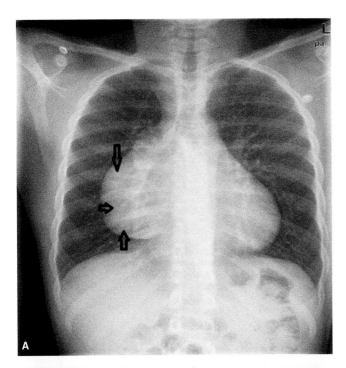
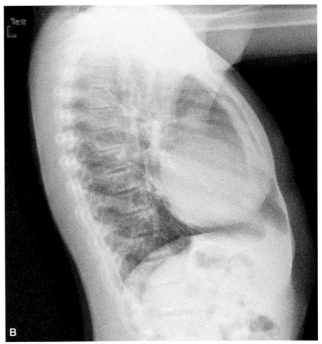
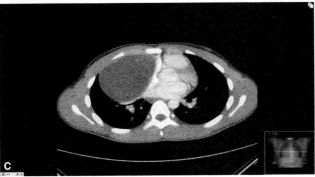

FIGURE 11.38 ■ Mediastinal Teratoma. (**A**) Posteroanterior radiograph of the chest in a 12-year-old boy presenting with chest pain demonstrates mediastinal mass (arrows) obscuring the right heart border. (**B**) Lateral radiograph of the chest shows mass to be anterior within the mediastinum. (**C**) CT scan of the chest shows large cystic mass in anterior mediastinum. At open thoracotomy, the cystic mass had "whitish curds associated with hair" consistent with teratoma; the diagnosis was later confirmed by pathology. The 4 Ts make up the mnemonic for anterior mediastinal masses: (1) thymus, (2) teratoma (germ cell), (3) thyroid, and (4) "terrible" lymphoma. (Photo contributor: John Amodio, MD.)

value (secondary to bleeding into the mass) and thrombocytosis (often seen in malignancies). Additional tests include comprehensive metabolic panel, LDH, ESR, and levels of AFP, HCG, and CA-125. Radiographic studies include MRI of the abdomen and pelvis, CXR, and CT scan. Surgical and hematology consultations should be obtained, and the patient should be admitted. Treatment is surgical resection of the tumor followed by chemotherapy for malignant tumors. Chemotherapeutic agents include cisplatin, vinblastine, bleomycin, and etoposide. Radiation therapy is avoided if possible for preservation of fertility.

Pearls

1. Abdominal mass, pain, and irregular menstrual periods need immediate abdominal and pelvic US for evaluation.
2. Ovarian tumors may rupture and present as acute abdomen and peritonitis.
3. Increased HCG in choriocarcinoma may result in a falsely positive pregnancy test.
4. The aim of treatment of ovarian tumors is cure with development of normal puberty and preservation of future fertility.

Clinical Summary

Osteosarcoma is the most common type of bone tumor, followed by Ewing sarcoma, with a peak incidence at age 16 years in girls and 18 years in boys. Derived from the mesenchyme, it occurs in the metaphyseal portions of rapidly growing bones such as the distal femur, proximal tibia, and proximal humerus; 5% are multifocal. It can also develop in the bones of the pelvis, chest wall, head and neck, and soft tissues. The axial skeleton is rarely affected. Etiology is undetermined, but there is a strong association with radiation, treatment with alkylating agents, hereditary retinoblastoma, and Li-Fraumeni syndrome. The majority of the patients present with dull aching pain at the site of the lesion that frequently begins after an incidental injury. Constitutional symptoms of fever and weight loss are rare but may occur in patients with metastasis, especially to lungs. A soft tissue mass or deformity is noted over the primary site, and there may be erythema, edema, tenderness, or limitation of movement. Painful limp that increases with weight bearing is a common finding.

Regional and distant lymph nodes are not enlarged. The average duration of symptoms is about 3 months.

Emergency Department Treatment and Disposition

The initial evaluation of suspected osteosarcoma includes plain radiographs of the involved site and chest (90% of the metastases are to the lungs). Laboratory studies include CBC, ESR, comprehensive metabolic panel, and serum phosphorus. Serum values of alkaline phosphatase and LDH may be elevated. Common radiographic findings are destruction of the bone with lytic lesions. Periosteal new bone formation with lifting of the cortex (Codman triangle) is a characteristic finding. As the tumor erodes the medullary cavity, a soft tissue mass is observed and a pathologic fracture may be seen. Ossification of the soft tissue can be seen in a radial or sunburst pattern. These findings are seen in the metaphyseal region of the long bones as opposed to Ewing sarcoma, which occurs

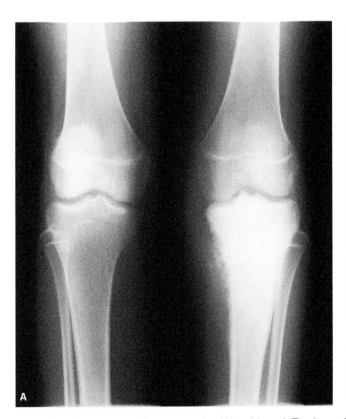 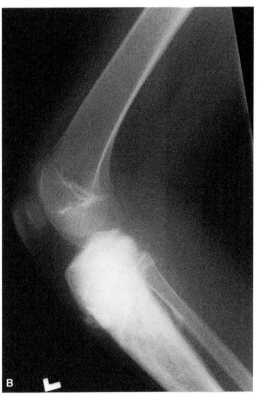

FIGURE 11.39 ■ Osteosarcoma. Anteroposterior (**A**) and lateral (**B**) views of the knee show osteosclerosis of the left tibial metaphysis with periosteal reaction and classical "sunburst" appearance representing breakout of bone-producing tumor into the soft tissues.

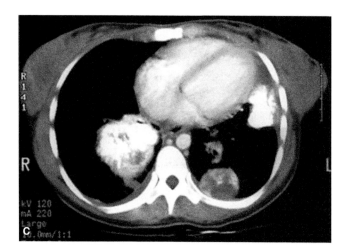

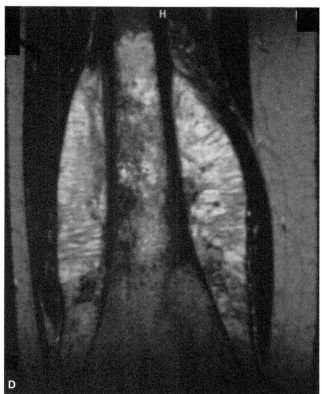

FIGURE 11.39 ■ (*Continued*) (**C**) CT scan of the chest in a patient with osteosarcoma showing large osseous metastases to the lungs. (**D**) MRI of distal femur. T2-weighted image shows bright signal in the medullary region of the femur with extension on either side of the bone, compatible with osteosarcoma invasion of adjacent soft tissues. (Photo contributor: John Amodio, MD.)

in the diaphysis. Additional radiographic studies include MRI to assess the intraosseous extent of the tumor and chest CT for the lung metastasis. These studies are essential in planning surgery. Radionuclide bone scan is indicated to detect skip lesions and distant bone metastasis. Patient should be admitted after consultations with orthopedic surgeon, oncologist, and radiologist for further workup and management. Although the radiographic findings are highly suggestive, a biopsy is always required to confirm the diagnosis. Biopsy should be done by the same orthopedic surgeon who will later do the definitive surgery. It can be a fine-needle biopsy or core or open biopsy. Treatment includes preoperative chemotherapy followed by amputation or limb salvage surgery and postoperative chemotherapy. There is no role for radiation in the treatment of osteosarcoma. Chemotherapeutic agents include methotrexate, doxorubicin, cisplatin, ifosfamide, and etoposide.

Echocardiogram is needed before chemotherapy because some chemotherapy drugs are cardiotoxic. The most important prognostic factor is the degree of tumor necrosis in response to preoperative chemotherapy. Overall survival is 70%.

Pearls

1. Osteosarcoma is the most common malignant bone tumor in children and adolescents, with a peak incidence in the second decade of life.

2. Pathologic fracture occurring with minor trauma is suggestive of an underlying bone pathology, including malignant bone tumors.

3. The appearance of the bone lesion in osteosarcoma may be mixed lytic and blastic, with a characteristic sunburst pattern of new bone formation.

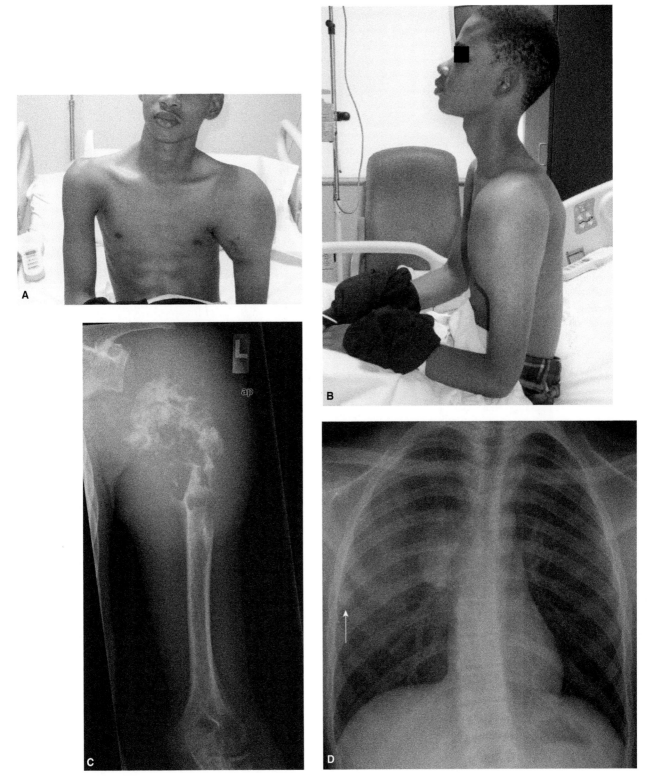

FIGURE 11.40 ▪ Osteosarcoma. (**A, B**) Progressive swelling that occurred over 9 months is seen around the left shoulder in this 17-year-old adolescent boy. Biopsy (scar seen) confirmed the diagnosis of osteogenic sarcoma. (**C**) Anteroposterior view of the left humerus shows a predominately lytic lesion of the proximal shaft with bone formation within the soft tissues. (**D**) Chest radiograph of the same patient shows a dense nodule in the right lung (arrow) and a right hilar mass, compatible with osteosarcoma metastasis. (Photo contributors: Haamid Chamdawala, MD [A, B], and John Amodio, MD [C, D].)

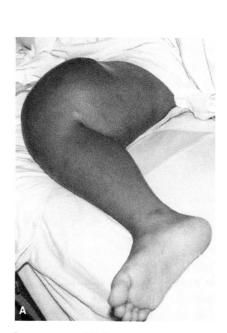

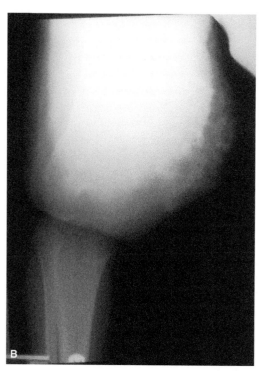

FIGURE 11.41 ■ Osteosarcoma. (**A**) Osteosarcoma of distal femur in a 14-year-old girl with an enlarging mass of 8 months in duration. (**B**) Frontal radiograph demonstrates a large lesion along the medial metaphysis. There is abundant calcification with an ill-defined cortex and significant soft tissue swelling. (Photo contributor: Binita R. Shah, MD [A], and [B] reproduced with permission from Shah BR, Laude TL. *Atlas of Pediatric Clinical Diagnosis*. WB Saunders; Philadelphia, PA, 2000.)

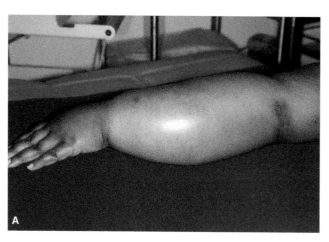

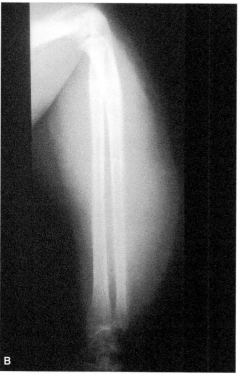

FIGURE 11.42 ■ Osteosarcoma Versus Lymphedema. (**A**) Massive enlargement of the forearm is seen in an 11-year-old adolescent girl who was mistakenly diagnosed as having lymphedema and sent home without any diagnostic workup. This progressive enlargement occurred over a period of 2 months. Tumor biopsy confirmed the diagnosis of osteosarcoma. (**B**) Radiograph showing marked soft tissue swelling with associated "sunburst" periosteal reactions.

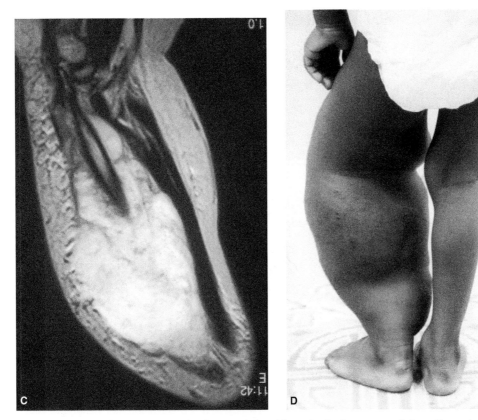

FIGURE 11.42 ■ (*Continued*) (**C**) T2 MRI showing increased signal intensity in the marrow of the radius and within the subcutaneous fat surrounding the tumor. (**D**) Lymphedema in a 4-year-old child. Note the swelling of the entire lower extremity that has been progressively increasing since birth. Lymphedema is the accumulation of interstitial fluid secondary to obstruction of lymphatic flow, and the most common location of lymphedema is the lower extremity. (Photo contributor: Binita R. Shah, MD.)

EWING SARCOMA

Clinical Summary

Ewing sarcoma is the second most common primary bone tumor in children and adolescents; it has a peak incidence between 10 and 15 years of age. The majority arises in a bone, but extraosseous tumors may occur in soft tissues and neural crest. They typically occur in the diaphysis of long bones, chest wall, paraspinal region, scapula, vertebrae, and pelvis. The Ewing sarcoma family of neoplasms includes the primitive neuroectodermal tumors with similar chromosomal translocations involving the *EWS* gene on chromosome 22q12. It is a small round cell tumor with rosette formation. The signs and symptoms are related to the site of origin. Patients present with bone pain or symptoms related to a mass. The pain may

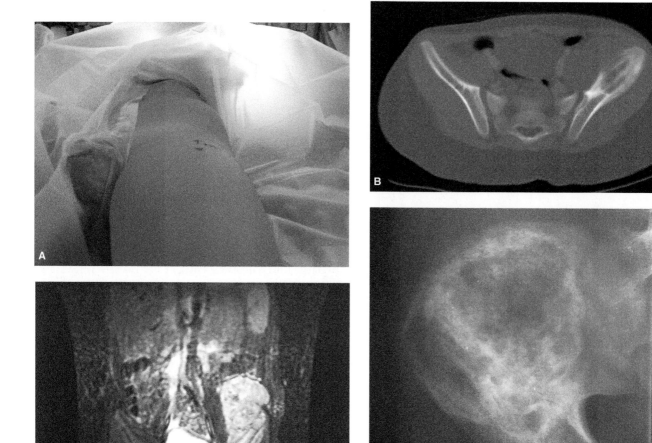

FIGURE 11.43 ■ Ewing Sarcoma. (**A**) Pain and swelling around the left hip and upper thigh were the presenting complaints of this adolescent patient. (**B**) CT image showing the classic "onion skin" appearance of the left pelvis. (**C**) MRI showing area of high signal of the left iliac bone, representing tumor, extending into adjacent soft tissues. (**D**) Anteroposterior view of the right pelvis and hip from a different patient demonstrates a large, mixed sclerotic and lytic lesion involving the right iliac bone. Ewing sarcoma was confirmed by biopsy. (Photo contributors: Mihir Thacker, MD [A–C], and John Amodio, MD [D].)

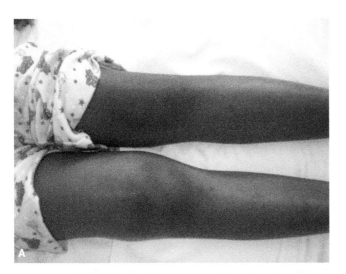

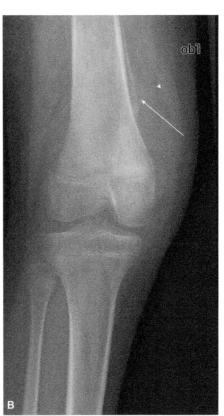

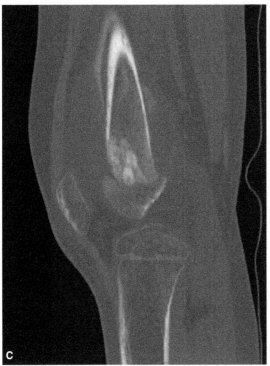

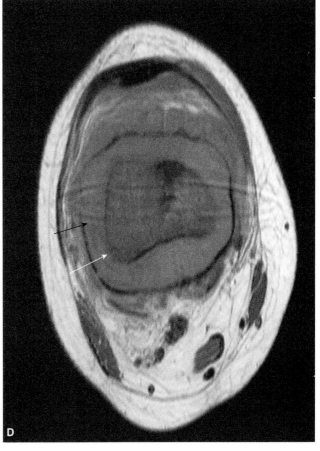

FIGURE 11.44 ■ Osteosarcoma; Differential Diagnosis of Ewing Sarcoma. (**A**) Swelling of the knee and pain were the presenting complaints of this 12-year-old adolescent girl who was seen twice in the ED and sent home without any radiographic studies. (**B**) Frontal view of the knee shows area of sclerosis in the metaphysis of the distal femur with a Codman triangle (arrow). Findings are consistent with osteosarcoma. The presence of sclerosis and the lack of a permeative appearance (moth-eaten) distinguishes this lesion from Ewing sarcoma. (**C**) Sagittal CT scan of the same knee shows marked area of sclerosis in the distal metaphysis, a Codman triangle, and soft tissue density surrounding the distal femur. (**D**) Axial T1-weighted MRI of the knee demonstrates bone marrow invasion (white arrow) by tumor surrounded by soft tissue tumor (black arrow). (Photo contributors: Silvia Delgado-Villalta, MD [A], and John Amodio [B–D].)

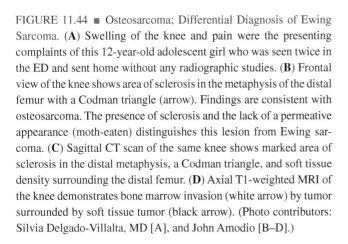

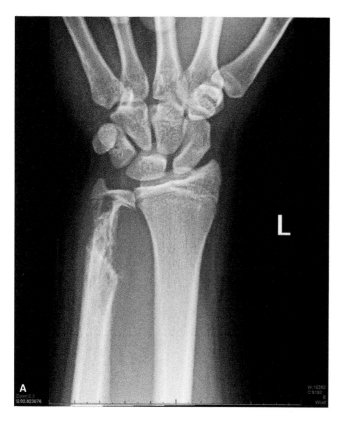

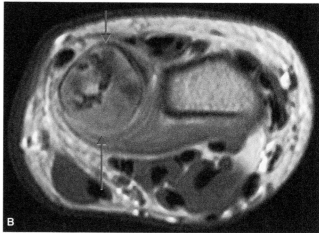

FIGURE 11.45 ■ Osteosarcoma. Differential Diagnosis of Ewing Sarcoma. (**A**) Anteroposterior radiograph of the left wrist showing a permeative pattern of destruction in the distal metaphysis of the ulna in this 14-year-old boy with a history of left arm pain for a few weeks. (**B**) Postgadolinium axial T1-weighted MRI showing an enhancing soft tissue mass (arrows) surrounding and destroying the distal left ulna. (Photo/legend contributors: Mario Peichev, MD, and Eric Minkin, MD.)

be severe enough to wake up the child from sleep. The swelling is tender and erythematous. A fracture may be present within the bony involvement. Serum LDH values are elevated. Metastasis is seen in 25% of patients at diagnosis, and sites include lungs, bone, bone marrow, and lymph nodes. Fever, anemia, and pancytopenia (bone marrow infiltration) may occur. Differential diagnosis of bone pain related to malignancies includes osteogenic sarcoma, leukemia, lymphoma, and neuroblastoma.

Emergency Department Treatment and Disposition

All clinically suspected cases of a malignant bone tumor require hospitalization for further workup and management by a multidisciplinary team, including hematology/oncology, radiology, orthopedic, and radiation oncology services. The plain radiographs of the involved site show cortical destruction and onion skin periosteal reaction, which is highly suggestive of a malignant bone tumor. Laboratory studies include CBC with a differential, comprehensive metabolic panel, ESR, and LDH. Additional studies include MRI of the involved site, chest CT for the lung metastasis, bone marrow aspiration, and biopsy of the mass. Treatment of localized disease is surgery and radiotherapy for nonresectable or inadequately resected tumors. Neoadjuvant chemotherapy is necessary for extensive disease. Chemotherapeutic agents include vincristine, doxorubicin (Adriamycin), etoposide, cyclophosphamide, and ifosfamide. Prognosis depends on the tumor size, location, stage, surgical resection, and response to chemotherapy.

Pearls

1. Ewing sarcoma is unusual in African Americans.
2. Bone pain severe enough to wake up a child from sleep deserves further evaluation.
3. Radiographic appearance of Ewing sarcoma is a primarily lytic bone lesion with a characteristic onion-skinning periosteal reaction.

Chapter 12

RHEUMATOLOGY

Julie Cherian
Farzana Nuruzzaman
Sarah F. Taber

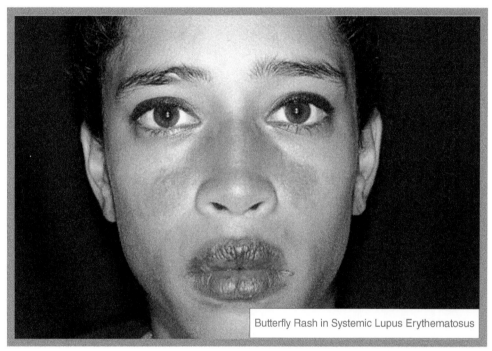

Butterfly Rash in Systemic Lupus Erythematosus

(Photo contributor: Binita R. Shah, MD)

The authors acknowledge the special contributions of Binita R. Shah, MD, to prior editions.

KAWASAKI DISEASE

Clinical Summary

Kawasaki disease (KD; also known as mucocutaneous lymph node syndrome) is a self-limited, medium-vessel vasculitis of unknown etiology. Prompt diagnosis and treatment prevent complications of KD, which include endothelial cell injury mainly in medium-sized arteries (in particular, coronary arteries) and systemic inflammation in multiple organs during the acute febrile phase of the disease. The risk of coronary artery aneurysm (CAA) is decreased from 25% to 4% by the timely administration of IV immunoglobulin (IVIG).

KD occurs in all ethnic groups; however, incidence is highest in Asians (in particular East Asians) and Pacific Islanders and is more common in boys compared to girls. In the continental United States, the incidence of KD is about 25 per 100,000 in children <5 years old. Clinical and epidemiologic features strongly implicate an infectious etiology, although no specific infectious trigger has been identified. Diagnosis of KD is largely based on clinical criteria, as summarized in Table 12.1, and exclusion of other similar disease presentations. Clinical features include extreme irritability, aseptic meningitis (50%), urethritis (sterile pyuria, 70%), hepatic dysfunction (40%), hydrops of gallbladder, diarrhea, vomiting, abdominal pain, arthritis or arthralgia (knees, ankles, hips), uveitis, pneumonitis, testicular swelling, peripheral gangrene, erythema, or induration at bacillus Calmette-Guérin (BCG) inoculation site.

KD should be considered in any child with prolonged unexplained fevers, but particularly in infants <6 months of age with fevers and irritability. Approximately 10% of children who develop CAA never meet criteria for KD. Clinicians should have a high index of suspicion because established clinical criteria do not, unfortunately, reliably identify all children with KD.

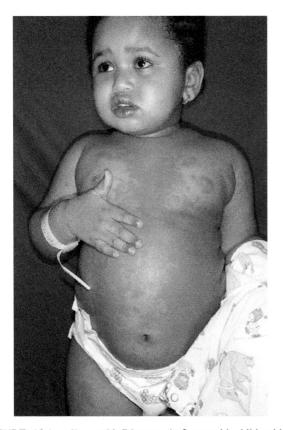

FIGURE 12.1 ■ Kawasaki Disease. A 3-year-old child with a history of high fever of 6 days in duration associated with diffuse erythematous maculopapular rash, red lips, and bilateral conjunctival injection. (Photo contributor: Binita R. Shah, MD.)

Emergency Department Treatment and Disposition

Obtain CBC (normal to elevated WBC count with a predominance of polymorphonuclear leukocytes and normocytic anemia), erythrocyte sedimentation rate (ESR), and C-reactive protein (CRP; usually elevated), liver enzymes (elevated with hypoalbuminemia), and urinalysis (sterile pyuria and proteinuria). Platelet counts are usually normal at onset of disease. Significant thrombocytosis (platelet count up to 1 million) occurs in the second week of illness and may indicate a longer duration of symptoms.

Be mindful of thrombocytopenia, anemia, or hyperferritinemia (>1000 ng/mL) because this may indicate early macrophage activation syndrome (see page 589), an emergent complication of KD. If clinically indicated, perform a lumbar puncture; CSF will show mild pleocytosis with normal glucose and usually normal protein. Obtain chest radiograph to look for cardiomegaly and an ECG for evidence of myocarditis, pericarditis, or arrhythmias. Admit patients with clinical diagnosis of KD or suspected incomplete KD (see page 567), for continuous cardiac monitoring and to initiate treatment with IVIG (2 g/kg; given as a single dose over 8–12 hours) and anti-inflammatory dose aspirin (80–100 mg/kg/day divided in 4 doses; given until patient is afebrile for at least

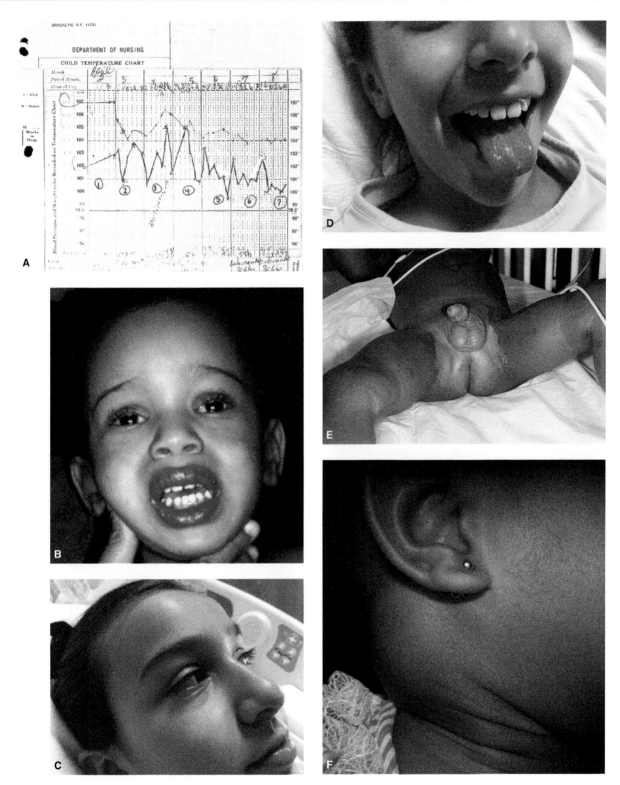

FIGURE 12.2 ■ Features of Kawasaki Disease (KD; Different Patients with KD). (**A**) Temperature curve in a typical untreated case of KD. With the administration of IV immunoglobulin on the seventh day of hospitalization (diagnosis of KD entertained), temperature returned to normal. (**B**) Red lips with fissuring, giving the appearance of red lipstick. (**C**) Nonexudative limbic-sparing conjunctivitis. (**D**) Red strawberry tongue. (**E**) Perineal desquamation seen in this 18-month-old infant with KD on the fourth day of illness. (**F**) Cervical adenopathy. (Photo contributors: Binita R. Shah, MD [A, B, E, F], and Julie Cherian, MD [C, D].)

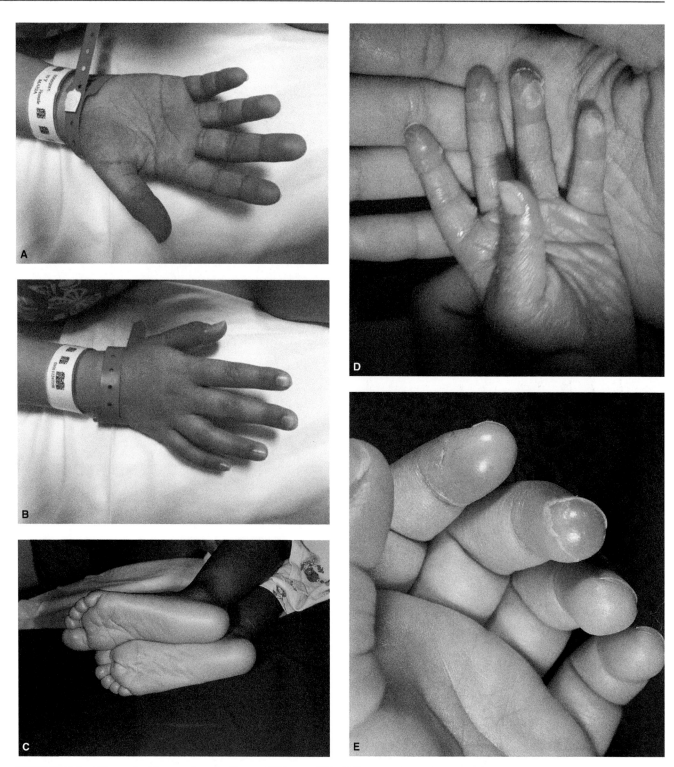

FIGURE 12.3 ■ Extremity Changes Seen in Kawasaki Disease (KD; Different Patients with KD). (**A, B**) Erythema and edema of the hands seen during acute phase of illness. (**C**) Erythema of the soles seen during acute phase of illness. (**D**) Erythema of the palm with desquamation of fingers, seen on the eighth day of illness (subacute phase; patient's hand against mother's hand). (**E**) Desquamation of the fingers on the 12th day of illness (subacute phase). (Photo contributors: Julie Cherian, MD [A, B], and Binita R. Shah, MD [C, D, E].)

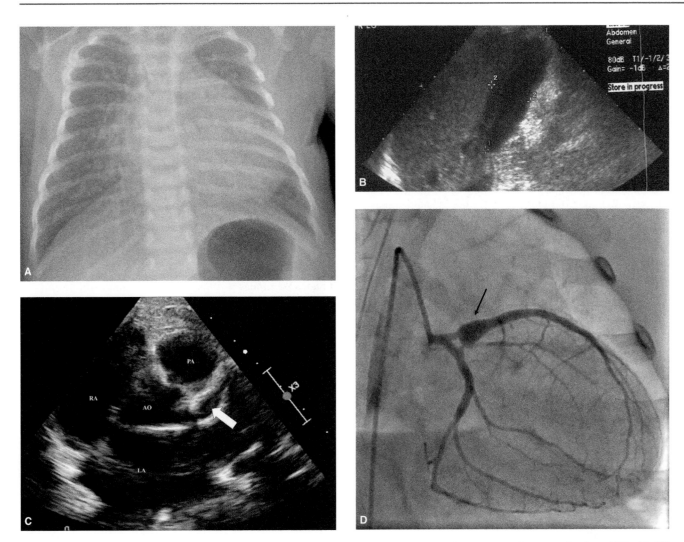

FIGURE 12.4 ▪ Kawasaki Disease (KD). (**A**) Frontal projection shows cardiomegaly and pulmonary vascular congestion in a child with KD presenting with evidence of myocarditis. During acute phase of KD, pericardium, myocardium, endocardium, cardiac valves and coronary arteries may be involved. (**B**) Sonogram of the right upper quadrant shows thick-walled, dilated gallbladder. Acute acalculous hydrops occurs in approximately 15% of patients during the first 2 weeks of the illness. (**C**) Coronary artery aneurysm (CAA). A 2-dimensional echocardiogram in a 5-year-old child with KD showing aneurysm of the left main coronary artery (arrow). AO, aorta; LA, left atrium; PA, pulmonary artery; RA, right atrium. (**D**) Angiogram of the left coronary artery in the same child as in part C. Arrow indicates left CAA. (Photo contributors: Rafael Rivera, MD [B], and Sushitha Surendran, MD [A, C, D].)

3–4 days) followed by antithrombotic dose aspirin (3–5 mg/kg/day as a single dose given until platelet count, ESR, and echocardiogram [ECHO] are normal). Low-dose aspirin therapy is continued indefinitely if a coronary artery abnormality is discovered. Consult cardiology on admission. Patient needs a 2-dimensional ECHO at baseline and during subsequent follow-up visits. If the diagnosis of KD is not certain or if the patient is not responding to conventional therapy, consultation with infectious disease or rheumatology is recommended.

TABLE 12.1 ■ CLINICAL FEATURES OF KAWASAKI DISEASE

Diagnosis is established clinically by:

Fever: high and unremitting (lasting ≥5 days, 4 days if the fever responds to IV immunoglobulin; unresponsive to antipyretics and antibiotics)

a. Presence of fever and at least 4 of the 5 criteria listed below not explained by another disease entity, *or*
b. Presence of fever and at least 3 of the 5 criteria listed below, and evidence of coronary artery abnormalities
   1. *Skin rash:* polymorphic (morbilliform, maculopapular, scarlatiniform, or erythema multiforme–like; nonvesicular); nonvesicular; commonly seen on trunk and extremities
   2. *Mucous membrane changes* (at least 1 of the following): erythematous or fissured lips; erythema of buccal mucosa and pharynx; "strawberry" tongue
   3. *Conjunctivitis:* bilateral limbic sparing bulbar involvement; nonexudative
   4. *Changes in distal extremities* (at least 1 of the following): erythema of palms or soles; indurative edema of hands or feet; periungual desquamation of fingers and toes (1–3 weeks after onset of illness)
   5. *Cervical lymphadenopathy* (least constant finding): unilateral; at least 1 node ≥1.5 cm in diameter; nonpurulent

Clinical phases (after onset of illness):

- *Acute febrile phase:* up to 1–2 weeks (fever and other acute signs)
- *Subacute phase:* up to 2–4 weeks (fever abated, desquamation, thrombocytosis, development of CAA
- *Convalescent phase:* up to 6–8 weeks (illness disappears, erythrocyte sedimentation rate and C-reactive protein return to normal, most children are asymptomatic, may have Beau lines [horizontal ridging of the nails])

Pearls

1. KD is the leading cause of acquired heart disease in children in developed countries. It is the most common systemic vasculitis seen in children.
2. Boys <1 year of age have the highest risk of developing CAA.

TABLE 12.2 ■ DIFFERENTIAL DIAGNOSIS OF KAWASAKI DISEASE

- Scarlet fever
- Viral infections (eg, measles, Epstein-Barr virus, enterovirus, adenovirus)
- Staphylococcal or streptococcal toxic shock syndrome
- Staphylococcal scalded skin syndrome
- Rocky Mountain spotted fever
- Shock/sepsis
- Bacterial adenitis/retropharyngeal phlegmon
- Aseptic meningitis
- Leptospirosis
- Hypersensitivity drug reactions (eg, Stevens-Johnson syndrome, erythema multiforme)
- Systemic-onset juvenile idiopathic arthritis
- Other vasculitides
- Mercury poisoning

3. Administration of IVIG in the acute phase (within 10 days of onset of fever) significantly reduces the prevalence of coronary artery dilation and aneurysms.
4. Perineal desquamation seen within the first week of illness in a highly febrile infant or child is an important early diagnostic clue.
5. A normal ECHO in the first week of illness does not rule out KD.
6. Leukopenia and a normal ESR in an infant or a child with fever, rash, and red eyes does not suggest a laboratory profile compatible with KD (suggests a viral infection).
7. Acute adenoviral infection shares many features of KD. Purulent conjunctivitis and exudative pharyngitis favor adenoviral infection, whereas perineal desquamation, extremity changes, and sterile pyuria point to KD.
8. Exudative conjunctivitis, Koplik spots, cough, and rash starting on face behind the ears and then becoming confluent and fading with a brownish hue are indicative of measles. KD rash is most prominent on the trunk and extremities and fades abruptly without residua. Perineal desquamation is a feature of KD and is not seen in measles.

Clinical Summary

Incomplete KD refers to children with symptoms suggestive of KD who fail to meet sufficient clinical criteria. This is in contrast to atypical KD, where all criteria are met but patients present with unusual features or complications. Incomplete KD is most commonly seen in young infants (<6 months old) and in older children (>5 years of age). Patients with incomplete KD do not have atypical features; rather, they do not fulfill the required criteria to confidently make the diagnosis of KD. Patients may present with high fevers for >5 days but have met <4 clinical criteria (see Table 12.1). Making a timely diagnosis of incomplete KD can be challenging, and these patients are at highest risk for coronary artery lesions and sudden cardiac death partly due to the delay in diagnosis.

Emergency Department Treatment and Disposition

Laboratory findings are similar, it should be noted, in both classic and incomplete KD (see KD, page 562, for more details). Incomplete KD can be considered in patients with a high clinical suspicion with elevated ESR and CRP and ≥3 supplemental laboratory findings or abnormal ECHO. The presence of mucous membrane changes is the most common clinical criterion seen in incomplete KD.

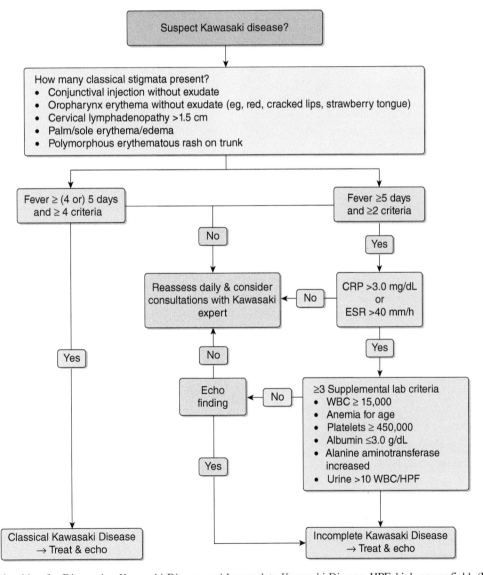

FIGURE 12.5 ■ Algorithm for Diagnosing Kawasaki Disease and Incomplete Kawasaki Disease. HPF, high-power field. (Reproduced with permission from Tenenbein M, Macias CG, Sharieff GQ, et al. *Strange and Schafermeyer's Pediatric Emergency Medicine*. 5th ed. McGraw-Hill Education; New York, NY, 2019.)

Pearls

1. A negative ECHO does not rule out incomplete KD.
2. Infants <1 year old may have prolonged fever and irritability as the only presenting signs and are at highest risk for coronary abnormalities. Consider incomplete KD in any infant (<6 months old) with prolonged and unexplained fever lasting for >5 days even in the absence of other clinical criteria.
3. Children with incomplete KD are more likely to be diagnosed later in the course of their disease.
4. Early diagnosis and prompt initiation of treatment with IVIG will result in improved outcomes.

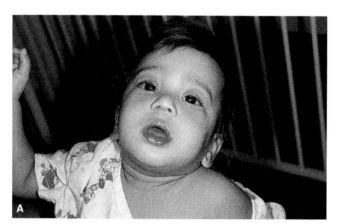

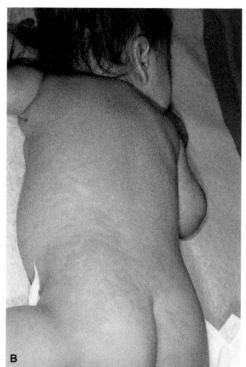

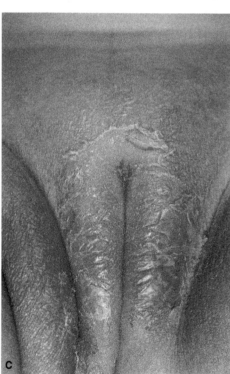

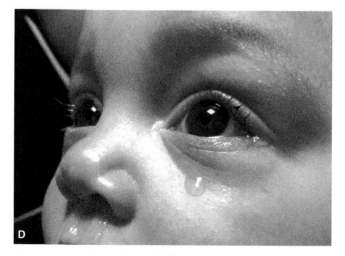

FIGURE 12.6 ■ Incomplete Kawasaki Disease (KD). Red lips (**A**), erythematous maculopapular rash (**B**), and perineal desquamation (**C**) in an infant presenting with fever (9 days in duration) not responding to either antibiotic (given for otitis media) or antipyretic therapy. This infant lacked extremity and eye findings and cervical adenopathy. (**D**) Nonexudative limbic sparing conjunctivitis is shown in another infant presenting with persistent fever later diagnosed with incomplete KD.

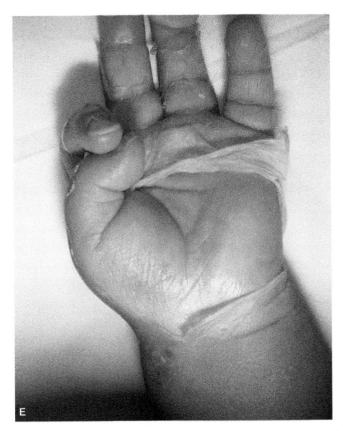

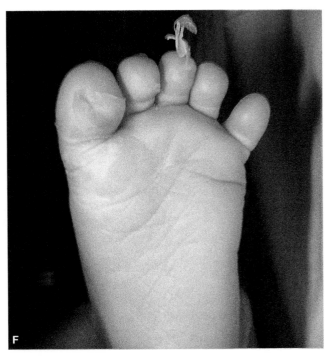

FIGURE 12.6 ■ (*Continued*) (**E, F**) Desquamation of the hand and foot are shown in an infant (not suspected of having KD) who remained extremely irritable and highly febrile and did not respond to IV antibiotics given for a clinical diagnosis of sepsis (all cultures negative). Prolonged fever followed by peripheral desquamation is among the most common signs of incomplete KD. (Photo contributors: Binita R. Shah, MD [A, B, C, E, F], and Ameer Hassoun, MD [D].)

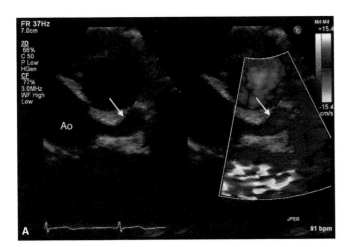

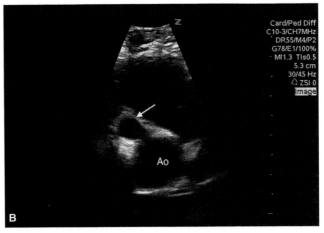

FIGURE 12.7 ■ Incomplete Kawasaki Disease (KD). (**A**) Transthoracic echocardiogram parasternal short axis view with 2-dimensional (2D) and color flow images in an 18-month-old infant with incomplete KD refractory to IVIG therapy. A giant fusiform aneurysm of the left main coronary artery (arrows) is seen. Ao, aorta. (**B**) Transthoracic echocardiogram parasternal short axis view 2D image in the same patient. Giant proximal right coronary artery aneurysm is seen (arrow). (Photo contributor: Kathleen E. Walsh-Spoonhower, MD.)

SYSTEMIC LUPUS ERYTHEMATOSUS

Clinical Summary

Systemic lupus erythematosus (SLE) is a multisystem auto-immune disease of complex etiology, characterized by production of autoantibodies and protean clinical manifestations. There is a genetic predisposition, making the disease more common and severe in African Americans, Latinos, and Asian Americans. Environmental (sunlight exposure) and hormonal factors also play a role. There is female predominance, and onset is usually after puberty. Certain drugs can lead to drug-induced SLE (eg, minocycline, hydralazine). Children with SLE may have an indolent presentation characterized by fevers, fatigue, and musculoskeletal complaints, or they may be acutely ill with life-threatening manifestations including renal failure, stroke, pulmonary hemorrhage, pancreatitis, psychosis, and cardiac tamponade. Patients may present with macrophage activation syndrome (MAS), with low cell counts, ESR, and fibrinogen, and elevated ferritin, liver function tests, lactate dehydrogenase (LDH), and D-dimer. Morbidity is often related to nephritis, neuropsychiatric involvement,

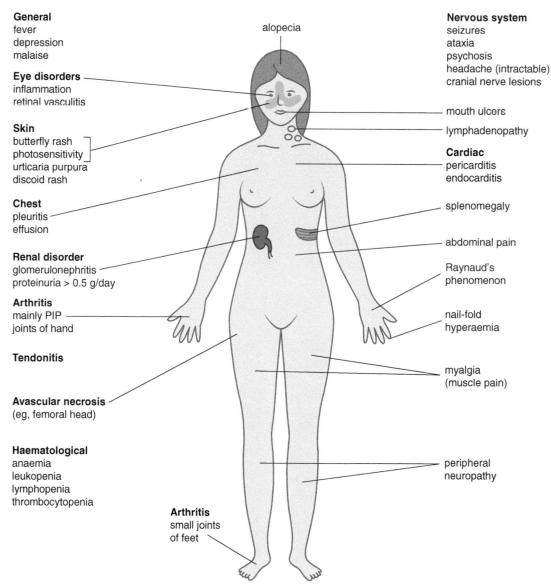

General
fever
depression
malaise

Eye disorders
inflammation
retinal vasculitis

Skin
butterfly rash
photosensitivity
urticaria purpura
discoid rash

Chest
pleuritis
effusion

Renal disorder
glomerulonephritis
proteinuria > 0.5 g/day

Arthritis
mainly PIP
joints of hand

Tendonitis

Avascular necrosis
(eg, femoral head)

Haematological
anaemia
leukopenia
lymphopenia
thrombocytopenia

Arthritis
small joints
of feet

alopecia

Nervous system
seizures
ataxia
psychosis
headache (intractable)
cranial nerve lesions

mouth ulcers

lymphadenopathy

Cardiac
pericarditis
endocarditis

splenomegaly

abdominal pain

Raynaud's
phenomenon

nail-fold
hyperaemia

myalgia
(muscle pain)

peripheral
neuropathy

FIGURE 12.8 ■ Clinical Features of Systemic Lupus Erythematosus. (Reproduced with permission from Murtagh J, Rosenblatt J, Coleman J, et al. *Murtagh's General Practice.* 7th ed. McGraw-Hill Education; New York, NY, 2018.)

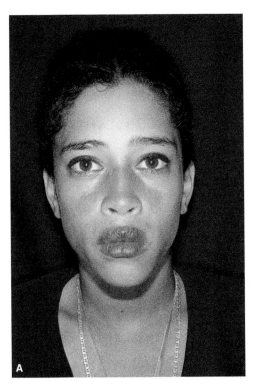
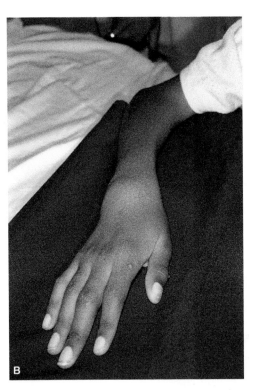

FIGURE 12.9 ▪ Systemic Lupus Erythematosus (SLE). (**A**) The butterfly rash, an erythematous macular blush or raised papules with fine scaling, is usually quite well demarcated. It is characteristically symmetrical, over both malar eminences and over the bridge of the nose, sparing the nasolabial folds. Malar rash is highly suggestive but not pathognomonic for SLE and may be seen in other rheumatologic diseases. The rash is photosensitive and may be precipitated by exposure to sunlight. (**B**) Arthritis of SLE. Arthralgias and arthritis are frequent presenting manifestations of SLE. Arthritis is polyarticular and may affect both large and small joints. (Photo contributor: Binita R. Shah, MD.)

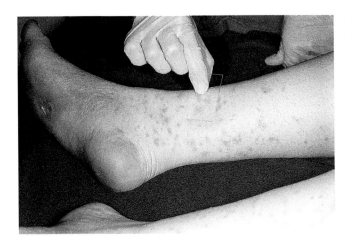

FIGURE 12.10 ▪ Systemic Lupus Erythematosus (SLE). Non-blanching lesions (petechiae and purpura with vasculitis) and ulcer on the sole are shown in an adolescent girl with SLE. (Photo contributor: Binita R. Shah, MD.)

infections, and therapeutic complications. Diagnosing pediatric SLE requires a high degree of clinical suspicion, and many children are initially misdiagnosed and mismanaged.

Emergency Department Treatment and Disposition

Obtain CBC with differential, platelet count, ESR, comprehensive metabolic panel, serum complements C3 and C4 (commonly reduced, especially with renal lupus), CRP, and urinalysis. If clinically indicated, obtain ECG (pericarditis), ECHO, and a CXR to look for pericardial effusion, pleural effusion, or other lung or cardiac involvement. In a patient with positive antiphospholipid antibodies, consider thrombotic events including venous sinus thrombosis, deep vein

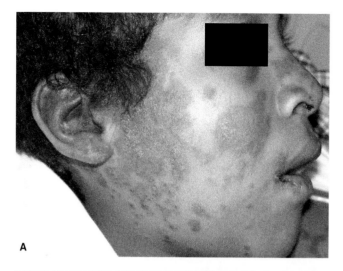

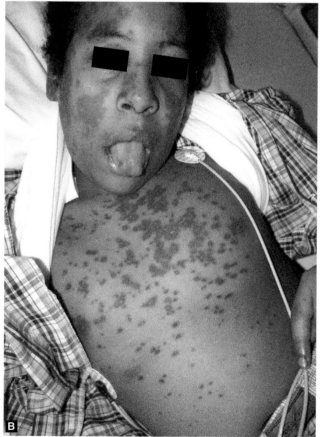

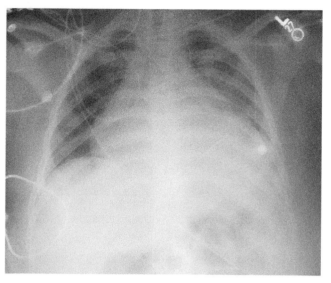

FIGURE 12.12 ▪ Systemic Lupus Erythematosus (SLE) with Serositis. Frontal view of the chest shows cardiomegaly that was secondary to a large pericardial effusion in an adolescent patient with SLE requiring sternotomy for a pericardial window. (Photo contributor: John Amodio, MD.)

FIGURE 12.11 ▪ Systemic Lupus Erythematosus. (A) An 8-year-old male with discoid lesions consisting of purple erythematous plaques with overlying scale seen on the ear and lateral cheek. (B) Malar cheek rash with scaling and erythema, papules, and coalescing red to purple discoid plaques are seen on the chest. Note ulceration of the tongue. (Photo contributor: Binita R. Shah, MD.)

thrombosis (DVT), and pulmonary embolism. Immunologic tests, including antinuclear antibody (ANA); anti–double-stranded DNA (anti-dsDNA); antibodies to Sm nuclear antigen, Ro, La, and RNP; and antiphospholipid antibodies, may help make the diagnosis. Many patients are immunosuppressed due to treatment; consider comprehensive infectious workup including blood, urine, and CSF cultures if indicated. Patients with concern for MAS (shock, bleeding, fevers, mental status changes) should have full MAS labs sent in addition to the above, including D-dimer, fibrinogen, coagulation profile, LDH, and ferritin.

Admit all patients with nephritis, pericarditis, CNS lupus, and complications of therapy such as infection with neutropenia. Patients may be on chronic high doses of steroids and may require stress-dose hydrocortisone. Consult rheumatology and other specialty services as appropriate. Refer stable patients to a pediatric rheumatologist for long-term management. Treatment options include NSAIDs, antimalarial drugs (eg, hydroxychloroquine), immunosuppressive agents (eg, cyclophosphamide, mycophenolate mofetil, and rituximab), and systemic corticosteroids in daily or pulse doses.

TABLE 12.3 ■ CLINICAL FEATURES OF SYSTEMIC LUPUS ERYTHEMATOSUS

The American College of Rheumatology classification of SLE requires the *presence of 4 of the following 11 criteria* (a person is said to have SLE if any 4 or more of the 11 criteria are present, *serially or simultaneously,* during an interval of observation).

1. Photosensitivity (skin rash as a result of an unusual reaction to sunlight)
2. Malar rash (affects ~60% of patients; butterfly distribution on face, spares nasolabial folds; macular erythematous blush or erythematous papules)
3. Oral or nasopharyngeal ulcers (affects ~85% of patients; painless)
4. Discoid lupus (uncommon in children; deeper lesions showing atrophy, adherent scales, hyper- and hypopigmentation, erythema, scarring; most common on face and scalp)
5. Arthritis (affects ~15% of patients; nonerosive arthritis involving small joints of hands or large joints, characterized by tenderness, swelling, or effusion)
6. Serositis (pleurisy, pericarditis, ascites)
7. Renal lupus (affects ~50%–90% of children; diagnosed by persistent proteinuria >0.5 g/d or 3+ if quantitation not performed, RBCs and cellular casts in urine)
8. CNS lupus (eg, psychosis, seizures, encephalopathy, myelitis, coma, stroke, peripheral neuropathy, migraines)
9. Hematologic lupus (anemia [hemolytic with positive direct Coombs test or anemia of chronic disease], leukopenia, lymphopenia, thrombocytopenia)
10. Positive antinuclear antibody
11. Immunologic tests (anti-dsDNA, anti-Sm, antiphospholipid antibodies)

Other Clinical Features of SLE

Alopecia, Raynaud phenomenon, vasculitis with palpable purpura and petechiae, urticaria, angioedema, vesicobullous SLE, deep vein thrombosis, cerebrovascular accidents, digital ulceration, fever, myalgia, arthralgia, poor weight gain, depression, hepatosplenomegaly, lymphadenopathy

Pearls

1. The most common clinical presentations of SLE are cutaneous, renal, hematologic, and musculoskeletal. Consider SLE in the differential diagnosis of many signs and symptoms ranging from fevers of unknown origin to arthralgia, anemia, and nephritis. Patients may have a prolonged course with multiple ED visits for fever and malaise or may be acutely ill at presentation.

2. CNS lupus may present with psychosis and seizures.

3. Patients with antiphospholipid antibodies may have thrombotic events including DVT, stroke, and pulmonary embolism.

4. Patients on long term steroids may require stress dosing and patients on any immunosuppressant (including steroids) may require treatment for sepsis or other severe infections.

Clinical Summary

Neonatal lupus (NL) is caused by transplacental passage of maternal autoantibodies to the fetus and is characterized by skin lesions, congenital heart block (CHB; prolongation of PR interval to complete heart block), cytopenias, and/or hepatic involvement. The majority of antibodies are maternal anti-Ro (also known as SSA) and/or anti-La (also known as SSB). Mothers of babies with NL may have clinical features of either Sjögren syndrome or SLE or may be asymptomatic. Skin lesions occur in 15% to 25% of affected infants and are either present at birth or appear later with sun exposure. Erythematous annular or elliptical macules with slight central atrophy and raised active margins are seen primarily in the periorbital region and scalp but may be present in other areas as well. The rash may be confused with other, more common rashes of infancy. Lesions disappear in 6 to 8 months, usually without scarring or atrophy. Complete heart block may be diagnosed in utero or at birth, and the infant may be asymptomatic, may require a pacemaker, or may develop signs of congestive heart failure. Other arrhythmias, cardiomyopathy, and endocardial fibroelastosis may also develop in these infants. Other findings of NL include anemia, leukopenia, thrombocytopenia, hepatomegaly, and cholestatic hepatitis. Infants with NL may be at risk of developing other autoimmune diseases during childhood or adolescence.

Emergency Department Treatment and Disposition

Obtain CBC with differential and platelet count, comprehensive metabolic panel, CXR, and ECG. Additional tests include anti-Ro/SSA, anti-La/SSB, and antinuclear antibody. Admit all symptomatic infants (eg, those with CHB or signs of congestive heart failure, severe cytopenias, or significant liver involvement) for further management. Refer asymptomatic patients to cardiology for follow-up and to dermatology, if the diagnosis is unclear. For cutaneous lesions, sunscreen, protective clothing, and mild topical corticosteroids may be used. Refer the mother to a rheumatologist for the workup for SLE or other connective tissue disease.

Pearls

1. The skin lesions of NL are benign and self-resolve. The most serious manifestation is CHB, which is permanent. Patients may also have cytopenias and liver involvement, which are typically mild but may be severe.
2. Periorbital "owl-eye" appearance of the facial rash is an important clue for the diagnosis.
3. The NL rash is often misdiagnosed as seborrheic or atopic dermatitis, psoriasis, or tinea (faciei or corporis).
4. The presence of anti-Ro/SSA antibodies in the infant or mother confirms the diagnosis of NL in patients with typical rash or cardiac involvement.

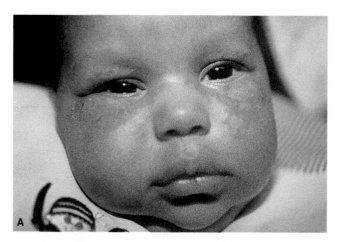

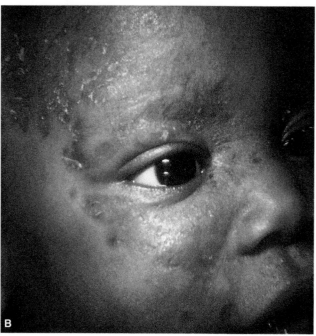

FIGURE 12.13 ■ Neonatal Lupus (NL). (**A, B**) Characteristic periorbital "owl-eye" appearance with erythematous, scaly, and atrophic changes in 2 different infants with NL. (Photo contributor: Binita R. Shah, MD.)

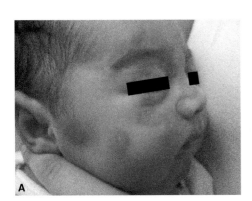
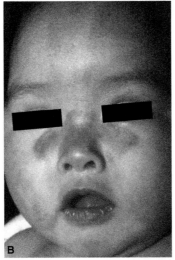
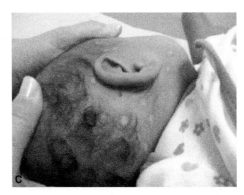

FIGURE 12.14 ■ Neonatal Lupus (NL). (**A**) Erythematous annular plaques with scaling are seen around the periorbital area and face in a neonate with NL. (**B**) A butterfly rash involving both malar eminences and the bridge of the nose is seen in an infant with NL. (**C**) Annular plaques with hypopigmentation are seen in an infant with NL. (Photo contributors: Ee Tay, MD [A], Binita R. Shah, MD [B], and Sharon A. Glick, MD [C].)

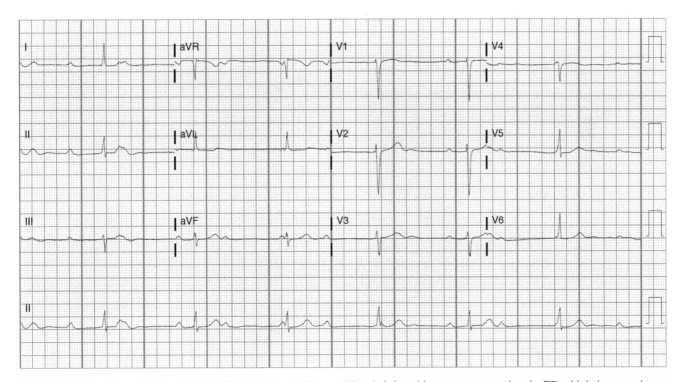

FIGURE 12.15 ■ Complete Heart Block (CHB) in Neonatal Lupus (NL). A 6-day-old neonate presented to the ED with lethargy and poor feeding. This 12-lead ECG shows a CHB with a ventricular rate of 40 bpm. Mother had a history of systemic lupus erythematosus. Infants with CHB may require a pacemaker. First- or second-degree heart block found at birth can progress to CHB; however, if there is no evidence of any heart block in utero or at birth, there is little risk of later cardiac involvement in such patients. (Photo contributor: Sushitha Surendran, MD.)

Clinical Summary

Raynaud phenomenon (RP; also known as Raynaud syndrome) is an exaggerated vasospastic response most commonly affecting the arterioles of the hands. RP is classified as *primary* when there is no underlying cause or *secondary* when it is associated with systemic disease (eg, SLE, scleroderma, polymyositis/dermatomyositis, rheumatoid arthritis, mixed connective tissue disease, Sjögren syndrome) or vascular disease. Primary RP is more common and seen in girls more often than boys. Physical examination is normal between attacks. Secondary RP may be associated with typical findings of underlying disease. Diagnosis is made by a history of episodic well-demarcated digital discoloration induced by cold exposure or stress with delayed recovery of vascular flow. Differential diagnosis of RP includes acrocyanosis (usually painless, persistent cyanosis of distal extremities due to

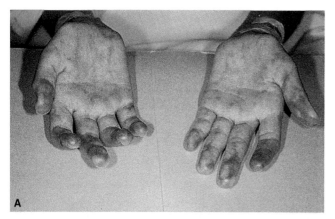

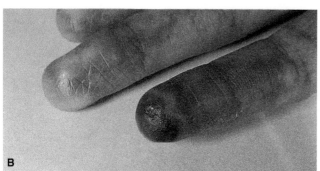

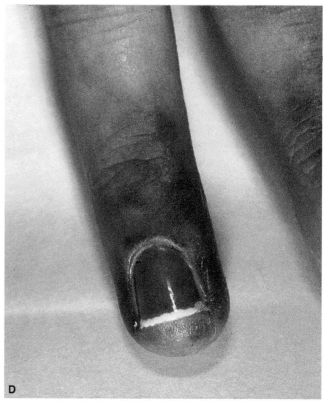

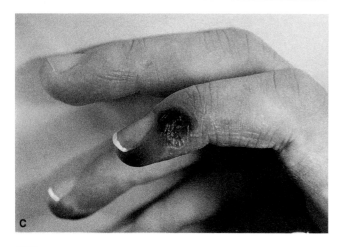

FIGURE 12.16 ■ Raynaud Phenomenon (RP). (**A**) A 15-year-old adolescent girl, diagnosed with SLE 2 years ago, presented with these changes in the fingers of both hands associated with severe pain. She moved 2 weeks prior to the appearance of this discoloration from Colombia to New York City during extremely cold weather. She started experiencing pain and tingling in both hands 6 days before this presentation; the color change in the fingers progressed from white to blue to patchy red with ulcerations on the fingertips. She also had a malar rash. (**B**) Close-up of the fingers, showing cyanosis, ulceration, and hyperemia. (**C**) Close-up of the fingers showing the ulceration (1 × 1 cm) on the distal phalanx and cyanosis. (**D**) Close-up of nail showing duskiness. (Photo contributor: Binita R. Shah, MD.)

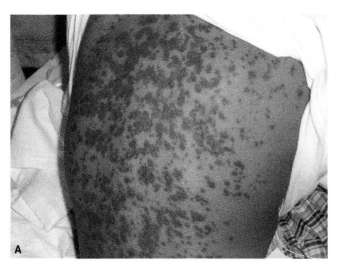
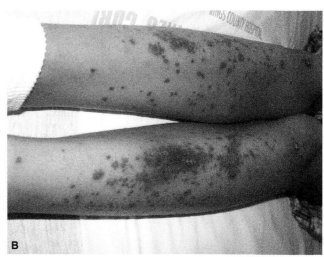

FIGURE 12.17 ■ Systemic Lupus Erythematosus (SLE). The most common cause of secondary Raynaud phenomenon (RP) is connective tissue diseases. About 20% or more of SLE patients have secondary RP, which may precede other signs and symptoms of SLE by months or years. Shown here is a patient with SLE with widespread purple papules and plaques with overlying scale on the back (**A**) and legs (**B**). This patient had extensive lesions of lupus on the face and trunk (see Figure 12.11). (Photo contributor: Shyam Sathanandam, MD.)

TABLE 12.4 ■ CLINICAL FEATURES OF RAYNAUD PHENOMENON

Precipitating factors for RP:
- Cold ambient temperature
- Emotional stress
- Drugs (eg, tobacco, caffeine, antihistamines, decongestants, amphetamines, cocaine, ergots)

Color changes: triphasic, biphasic, or monophasic.

Classic *triphasic color response*
- Pallor (initial spasm leading to decreased cutaneous blood flow), affected digits cold, numb, painful
- Cyanosis (blue-purple discoloration resulting from deoxygenated venous blood in capillary bed)
- Hyperemia (red color with resolution of vasospasm, increased blood flow with reopening of digital arteries with resultant blushing)

Biphasic color changes may be white to red or blue to red

Monophasic color changes are white or blue or a mottled appearance

Primary RP	*Secondary RP*
• Symmetric, bilateral, episodic attacks	• Asymmetric, painful attacks
• Absence of tissue necrosis in distal extremities	• Ischemia proximal to fingers and toes
• Normal nailfold capillaroscopy	• Abnormal nailfold capillaroscopy
• Negative ANA and normal ESR	• Abnormal lab parameters consistent with underlying vascular or autoimmune disorder

exaggerated vasomotor response that can occur at any age), chilblains or perniosis (painful, erythematous papules or nodules, induced by cold without blanching), and frostbite (see Figures 18.5 to 18.8).

Emergency Department Treatment and Disposition

Diagnosis of RP may be made with characteristic history alone. History may be suggestive of underlying connective tissue disease or possible associated or precipitating factors. Examine BP, pulses, and nailfold capillaroscopy to suggest systemic disease in secondary RP. If there is clinical suspicion of a secondary cause of RP, obtain a CBC, electrolytes, renal and liver function, urinalysis, complement (C3 and C4), and ANA. Refer patient to rheumatology for further diagnostic workup if secondary RP is suspected. Educate patients about avoidance of potential triggers including cold exposure, smoking, and stress. Outpatient management includes pharmacologic treatments including calcium channel blockers (eg, nifedipine), phosphodiesterase inhibitors (eg, sildenafil), pentoxifylline, and topical nitroglycerin.

Admit patients with severe digital ischemia, uncontrolled pain, or impending digital amputation. Immediate evaluation to identify reversible vascular and coagulation defects is critical. Control pain with narcotic analgesic or regional nerve block. Aggressive vasodilator therapy and antiplatelet therapy can be used initially to restore blood flow. Transdermal nitroglycerin, sympatholytic agents, or even heparin is suggested if digital ischemia progresses. Sympathectomy, vascular reconstruction, or even surgical amputation may be required.

Pearls

1. Patients with RP classically describe triphasic color changes in the digits; however, not every patient has all 3 phases.
2. Ulcerations and areas of digital gangrene can be seen in severe cases.

Clinical Summary

Juvenile dermatomyositis (JDM) is a systemic disease with chronic inflammation of striated muscle and skin leading to primarily proximal muscle weakness and characteristic skin rashes, but it can affect any organ. Preceding infection, stress, and ultraviolet light exposure in genetically predisposed individuals lead to an immune complex–mediated vasculopathy, autoantibody production, and a pronounced type I interferon response. Childhood-onset disease typically occurs between age 5 and 14 years, with a median age of 7 years. There is a 2:1 female predominance in JDM, and it typically presents with an insidious onset of malaise, fatigue, weight loss, photosensitive rashes, and proximal muscle weakness. Up to a third of children may have more acute onset of proximal muscle weakness. Children may show Gower or Trendelenburg signs. The Bohan and Peter Classification Criteria have been used for diagnosis. Differential diagnosis includes other causes of muscle weakness in children. Diagnostic delay and untreated disease lead to calcinosis, a major source of morbidity. In contrast to adult-onset dermatomyositis, there is no increased risk of malignancy in children with JDM.

Emergency Department Treatment and Disposition

Assess airway muscle involvement by monitoring ventilatory effort and swallowing. Suctioning and respiratory assistance may be needed. Evaluate for internal organ involvement as appropriate including respiratory insufficiency, myocarditis, and acute gastrointestinal (GI) ulceration with perforation. Admit patients with respiratory difficulty or those at risk for aspiration, patients with acute onset of muscle weakness, or patients with acute manifestations of internal organ involvement after appropriate consultations (eg, surgery and gastroenterology for acute GI ulceration with perforation).

Acute treatment for moderate to severe JDM includes pulse dose steroids to gain rapid control and minimize long-term corticosteroid exposure. Consult rheumatology and neurology as indicated.

Obtain muscle enzymes (eg, creatine kinase, aspartate aminotransferase, LDH, aldolase) and von Willebrand factor (marker of endothelial damage that may be elevated in active disease). Immunologic tests including ANA, anti-Jo-1,

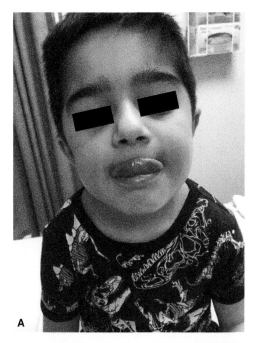

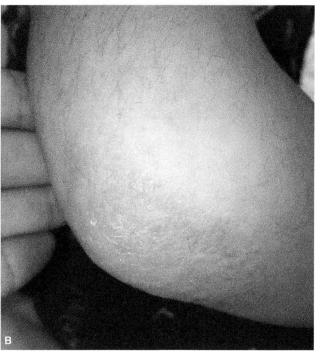

FIGURE 12.18 ■ Dermatomyositis. A 5-year-old boy with a 2-month history of nonresolving facial rash (**A**) and Gottron sign, an erythematous papulosquamous eruption overlying extensor aspects of elbow (**B**). He also had muscle weakness associated with muscle enzyme elevations. The rash on the elbow can mimic psoriasis and can also be seen over knees and medial malleoli. (Note: There is no pathology on the tongue; he is just sticking his tongue out at you!) (Photo contributor: Christy Beneri, MD.)

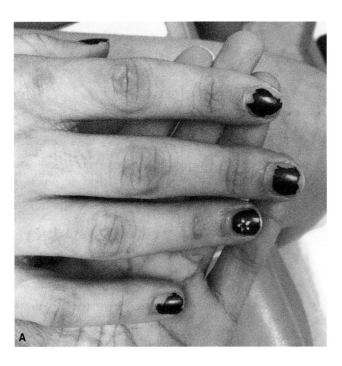

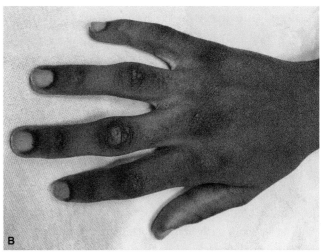

FIGURE 12.19 ■ Gottron Papules; Dermatomyosis. (**A**) Gottron papules are shown in a 14-year-old girl presenting with a facial rash and rash overlying the knuckles of her hands associated with mild muscle weakness. (**B**) Gottron papules are shown in a 17-year-old male with insidious 9-month history of worsening muscle weakness and rash on his eyelids and over the knuckles of his hands. (Photo contributors: Julie Cherian, MD [A], and Farzana Nuruzzaman, MD [B].)

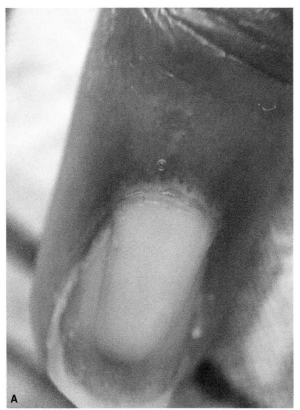

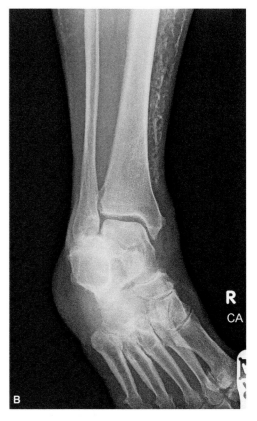

FIGURE 12.20 ■ Dermatomyosis. (**A**) Capillaroscopy examination showing dilatation, tortuosity, and drop-out of nailfold capillaries in a 17-year-old female who presented at age 14 with muscle weakness, rash, and Raynaud phenomenon. (**B**) Oblique view of the right ankle demonstrates multiple, relatively linear soft tissue calcifications secondary to dermatomyosis (Photo contributors: David Fernandez, MD, PhD [A], and John Amodio, MD [B].)

TABLE 12.5 ■ JUVENILE DERMATOMYOSITIS: CRITERIA FOR THE DIAGNOSIS OF DERMATOMYOSITIS AND POLYMYOSITIS

Definite disease: for dermatomyositis, inclusion of the rash and presence of 3 other criteria; for polymyositis, exclusion of rash and presence of the other 4 criteria.

Probable disease: for dermatomyositis, inclusion of the rash and presence of 2 other criteria; for polymyositis, exclusion of rash and presence of 3 other criteria.

1. Symmetric, often progressive proximal and axial weakness
2. Characteristic rashes of dermatomyositis (required)
   a. Scaly, erythematous papules over the metacarpophalangeal or interphalangeal joints, elbows, knees, or medial malleoli (Gottron papules) OR
   b. Purplish or erythematous discoloration of the eyelids (heliotrope rash)
3. Elevation of serum levels of muscle-associated enzymes, including creatine kinase, aldolase, lactate dehydrogenase, transaminases
4. Characteristic electromyographic changes in a triad, including:
   a. Short-duration, small, low-amplitude polyphasic potentials
   b. Fibrillation potentials, positive sharp waves, and insertional irritability, present even at rest
   c. Bizarre high-frequency repetitive discharges
5. Evidence of chronic inflammation on muscle biopsy, including the presence of necrosis of type I and type II muscle fibers, degeneration and regeneration of myofibers with variation in myofiber size, perivascular and interstitial infiltration of mononuclear cells, and perifascicular atrophy

These criteria require exclusion of all other forms of myopathies.
Data from Bohan A, Peter JB. Polymyositis and dermatomyositis (first of two parts). *N Engl J Med.* 1975;292:344-347. Bohan A, Peter JB. Polymyositis and dermatomyositis (second of two parts). *N Engl J Med.* 1975;292:403-407.
Reproduced from Kline MW, Blaney SM, Giardino AP, et al. *Rudolph's Pediatrics.* 23rd ed. McGraw-Hill Education; New York, NY, 2017, Table 202.4.

anti-synthetase, anti-Mi2, and anti-SRP antibodies may also be sent. Edema on T2-weighted MRI of affected limbs suggests active disease, whereas fibrosis, atrophy, and fatty infiltration on T1-weighted MRI indicates chronic disease.

Radiographs may also show calcinosis. Refer stable patients to a pediatric rheumatologist for long-term management. Treatment options for steroid-sparing agents include methotrexate and IVIG.

TABLE 12.6 ■ DIFFERENTIAL DIAGNOSIS OF JUVENILE DERMATOMYOSITIS

Infectious myopathies
- Viral: enterovirus, coxsackie, influenza
- Bacterial: *Staphylococcus, Streptococcus*
- Parasitic: trichinosis, toxoplasmosis, Lyme borreliosis

Other idiopathic inflammatory myopathies, such as juvenile polymyositis

Noninflammatory myopathies
- Congenital myopathies
- Muscular dystrophies
- Metabolic myopathies, such as lipid disorders or glycogen storage diseases
- Endocrinopathies
- Drug-induced myopathy
- Toxins, such as botulinum, insecticides

Other systemic rheumatic diseases, such as MCTD, vasculitis, SLE

Abbreviation: MCTD, mixed connective tissue disease.

Pearls

1. Consider pharyngeal, hypopharyngeal, and palatal muscle involvement in patients presenting with changes in phonation, nasal speech, regurgitation, or difficulty swallowing.
2. Patients with vasculopathy may present with mesenteric infarction, leading to melena or hematemesis and GI perforation.
3. Calcinosis can lead to cellulitis and cause flexion contractures.
4. Amyopathic dermatomyositis, characterized by only skin manifestations, can occur rarely in the pediatric population.
5. Patients with JDM have an increased risk of X-linked agammaglobulinemia.

JUVENILE IDIOPATHIC ARTHRITIS

Clinical Summary

Chronic arthritis in childhood is a genetically diverse group of systemic inflammatory diseases affecting joints and other structures. Juvenile idiopathic arthritis (JIA) is the current terminology established by the International League of Associations for Rheumatology to classify idiopathic chronic arthritides of childhood that can have both quiescent periods and intermittent flares. Arthritis is defined as pain, swelling, or limitation of motion in a joint and is associated with morning stiffness. JIA must begin before the 16th birthday and persist for at least 6 weeks and be of unknown etiology. Pathogenesis is thought to be related to alterations of adaptive immunity, genetic factors, and environmental triggers. IgA deficiency, HLA-B27 positivity, and family history of psoriasis or inflammatory bowel disease are associated with prolonged or recurrent arthritis.

Typical presentations of the different subtypes are listed in Table 12.7. These subtypes affect prognosis and different responses to medications.

Treatment may include NSAIDs, intra-articular steroids, systemic corticosteroids, disease-modifying antirheumatic drugs (DMARDs), and biologic agents, depending on subtype. Untreated JIA can lead to irreversible joint damage in the growing skeleton of children; thus, diagnosis and referral to pediatric rheumatology outpatient care are critical. Complications include uveitis, limb-length discrepancy, and bony

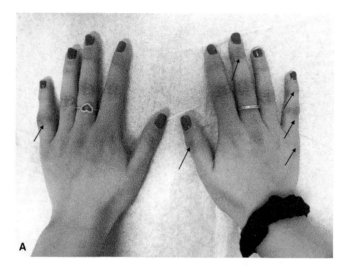

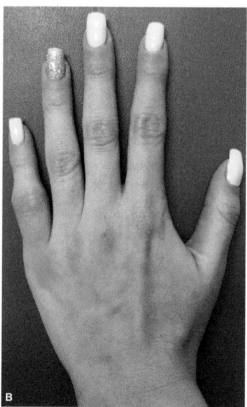

FIGURE 12.22 ■ Polyarticular Juvenile Idiopathic Arthritis. (**A**) Arthritis of bilateral proximal interphalangeal (PIP; fifth fingers), distal interphalangeal (DIP; right fifth, third, and first fingers), and metacarpophalangeal (right fifth finger) joints is shown in this 16-year-old girl with a several-month history of finger pain and ankle pain. Labs notable for rheumatoid factor (RF)/cyclic citrullinated peptide (CCP) positivity, anemia, and elevated ESR. (**B**) Arthritis of left fifth PIP and DIP is shown in this 15-year-old girl with a several-month history of multiple finger pains and morning stiffness. She was found to be RF/CCP positive. This image is after treatment with methotrexate, and eventually, she required biologic therapy due to persistent arthritis. (Photo contributor: Farzana Nuruzzaman, MD.)

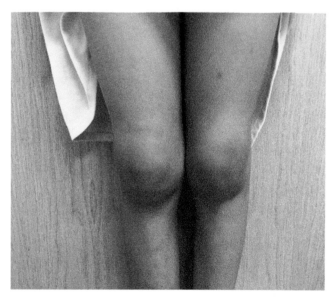

FIGURE 12.21 ■ Oligoarticular Juvenile Idiopathic Arthritis. An 8-year-old girl presented with joint pain, swelling, and morning stiffness for a few months. She was found to be ANA positive. She was previously treated with methotrexate. She is shown here with a flare of bilateral knee arthritis. (Photo contributor: Farzana Nuruzzaman, MD.)

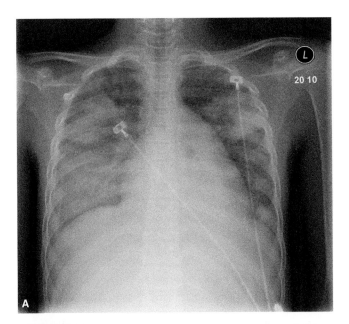

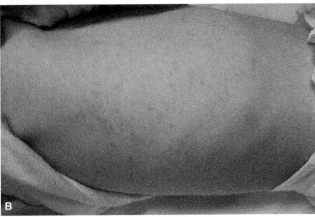

FIGURE 12.23 ■ Systemic-Onset Juvenile Idiopathic Arthritis (JIA). (**A**) Single anteroposterior view of the chest demonstrates patchy airspace opacities and right pleural effusion in a patient with JIA. (**B**) Salmon-pink rash in systemic-onset JIA. (Photo contributor: John Amodio, MD [A], and [B] reproduced with permission from Kline MW, *Rudolph's Pediatrics*. 23rd ed. McGraw-Hill Education; New York, NY, 2018.)

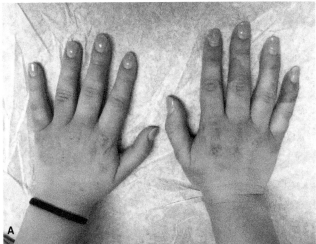

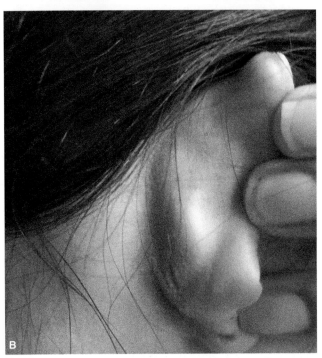

FIGURE 12.24 ■ Psoriatic Arthritis. (**A**) Symmetrically distributed, sharply demarcated erythematous psoriatic plaques overlying the dorsum of hands and arthritis of metacarpophalangeal joints are seen in this 13-year-old girl with psoriasis presenting with finger pain and swelling. (**B**) Psoriasis behind ear is seen in the same patient. (Photo contributor: Farzana Nuruzzaman, MD.)

deformities such as joint subluxation, cervical spine fusion, or micrognathia from temporomandibular joint involvement.

Emergency Department Treatment and Disposition

For Patients Suspected of Having Juvenile Idiopathic Arthritis

It is essential to exclude other potential etiologies, including trauma and infectious, orthopedic, and oncologic (eg, leukemia) causes of limb pain, before the diagnosis of JIA can be made.

A consistent history and examination usually makes the diagnosis of JIA once alternate diagnoses are excluded. Laboratory tests such as CBC with differential, ESR, and comprehensive metabolic panel can be useful in assessing disease

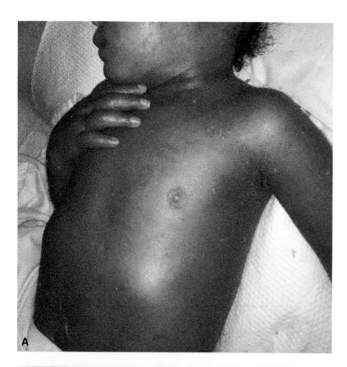

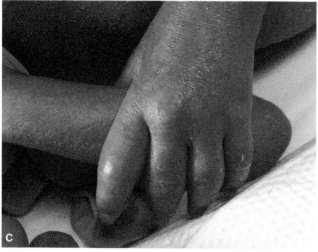

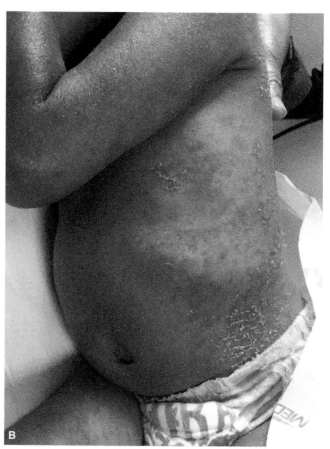

FIGURE 12.25 ■ Erythrodermic Psoriasis with Arthritis. (**A, B**) This 3-year-old girl was admitted with erythroderma that was mistaken as staphylococcal scalded skin syndrome, for which she received antibiotics in the ED (**A**, picture taken on the day of admission; and **B**, picture taken on day 5 of hospitalization). She had received systemic steroids 4 days prior to this admission for this rash that was thought to be atopic dermatitis. Acute psoriasis was confirmed by skin biopsy, and she was started on methotrexate with improvement of the arthritis. Subsequently she was treated with Enbrel, and her skin is now clear without arthritis. (**C**) Sausage-shaped fingers. (Photo contributors: Rachel Levene, MD [A], and Sharon A. Glick, MD [B, C].)

activity. Immunologic tests include ANA, rheumatoid factor, and anti-cyclic citrullinated peptide antibodies. Radiographs for JIA early in presentation may be normal or only show periarticular swelling. Late findings include joint space narrowing, osteopenia, and joint destruction. Musculoskeletal US with Doppler can be used to assess thickened synovial membrane, effusion, and hyperemia. Optimal long-term management necessitates referral to pediatric rheumatology.

Untreated JIA can lead to Baker cyst formation (popliteal synovial cyst), which may dissect from the knee to the calf, causing redness, swelling, and a positive Hoffman sign, mimicking a DVT of the lower extremity. Complications of an enlarged or ruptured cyst may lead to venous obstruction, nerve entrapment, or acute compartment syndrome, if severe. A ruptured cyst can also lead to ecchymosis below the medial malleolus ("crescent sign"). Similarly, a bicipital synovial

TABLE 12.7 ■ JUVENILE IDIOPATHIC ARTHRITIS (JIA)

Type	Frequency	Age at Onset	Gender	Arthritis	Joints
Systemic arthritis	10%–20%	Childhood	F = M	Symmetrical Polyarticular	Large and small
Oligoarthritis	50%–60%	Early childhood(<6y)	F >>> M	Asymmetric	Lower extremities
RF [+] polyarthritis	5%–10%	Late childhood/ adolescence	F >> M	Symmetric	Small joints (+/– large joints)
RF [−] polyarthritis	20%–30%	Childhood	F >> M	Asymmetric or symmetric	Large and small
Enthesitis-related arthritis	1%–7%	Late childhood/ adolescence	M >> F	Oligoarticular	Lower extremities Axial skeleton SI joints
Psoriatic arthritis Undifferentiated arthritis	2%–15% 11%–21%	Childhood		Asymmetrical Oligoarticular	Small and large

ILAR, International League of Associations for Rheumatology; RF, rheumatoid factor.
Reproduced with permission from Tenenbein M, Macias CG, Sharieff GQ, et al. *Strange and Schafermeyer's Pediatric Emergency Medicine*. 5th ed. McGraw-Hill Education; New York, NY, 2019.

cyst may cause acute painful upper arm swelling. Treatment includes rest, elevation, and analgesics. Arthrocentesis and intra-articular steroid injections by orthopedic surgeons and/or rheumatologists can also be considered for severe cases.

A child with uncontrolled JIA may also develop tenosynovitis of the superior oblique muscle, leading to inability to elevate the eye, particularly when adducted (acquired Brown syndrome). Treatment of this type of tenosynovitis includes NSAIDs, oral steroids, or steroids injected into the superonasal orbit around the trochlea by an ophthalmologist.

A child with unrecognized JIA may also develop an indolent chronic anterior uveitis and present with difficulties in vision. Diagnosis requires slit-lamp examination by an ophthalmologist as it can lead to eventual cataracts, glaucoma, band keratopathy, and even blindness if not recognized in a timely fashion. Treatment includes steroid eye drops, mydriatics, DMARDs, and biologic agents.

For Patients with a Known Diagnosis of Juvenile Idiopathic Arthritis

If a patient with JIA who is on immunosuppressive therapy presents with a fever, obtain a CBC with differential, microbial cultures, and viral studies to look for underlying infection. The patient may need hospitalization for antimicrobial therapy and infectious disease consultation.

In a child with systemic-onset JIA who presents with a fever, additionally consider a flare of the disease itself or MAS (see page 589). It may be difficult to distinguish infection from disease flares or MAS, and therefore, both should be considered and possibly treated. Consider evaluation for internal organ involvement in patients with systemic-onset JIA based on other presenting complaints. Initial treatment for systemic-onset JIA usually includes corticosteroids. Further management and consultations are indicated based on involved organ system—for example, drainage of pericardial effusions, diuretics, afterload-reducing agents, and management of arrhythmias for myocarditis; oxygen and management of superinfections for pleuritis; and RBC transfusions for anemia.

A child with severe and longstanding disease from JIA may present with bony deformities that may affect certain ED procedures. Cervical spine arthritis can present with atlantoaxial instability (seen on flexion-extension neck radiographs), leading to neurologic deficits. Temporomandibular joint arthritis suggested by jaw pain, difficulty chewing, and facial asymmetry can cause micrognathia. Both atlantoaxial instability and micrognathia may make tracheal intubation difficult. Micrognathia may impede nutrition, causing failure to thrive.

Pearls

1. JIA is a diagnosis of exclusion.
2. Bone pain, particularly pain out of proportion to physical exam, is *not* typical of JIA.
3. JIA usually does not present with fever or rash except in patients with systemic-onset arthritis.
4. In patients with systemic-onset JIA, MAS should be suspected in extremely ill-appearing children with recurring fevers.
5. Patients with JIA on immunosuppressive therapies presenting with fever need a thorough evaluation for underlying infection.
6. Children with JIA should be screened for asymptomatic uveitis.

Clinical Summary

Granulomatosis with polyangiitis (GPA; formerly known as Wegener granulomatosis) is a rare small-vessel vasculitis that is often associated with antineutrophil cytoplasmic antibodies (ANCA). The disease occurs in the second decade of life with a female preponderance. The diagnosis is made based on clinical features, serologic markers, and histopathologic findings. Clinical features are characterized by pulmonary-renal vasculitis. The spectrum of pulmonary involvement may include chronic cough (61%), shortness of breath (49%), and hemoptysis or alveolar hemorrhage (42%). Pulmonary hemorrhage may be the initial presenting symptom. European League Against Rheumatism criteria are used for the diagnosis (GPA likely with 3 of 6 criteria met) and include:

1. Upper airway involvement (chronic nasal discharge, recurrent epistaxis, nasal septal perforation, saddle nose deformity)
2. Pulmonary involvement (CXR or chest CT demonstrating nodules, cavities, or infiltrates)
3. Renal involvement (proteinuria, hematuria/RBC casts, necrotizing pauci-immune glomerulonephritis)
4. Granulomatous inflammation (granulomatous inflammation within wall of artery or in perivascular or extravascular area of artery or arteriole)
5. Laryngotracheobronchial stenosis (subglottic, tracheal, or bronchial stenosis)
6. ANCA positivity by immunofluorescence microscopy (MPO/P ANCA or PR3/C ANCA)

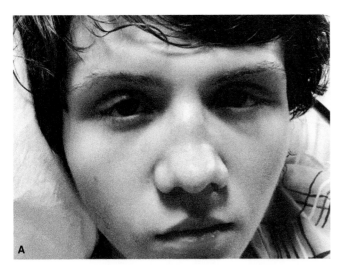

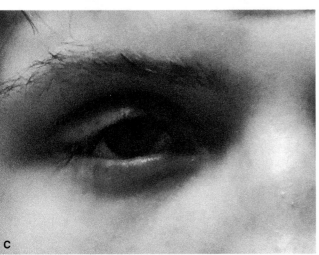

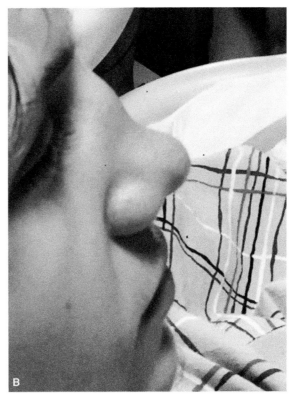

FIGURE 12.26 ■ Granulomatosis with Polyangiitis (GPA). (**A, B**) Saddle nose deformity is seen in this 18-year-old man with GPA. He had several bouts of sinusitis and cough for months prior to the diagnosis. He went to his college health office for a CXR due to worsening cough and was found to have cavitary lung nodules (see Figure 12.27) and thus referred to ED for possible tuberculosis but instead was found to have GPA. (**C**) Dacryoadenitis. Inflammatory enlargement of the lacrimal gland is shown in the same patient. (Photo contributor: Julie Cherian, MD.)

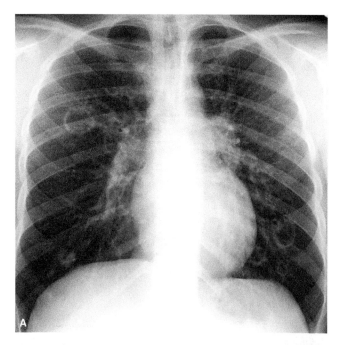

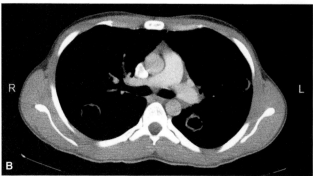

FIGURE 12.27 ▪ Granulomatosis with Polyangiitis (GPA). (**A**) Frontal view of the chest demonstrates multiple cavitary lesions bilaterally. (**B**) Axial view of the CT scan of the chest demonstrates multiple cavitary nodules in the same patient (see Figure 12.26). These studies were performed due to chronic cough. (Photo contributor: Julie Cherian, MD.)

Additional features include dacryocystitis, auditory involvement/hearing loss, and proptosis associated with periorbital tumor and lung nodules. If a firm diagnosis is difficult to make and if the disease is limited to only 1 organ system (ie, lungs), biopsy of the lung nodule is recommended for confirmatory diagnosis. Although a rare vasculitis in children, prompt recognition of the disease and initiation of treatment improves outcomes.

Differential diagnosis for GPA includes infections (eg, mycobacteria, fungi, or helminths), neoplastic diseases, and rheumatologic disease (eg, sarcoidosis, SLE, mixed connective tissue disease, polyarteritis nodosa, microscopic polyangiitis, anti–glomerular basement membrane disease, and ANCA-positive ulcerative colitis).

Emergency Department Treatment and Disposition

Initial stabilization followed by hospitalization is needed for patients presenting with acute respiratory insufficiency related to pulmonary hemorrhage. A CBC may show leukocytosis, normochromic normocytic anemia, and thrombocytosis. ESR and CRP levels may be elevated. Urinalysis may show proteinuria, microscopic hematuria, and RBC casts indicating glomerular disease. Rheumatologic testing that may be positive includes ANA, antiphospholipid antibodies, and ANCA positivity. von Willebrand factor antigen may be elevated in vasculitis and is an indicator of endothelial damage. Abnormalities in the CXRs are commonly seen (~78%). The most common abnormality is lung nodule rather than fixed infiltrates. Other findings include cavitations, pleural effusions, and pneumothoraces. Small nodules and linear opacities are better visualized by high-resolution CT of the chest. Pulmonary hemorrhage is suggested by the halo sign (rim of ground glass opacities around a lung lesion) on high-resolution CT. MRI is an excellent modality in evaluating mucosal and soft tissue disease. In particular, it is useful for evaluating changes that affect the nose, orbits, mastoids, and upper airways (subglottic stenosis). A prompt consultation with a rheumatologist is required in all suspected cases of GPA for rapid aggressive therapy with corticosteroids and further immunosuppression.

Pearls

1. Patients presenting with pulmonary hemorrhage may be acutely ill, and this may be the initial presentation of GPA. Clinicians must have a high index of suspicion for this diagnosis.
2. Diagnosis of GPA is challenging and relies on both clinical and serologic features of the disease, which includes pulmonary-renal vasculitis and ANCA positivity.
3. If GPA is suspected, a careful upper respiratory tract history and ENT evaluation may be considered.
4. Saddle nose deformity may be a significant clinical finding that may occur due to longstanding disease causing nasal cartilage damage. Renal involvement may present subsequent to respiratory manifestations. However, limited GPA (with only upper respiratory symptoms) may occur rarely in children compared to adults.

Clinical Summary

Macrophage activation syndrome (MAS) is a potentially life-threatening complication related to an underlying rheumatic disease. It is most commonly seen in systemic-onset JIA (7%–17%), SLE (1%), and KD. It occurs with equal frequency in males and females and has no predilection for ethnicity or age. Although the exact etiology is not known, Ebstein-Barr virus, cytomegalovirus, herpesvirus, or bacterial infections can be triggers. Changes in therapy of rheumatic disease have also been associated with the development of MAS in these patients.

MAS is thought to result from uncontrolled activation and expansion of macrophages and T cells leading to a cytokine storm. It closely resembles hemophagocytic lymphohistiocytosis (HLH) and is sometimes thought of as a secondary HLH. In initial presentations involving young children (age <5 years), consideration must also be given to familial or primary HLH that encompasses a variety of rare autosomal recessive immune defects.

Children with MAS typically present with prolonged unexplained fevers, hepatosplenomegaly, lymphadenopathy, severe cytopenias, transaminitis, disseminated intravascular coagulopathy (DIC), and a significant hyperferritinemia. It

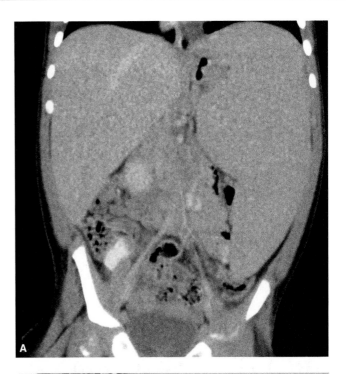

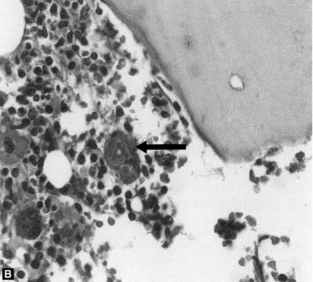

FIGURE 12.29 ■ Macrophage Activation Syndrome (MAS). (**A**) Massive hepatosplenomegaly is seen in this 2-year-old girl who presented with a 6-month history of daily unremitting fevers. She also had rash, leukopenia, and thrombocytopenia associated with elevated inflammatory markers. She presented to the ED with massive abdominal distention, pain, and constipation. (**B**) Bone marrow biopsy was done because the initial presentation was concerning for a leukemia. Biopsy revealed hemophagocytosis of red blood cells by macrophages. She was subsequently diagnosed as having MAS related to systemic-onset JIA. (Photo contributors: Julie Cherian, MD [A], and Tahmeena Ahmed, MD [B]).

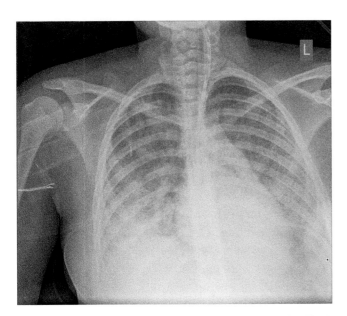

FIGURE 12.28 ■ Macrophage Activation Syndrome (MAS). Single anteroposterior view of the chest demonstrates diffuse airspace disease compatible with pulmonary hemorrhage in a patient presenting with MAS due to systemic JIA (Photo contributor: John Amodio, MD.)

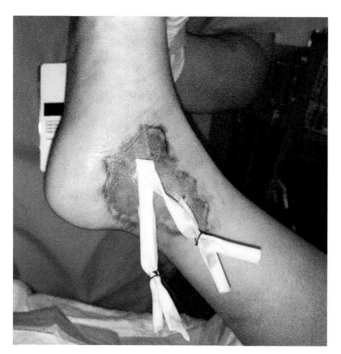

FIGURE 12.30. ■ Purpura; Macrophage Activation Syndrome (MAS). Purpura at the medial malleolus of a 6-year-old girl initially thought to be septic. The patient presented with unremitting quotidian fevers with pancytopenia and disseminated intravascular coagulopathy. A bone marrow was done to evaluate concerns for malignancy that demonstrated massive amounts of macrophages engulfing various cells. The patient was later diagnosed with MAS due to systemic-onset JIA. (Photo contributor: Julie Cherian, MD.)

is often mistaken for sepsis. A clinician should have a high index of suspicion for MAS. Diagnostic criteria have been validated for HLH, but the criteria have been shown to have a low sensitivity in MAS. Diagnosis of MAS is largely based on clinical vigilance and trending characteristic laboratory features because there are no validated diagnostic criteria. Currently consensus guidelines are being validated for MAS.

Emergency Department Treatment and Disposition

Prompt recognition and diagnosis are crucial because MAS is a life-threatening condition with a high mortality rate (20%). Patients may present as acutely pancytopenic, and the differential includes infectious etiologies, malignancy, and rheumatic disease. Laboratory tests include CBC with differential and peripheral smear, reticulocytes, ESR, CRP, comprehensive metabolic panel, ferritin, fibrinogen, PT, PTT, and D-dimer. In patients with active underlying rheumatic disease, MAS should be considered in patients with a decreasing ESR (sign of consumptive coagulopathy and hypofibrinogenemia) and a decreasing platelet count in light of elevated CRP, LDH, D-dimer, triglycerides, and ferritin (typically >10,000 ng/mL). Initial stabilization, hospitalization, and multidisciplinary consultations, as indicated (eg, rheumatology, hematology), are required because the clinical picture can rapidly progress to multiorgan failure. Symptoms may progress to a hemorrhagic DIC-like syndrome, and patients may develop petechiae, purpura, ecchymosis, or spontaneous bleeding. Patients can also present with a wide array of CNS involvement and may become encephalopathic.

This overwhelming multisystem inflammatory process can be a therapeutic challenge. A bone marrow biopsy may be required to rule out malignancy prior to starting appropriate therapy. Hemophagocytosis can be seen on bone marrow, but results are typically variable early in the disease course. This finding on bone marrow is not essential for diagnosis and serves to exclude other etiologies such as a malignant process. The initial mainstay of therapy is pulse doses of methylprednisolone (30 mg/kg/dose). Other immunosuppressive agents such as cyclosporine, anakinra, or etoposide may be used in conjunction with steroids.

Pearls

1. MAS is a rheumatologic emergency. Prompt recognition and aggressive treatment are paramount as it can result in extreme morbidity and high fatality.
2. MAS is most commonly associated with systemic-onset JIA but can also be seen in SLE and KD.
3. Triggers that may induce MAS in patients with rheumatic disease include infections and changes in medications.
4. MAS may be the initial presenting sign of an undiagnosed rheumatic disease.
5. A paradoxical decrease in ESR levels with other high inflammatory markers and hyperferritinemia should alert physicians to severe MAS.

Clinical Summary

Lyme disease (borreliosis or Lyme borreliosis) is a spirochetal infection transmitted by ticks infected with *Borrelia* species (*B burgdorferi* in the United States; *B burgdorferi*, *B afzelii*, *B garinii*, and *B spielmanii* in Europe and Asia). There is a biphasic peak of incidence in school-age children and adults age 40 to 74 years old. The most characteristic and earliest manifestation is erythema migrans (EM; ~90% of children), occurring days to several weeks after inoculation. Multiple lesions are cutaneous markers of disseminated disease resulting from hematogenous spread of spirochete. Acute peripheral facial palsy is the most frequent manifestation of neuroborreliosis in childhood, and bilateral facial palsy is pathognomonic. Varying degrees of reversible atrioventricular block (first, second, or third degree) are the most frequent manifestation of Lyme carditis, although this is rare in children. After EM, arthritis is the most common late manifestation of Lyme borreliosis in children, occurring months after infection. Diagnosis is made clinically (see Table 12.8).

Emergency Department Treatment and Disposition

Remove any ticks that are still attached promptly (transmission of *B burgdorferi* requires attachment for >48 hours). *Do not squeeze* the body of the tick during removal. Grasp the

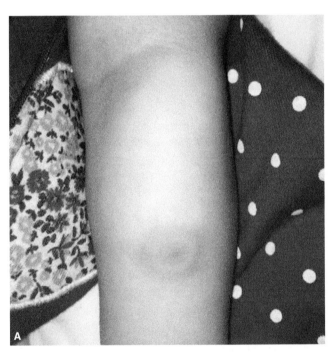
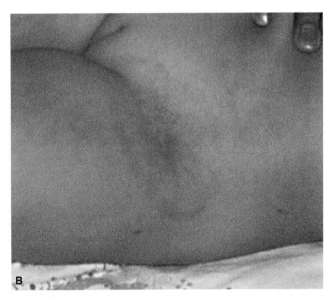
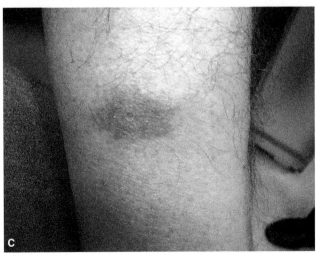

FIGURE 12.31 ■ Erythema Migrans (EM) in Lyme Disease. Three different patients with EM with a confirmed diagnosis of Lyme disease are shown. EM lesions can gradually expand and may reach >12 inches in diameter, if untreated. Differential includes tinea corporis, herald patch (pityriasis rosea), cellulites, nummular eczema, granuloma annulare, erythema multiforme, other arthropod or spider bite, fixed drug eruption, and urticaria. (**A**) EM is seen in this 18-month-old girl whose possible exposure was while playing in the grass in Brooklyn, New York. (**B**) Target-shaped erythematous lesion in a girl from New Jersey. (**C**) An erythematous plaque seen on the lower leg in a patient from Brooklyn, New York. (Photo contributors: Moshe Kupferstein, DO [A], Bipin Patel, MD [B], and Morgan Rabach, MD [C].)

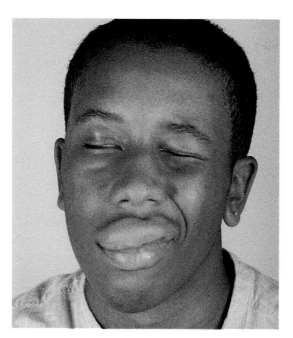

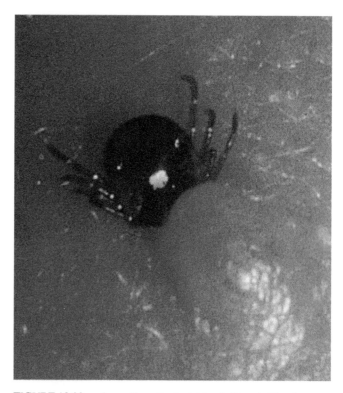

FIGURE 12.32 ■ Peripheral Seventh Nerve Palsy. Acute peripheral facial palsy (clinically indistinguishable from Bell palsy) may be the presenting as well as the only manifestation of Lyme disease. Usually it lasts from 2 to 8 weeks and generally resolves completely. Antibiotics do not hasten the resolution but are given to prevent other complications of disseminated Lyme disease. Also note the markedly swollen upper lip (angioedema) in this patient following an arthropod bite. (Photo contributor: Binita R. Shah, MD.)

FIGURE 12.33 ■ Lyme Borreliosis. A blood-distended *Ixodes scapularis* nymph (also known as the black-legged or deer tick) feeding on human skin. *Borrelia* transmission usually occurs after prolonged attachment and feeding (>48 hours). (Reproduced with permission from Kane KS, Nambudiri VE, Stratigos AJ. *Color Atlas & Synopsis of Pediatric Dermatology*, 3rd ed. McGraw-Hill Education; New York, NY, 2017.)

tick with a pair of fine tweezers as close to the skin as possible and remove the tick by gently pulling straight out and *not* with a twisting motion. Protect the fingers with gloves or tissue and wash hands thoroughly after tick removal.

Routine laboratory tests are rarely useful in making the diagnosis. Obtain CBC (normal or elevated WBC), ESR (usually elevated), and ECG, if clinically indicated. In patients with meningitis, CSF examination shows mild lymphocytic pleocytosis. An enzyme-linked immunosorbent assay (ELISA) is the most common initial serologic test used to support the diagnosis (false-positive ELISA testing occurs with other borrelial or spirochetal diseases). Positive Western blot tests in patients with positive or equivocal ELISA tests confirm the diagnosis.

Admit patients with meningitis, encephalitis, or carditis after consultations with neurology, cardiology, and infectious disease, as clinically indicated. Refer to the guidelines published by Infectious Diseases Society of America for the treatment of Lyme disease in the United States, which is varied according to disease manifestation, and refer to primary care physician for follow-up.

Pearls

1. Lyme disease is the most common vector-borne disease in the United States and Europe.
2. Prophylactic antibiotics are not indicated after tick bite.

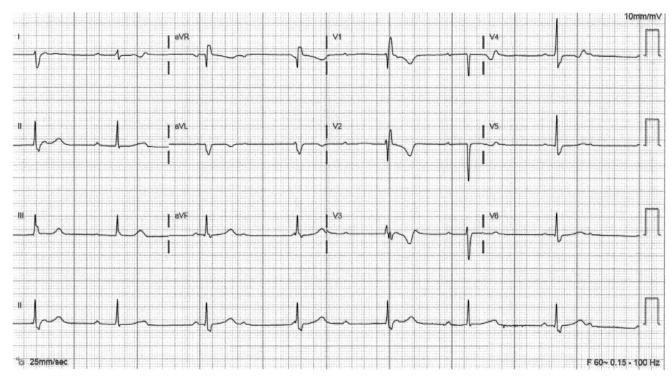

FIGURE 12.34 ■ Lyme Carditis Presenting with Complete Heart Block (CHB). ECG showing CHB (note atrioventricular [AV] dissociation) with intermittent junctional escape beats, heart rate of 43 bpm, and right axis deviation in an 18-year-old man presenting to the ED for knee pain lasting for 4 weeks. There was no history of tick bite; however, the patient resided in an endemic area for Lyme disease. Lyme carditis can present with varying degrees of AV conduction delay. It may also cause pericarditis, endocarditis, myocarditis, pericardial effusion, myocardial infarction, coronary artery aneurysm, tachyarrhythmias, and congestive heart failure. CHB is transient and usually resolves within 1 week, whereas lesser conduction disturbances usually resolve within 6 weeks. (Photo/legend contributors: Rabia Malik, MD, and Sushitha Surendran, MD.)

TABLE 12.8 ■ CLINICAL SIGNS OF LYME DISEASE

	Skin and Joints	Nonspecific Signs	CNS Signs	Cardiac Signs
Stage 1: Early localized disease	Erythema migrans (EM) 7–14 days after tick bite (can occur 3–30 days after bite) Red macule at site expands into enlarging ring over days to weeks Lesion annular or target-shaped flat lesion without scales or vesicles at the periphery, blanches with pressure and has variable degrees of central clearing, may be pruritic Lesion usually fades within 3–4 weeks (even in untreated patients)	Fever, headache, myalgia, arthralgia, fatigue, lymphadenopathy		
Stage 2: Early disseminated disease	Multiple EM lesions	Fever, headache, myalgia, arthralgia, fatigue, lymphadenopathy	Seventh nerve palsy, meningitis	Heart block, myopericarditis
Stage 3: Late disease: arthritis	Usually mono- or oligoarticular swelling and tenderness (knee most common) Seen weeks to months after tick bite May occur without a prior history of earlier stages of illness (including EM)			

Chapter 13

NEUROLOGY

Geetha Chari
Vikas S. Shah

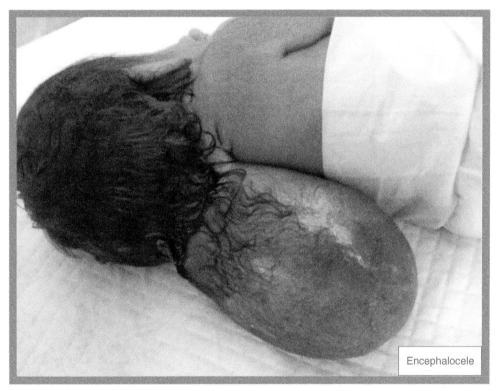

Encephalocele

(Photo contributor: Prerna Batra, MD)

The authors acknowledge the special contributions of Binita R. Shah, MD, to prior edition.

BACTERIAL MENINGITIS

Clinical Summary

Meningitis is inflammation of the membranes (dura, pia mater, and arachnoid) surrounding the brain and spinal cord. Bacterial meningitis most commonly results from seeding of the leptomeninges from a distant focus (hematogenous spread), direct extension from contiguous focus (eg, sinusitis, otitis media, mastoiditis), or by direct invasion (eg, head trauma). Etiologies in the neonatal period include group B streptococci, gram-negative enteric bacilli (*Escherichia coli, Enterobacter* spp.), and *Listeria monocytogenes*. Etiologies from age 1 to 3 months include group B *Streptococcus*, gram-negative bacilli, *Streptococcus pneumoniae,* and *Neisseria meningitides*. Etiologies in infants >3 months include *S pneumoniae, N meningitidis*, group B *Streptococcus*, gram-negative bacilli, and *Haemophilus influenzae* type b (Hib; unvaccinated children).

In patients with ventriculoperitoneal (VP) shunts, coagulase-negative *Staphylococcus epidermidis* and *Staphylococcus aureus* are common pathogens. Tuberculous meningitis presents with a gradual onset (several weeks). Low-grade fever, weight loss, adenopathy, vomiting, lethargy, cranial nerve palsies, and coma are common presentations. Differential diagnosis includes viral meningitis, subarachnoid hemorrhage (ruptured arteriovenous malformation/aneurysm), parameningeal/paraspinal infection (eg, brain abscess, subdural or

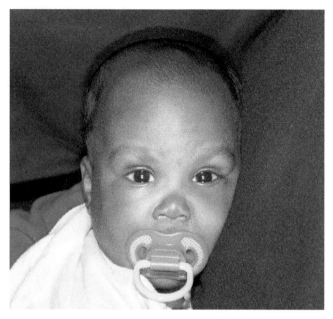

FIGURE 13.2 ■ Bulging Anterior Fontanelle as a Presenting Sign of Meningitis. The anterior fontanelle is normally open in infants (usually closes between 9 and 18 months) and is pulsatile and slightly depressed in an infant in an upright position. The anterior fontanelle may appear full in an infant lying in a supine position or during crying. A bulging anterior fontanelle suggests increased intracranial pressure from any etiology (eg, meningitis, tumor, hydrocephalus). (Photo contributor: Binita R. Shah, MD.)

epidural abscess), retropharyngeal abscess, and trauma (eg, abusive head trauma, subdural or epidural hematoma).

Emergency Department Treatment and Disposition

Stabilization of the patient and continuous cardiopulmonary monitoring are encouraged. Shock should be identified and addressed appropriately and expeditiously. Patients not in shock should receive IV fluid at maintenance with 0.9% NaCl solution because of possible syndrome of inappropriate antidiuretic hormone. Diagnosis is made with evaluation of CSF with lumbar puncture (LP). Head CT scan *is not required routinely* before LP when there is a clinical diagnosis of uncomplicated meningitis or no signs or symptoms of increased intracranial pressure (ICP). If focal neurologic signs are present (eg, papilledema) or vital signs are suggestive of increased ICP (hypertension, bradycardia, or abnormal respirations), begin antibiotics and obtain a CT scan before performing LP. Antigen detection tests (eg, latex agglutination) may help in

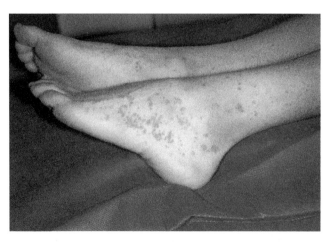

FIGURE 13.1 ■ Bacterial Meningitis Presenting with Purpura. An adolescent patient with AIDS presented with high fever, neck stiffness, and signs of septic shock with purpuric lesions (photograph taken on second day of hospitalization). Both blood and CSF cultures were positive for *S pneumoniae*. (Photo contributor: Binita R. Shah, MD.)

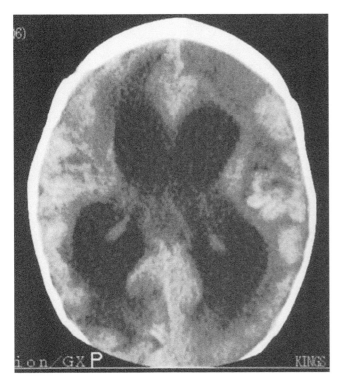

FIGURE 13.3 ■ Hydrocephalus; Complication of Bacterial Meningitis. A CT scan of the head shows moderate to severe hydrocephalus with periventricular transudation around the lateral ventricles and abnormal sulcal thickening along the parietal region due to subarachnoid exudates. This 10-month-old infant remained persistently febrile on amoxicillin for a presumed pneumonia. Her blood and CSF cultures were positive for *S pneumoniae* that showed intermediate resistance to penicillin and cefotaxime but was sensitive to vancomycin. (Photo contributor: Binita R. Shah, MD.)

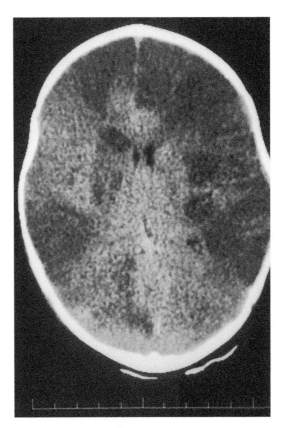

FIGURE 13.4 ■ Neurologic Sequelae; Bacterial Meningitis. A noncontrast head CT scan shows multiple hypodense areas (left > right) over the frontal and parietal regions, with additional areas of hypodensity in the right deep white matter and basal ganglia indicative of multiple infarcts in an infant with group B streptococcal meningitis. (Photo contributor: Binita R. Shah, MD.)

partially treated meningitis. Order India ink stain for immunocompromised patients and acid-fast stain when tuberculous meningitis is suspected. A CBC count with differential of WBCs, blood and CSF cultures, serum electrolytes, and glucose should be ordered. Place a 5-tuberculin-unit purified protein derivative tuberculin test on the forearm of all patients in whom tuberculosis is suspected. Treat patients <4 weeks of age empirically with ampicillin *and* cefotaxime *or* ampicillin and an aminoglycoside (eg, gentamicin). Consider antiviral therapy if herpes is suspected. Treat patients >4 weeks of age empirically with vancomycin *and* cefotaxime *or* ceftriaxone. Offer antibiotic prophylaxis to close contacts

for exposure to Hib and *N meningitides.* Adjunctive therapy with dexamethasone is beneficial for treatment of infants and children with Hib meningitis to diminish the risk of hearing loss, if administered before or concurrently with the first dose of antimicrobial agent(s). Use of dexamethasone as an adjunctive therapy with suspected or proven pneumococcal meningitis for infants and children remains controversial, and data are not sufficient to make a routine recommendation for children. Admit patients with a clinical diagnosis; admit those with septic shock requiring resuscitation to the pediatric ICU (PICU). Use standard and droplet precautions for the first 24 hours after institution of appropriate antibiotics.

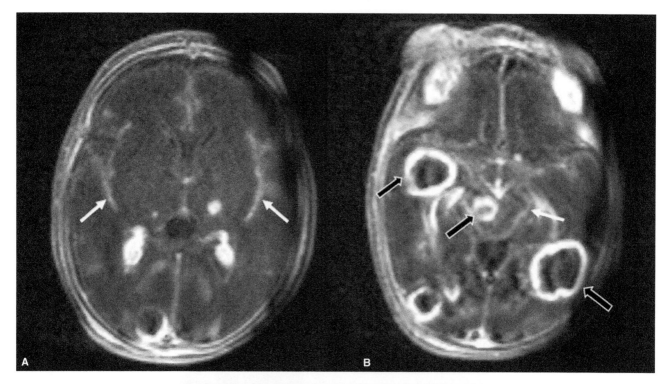

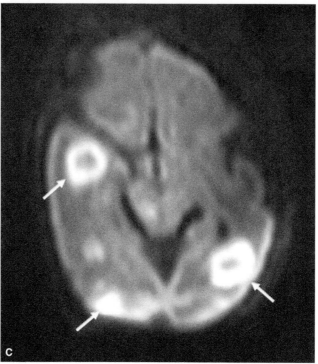

FIGURE 13.5 ■ Meningitis and Brain Abscesses. (**A and B**) Axial T1-weighted postcontrast images in a 2-month-old baby boy with meningitis demonstrate abnormal leptomeningeal enhancement (white arrows) within the sulci and fissures and surrounding the brainstem, consistent with meningitis. There are multiple rim-enhancing lesions (black arrows) in the cerebral hemispheres and brainstem consistent with brain abscesses. (**C**) The abscesses demonstrate high signal on diffusion-weighted images due to restricted water diffusion in pus (white arrows). (Photo contributor: Vinodhkumar Velayudhan, DO.)

TABLE 13.1 ■ SIGNS AND SYMPTOMS OF MENINGITIS

Neonate *(signs and symptoms are often subtle and nonspecific)*
- Fever or hypothermia
- Poor suck/poor feeding
- CNS: Lethargy or irritability, seizures
- Weak or high-pitched cry
- Apnea or respiratory distress
- Septic shock

Infants
- Fever, vomiting.
- CNS: Lethargy or irritability, coma, seizures
- Bulging anterior fontanelle
- Petechiae or purpura
- Septic shock

Older child
- Fever, headache, photophobia
- CNS: Lethargy, confusion or coma, seizures, focal neurologic findings
- Petechiae or purpura
- Septic shock
- Ataxia (labyrinthine dysfunction or vestibular neuronitis)
- Signs of meningeal irritation
  1. Nuchal rigidity or meningismus (neck resists passive flexion)
  2. Kernig sign (attempt to passively extend the knee while patient is seated is met with resistance in the presence of meningitis)
  3. Brudzinski sign (passive flexion of the neck with the patient in a supine position results in spontaneous flexion of the hips and knees)

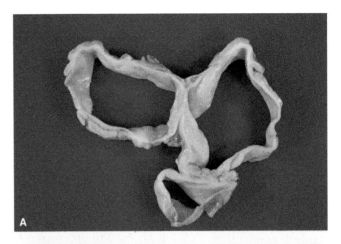

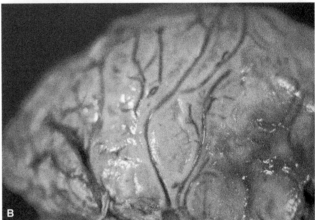

FIGURE 13.6 ■ Bacterial Meningitis. **(A)** Severe Hydrocephalus; Complication of Bacterial Meningitis. This autopsy photograph shows marked dilation of the ventricular system and prominent thinning of the cerebral mantle in a child who developed hydrocephalus requiring a ventriculoperitoneal shunt after group B streptococcal meningitis. **(B)** Dorsal surface of the brain at autopsy showing purulent exudate in the subarachnoid space. Highlighting of vessels by pus is prominent. (Photo contributor: Chandrakant Rao, MD.)

TABLE 13.2 ■ CSF FINDINGS IN MENINGITIS

Type of Meningitis	Leukocytes (Number)	Glucose	Protein	Gram's Stain
Bacterial	Neutrophils (hundreds to thousands)	Low	High	Often positive
Viral	Lymphocytes (hundreds)	Normal	Slightly high	Negative
Tuberculous	Lymphocytes (hundreds)	Low	High	Negative
Cryptococcal	Lymphocytes (few to hundreds)	Low	Normal or high	Negative
Parameningeal Brain abscess Subdural abscess	Lymphocytes (few)	Normal	High	Negative

Reproduced with permission from Finberg L, Kleinman RE. *Saunders Manual of Pediatric Practice,* 2nd ed. WB Saunders; Philadelphia, PA, 2002.

Pearls

1. Meningitis is a life-threatening medical emergency; maintain a high index of suspicion for all patients with signs and symptoms.

2. Absence of meningeal signs in infants <18 months old does *not* exclude meningitis. In this age group, such signs are often not present, and when seen, usually represent a very late finding.

3. Stiff neck is a pathognomonic sign of meningeal irritation from a purulent exudate or hemorrhage in the subarachnoid space.

4. CSF examination is the gold standard for diagnosis; *always perform LP* when there is any suspicion of meningitis. Neutrophils may predominate early even in viral meningitis. Decreased CSF glucose may also occur in mumps, herpes meningoencephalitis, and tuberculous meningitis.

5. Petechiae or purpura are seen in only 70% of cases of meningococcemia. Patients with meningococcal meningitis may also lack CSF abnormalities on initial LP even with a positive CSF culture. Consider infections caused by *N meningitides* even in the absence of skin lesions or CSF abnormalities.

6. Seizures are seen in about 20% to 30% of patients with bacterial meningitis; consider meningitis in children presenting with seizures associated with fever.

7. Avoid delays in initiating antibiotic therapy while awaiting completion of diagnostic studies.

8. Failure to diagnose meningitis in a timely manner is a leading cause of malpractice litigation in pediatrics.

Clinical Summary

Sustained elevations in intracranial pressure (ICP) may permanently retard normal brain function. By volume, skull contents consist of brain (80%), blood (10%), and CSF (10%), and this volume is fixed. Increases in one component therefore must be compensated by a decrease in the others (Monroe-Kellie hypothesis); otherwise, there will be an increase in ICP leading to brain compression, especially if the cranial vault is noncompliant. Normal values for ICP vary according to age and body position (normal <20 mm Hg). Patients with elevated ICP may be asymptomatic or present with nausea, headache, blurry vision, weakness, vomiting, or seizures. Clinical signs may be present, including tachycardia or bradycardia,

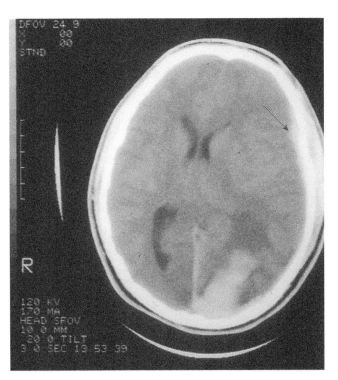

FIGURE 13.8 ■ Hemorrhagic Stroke (Intraparenchymal Bleed) with Transtentorial and Subfalcine Herniation. A noncontrast CT scan of the head shows left parieto-occipital intraparenchymal bleeding with left frontoparietal subdural hematoma (arrow). The basal cisterns are obscured with a significant mass effect with evidence of transtentorial and subfalcine herniation in an adolescent patient brought to the ED with Cushing triad. He was found unresponsive with mouth frothing and urinary incontinence in his bed. About 12 hours before this, he complained of a severe headache. He was intubated, hyperventilated, and given a dose of mannitol before this CT scan. (Photo contributor: Vikas S. Shah, MD.)

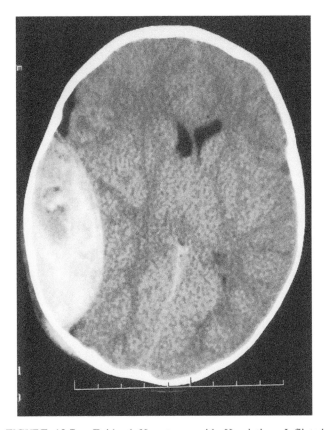

FIGURE 13.7 ■ Epidural Hematoma with Herniation; Inflicted Head Trauma. A noncontrast CT scan of the head shows a large right temporoparietal lenticular extradural hematoma with heterogenous density. There is a mass effect on the adjacent parieto-occipital lobe with evidence of subfalcine herniation, and a midline shift from right to left. This 4-month-old infant was brought to the ED with vomiting, inability to arouse, and vital signs showing Cushing triad. His mother subsequently confessed to shaking him violently and throwing him against the wall because he would not stop crying. (Photo contributor: Vikas S. Shah, MD.)

bradypnea, hypertension, focal neurologic deficits, bulging fontanel or widening diathesis of cerebral sutures in infants, doll's eye, papilledema, retinal hemorrhages, and unequal pupils.

Emergency Department Treatment and Disposition

Sustained ICP elevations (>20 mm Hg) need to be treated aggressively, and management is dependent on etiology. The factors contributing to ICP, including cerebral blood flow (CBF), cerebral perfusion pressure (CPP), and mean arterial pressure (MAP), guide treatment. As CBF increases, ICP increases. CBF is autoregulated under a wide range of CPP and remains relatively constant. CPP is the difference

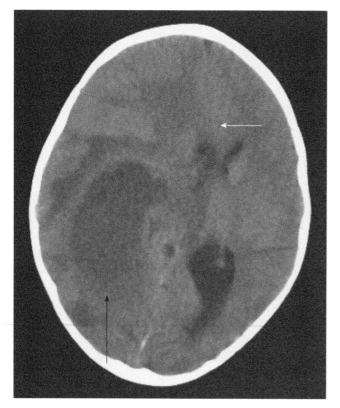

FIGURE 13.9 ■ Brain Tumor Presenting with Increased Intracranial Pressure. An axial head CT image shows a large right-sided cerebral hemisphere mass with vasogenic edema (black arrow), right to left subfalcine (white arrow), transtentorial, and right uncal herniation with obliteration of the right lateral ventricle in a 2-year-old child presenting with seizures, unsteady gait, and excessive sleepiness. (Photo contributor: Vikas S. Shah, MD.)

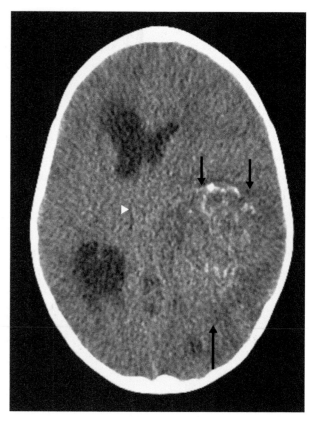

FIGURE 13.10 ■ Brain Tumor Presenting with Increased Intracranial Pressure. An axial head CT image shows a large lobulated supratentorial mass with calcifications (black arrows), surrounding vasogenic edema, a midline shift (arrowhead), and compression of anterior horn of left lateral ventricle with hydrocephalus in a 2-year-old child presenting to ED with Cushing triad and lethargy. Subsequently, patient developed signs of herniation requiring intubation, mannitol, and ventricular drain by neurosurgeon. (Photo contributor: Vikas S. Shah, MD.)

between MAP and ICP. When ICP is not immediately available, central venous pressure (CVP) can be used as a surrogate for ICP to calculate CPP. In adolescents and adults, CPP ranges between 70 and 90 mm Hg when MAP is between 60 and 150 mm Hg. In children, the CPP is 50 to 70 mm Hg. From these relationships, to maintain constant CBF and ICP, constant CPP must be maintained.

Adhere to Pediatric Advanced Life Support and Advanced Trauma Life Support guidelines and mitigate any factors that may further compromise CPP. If ICP elevation is from trauma, immobilize the cervical spine and intubate trachea under rapid sequence protocol, especially if Glasgow Coma Scale score is <8. Initiate mechanical ventilation and maintain normal ventilation ($Paco_2$ between 35 and 40 mm Hg), optimize oxygenation by maintaining Pao_2 >110 mm Hg, and maintain normal acid-base status. Hyperventilation ($Paco_2$ <35 mm Hg) and hypoventilation are to be avoided unless there

is active cerebral herniation. Hypoventilation and hypoxemia cause vasodilation and lead to an increase in CBF, leading to increased ICP. Hyperventilation leads to vasoconstriction of the cerebral vasculature, leading to ischemia from decreased blood flow. When maximizing oxygenation, minimize positive end-expiratory pressure to avoid decreases in venous drainage, which increase ICP and reduce cerebral perfusion. Avoid hyperoxia (ie, PaO_2 >110 mm Hg). Intubation raises ICP and negatively affects CPP. To minimize this, sedate the patient with fentanyl and etomidate and use lidocaine prior to intubation. Use short-acting drugs whenever possible to allow for accurate and frequent assessment of neurologic status. When a patient with increased ICP requires tracheal intubation, placement of an ICP monitor is recommended. Head of

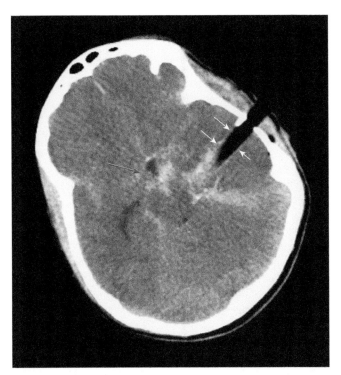

FIGURE 13.11 ■ Traumatic Subarachnoid Hemorrhage with Increased Intracranial Pressure (ICP). A noncontrast head CT scan shows extensive subarachnoid hemorrhage with obliteration of the basal CSF cisterns (red arrow) indicative of increased ICP in a 12-year-old boy brought to the ED with a penetrating brain trauma (a foot-long wooden stick into the left temporal region). Blood can also be seen around the foreign object penetrating the left temporal region (white arrows). (Photo contributor: Geetha Chari, MD.)

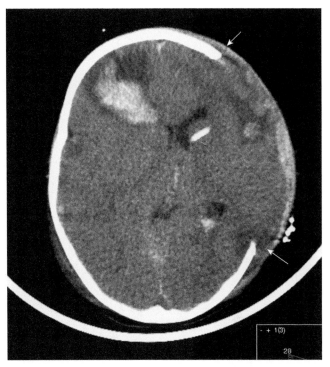

FIGURE 13.12 ■ Intraventricular Drain and Hemicraniectomy; Increased Intracranial Pressure (ICP). Noncontrast head CT scan shows a large left craniectomy, left ventricular drain (red arrow), bulging of the brain through the craniectomy site (white arrows), and a right frontal hematoma in a 5-year-old boy who was struck by a motor vehicle. He was taken to the operating room from the ED for emergent treatment of raised ICP with hemicraniectomy and intraventricular drain. (Photo contributor: Vikas S. Shah, MD.)

bed should be elevated to 30 degrees and placed in midline position if there are no contraindications.

Maximization of CPP is dependent on augmenting MAP and minimizing ICP and requires that central venous volume be optimized. If CVP is decreased, resuscitate the patient with crystalloid. If the CVP is adequate and the MAP remains low, to maintain adequate CPP, initiate inotropes and vasotropes. Femoral vein cannulation is preferable for central access as placement of catheter in the superior circulation may retard cerebral venous drainage and decrease CPP. Consult neurosurgery immediately. Order noncontrast head CT to aid in diagnosis and management. Address factors that worsen ICP (see Table 13.3).

If herniation is suspected (unequal pupil size, irregular respiration, hypertension, altered respirations and bradycardia, abnormal CT), prompt attention is warranted. In this case, implement the above recommendations and administer

bolus of 3% normal saline or mannitol. Renal failure, severe dehydration, cerebral hemorrhage, and pulmonary edema are contraindications for administration of mannitol. If an intraventricular catheter is in place, diversion of CSF externally may decrease ICP. Hyperosmolar therapy with 3% normal saline can be initiated in the ED; however, electrolyte goals may not be achieved until much later.

Pearls

1. The Cushing triad (bradycardia, bradypnea, and hypertension) need not be present concomitantly in pediatric patients with increased ICP.

2. Goal of increased ICP management is to maintain adequate CPP.

3. Administer short-acting pharmaceuticals for sedation, analgesia, and paralysis whenever possible.

TABLE 13.3 ■ CAUSES OF RAISED INTRACRANIAL PRESSURE

Brain	Traumatic brain injury
	Neoplasm
	Seizure
	Infection
	Meningitis
	Encephalitis
	Brain abscess
	Vasculitis
	Systemic lupus erythematosus
	Anoxic injury
Blood	Ruptured aneurysm
	Subdural hematoma
	Epidural hematoma
	Venous thrombosis
CSF	Aqueductal stenosis
	Decreased resorption
	Arachnoid villi blockage
	Increased production
	Choroid plexus tumor
Additional factors	Fever
(Few examples)	Pain
	Inadequate sedation/agitation
	Increased CO_2
	Acidosis

Clinical Summary

Alteration in the level of consciousness (LOC) is a common presentation in the ED and is a vague term that requires evaluation to be specified. Consciousness requires both cerebral hemispheres and the brainstem ascending reticular activating system to be functional. The spectrum of altered consciousness includes lethargy, confusion, delirium, obtundation, stupor, and coma, and causes of altered LOC include a wide spectrum of disorders.

Emergency Department Treatment and Disposition

Obtain a history and vital signs with attention to possible causes. Fever suggests infectious etiology (eg, encephalitis, meningitis). Hypothermia may indicate metabolic conditions or toxic ingestions. Tachypnea is seen in hypoxia, sepsis, acidosis, and toxin ingestion. CNS involvement with increased ICP and herniation will cause Cheyne-Stokes respiration. General examination may show signs of trauma and infection. A brief focused neurologic examination can reveal significant information. Use the Glasgow Coma Scale to measure LOC;

using the parameter of motor response to pain helps to also determine any focal weakness. Obtain fingerstick blood glucose, metabolic panel (eg, electrolytes, BUN, creatinine, calcium, liver enzymes, magnesium, phosphate), CBC, arterial blood gas analysis, and urinalysis. Monitor cardiorespiratory status and stabilize patient with evaluation and maintenance of ABCs (airway, breathing, and circulation). If trauma is suspected, immobilize cervical spine until cervical trauma is ruled out. Administer IV dextrose 25%, if fingerstick glucose is not available to confirm hypoglycemia. Administer thiamine 100 mg IV to adolescents if alcohol intoxication or thiamine-deficient states are suspected. If clinically indicated, administer naloxone for opioid intoxication. Order urgent head CT if symptoms and signs of raised ICP are present or if no metabolic cause is identified. Perform an LP if

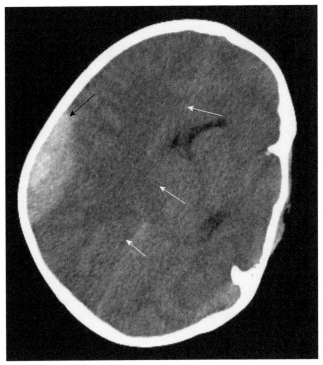

FIGURE 13.14 ■ Epidural Hematoma Following a Trivial Fall. A noncontrast head CT scan shows a biconvex hyperdense extra-axial collection in the right parietal region, characteristic of an epidural hematoma (black arrow), with edema of the white matter of the right cerebral hemisphere and midline shift (white arrows). This 2-year-old child presented to ED following a fall from a short flight of stairs with no loss of consciousness. After a lucid interval, he developed lethargy. (Photo contributor: Geetha Chari, MD.)

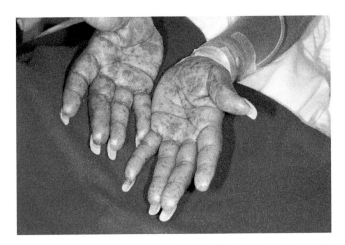

FIGURE 13.13 ■ Purpura and Septic Shock Presenting with Obtundation. A 21-year-old patient presented with fever and rapidly spreading purpuric rash and shock (unresponsiveness to stimuli, hypotension, poor capillary refill with cold and clammy extremities, and decreased urine output). Her blood culture grew *Neisseria meningitidis* type B. This photograph was taken on the third day of the hospitalization. (Photo contributor: Binita R. Shah, MD.)

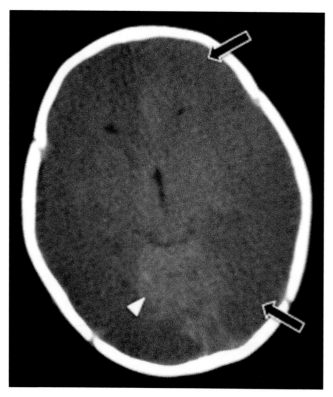

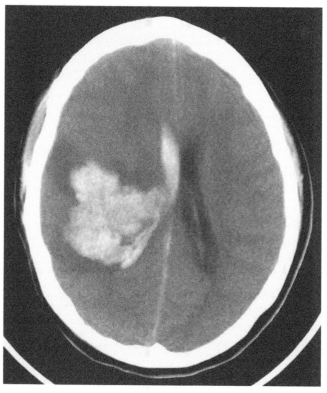

FIGURE 13.15 ■ Global Anoxic Ischemic Brain Injury. A 4-month-old baby boy was brought in for vomiting and lethargy and was suspected to have nonaccidental trauma. Axial CT demonstrates diffuse hypodensity and loss of gray-white differentiation with effacement of the sulci and fissures involving the cerebral hemispheres bilaterally (black arrows) consistent with cerebral edema. There is relatively increased attenuation of the cerebellum (white arrowhead), termed the *cerebellar reversal sign*, which carries a poor prognosis and is indicative of irreversible brain injury. (Photo contributor: Vinodhkumar Velayudhan, DO.)

FIGURE 13.16 ■ Hemorrhagic Stroke (Intraparenchymal Hemorrhage). A noncontrast axial CT image of the head shows a large area of hyperdensity (hematoma) involving the right parietal area with surrounding hypodensity (representing associated edema) and intraventricular extension to the right lateral ventricle. A mass effect with a significant right-to-left midline shift is also seen. This adolescent girl presenting with headache, stiff neck, and fever was diagnosed as having aseptic meningitis (CSF: RBCs 720/mm^3, WBCs 11/mm^3, normal protein, and glucose with negative culture). With clinical improvement, she was discharged after 48 hours. Within 8 hours after discharge, she complained of severe headache followed by seizures. On arrival to the ED, she was comatose with these CT findings. (Photo contributor: Binita R. Shah, MD.)

infectious etiology is considered. Initiate specific therapy for various causes based on the assessment (eg, antibiotics for meningitis, anticonvulsants for seizures, correction of electrolyte and acid-base imbalance, antidote for toxic overdose). Obtain specific consultations depending on the etiology of the coma (eg, neurosurgery for intracranial bleed, poison control for toxic ingestion, neurology for stroke). After initial stabilization, admit to ICU for continuous monitoring and further management.

Pearls

1. Altered mental status has a very wide differential diagnosis; it is essential to treat the underlying cause.

2. Pupillary assessment can help differentiate metabolic and structural causes of coma; reactive pupils suggest metabolic causes, while asymmetric or absent pupillary responses suggest trauma.

3. Features of increased ICP and herniation include headache, vomiting, altered mental status, Cushing triad (systolic hypertension, bradycardia, bradypnea), and unequal pupils.

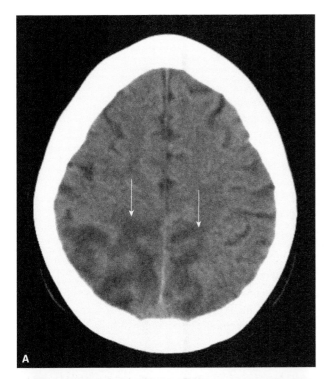

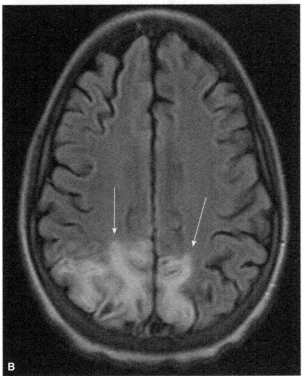

FIGURE 13.17 ■ Hypertensive Encephalopathy (Posterior Reversible Leukoencephalopathy Syndrome [PRES]). (**A**) A noncontrast head CT scan reveals hypodensity in the posterior white matter of both hemispheres in a 7-year-old girl with hypertensive encephalopathy with hemolytic uremic syndrome. These findings are characteristic of hypertensive encephalopathy. (**B**) Axial FLAIR MRI shows hyperintensities in the occipital white matter (white arrows). (Photo contributor: Steve Pulitzer, MD.)

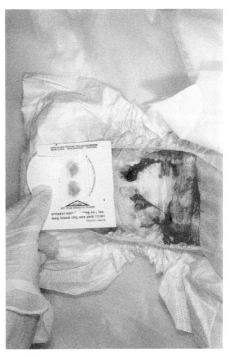

FIGURE 13.18 ■ Currant Jelly Stool; Intussusception Presenting with "Neurologic" Signs. This currant jelly stool was passed by an 8-month-old infant brought to the ED with vomiting, extreme lethargy, and intermittent episodes of crying. He responded with a very weak cry to any painful stimuli and fell back to sleep as soon as stimulus was withdrawn. He had ileocolic intussusception that required surgical reduction. "Neurologic" signs of intussusception (often misdiagnosed as sepsis or a postictal state) include lack of interaction, extreme lethargy, coma or shock-like state, apnea, seizures and seizure-like activity, opisthotonic posturing, weak cry, hypotonia, or pinpoint pupils. (Photo contributor: Binita R. Shah, MD.)

TABLE 13.4 ■ DEFINITIONS OF ALTERED LEVELS OF CONSCIOUSNESS

Lethargy	Reduced wakefulness, lack of interest in environment; arousable and able to communicate
Confusion	Inattentiveness, mental slowness, dulled perception, and incoherence
Delirium	Confusion with hallucinations and motor abnormalities (such as tremors or myoclonus), agitation that may alternate with drowsiness
Obtundation	Severe blunting of awareness with decreased response to stimuli
Stupor	Unresponsiveness from which the individual can be aroused only temporarily by vigorous and repeated stimuli
Coma	Unresponsiveness from which the patient cannot be aroused by verbal, tactile, or painful stimuli

TABLE 13.5 ■ ETIOLOGY AND DIFFERENTIAL DIAGNOSIS OF ALTERED MENTAL STATUS

Mnemonic: COMATOSE PATIENT

C: Carbon monoxide poisoning

O: Overdose (anticholinergics, phencyclidine, amphetamines, sedative hypnotics, narcotics, organophosphates, salicylates, iron)

M: Metabolic: electrolytes/ions (hypernatremia or hyponatremia, hypercalcemia or hypocalcemia, hypermagnesemia or hypomagnesemia, hypophosphatemia)

A: Abuse, alcohol, asphyxia (airway obstruction, drowning), anemia (acute/severe; impaired oxygen delivery), autoimmune (NMDA receptor antibody encephalitis)

T: Trauma (head: hematomas [intracerebral, subdural, epidural], cerebral edema, severe concussion, contusion, laceration)

O: Organic acidurias, inherited hyperammonemia, and other inborn errors of metabolism

S: Seizures (postictal), nonconvulsive status epilepticus
    Stroke (thromboembolism, arteriovenous malformations)
    Shunt failure (ventriculoperitoneal shunt infection/obstruction)
    Shock (hypovolemic, septic, cardiogenic, neurogenic)

E: Encephalopathy (Reye syndrome, hepatic, uremic, hypertensive, lead, hypoxic ischemic [drowning, strangulation])

P: Psychogenic/pseudocoma (conditions mimicking coma: conversion reaction, malingering, catatonia)

A: Acidosis: metabolic (eg, methanol, ethylene glycol, or salicylate intoxication); respiratory (eg, sedative hypnotic intoxication)
    Alkalosis: respiratory (eg, hepatic encephalopathy, salicylate intoxication)

T: Tumor (increased ICP, hemorrhage, secondary hydrocephalus)

I: Insulin (too little/too much: diabetic ketoacidosis/hypoglycemia)
    Infection (meningitis, sepsis, encephalitis, brain abscess, empyema [epidural/subdural])
    Intussusception

E: Endocrine (hyperfunction or hypofunction)
    Thyroid (myxedema or thyrotoxicosis)
    Adrenal (Addison or Cushing disease)
    Parathyroid (hypoparathyroidism or hyperparathyroidism)

N: Narcosis (hypercapnia [eg, pickwickian syndrome])

T: Temperature (hypothermia, hyperthermia/heat stroke, malignant hyperthermia)

Reproduced with permission from Finberg L, Kleinman RE. *Saunders Manual of Pediatric Practice,* 2nd ed. WB Saunders; Philadelphia, PA, 2002.

TABLE 13.6 ■ COMMON CAUSES OF ALTERED LEVEL OF CONSCIOUSNESS

Commonly Used Mnemonic: TIPS from Vowels

T Trauma, tumor

I Insulin-hypoglycemia, intussusception

P Poisons

S Shock

A Alcohol, abuse

E Epilepsy, encephalopathy

I Infection, inborn errors

O Opiates

U Uremia

Clinical Summary

Febrile seizures are an age-related phenomenon in which a child between 6 months and 5 years of age has fever and a generalized seizure not associated with CNS infection or any other definable cause (eg, metabolic abnormality) or previous history of afebrile seizures. Types of febrile seizures are listed in Table 13.7.

Emergency Department Evaluation and Disposition

Strongly consider performing LP in infants <12 months of age. Between ages 12 and 18 months, LP should be considered. After the age of 18 months, LP is not routinely warranted, but should be done if meningeal signs are present. Obtain laboratory studies (eg, CBC, chemistry) based on clinical evaluation. Treat ongoing seizure activity with benzodiazepine IV

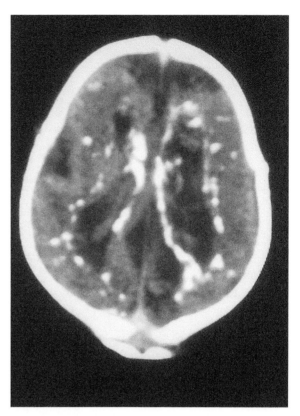

FIGURE 13.20 ■ Convulsion Associated With Fever; Intrauterine Cytomegalovirus (CMV) Infection. A noncontrast CT scan of the head shows extensive periventricular and intraparenchymal calcifications characteristic of prenatal CMV infection in an infant brought to the ED with a febrile seizure followed by loss of consciousness. Infant was also globally delayed with microcephaly. (Photo contributor: Binita R. Shah, MD.)

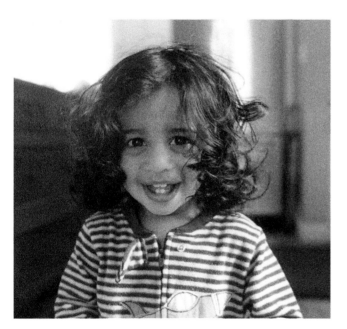

FIGURE 13.19 ■ A Toddler Presenting to the ED with a Recent History of a Simple Febrile Seizure. This toddler was brought to the ED following a very brief febrile seizure at home. His examination did not show any postictal neurologic deficits (overwhelming majority of febrile seizures terminate before presentation to the ED as seen in this toddler). In the absence of clinical signs or symptoms suggestive of CNS infection, such patients can be safely discharged home (once the etiology of fever has been determined). Discharge instructions include fever management, education about the possibility of recurrence of febrile seizures, and first aid management of seizures. (Photo contributor: Kunal M. Shah, MD.)

or rectally. The rectal preparation comes in a predosed syringe (2.5, 5, 10, 15, and 20 mg), making it easy to deliver. Absorption is rapid and effective in interrupting seizure clusters or repetitive seizures. Give antipyretics to make the child more comfortable.

Neither continuous nor intermittent anticonvulsant therapy is recommended for children with 1 or more simple febrile seizures. When the risk of recurrence is high, intermittent oral diazepam at onset of febrile illness may be effective in preventing recurrence. Risk factors for recurrence include early age at first onset, epilepsy or febrile seizures in a first-degree relative, day nursery (increased frequency of febrile episodes), or a first complex febrile seizure. In the absence of risk factors and age >15 months, recurrence is 10% in 18 months. In the presence of 1 to 2 risk factors, recurrence is 25% to 50%; with 3 or more factors, risk is 50% to 100%. Neuroimaging and electroencephalogram (EEG) are not recommended routinely after the first febrile seizure.

TABLE 13.7 ■ TYPES OF FEBRILE SEIZURES

	Ictal Features	Duration	Postictal Features	Recurrence
Simple	Tonic, clonic, tonic-clonic, rarely atonic	<15 min	None	None within 24 hours
Complex	Focal onset	>10–15 min		Within 24 hours
Status epilepticus	Tonic, clonic, tonic-clonic, rarely atonic	30 min or longer or a series of short seizures, without regaining consciousness in between		
	Focal onset			

Pearls

1. Febrile seizures are common in young children (2%–5%) and generally benign with an overall excellent prognosis in most cases.

2. Aim treatment at determining cause of fever and terminating seizure activity.

3. Strongly consider LP in children <18 months of age, as meningitis may present with fever and seizures without meningeal signs in this age group.

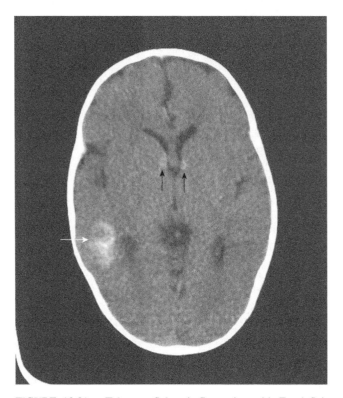

FIGURE 13.21 ■ Tuberous Sclerosis Presenting with Focal Seizure; Differential Diagnosis of Complex Febrile Seizures. A noncontrast CT scan of head shows a high-density lesion in the right posterior temporal region (white arrow) suggestive of a tuber, with 2 small lesions next to the foramen of Monroe of the lateral ventricles (black arrows), suggestive of subependymal nodules in a 4-month-old infant presenting with focal seizures and fever due to acute gastroenteritis. This infant had multiple hypopigmented skin lesions, a finding characteristic of tuberous sclerosis. (Photo contributor: Geetha Chari, MD.)

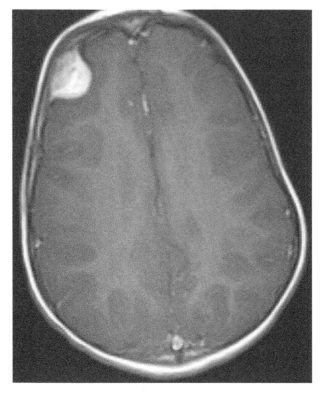

FIGURE 13.22 ■ Brain Tumor Presenting with Focal Seizure; Differential Diagnosis of Complex Febrile Seizures. A 22-month-old toddler presented with several episodes of left-sided focal seizures with generalization, with each episode lasting for about 3 to 5 minutes. A noncontrast CT scan of the brain showed a right frontal extra-axial mass with peripheral curvilinear calcification. His contrast-enhanced axial T1-weighted MRI showed an enhancing extra-axial right frontal mass with "dural tail" anteriorly and posteriorly. Histopathology confirmed histiocytosis. (Photo contributor: Binita R. Shah, MD.)

Clinical Summary

Seizures result from abnormal and excessive synchronized neuronal firing and are characterized by intermittent, stereotypical, usually unprovoked disturbances in consciousness, behavior, emotion, motor function, or sensation. Convulsion is a lay term used to describe excessive, abnormal muscle contractions, usually bilateral, which may be sustained or uninterrupted. Epilepsy is the occurrence of recurrent unprovoked seizures. Aura is the portion of the seizure experienced before consciousness is lost and for which memory is retained. When aura occurs alone, it constitutes a focal seizure with retained awareness, formerly called simple partial seizure. Automatism is a more or less coordinated, repetitive, motor activity that usually occurs during altered consciousness that is not usually remembered by the patient and may resemble a voluntary movement or inappropriate continuation of ongoing preictal motor activity. Generalized tonic-clonic seizures and focal seizures constitute 75% of all the seizure types in childhood followed by absence epilepsy (15%) and other generalized epilepsies including catastrophic syndromes (10%).

Symptomatic seizures follow a triggering event such as fever, head trauma, electrolyte imbalance, hypo- or hyperglycemia, meningitis, or encephalitis. Seizures must be differentiated from other paroxysmal disorders that occur commonly in children. Some examples include episodes without alteration in consciousness like tics, rhythmic motor habits or mannerisms, shuddering spells, rigors (with any febrile illness), jitteriness (newborn period), hypnagogic jerks (sleep myoclonus), benign myoclonus of infancy, benign paroxysmal vertigo, gastroesophageal reflux, cardiac dysrhythmias, Munchausen syndrome by proxy, and nonepileptic (pseudo) seizures. Episodes associated with change in consciousness may also be mistaken for complex partial seizures (eg, delirium with any febrile illness, syncope, cyanotic breath-holding attacks, pallid syncopal attacks, night terrors, migraine [the aura or confusional and basilar artery variants], or narcolepsy).

Emergency Department Evaluation and Disposition

Obtain a detailed history and neurologic examination, and determine if a seizure has occurred or not and the possible cause of the seizure. Order tests based on history or

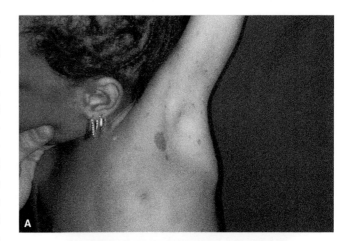

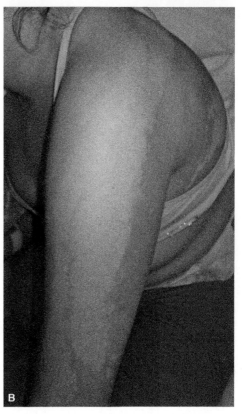

FIGURE 13.23 ■ Neurocutaneous Manifestations Seen in Seizures and Epilepsy. (**A**) Crowe sign and café-au-lait spots in neurofibromatosis. Tiny freckle-like lesions in the axillae are highly characteristic of neurofibromatosis. These lesions were seen in a 6-year-old girl who presented with one episode of afebrile seizure. (**B**) Hypomelanosis of Ito. Linear areas of hypopigmentation that usually follow the lines of Blaschko are typically seen in hypomelanosis of Ito. These were present in a 11-year-old girl with history of intractable epilepsy and intellectual disability. (Photo contributors: Binita R. Shah, MD [A], and Geetha Chari, MD [B].)

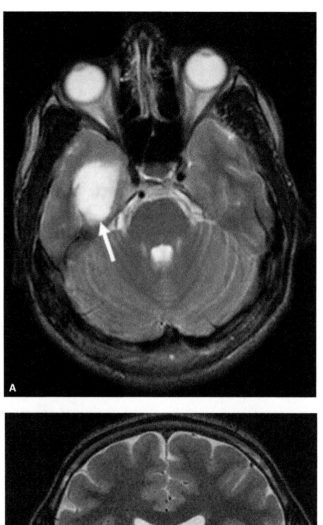

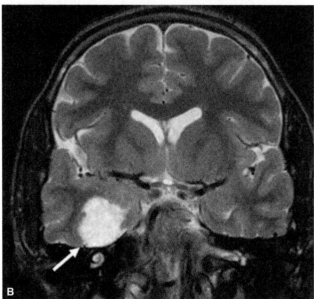

FIGURE 13.24 ■ Dysembryoplastic Neuroepithelial Tumor (DNET). Axial (**A**) and coronal (**B**) T2-weighted images demonstrate a hyperintense cystic-appearing mass centered within the inferior right temporal lobe cortex (white arrows). The cortical involvement, location within the temporal lobe, and bubbly or cystic appearance in a child or young adult are classic for DNET. (Photo/legend contributors: Geetha Chari, MD, and Vinodhkumar Velayudhan, DO.)

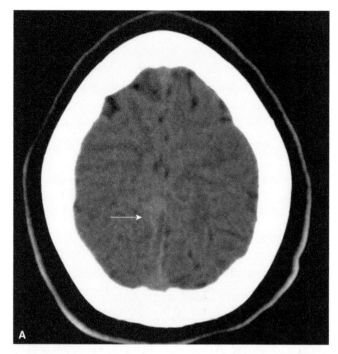

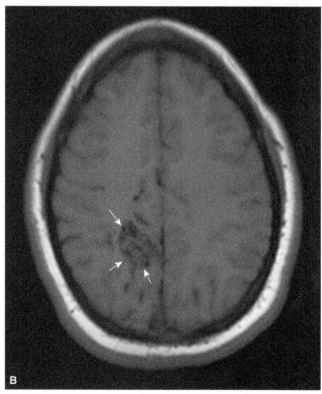

FIGURE 13.25 ■ Arteriovenous (AV) Malformation Presenting with Seizures. (**A**) A noncontrast head CT scan shows a suspicious high-density region in the right parietal region (arrow) in an adolescent girl with a new-onset generalized tonic-clonic seizure during sleep. (**B**) An axial T1-weighted MRI of the brain shows the classic serpiginous flow voids (arrows) of an AV malformation in the right parietal region. (Photo contributor: Geetha Chari, MD.)

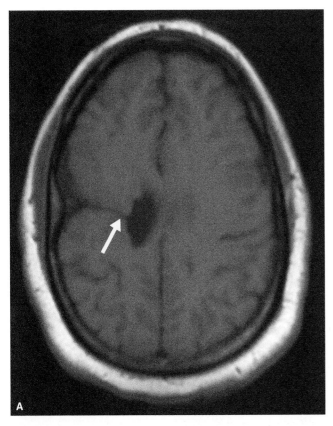
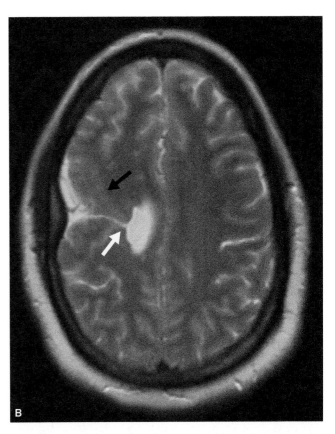

FIGURE 13.26 ■ Closed-Lip Schizencephaly. A 4-year-old girl presented with new onset of focal motor seizures. Axial T1- (**A**) and T2-weighted images (**B**) demonstrate a cleft extending from the cortical surface of the right parietal lobe into the right lateral ventricle (white arrows) that is lined by gray matter (black arrow, **B**), consistent with schizencephaly. The gray matter lining the cleft differentiates schizencephaly from encephalomalacia, porencephaly, or other pathology that may produce a cleft. (Photo contributor: Vinodhkumar Velayudhan, DO.)

clinical findings (eg, vomiting, diarrhea, dehydration, or failure to return to baseline alertness) and toxicology screening (if possibility of drug exposure or substance abuse). Consider LP if there is concern for meningitis or encephalitis. CT scan is not routinely indicated for evaluation of new-onset seizure unless abnormal neurologic examination, predisposing history, or focal-onset seizure suggests an acute management intervention is required. An EEG is recommended as part of the neurodiagnostic evaluation of the child with an apparent first unprovoked seizure; however, it is not required in the ED and may be performed nonemergently unless the child is in status epilepticus.

Children with new-onset unprovoked seizures do not require hospitalization and should be referred to their primary care physician for follow-up. The majority will have few or no recurrences (risk of recurrence is ~40%, which rises to 80% after a second unprovoked seizure). About 75% of all recurrences occur within 6 months, and very few occur after 2 years. Treatment with anticonvulsants may be considered in circumstances where the benefits of reducing the risk of a second seizure outweigh the risks of pharmacologic and psychosocial side effects. Consult neurology to assist in such decisions.

Pearls

1. MRI is the preferred neuroimaging modality for unprovoked new-onset seizures.

2. Obtain emergent head CT in any child exhibiting a postictal focal deficit (Todd paresis) not quickly resolving or who has not returned to baseline within several hours after the seizure.

3. Long-term anticonvulsant therapy is not routinely started in a child with the first unprovoked seizure.

Clinical Summary

Status epilepticus is a condition resulting either from the failure of the mechanisms responsible for seizure termination or from the initiation of mechanisms that lead to abnormally prolonged seizures. It is a condition that can have long-term consequences including neuronal death, neuronal injury, and alteration of neuronal networks, depending on the type and duration of seizures. A more practical definition is a generalized convulsive seizure longer than 5 minutes in duration, because the vast majority of self-limiting generalized seizures stop 2 to 3 minutes after onset, and almost all cease within 5 minutes. Acute repetitive seizures are those that recur at frequent intervals, with full recovery between seizures. Seizure clusters may occur regularly at certain times in some patients (eg, around menstruation). Status epilepticus may be convulsive (focal or generalized tonic clonic) or nonconvulsive (including absence and focal onset).

Status epilepticus may be the initial manifestation in one-third of epilepsy cases. One-third of status cases occur in previously diagnosed epilepsy. One-third occur as a result of an acute isolated brain insult. Status epilepticus is more common in infants and young toddlers, and >50% of cases occur in those <3 years of age.

In patients with epilepsy, common causes of status epilepticus include low anticonvulsant levels, sudden withdrawal of antiepileptic medications, failure to adhere to medication regimen, and drug interactions. Other causes include fever, toxic causes (alcohol, drugs, poisons), CNS infections (eg,

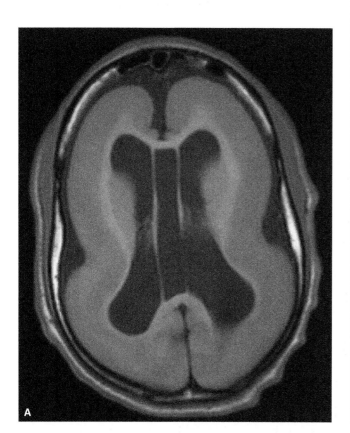 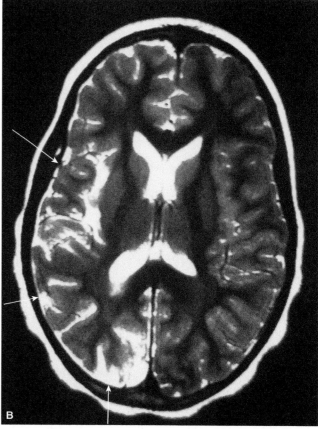

FIGURE 13.27 ■ Status Epilepticus from Different Etiologies. (**A**) Cortical malformations presenting with status epilepticus. Axial T1-weighted MRI of brain shows lissencephaly (a major malformation of cortical development characterized by smooth brain, without sulci and abnormal thickened cortex with enlarged ventricles) in an adolescent boy with status epilepticus due to low anticonvulsant levels. He had microcephaly with severe cognitive and motor impairment. (**B**) Autoimmune encephalitis presenting with status epilepticus. The T2-weighted MRI shows atrophy of the right hemisphere, with excessive CSF spaces (arrows) in a child brought in with epileptica partialis continua, with continuous clonic jerks of the left hand, and mild left hemiparesis. Together with the history, the imaging findings are suggestive of Rasmussen encephalitis. (Photo contributor: Geetha Chari, MD.)

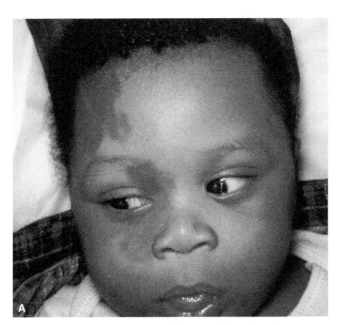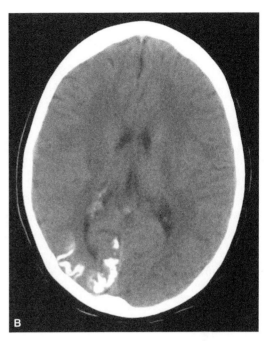

FIGURE 13.28 ■ Sturge-Weber Syndrome (SWS). (**A**) Port-wine stain (PWS). PWS is seen in a patient who was brought to the ED with status epilepticus. The most common location of a PWS is the face. (PWS may also get confused with a red or purple bruise of inflicted injury, especially when it is very extensive, as in this case). When a PWS is localized to the trigeminal area of the face (especially upper eyelid and forehead), a diagnosis of SWS must be considered. (**B**) Noncontrast CT of the head showing "tram-track" calcifications of the right occipital cortex with atrophy. An enlarged right-sided choroid plexus is also noted, which may be secondary to an angioma. (Photo contributor: Binita R. Shah, MD.)

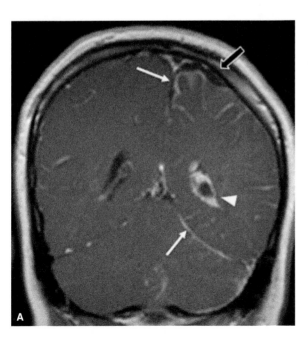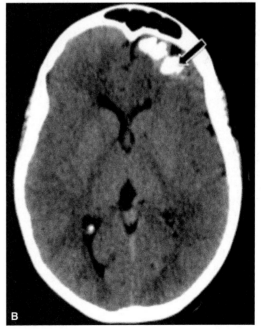

FIGURE 13.29 ■ Sturge-Weber Syndrome (SWS). (**A**) Coronal T1-weighted postcontrast image demonstrates mild atrophy of the left cerebral hemisphere with sulcal widening (black arrow), abnormal enhancement due to increased vascularity extending over the gyri and into the sulci (white arrows), and an enlarged choroid plexus in the left lateral ventricle (arrowhead). (**B**) Noncontrast CT image demonstrates cortical calcifications in the left frontal lobe (black arrow) in an adolescent girl presenting with focal seizures. She also had port-wine hemangiomas over the left side of her face. (Photo/legend contributors: Geetha Chari, MD, and Vinodhkumar Velayudhan, DO.)

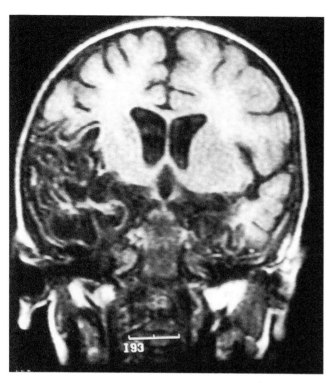

FIGURE 13.30 ■ Herpes Encephalitis. An 18-month-old child was brought in with status epilepticus. History was positive for herpes simplex virus encephalitis at the age of 6 months. This patient cannot talk or sit and has developed choreoathetoid movements and seizures with extension of the legs and flexion of the arms. MRI showed encephalomalacia of the right temporoparietal lobe. (Photo contributor: Geetha Chari, MD.)

herpes encephalitis), trauma, stroke, acute hydrocephalus, electrolyte imbalance (hypoglycemia, hyponatremia, hypocalcemia), and progressive degenerative disorders.

Emergency Department Evaluation and Disposition

The first step in management is ensuring the ABCs of life support; monitor vital signs, pulse oximetry, and ECG.

TABLE 13.8 ■ GUIDELINES FOR MANAGEMENT OF STATUS EPILEPTICUS

1. Emergently give IV anticonvulsant therapy when seizures continue for 2 minutes or longer:
   - Benzodiazepines (first medication of choice): lorazepam or diazepam (if IV access is not achieved, give rectal diazepam or intranasal midazolam)
   - If seizures still continue: fosphenytoin IV loading dose, valproic acid IV, or levetiracetam IV
   - If seizures continue (patient in refractory status epilepticus): phenobarbital given IV
2. Consider intubation and mechanical ventilation
3. For patients who continue to seize: begin continuous infusion of sedative medications: midazolam, propofol, or pentobarbital

Administer anticonvulsants to stop the seizure safely and quickly while minimizing treatment-related morbidity. Pay close attention to the systemic effects of status epilepticus and the side effects of treatment (sedation, cardiovascular and respiratory compromise). Obtain a fingerstick glucose test as soon as possible to detect hypoglycemia and administer IV glucose if hypoglycemia is found or suspected. In adolescents, administer IV thiamine 100 mg first. Take blood for CBC, chemistries, toxicology screening, and anticonvulsant levels, if applicable. Watch for hyperthermia, which can occur secondary to prolonged seizure activity. If available, use continuous bedside EEG to monitor therapy. Admit patient to ICU for further management and monitoring.

Pearl

1. Identify the cause and precipitating factors and provide specific antidote if a cause is known (eg, pyridoxine for status epilepticus due to isoniazid overdose).

Clinical Summary

Stroke is the sudden occlusion or rupture of cerebral blood vessels resulting in focal cerebral damage causing clinical neurologic deficits. Strokes in children are relatively rare, and diagnosis is frequently delayed. Stroke is either ischemic (either arterial embolic or thrombotic or venous sinus thrombosis) or hemorrhagic. Risk factors for stroke in children include cardiac abnormalities (eg, atrial septal defect, ventricular septal defect, cyanotic heart disease, myocarditis,

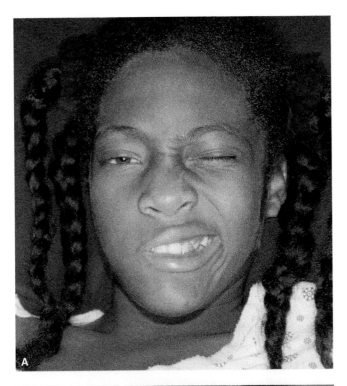

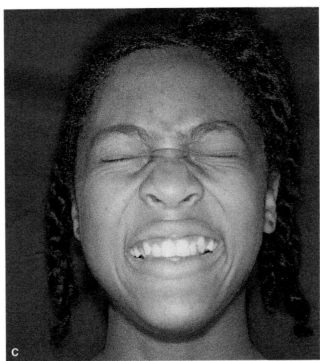

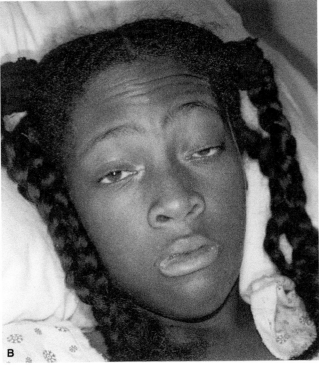

FIGURE 13.31 ■ Right Facial Palsy (Central Facial Palsy or Upper Motor Neuron Palsy) Presenting with Stroke. (**A**) Asymmetric movements of facial muscles, inability to close right eye (but not left), deviated angle of the mouth, and flattening of the right naso-labial fold. (**B**) Ability to wrinkle the forehead equally bilaterally and raise eyebrows symmetrically is preserved. Right-sided facial weakness involving lower part of face with sparing of upper part (forehead) are classic findings for upper motor neuron facial palsy. (**C**) Full recovery (after 6 months) from the right facial palsy with symmetrical smile and ability to close eyes bilaterally. This patient had a history suggestive of a thrombotic ischemic stroke (see also Figure 13.32). (Photo contributor: Binita R. Shah, MD.)

617

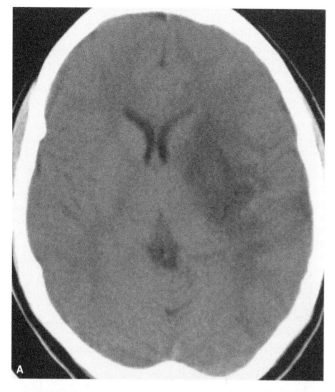

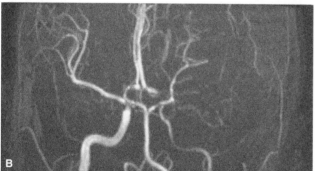

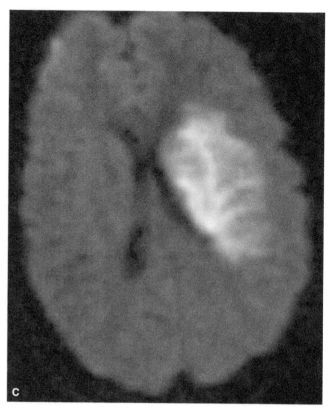

FIGURE 13.32 ■ Ischemic Stroke; Middle Cerebral Artery (MCA) Infarct. (**A**) A Noncontrast head CT of the patient in Figure 13.31) shows left MCA infarct (area of low attenuation) involving left lentiform nucleus parietal cortex. There is evidence of mass effect with mild midline shift toward the right and mild compression of the left lateral ventricle. Other findings included left MCA hyperdense and infarct areas involving left frontal temporal lobes including basal ganglia. (**B**) MRI and MRA with gadolinium reveals decreased flow in left internal carotid artery (along its entire course) and MCA with nonvisualization of sylvian branches. (**C**) Diffusion-weighted image reveals large acute MCA infarct in left basal ganglia and parietal lobe. (Photo contributor: Binita R. Shah, MD.)

endocarditis, arrhythmias), vascular abnormalities (eg, vasculitis, lupus, moyamoya, Ehler-Danlos syndrome, fibromuscular dysplasia, atrioventricular malformation, Sturge-Weber syndrome), hematologic disorders (eg, sickle cell disease, protein C or S deficiency, antithrombin III deficiency, thrombocytopenia), metabolic disorders (eg, homocystinuria, organic acidurias, mitochondrial disorders), trauma (eg, child abuse, arterial dissection, blunt cervical arterial trauma, intraoral trauma), or systemic disorders (eg, diabetes mellitus, hypertension). Typically, stroke is an acute neurologic event manifesting as hemiparesis with or without seizures, which are relatively frequent at stroke onset in children compared

to adults. Seizures, fever, headache, and lethargy occur more commonly in younger children. Dystonia is more common in children with basal ganglia infarction. Neonatal strokes manifest with persistent acute focal seizures.

Emergency Department Treatment and Disposition

Consult neurology emergently for a child with a sudden-onset focal neurologic deficit, as stroke in children may have many causes, is difficult to diagnose, and may have therapeutic

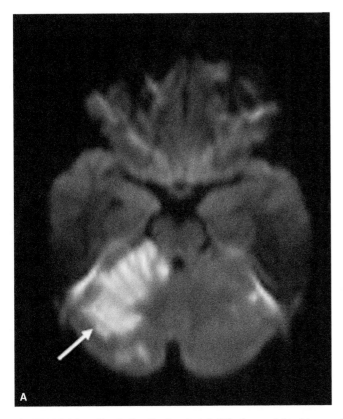 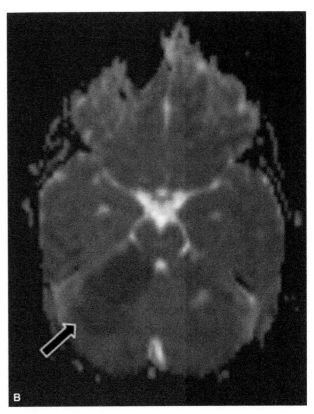

FIGURE 13.33 ■ Cerebellar Stroke. Axial diffusion-weighted image (**A**) demonstrates high signal (white arrow) with corresponding low signal (black arrow) on the apparent diffusion coefficient map (**B**) consistent with restricted water diffusion due to acute ischemia. Diffusion-weighted images are the most sensitive MRI sequence for acute stroke and can detect ischemia within minutes. These findings were seen in an 8-year-old boy presenting with unsteadiness of gait for one day. (Photo contributor: Vinodhkumar Velayudhan, DO.)

implications. Obtain an emergent head CT to look for fresh blood and subarachnoid hemorrhage. CT findings of ischemic stroke appear as low density fitting a vascular territory (findings similar to adults). Hemorrhagic infarcts have additional high-density components. MRI is more sensitive than CT in detecting small and multiple infarcts. Diffusion-weighted imaging and perfusion-weighted imaging have improved early detection and specificity of ischemic injury. Perform magnetic resonance angiography (MRA) at the same time as MRI because it adds valuable information regarding the cerebral arteries and angiomatous malformations. MRA is noninvasive and correlates well with conventional angiography. Magnetic resonance venography is the diagnostic study of choice in sinovenous thrombosis. Helical CT angiography can provide diagnostic information; however, exposure to excessive radiation in children is of concern. When dissection is suspected, conventional angiography is the criterion standard.

Thrombolytic agents (tissue plasminogen activator) have been effective in adults when administered within 3 hours of onset of stroke symptoms. Use of thrombolytic agents in children with arterial ischemic stroke has been rare; however, accumulating experience with antithrombotic and anticoagulant treatment in children suggests that these agents can be safely used. Hospitalize patients to ICU for monitoring and ongoing care.

Pearls

1. Recognize *stroke* means *brain attack*.
2. Differentiate ischemic from hemorrhagic stroke. In children, ischemic and hemorrhagic stroke are similar in frequency, unlike adults.
3. Quickly assess if patient is a candidate for thrombolytic therapy (time is of essence: within 3 hours).
4. Consider antithrombotic, anticoagulant, or anticonvulsant administration.

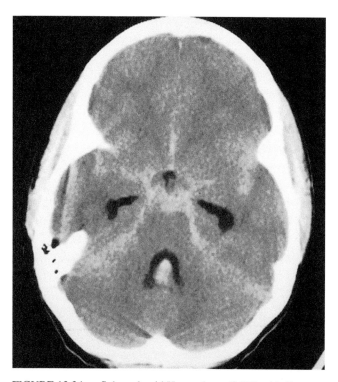

FIGURE 13.34 ■ Subarachnoid Hemorrhage (SAH) with Communicating Hydrocephalus. A noncontrast CT scan of the brain shows SAH in basal cisterns, sylvian fissures, and intraventricular blood in the fourth ventricle with associated hydrocephalus (ventricles uniformly dilated out of proportion to sulci suggestive of communicating hydrocephalus). Severe headache followed by vomiting and unresponsiveness were presenting complaint of this girl. (Photo contributor: Binita R. Shah, MD.)

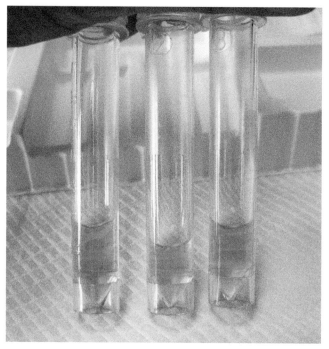

FIGURE 13.35 ■ CSF Examination in Subarachnoid Hemorrhage (SAH). A lumbar puncture is performed if the CT scan fails to confirm the clinical diagnosis of SAH. In stroke, CSF exam usually reveals markedly elevated pressure and is grossly bloody (as seen in all tubes) containing 100,000 to >1 million RBCs/cm³. The supernatant of centrifuged CSF becomes xanthochromic within several hours due to breakdown of hemoglobin from RBCs. WBCs in the CSF are in the same proportion to RBCs as in peripheral blood. Presence of blood in the CSF may produce chemical meningitis and pleocytosis (several thousand WBCs) during first 48 hours and reduction of CSF glucose (usually 4–8 days after hemorrhage). CSF glucose is normal in absence of pleocytosis. (Photo contributor: Binita R. Shah, MD.)

Clinical Summary

Neurocysticercosis is a CNS infestation by the larval stage of *Taenia solium* (tapeworm), resulting from ingestion of *T solium* eggs. Symptoms depend on the number, stage, and localization of parasites in the nervous system and the severity of the host's immune response to the parasite. Seizures are the most common presentation, occurring in about 70% of patients. Increased ICP may result from hydrocephalus (meningeal infestation results in arachnoiditis and adhesions leading to obstruction or from ventricular cysts), pseudotumor, giant cysts, or cysticercal encephalitis. Focal neurologic deficits may result from direct compression by the cysts or transiently secondary to seizures (Todd phenomenon). Spinal cord may also be involved, more commonly with leptomeningeal larval infestation, whereas intramedullary involvement is uncommon. Consider diagnosis of neurocysticercosis in any patient with new onset of focal-onset or secondarily generalized seizures, especially if the patient has either recently migrated or recently traveled to one of the endemic regions.

Emergency Department Treatment and Disposition

Use noncontrast head CT to detect calcifications, which are present in 50% of the cases. Cysts appear as small, round, low-density lesions, with an eccentric hyperdense mural nodule (scolex). Edema around the lesion indicates a dying cyst. Use of contrast causes ring enhancement. The most common

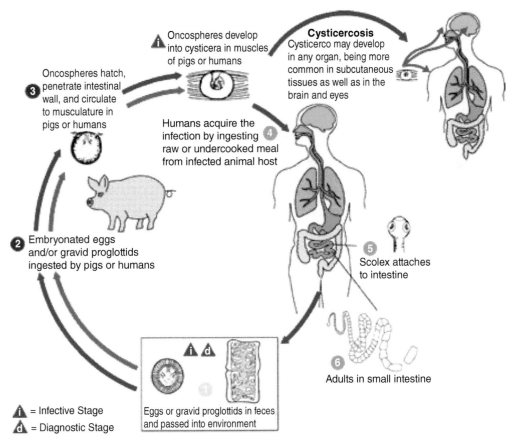

Oncospheres develop into cysticera in muscles of pigs or humans

Cysticercosis
Cysticerco may develop in any organ, being more common in subcutaneous tissues as well as in the brain and eyes

3 Oncospheres hatch, penetrate intestinal wall, and circulate to musculature in pigs or humans

Humans acquire the infection by ingesting **4** raw or undercooked meal from infected animal host

2 Embryonated eggs and/or gravid proglottids ingested by pigs or humans

5 Scolex attaches to intestine

6 Adults in small intestine

Eggs or gravid proglottids in feces and passed into environment

= Infective Stage
= Diagnostic Stage

FIGURE 13.36 ■ Life Cycle of Tapeworms (Taeniasis and Cysticercosis). Cysticercosis is infection with the larval stages of the parasitic cestode *Taenia solium* shed in the feces of a human tapeworm carrier (1), which are ingested by humans or pigs (2). Humans are infected by ingestion of contaminated pork or autoinfection. In the latter, a human ingests eggs through fecal contamination or from proglottids carried into the stomach by reverse peristalsis. Once eggs are ingested, oncospheres hatch in the intestine (3), invade the intestinal wall, and migrate to striated muscles, as well as the brain, liver, and other tissues, where they develop into cysticerci (4 and 5). In humans, cysts in the brain can cause neurocysticercosis. (Reproduced with permission from Centers for Disease Control and Prevention. DPDx: Taeniasis: www.cdc.gov/dpdx/taeniasis/index.html.)

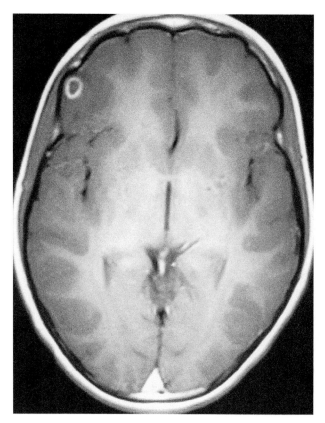

FIGURE 13.37 ■ Ring-Enhancing Cortical Lesion of Neurocysticercosis. Axial T1-weighted gadolinium-enhanced MRI shows solitary ring-enhancing lesion in right frontal cortex a child presenting with new-onset partial complex seizures. (Photo contributor: Binita R. Shah, MD.)

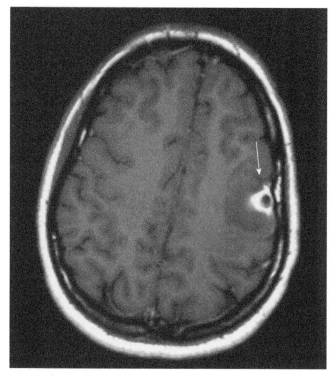

FIGURE 13.38 ■ Neurocysticercosis. An axial T1-weighted MRI with contrast reveals ring-enhancing lesion, with surrounding edema (arrow) indicative of a dying cyst. This patient presented with new-onset focal seizures. (Photo contributor: Geetha Chari, MD.)

finding of neurocysticercosis in a patient with seizures is a single small enhancing lesion. Multiple cysts ("starry night") may be seen in some patients. Extensive edema is seen with an encephalopathic presentation. Brain MRI is useful for assessing the degree of infection and location and evolutionary stage of the disease, and helps to identify lesions in the brainstem, cerebellum, base of the brain, eye, and spinal cord; however, it will not pick up small calcifications. Differential diagnoses of the imaging findings include tuberculoma, brain abscess, fungal abscess, toxoplasmosis, brain tumor, and infectious vasculitis. Immunologic testing may be performed using serum or CSF. Enzyme-linked immunoelectrotransfer blot is a very sensitive and specific test; however, >30% of patients with a single brain lesion may test negative.

Admit patients with signs of increased ICP, hydrocephalus, or encephalitic presentation. Consult neurology for treatment, which depends on the lesion type. Antiparasitic medications (cysticidal drugs) include albendazole and praziquantel.

Albendazole has been shown to be superior to praziquantel, and a 1-week course of therapy is adequate. Treatment of a single solitary calcified lesion is controversial. Use corticosteroids in combination with cysticidal drugs in cases with arachnoid involvement, encephalitic presentation, multiple live cysts, spinal cysts, and ventricular cysts. Consult neurosurgery for shunt placement if hydrocephalus is present.

Pearls

1. Neurocysticercosis is a parasitic infestation of the CNS and the most common cause of acquired epilepsy worldwide.
2. Cysticercosis is endemic in various regions in the world including Latin America, India, Africa, and China.
3. Seizures are the most common presentation.
4. Neuroimaging is the main diagnostic investigation.

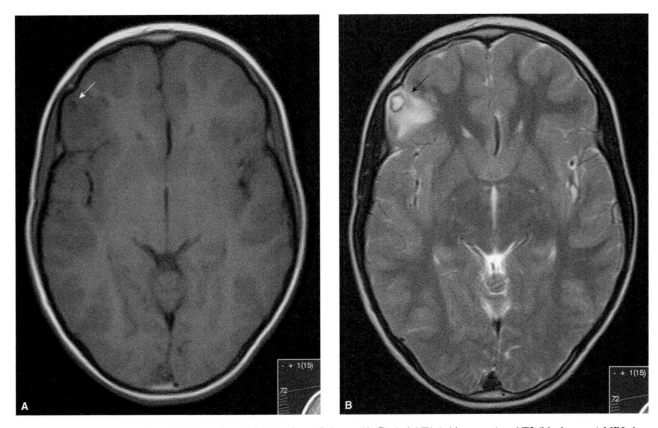

FIGURE 13.39 ■ Neurocysticercosis Presenting with New-Onset Seizure. (**A, B**) Axial T1 (white arrow) and T2 (black arrow) MRI shows a small round lesion with surrounding edema in a 13-year-old boy presenting with history of seizures. He had recently migrated from Haiti. His CSF was positive for cysticercus antibody. (Photo contributor: Geetha Chari, MD.)

Clinical Summary

Bell palsy is an idiopathic condition characterized by a lower motor neuron (peripheral) facial neuropathy and is almost always unilateral. The facial nerve has a long intracranial and extracranial course beginning in the pons at the facial nerve nucleus and ending in the parotid gland. Etiology of facial neuropathy is varied, and evidence of other neurologic symptoms and signs is often seen. Isolated facial nerve involvement is seen in Ramsay-Hunt syndrome secondary to herpes zoster infection. The typical presentation of Bell palsy is sudden-onset unilateral facial paresis that evolves rapidly and maximizes within 2 days. Associated symptoms include hyperacusis, decreased production of tears, and altered taste. Ear pain or fullness and mild facial pain may be present. Severe pain should raise the suspicion of Ramsay-Hunt syndrome. Neurologic examination reveals isolated lower motor neuron facial weakness with inability to wrinkle the forehead, impaired closure of the eye, drooping of the brow and corner of the mouth, and difficulty closing the mouth. Bell phenomenon (upward eye movement on attempted eye closure) is seen because of incomplete closing of the eye.

Emergency Department Treatment and Disposition

Examine the ear canal, palate, and tongue. Vesicles suggest Ramsay-Hunt syndrome and opacity of the tympanic membrane, granulations and polyposis suggest middle ear pathology. Check for skin lesions such as erythema migrans, which suggest Lyme disease as a cause (isolated unilateral or bilateral peripheral facial palsy could be a manifestation of Lyme disease). If there are no other findings besides unilateral facial paresis, a diagnosis of Bell palsy can be made clinically, and no further workup may be required in the ED. Provide treatment to hasten recovery and prevent corneal complications. Use lubricating eye drops, applied several times daily to protect the cornea from drying and abrasion due to impaired eye closure. Use a lubricant eye ointment, and tape the eye shut at night. Do not use gauze as it can dry the eye further by a wicking effect of the gauze. Give oral prednisone 1 mg/kg/day for 5 to 7 days and then taper over next 5 days and discontinue. Steroids should ideally be given within the first 72 hours of symptom onset. The role of antiviral agents (eg, Acyclovir) in Bell palsy is not clear. Most patients start to improve with

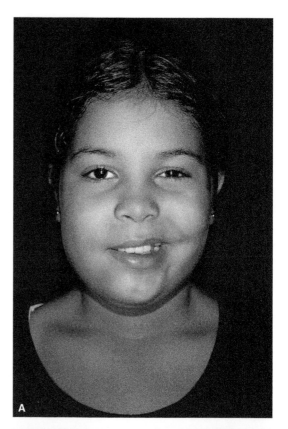

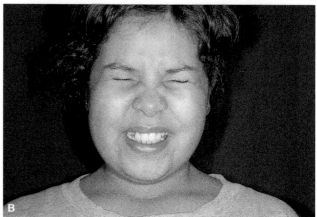

FIGURE 13.40 ■ Right-Sided Bell Palsy. (**A**) Bell palsy is a clinical diagnosis. Ask the patient to smile, close eyes, raise eyebrows, and whistle or puff out the cheeks. Facial muscle paresis, facial asymmetry, drooling, widened palpebral fissure, smooth forehead, and flattened nasolabial fold are characteristic findings. (**B**) Complete recovery from facial palsy. These 2 photographs were taken 8 weeks apart in this otherwise healthy adolescent girl with Bell palsy. (Photo contributor: Binita R. Shah, MD.)

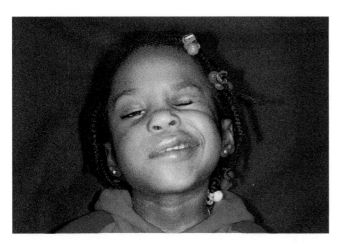

FIGURE 13.41 ■ Right-Sided Facial Palsy Secondary to Rhabdo-myosarcoma. Sudden onset of right lower motor neuron facial palsy was a presenting compliant in this 3-year-old girl who also had a history of intermittent bloody otorrhea from her right ear of 5 days in duration. She denied any history of fever, earache, headache, or vertigo. Her right tympanic membrane showed perforation with bloody discharge. A noncontrast CT scan of her temporal bone showed presence of external canal soft tissue mass on the right side extending in the middle ear cavity and mastoid cells associated with bony erosion of the mastoid cells. (Photo contributor: Binita R. Shah, MD.)

or without treatment in 2 weeks, and complete recovery may occur in 2 to 3 months.

Pearls

1. Differentiate Bell palsy, which causes a complete unilateral involvement of the face, from upper motor neuron (central) facial paresis, which spares the forehead.
2. Bilateral facial palsy is seen in Lyme disease, Miller-Fisher syndrome, Guillain-Barré syndrome, HIV, meningitis, and pontine lesions.

Clinical Summary

Headache in children and adolescents is common and may be a primary disorder, such as migraine or tension-type headache, or secondary to a systemic illness or a CNS disorder. Migraine is seen in about 10% of children aged 5 to 15 years and has a genetic component, with history of migraine reported in at least 1 parent in 90% of cases. Headaches can present as acute generalized, acute localized, recurrent acute, chronic nonprogressive, and chronic progressive forms. Raised ICP is of major concern when a child presents to the ED with headaches. Signs and symptoms suggestive of intracranial pathology include morning headache on wakening, aggravation by sneezing/coughing, recurrent localized headache, persistent vomiting, progressive frequency or severity, diplopia, papilledema, strabismus, focal neurologic deficit, and macrocephaly.

Signs suggestive of increased ICP include new-onset sixth nerve palsy (unilateral or bilateral), which is a false localizing sign. Third nerve palsy is more ominous (ptosis, abduction, and dilated pupil), suggesting uncal herniation. Downward deviation of both eyes (sunsetting) indicates impaired upgaze due to pressure on the tectum of the midbrain, seen in central herniation. Central upward herniation due to pressure from the posterior fossa can cause reverse sunsetting, with impaired downgaze.

Uncal herniation causes declining consciousness, dilated and fixed ipsilateral pupil, decerebrate rigidity, increased blood pressure, bradycardia, and respiratory irregularity. Central transtentorial herniation causes declining consciousness, decerebrate or decorticate rigidity, impaired upward gaze, irregular respiration, and papillary constriction or dilation. Cerebellar herniation will lead to decreased LOC, impaired upgaze, irregular respiration, lower cranial nerve palsies, neck stiffness, or head tilt. Headaches due to ominous conditions leading to increased ICP almost always have abnormal findings on examination.

Emergency Department Treatment and Disposition

Take a detailed history with attention to the duration (days, weeks, months, years); location (frontal, occipital, hemicranial, bitemporal); timing (on awakening, morning, afternoon, evening, from sleep); quality (eg, throbbing, pulsatile, pressure, tight band); frequency (daily, weekly, monthly); and

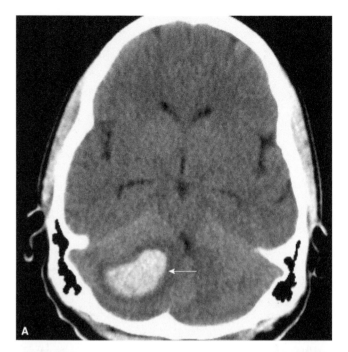

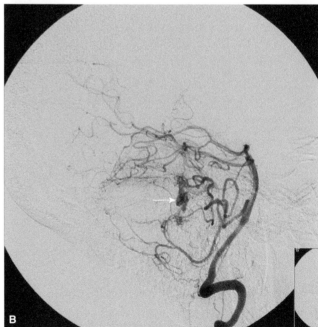

FIGURE 13.42 ■ Acute Hematoma from Ruptured Arteriovenous (AV) Malformation. (**A**) A precontrast head CT reveals hyperdense lesion in right cerebellum (arrow) consistent with acute hematoma in a 12-year-old with headache, vomiting, dysarthria, and ataxia. (**B**) Vertebral angiogram shows small AV malformation (arrow). (Photo contributor: Geetha Chari, MD.)

severity (mild, moderate, severe; scale 1–10) of the headaches. Note any visual symptoms (flashing lights, double vision, scotomas, obscurations) or nausea or vomiting, photophobia or phonophobia, and relieving factors (eg, analgesics, sleep).

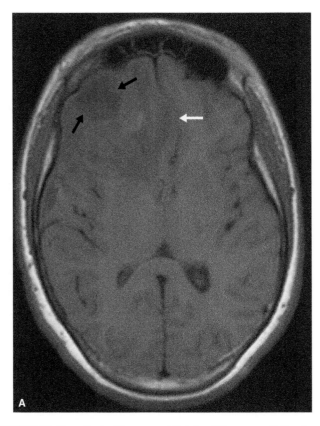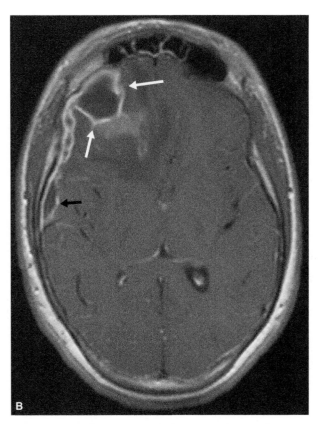

FIGURE 13.43 ■ Brain Abscess and Subdural Empyema Following Sinusitis. (**A**) An axial T1-weighted MRI reveals a hypointense lesion in the right frontal region (black arrows) with surrounding vasogenic edema and midline shift (white arrow) in a 14-year-old adolescent presenting with headache, vomiting, and new-onset secondarily generalized seizure following recent sinusitis. (**B**) Postcontrast axial MRI shows abscess with ring enhancement (white arrows) and a subdural empyema (black arrow). (Photo contributor: Geetha Chari, MD.)

Perform a careful neurologic examination including mental status assessment and fundus exam, and check cranial nerves, motor function, cerebellar functions, and gait evaluation.

Obtain a head CT for the first or "worst" headache, progressive symptoms, macrocephaly, any abnormality on neurologic examination, presence of VP shunt, age <3 years, pain in the occipital region, nuchal rigidity, or suspicion of hemorrhage. Neuroimaging is usually not necessary in a patient with typical migraine or tension-type headache. Use brain MRI in a nonemergent situation, as it provides better information about areas such as the posterior fossa, craniocervical junction, and sellar region. Use contrast when infection, inflammation, or mass lesion is suspected. Perform an LP if infection is suspected or pseudotumor is a consideration, and measure opening pressure of CSF to confirm the diagnosis.

Management depends on the underlying cause. NSAIDs (ibuprofen or naproxen) can help abort most migraine headaches, if acetaminophen does not help. Triptans are approved for abortive treatment of uncomplicated migraine in children over the age of 12 years.

Pearls

1. Majority of children with headaches *do not* have organic intracranial pathologies.
2. Neuroimaging is not indicated in all patients presenting with headache to the ED.
3. Increased ICP will manifest abnormalities on neurologic examination.
4. The American Academy of Neurology practice parameter for evaluating recurrent headaches in children states that presence of a space-occupying lesion is suggested by headache lasting <1 month, absence of family history of migraine, abnormal neurologic findings on examination, gait abnormality, and occurrence of seizures.

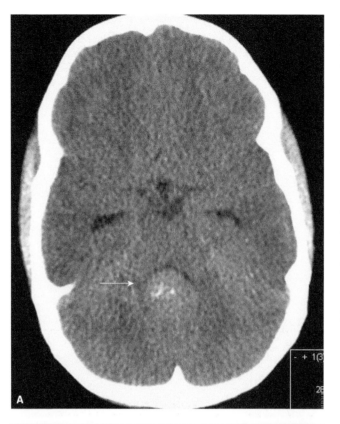

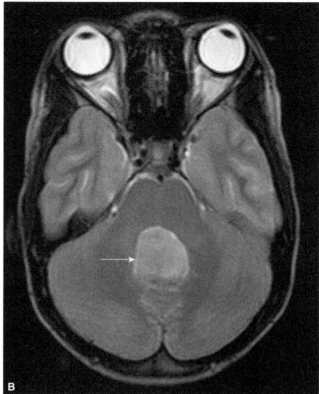

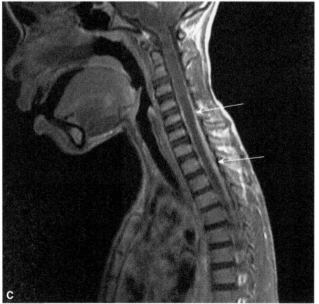

FIGURE 13.44 ■ Brain Tumor; Medulloblastoma. (A) A non-contrast CT reveals a poorly defined mass in the posterior fossa (white arrow), with specks of calcification, and compression of the fourth ventricle in an 8-year-old child with longstanding history of "migraines" with recent headache lasting several days and associated with vomiting. (B) Axial T2-weighted MRI reveals hyperintense mass in midline of posterior fossa blocking the fourth ventricle (white arrow). (C) Postcontrast spine MRI shows diffuse meningeal enhancement (white arrows) suggestive of meningeal spread of tumor. These findings suggest aggressive medulloblastoma with meningeal spread. (Photo contributor: Geetha Chari, MD.)

Clinical Summary

Brain tumors are the most common solid tumors in childhood and the second most frequent malignancy (next to leukemia) in children. Posterior fossa tumors account for nearly 85% of tumors in children >1 to 2 years old and include medulloblastoma, cerebellar astrocytoma, ependymoma, and brainstem

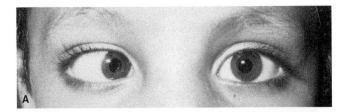

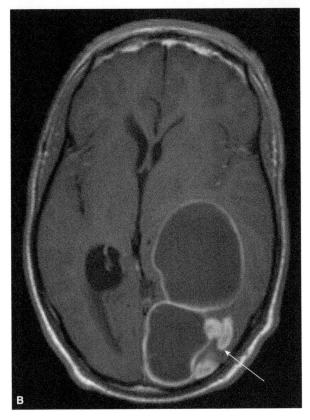

FIGURE 13.45 ■ Supratentorial Brain Tumor; Ganglioglioma. (**A**) An adolescent boy presented with severe headache, vomiting, and a right-sided sixth cranial nerve palsy. The sixth nerve has the longest intracranial course, which makes it vulnerable to raised intracranial pressure (ICP). Even though it is one of the earliest signs of raised ICP, it is a false localizing sign, because it does not suggest necessarily that the lesion is in the brainstem, where the sixth nerve nucleus lies. (**B**) Axial T1 MRI with contrast reveals a cystic tumor with an enhancing solid component (arrow). Pathology revealed an anaplastic ganglioglioma. (Photo contributors: Shahina Qureshi, MD [A], and Geetha Chari, MD [B].)

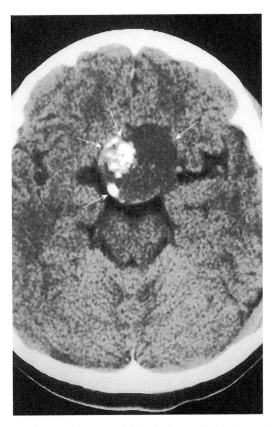

FIGURE 13.46 ■ Supratentorial Brain Tumor; Craniopharyngioma. A CT scan of the head shows a round cystic midline mass (arrows) in the suprasellar region, with areas of hyperdensity indicative of calcification, characteristic of craniopharyngioma in a 12-year-old girl presenting with visual field defects. (Photo contributor: Binita R. Shah, MD.)

glioma. Supratentorial tumors are less common and include astrocytoma, oligodendroglioma, pineal tumors, ganglioglioma, and sellar and suprasellar tumors. Clinical manifestations depend on tumor location and whether it is slow growing or rapidly expanding. In rare instances, with tumors in infancy, enlarging head circumference may be the presenting feature. More commonly, symptoms of increased ICP including headache, vomiting, impaired vision, and alteration in consciousness are seen. Signs of increased ICP are sixth nerve palsy (false localizing sign) and papilledema. Depending on the location, other neurologic signs may develop, such as cranial nerve deficits, spasticity, hyperreflexia, ataxia, and dysmetria. Seizures may be seen in tumors involving the cerebral hemispheres but are not common (<1% of new-onset seizures result from a brain tumor).

Cerebellar astrocytomas are slow-growing tumors, characterized by a large cystic lesion with a mural nodule. Symptoms include insidious and intermittent headaches, unsteady

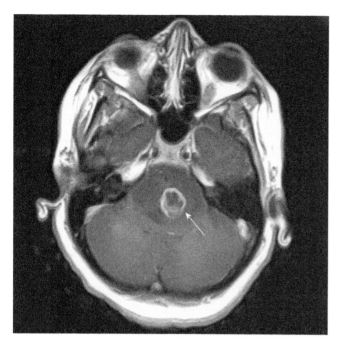

FIGURE 13.47 ■ Posterior Fossa Tumor; Pontine Glioma. T1 axial postcontrast MRI reveals diffuse hypointense enlargement of pons, with area of increased hypointensity with ring enhancement (arrow), in a 12-year-old adolescent with history of unsteady gait, intermittent vomiting, and headache. Imaging is consistent with a pontine glioma, with central necrosis. (Photo contributor: Geetha Chari, MD.)

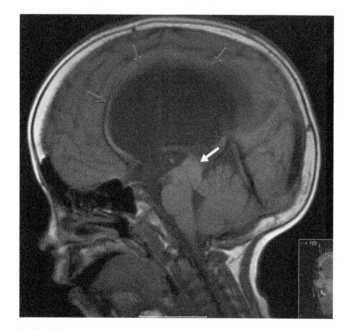

FIGURE 13.48 ■ Midbrain Tumor. A sagittal T1 noncontrast MRI reveals isointense enlargement of midbrain (white arrow), with compression of aqueduct leading to ventricular enlargement (red arrows) in an 8-year-old with developmental delay and large head. These findings are fairly typical for a low-grade midbrain tumor. (Photo contributor: Geetha Chari, MD.)

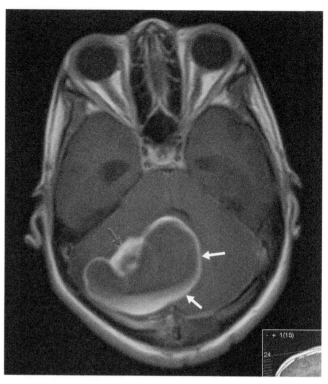

FIGURE 13.49 ■ Posterior Fossa Tumor; Cerebellar Astrocytoma. An axial T1-weighted MRI with contrast reveals a large cystic tumor (white arrows) with a mural nodule that enhances with contrast (red arrow), typical of a cerebellar astrocytoma in a 10-year-old child with headache and difficulty walking. (Photo contributor: Geetha Chari, MD.)

gait, and vomiting. Papilledema, ataxia (mild or severe), and dysmetria may be present. Cranial nerve palsies, head tilt, and neck stiffness may be present in advanced tumors. Medulloblastomas are rapidly growing tumors in the vermis or fourth ventricle extending into cerebellar hemispheres and presenting with vomiting (most common initial symptom), headache, unsteady gait, and torticollis. Examination reveals papilledema, with truncal ataxia and dysmetria. Ependymomas are slow-growing tumors in the fourth ventricle presenting with increased ICP, hydrocephalus, unsteady gait, neck pain or stiffness, nystagmus, and cranial nerve dysfunction. Medulloblastomas and ependymomas tend to seed the subarachnoid space, leading to metastases in the spinal cord and ventricular system. Brainstem gliomas are diffuse infiltrating tumors predominantly involving the pons and present with bilateral cranial nerve palsies, with corticospinal involvement such as hemiplegia and ataxia, dysphagia, and hoarseness. Signs of increased ICP are not seen early in the course. Vomiting can be present because of irritation of the emetic center in the brainstem.

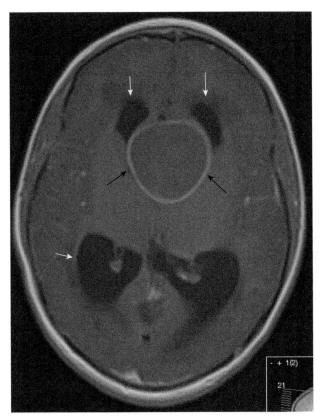

FIGURE 13.50 ■ Pituitary Gland Tumor with Obstructive Hydro-cephalus. Axial T1-weighted MRI reveals a large cystic tumor aris-ing from pituitary gland with ring enhancement on contrast (black arrows) and associated obstructive hydrocephalus (white arrows) in a 14-year-old adolescent with headache, vomiting, and lethargy with difficulty to arouse and visual field defects. (Photo contributor: Geetha Chari, MD.)

Tumors involving the cerebral hemispheres are less com-mon, and depending on the site of involvement, the presenting features vary. Midline tumors involving the pineal gland, mid-brain, and thalami tend to obstruct the CSF pathways leading to hydrocephalus and increased ICP. Tumors involving the pituitary and hypothalamus present with endocrine distur-bances and visual field defects.

Differential diagnosis includes other space-occupying lesions (eg, brain abscess, tuberculomas), postinfectious conditions (eg, acute disseminated encephalomyelitis with symptoms of encephalopathy and raised ICP), and idiopathic intracranial hypertension (pseudotumor cerebri) presenting with increased ICP with normal neuroimaging.

Emergency Department Treatment and Disposition

Obtain a head CT scan that helps to screen for large space-occupying lesions and hydrocephalus. For more optimal diagnosis, brain MRI, with and without contrast, is essential. Management in the ED includes stabilization of the patient, with symptomatic treatment. Consult neurology and neu-rosurgery and admit to ICU or a monitored bed for further management.

Pearls

1. The presenting symptoms of brain tumors can be nonspe-cific; thus, a high index of suspicion is necessary.
2. Consider brain tumors in the differential for any child presenting with increased ICP of unclear etiology.

Clinical Summary

Hydrocephalus is accumulation of excess CSF in the intracranial space and is classified as communicating (when CSF communicates through the ventricular system and subarachnoid space) or noncommunicating (when there is a block within the system). Causes of communicating hydrocephalus include meningeal fibrosis or obstruction (due to inflammatory or infectious conditions), posthemorrhagic or neoplastic infiltration, and less commonly, excessive production of CSF (choroid plexus tumor). Noncommunicating or obstructive hydrocephalus can result from aqueductal stenosis (congenital or secondary to compression from mass lesions), congenital malformations (eg, Arnold-Chiari or Dandy-Walker malformation), or vein of Galen aneurysm. Presenting symptoms depend on the age and cause of hydrocephalus, which can be acute or longstanding. Enlarging head circumference is the most common presenting feature in young infants. Acute

signs of increased ICP in infants can be very nonspecific, such as irritability, poor feeding, vomiting, and lethargy, with bulging fontanel on examination. When hydrocephalus develops gradually, enlarging head size may be the only symptom. On examination, besides increased head circumference, frontal or parietal bossing, wide or bulging anterior fontanel, separation of sutures, prominent scalp veins, sunsetting sign, head lag, spasticity, and brisk deep tendon reflexes may be present.

In older children, symptoms are those of increased ICP, such as headache and vomiting, with lethargy, if the presentation is acute. On examination, papilledema may be seen, with increased tone and brisk reflexes. If the hydrocephalus is secondary to a mass lesion or tumor, focal neurologic signs are present depending on the site of the lesion. Sixth nerve palsy is a common finding (a false localizing sign). Paralysis of upgaze or Parinaud syndrome is a relatively specific sign of compression of the tectum of the midbrain. This is equivalent to the sunsetting sign seen in young infants.

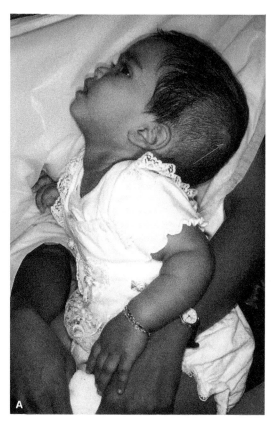
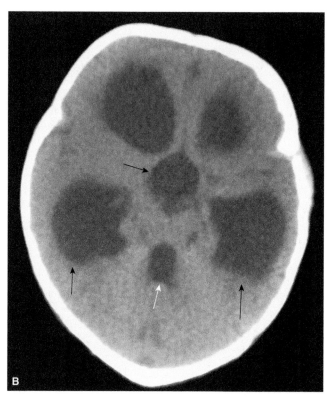

FIGURE 13.51 ■ Aqueductal Stenosis Leading to Hydrocephalus. (**A**) Increasing head size since birth was seen in this infant requiring shunt placement (arrow). (**B**) CT scan of the head reveals enlargement of lateral and third ventricles (black arrows) and relatively normal size of fourth ventricle (white arrow), suggestive of congenital aqueductal stenosis.

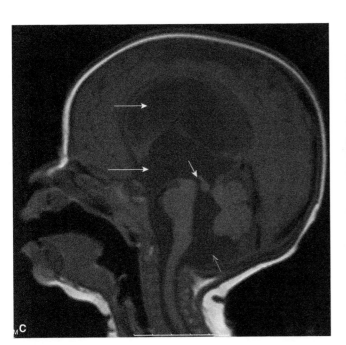

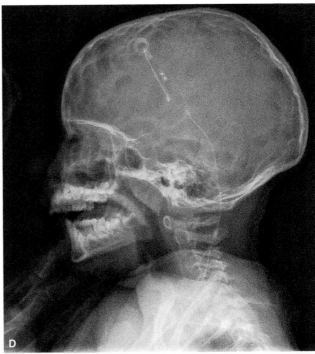

FIGURE 13.51 ■ (*Continued*) (**C**) Sagittal T1 MRI shows enlarged third ventricle (white arrows), small aqueduct (yellow arrow), and mildly enlarged fourth ventricle with enlarged cisterna magna (red arrow). (**D**) Chronic hydrocephalus. Lateral view of the skull in a child demonstrates a right-sided ventriculoperitoneal shunt catheter and copper-beaten skull deformity, compatible with chronic hydrocephalus. (Photo contributors: Geetha Chari, MD [A–C], and Stuart A. Bradin, DO [D].)

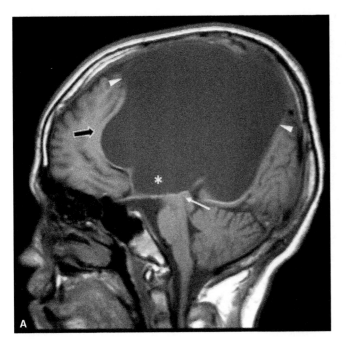

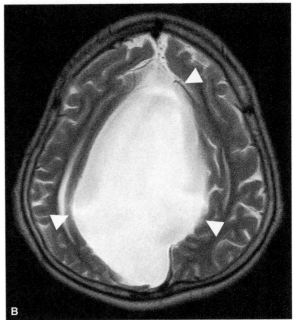

FIGURE 13.52 ■ Multiple Congenital Brain Malformations with Severe Hydrocephalus. These images were obtained from a 12-year-old boy (an emigrant presenting to the ED for headache). His head circumference was 60 cm. Sagittal T1-weighted image (**A**) and axial T2-weighted image (**B**) demonstrate aqueductal stenosis (white arrow) with marked dilatation of the third ventricle (asterisk) and lateral ventricles (white arrowheads). A large interhemispheric cyst is present, likely also contributing to hydrocephalus, along with dysgenesis of the corpus callosum (black arrow) and an absent septum pellucidum. (Photo/legend contributors: Geetha Chari, MD, and Vinodhkumar Velayudhan, DO.)

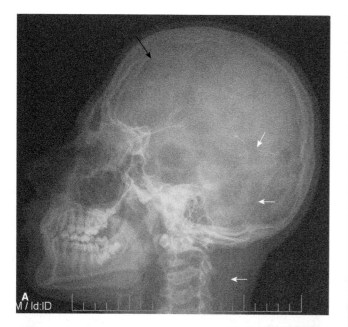

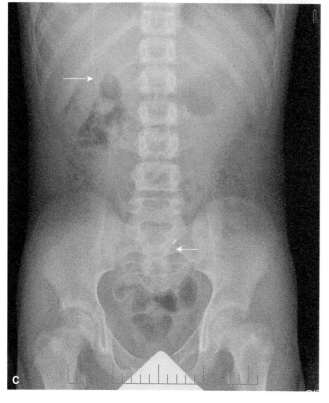

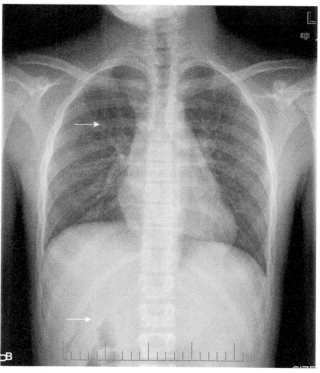

FIGURE 13.53 ■ Shunt Series. A 15-year-old boy presented with intermittent headaches and a history of ventriculoperitoneal (VP) shunt that was inserted in infancy but never revised. Shunt series was obtained. Lateral view of the skull demonstrates microcephaly, fusion of all of the sutures, and a copper-beaten appearance of the skull (black arrow), compatible with chronic hydrocephalus. VP shunt catheter (white arrows) is noted over the parieto-occipital region (**A**). Frontal view of the chest shows VP shunt catheter traversing the right hemithorax. The catheter is intact (**B**). Frontal view of the abdomen shows VP shunt catheter coiled in the pelvis. The catheter is intact (**C**). (Photo contributor: John Amodio, MD.)

Emergency Department Treatment and Disposition

Obtain a noncontrast head CT to confirm the presence of hydrocephalus, and in acute presentations, identify conditions such as posthemorrhagic hydrocephalus (eg, following traumatic or spontaneous subarachnoid hemorrhage) and determine whether surgical treatment is needed. Order brain MRI with and without contrast to determine etiology. Low-grade midbrain tumors (eg, tectal glioma) can cause aqueductal stenosis and are not readily identified on CT. Brain MRI will also show other mass lesions, such as posterior fossa

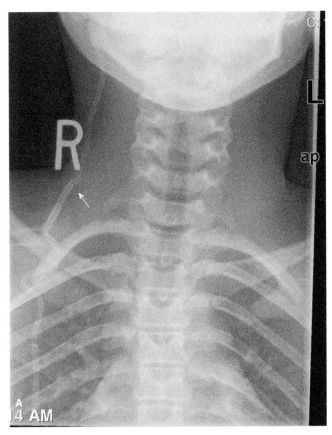

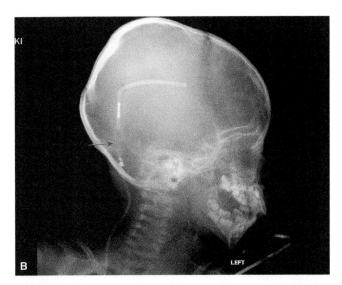

FIGURE 13.54 ■ Shunt Fracture. (**A**) A 10-year-old girl presented with symptoms of shunt obstruction. Radiograph reveals a ventriculoperitoneal (VP) shunt catheter fracture at the level of the neck (arrow). (**B**) Radiolucent VP shunt valve mistaken for shunt discontinuity. Lateral projection of the skull demonstrates a VP shunt catheter in place. Note the radiolucent area of the catheter (red arrow), which represents the shunt valve. This radiolucent area may be misinterpreted as a shunt disconnection. A copper-beaten appearance of the frontal calvarium, a radiographic sign of chronic hydrocephalus, is also noted in this 7-year-old girl presenting with fever and vomiting with a history of VP shunt. (Photo contributors: Geetha Chari, MD [A], and John Amodio, MD [B].)

tumors (eg, medulloblastoma, ependymoma, astrocytoma), not seen well on CT, which does not delineate structures well in the posterior fossa.

Management includes drainage of the CSF and treatment of the cause (eg, tumor resection). Surgical diversionary procedures help drain CSF from the enlarged ventricles. Third ventriculostomy is an option to manage hydrocephalus secondary to aqueductal stenosis. Most commonly, a VP shunt is placed. Programmable shunts can be adjusted to the required pressure for optimal drainage using a magnetic programming device to set the appropriate pressure level. After placement, shunt infection and obstruction are of concern. Shunt infection usually presents in the first 2 months after the insertion of the shunt. Besides fever, there may be redness and swelling around the shunt tubing. An infected shunt can become

obstructed, leading to features of increased ICP. The neurosurgeon may perform a shunt tap under strict aseptic conditions to draw CSF from the proximal tubing to determine presence of infection.

Shunt obstruction can occur without infection at any time after insertion and may be proximal or distal. Proximal obstruction may be due to entangled choroid, or the shunt end may have migrated out of the ventricles into the parenchyma. Distal obstruction in the peritoneal cavity can be secondary to fibrosis, formation of a pseudocyst, or peritonitis. Breakage of shunt tubing is an uncommon cause of shunt malfunction, and a shunt series can be performed to evaluate the shunt integrity when obstruction or malfunction is suspected by obtaining radiographs of the skull, chest, and abdomen. Head CT should be done to evaluate ventricular size compared to prior

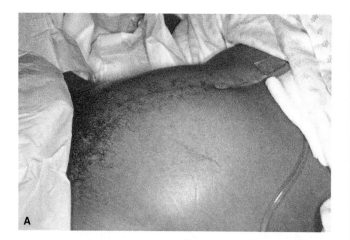

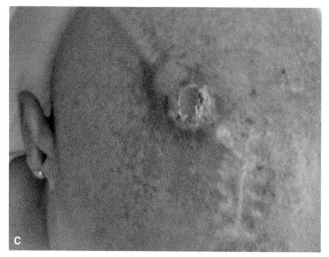

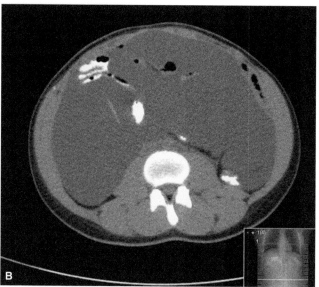

FIGURE 13.55 ■ Shunt-Related Complications. (**A**) CSF ascites. A 9-year-old girl (with premature adrenarche) presented with abdominal distension and vomiting, with previous history of a ventriculoperitoneal (VP) shunt for hydrocephalus. (**B**) Abdominal CT scan reveals VP shunt catheter tip in abdomen, embedded within a large collection of CSF (CSF-oma) because of poor peritoneal absorption. (**C**) VP shunt eroding through the skin is seen in this 10-year-old boy, who had a VP shunt since early childhood without any recent revision. He was taken to the operating room for shunt revision. (Photo contributors: Binita R. Shah, MD [A], Sharon Yellin, MD [B], and Stuart A. Bradin, DO [C].)

scans to determine the degree of obstruction. Sometimes, the size of the ventricles may not show any change, but the child is symptomatic. This can be due to poor compliance of the ventricular lining ("stiff ventricle syndrome"). Overdrainage of the CSF can lead to collapse of the ventricles with symptoms of increased ICP ("slit ventricle syndrome").

Pearls

1. Hydrocephalus can present at any age, and it is important to determine the cause.

2. Head CT is useful for emergent evaluation and management, but MRI is the imaging mode of choice to determine the etiology.

3. A CT scan is *not* necessary every time a child with a VP shunt presents to the ED, unless obstruction or malfunction is strongly suspected. Recent availability of focused MRI with limited scans to evaluate shunt malfunction offers a good alternative to avoid radiation.

Clinical Summary

Patients with spinal cord conditions present with paraparesis or quadriparesis, sensory disturbances, back pain, bladder and bowel dysfunction, autonomic dysfunction, and change in reflexes. Cranial nerves are typically not involved. In toddlers, the most common complaint is refusal to stand or walk, suggesting an acute process that results from weakness and/or pain. Older children present with difficulty walking, sensory complaints, and bladder distension. Typical neurologic findings include relatively symmetric weakness of lower extremities (upper extremity weakness also is present with cervical spine involvement), hyperreflexia, and a sensory level. In an acute presentation, areflexia due to spinal shock may be present.

Acute nontraumatic spinal cord lesions include transverse myelitis, infections such as diskitis, epidural abscess, tuberculous osteomyelitis (Potts disease), and myelitis due to herpes zoster. Spinal cord tumors such as astrocytoma, ependymoma, or neuroblastoma can present with subacute or chronic course of pain and weakness, with bladder and bowel involvement. Congenital malformations (eg, syringomyelia, arachnoid cyst, Chiari malformation, tethered cord, or spinal dysraphism) have a more chronic indolent course. Vascular conditions (eg, arteriovenous malformation, angiomas) may present acutely or with a gradual onset.

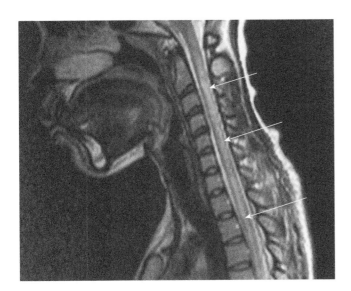

FIGURE 13.56 ■ Neuromyelitis Optica (NMO). MRI reveals a long hyperintense lesion on T2 sagittal image (arrows) in a 19-year-old patient with a rapidly progressive weakness and decreased sensation of lower and upper extremities. NMO IgG antibody (antibody to aquaporin 4 receptor) was positive, confirming the diagnosis. (Photo contributor: Geetha Chari, MD.)

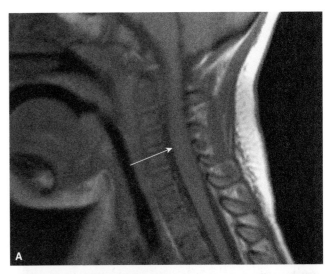

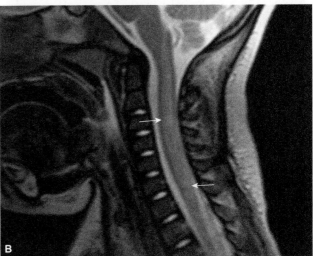

FIGURE 13.57 ■ Longitudinally Extensive Transverse Myelitis (LETM). (**A, B**) Sagittal T1-weighted MRI shows swelling of cord (white arrow; **A**) with variable increased T2 signal intensity within the cord extending from the medulla down to the upper thoracic level (white arrows; **B**) in a 13-month-old toddler who stopped walking followed by inability to hold her head up. The findings are characteristic of LETM. (Photo contributor: Geetha Chari, MD.)

Acute spinal cord lesions are a neurologic emergency. A complete history and pertinent neurologic evaluation can point to a diagnosis. Of concern is diagnosis of cord compression mandating emergent management, which is of utmost importance for neurologic recovery. Extramedullary lesions (either intradural or extradural) lead to cord compression. Extradural lesions include tumors such as neuroblastomas, ganglioneuromas, or sarcomas; epidural abscess; hematoma; or metastases. Intradural lesions include neurofibromas, lipomas, angiomas, or meningiomas. Tumors within the spinal

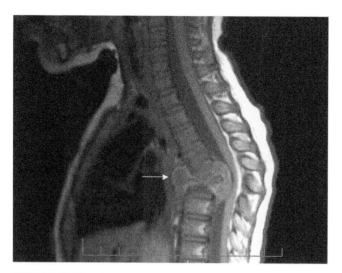

FIGURE 13.58 ■ Epidural Abscess with Spinal Cord Compression. An 18-month-old toddler who refused to walk, with a "lump" on his back and low-grade fever. Sagittal T1-weighted MRI reveals kyphosis with collapse of vertebral body and a circumscribed lesion from the prevertebral region (arrow) into the epidural space compressing the spinal cord that showed ring enhancement following contrast. Surgical intervention revealed abscess due to *Staphylococcus aureus.* (Photo contributor: Geetha Chari, MD.)

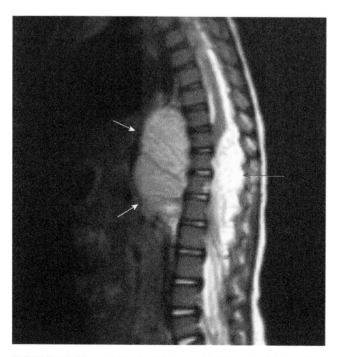

FIGURE 13.59 ■ Abdominal Mass with Intraspinal Extension. Sagittal T2-weighted MRI reveals large abdominal mass (white arrows) with intraspinal extension (red arrow) in a 4-year-old child with abdominal distension, vomiting, and inability to walk. Excision revealed a lipoblastoma. (Photo contributor: Geetha Chari, MD.)

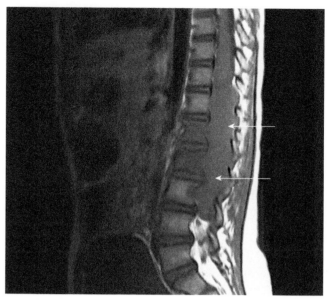

FIGURE 13.60 ■ Intramedullary Spinal Cord Tumor. Sagittal T1-weighted MRI reveals space-occupying lesion in lower thoracic and lumbar spinal canal involving the spinal cord and roots (arrows) in a 4-year-old child with progressive gait difficulty and bladder and bowel dysfunction. There is replacement of adjacent bone marrow in the region of tumor. Pathology revealed ependymoma. (Photo contributor: Geetha Chari, MD.)

cord (intramedullary) include astrocytomas and ependymomas. Tumors tend to progress slowly over weeks to months. Vascular conditions such as spinal cord infarction (although uncommon) have the most rapid course, progressing in <4 hours.

Idiopathic acute transverse myelitis is a demyelinating condition (diagnosis of exclusion). Spinal cord involvement typically is short (1–2 segments). Longitudinally extensive transverse myelitis (LETM), more common in younger children, refers to involvement extending beyond 3 segments. LETM is characteristic of neuromyelitis optica in adolescents and adults. Multiple sclerosis can also cause a demyelinating lesion and is seen more often in children >12 years of age. Acute disseminated encephalomyelitis presents with lesions both in the CNS and spinal cord. Demyelinating disorders tend to progress quickly and symptoms may be present for less than a week, usually 2 to 4 days. Conditions presenting similar to transverse myelitis include systemic autoimmune disorders (eg, lupus, mixed connective tissue disease) and postinfectious diseases (eg, Lyme disease, Epstein-Barr virus [EBV], *Mycoplasma*, herpes simplex virus, cytomegalovirus). Guillain-Barré syndrome can be in the differential, but the presence of a sensory level rules this condition out.

Emergency Department Treatment and Disposition

Order spinal MRI with and without contrast to identify spinal pathology that is intra- or extramedullary. Extramedullary (intradural/extradural) lesions may require immediate neurosurgical intervention. Transverse myelitis typically reveals swelling of the cord, with high T2 signal intensity lesion within the spinal cord, with patchy enhancement following contrast. If the spinal cord reveals transverse myelitis, order MRI of the brain to exclude lesions in the brain and optic nerves. Perform an LP if there are no structural lesions. Transverse myelitis is associated with mildly elevated protein, mild lymphocytic predominance, and presence of myelin basic protein. If postinfectious etiology is suspected, order appropriate tests (eg, Lyme titers, EBV, *Mycoplasma*, herpes simplex virus PCR).

Admit patient to ICU or a monitored bed because symptoms may continue to progress. Cord compression due to structural lesions requires urgent neurosurgical intervention. Catheterize patient with bladder distension. Transverse myelitis is treated with high-dose IV methylprednisolone, and for severe cases, IV immune globulin (IVIG) and plasmapheresis are other options.

Pearls

1. Absent reflexes can be a sign of spinal shock.
2. Cord compression due to structural lesions requires urgent neurosurgical evaluation.

GUILLAIN-BARRÉ SYNDROME

Clinical Summary

Guillain-Barré syndrome (GBS) is an immune-mediated disease directed against the peripheral nervous system myelin, with or without involvement of the axon. The main presenting feature is weakness, initially distal and symmetric, that can rapidly progress within 24 hours to ascending weakness and bulbar involvement, requiring ventilatory assistance. Facial involvement is bilateral in 50% of cases, and lower motor neuron facial weakness can be seen. Ptosis and extraocular weakness, unsteady gait, and areflexia are characteristics of a variant of GBS, called Miller-Fisher syndrome. The course consists of progressive weakness, which reaches a maximum in the first 2 weeks of the illness in >50% of the individuals. Recovery begins gradually 2 to 4 weeks after progression. Vague insidious sensory symptoms are often present at onset, with fleeting paresthesias and muscle tenderness. Younger children complain of pain. Recent history of viral illness may often be present. Neurologic examination reveals diffuse weakness (distal more than proximal), with prominent areflexia. Autonomic dysfunction is common, with tachycardia, BP instability (hypo- or hypertension), abdominal pain, and bowel or bladder incontinence.

Emergency Department Treatment and Disposition

Ascending weakness and vague sensory complaints should raise the suspicion of GBS. Admit all patients with clinically suspected GBS to the ICU in case rapid progression of weakness and autonomic instability require appropriate supportive care and treatment with IVIG. Measure and monitor vital capacity to check for bulbar involvement, which may require intubation and ventilation. Perform LP if the illness has been present for >1 week. Elevated protein in CSF with normal (<10) cell count (albuminocytologic dissociation) is diagnostic after the first week of illness (earlier CSF tests may be normal). Order CBC, comprehensive metabolic panel, and tests for postinfectious etiology (eg, EBV, *Mycoplasma*, *Campylobacter jejuni*, Lyme titers). Spine MRI with contrast may reveal enhancement of the nerve roots. Nerve conduction studies (performed after hospitalization) aid in confirmation of GBS.

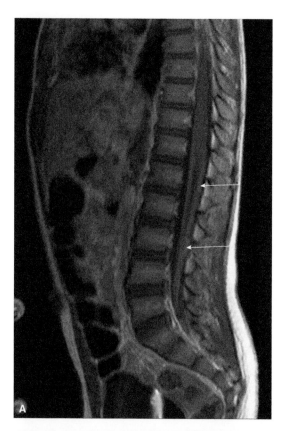

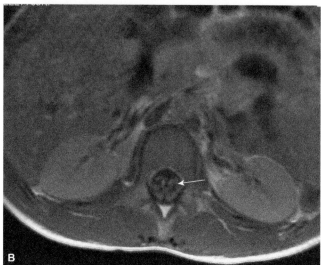

FIGURE 13.61 ■ Guillain-Barré Syndrome. (**A, B**) Sagittal and axial T1-weighted MRI of the lumbosacral spine reveals enhancement of the spinal roots after contrast administration (arrows), which can be seen in Guillain-Barré syndrome. (Photo contributor: Geetha Chari, MD.)

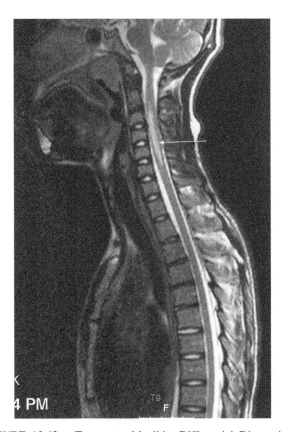

FIGURE 13.62 ■ Transverse Myelitis; Differential Diagnosis of Guillain-Barré Syndrome. A sagittal T2-weighted MRI of cervical spine shows a hyperintense lesion (arrow) within the spinal cord from C2 to C5, suggestive of transverse myelitis in a 14-year-old boy presenting with weakness of lower extremities followed by weakness of upper extremities over a period of 2 to 3 days. (Photo contributor: Geetha Chari, MD.)

Pearls

1. GBS is also known as acute inflammatory demyelinating polyneuropathy.
2. Rapid symmetric ascending weakness with areflexia is the hallmark of GBS.
3. Autonomic instability can be prominent.

Clinical Summary

Myasthenia gravis (MG) is a group of disorders of neuromuscular transmission, differing in age of onset and clinical features. Most commonly, it is autoimmune in etiology and characterized by fluctuating asymmetric weakness and fatigue, involving extraocular, oropharyngeal, neck, and/or skeletal muscles, with normal sensation and reflexes.

Ptosis or ophthalmoplegia (90% of patients) is the most prominent clinical feature, and ptosis is often asymmetric and variable. Extraocular muscle weakness is the only manifestation in 10% to 15% of patients. Over 50% of children presenting with ocular symptoms progress to systemic or bulbar weakness in 2 years. Bulbar weakness, seen in 75% of patients, presents with drooling, slow chewing and swallowing, nasal voice, or poor cough. Facial weakness can be present. Diffuse muscle weakness (prominently proximal) presents as fatigability and inability to run, climb stairs, and keep up with peers. Weakness of diaphragm and respiratory muscles may cause respiratory failure. Spontaneous remission of symptoms (often transient) can occur, and symptoms can recur after a period of time. MG can be graded clinically by the Osserman scale as follows:

- Grade I—weakness restricted to extraocular muscles
- Grade II—generalized weakness (mild IIa, moderate IIb)
- Grade III—severe generalized weakness
- Grade IV—life-threatening weakness of respiratory musculature (myasthenic crisis)

Diagnosis is essentially clinical, and confirmatory tests include immunologic studies (acetylcholine receptor antibodies and muscle-specific kinase antibodies; a large proportion of pediatric patients may be seronegative), electrophysiologic studies (electromyography/nerve conduction), and pharmacologic testing (eg, edrophonium).

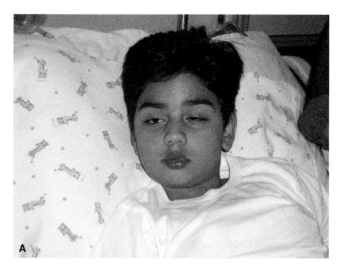

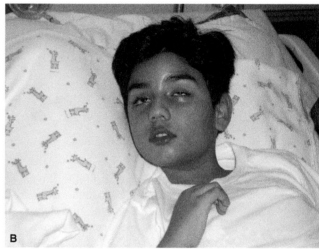

FIGURE 13.63 ■ Myasthenia Gravis. This is a 6-year-old boy who presented with difficulty keeping his eyes open and problems with swallowing. Bilateral ptosis is evident, worse on the left, with weakness of the left lateral rectus on eye movements seen looking straight (**A**) and looking up (**B**). (Photo contributor: Radha Giridharan, MD.)

Emergency Department Treatment and Disposition

Suspect MG if a child presents to the ED with generalized weakness or more acutely with respiratory distress. Take a careful clinical history for prior symptoms especially when neurologic examination reveals abnormalities only in the motor system, with normal mental status; normal pupillary response; normal deep tendon reflexes, sensation, and coordination; and a normal general examination. Assess vital signs including respiratory status, and obtain vital capacity in cooperative patients, if possible. Provide respiratory support, either noninvasive (continuous positive airway pressure/bilevel positive airway pressure) or invasive (intubation), as needed in the ED.

Consult neurology for bedside edrophonium testing. Edrophonium is a short-acting (5 minutes) inhibitor of acetylcholinesterase and improves neuromuscular transmission. After an initial test dose, give edrophonium via IV and monitor symptoms for improvement. Keep atropine available to counteract any adverse events such as bradycardia, abdominal cramps, and worsening of oropharyngeal weakness. Alternatively, neostigmine can be given subcutaneously or intramuscularly with effect lasting up to 4 hours. Side effects are similar to edrophonium.

Intubate patients with significant weakness and respiratory compromise. Admit to the ICU for ventilator management and further care, including IVIG or plasma exchange for very weak patients. Treat mildly affected patients with oral pyridostigmine (Mestinon). Long-term therapy includes use of immunosuppressants (eg, prednisolone, azathioprine, cyclosporine). Thymectomy may help some of the patients.

Pearls

1. MG is characterized by weakness and easy fatigability with diurnal variation; symptoms are less severe on awakening and become more obvious as the day progresses.
2. Ptosis and extraocular muscle involvement may be the only manifestations.
3. Pupillary reaction is always normal.
4. Bulbar and respiratory muscle involvement can cause myasthenic crisis.
5. Edrophonium testing is a useful bedside diagnostic tool.

Clinical Summary

Infantile botulism is a rare life-threatening neuromuscular condition, caused by ingestion of Clostridium botulinum spores. It is more common in certain geographic areas (eg, California Pennsylvania, New Jersey) presumably due to higher concentrations of botulinum spores in soil. When these spores are ingested, they germinate and multiply in the gastrointestinal tract, and release the botulinum neurotoxin into the bloodstream. The toxin binds irreversibly to the cholinergic receptors of the presynaptic membrane of the neuromuscular junctions, which leads to failure of neuromuscular transmission and resultant flaccid paralysis.

Infantile botulism typically affects children less than 1 year of age, majority between 1 to 6 months. Ingestion of contaminated honey or corn syrup have been implicated in many cases. However, a definite etiology may not be determined in a large number of patients. The American Academy of Pediatrics recommends against feeding honey or corn syrup to infants less than 12 months old.

The most common presenting symptom is constipation. This is followed by lethargy, decreased appetite and diminished spontaneous activity, which progress to generalized weakness, loss of head control, hypotonia, hypoventilation and apnea. Neurologic exam reveals symmetric bulbar involvement including ptosis, sluggishly reacting pupils, decreased eye movements, facial weakness, poor suck and decreased gag reflex. Generalized weakness and hypotonia are seen. Deep tendon reflexes may be present initially followed by hyporeflexia. The baby is otherwise afebrile. Since botulinum toxin does not cross the blood-brain barrier, the mental status usually is not affected unless baby develops respiratory insufficiency. Respiratory failure invariably develops, requiring mechanical ventilation. Autonomic disturbance such as decreased heart rate variability can occur.

Diagnosis is made by the clinical history and confirmatory tests. Definitive diagnosis is by detection of the botulinum toxin in the stool sample using a toxin neutralization bioassay. The diagnosis is made by demonstrating botulinum toxin or botulinum toxin-producing organisms in feces or enema fluid or toxin in serum. Nerve conduction studies and electromyography can be helpful in confirming the diagnosis and ruling out other conditions. Incremental compound muscle action potential response to high frequency stimulation, with brief small amplitude abundant motor action potentials following muscle stimulation are characteristic findings.

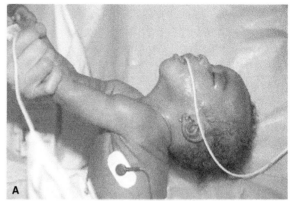
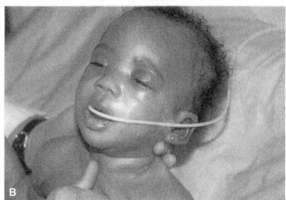

FIGURE 13.64 ■ Infant Botulism. (**A**) A 12-week-old infant was brought to the ED with lethargy, poor feeding, and constipation. She was found to have hypotonia and head lag and underwent diagnostic workup to exclude sepsis. She remained hospitalized and treated with broad-spectrum antibiotics and nasogastric feedings. All the repeated cultures including blood, urine, and CSF were negative when a diagnosis of infant botulism was entertained on the 10th day of hospitalization (when these images were also taken). *Clostridium botulinum* organisms and type B neurotoxin were identified in her stool. No source of exposure to *C botulinum* spores was identified. (**B**) Ptosis and expressionless face are seen despite painful stimulation applied to the chest. She required hospitalization for 6 weeks, mainly for nutritional support, but she recovered completely in 8 weeks. (Reproduced with permission from Shah BR, Laude TA. *Atlas of Pediatric Clinical Diagnosis*. WB Saunders; Philadelphia, PA, 2000.)

Differential diagnoses include Guillain-Barre syndrome, poliomyelitis, myasthenia gravis, spinal muscular atrophy type 1, tick paralysis, metabolic disorders and meningitis.

Emergency Department Treatment and Disposition

Botulism should be suspected in young infants presenting with constipation, lethargy and generalized weakness. Obtain

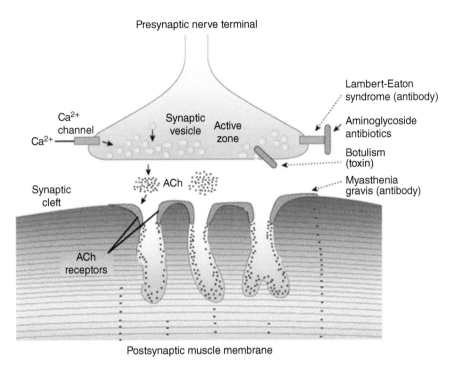

Presynaptic nerve terminal

FIGURE 13.65 ▪ Sites of Involvement in Disorders of Neuromuscular Transmission. Left: Normal transmission involves depolarization-induced influx of calcium (Ca^{2+}) through voltage-gated channels. This stimulates release of acetylcholine (ACh) from synaptic vesicles at the active zone and into the synaptic cleft. ACh binds to ACh receptors and depolarizes the postsynaptic muscle membrane. Right: Disorders of neuromuscular transmission result from blockage of Ca^{2+} channels (Lambert-Eaton syndrome or aminoglycoside antibiotics), impairment of Ca^{2+}-mediated ACh release (botulinum toxin), or antibody-induced internalization and degradation of ACh receptors (myasthenia gravis). (Reproduced with permission from Simon RP, Aminoff MJ, *Greenberg: Clinical Neurology*, 10th ed. McGraw-Hill Education; New York, NY, 2018.)

a careful history, including the feeding history. A rapid thorough neurological examination, which reveals sluggish pupillary response, expressionless face, generalized weakness and hypotonia, should suggest the possibility of botulism. Vital signs should be closely monitored, as the infant may require to be intubated and mechanically ventilated. Obtain routine labs, which are typically normal, to rule out other diagnoses. Stool specimen should be collected, if possible, with adequate precautions in view of the presence of toxin, and sent for testing before treatment is started.

Neurology consultation should be obtained and the baby should be admitted to the pediatric ICU. Further management in the PICU will include IV administration of Human Botulism Immune Globulin (BIG-IV; BabyBIG). It is licensed by FDA for the treatment of infant botulism caused by *C botulinum* type A or type B. BabyBIG is produced and distributed by the California Department of Public Health (www.infantbotulism.org). Adequate ventilatory support and prevention of secondary infections are important. Antibiotic use should be judicious, since clostridicidal antibiotics can increase toxin release and cause further clinical deterioration. BabyBIG is first-line therapy and significantly decreases days of mechanical ventilation, days of ICU stay including total length of hospital stay. Prognosis for recovery is excellent. Mortality rate is less than 1%, when recognized and managed appropriately.

Pearls

1. Infantile botulism is characterized by constipation, increasing lethargy and generalized weakness, and is caused by ingestion of Clostridium botulinum spores.
2. Ptosis and sluggishly reacting pupils, facial weakness with depressed gag are typical features.
3. Mechanical ventilation is often required.
4. IV Botulinum immunoglobulin is the definitive treatment.
5. Prognosis for recovery is excellent.

Chapter 14

ENDOCRINOLOGY

Glenn D. Harris
Irma Fiordalisi
Scott M. Thomas

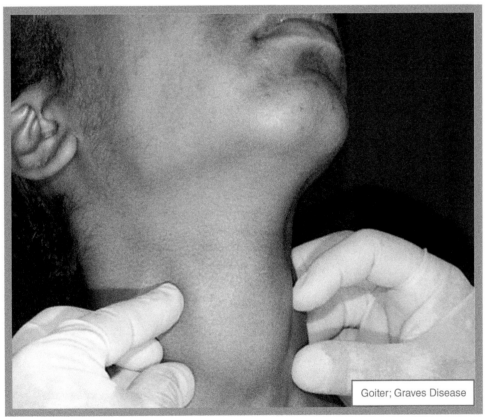

Goiter; Graves Disease

(Photo contributor: Binita R. Shah, MD)

The authors acknowledge the special contributions of Irene Mamkin, MD, and Sonal Bhandari, MD, to prior edition.

DIABETIC KETOACIDOSIS

Diabetic ketoacidosis/ketoacidemia (DKA) is a life-threatening metabolic disturbance caused by an absolute or relative insulin deficiency resulting in ketone body production and decreased serum total CO_2 concentration. DKA occurs most commonly in type 1 diabetic patients, but may also occur in type 2 diabetic patients.

Insulin deficiency results in hyperglycemia, glycosuria, and intracellular starvation, leading to release of counter-regulatory hormones (catecholamines, glucagon, cortisol, and growth hormone). This triggers lipolysis, proteolysis, glyco-genolysis, gluconeogenesis, and insulin resistance. Glycoge-nolysis and gluconeogenesis exacerbate the already-present

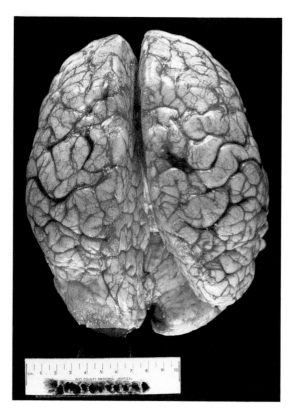

FIGURE 14.2 ■ Brain Swelling Seen at Autopsy; Diabetic Ketoaci-dosis (DKA). A dorsal view of the brain shows severe brain swelling with flattened gyri and effaced sulci. Evidence of brain swelling with herniation was seen on the brain's ventral surface. Pretreatment brain herniation is rare, but brain swelling prior to treatment (incompletely understood cause[s]) appears common among pediatric patients with DKA. This 17-year-old known diabetes patient collapsed at home and developed hypertension, bradycardia, and agonal respirations on arrival of first responders. Such patients underscore the need for careful volume resuscitation, fluid and electrolyte management, and timely administration of insulin in those with DKA, because they likely present with some degree of brain swelling even before treat-ment begins. (Photo contributor: M.G.F. Gilliland, MD.)

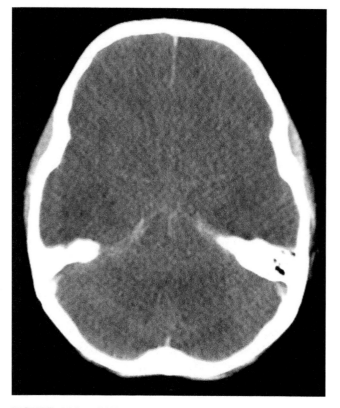

FIGURE 14.1 ■ Diffuse Brain Swelling; Diabetic Ketoacidosis. A noncontrast head CT scan shows obliteration of all CSF spaces including ventricles and basal cisterns with blurring of the margins of gray and white matter, typical for diffuse cerebral edema and her-niation around the brainstem. These findings were seen in a patient with new-onset diabetes who initially presented with a normal men-tal status, severe ketoacidemia without shock, and received isotonic saline 60 mL/kg over 2 hours. Progressively diminished arousabil-ity and hypertension were unrecognized signs of raised intracranial pressure until irregular respirations and a decrease in heart rate ensued. (Photo contributor: Geetha Chari, MD.)

hyperglycemia. A negative cycle of progressive ketoacidemia, hyperglycemia, dehydration, electrolyte losses, and possible brain swelling may result in death.

Clinical Summary

Key findings include all or some of the following: polyuria/incontinence, polydipsia, polyphagia (inconsistent), nocturia/enuresis, varying degrees of dehydration, weight loss, abdom-inal pain, nausea, vomiting, hyperventilation, Kussmaul breathing (which is clinically visible and may be confused with

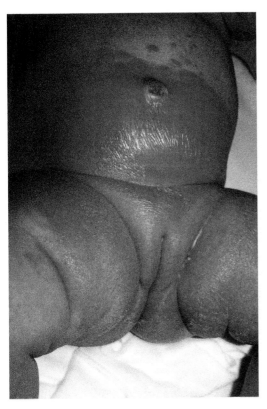

FIGURE 14.3 ■ Candidiasis as a Presenting Sign of Diabetes. Extensive candidiasis involving perianal and inguinal areas with extension to the abdomen and thighs was seen in this infant presenting with diabetic ketoacidosis. Perineal *candidiasis* in a diapered infant can occur at any age. However, severe, recurrent, or intransigent *candidiasis* despite appropriate treatment and/or presence of oral candidiasis (uncommon after 12 months of age) should alert the physician to the possibility of diabetes mellitus or immune deficiency. (Photo contributor: Binita R. Shah, MD.)

respiratory distress from primary respiratory diseases such as pneumonia), subnormal body temperature (in severe DKA; may also occur in sepsis), altered mental status (which may be caused by shock, profound ketoacidemia, or raised intracranial pressure [ICP]), the fruity odor of ketones on the breath, and *Candida* infections (eg, vaginitis or perineal yeast). Typical laboratory findings include hyperglycemia (may be only modest with serum glucose <300 mg/dL), glycosuria, ketonemia, ketonuria, metabolic acidosis/acidemia, and compensatory hypocarbia. Other abnormalities may include apparent or actual hyponatremia, hypernatremia, hypokalemia, hypophosphatemia, hypomagnesemia, increased serum urea nitrogen, increased serum creatinine, hypertriglyceridemia, and increased serum amylase. Increased lipase in the absence

of pancreatitis may occur. Initially, potassium, magnesium, and phosphorus may be increased or normal; however, close monitoring is required because serum concentrations of these salts may decrease significantly with treatment as these ions move intracellularly, and total-body depletion of one or more of these ions may become manifest.

Importantly, the degree of dehydration varies among patients with DKA. Severe DKA (ie, severe ketoacidemia) does not necessarily mean that severe dehydration is present; the degree of ketonemia and the degree of dehydration should be individually assessed. Raised ICP is the most common cause of morbidity and mortality; monitoring for neurologic symptoms of cerebral edema (brain swelling) is essential. Avoid excessive volume administration, which can exacerbate ICP. Efforts to assign a volume of deficit should be made (Table 14.1).

Emergency Department Treatment and Disposition

Airway, breathing, and circulation must be addressed. In rare cases where tracheal intubation is indicated, it should be accomplished using techniques that are protective for patients at risk for raised ICP. In addition, such patients are often profoundly hypocarbic (some patients have $PaCO_2$ values in the single digits). This degree of compensatory hyperventilation should be maintained once the patient is intubated to avoid further decreases in blood and possibly CSF pH, since CSF acidosis may contribute to brain swelling.

If shock is present, emergency volume resuscitation is required (Figure 14.6 and Table 14.1). A requirement for >20 mL/kg of isotonic saline resuscitation fluid is uncommon, and the need for emergency volumes in excess of 20 to 30 mL/kg of *ideal* body weight should raise suspicion of significant complicating illnesses (eg, septic shock, pancreatitis, severe enteritis). Severe ketonemia causes vasoconstriction. Cool, sometimes mottled skin may be attributable to a very low blood pH rather than hypovolemia. For this reason, if foot pulses are strong and blood pressure is appropriate but skin remains cool and/or mottled despite 10 to 20 mL/kg of resuscitation fluid in the presence of severe acidemia, further bolus volume resuscitation may not be warranted. In these cases, insulin and rehydration therapy are recommended with serial reassessments; impaired perfusion should resolve as ketonemia is corrected with insulin and rehydration. For

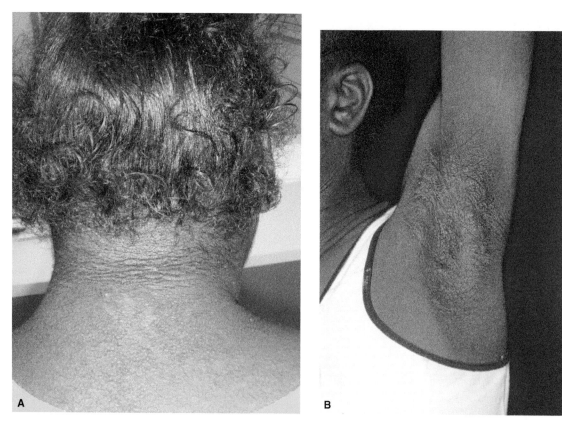

FIGURE 14.4 ▪ Acanthosis Nigricans and Diabetes. (**A, B**) Acanthosis nigricans is a cutaneous finding of abnormal texture ("velvety") with darkened pigmentation of the skin that occurs in neck and flexural skin folds, most often associated with insulin resistance. In pediatric patients, it is most commonly associated with obesity and type 2 diabetes or an increased risk for developing this disease. (Photo contributors: Amrit P. Bhangoo, MD [A], and Binita R. Shah, MD [B].)

the remainder of hydration, use solutions as described in Figure 14.6.

Monitor closely for signs of raised ICP, including altered mental status (including lethargy), age-inappropriate bed wetting, headache, hypertension, bradycardia (or relative bradycardia for the clinical situation), pupillary sluggishness or unresponsiveness, anisocoria, new focal neurologic signs, and/or seizures. If raised ICP is suspected, treat with hypertonic (20% or 25%) mannitol 0.5 to 1 g/kg over 20 minutes and evaluate the patient for a decrease in volume delivery (ie, consider a decrease in the rate of IV fluid infusion). If hemodynamic instability is present, infusion of 3% NaCl (3–10 mL/kg) may be an alternative to use of hypertonic mannitol (an osmotic diuretic). Tracheal intubation with an appropriate degree of hyperventilation may also be required.

Initiate treatment with insulin as soon as possible (by the end of the first treatment hour) by continuous IV infusion of regular human insulin 0.1 unit/kg of *actual* (not ideal) body weight per hour. An improvement in the base deficit by approximately 1 mEq/L/h indicates appropriate insulin dosing and delivery. Failure to achieve this goal suggests an inadequate insulin dose or a problem with insulin delivery (eg, adsorption of insulin to IV tubing, infiltrated IV site, malfunction of the IV pump). If insulin delivery is ensured, the insulin dose should be increased by increments of 100% if ketoacidosis is not improving. If the patient is using an insulin pump and presents with DKA, discontinue the insulin pump and treat DKA with continuous IV insulin even if the pump appears to be functioning. In order to achieve an appropriate and gradual decline in serum osmolality, note that the serum concentration of sodium should increase by 1 to 2 mEq/L for every 100 mg/dL decline in the serum glucose. If this rate of rise in sodium is not achieved, consider decreasing the rate of volume administration. If this rate of rise in sodium

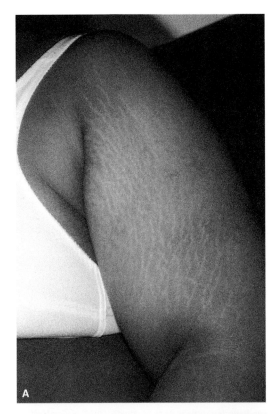

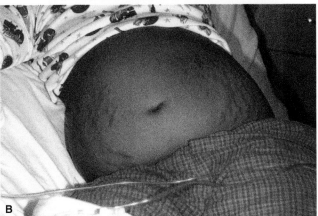

FIGURE 14.5 ▪ Obesity and Diabetes. (**A, B**) Obesity is a risk factor for type 2 diabetes, and patients may present with hyperosmolar hyperglycemic syndrome. Two different patients with diabetes with obesity and striae are shown. Striae (stretch marks) occur due to a rapid stretching of the skin (eg, rapid weight gain), and most common locations are abdomen, breasts, hips, thighs, buttocks, and flank. Striae appear as parallel streaks of red, thinned skin that becomes white and scar-like in appearance over time. (Photo contributor: Binita R. Shah, MD.)

concentration is exceeded, the rate of volume delivery may need to be increased.

Although DKA is most commonly triggered by treatment noncompliance, it is also important to rule out triggers including insulin pump malfunction, infections, acute abdominal processes, depression, behavioral disorders, illicit drug use, pregnancy, psychosocial problems, and physical and sexual abuse.

After stabilization in the ED, patients should be admitted to a pediatric ICU or alternative unit capable of close metabolic and neurologic monitoring. The diabetes team should be contacted as soon as feasible regarding hospital admission.

Hyperglycemic hyperosmolar syndrome (HHS; formerly hyperosmolar nonketotic coma), historically seen only in adult patients, is increasingly recognized in the pediatric population, most frequently among patients with type 2 diabetes. While some degree of overlap with the features of DKA occurs, these patients typically present with more severe dehydration, circulatory impairment, and alterations in mental status but with a lesser degree of ketosis/acidosis (Table 14.3). Initial volume resuscitation to restore peripheral perfusion may be accompanied by a marked decrease in serum glucose; therefore, initiation of insulin therapy warrants caution to avoid a precipitous decrease in osmolality. Due to a lesser degree of acidemia yet greater degree of dehydration as compared to that seen in DKA, patients with HHS usually require a smaller dose of insulin (eg, 0.025–0.05 units/kg/h) but greater volume of IV fluid as compared to DKA patients. We do not recommend mL/mL replacement of urine output; we recommend close cardiovascular monitoring and monitoring of input and output data to ensure that rehydration progresses appropriately.

Patients with HHS should be also admitted to a pediatric ICU where close metabolic, neurologic, and cardiovascular monitoring can be accomplished. Morbidity and mortality are usually associated with the effects of hyperosmolality and dehydration rather than brain swelling as seen in DKA.

TABLE 14.1 ■ HOW TO ESTIMATE DEGREE OF DEHYDRATION (VOLUME OF DEFICIT) IN DKA

Guidelines	Mild	Moderate	Severe
	Degree of Dehydration		
Volume of deficit (mL/kg)*			
>2 years	30	60	≥90
≤2 years	50	100	≥150
Clinical measures			
Peripheral perfusion[†]			
Palpation of peripheral pulses (pulse volume)	Normal	Normal to decreased	Decreased to absent
Capillary refill time (s)[‡]	<2	2–3	≥3
Skin temperature (tactile)	Normal	Normal to cool	Cool to cold
Heart rate	Normal to mildly increased	Moderately increased	Moderately to severely increased
BP	Normal	Normal to increased	Decreased to increased
BUN (mg/dL)	Normal to mildly increased eg, <20	Mildly increased eg, 20–25	Moderately to severely increased, eg, >30
Predicted Na+ (mEq/L)[§]	Usually normal	Usually normal	Normal to increased
Glucose (mg/dL)	Mildly increased eg, ~400	Moderately increased eg, ~600	Severely increased eg, >800

*Use actual weight for normally nourished patients; for obese patients, use ideal body weight.

[†]If peripheral (foot) pulses are easily palpable on presentation but skin is cool to cold and capillary refill time is delayed, we give 0.9% NaCl 10 mL/kg. If the patient has easily palpable peripheral (foot) pulses with cool to cold skin and delayed capillary refill *after* up to 20 mL/kg resuscitation fluid has been given, these findings are most likely due to severe ketonemia. Treatment with insulin and serial reassessments, not necessarily more resuscitation fluid, should be considered.

[‡]Capillary refill time is modified by the hypertonic state. Capillary refill time between 2 and 3 seconds suggests moderate to severe dehydration.

[§]Predicted Na (mEq/L) = Na (mEq/L + {1.6 × ([glucose mg/dL − 100]/100)}

Reproduced with permission from Harris GD, Fiordalisi I, Harris WL, et al. Minimizing the risk of brain herniation during treatment of diabetic ketoacidemia: a retrospective and prospective study. *J Pediatr.* 1990 Jul;117(1 Pt 1):22-31.

TABLE 14.2 ■ RECOMMENDED LABORATORY STUDIES IN THE ED

Initial	Minimum Frequency
Bedside blood glucose	Hourly
Urine glucose and ketones	As needed
Serum	
Glucose	Every 2 hours
Electrolytes	Every 2 hours
Urea nitrogen and creatinine	Every 2 hours
Potassium	May be required hourly if K+ is low, or if in the normal range in the presence of severe acidemia.
Magnesium	Usually every 4–6 hours; hypomagnesemia may not be evident prior to treatment but may become manifest with volume repletion. Mg depletion may confound potassium depletion, since Mg is needed for renal tubular reabsorption of K+.
Phosphorus	Usually every 4–8 hours; hypophosphatemia may become evident only during treatment. Phosphorus <1 mg/dL is associated with respiratory failure.
Blood gases	Hourly in very sick patients; these can be venous if obtained from a freely flowing vein without prolonged application of a tourniquet. The base deficit should decrease by at least 1 mEq/L/h if an effective dose of insulin is being delivered.

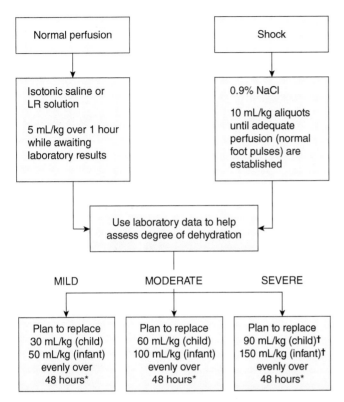

*Electrolyte content of rehydration solutions in the first 12–18 hours:
Child (> 2 yr): Lactated Ringer's solution plus K⁺. Alternatively, a solution containing NaCl 100 mEq/L plus NaHCO₃ or Na-acetate 25 mEq/L plus K⁺ can be used.
Infant (≤ 2 yr): NaCl 0.45% **PLUS** NaHCO₃ or Na-acetate 25 mEq/L (total Na⁺ 102 mEq/L)
  PLUS K⁺
Potassium: K⁺: usually 40 mEq/L (usually half as acetate, half as phosphate)
  K⁺ should be withheld if there is ECG evidence of hyperkalemia, K⁺ ≥ 6.0, or anuria
Glucose: Added to the rehydration solution as 5% dextrose (or greater) once serum glucose is < 300 mg/dL.
†In severe dehydration, volumes of deficit may exceed these estimates

FIGURE 14.6 ■ Initial Fluid Therapy for DKA. LR, Lactated Ringer's.

Pearls

1. Monitor closely for altered mental status and other signs of cerebral edema or increased ICP; treat suspected raised ICP with mannitol and/or hypertonic saline. Brain imaging should be obtained in any patient who does not respond promptly and completely with treatment.

2. Do not assume that severe acidemia is necessarily associated with severe dehydration or that the parched oral mucosa commonly seen with Kussmaul breathing and severe acidemia is indicative of severe dehydration.

Feature	DKA	HHS
Age	Any age	Usually > 9 years
Diabetes type	Type 1 > type 2	Type 2 > type 1
Obesity	Often in type 2 diabetes mellitus	Very common
Mental status	Normal to altered	Altered
Glucose (mg/dL)	Usually >200	>600
Total CO₂ (mEq/L)	≤15	Usually >15
Acidosis	Ketoacidosis	Lactic acidosis
Degree dehydration	Mild to severe	Severe
Urine/serum ketones	Moderate to large	Small to absent
Effective osmolality (Eosm)*	Increased (mild to moderate)	Increased (severe; >320)
Most frequent cause of death	Brain herniation	Multiple organ failure

*Eosm (mOsm/kg) = 2[Na] in mEq/L + ([glucose] in mg/dL ÷ 18).

3. Fluid and electrolyte administration should be based on ideal body weight. Insulin dose should be based on actual body weight. All patients with DKA should be NPO.

4. Give emergency volume resuscitation only in the presence of shock.

5. Concomitant illness (eg, pancreatitis, sepsis, acute abdomen) may be present but masked.

6. All patients should receive a continuous infusion of insulin in effective doses by the end of the first treatment hour (after shock, if present, is treated). Deep IM administration of regular insulin 0.1 units/kg given hourly may be used as a bridge to continuous IV infusion in situations where IV access or appropriate monitoring cannot be optimally achieved (eg, certain transport situations).

7. Avoid antiemetics because these can mask the neurologic status; vomiting and abdominal pain caused by DKA resolve with insulin and fluid administration. If vomiting and abdominal pain continue after 1 to 2 hours of appropriate treatment, consider confounding illness.

8. In order that insulin can continue to correct ketoacidosis without high risk of hypoglycemia, glucose delivery should be increased (rather than decreasing the insulin dose) once glucose is <250 to 300 mg/dL.

ADDISON DISEASE

Clinical Summary

Addison disease, or primary adrenal insufficiency, is often unrecognized in its early stages, and it may present with a life-threatening crisis. Presenting symptoms are often vague, including fatigue, weakness, abdominal pain, vomiting, diarrhea, salt craving, behavior changes, and depression. Signs can include postural hypotension, weight loss, or increased pigmentation, especially of skin creases, buccal mucosa, and nail beds. Addisonian crisis may be precipitated by infection, surgery, trauma, or emotional stress, and constitutes a medical emergency. Iatrogenic causes include failure to increase steroid dose and bilateral removal of the adrenals. Patients with Addison disease may present with hyponatremia, hyperkalemia, hypoglycemia, eosinophilia, or lymphocytosis, and they will have low adrenocorticotropic hormone (ACTH)–stimulated cortisol responses.

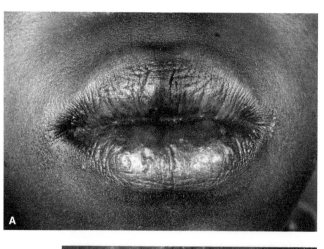

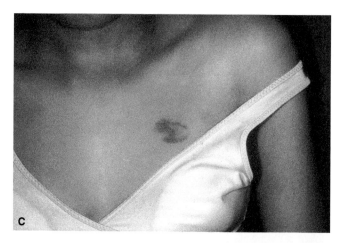

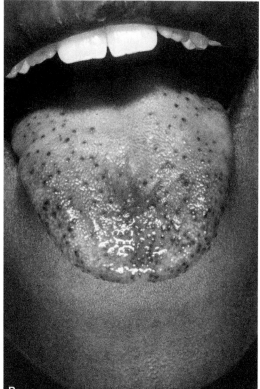

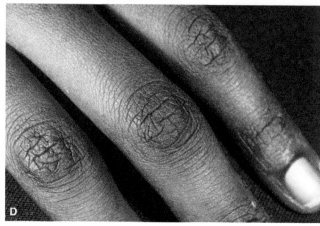

FIGURE 14.7 ■ Addison Disease. Black pigmentation of the lips (**A**), spotty pigmentation of the tongue (**B**), pigmentation of the scar (**C**) from bite mark by classmate 2 months earlier, and pigmentation of the knuckles (**D**) are seen in a 14-year-old girl presenting with weight loss, anorexia, and progressive weakness of a few months in duration. (Reproduced with permission from Shah BR, Laude TL. *Atlas of Pediatric Clinical Diagnosis*. WB Saunders; Philadelphia, PA, 2000.)

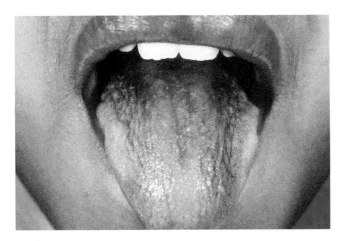

FIGURE 14.8 ■ Black Tongue Secondary to Bismuth Subsalicylate. Pigmentation of the tongue (which is smooth without enlargement of filiform papillae) is seen in a patient following ingestion of bismuth subsalicylate (Pepto-Bismol). When a small amount of bismuth combines with trace amounts of sulfur in the saliva and gastrointestinal tract, a black-colored bismuth sulfide is formed. The discoloration is temporary and harmless and can last several days even after stopping Pepto-Bismol. (Photo contributor: Binita R. Shah, MD.)

Causes of Addison disease can be divided into 3 main categories: adrenal hypoplasia, adrenal destruction, and impaired steroid production. Excluding congenital adrenal hyperplasia presenting in the neonatal period, the most common cause of primary adrenal insufficiency is autoimmune

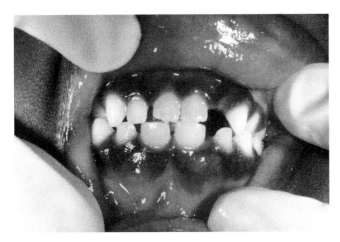

FIGURE 14.9 ■ Physiologic Pigmentation. Physiologic (normal) pigmentation of gums is shown in an African American child. Such pigmentation may be difficult to differentiate from Addition disease; however, a recent and progressive increase in pigmentation associated with symptoms of adrenal insufficiency is highly suggestive of gradual adrenal destruction. Physiologic pigmentation also remains indefinitely. The hyperpigmentation seen with Addison disease improves with steroid therapy. (Photo contributor: Binita R. Shah, MD.)

disease, and adrenal insufficiency is included in both poly-endocrinopathy syndrome types 1 and 2. Historically, tuberculosis was the most common cause of Addison disease worldwide, and it remains an important etiology outside of the United States, particularly in the developing world. Other causes include adrenal metastasis, hemorrhage, drugs, infections, and amyloidosis.

Emergency Department Treatment and Disposition

Because Addison disease presents with vague symptoms and potential life-threatening complications, clinicians should keep a high index of suspicion for this entity. Patients with suspected Addison disease presenting to the ED should have a random cortisol measured prior to stress dose steroids being given (100 mg/m² or rough estimate as follows: 25 mg for infants, 50 mg for small children, and 100 mg for adolescents). Patients with Addisonian crisis require aggressive fluid resuscitation for the treatment of hypotension and shock and likely require ICU-level care for cardiovascular monitoring. Initial testing may include morning (8:00 AM) serum cortisol, ACTH, electrolyte, renin, and aldosterone levels.

Pearls

1. Maintain a high index of suspicion for Addison disease in patients with vague complaints, especially if they have increased pigmentation of the skin or buccal mucosa.
2. Hyperpigmentation may be equally intense over entire body or accentuated in sun-exposed areas. Failure of a suntan to disappear may be an important clue.
3. Addison disease is most commonly an autoimmune disease; consider tuberculosis in patients with travel to endemic areas.
4. Patient's in Addisonian crisis need IV fluid resuscitation, followed by glucocorticoid replacement. Mineralocorticoid replacement can be delayed.
5. Ideally, a cortisol level should be obtained prior to glucocorticoids being given.

CONGENITAL ADRENAL HYPERPLASIA

Clinical Summary

Congenital adrenal hyperplasia (CAH) is the most common cause of ambiguous genitalia, and it is caused by a disruption in the biosynthesis of steroids from cholesterol. It is part of routine neonatal screening in all 50 states, which detects elevation in 17-hydroxyprogesterone. Nearly all cases are caused by a deficiency in either 21-hydroxylase (90%–95% of cases) or 11β-hydroxylase (up to 5% of cases). Several other enzyme defects have been implicated as the cause of remaining cases. CAH can be divided into salt-wasting and non–salt-wasting varieties. In absence of routine screening, patients with salt-wasting forms are typically identified earlier, in the first months of life, and may present with severe hyponatremic dehydration and shock. Symptoms of salt wasting may include poor appetite, lethargy, vomiting, and failure to thrive, and may be mistaken for other entities such as pyloric stenosis or formula intolerance. Females with either salt-wasting or non–salt-wasting varieties typically are identified in the first months because of the ambiguous genitalia noted at birth. Males with non–salt-wasting varieties may go unidentified due to their normal genitalia and absence of symptoms. In addition, mild forms of CAH may present later in life during times of stress such as illness, surgery, or trauma. Patients with suspected CAH should have a metabolic panel, 17-hydroxyprogesterone, and aldosterone panel drawn as part of their laboratory evaluation.

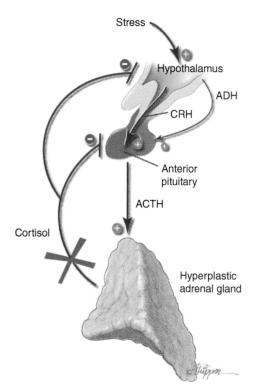

FIGURE 14.10 ■ Impaired Cortisol-Mediated Negative Feedback due to Congenital Adrenal Hyperplasia (CAH) on the Hypothalamic–Pituitary–Adrenal Axis. The CAHs are a group of adrenal disorders characterized by histologic alterations of adrenal cortical tissue secondary to chronic overstimulation by elevated levels of ACTH due to a defect in the pathway that converts cholesterol into cortisol. In most forms of CAH, the enzymatic defect blocks cortisol synthesis, impairing cortisol-mediated negative feedback control of ACTH secretion. The constant unsuccessful ACTH stimulation of the adrenals to produce cortisol causes the adrenals to increase in size. ACTH, adrenocorticotropic hormone; ADH, antidiuretic hormone; CRH, corticotrophin-releasing hormone. (Reproduced with permission from Sarafoglou K, Hoffmann GF, Roth KS. *Pediatric Endocrinology and Inborn Errors of Metabolism*, 2nd ed. McGraw-Hill Education; New York, NY, 2017.)

Emergency Department Treatment and Disposition

Salt wasting crisis due to CAH is a medical emergency and may present with shock that should be promptly recognized in the ED and requires immediate resuscitation with isotonic IV fluids. Electrolyte abnormalities, particularly hyponatremia and hyperkalemia, along with hypoglycemia should be assessed and treated as appropriate. Glucocorticoids should be initiated early, based on the presumptive diagnosis of CAH, because delaying treatment may be life threatening. Stress doses of injectable glucocorticoids should be given IV in the ED (dose: 2 mg/kg, or a rough estimate as follows: 25 mg for infants, 50 mg for small children, and 100 mg for adolescents). Patients with salt wasting crisis should be admitted to the pediatric ICU, and endocrinology should be consulted for further evaluation and management.

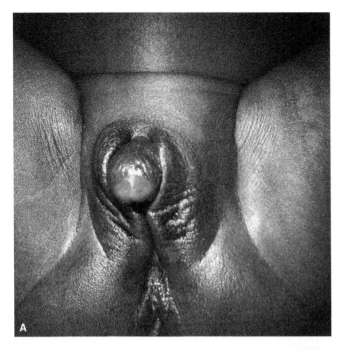

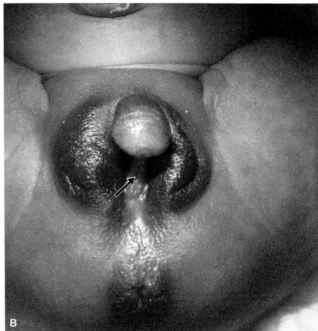

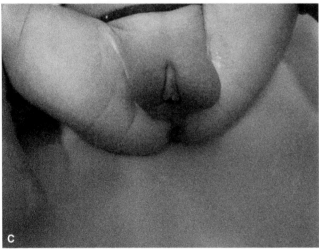

FIGURE 14.11 ■ Ambiguous Genitalia. (**A, B**). Two different female neonates (46,XX) with virilizing congenital adrenal hyperplasia are seen with an enlarged clitoris (phallus-like structure), genital hyperpigmentation, empty labioscrotal folds, and a single perineal opening (common opening of vagina and urethra; arrow) into urogenital sinus are shown. Most frequent cause of ambiguous genitalia is CAH due to 21-hydroxylase (OH) deficiency. Females with classic 21-OH deficiency (salt-losing type) tend to show a greater degree of virilization than those with non–salt-losing type. (**C**) A female neonate presenting with adrenal crisis is seen with an enlarged clitoris, genital hyperpigmentation, and labioscrotal folds. (Reproduced with permission from Shah BR, Laude TL. *Atlas of Pediatric Clinical Diagnosis*. WB Saunders; Philadelphia, PA, 2000 [A, B], and Raj Pal Singh, MD [C].)

Pearls

1. Consider CAH in patients with hypotension and shock after seemingly minor stress.
2. Ideally, obtain cortisol level prior to giving glucocorticoids.
3. Glucocorticoid dosing can be estimated as 25 mg for infants, 50 mg for small children, and 100 mg for adolescents.
4. Injectable glucocorticoids and IV fluid replacement are the mainstay of therapy in the ED.
5. Consider potential causes of physiologic stress, such as trauma or sepsis, in patients with salt-wasting crisis and evaluate and treat as appropriate.

Clinical Summary

Hypothyroidism can be caused by disease of the thyroid gland itself (eg, Hashimoto thyroiditis), treatment of hyperthyroidism (eg, antithyroid medications), medications (eg, lithium), or pituitary or hypothalamic disorders (eg, tumors, radiation therapy). In the United States, hypothyroidism is most commonly an autoimmune disease. Adolescents are more commonly affected than young children, and girls are more often affected than boys. Worldwide, hypothyroidism is often caused by a dietary iodine deficiency, especially in areas where the soil has a low iodine content. Hypothyroidism often presents with vague symptoms such as fatigue, exhaustion, lethargy, cold intolerance, or constipation. Physical exam findings include thyroid enlargement, thinning of the lateral eyebrow, dry skin, brittle hair, or facial swelling. Patients may also demonstrate a decrease in growth velocity, weight gain, or delayed pubertal development. If hypothyroidism is severe and untreated, patients may develop myxedema—a nonpitting edema. Other signs and symptoms in severe hypothyroidism include hyporeflexia, pericardial effusion with associated hypotension, bradycardia, hypothermia, and even coma.

Emergency Department Treatment and Disposition

Patients with acquired hypothyroidism, in whom thyroid-stimulating hormone (TSH) and free T_4 are available, can be started on thyroid replacement therapy and managed as outpatients in consultation with endocrinology. Patients with myxedema and other signs of severe hypothyroidism have a life-threatening condition and admission to an ICU is warranted. Workup should include assessing serum electrolytes and cortisol and for other endocrinopathies.

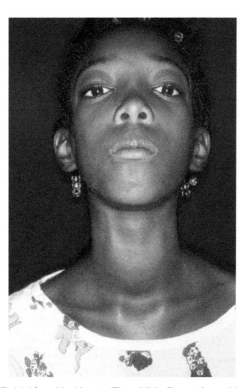

FIGURE 14.12 ■ Hashimoto Thyroiditis Presenting with Goiter. One of the most common clinical manifestations of Hashimoto thyroiditis is goiter. The thyroid is usually diffusely enlarged, symmetrical, freely moveble and nontender without any signs of local inflammation. It usually feels firm but may be nodular and the size varies among patients. (Photo contributor: Binita R. Shah, MD.)

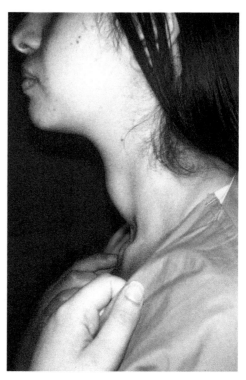

FIGURE 14.13 ■ Hashimoto Thyroiditis Presenting with Goiter. A firm, nontender goiter discovered incidentally during examination is a common presentation as seen in this adolescent girl. Most patients at presentation are euthyroid, some have evidence of subclinical or overt hypothyroidism, and less commonly, a few are hyperthyroid (Hashitoxicosis [thyroid hormone release due to inflammatory process]; see also Figure 14.21). The majority of patients with Hashimoto thyroiditis will develop frank hypothyroidism at some point in their life. (Photo contributor: Binita R. Shah, MD.)

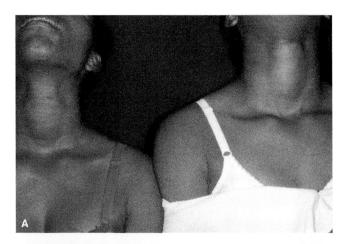

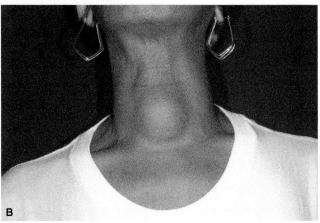

FIGURE 14.14 ■ Hashimoto Thyroiditis Presenting with Goiter. Familial clusters of Hashimoto thyroiditis are common. About 30% of patients with Hashimoto thyroiditis have family members with thyroid disease. Two sisters (**A**) and the mother (**B**) are seen with goiters. (Photo contributor: Binita R. Shah, MD.)

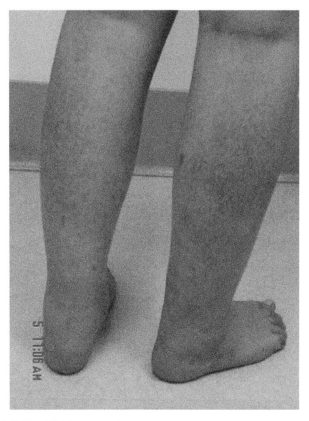

FIGURE 14.15 ■ Myxedema. Edema of hypothyroidism in adolescent girl presented for evaluation of her fatigue and weight gain. Edema of hypothyroidism is nonpitting with yellowish and waxy-appearing skin. (Photo contributor: Svetlana Ten, MD.)

Pearls

1. Consider hypothyroidism in patients presenting with vague symptoms such as fatigue, weakness, or lethargy.
2. The most common cause of hypothyroidism in children and adolescents is Hashimoto thyroiditis (also known as lymphocytic or autoimmune thyroiditis).
3. Hypothyroidism is associated with other autoimmune diseases, including diabetes mellitus, adrenal insufficiency, vitiligo, hypoparathyroidism, inflammatory bowel disease, and juvenile arthritis.
4. Myxedema is a life-threatening condition requiring intensive care and prompt thyroid replacement.

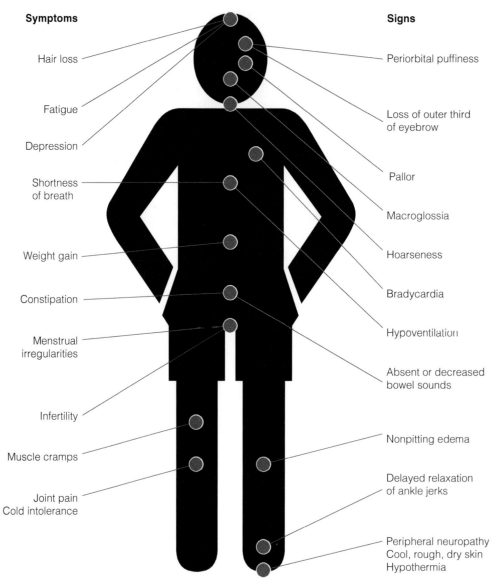

FIGURE 14.16 ■ Symptoms and Signs of Hypothyroidism. (Reproduced with permission from Cydulka RK, Fitch MT, Joing SA, et al. *Tintinalli's Emergency Medicine Manual,* 8th ed. McGraw-Hill Education; New York, NY, 2017.)

Clinical Summary

The most common cause of hyperthyroidism in children is Graves disease. Hyperthyroidism presents with symptoms including palpitations, anxiety, fatigue, weakness, weight loss, heat intolerance, increased bowel movement frequency, and pain or fullness in the anterior neck. Signs can include tachycardia, hypertension, muscle weakness, hyperactivity, eyelid retraction, and proptosis, all of which are caused by the excessive release of thyroid hormones. Thyroid storm is the severe, potentially life-threatening version of excessive thyroid hormone and presents with fever (almost invariably present; often severe and in excess of temperature elevation expected from the intercurrent illness), tachycardia (out of proportion to the degree of fever), and acute metabolic encephalopathy (extreme restlessness, agitation, psychosis, delirium, confusion, stupor, or coma).

Laboratory evaluation should include TSH, free T_4 and T_3, and thyroid antibodies (antithyroid peroxidase antibody and thyroid-stimulating immunoglobulins). In thyrotoxicosis, TSH will be suppressed to almost undetectable levels, and free T_4 and/or T_3 will be elevated. High thyroid-stimulating antibody titers indicate Graves disease, although some patients with Graves disease may be seronegative. Hyperthyroidism may precipitate arrhythmias or congestive heart failure, so an ECG and CXR should be obtained, particularly in the setting of hypertension, tachycardia, and dyspnea. Alternatively, dyspnea may be caused by muscular weakness and not as a cardiac complication. A pregnancy test should be obtained for all postmenarchal adolescent females both to rule out rare causes of thyrotoxicosis secondary to extreme elevation of human chorionic gonadotropin levels and pre-radioiodine exposure when needed.

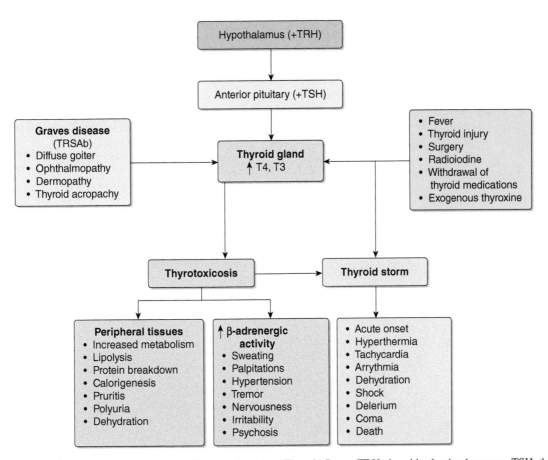

FIGURE 14.17 ■ Etiology and Pathophysiology of Thyrotoxicosis and Thyroid Storm. TRH, thyroid-releasing hormone; TSH, thyroid-stimulating hormone; TRSAb, Thyrotropin receptor-stimulating antibodies. (Reproduced with permission from Tenenbein M, Macias CG, Sharieff GQ, et al. *Strange and Schafermeyer's Pediatric Emergency Medicine,* 5th ed. McGraw-Hill Education; New York, NY, 2019.)

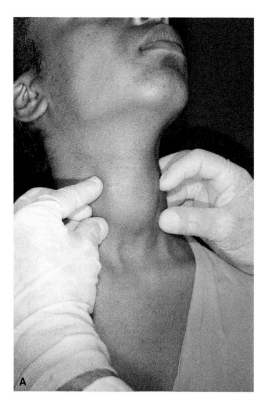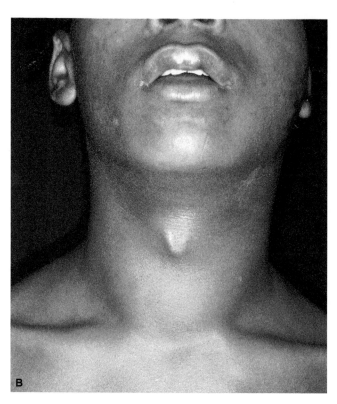

FIGURE 14.18 ■ Goiter; Graves Disease. Most cases of thyroid storm are secondary to Graves disease. (**A**) Goiter, a feature of Graves disease, will be seen in most patients with thyroid storm. Sudden onset of hyperpyrexia, palpitations, profuse sweating, and extreme restlessness were the presenting signs of this adolescent girl known to have Graves disease. (**B**) A diffuse, firm, nontender, symmetrically enlarged thyroid gland that moved with swallowing were noted in this adolescent male patient. A bruit was also heard over the enlarged gland. The female-to-male ratio of Graves disease is 5:1. (Photo contributor: Binita R. Shah, MD.)

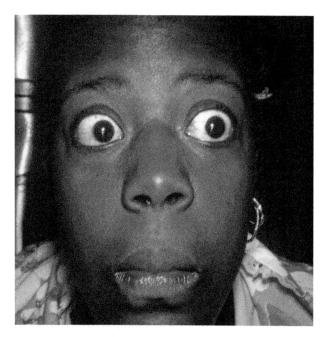

FIGURE 14.19 ■ Exophthalmos; Graves Disease. Retraction of the upper eyelids and infrequent blinking associated with exophthalmos were seen in this adolescent girl with Graves disease. Pain, chemosis, lid erythema, decreased visual acuity, and decreased extraocular movements are the other findings of Graves disease ophthalmopathy. (Photo contributor: Binita R. Shah, MD.)

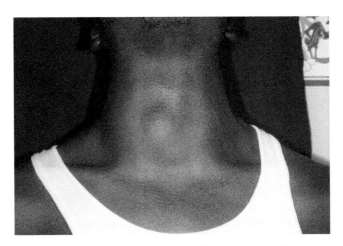

FIGURE 14.20 ■ Multinodular Goiter Presenting with Thyrotoxicosis. Patients with multinodular goiter may present with a very large goiter that is soft and not painful either with or without palpable nodules. (Photo contributor: Binita R. Shah, MD.)

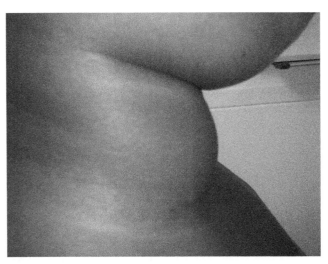

FIGURE 14.21 ■ Hashitoxicosis Presenting with Goiter. This adolescent girl presented with a chief complaint of swelling in the neck. She had positive thyroid antiperoxidase antibodies. She also gave a history of nervousness, increased sweating, and palpitations suggestive of hyperthyroiditis. Patients with Hashimoto thyroiditis can present with signs of thyrotoxicosis that are usually transient. (Photo contributor: Amrit P. Bhangoo, MD.)

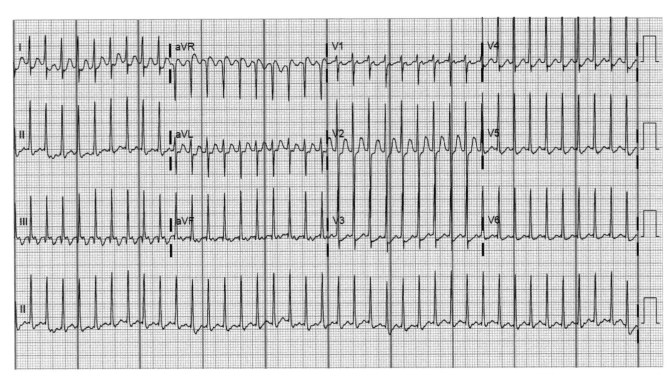

FIGURE 14.22 ■ Supraventricular Tachycardia (SVT) with Thyrotoxicosis. Palpitations and sweating were the presenting complaint of this adolescent girl whose ECG showed narrow complex tachycardia consistent with SVT. She also gave a history of weight loss, polymenorrhea, and heat intolerance. She was diagnosed as having Graves disease. (Photo contributor: Shyam Sathanandam, MD.)

Emergency Department Treatment and Disposition

Patients with thyroid storm should initially be admitted to the ICU. Initial management will include initiating β-blockers and antithyroid medications—methimazole or propylthiouracil (PTU). PTU currently has a black box warning for its association with liver failure in some patients; thus, methimazole is currently considered the first-line therapy. PTU does not cross the placenta and is preferred in pregnant patients with hyperthyroidism, particularly in the first trimester where methimazole may have teratogenic effects. Further supportive care may include treating hyperpyrexia, treatment of the precipitating event, and correction of fluid deficits. Patients with thyrotoxicosis who are not in thyroid storm generally do not require hospital admission, and, if stable, can be referred to endocrinology for outpatient follow-up. Radioactive iodine and thyroidectomy are additional potential therapies that are part of the long-term management of patients with hyperthyroidism but are not part of the emergent treatment.

Pearls

1. The terms hyperthyroidism, thyrotoxicosis, and thyroid storm describe the continuum of disease that results from hyperfunction of the thyroid gland.

2. Propranolol, IV fluids, antithyroid medication, and supportive measures are the mainstays of therapy for hyperthyroid patients presenting in thyroid storm.

3. Graves disease typically presents with hyperthyroidism, although patients may also be hypo- or euthyroid. In addition, up to 5% of patients may be seronegative for antithyroid antibodies.

4. Graves disease is the most common cause of thyrotoxicosis and may typically presents with goiter and ophthalmopathy, such as eyelid retraction, periocular edema, proptosis, or diplopia.

Chapter 15

GASTROINTESTINAL DISORDERS

Sandra Herr
Cole Condra

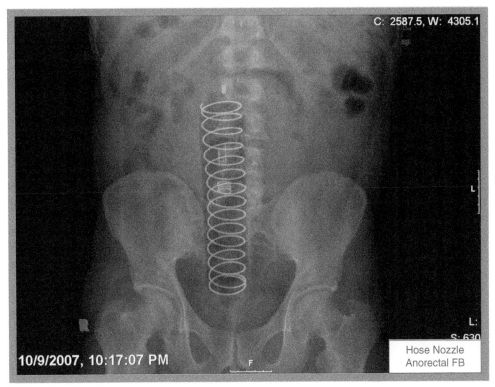

(Photo contributor: Mark Silverberg, MD)

The authors acknowledge the special contributions of Kanwal S. Chaudhry, MD, to prior edition.

ESOPHAGEAL FOREIGN BODIES

Clinical Summary

One of the most common gastrointestinal (GI) emergencies are ingested foreign bodies (FBs). Fortunately, most FBs pass through the GI tract spontaneously and require minimal medical intervention. In young children, typical swallowed FBs include coins, beads, button batteries, and toys, typically anything within reach. Accidental FB ingestions in adolescents are typically a result of a partially digested food bolus that becomes lodged in the esophagus. Unfortunately, some FB ingestions are intentional for various psychiatric reasons, and these ingestions may include sharp and potentially harmful objects (eg, razors, glass). The pediatric patient with an FB ingestion may be asymptomatic; however, a patient with a lodged FB in the esophagus often presents with drooling, excessive salivation, voice changes, vomiting, or respiratory symptoms.

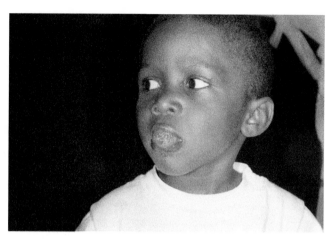

FIGURE 15.1 ■ Drooling as a Presenting Sign of an Esophageal Foreign Body (FB). An afebrile child presented with a sudden onset of drooling and inability to eat solid foods. There was no witnessed episode of choking, gagging, or any FB ingestion. An esophageal FB was suspected based on the history and subsequently confirmed (see Figure 15.2C). Drooling is a very common and consistent sign seen with a high-grade esophageal obstruction. (Photo contributor: Binita R. Shah, MD.)

TABLE 15.1 ■ NONSPECIFIC SIGNS AND SYMPTOMS AND COMPLICATIONS OF RETAINED ESOPHAGEAL FOREIGN BODIES (FB)

Nonspecific Signs/ Symptoms of Esophageal FB	Complications of Retained Esophageal FB
• Fever	• Mucosal abrasions or ulcerations
• Pain	• Necrosis (ie, button batteries)
• Neck mass	• Airway obstructions
• Crepitus	• Lobar atelectasis
• Shock secondary to perforation	• Regurgitation and aspiration of FB
	• Extraluminal migration
• Vomiting	• Esophageal stricture formation
• Respiratory symptoms	• Esophageal diverticula
	• Esophageal perforation
• Cough	• Abscess formation
• Wheezing	• Mediastinitis
• Stridor	• Pericarditis
	• Pericardial tamponade
	• Pneumothorax
	• Pneumomediastinum
	• Tracheoesophageal fistula
	• Esophageal-aortic fistula
	• Death

Emergency Department Treatment and Disposition

After stabilizing the patient, the first treatment priority is identifying the location of the FB. The location of a metallic FB may be found through the use of a hand-held metal detector. However, the most common technique for detection of radiopaque FBs is radiography. Plain-film imaging of the entire GI tract is often used to avoid missed FBs. Obtain anteroposterior and lateral CXRs if the FB is above the diaphragm to determine if it is in the trachea or esophagus and whether there is >1 FB (eg, 2 or more coins stacked together). If the FB is suspected to be radiolucent and perforation is *not* a concern, contrast esophagram may be useful. Consider CT scan with coronal and sagittal reconstructions if the FB is thought to have migrated to the extraluminal space or perforation or fistulas are suspected.

Objects lodged in the proximal esophagus may threaten the airway and should be removed promptly. Options for removal of an esophageal FB in place for <24 hours include endoscopy, extraction by Foley catheter, or advancement with a bougie dilator. Use endoscopy to emergently remove FB if it

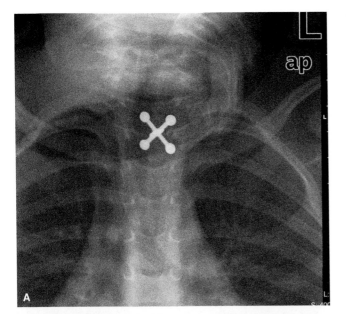

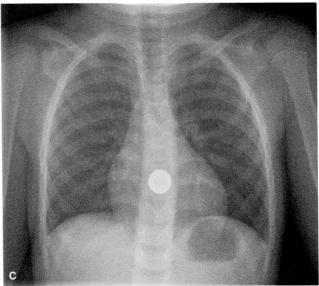

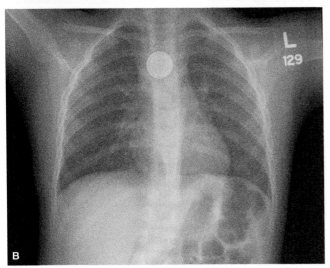

FIGURE 15.2 ■ The 3 Most Common Locations Where an Esophageal Foreign Body (FB) Becomes Lodged (Sites of Normal Anatomic Narrowing of the Esophagus). (**A**) *Proximal esophagus* at the thoracic inlet (defined as the area between the clavicles on a CXR) is the *most common location of entrapment*. Frontal projection of the neck shows a jack in upper thoracic esophagus. (**B**) *Mid-esophagus* at the level of the carina. Frontal projection of the chest shows a battery within the esophagus at the level of the aortic arch. (**C**) *Distal esophagus* just proximal to the gastroesophageal junction. Frontal projection of the chest shows a coin in region of the distal esophagus. (Photo contributor: John Amodio, MD.)

poses a risk of corrosive injury (button battery) or risk of perforation (sharp objects). Prompt endoscopic evaluation is also necessary (even if the radiographs are unrevealing) in symptomatic patients (eg, respiratory distress or difficulty managing secretions). Rigid endoscopy with forceps extraction under general anesthesia is the standard method for removal of objects that may be sharp or are embedded in the mucosa as well as objects that may have been in place for a prolonged period or for patients with previous esophageal disease or GI surgeries. This method provides a controlled setting with airway management and direct visualization of the esophagus

to identify and delineate any mucosal injury or esophageal pathology. Expectant management may be considered for asymptomatic healthy patients with a noncorrosive FB in the esophagus for <24 hours. Allow the patient to eat or drink and repeat the radiographs in a few hours to ensure spontaneous passage through the lower esophageal sphincter (LES). If the FB fails to progress beyond the LES or food is not tolerated, the patient is a candidate for endoscopic removal of the FB. The use of glucagon cannot be recommended because of the lack of evidence of efficacy in children, in addition to the risk of inducing nausea and vomiting.

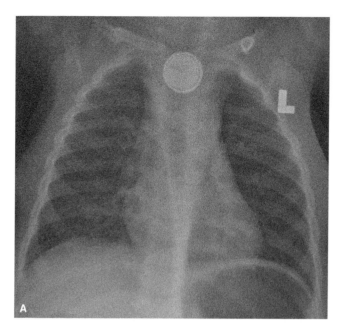
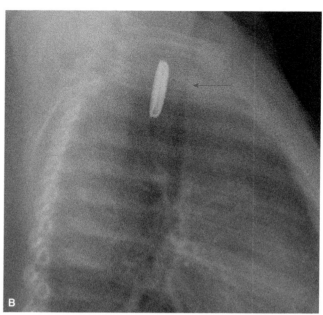

FIGURE 15.3 ▪ Classic Orientation of an Esophageal Foreign Body on Radiographs. (A) Frontal view of chest shows a battery lodged in the esophagus at thoracic inlet. The battery (or coin) in the esophagus will lie in coronal plane (ie, battery seen as a disk on a frontal view) because the opening into the esophagus is much wider in this orientation. (B) Note sagittal orientation of battery on a lateral film (ie, battery seen from the side and posterior to tracheal air column). Narrowing of trachea at the level of battery is seen (arrow). (Photo contributor: John Amodio, MD.)

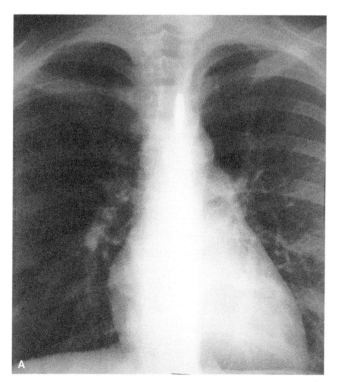
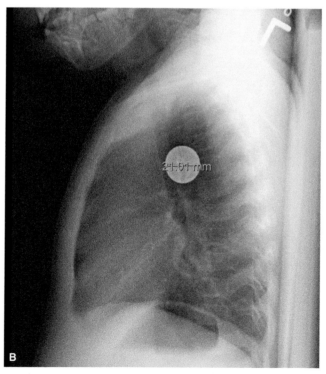

FIGURE 15.4 ▪ Esophageal Foreign Body (FB) Mimicking a Tracheal FB. Frontal view of the chest showing a coin at the thoracic inlet. When an FB gets lodged in the trachea, the orientation of the FB is typically *opposite* that seen with an esophageal FB. With the configuration of the tracheal rings and with incomplete cartilage posteriorly, a coin in the trachea appears in the sagittal orientation (ie, the coin is seen from the side) in a frontal view (A), and in the coronal orientation (ie, the coin is seen as a disk) on a lateral view (B). However, as seen here, this rule is not always correct; these radiographs actually show an impacted esophageal coin that mimics the orientation that is classically seen with a coin lodged in the trachea. (Photo contributor: Binita R. Shah, MD.)

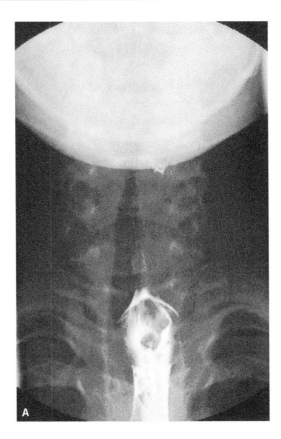

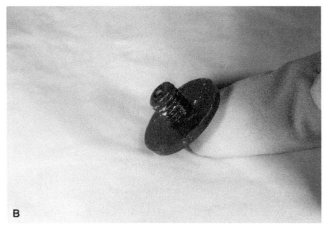

FIGURE 15.5 ■ Radiolucent Esophageal Foreign Body. (**A**) This 8-year-old child presented with drooling 12 hours after swallowing a piece of a toy; he was initially sent home from the ED when the chest and neck x-rays were normal. He later returned due to persistent symptoms, and a limited contrast esophagram showed a disc-like structure with a central protrusion at the level of T1–T2 in the upper thoracic esophagus without any evidence of perforation or obstruction. (**B**) A plastic toy that was removed by direct endoscopy under general anesthesia is shown. (Photo contributor: Binita R. Shah, MD.)

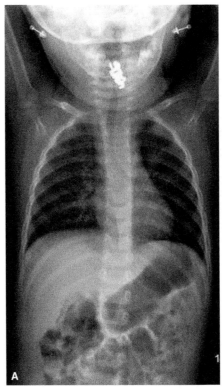

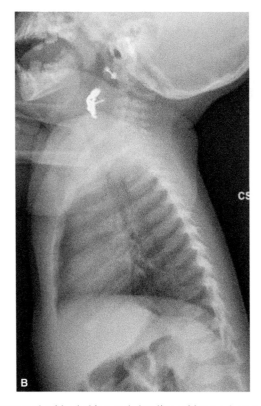

FIGURE 15.6 ■ Stick-pin ingestion. This 18-month-old toddler presented with choking and drooling without a known FB ingestion. (**A**) Anteroposterior radiograph shows the radiopaque FB at the thoracic inlet. (**B**) The lateral radiograph shows the pin extending posteriorly from the body of the pin. The pin was removed endoscopically; it was embedded in the posterior wall of the esophagus, but no definite perforation was identified. (Photo contributor: Sandra Herr, MD.)

Pearls

1. Coins are the most commonly lodged esophageal FBs in children. A preceding history of ingestion may or may not be present.

2. The most common symptoms of ingested FB are drooling, excessive salivation, dysphagia (refusing solids), retching, hoarseness, vomiting, or respiratory.

3. The 3 most common locations for entrapment of an FB are: (1) proximal esophagus at the cricopharyngeus muscle (C6) or upper esophageal sphincter, (2) mid-esophagus at the level of the aortic arch (T4), and (3) distal esophagus (gastroesophageal junction).

4. If the FB is lodged in an unusual location (ie, other than the normal anatomic narrowing sites), suspect underlying esophageal disease.

5. If the duration of lodged FB is unknown, it should be removed by rigid endoscopy under general anesthesia.

6. Eighty percent of ingested FBs occur in children <5 years of age, with the peak incidence between 6 months and 3 years of age.

Clinical Summary

FB ingestion is more common in pediatric or psychiatric patients, but it can be seen in all age groups. Anorectal FBs are most often seen in adolescents as a result of retrograde introduction due to sexual practices (see Figures 15.10 to 15.12). "Stuffing" drug packets (hurried ingestion of poorly prepared packages) to avoid law enforcement or carefully "packing" packets to smuggle drugs (heroin and cocaine being the most common drugs) across borders are other examples of ingested FBs. The size and shape of the FB will determine where it might get lodged. Some common narrow sites are pylorus, duodenum, ligament of Treitz, ileocecal valve (most clinically significant), appendix, hepatic and splenic flexures, and rectum. However, congenital or acquired narrowing in the GI tract (eg, webs, diaphragms, strictures, or diverticula) may also become a site for impaction of the FB.

Patients present with variable symptoms ranging from none (history of a swallowed FB, incidental finding on imaging done for other reasons, or an FB passed in the stool) to abdominal pain, vomiting, fever, abdominal distention, or abdominal mass (ie, bezoars). Patients may also present with sudden onset of choking, coughing, or gagging.

Emergency Department Treatment and Disposition

Endoscopic removal of FBs is indicated for any sharp object located before the duodenal sweep; in addition, any large object >3 cm in length in children <1 year old (or >5 cm in patients >1 year old) should be removed via endoscopy because its length makes it unlikely to pass the pylorus. Once an object has passed the ligament of Treitz, it cannot be retrieved endoscopically.

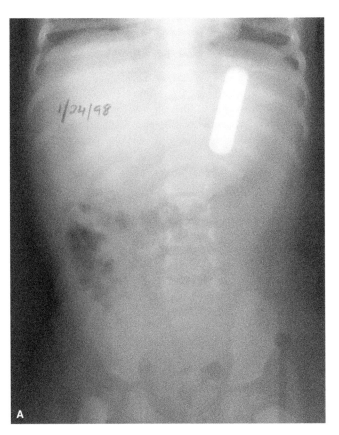
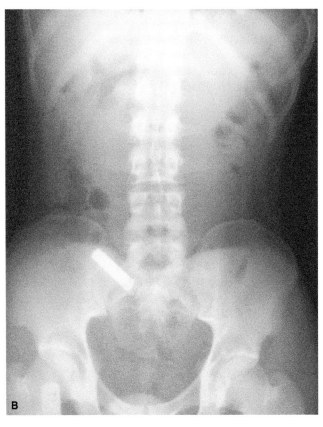

FIGURE 15.7 ■ Cylindrical Battery Ingestions. (**A**) Frontal view of the abdomen showing a cylindrical battery lodged in the stomach of a 5-month-old infant incidentally noted on a chest radiograph obtained for a suspected pneumonia. Because the exact time of ingestion was unknown and the battery failed to progress beyond the stomach (arrested transit) on serial radiographs over 72 hours, it was removed endoscopically and turned out to be a severely corroded AAA battery. (**B**) A completely asymptomatic adolescent psychiatric patient confessed to intentionally swallowing a battery 24 hours before this radiograph was obtained. He passed the battery in his stool 48 hours later. (Photo contributor: Binita R. Shah, MD.)

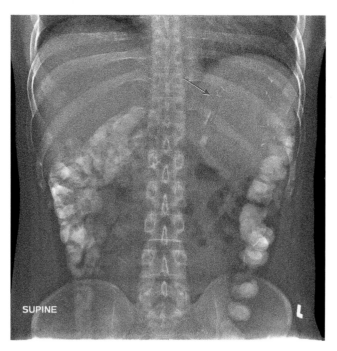

FIGURE 15.8 ■ Pencil Ingestion. Anteroposterior view of the abdomen shows a pencil in the region of the stomach (arrow) in a patient who had a history of many similar episodes of ingesting foreign objects. Staples and evidence of contrast from the prior study are also seen. (Photo/legend contributors: Kanwal Chaudhry, MD, and John Amodio, MD.)

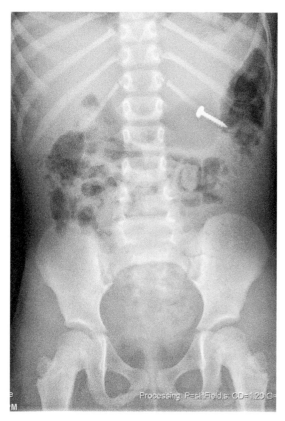

FIGURE 15.9 ■ Screw Ingestion. Anteroposterior view of the abdomen shows a screw in the region of the stomach. Ingested objects visualized within the stomach such as coins or bearings can be allowed to pass through the GI tract if they are small enough to fit through the pylorus. This screw required removal endoscopically. (Photo/legend contributors: Mark Silverberg, MD, and John Amodio, MD.)

Expectant management is recommended for all other FBs that have passed the esophagus. Most will pass through the GI tract in 4 to 6 days; however, some may take as long as 3 to 4 weeks. Repeat radiographs as an outpatient are not routinely indicated. Educate parents about warning signs of obstruction or perforation (eg, abdominal pain, vomiting, fever, or hematemesis). Admit body stuffers and packers to monitor for signs of toxicity as well as for passage of the packets. Whole-bowel irrigation and laxatives can be used to facilitate passage; however, endoscopic removal of packets is not advised because of the risk of rupture. Signs or symptoms of obstruction or perforation should prompt emergent surgery consult.

Pearls

1. Coins are the most commonly swallowed FBs by children.
2. Most FBs that pass the esophagus will pass through the remainder of the GI tract without complications.
3. Child neglect should be suspected in a child with repeated history of FB ingestion.
4. Ingestion of unusual FBs may suggest an underlying psychiatric illness.

Clinical Summary

Anorectal FBs result from retrograde introduction (eg, as a sexual practice or as a "mule" for smuggling) or, less commonly, an FB ingestion that lodges in the lower GI tract. Patients may present with vague symptoms (including rectal bleeding or constipation) rather than providing a history of inserting a rectal FB because of embarrassment. It is important to approach patients in a very nonjudgmental manner so they may feel comfortable and share the information regarding the events surrounding the FB or any attempts at self-removal.

Emergency Department Treatment and Disposition

Identify the type, size, shape, position, number of FBs, and the length of time/duration of FB before attempting its removal.

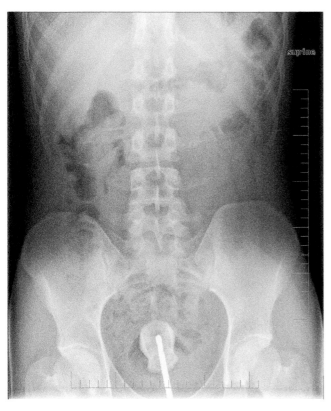

FIGURE 15.10 ■ Screwdriver; Anorectal Foreign Body (FB). Anteroposterior view of the abdomen shows a screwdriver in the region of the rectum. It is often difficult to get a good history from patients complaining of rectal pain because they are embarrassed or unwilling to be truthful. However, missing an FB like this could have grave consequences if it were to cause perforation. Because this FB was lodged just inside the anal sphincter, it was easily removed manually. (Photo contributor: Mark Silverberg, MD.)

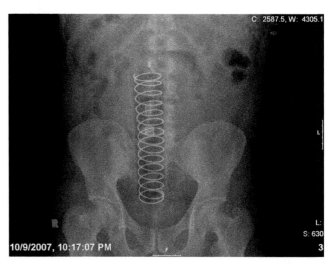

FIGURE 15.11 ■ Hose Nozzle; Anorectal Foreign Body (FB). Anteroposterior view of the abdomen shows a hose nozzle in the rectosigmoid. Anything that fits within the rectum can become lodged there. Objects that are made from plastic or wood can be difficult to see radiographically, although this metal spring–encircled garden hose is readily seen. Because of the large nature and irregular shape of this FB, it was removed under general anesthesia in the operating room. (Photo contributor: Mark Silverberg, MD.)

Defer the rectal examination until the location and type of FB are determined (risk of breaking fragile objects like light bulbs or pushing the FB deeper or injury to examining physician from a sharp FB). Obtain plain abdominal or pelvic

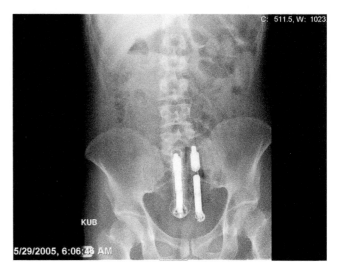

FIGURE 15.12 ■ Vibrators; Anorectal Foreign Body (FB). Anteroposterior view of the abdomen shows 2 vibrators in the region of the rectosigmoid. FBs can often be recognized by their silhouette. These 2 vibrators have a very distinct shape and can be easily identified. In this case, the treating physician was able to grab 1 of the vibrators with his fingers and pulled it out, allowing the second one to slide out easily. (Photo contributor: Mark Silverberg, MD.)

radiographs to detect radiopaque FBs. If indicated, additional views may be obtained to detect free air under the diaphragm or along the psoas muscle (suggests anorectal perforation). Treatment depends on the location and type of the FB. Most are in the rectal ampulla and easily palpated with a digital rectal exam or visualized with anoscopy. These can be removed in the ED with procedural sedation by digital extraction or with an anoscope or vaginal speculum for visualization of FB followed by forceps-aided removal. Sphincter relaxation with local anesthetic infiltration is key. The distal end of the FB may adhere to the rectal mucosa, creating a vacuum effect impeding its withdrawal. In these instances, a Foley catheter may be passed beyond the FB; insufflate air to break the vacuum, inflate the Foley balloon, and remove the FB. Once the FB has been removed, a sigmoidoscopy should be performed to look for mucosal tears and perforations, and follow-up radiographs should be taken to exclude free air. Consult surgery if there is a risk of perforation (glass or object with sharp edges) or the object is difficult to remove. Such patients may require laparotomy or sigmoidoscopy with forceps-aided removal of the FB.

Pearls

1. Anorectal FBs have to be removed to prevent complications such as bleeding, intestinal obstruction, perforation, and/or sepsis.

2. *Caution:* Use of enemas or cathartics to facilitate passage of an anorectal FB may increase the risk of perforation (especially with sharp FBs).

Clinical Summary

Button batteries are a frequently ingested item and are often ingested accidentally in young children. Common sources of the battery include child's own hearing aid, remote controls, toys, games, watches, and calculators. Eighty percent of patients remain asymptomatic, and the majority pass the battery within 48 to 96 hours. However, if the battery becomes lodged in the esophagus, it can result in esophageal mucosal injury, leading to ulceration, perforation, stricture, or liquefaction necrosis (from the electrical current). Longer retention can result in direct pressure necrosis and leakage of caustic material. Symptoms of a button battery impacted in the esophagus may include drooling, gagging, vomiting, refusing food, or respiratory symptoms (eg, stridor, wheezing, cough). A button battery causing GI tract injury may present with abdominal pain, vomiting, fever, or hematochezia.

Emergency Department Treatment and Disposition

An algorithm for the evaluation and treatment of suspected or confirmed button battery ingestion is developed and published by National Capital Poison Center, Washington, DC (https://www.poison.org/battery/guideline).

Obtain radiographs of the neck, chest, and abdomen to locate the battery. On an anteroposterior view, the battery will have a double density shadow, and on the lateral view, the edge of the battery will have a step-off. Remove batteries in the nasal passage, external auditory canal, or esophagus emergently. Use endoscopy for removal of batteries lodged in the esophagus since serious burns can develop as soon as 2 hours after ingestion. However, once the battery has passed into the stomach, the asymptomatic pediatric patient can be managed conservatively. Repeat radiographs should be obtained

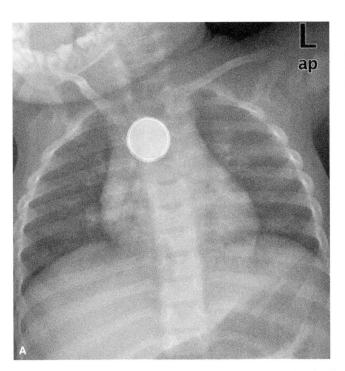

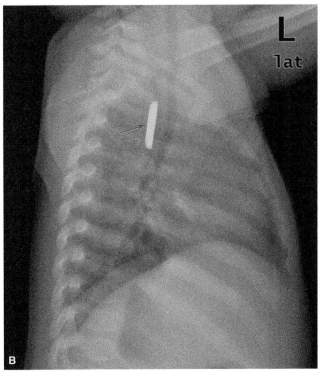

FIGURE 15.13 ■ Button Battery Ingestion and Spondylodiscitis (Complication of Battery Ingestion). (**A**) Frontal view of the chest shows battery in the esophagus at the level of the aortic arch. Note that the orientation of the negative pole cannot be determined by the frontal projection. (**B**) Lateral view of the chest shows battery within the esophagus at the level of the aortic arch. Note that the smaller negative side of the battery (arrow) is posteriorly oriented (negative pole of the battery facing posteriorly on the CXR puts the patient at risk of spondylodiscitis and anteriorly facing negative pole puts the patient more at risk for tracheoesophageal fistula or esophagoaortic fistula).

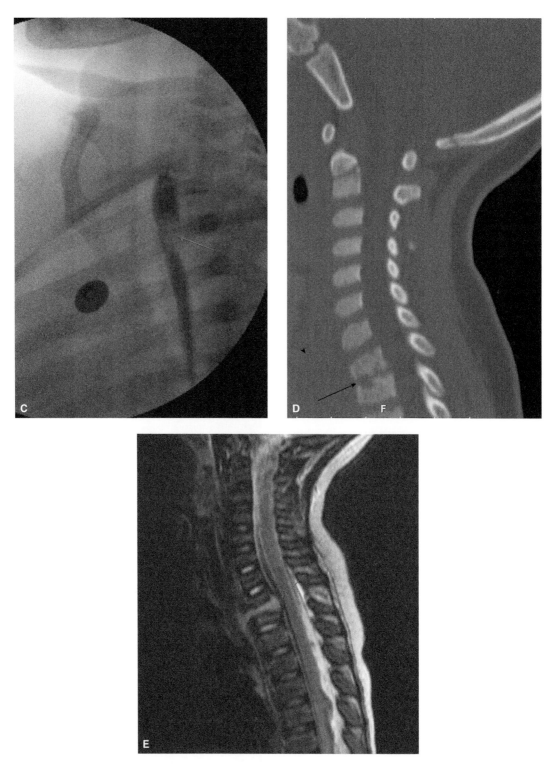

FIGURE 15.13 ▪ *(Continued)* **(C)** A filling defect is noted within the barium-filled esophagus (arrow), found to be an inflammatory polyp at endoscopy. This study was performed 48 hours following the removal of the battery. **(D)** Five weeks after the battery removal, the same patient presented to the ED with new onset of torticollis. Sagittal reconstruction of the cervical spine shows disc space loss and vertebral end plate irregularity at T1–T2 level (arrow) compatible with spondylodiscitis. **(E)** Sagittal T2 image of the cervical spine shows abnormal signal of the disc space at T1–T2 level (arrow) compatible with spondylodiscitis. There is mild impingement upon the thecal sac. ([A, E] Reproduced with permission from Tan A, Wolfram S, Birmingham M, et al. Neck pain and stiffness in a toddler with history of button battery ingestion. *J Emerg Med.* 2011;Aug;41(2):157–160. [B, C, D] Photo contributors: John Amodio, MD.)

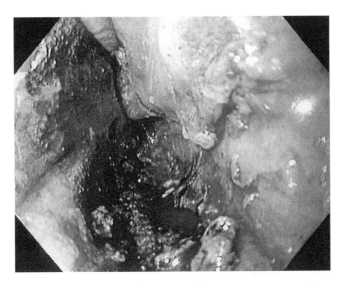

FIGURE 15.14 ▪ Battery Ingestion: Endoscopic Findings. Severe circumferential esophageal burn with necrosis and significant edema of surrounding mucosa are noted at the level of the cricopharyngeus after removal of a battery (about 7 hours after ingestion). This 8-year-old girl presented at a rural hospital with abdominal and chest pain following ingestion of a button battery, which was noted at the gastroesophageal junction on the initial chest radiograph. She subsequently vomited, and a repeat radiograph showed battery in the esophagus at the thoracic inlet. Her transfer to the treating institution took about 6 hours. Following the removal of the battery, esophagram did not show any perforation. However, 1 month later, she developed intermittent dysphagia, and a repeat esophagram showed a circumferential esophageal stricture at the level of the cricopharyngeus requiring balloon dilation. (Photo contributor: Stephen E. Nanton, MD.)

in 4 days after ingestion (or sooner if symptoms develop). Educate parents on signs of perforation (pain, vomiting, or blood in stools). Batteries that remain in the stomach for >4 days should be removed via endoscopy, even if the patient is asymptomatic. If the patient presents with signs of perforation (abdominal pain, vomiting, fever, or bleeding), surgical intervention is indicated.

Pearls

1. Button batteries lodged in the esophagus can cause severe tissue damage within 2 hours of ingestion.
2. Hospitalize all patients with batteries lodged in the esophagus or with evidence of complications related to ingestion.
3. Button batteries lodged in the ear, nose (see Figure 9. 28) or vagina (see Figure 10.37) can cause tissue necrosis and must be removed emergently.
4. Routine use of steroids or antibiotics is not recommended.
5. Do *not* induce vomiting!
6. Removal via Foley catheter should be avoided (does not allow direct visualization, risk of esophageal perforation may be increased, and the battery may be aspirated during retrograde movement).
7. Batteries that have passed into the stomach do not require urgent removal; if they remain in the stomach beyond 4 days, endoscopic retrieval should be performed.

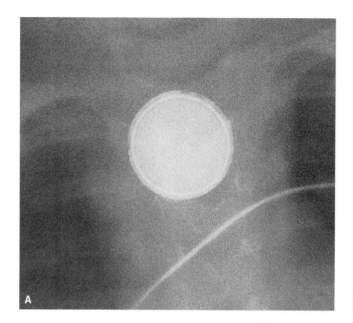
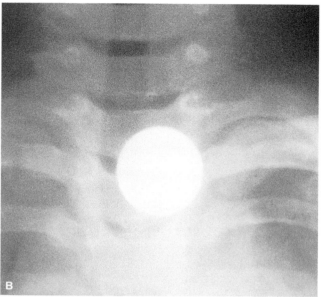
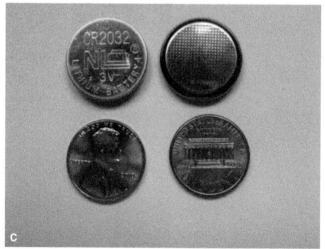

FIGURE 15.15 ■ Interpreting Radiography in Battery and Coin Ingestion. (**A, B**) Compare the close-ups of a battery with a coin from 2 different patients clearly demonstrating the radiographic differences. Battery has a lucent center and double ring or halo appearance, and coin has a homogenous density with smooth edges. (**C**) Compare the size and appearance of a button battery with that of a penny. (Photo contributor: Binita R. Shah, MD.)

Clinical Summary

In countries where fish and chicken are one of the major dietary resources, children commonly swallow fish or chicken bones, and with impacted swallowed bones, patients present with "something" stuck in the throat or throat pain while eating. Most bones become lodged at the base of the tongue, at the tonsillar level, or in the posterior pharyngeal wall or vallecula. Symptoms are often due to minor mucosal injury (eg, abrasion or laceration). A lateral plain radiograph with soft tissue technique may show the presence of a bone. Plain radiographs are not always useful. Salmon, mackerel, and trout bones are radiolucent; cod, haddock, and halibut are radiopaque. However, the radiograph may still be negative, and an actual bone is identified in only 20% to 30% of such patients.

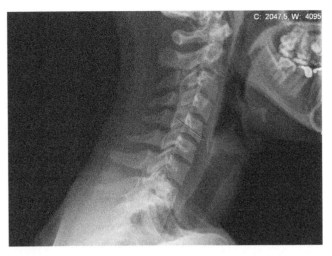

FIGURE 15.17 ■ Retained Goat Bone. Lateral view of the neck shows a goat bone (arrow) in the cervical esophagus in a patient presenting with throat pain that began while eating curried goat. The bone was removed under sedation. (Photo/legend contributors: Mark Silverberg, MD, and John Amodio, MD.)

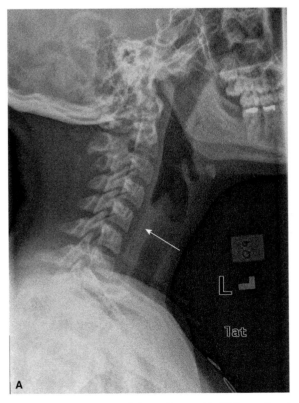

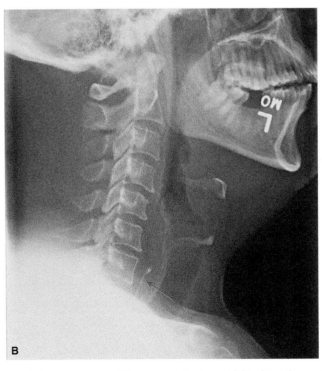

FIGURE 15.16 ■ Retained Chicken Bones. (A, B) Lateral projections of the neck from 2 different patients show chicken bone (arrows) in the lower cervical esophagus. (Photo/legend contributors: Mark Silverberg, MD [A], Kanwal Chaudhry, MD, and John Amodio, MD [B].)

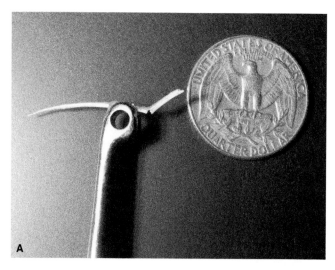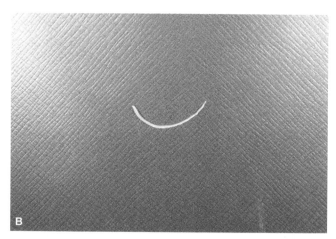

FIGURE 15.18 ■ Retained Fish Bones. (**A**) This fishbone was retrieved from the vallecula of a young patient who was eating snapper. Sedation with ketamine was required to pull it out using direct laryngoscopy and Magill forceps. (**B**) An adolescent girl presented with a complaint of something stuck in back of her throat after eating fish for dinner. Radiographs of the neck and chest were negative for the presence of any radiopaque foreign body. This impacted fish bone was removed by direct laryngoscopy from the hypopharynx. Chicken or fish bones are often poorly visualized because of their varying degree of calcification. Only 29% to 50% of endoscopically proven bones are seen on plain radiographs. (Photo contributors: Mark Silverberg, MD [A], and Binita R. Shah, MD [B].)

Emergency Department Treatment and Disposition

Direct inspection of oropharynx and hypopharynx is used to make the diagnosis. Specialty consultation should be obtained for endoscopic visualization and removal of the offending agent. Local anesthetic spray may aid in the evaluation and removal of a retained bone, or patients may require sedation or general anesthesia.

Pearls

1. Retained bones commonly become impacted at the tonsils, base of tongue, and/or posterior pharyngeal wall.
2. Retained bones rarely pass spontaneously once lodged in the mucosa and usually require removal.
3. Plain radiographs are usually not useful because fish or chicken bones are poorly visualized on radiographs because of their varying degrees of calcification.

Clinical Summary

Young children tend to ingest toys and coins, whereas adolescents often intentionally ingest sharp objects such as razors, safety pins, and sewing needles.

Emergency Department Treatment and Disposition

Treatment depends on the location of the FB and patient's presentation. Any sharp object lodged in the esophagus necessitates subspecialty consultation for emergent endoscopic removal. Surgical consultation for possible laparotomy is indicated in patients with symptoms of perforation (fever, abdominal pain, vomiting, or GI bleeding). The majority of sharp objects that enter the stomach pass through the remaining GI tract without any problem. However, the risk of complications in such patients is high (about 35%). Remove sharp objects in the stomach or proximal duodenum (before the duodenal sweep) endoscopically if it can be done safely. Manage patients who have ingested other sharp objects (beyond the duodenal sweep [first and second part of the duodenum]) conservatively with daily radiographs over 3 days as long as they remain asymptomatic. If the FB does not progress in 3 days, surgical retrieval by laparotomy is recommended.

Pearls

1. Ingested sharp objects proximal to the duodenal sweep should be emergently removed via endoscopy.
2. Ingested sharp objects beyond the duodenal sweep should be evaluated with daily radiographs and removed if there is no progress through the GI tract after 3 days.

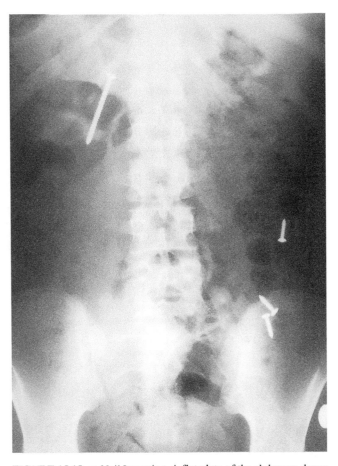

FIGURE 15.19 ■ Nail Ingestion. A flat plate of the abdomen shows several nails scattered throughout the intestines that were intentionally ingested by an adolescent psychiatric patient. She remained asymptomatic and passed them over a period of 72 hours. (Photo contributor: Binita R. Shah, MD.)

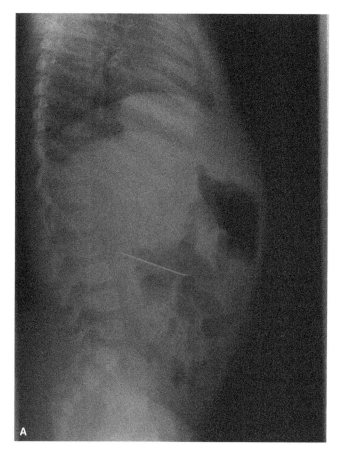

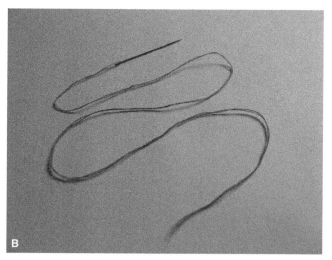

FIGURE 15.20 ■ Needle Ingestion. Lateral view of the abdomen shows a sewing needle in the midabdominal region (**A**) in a 9-month-old infant presenting with a history of choking and gagging. The infant had normal abdominal examination. During endoscopy, the needle was found to be embedded in the mucosa in the second part of duodenum and was not removed because of the risk of further injuries. (**B**) Subsequently, a rusted needle measuring 3.9 cm with a green thread measuring 37 cm in length was removed at laparotomy. (Photo/legend contributors: Ambreen Khan, MD, and John Amodio, MD.)

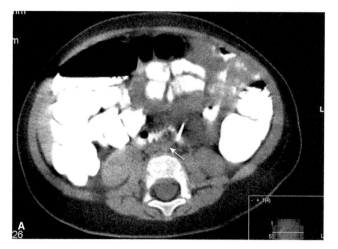

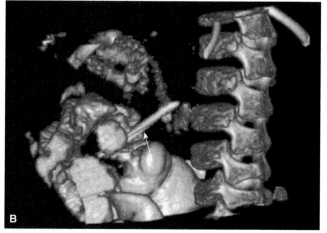

FIGURE 15.21 ■ Perforation of Duodenojejunal Junction with Needle. (**A**) CT scan shows sewing needle (same patient; Figure 15.20) has perforated the duodenum and lies adjacent to the aorta (arrow). (**B**) CT surface-rendered image, in the coronal plane, shows needle (white arrow) outside of the bowel. (Photo contributor: John Amodio, MD.)

Clinical Summary

High-powered magnets are now common household objects and are often within easy reach of an exploring toddler. Two (or more) strong magnets (or 1 magnet and a second metallic FB) may attract across layers of bowel, resulting in pressure necrosis, perforation, and/or intestinal obstruction.

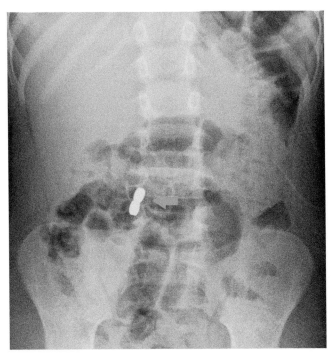

FIGURE 15.22 ■ Magnet Ingestion. A 6-year-old child presented to the ED after ingestion of foreign objects. Frontal view of the abdomen demonstrated 2 rounded radiopaque foreign bodies in a close approximation to each other within the small bowel, compatible with magnets (blue arrow). This was confirmed at the surgery. (Photo contributors: Jonathan N. Stern, MD, and Jeremy Neuman, MD.)

Emergency Department Treatment and Disposition

Suspected magnet ingestion requires immediate medical evaluation. Plain radiographs should be obtained to determine the location of the magnet(s). Ingestion of a single magnet, although less concerning, is still not without risk. Although conservative management is acceptable (serial radiographs), endoscopic removal should be considered if the magnet is in the esophagus or stomach. Unfortunately, x-rays often cannot determine if bowel wall is compressed between 2 magnets. As such, in the case of ingestion of multiple magnets (or a single magnet and a metal object), the location of the FBs is once again key. Magnets in the esophagus or stomach should be removed as soon as possible. For those magnets beyond the duodenal sweep in an asymptomatic pediatric patient, the management can vary. Often these patients are admitted for observation and serial examinations or radiographs every 4 to 6 hours. Surgical intervention is indicated in any patient who develops GI symptoms or in patients with magnets that do not progress on serial radiographs.

Pearls

1. Magnet ingestion is a medical emergency that requires immediate identification of the number and location of the magnet(s) and any other metallic FB.
2. Magnets located proximal to the duodenal sweep should be emergently removed via endoscopy.
3. A patient who ingested magnets now located beyond the duodenal sweep should be admitted for observation and serial radiographs with the potential for emergent surgical intervention.

Clinical Summary

Hematemesis is the vomiting of red blood or coffee-ground–like material, and it is usually due to a lesion or complication proximal to the ligament of Treitz in the duodenum. The etiology of hematemesis varies based on the age of presentation. The most common cause of bright red blood in the emesis of neonates is actually swallowed maternal blood. Other causes of hematemesis in neonates include bleeding due to congenital anomalies and vitamin K deficiency. The causes of upper GI bleeding in children and adolescents mirror those of adults. These include erosion of esophageal and stomach mucosa (esophagitis, ulcers/gastritis), lodged FB in esophagus (see above), esophageal varices (pediatric patients with chronic liver disease), and Mallory-Weiss tears due to forceful retching. One of the more common causes of bloody emesis in children is epistaxis or oropharyngeal bleeding due to trauma, infection, or inflammation.

Emergency Department Treatment and Disposition

The evaluation of the pediatric patient with suspected upper GI bleeding should begin with an assessment of hemodynamic stability (including vital signs, mental status, and

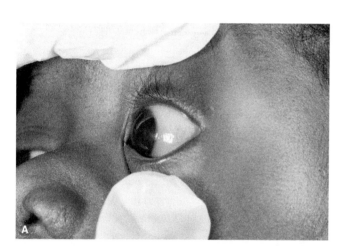
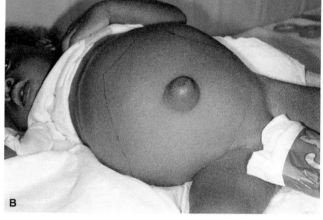
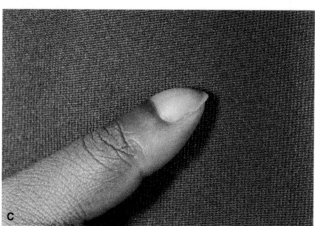
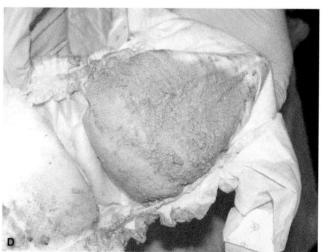

FIGURE 15.23 ■ Biliary Atresia with Portal Hypertension. Marked jaundice (**A**) and hepatosplenomegaly with ascites (**B**), clubbing (**C**), and clay-colored stool (**D**) are seen in a patient with untreated biliary atresia with portal hypertension and esophageal varices. In such children, sudden massive hemorrhage may result from rupture of varices. (Photo contributor: Binita R. Shah, MD.)

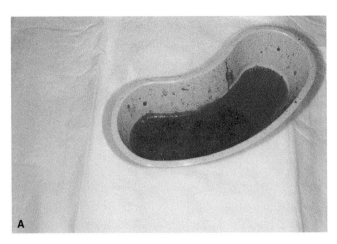
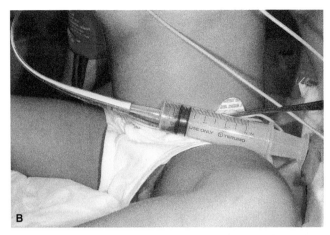

FIGURE 15.24 ■ Upper Gastrointestinal Tract Bleeding: Peptic Ulcer Disease. An 8-year-old child was brought to the ED with a sudden history of vomiting blood. Nasogastric lavage showed fresh blood (**A**). He was lavaged with room-temperature normal saline. Coffee-ground–appearing material is seen during lavage (**B**). Endoscopic examination showed the presence of gastritis (due to *Helicobacter pylori*) and superficial ulcers. His father also had peptic ulcer disease. (Photo contributor: Binita R. Shah, MD.)

capillary refill). Further physical exam elements should include careful inspection of the skin and mucosa for the presence or absence of ecchymosis, petechiae, or mucosal bleeding due to bleeding disorder. Rectal examination should be undertaken with testing of stool for blood (likely positive if

bleeding is subacute or chronic). Diagnostic studies include testing of the emesis using a Gastroccult card to determine if the specimen contains hemoglobin. In neonates, an Apt-Downey test should be performed on blood-tinged emesis to determine if the specimen contains swallowed maternal blood

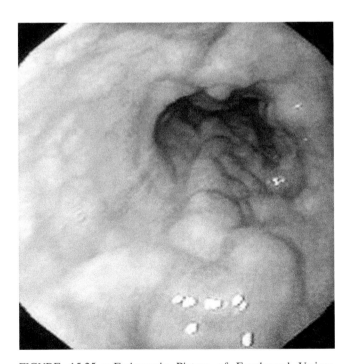
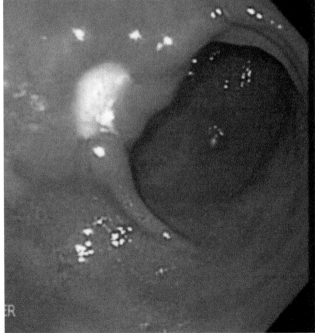

FIGURE 15.25 ■ Endoscopic Picture of Esophageal Varices. Endoscopy was performed on this child with a history of biliary atresia and portal hypertension after an episode of hematemesis. Extensive submucosal varices are visualized throughout the esophagus. (Photo contributor: Angela Jeffries, MD.)

FIGURE 15.26 ■ Endoscopic Picture of Gastric Ulcer. This adolescent male presented with coffee-ground emesis and mild anemia. Gastric lavage produced moderate volume of coffee-ground material, and endoscopy confirmed the diagnosis of gastric ulceration. (Photo contributor: Angela Jeffries, MD.)

versus the infant's blood. Lab testing may include a CBC, coagulation studies, and liver function testing. In the setting of significant upper GI bleeding, a type and screen should be obtained for potential transfusion. Nasogastric lavage (with large-bore Salem Sump tube) identifies blood in the stomach and helps to determine if the bleeding is continuous or has ceased; however, it has no benefit in the control of bleeding. Plain radiographs may be useful to determine the presence of an esophageal FB and to exclude free air due to perforation. Barium studies should be avoided in the setting of upper GI bleeding due to their interference with subsequent endoscopy. The definitive evaluation of a pediatric patient with upper GI bleeding must involve endoscopic examination. Treatment for GI bleeding should include pharmacologic interventions (H_2 blockers, sucralfate, or proton pump inhibitors) and antiemetics such as ondansetron (swallowed blood can cause nausea).

If the bleeding is significant and difficult to control, an octreotide drip can be administered with an initial bolus of 1 to 2 µg/kg and then a continuous infusion at 1 to 2 µg/kg/h.

Pearls

1. Hematemesis in neonates is often due to swallowed maternal blood and can be identified using the Apt-Downey test.

2. One of the most common causes of pediatric hematemesis is swallowed blood from epistaxis or oropharyngeal sources; evaluate the naso- and oropharynx as part of your physical examination.

3. Swallowed blood causes nausea and vomiting, necessitating the use of antiemetics and H_2 blockers or proton pump inhibitors.

Clinical Summary

Pancreatitis is a relatively uncommon diagnosis in children compared to their adult counterparts; however, due to this fact and its vague presentation, pancreatitis can often go undiagnosed. Pancreatitis in the pediatric population is often infectious in etiology (coxsackie virus) or related to blunt trauma (eg, bicycle handlebars) transmitted directly to the organ. Other causes include genetic conditions (cystic fibrosis) and certain medications. The more common adult causes of pancreatitis (eg, obstructive, alcohol use) are extremely rare in pediatrics. Most patients with acute pancreatitis present with a progressive onset of severe, sharp, constant epigastric abdominal pain associated with nausea and vomiting. The vomiting is usually nonbloody and nonbilious. Fever may be present, especially in those cases with an infectious etiology. Physical exam findings are often negative with the exception of epigastric abdominal tenderness. Although guarding of the abdomen is often present, rebound tenderness associated with peritoneal inflammation is rare. Since pediatric pancreatitis due to obstructions in the biliary tree is uncommon, physical exam findings such as jaundice, scleral icterus, and arrest of respiratory inspiration with deep palpation of the right upper quadrant of the abdomen (Murphy sign) are rarely found.

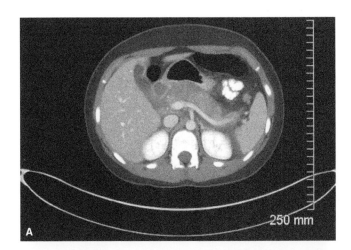

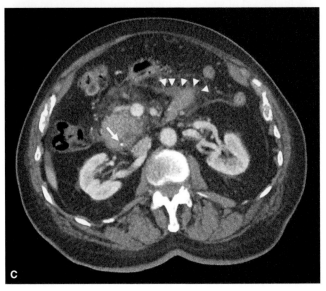

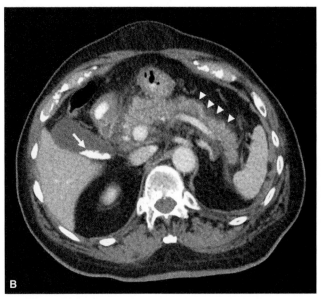

FIGURE 15.27. ■ Pancreatitis and Gallstone Pancreatitis. (**A**) A 16-year-old girl presented with 2 weeks of upper abdominal pain, nausea, and vomiting with mildly elevated serum transaminases and lipase of 6000 U/L. An axial view of CT image shows heterogeneous appearance of the pancreas with low density in the tail and body regions and peripancreatic fat stranding consistent with pancreatitis. (**B, C**). A 25-year-old man presented with 2 days of abdominal pain, nausea, and vomiting (serum lipase of 11,000 U/L, aspartate aminotransferase of 254 U/L, and total bilirubin of 2.0 mg/dL). (**B**) Axial postcontrast CT image shows peripancreatic fat stranding (arrowheads) and layering stones in the gallbladder (arrow). (**C**) Mesenteric fluid (arrowheads) and 2-mm stone in the distal common bile duct (arrow). These findings are consistent with gallstone pancreatitis. (Photo contributors: Philip Dydynski, MD [A], and Jesse Chen, MD [B, C].)

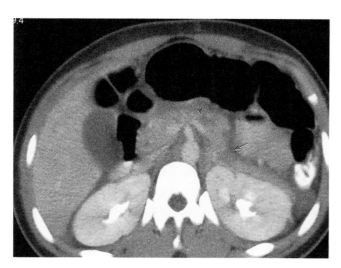

FIGURE 15.28 ▪ Pancreatic Laceration. An axial CT scan demonstrates 2 pancreatic fractures (arrows) and surrounding pancreatic fluid in a child who fell over handle bars. Pancreatic duct was shown to be intact on magnetic resonance cholangiopancreatography. Intrusion-type injuries (punch, kick, fall onto a pointed or irregular object) to the upper abdomen commonly impact the duodenum, pancreas, and left lobe of the liver. Pancreatic and bowel injuries often present with delayed and progressive symptoms hours to days after the initial injury. (Photo contributor: John Amodio, MD.)

Emergency Department Treatment and Disposition

The symptoms of pancreatitis (fever, vomiting, abdominal pain) can be found in many disease processes; as such, the inclusion of pancreatitis in the differential of the pediatric patient with these symptoms is imperative in order to make the diagnosis. Laboratory evaluation for the ill-appearing vomiting pediatric patient with abdominal pain should include testing for pancreatic enzymes. Classically, amylase and lipase are obtained in patients with suspected pancreatitis. Amylase rises within 6 to 12 hours after onset of pancreatitis; however, amylase has a short half-life (10 hours) and may be falsely normal in patients with pain for >24 hours. Lipase rises 4 to 8 hours after initial symptoms and does not normalize for up to 14 days. Since lipase elevation occurs earlier and lasts longer that amylase, obtaining a lipase alone is often sufficient for testing for medical causes of pancreatitis in the pediatric population. Additional laboratory testing should include evaluation for hyperbilirubinemia and transaminitis. Abdominal US is the preferred initial imaging modality in pediatrics, but CT may be necessary in some patients.

In the ED, pediatric patients with pancreatitis should be placed on gut rest and provided IV fluids (and fluid resuscitation when indicated). If the cause of pancreatitis is suspected to be medication induced, removal of the offending agent is required. IV analgesia is imperative; however, there is debate about the preferred medication for pain associated with pancreatitis. Although morphine can theoretically increase spasm at the sphincter of Oddi, opioids are the most common analgesics used in pediatric pancreatitis patients. Antibiotics are not indicated in the initial management of pancreatitis. Almost all patients with pancreatitis require hospital admission.

Pearls

1. The etiology of pancreatitis in pediatrics (infectious, trauma) differs from that of adults.
2. A high level of suspicion for pancreatitis should be present in the febrile, vomiting pediatric patient with abdominal pain.
3. Although amylase is useful in the evaluation of acute traumatic injury to the pancreas, a lipase level is more sensitive and specific for acute pancreatitis.

Clinical Summary

Biliary colic is the pain associated with obstruction of the biliary tree with stones originating from the gallbladder. Historically, cholecystitis due to cholelithiasis is uncommon in pediatrics outside of certain patient populations (eg, sickle cell disease, spherocytosis); however, this diagnosis is increasing in part due to worsening modern diets and pediatric obesity. A classic symptom of biliary colic is acute onset of sharp pain in the right upper quadrant (RUQ) of the abdomen (usually following a fatty meal). The patient is often restless, trying to find a comfortable position, but unfortunately, the pain does not improve with position changes. Nausea and vomiting can be present but are not as severe or intense as in pancreatitis. Jaundice can be present in up to 25% of patients. Physical

examination should include testing of Murphy sign (arrest of inspiration with deep palpation of the RUQ).

Emergency Department Treatment and Disposition

Patients with suspected biliary colic should be made NPO and begun on IV fluids. Pain management can be provided by using either ketorolac or opioids. Laboratory testing is often nonspecific in biliary colic. Although biliary obstruction can cause transaminitis and elevation in pancreatic enzymes, these tests are often normal. Serum bilirubin may be elevated but is often <4 mg/dL. Abdominal plain films are not useful. Gallbladder disease (including cholecystitis) is best visualized on limited abdominal US of the RUQ. Unfortunately, US imaging of the gallbladder is best performed on patients with at least 8 hours of fasting—a patient population that rarely presents to the ED. Patients with suspected or confirmed biliary colic can often be discharged from the ED with outpatient follow-up if pain is well controlled and there is no sign of cholangitis (ascending biliary infection most common in pediatric patients status postoperative repair of biliary atresia). Patients with documented cholecystitis require prompt surgical consultation.

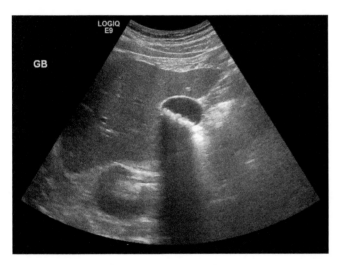

FIGURE 15.29 ■ US Image of Multiple Gallstones. This 16-year-old girl presented with 2 weeks of worsening right-sided upper abdominal pain, nausea, and vomiting. US shows echogenic foci and posterior shadowing consistent with multiple gallstones. There is no wall thickening or surrounding fluid to suggest cholecystitis. (Photo contributor: Jesse Chen, MD.)

Pearls

1. Cholecystitis due to cholelithiasis is associated with hematologic diseases such as sickle cell anemia and hereditary spherocytosis.
2. Acute biliary colic is increasingly being seen in pediatrics secondary to a rise in prevalence of obesity.
3. US evaluation of biliary colic is ideal but best performed after at least 8 hours of fasting.

INFLAMMATORY BOWEL DISEASE EXACERBATIONS

Clinical Summary

Inflammatory bowel disease (IBD) includes 2 chronic GI disorders: ulcerative colitis and Crohn disease. Although both involve mucosal inflammation, ulcerative colitis is localized to the colon, whereas Crohn disease can manifest anywhere in the GI tract. The most common presenting symptoms of IBD in the ED include diarrhea, rectal bleeding, weight loss, and abdominal pain. Pain is often colicky, and the abdominal exam may include guarding and even peritoneal signs such as rebound tenderness. A thorough physical exam must include a rectal exam; not only is the evaluation for rectal bleeding imperative, but perianal changes (ulcers, fistulas, skin tags) in Crohn disease can precede intestinal manifestations by several years. Although rare in pediatrics, patients with IBD can develop toxic megacolon. Toxic megacolon is significant colonic distension (usually transverse colon) due to extensive inflammation and can result in perforation and sepsis. Patients with Crohn disease may also have extraintestinal manifestations of the disease including arthritis, erythema nodosum, and uveitis. Since the mean age of diagnosis of IBD is 12.5 years of age (with a median of 15 years), preteens and adolescents with these signs and symptoms should be evaluated for IBD.

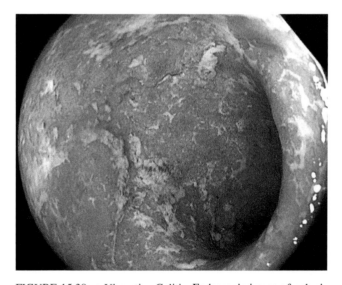

FIGURE 15.30 ■ Ulcerative Colitis. Endoscopic image of colonic inflammation in a patient with chronic diarrhea, hematochezia, and weight loss. Multiple areas of ulceration (white lesions) are seen throughout the colonic mucosa. Findings and biopsy results confirmed a new diagnosis of ulcerative colitis. (Photo contributor: Angela Jeffries, MD.)

Emergency Department Treatment and Disposition

Pediatric patients who present with weight loss, abdominal pain, diarrhea, and/or rectal bleeding should be evaluated for suspected inflammatory bowel disease. The initial evaluation should include a rectal exam for occult (or frank) blood and perianal disease. Laboratory testing will assist in determining the likelihood of the diagnosis of IBD. Patients with an IBD exacerbation may have anemia of chronic disease (normocytic) and leukocytosis on a CBC. Electrolytes and liver function testing may reveal hypoalbuminemia. The laboratory hallmark of IBD (although nonspecific) is elevated inflammatory markers including erythrocyte sedimentation rate (ESR) and C-reactive protein (CRP). Fluid resuscitation and gut rest should be implemented as soon as possible in the ED. Treatment with pain medications such as opioids may be necessary as well. Abdominal imaging with plain radiographs is of little benefit unless the patient has exam findings consistent with obstruction (and/or concern for toxic megacolon). Although CT evaluation of the abdomen/pelvis with IV and oral contrast may show inflammation and mucosal thickening, this mode of imaging should only be used in consultation with a pediatric gastroenterologist. The gold standard for confirmatory diagnosis of IBD is endoscopy, and prompt endoscopic evaluation should replace advanced radiographic imaging. Patients with a new diagnosis of IBD in the ED are often admitted for further evaluation and initial treatment.

Patients with a known diagnosis of IBD who present with GI symptoms should be evaluated and treated for a presumed IBD exacerbation. Once labs have been obtained and fluids provided, the ED provider should discuss further care with the patient's gastroenterologist. Medication adjustments (including steroids, immunomodulators, etc) may be possible and may allow discharge of the patient with close follow-up.

Pearls

1. There should be a high level of clinical suspicion for IBD in the adolescent with abdominal pain, diarrhea, weight loss, and rectal bleeding.
2. Abnormal physical exam findings outside of the abdomen (uveitis, arthritis, rash, perianal disease) are often associated with Crohn disease.
3. The hallmark of the laboratory evaluation of IBD is elevated inflammatory markers such as ESR and CRP.

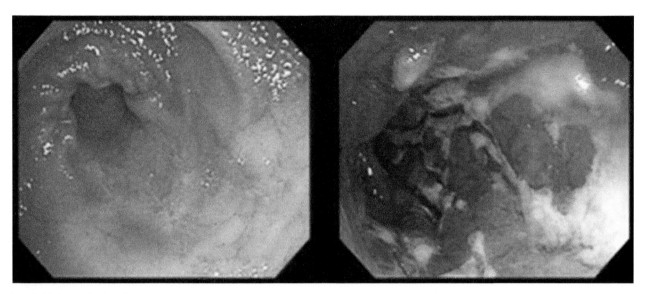

FIGURE 15.31 ■ Crohn Disease. Endoscopic image of small bowel mucosal lesions in a 12-year-old girl with recurrent abdominal pain and fever, poor weight, gain and erythema nodosum rash. Crohn disease can affect any portion of the GI tract and is associated with inflammation, narrowing, and/or ulcerative lesions. The endoscopic findings along with biopsy results confirmed a new diagnosis of Crohn disease. (Photo contributor: Angela Jeffries, MD.)

Clinical Summary

Constipation is passing of hard/lumpy, large-diameter, or pellet-like stools <3 times a week. It is often associated with pain or excessive straining and may be a presenting symptom of medication use or underlying diseases such as Hirschsprung disease, hypothyroidism, or spina bifida occulta. Patients may present with straining, crampy abdominal pain, anorexia, nausea/vomiting, tenesmus, blood-streaked stools, or encopresis (fecal soiling associated with solidified fecal impaction). Many young boys present with penile pain as a result of the stool burden compressing the dorsal penile nerve intra-abdominally via the pudendal canal. Constipation may lead to recurrent UTIs, especially in young female patients. Rectal exam may reveal a tight anal canal with an empty rectal vault.

Emergency Department Treatment and Disposition

The majority of patients with constipation do not require hospitalization and can be managed as outpatients. For fecal impaction or extreme abdominal pain, an infusion of an enema via rectum can begin the process of bowel cleanout if there is a large volume of stool in the descending and rectosigmoid colon. Almost all patients with constipation should

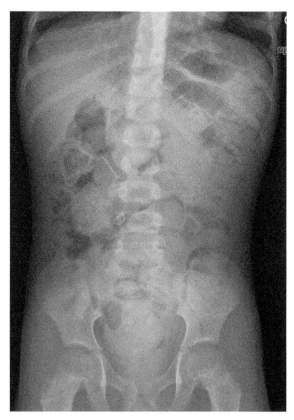

FIGURE 15.33 ■ Constipation. Frontal view of the abdomen shows a large amount of stool in the colon, compatible with constipation. (Photo contributor: John Amodio, MD.)

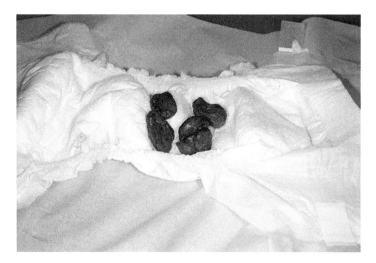

FIGURE 15.32 ■ Constipation. Passing lumpy or hard, large-diameter stools, pellet-like stools or passing fewer than 3 stools per week associated with pain or excessive straining are features of constipation. Excessive crying and passing hard stools were the complaints in this 18-month-old infant presenting with fecal impaction. During his rectal examination, very hard stool was felt in the ampulla, and after manual disimpaction, he passed this stool. (Photo contributor: Binita R. Shah, MD.)

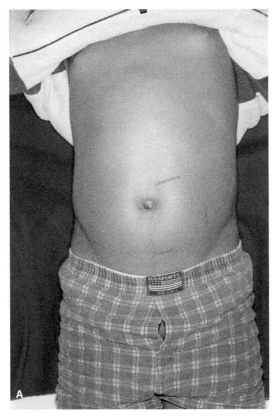
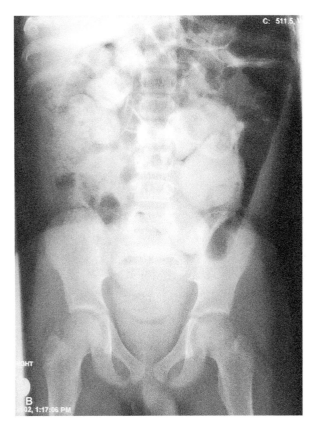

FIGURE 15.34 ■ Hirschsprung Disease. (**A**) Abdominal distension is seen in this 10-year-old boy presenting with abdominal pain, vomiting, and a chronic history of constipation since 3 weeks of age. He had a very protuberant abdomen with a palpable abdominal mass (shown by the marks) in the left lower quadrant. He had received numerous enemas and suppositories in various EDs for fecal impaction and had missed appointments for rectal biopsy. (**B**) Frontal radiograph of the abdomen shows gross dilation of the rectum and sigmoid colon secondary to distal rectal obstruction. Also seen is mild dilation of more proximal colonic loops. A rectal biopsy confirmed the diagnosis of an aganglionic segment in the rectosigmoid region. (Photo contributor: Binita R. Shah, MD.)

be begun on maintenance therapy daily to improve bowel function and thorough stooling. One of the most commonly used medications is the nonstimulant, high-density molecule laxative polyethylene glycol (PEG 3350). Daily dosing of polyethylene glycol minimizes absorption of water and forces more water to remain in the colon, leading to a softer stool. A high-fiber diet should be encouraged, along with increased water intake and increased physical activity. Refer patients with suspected Hirschsprung disease to a gastroenterologist or surgeon for a rectal biopsy.

Pearls

1. Abdominal radiographs should not be routinely performed for constipation.
2. Oral fluids, high-fiber diet, behavioral modification, and treating the underlying aggravating factors are key in treating constipation.
3. Delayed stooling at birth, an absence of hard stool in the rectal vault, and expulsion of foul-smelling liquid stool are features of HD.

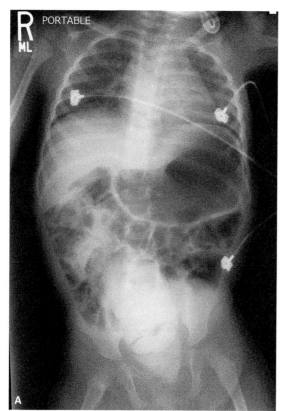

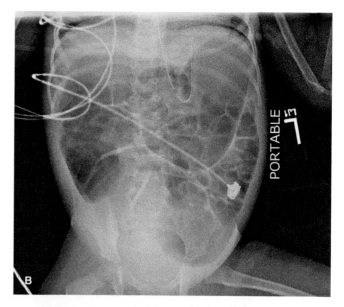

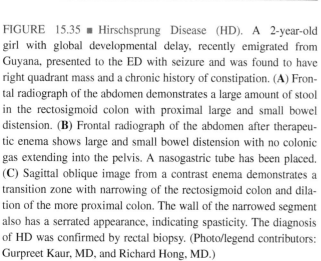

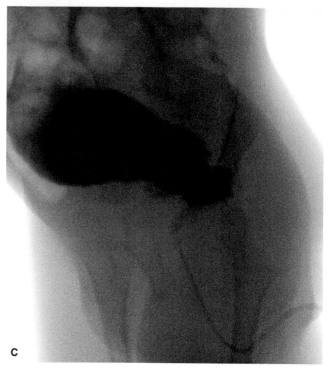

FIGURE 15.35 ■ Hirschsprung Disease (HD). A 2-year-old girl with global developmental delay, recently emigrated from Guyana, presented to the ED with seizure and was found to have right quadrant mass and a chronic history of constipation. (**A**) Frontal radiograph of the abdomen demonstrates a large amount of stool in the rectosigmoid colon with proximal large and small bowel distension. (**B**) Frontal radiograph of the abdomen after therapeutic enema shows large and small bowel distension with no colonic gas extending into the pelvis. A nasogastric tube has been placed. (**C**) Sagittal oblique image from a contrast enema demonstrates a transition zone with narrowing of the rectosigmoid colon and dilation of the more proximal colon. The wall of the narrowed segment also has a serrated appearance, indicating spasticity. The diagnosis of HD was confirmed by rectal biopsy. (Photo/legend contributors: Gurpreet Kaur, MD, and Richard Hong, MD.)

Clinical Summary

Lower GI bleeding (LGIB) is bright red blood or dark, tarry stools from the rectum. Bleeding proximal to the ileocecal valve usually produces melena (tarry stools) and bleeding distal to it usually produces hematochezia (bloody stools); extremely brisk bleeding from the more proximal bowel can be the exception, resulting in bright red blood per rectum. The most common cause of LGIB in neonates is anal fissure. However, necrotizing enterocolitis, intestinal malrotation, and midgut volvulus should be suspected in a neonate with bilious emesis, abdominal distention, and/or rectal bleeding.

Infants and toddlers (1 month to 2 years old) with blood in the stool should be evaluated for anal fissures as well. However, an increasing number of infants are developing milk protein–induced colitis, which is an inflammatory reaction caused by ingestion of cow's milk or soy proteins in formula or via mom's diet in breast-fed infants. This inflammation can result in sloughing of mucosa, leading to a distended abdomen

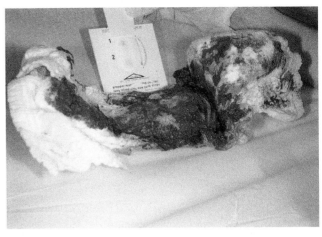

FIGURE 15.37 ■ Ingestion of Beets Presenting with "Bloody" Stool. Red "bloody" stool was passed by this completely asymptomatic toddler, who was rushed to the ED by a very frightened mother. As shown, a stool guaiac test was negative. The mother gave a history of feeding him beets for the past 2 days. This is a good example of how a lot of unnecessary and some potentially dangerous tests can be avoided with a thorough history and negative guaiac test in a well-appearing infant. (Photo contributor: Binita R. Shah, MD.)

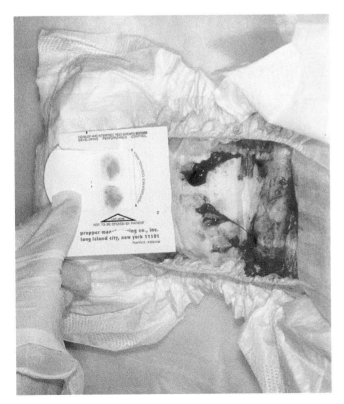

FIGURE 15.36 ■ Bleeding per Rectum: Intussusception. This currant jelly stool was passed by an 8-month-old infant brought to the ED with complaints of vomiting, lethargy, and intermittent episodes of crying of 12 hours in duration. He had ileocolic intussusception that was not able to be reduced by barium enema and required surgical reduction. (Photo contributor: Binita R. Shah, MD.)

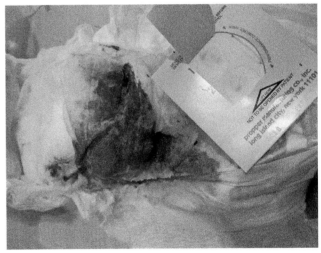

FIGURE 15.38 ■ Cefdinir–Iron Interaction Presenting with "Bloody" Stool. Sudden passing of grossly red "bloody" stool was the presenting complaint of this otherwise completely asymptomatic 2-year-old child who was receiving cefdinir for a urinary tract infection and Peptamen Jr. (supplemental elemental diet containing iron). "Bloody" stool tested negative for occult blood. Formation of a nonabsorbable complex in the GI tract between cefdinir or its breakdown products and iron (commonly found in infant formula) leads to reddish color. Even though this drug–diet interaction is not harmful, families may request changing to another oral antibiotic medication because the stool color is distressing. (Photo contributor: Haamid Chamdawala, MD.)

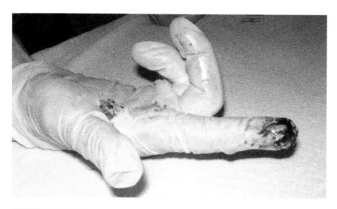

FIGURE 15.39 ■ Melena. Melena is dark stool found in the setting of GI bleeding. As blood is broken down, it appears blacker. It can be mixed with undigested blood and may have a maroon color (as seen here). (Photo contributor: Mark Silverberg, MD.)

and hematochezia. Although intussusception can present with bloody stools and even frank "currant jelly" stool, these signs are a late finding in intussusception.

The most frequent causes of LGIB in children (>2 year old) are infectious colitis and anal fissures. Infectious etiologies (ie, *Campylobacter, Salmonella, Shigella,* or *Yersinia*) usually cause hematochezia. Pediatric patients with an LGIB and a history of recent antibiotics should be evaluated for *Clostridium difficile* enteritis; however, it is important to remember that *C difficile* can be normal gut flora in infants under 1 year of age. Other diagnoses in children that cause LGIB include inflammatory bowel disease (ulcerative colitis, Crohn disease), juvenile polyps, Meckel diverticulum, Henoch-Schönlein purpura (vasculitis of the GI tract), and hemolytic uremic syndrome (thrombosis of small mucosal vessels). Finally, constipation with hard or firm stools may cause small amounts of rectal bleeding as well.

Emergency Department Treatment and Disposition

A thorough history and physical exam will often direct the appropriate evaluation and narrow the differential diagnosis in the pediatric patient with suspected LGIB. Historical elements such as the duration, amount, and color of bleeding are key. In addition, the consistency of stool could direct the provider toward anything from infectious causes to constipation. In the pediatric patient presenting with presumed LGIB, the initial evaluation should include guaiac testing of the stool to confirm the presence of blood. There are many foods and medicines that can give stool a red or black appearance that

TABLE 15.2 ■ GASTROINTESTINAL (GI) BLEEDING

Character of Bleeding
- High rate of bleeding: "Hawaiian punch" emesis, maroon stool with clots (blood is a cathartic)
- Lower rate of bleeding: Coffee-ground emesis (fresh blood changes to brown in an acid environment), melena

Types of Bleeding
- *Hematemesis*: Upper GI bleeding
- *Melena*
  1. Black, tarry stool usually with a distinct odor
  2. Blood present in the GI tract for a prolonged period; degradation of hemoglobin by colonic bacteria
  3. Blood usually from lesions proximal to the ileocecal valve and often above the ligament of Treitz
- *Hematochezia*
  1. Bright red blood per rectum *or* maroon-colored stool usually from colonic source
  2. Rarely upper GI hemorrhage with very rapid GI transit time
- *Occult blood*
  1. Presence of blood in the stool that is not grossly detectable
  2. False-positive results: meat, ferrous sulfate, fresh red berries, tomatoes, turnips, horseradish
  3. False-negative results: vitamin C, outdated reagent or card

can be mistaken for hematochezia or melena. These items include foods with red dyes (fruit punch, popsicles), beets, and licorice. Medications such as cefdinir can cause red-colored stool, whereas iron, activated charcoal, and bismuth (Pepto-Bismol) can cause black stools that may be misinterpreted as melena.

As with upper GI bleeds, patients with suspected LGIB should initially be assessed for hemodynamic stability. Hemodynamically unstable patients (eg, abnormal vital signs, orthostatic changes in heart rate and BP, mental status changes, peripheral vasoconstriction, diaphoresis) require 2 large-bore IV lines for boluses of normal saline or lactated Ringer's solution, cardiac and pulse oximetry monitoring, and oxygen therapy. Emergent specialty consultation and admission are indicated for these patients. Laboratory evaluation should include CBC, coagulation profile, electrolytes with liver function testing, and blood type and screen. In the stable patient with suspected LGIB, stool cultures and testing for *C difficile* can help exclude infectious etiology of the bleeding. In patients with suspected IBD, inflammatory lab markers

TABLE 15.3 ■ ETIOLOGY AND DIFFERENTIAL DIAGNOSIS OF GASTROINTESTINAL (GI) BLEEDING

Age	Upper GI Bleed	Lower GI Bleed
Birth to 1 month	Idiopathic	Anal fissure
	Gastritis	Upper GI bleeding
	Stress ulcers	Midgut volvulus
	Esophagitis	Necrotizing enterocolitis
	Swallowed maternal blood	Swallowed maternal blood
	Congenital blood dyscrasia	Infectious colitis
	Arteriovenous (AV) malformation	Milk allergy
		Blood dyscrasia
		Intestinal duplication
1 month to 1 year	Gastritis	Anal fissure
	Esophagitis	Intussusception
	Stress ulcer	Meckel diverticulum
	Mallory-Weiss tear	Infectious diarrhea
	Vascular malformation	Milk allergy
	Intestinal duplication	Intestinal duplication
	Munchausen syndrome by proxy	Pseudomembranous colitis
1 to 12 years	Esophageal varices	Polyps
	Peptic ulcer disease	Anal fissure
	Stress ulcer	Infectious diarrhea
	NSAIDs	Meckel diverticulum
	Gastritis	Henoch-Schönlein purpura (HSP)
	Mallory-Weiss tear	Hemolytic uremic syndrome (HUS)
	Foreign body	Intussusception
	Esophagitis	Pseudomembranous colitis
		Perianal streptococcal dermatitis
Adolescent	Peptic ulcer disease	Polyps
	Gastritis	Anal fissure
	Esophageal varices	Hemorrhoids
	Mallory-Weiss tear	Inflammatory bowel disease (IBD)
	Esophagitis	Infectious disease
	Stress ulcer	Foreign body

(ESR and CRP) should be obtained. Abdominal radiographs should be obtained in almost all patients with LGIB. US is the gold standard for the diagnosis of intussusception and can also help assess for malrotation through the relationship of the superior mesenteric vein and artery.

Pearls

1. The first step in the evaluation of a patient with suspected LGIB is confirming the presence of blood by guaiac testing since there are many causes of factitious blood in the stool.

2. Milk protein–induced colitis is a common cause of bloody stool in infants and should be treated with an amino acid–based formula or elimination of dairy from the breast-feeding mother's diet.

3. Meckel diverticulum will cause asymptomatic, painless rectal bleeding, which may present chronically or acutely with massive bleeding and is most common in children under 2 years of age.

Chapter 16

NEPHROLOGY

Anil K. Mongia
Manju Chandra

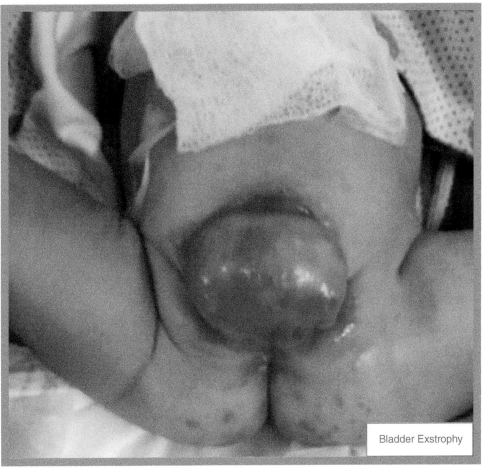

Bladder Exstrophy

(Photo contributor: Abhijeet Saha, MD)

The authors acknowledge the special contributions of Anup Singh, MD, to prior edition.

Clinical Summary

Healthy children normally have protein in their urine, with a protein excretion rate of <4 mg/m²/h or <100 mg/m²/day throughout childhood. The upper limit of normal protein excretion is up to 150 mg/day. Albumin, relatively small in molecular size, tends to be the dominant constituent, and

Tamm-Horsfall protein, a mucoprotein produced in the distal tubule, makes up the remainder.

Proteinuria in children can be transient, orthostatic, or pathologic. Transient proteinuria (often associated with fever or exercise) does not indicate underlying renal disease. Orthostatic proteinuria (elevated protein excretion when the subject is upright but normal protein excretion in recumbent position) occurs most commonly in school-aged children and rarely exceeds 1 g/m²/day. These patients do not have hematuria and have normal values of estimated glomerular filtration rate and C3 complement. Pathologic proteinuria is likely if

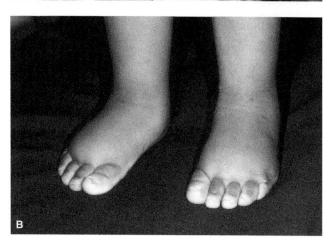

FIGURE 16.1 ■ Nephrotic Syndrome (NS) Presenting with Edema and Proteinuria. (A, B) An 18-month-old child presented with periorbital and facial edema (A) and edema of the feet (B). Urinalysis showed 4+ proteinuria associated with hypoproteinemia. He was clinically diagnosed as minimal change NS. (Reproduced with permission from Shah BR, Laude TL, *Atlas of Pediatric Clinical Diagnosis*. WB Saunders; Philadelphia, PA, 2000.)

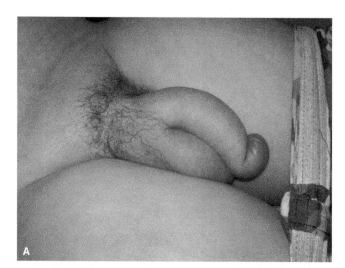

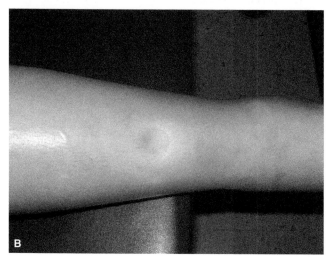

FIGURE 16.2 ■ Nephrotic Syndrome (NS) Presenting with Edema and Proteinuria. (A) This adolescent male with NS presented with anasarca, hypoproteinemia, and heavy proteinuria. He had edema involving the scrotum, shaft, and foreskin of the penis. (B) Pitting edema is demonstrated here on the shin (edema of hypothyroidism or lymphedema is nonpitting). (Photo contributor: Mark Silverberg, MD.)

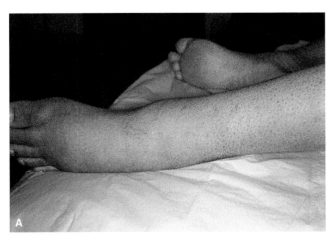
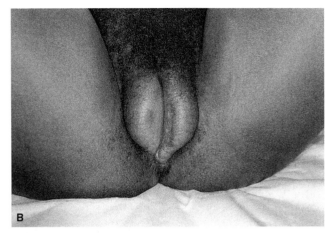

FIGURE 16.3 ▪ Severe Edema Associated with Heavy Proteinuria. (**A, B**) Severe edema of the lower extremity and edema of the vulva are seen in an adolescent girl who had hypoalbuminemia, heavy proteinuria, microscopic hematuria, and hypertension. Renal biopsy confirmed diagnosis of focal segmental glomerulosclerosis. (Photo contributor: Binita R. Shah, MD.)

proteinuria is associated with hematuria and/or the first morning urine protein-to-creatinine ratio is >0.2 in older children. Nephrotic-range proteinuria is defined as levels >40 mg/m^2/h in 24 hours.

Emergency Department Treatment and Disposition

Take a complete history and physical examination including BP in a patient with proteinuria. In general, urinalysis showing mild proteinuria (trace to 1+) during acute illness does not necessarily indicate renal disease unless there are other symptoms and signs pointing to renal disease. Discharge patients with mild proteinuria who have normal BP, urine output and, urine sediment, and absence of systemic symptoms. For patients with moderate to severe proteinuria (3+ or 4+), obtain serum albumin, BUN, creatinine, cholesterol, and electrolytes. In patients with concomitant microhematuria, obtain serum C3/C4 complement, antinuclear antibody, and serologies for hepatitis B and C and HIV as clinically indicated. Obtain renal US to exclude underlying renal disease, renal hypodysplasia,

or solitary functioning kidney. Consult pediatric nephrology for further evaluation if any of the studies are abnormal. Hospitalize patients with nephrotic syndrome associated with significant anasarca or hypertension (HTN), especially with the first episode.

Pearls

1. Proteinuria is not an uncommon finding in children. It may be transient, orthostatic, or persistent. Persistent proteinuria can be the first clue to a significant renal parenchymal disease.

2. Transient mild proteinuria can occur with fever, exercise, and congestive heart failure.

3. Evaluate urine specific gravity since 1+ proteinuria in a dilute urine of specific gravity 1.010 is more significant than in a concentrated urine of specific gravity 1.030.

4. Hematuria associated with proteinuria generally reflects underlying urinary tract problem.

5. Heavy proteinuria (3+ or 4+ in urinalysis) is the hallmark of nephrotic syndrome.

Clinical Summary

Gross hematuria is visible blood in urine and can occur with or without systemic signs and symptoms or urinary tract–related symptoms. Major causes of gross hematuria in children and adolescents include glomerulonephritis, UTI, hypercalciuria, nephrolithiasis, and trauma. Less common causes include urinary tract malignancy, exercise, angiomatous malformations of the collecting system, nutcracker syndrome (compression of left renal vein between the vertebrae and superior mesenteric artery), medullary sponge kidney, and sickle hemoglobinopathies.

In patients with glomerular disease, the urine is uniformly red, tea, or cola-colored or muddy green. In patients with vascular bleeding or urinary tract mucosal bleeding, the urine appears bright red. Terminal hematuria (ie, passage of a few drops of blood at the end of urination) reflects urethral bleeding from urethral obstruction (eg, from voluntary pelvic withholding maneuvers in response to overactive bladder

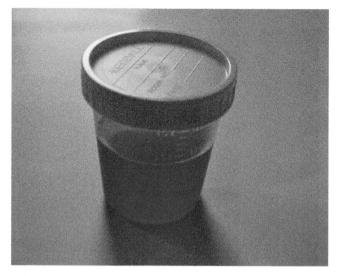

FIGURE 16.4 ■ Gross Hematuria; Hemorrhagic Cystitis. A child with hematuria at the end of micturition (terminal hematuria) due to hemorrhagic cystitis (adenovirus is a common etiology). Passage of blood clots and eumorphic erythrocytes are suggestive of a nonglomerular cause of hematuria. (Photo contributor: Anil Mongia, MD.)

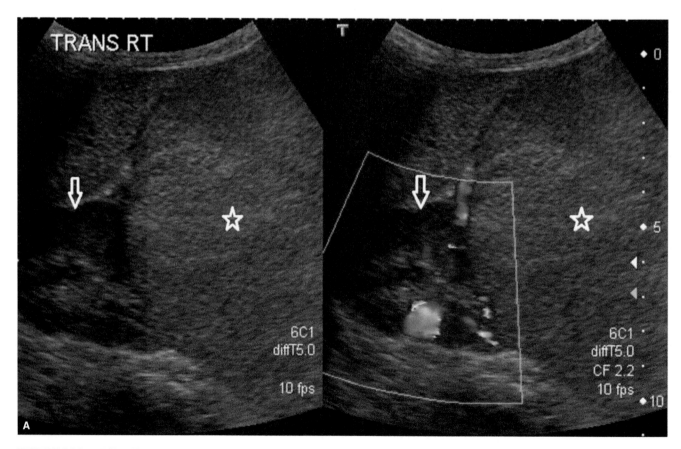

FIGURE 16.5 ■ Wilms Tumor (Nephroblastoma) Presenting with Hematuria. (**A**) Sagittal sonographic images of the right abdomen with and without Doppler demonstrate a large solid mass (star) arising off the inferior aspect of the kidney. Arrows point to normal renal parenchyma.

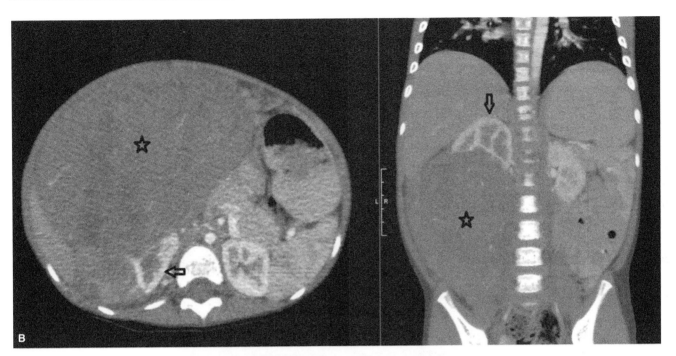

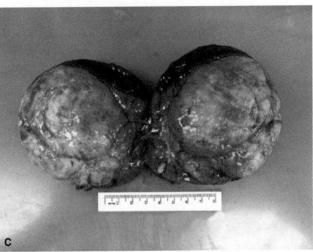

FIGURE 16.5 ■ (*Continued*) (**B**) Axial and coronal postcontrast CT images show the entirety of the large solid mass (star), which clearly arises from the right kidney. Arrows point to normal renal parenchyma. Neovascularity is seen within the mass (mimicking calcifications). (**C**) Cut section of the wilms tumor from the lower pole of kidney with the characteristic tan to gray color and well-circumscribed margins in a different patient presenting with hematuria. (Photo contributors: Jeremy Neuman, MD [A, B], and Shella Mongia, MD [C].)

or urethral stricture). Dysuria and urinary frequency suggest a UTI. Viral and chemical agents can cause a hemorrhagic cystitis that may be difficult to clinically distinguish from bacterial cystitis. Oliguria, edema, and HTN suggest an acute nephritic process. The most common causes of glomerulonephritis in children are acute poststreptococcal glomerulonephritis (APSGN) and IgA nephropathy. The former is generally associated with a preceding acute pharyngitis or impetigo, whereas the gross hematuria from IgA nephropathy generally occurs on the day of the URI or fever. Severe flank or upper back pain associated with gross hematuria strongly suggests nephrolithiasis.

Emergency Department Treatment and Disposition

In patients with gross hematuria, order CBC, BUN, serum creatinine, albumin, C3 and C4, urinalysis, and urine culture

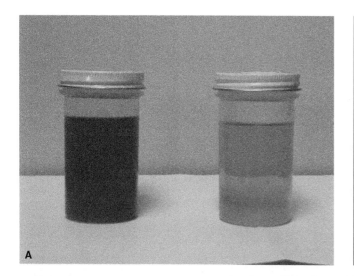

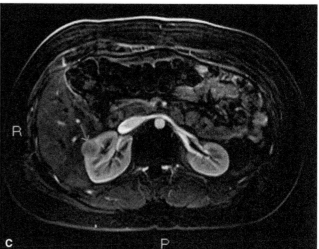

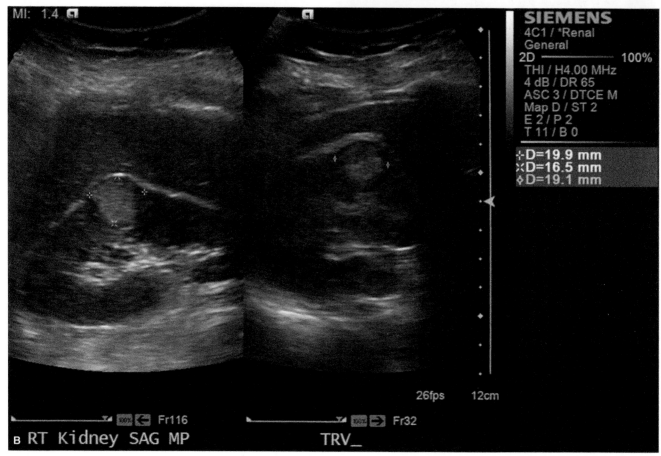

FIGURE 16.6 ■ Renal Cell Carcinoma Presenting with Hematuria. (**A**) Intermittent history of passing "red urine" for 3 months followed by passing "red urine" daily for a week was the presenting complaint of this 12-year-old patient. His reddish urine (shown with normal urine) was loaded with RBCs on microscopy. He was found to have renal papillary cell carcinoma. (**B**) Sagittal and transverse images of the right kidney in an 11-year-old patient demonstrates an echogenic round parenchymal mass approximately 2 cm in diameter (calipers). (**C**) Axial spoiled 3-dimensional gradient echo postgadolinium subtraction image demonstrates the enhancing right renal mass, consistent with neoplasm. Patient underwent partial nephrectomy, which showed chromophobe renal cell carcinoma, a rare subtype. Renal cell carcinoma is a rare yet known occurrence in children. (Photo contributors: Haamid Chamdawala, MD [A], and Daniel Eisman, MD, and Josh Greenstein, MD [B, C].)

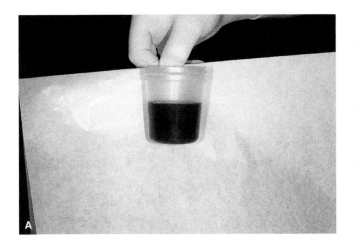

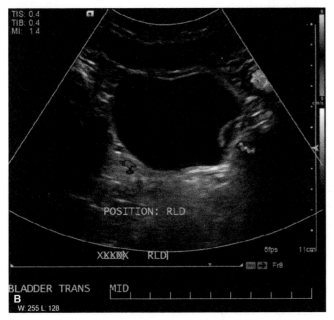

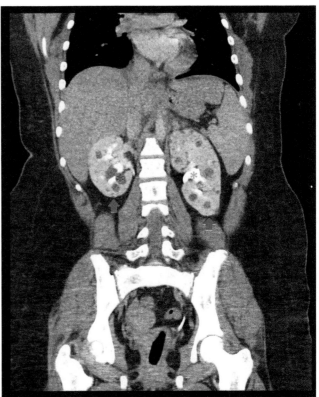

FIGURE 16.8 ■ Polycystic Kidney Disease (PKD). Coronal image of a contrast-enhanced CT scan showing bilateral kidneys (red arrows) of a 13-year-old girl with PKD. A cyst in the right kidney (red asterisk) remains dark relative to the normal kidney parenchyma. Contrast being excreted by the kidneys (blue asterisk) appears white in the renal collecting system. Hematuria, which is often gross, may be the presenting symptom in some patients and occurs at some time in the course in approximately 35% to 50% of patients with autosomal dominant PKD (ADPKD). This most likely occurs from rupture of the cyst into the collecting system. Conservative therapy consists of bedrest, hydration, and analgesics that should exclude NSAIDs. With unusual and severe bleeding, percutaneous arterial embolization or even nephrectomy may become necessary. Nephrolithiasis is another cause of hematuria in ADPKD patients. (Photo contributors: Amit Ramjit, MD, and Josh Greenstein, MD.)

FIGURE 16.7 ■ Hematuria. (**A**) Sickle cell disease. Sudden onset of painless gross hematuria was a presenting complaint of this adolescent patient with sickle cell anemia. Hematuria, also seen in sickle cell trait and Hb-SC disease, occurs because of ischemia in the renal papillae resulting in necrosis. Treatment is supportive, including adequate hydration and pain management. (**B**) Schistosomiasis. A 15-year-old adolescent boy, a recent immigrant from West Africa, presented with gross hematuria. Transverse sonogram of the bladder demonstrates a nonmobile mass along the left lateral wall. Patient had cystoscopy, and diagnosis of schistosomiasis was confirmed. This condition is commonly known as "male menarche" from human schistosomiasis. Bleeding is from release of eggs causing micro-perforations in the bladder mucosa and it is often recurrent. (Photo contributors: Binita R. Shah, MD [A], and Anil Mongia, MD [B].)

as indicated clinically. If there is low suspicion for a glomerular disease, order renal and bladder US to look for hydronephrosis, renal stone, tumor, or cysts. If CT scan is done for detection of nephrolithiasis, it is done without contrast injection. Send any stone collected for analysis. Order abdominal CT with contrast for patients with gross hematuria and a history of abdominal trauma to assess the injury and possible need for surgery. If blood is present at the urethral meatus, obtain retrograde urethrogram by injecting contrast with the syringe in the urethra before catheterization to evaluate for urethral injury.

Most children with hematuria do not require hospitalization. Admit patients with hematuria with HTN, oliguria, or pulmonary edema due to APSGN; hematuria due to renal injury from trauma; or hematuria due to papillary necrosis resulting from sickle cell hemoglobinopathy; also admit patients with nephrolithiasis and renal colic requiring IV hydration (eg, vomiting and poor intake) and pain management.

If history or physical examination is not suggestive of any obvious cause of hematuria, refer to a pediatric nephrologist for differentiation of glomerular versus nonglomerular origin of hematuria and further workup as indicated. If no cause is identified for persistent significant gross hematuria, obtain urology consultation for possible cystoscopy to identify unilateral bleeding from vascular malformations.

Pearls

1. Microscopic examination of the urine is required to confirm the presence of RBCs. Absence of RBCs in microscopic exam despite a positive dipstick for blood suggests hemoglobinuria or myoglobinuria.

2. An occasional RBC per high-power field (HPF) on microscopic examination of the urine may be seen in most children. Further testing is required if examination reveals >5 RBCs/HPF.

3. Tea- or cola-colored urine, RBC casts, and dysmorphic RBCs are pathognomonic for glomerular bleeding (eg, APSGN).

Clinical Summary

Nephrotic syndrome (NS) is characterized by proteinuria severe enough to cause hypoalbuminemia (serum albumin <2.5 g/dL), hypercholesterolemia, and edema. The nephrotic range of proteinuria is >40 mg/m^2/h (normal: <4 mg/m^2/h), which generally amounts to a urine protein-to-creatinine ratio of >2.0 in a random urine. Minimal change NS (MCNS) is the most common variety of primary idiopathic NS. Most patients with MCNS present with edema. Initially, edema is often mild and variable in distribution, being periorbital in the early morning hours. More severe degrees of edema may result in ascites, pleural effusions, scrotal or vulvar edema, and skin breakdown. Serum cholesterol level of 500 mg/dL is

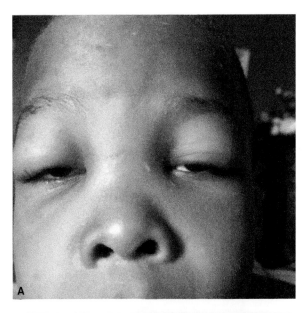

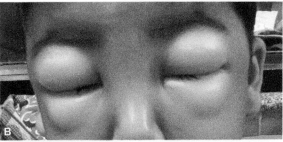

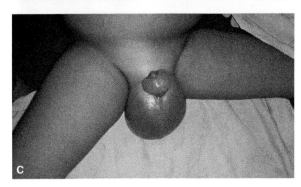

FIGURE 16.10 ■ Minimal Change Nephrotic Syndrome (MCNS). Two different children who were diagnosed as having MCNS and presenting with varying severity of periorbital edema are shown. Such periorbital edema, especially when mild, is often mistaken for an allergic reaction. Absence of itching and checking urine for proteinuria in such cases should alert a clinician to the possibility of nephrotic syndrome (NS). (**A**) This 3-year-old child had a 3-week history of periorbital swelling that was thought to be due to "allergies" for which he was given treatment by his primary care physician. His urinalysis in the ED showed proteinuria, which subsequently led to his diagnosis of NS. (**B, C**) A 6-year-old boy with severe periorbital edema and edema of the scrotum and penis with decreased urine output from MCNS. (Photo contributors: Anil Mongia, MD [A], and Abhijeet Saha, MD [B, C].)

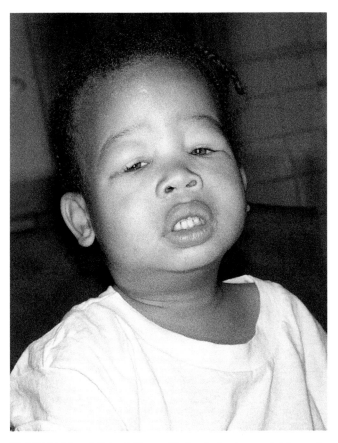

FIGURE 16.9 ■ Minimal Change Nephrotic Syndrome. A 15-month-old infant with periorbital/facial edema. This photo was taken soon after he woke up in the morning. Facial edema is usually seen on arising in the morning, and edema is gravity dependent; thus, early morning periorbital/facial edema may not be apparent by the time the child is seen later in the day. Edema also involves dependent areas such as feet, legs, scrotum (loose tissue with low interstitial tissue pressure), and sacrum. (Photo contributor: Binita R. Shah, MD.)

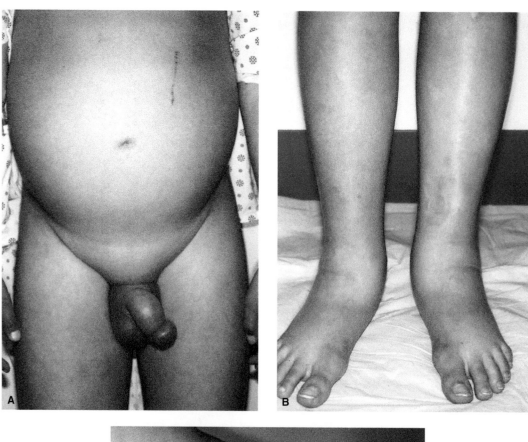

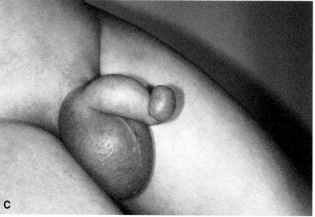

FIGURE 16.11 ■ Minimal Change Nephrotic Syndrome (MCNS). (**A–C**) Ascites, edema of the genitalia, bilateral edema of the lower extremity with ankle swelling, and pitting edema were seen in this child with steroid-responsive MCNS presenting with a relapse. (Photo contributor: Binita R. Shah, MD.)

not unusual at presentation of MCNS. Hypercholesterolemia resolves with complete remission of the NS. Children with NS are prone to develop cellulitis and spontaneous bacterial peritonitis (usually pneumococcal or due to *Escherichia coli*) and pneumococcal bacteremia. Patients with NS and primary peritonitis (especially when they present with an acute

abdomen) are not uncommonly misdiagnosed as having acute appendicitis.

Although NS is usually associated with avid sodium retention, serum sodium concentrations are low in some patients from water retention secondary to high antidiuretic hormone levels and spurious hyponatremia from high plasma lipids.

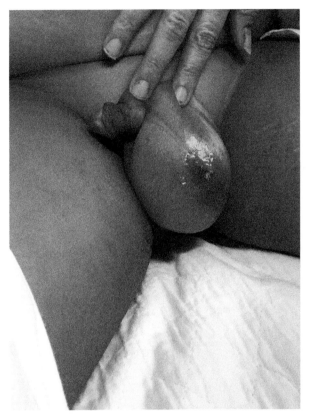

FIGURE 16.12 ■ Minimal Change Nephrotic Syndrome (MCNS). Scrotal swelling in a different child with MCNS. Notice some areas of discoloration, skin erosion, and cellulitis in the inferior part of scrotum. (Photo contributor: Anil Mongia, MD.)

Although the total serum calcium in patients with NS is often low, resulting from low level of protein-bound calcium, the level of free ionized calcium is usually normal. Patients with NS usually demonstrate laboratory features of a hypercoagulable state. Infants with NS may present with manifestations of acute cerebral dural sinus thrombosis since they are prone to thrombotic events from reduced intravascular volume and loss of anticoagulant factors in the urine. They may develop acute pulmonary embolism because of the predisposition to venous thrombosis. Acute renal vein thrombosis (uncommon) will present with a triad of flank pain, palpable renal enlargement, and gross hematuria.

Emergency Department Treatment and Disposition

Order CBC, BUN, serum creatinine, albumin, lipid profile, C3, and C4. Urinalysis is likely to show a high specific

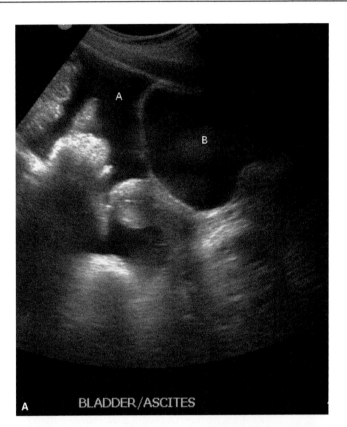

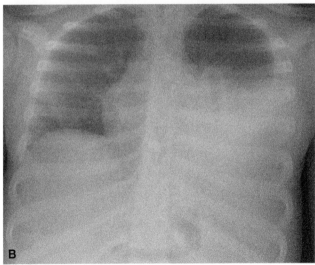

FIGURE 16.13 ■ Minimal Change Nephrotic Syndrome (MCNS). (**A**) Longitudinal sonographic image shows ascites (A). B, bladder. (**B**) Frontal view of the chest shows large left pleural effusion. (Photo contributor: John Amodio, MD.)

gravity (from intravascular volume depletion), heavy proteinuria, hyaline and fatty casts, and free lipid droplets. Microscopic hematuria can be seen in 20% of patients with MCNS. Consult pediatric nephrology for any child with suspected NS. Admit patients with evidence of acute peritonitis or severe anasarca. Consider admission for a first episode of nephrosis (provide education about the chronic relapsing nature of the disease, home monitoring of urine by dipstick, diet, and complications related to both the disease and therapy). Therapies include oral prednisone given daily for the first 4 to 6 weeks followed by prednisone every other day for the following 4 to 6 weeks, salt and fluid restriction, and diuretics (eg, furosemide) during periods of symptomatic edema as indicated. Diuretics are used judiciously and avoided in patients with a history of thromboembolic events. Antiplatelet drugs and/or anticoagulants are recommended for patients with thromboembolic events.

Pearls

1. Heavy proteinuria is the hallmark of NS. Proteinuria from other causes (eg, transient proteinuria associated with fever, dehydration, or exercise) or orthostatic proteinuria rarely exceeds 1 g per 24 hours and is not associated with edema.

2. Children with periorbital edema due to NS are often misdiagnosed as having allergic reaction on initial presentation. Absence of itching and a positive urine dipstick for proteinuria should alert to the possibility of NS in such children.

Clinical Summary

APSGN is characterized by abrupt onset of 1 or more features of acute nephritic syndrome: hematuria, proteinuria, volume overload, HTN, and azotemia. Children with APSGN are generally 6 to 12 years old and typically present with sudden onset of painless gross hematuria often described as "cola or tea colored." Patients may also present with acute dyspnea from pulmonary edema, headaches, seizure, or acute cortical blindness from the posterior reversible encephalopathy syndrome associated with parieto-occipital edema. Patients may be oliguric or even anuric. Edema from fluid retention is not generally periorbital, as seen in children with NS; however, the face may be swollen.

Pyoderma (impetigo) and pharyngitis are the most common antecedent infections. Streptococcal pharyngitis occurs more commonly in children between 5 and 15 years old during the winter and spring; impetigo occurs most commonly in summer and fall. There is a latent period between onset of primary infection and nephritis. With pharyngitis, the latent period is 7 to 14 days; with impetigo, the latent period is up to 6 weeks. Some children present with the disease without any identifiable prodrome due to the high incidence of streptococcal carriage (20%) in schoolchildren.

Differential diagnosis of acute glomerulonephritis includes other glomerulonephritides including IgA nephropathy, membranoproliferative glomerulonephritis, lupus nephritis, and

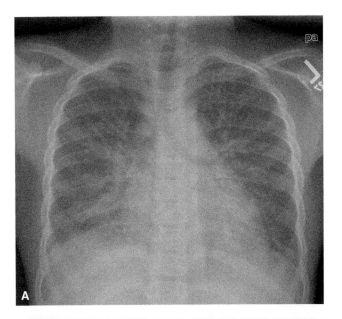

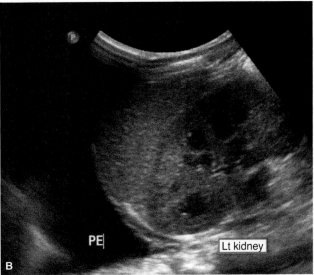

FIGURE 16.15 ■ Acute Poststreptococcal Glomerulonephritis (APSGN) Presenting with Congestive Heart Failure (CHF). (**A**) Frontal view of the chest shows cardiomegaly, increased bronchovascular markings, and bilateral pleural effusions compatible with CHF. (**B**) Sagittal sonographic image shows echogenic left kidney, compatible with medical renal disease. Note left pleural effusion (PE). This patient had microscopic hematuria with hypocomplementemia confirming a diagnosis of APSGN. (Photo contributor: John Amodio, MD; see also Figure 16.16.)

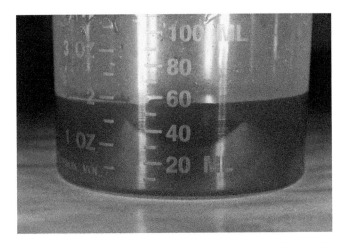

FIGURE 16.14 ■ Hematuria; Acute Poststreptococcal Glomerulonephritis. Tea- or cola-colored urine in an adolescent with a previous history of fever and sore throat is shown. He had hypertension and mildly raised creatinine. These findings and urinary RBC casts, dysmorphic RBCs, and proteinuria are suggestive of glomerular causes of hematuria. (Photo contributor: Binita R. Shah, MD.)

rapidly progressive glomerulonephritis. Patients with IgA nephropathy often present with sudden onset of gross hematuria during an episode of pharyngitis. This is in contrast to APSGN, in which hematuria occurs 1 to 3 weeks after an episode of pharyngitis. Acute IgA nephropathy can coexist

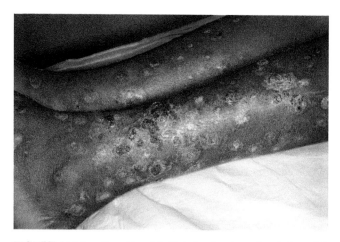

FIGURE 16.16 ■ Impetigo. Multiple healing impetigo lesions following arthropod bites are seen on both lower extremities of the same patient in Figure 16.15. (Photo contributor: Binita R. Shah, MD.)

with MCNS and present with HTN and edema. The prognosis of APSGN is excellent, with about 95% of patients recovering spontaneously and the gross hematuria disappearing in a few days. Microscopic hematuria may persist for up to 6 months. Serum C3 value is low at onset of APSGN and usually returns to normal in 6 to 8 weeks in APSGN, whereas persistent depression of C3 is seen in patients with membranoproliferative glomerulonephritis.

Emergency Department Treatment and Disposition

Obtain urinalysis in patients with edema, HTN, and red or brown urine. In patient with acute glomerulonephritis, urinalysis usually shows proteinuria, dysmorphic RBCs, many WBCs, and many mixed cellular and granular casts. Obtain serum creatinine, BUN, total protein, albumin, and cholesterol. BUN and serum creatinine are generally elevated in patients with APSGN. Serum total hemolytic complement (CH50) and C3 are low in almost all patients

in the first week of illness, but C4 is generally normal. As indicated, obtain throat culture, serum antistreptolysin titers, or Streptozyme test for evidence of recent streptococcal infection.

Treatment of APSGN is primarily supportive. Admit patients with obvious edema, HTN, azotemia, or signs of congestive heart failure. Consult pediatric nephrology. Restrict fluid intake to insensible water loss plus urine output and salt intake to one-third to one-half of the usual intake. Treat HTN by inducing diuresis with furosemide and using peripheral vasodilators such as hydralazine or nifedipine. Treat mild to moderate hyperkalemia with potassium restriction and induction of diuresis. Manage severe hyperkalemia with bicarbonate administration, insulin and glucose infusion, calcium gluconate infusion, and in patients with severe oliguria, hemodialysis.

Treatment with antimicrobials does not alter the course of established APSGN. Family members of patients with APSGN should be cultured for group A β-hemolytic *Streptococcus* if symptomatic with pharyngitis or during an epidemic of APSGN and treated if culture positive. Discharged patients should be referred to their primary care physician for a close follow-up.

Pearls

1. APSGN is a delayed nonsuppurative sequela of pharyngeal or skin infection by nephritogenic *Streptococcus pyogenes* strains.
2. APSGN is the most common type of acute glomerulonephritis and one of the most common glomerular causes of gross hematuria in children.
3. Acute nephritic syndrome associated with hypocomplementemia and antecedent streptococcal infection strongly suggests the diagnosis of APSGN.
4. The hallmark of APSGN is hematuria and minimal to moderate proteinuria. Multiple microscopic examinations may be needed to visualize RBC casts.

Clinical Summary

UTI may involve the kidneys (acute pyelonephritis) or the bladder (acute cystitis). Most UTIs are ascending infections that result from translocation of periurethral bacteria to the bladder and, in some cases, retrograde passage of the bacteria to the kidneys. Most UTIs in children are monomicrobic, with *E coli* (60%–80%) being the predominant organism followed by *Proteus, Klebsiella, Enterococcus,* and coagulase-negative staphylococci. The presenting signs and symptoms of UTI depend on the age of the patient, the presence of pyelonephritis, and the underlying voiding dysfunction that predisposed to the UTI. Older girls with acute cystitis related to overactive bladder may present with dysuria and worsening symptoms of the overactive bladder, including urinary frequency, urgency, urge incontinence, and suprapubic pain. Girls with UTI related to infrequent bladder emptying (≤3 times in 24 hours) may present with suprapubic or lower back pain and dysuria but are unlikely to manifest extreme urinary frequency urgency and urge incontinence. Infants with UTI more commonly present with nonspecific symptoms such as fever, irritability, poor feeding, diarrhea, and vomiting, similar to gastroenteritis. UTI in the first 3 months of life is associated with pyelonephritis in 70% of patients and accounts for majority of febrile episodes due to bacterial etiology in the first 12 weeks of life. Adolescents and young adults with acute pyelonephritis

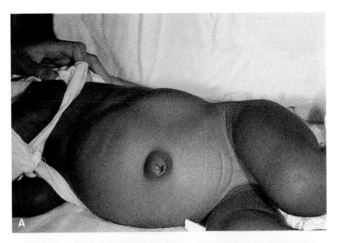

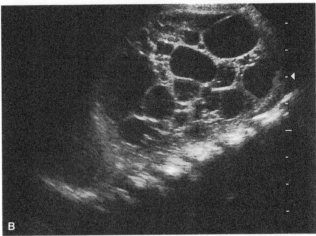

FIGURE 16.18 ■ Multicystic Dysplastic Kidney in a Patient Presenting with UTI. (**A**) A urinalysis showing positive nitrites and bacteriuria during the workup of fever without a source in this infant led to appreciating a left-sided abdominal mass that was not easily felt with infant in a supine position but became more obvious (as seen) in the lateral position. (**B**) Pelvic US reveals a large mass consisting of multiple noncommunicating cysts of varying sizes occupying the left renal fossa. No normal renal parenchyma is identified, and the mass has no solid structure. About 30% of patients with multicystic dysplastic kidneys have associated vesicoureteral reflux leading to UTI. (Photo contributor: Binita R. Shah, MD.)

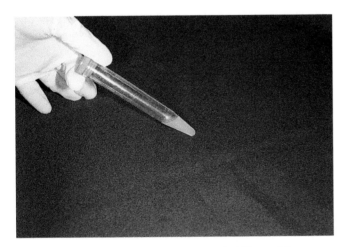

FIGURE 16.17 ■ Cloudy Urine in UTI. Irritability and fever were the presenting complaints of this 3-month-old uncircumcised infant presenting with hyperbilirubinemia with total bilirubin/direct bilirubin of 18/8 mg/dL. Catheterized urine had a cloudy appearance and was nitrite and leukocyte esterase positive with bacteriuria and pyuria. Subsequent urine culture was positive for *Escherichia coli.* (Photo contributor: Binita R. Shah, MD.)

present with fever, chills, and flank and upper back pain; they may not manifest any symptom of acute cystitis.

Emergency Department Treatment and Disposition

Take a thorough history of voiding and bowel-emptying habits in children with high suspicion of UTI. Physical examination

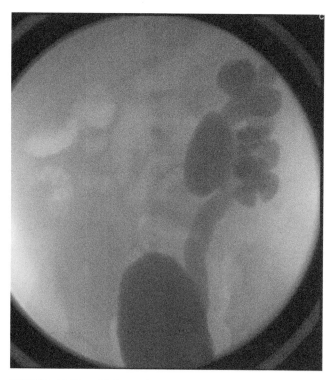

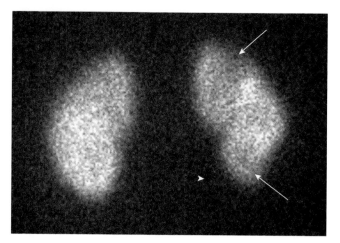

FIGURE 16.20 ■ Renal Scarring. A dimercaptosuccinic acid (DMSA) scan shows decreased uptake in upper and lower pole regions of the left kidney (arrows) compatible with renal scarring. The incidence of scarring is higher in children with recurrent UTIs. This emphasizes the importance of prevention of further episodes of UTI. (Photo contributor: John Amodio, MD.)

FIGURE 16.19 ■ Vesicourethral Reflux (VUR). Frontal projection of a voiding cystourethrogram shows grade IV reflux of contrast into the left ureter and collecting system. UTI is the most common reason for recognition of VUR. The most significant risk factor for acute pyelonephritis and renal scarring is VUR. (Photo contributor: John Amodio, MD.)

should include examination of the external genitalia for perineal erythema, labial adhesions, and smell of stagnant urine from urinary incontinence and examination of the lower back and feet for evidence of myelodysplasia. Obtain dipstick urinalysis and urine culture. Presence of both significant bacteriuria and leukocyturia (>5 WBCs/HPF) is needed for the diagnosis of UTI. Bladder catheterization provides the best urine specimen for culture. Urine from bagged and voided specimens has significant false-positive rates because of contamination with skin flora (up to 63% for the bag method). However, negative urine culture from bag specimen rules out bacterial UTI in the majority of cases. Pyuria with negative urine culture suggests viral infection, infection with fastidious organisms such as *Mycobacterium*, or noninfectious cystitis. Bacteriuria without pyuria may be seen in children with voiding dysfunction; it does not deserve antibiotic therapy, but the underlying voiding dysfunction should be addressed with appropriate therapy. Symptoms of urinary frequency, urgency, and urge incontinence do not always indicate acute

cystitis because these symptoms may result from overactive bladder as well. Children with overactive bladder often use pelvic-tightening maneuvers to abort unwanted bladder contractions and prevent incontinence. Constipation and stool withholding are common predisposing factors for UTI.

Management of UTI depends on the patient's age and whether pyelonephritis or cystitis is present. Admit patients who are <2 months of age, ill appearing, are vomiting, or have elevated serum creatinine for age. Febrile infants <2 months of age with suspected UTI are treated with broad-spectrum antibiotic coverage until culture results are available, at which time an appropriate antibiotic for the organism(s) found can be substituted. Common IV antibiotics used for treatment of UTI include ceftriaxone, cefotaxime, cefazolin, and gentamicin. Ampicillin should not be used as a first-line medication (resistance of *E coli* to ampicillin is as high as 30%–40% in some centers).

Common oral medications for treatment of cystitis in children include amoxicillin-clavulanate, cefazolin, cefixime, cefpodoxime, and trimethoprim-sulfamethoxazole. Patients generally show clinical improvement in 24 to 48 hours. When improvement does not occur in 24 to 48 hours, consider urinary tract abnormalities such as obstruction, infection of renal cyst, or perinephric abscess.

Treat children with cystitis with oral antibiotics for 7 days and discharge with instructions to follow up with their primary care physician. Urinary tract imaging, typically a renal and bladder US, is recommended in a febrile infant or young child between the ages of 2 months and 2 years with a first documented UTI. A voiding cystourethrogram is indicated in infants with abnormal renal US, recurrent UTIs, first infection with uncommon organism such as *Proteus* or *Klebsiella*, and poor urinary stream.

Pearls

1. About 8–10% of all febrile episodes in infants are due to serious bacterial infections, the majority (~75%) of which are UTIs.

2. Infants <2 year of age with fever without an apparent source should be evaluated for UTI.

3. UTIs are rare in boys after age 2 years. If present, they are generally associated with either anatomic urinary tract problems such as posterior urethral valve or ureteral dilatation or functional voiding dysfunction related to overactive bladder and stool withholding.

4. UTIs are uncommon in circumcised boys older than 6 months of age.

HEMOLYTIC UREMIC SYNDROME

Clinical Summary

Hemolytic uremic syndrome (HUS) is characterized by the triad of microangiopathic anemia, thrombocytopenia, and renal failure. It is generally classified as diarrhea associated (D+HUS) and atypical or sporadic HUS not associated with diarrhea (D–HUS). The typical form is most commonly caused by vascular endothelial damage from endotoxins

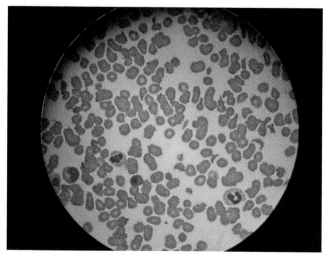

FIGURE 16.22 ■ Peripheral Blood Smear; Hemolytic Uremic Syndrome. The peripheral blood smear (×1000) shows schistocytes with characteristic sheared, triangular, or "helmet" shapes reflecting cells that have recently undergone fragmentation. Spherocytes are also seen. (Photo contributor: Scott T. Miller, MD.)

released by *E coli* O157:H7 and is one of the most common causes of renal failure in children younger than age 2 to 3 years. Boys and girls are affected equally. Typically, there is a prodromal illness, usually hemorrhagic colitis with abdominal pain, vomiting, and diarrhea, which may be bloody. The abdomen is often tender. D–HUS may follow an upper respiratory infection or pneumococcal pneumonia and is usually associated with dysregulation of the alternative complement pathway. CNS symptoms include drowsiness, lethargy, irritability, and seizures. Patients with HUS may manifest features of hepatitis or pancreatitis with endocrine and exocrine dysfunction. Oligoanuria with renal failure is common at presentation. There may be evidence of fluid overload, including HTN and congestive heart failure. Most patients look pale, and petechiae and ecchymosis may be present. BP is generally normal in D+HUS but is quite high in patients with D–HUS. All patients have microangiopathic hemolytic anemia with negative direct and indirect Coombs. Platelets are usually diminished to <100,000/μL. Peripheral smear shows fragmented and helmet-shaped RBCs. Haptoglobin is low, and indirect bilirubin and plasma lactate dehydrogenase are usually elevated. These patients have normal prothrombin time and partial thromboplastin time. Urinalysis shows hematuria, proteinuria, and cellular casts. Acute renal failure is manifested with oligoanuria, raised BUN and creatinine, and other features of renal failure, including hyperkalemia, hypocalcemia, and metabolic acidosis. Gastrointestinal

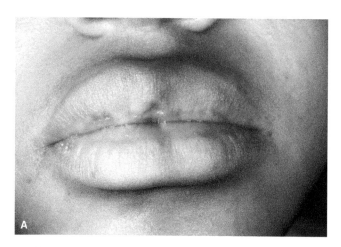

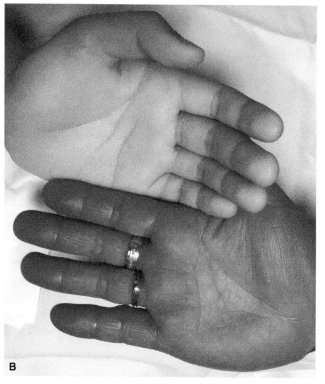

FIGURE 16.21 ■ Hemolytic Uremic Syndrome (HUS). Extreme pallor of the lips (**A**) and hand (**B**) is seen in an adolescent girl with HUS following episodes of bloody diarrhea. Her hemoglobin was 5 g/dL. (Photo contributor: Ameer Hassoun, MD.)

manifestation may be confused with intussusception, ulcerative colitis, rectal prolapse, or acute bacterial enterocolitis.

Emergency Department Treatment and Disposition

Consult pediatric nephrology as soon as the diagnosis is suspected and admit patient to ICU. Management is essentially supportive, including strict adherence to fluid and electrolyte balance. Begin aggressive fluid resuscitation if patients are dehydrated or hypotensive unless there is oliguria with HTN and edema, in which case fluids must be limited to insensible losses plus the urine output. Avoid addition of potassium to the IV fluids because rapid elevation in serum potassium can result from continued hemolysis. Packed RBC transfusion may be needed for hemoglobin concentration <6 g/dL. Platelet transfusion should be avoided except for an invasive procedure with risk of active bleeding. Dialysis should be instituted early in oliguric patients with therapy-resistant fluid overload, hyperkalemia, hyponatremia, or severe metabolic acidosis.

Pearls

1. Antibiotics given to treat hemorrhagic colitis predispose to the development of HUS because they increase the release of toxin produced by *E coli* O157:H7.
2. Drugs that reduce intestinal peristalsis are potentially harmful because they delay the elimination of bacterial toxin from the gut.
3. HUS may occur without preceding hemorrhagic colitis, in which case it may be related to the dysregulation of the alternative complement pathway.

Clinical Summary

Postrenal failure can result from obstruction of the urinary tract anywhere from the urethra to the pelvicalyceal system. Causes of obstruction include posterior urethral valves (PUV), ureteropelvic junction obstruction, ureterocele, phimosis, renal calculi, blood clots, bladder outlet obstruction, detrusor-sphincter dyssynergy of neurogenic origin, and retroperitoneal or intraabdominal tumor. A history of prenatal US demonstrating bilateral hydronephrosis and hydroureters suggests the presence of PUV or bilateral ureteropelvic junction obstruction. Male neonates with PUV may have a distended bladder, palpably large kidneys, and poor urinary stream, or may present with urosepsis. Older boys with PUV may present with UTI, urinary frequency, urgency incontinence, nocturnal enuresis, or HTN. Patients with ureteropelvic junction obstruction may present with recurrent flank pain especially after large fluid intake. Obstructive renal stones can cause gross hematuria or renal colic.

Emergency Department Treatment and Disposition

Obtain urinary tract US in suspected cases. Ureteropelvic junction obstruction is characterized by dilated renal pelvis and calyces without ureteral dilatation, whereas ureterovesical

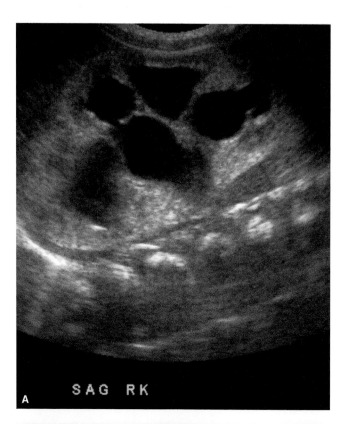

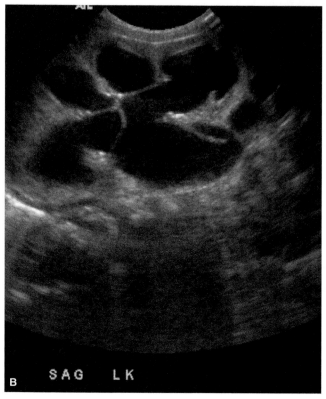

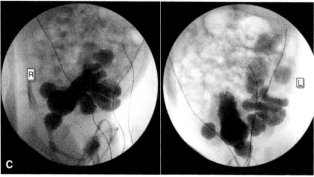

FIGURE 16.23 ■ Obstructive Uropathy. (**A, B**) Sagittal sonograms of the kidneys show bilateral hydronephrosis. (**C**) Bilateral oblique images from a voiding cystourethrogram demonstrate grade V reflux on the left. The hydronephrosis of the right kidney on sonography is secondary to obstruction at level of the ureterovesical junction. Note the trabeculated bladder and dilated posterior urethra, consistent with posterior urethral valves. (Photo/legend contributors: Mandakini Sadhir, MD/John Amodio, MD.)

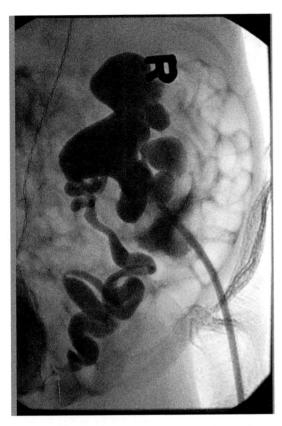

FIGURE 16.24 ■ Obstructive Uropathy. Right nephrostogram demonstrates marked hydroureteronephrosis down to the level of the ureterovesical junction, where there is narrowing and kinking of the distal ureter (arrow). (Photo contributor: John Amodio, MD.)

junction obstruction results in dilated renal pelvis as well as dilated ureter. In patients with PUV, the bladder has thick wall musculature, which may be trabeculated. In patients with dilated ureter, look for ureterocele in the bladder; the latter is generally associated with complete duplication of the ureters. Evaluate renal parenchyma for cortical thinning, dysplasia, and cysts.

Obtain CBC and basic metabolic panel. Look for evidence of renal failure suggested by elevated BUN and serum creatinine, hyperkalemia, and metabolic acidosis. Urine output and urinary sediment findings may be variable.

Admit patients with acute kidney injury. Management includes maintaining renal perfusion, restoration of fluid and electrolyte balance, controlling blood pressure, adjusting medications for the degree of renal impairment, and initiating dialysis if indicated. Specific therapy for postrenal failure depends on the site of obstruction and may include placement of an indwelling bladder catheter to bypass urethral obstruction, ureteral catheters (stents), or surgical diversion of the urine flow with vesicostomy or nephrostomy tubes. Obtain pediatric nephrology and urology consultations in all these cases.

Pearls

1. Consider urinary tract obstruction whenever the cause of acute kidney injury is not evident.
2. Sudden development of anuria should strongly suggest the possibility of total urinary obstruction.
3. Initial management of patients with suspected PUV involves insertion of a fine urethral catheter into the bladder; do not use a balloon type of catheter (Foley) because the catheter may become lodged in the posterior urethra and not drain freely.

Clinical Summary

Hypertensive emergency is defined by the presence of acute target-organ injury from rapid increase in BP. *Hypertensive urgency* is a term used to denote severe elevations of BP without any signs or symptoms of end-organ involvement. The severity of manifestations depends on the acuity and magnitude of BP elevation. The manifestation of hypertensive emergencies include hypertensive encephalopathy, cerebral infarcts or hemorrhage, acute renal failure, pulmonary edema, congestive heart failure, myocardial infarction, aortic dissection in older people, retinal exudates, hemorrhages, and papilledema. The most common symptoms of severe HTN in children are hypertensive encephalopathy manifested by headache, nausea, vomiting, mental confusion, blurred vision, agitation, or frank seizures. MRI of the brain may show edema of the white matter of the occipital and parietal areas of the brain perfused by the posterior brain circulation; it is generally referred to as posterior reversible encephalopathy syndrome.

Newborns and infants with severe HTN may present with congestive heart failure, respiratory distress, apnea, cyanosis,

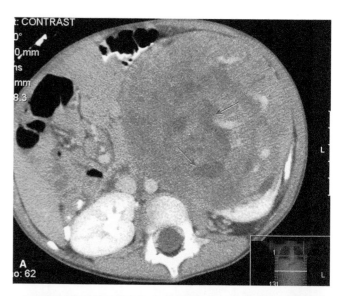

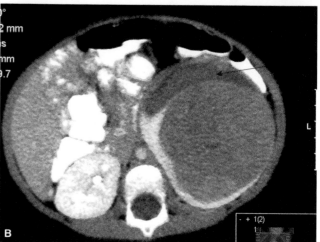

FIGURE 16.26 ■ Wilms Tumor Presenting with Hypertension and Abdominal Mass. (**A**) A large mass arising from left kidney containing areas of necrosis and hemorrhage (arrows). (**B**) Note area of subcapsular hemorrhage (arrow). Hypertensive emergencies usually occur in children with a known underlying renal disease; however, in some children, severe hypertension may be the first sign of renal disease. This child presented to ED with abdominal pain and vomiting. Examination revealed an irritable child with a BP of 183/110 mm Hg and abdominal distension with a mass. Such severe hypertension may be related to compression of normal renal parenchyma by the tumor and renin release from ischemic parenchyma. Patient underwent nephrectomy, and Wilms tumor was confirmed at pathology. (Photo contributor: John Amodio, MD.)

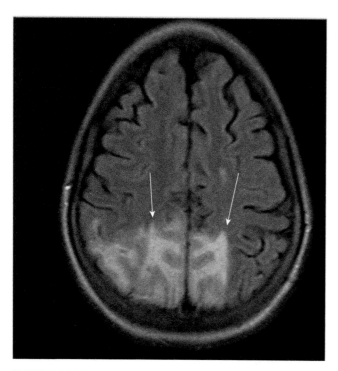

FIGURE 16.25 ■ Posterior Reversible Encephalopathy Syndrome (PRES). Axial FLAIR MRI image showing nearly symmetric, bilateral, confluent foci of T2/FLAIR hyperintense signal predominantly in the cerebral white matter in the occipital lobes in the posterior cerebral artery distribution without mass effect compatible with PRES. (Photo contributor: Steven Pulitzer, MD.)

extreme irritability, convulsions, or coma. Acute facial nerve paralysis may also be a manifestation of acute severe HTN in children.

The most common causes of acute hypertensive emergencies in children include: (1) acute poststreptococcal glomerulonephritis with fluid retention; (2) nondiarrheal sporadic

HUS; (3) sympathetic crisis from pheochromocytoma, substance of abuse such as cocaine, amphetamine, or phencyclidine, or withdrawal from high-dose clonidine; and (4) previous history of HTN and nonadherence to medications.

Emergency Department Treatment and Disposition

Patients with severe symptoms related to HTN need prompt treatment. However, lowering the BP too rapidly in those with longstanding HTN can lead to cerebrovascular and myocardial ischemia. Reduce BP by 25% of the planned BP reduction over the first 8 to 12 hours, a further 25% over the next 8 to 12 hours, and the final 50% over the 24 hours after that.

Obtain urinalysis, BUN, creatinine, electrolytes, plasma renin activity, plasma cortisol, and serum aldosterone. Presence of proteinuria and elevated serum creatinine and BUN will reflect kidney disease, whereas hypokalemia indicates primary or secondary hyperaldosteronism. Obtain CXR and an ECG to look for evidence of left ventricular hypertrophy from chronic HTN and cardiomegaly or pulmonary edema from acute severe HTN. Obtain a brain MRI in patients with abnormal neurologic findings. Consult pediatric nephrology and admit patient to ICU.

Choose antihypertensive medication based on etiology, side effect profile, and physician familiarity with the drug. The drugs that can be used parenterally include loop diuretics, direct vasodilators such as sodium nitroprusside and hydralazine, calcium channel blockers such as nicardipine, angiotensin-converting enzyme inhibitors such as enalaprilat, and adrenergic blockers such as labetalol and esmolol.

Sodium nitroprusside has a rapid onset and short duration of action. Prolonged administration (>24–48 hours) may cause nausea, vomiting, neurologic symptoms, dyspnea, and lactic acidosis due to accumulation of its metabolic end products composed of cyanide and thiocyanate.

Nicardipine, a calcium channel blocker, also has rapid onset and short duration of action and is given by continuous IV infusion. It may be more suitable for children with renal insufficiency.

Labetalol, a combined α- and β-blocker can be used as a bolus or as continuous infusion. The hypotensive effects of a single dose of IV labetalol administration appear within 2 to 5 minutes, peak at 5 to 15 minutes, and last up to 2 to 4 hours.

Adverse reactions include β-adrenergic blockage including bradycardia and bronchospasm. It is contraindicated in patients with acute left ventricular failure.

Esmolol is an ultra-short-acting, cardioselective β_1-adrenergic blocker that may be given by constant infusion (onset of action ~60 seconds and short duration of action of 10–20 minutes). Its rapid metabolism by an intracytoplasmic RBC esterase makes it well suited for critically ill patients with multiorgan failure.

Fenoldopam, a vascular dopamine receptor agonist, is also effective and suitable for hypertensive emergencies with renal insufficiency. Fifty percent of the maximal effect is seen within 15 minutes after commencing an IV infusion, with maximal BP reduction occurring at about 1 hour.

Use oral antihypertensive agents in children with mild manifestations of HTN and no evidence of active organ injury. Clonidine, an oral agent with a rapid onset of effect (about 15–30 minutes), is useful in the acute setting, particularly in hemodialysis patients. Clonidine is minimally removed by hemodialysis and does not require dose adjustment in renal failure. Somnolence and dry mouth are the most common adverse effects. Isradipine (dihydropyridine calcium channel blocker) is a useful oral antihypertensive with a rapid onset of action. It reduces BP within 1 hour of administration, with a peak effect in 2 to 3 hours. Isradipine has limited effects on myocardial contractility; thus it is a suitable agent for patients with myocardial dysfunction. The use of oral short-acting nifedipine is discouraged because it may cause severe hypotension, headaches, palpitations, and acute angina.

Pearls

1. Primary HTN rarely presents with hypertensive emergencies in children.
2. The younger the child and higher the BP readings, the more likely there is a secondary cause for HTN. Renal parenchymal or renal vascular causes of HTN outnumber all other causes of secondary HTN in children.
3. Infants with severe HTN can present with poor feeding, respiratory distress, and facial palsy.
4. In hypertensive children, always palpate femoral pulses and take BP readings in all 4 extremities during the initial evaluation to check for coarctation of the aorta or Takayasu arteritis.

Clinical Summary

Kidney stones in children are most commonly composed of calcium oxalate, with hypercalciuria and hypocitraturia being the 2 most common predisposing factors. Cystinuria and primary hyperoxaluria are autosomal recessive disorders that commonly present with kidney stones in infancy.

The classic presentation of renal colic from a stone obstructing the mid ureter is sudden onset of severe flank pain that radiates to the groin and is often associated with nausea and vomiting. A renal stone obstructing the ureteropelvic junction

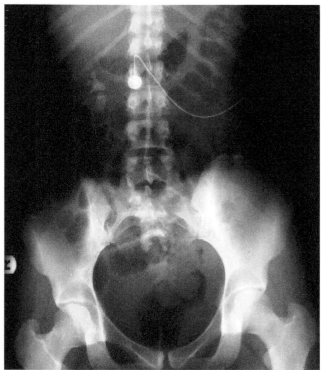

FIGURE 16.28 ■ Staghorn Calculus. A plain film of the abdomen shows calcification that conforms to the renal pelvis and collecting system, compatible with a staghorn calculus (arrow). (Photo contributor: Mark Silverberg, MD.)

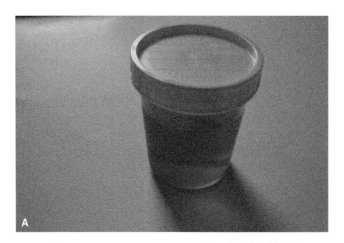

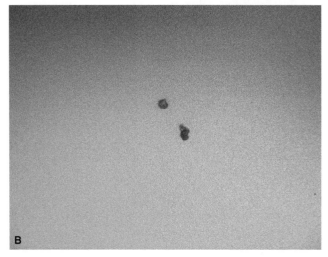

FIGURE 16.27 ■ Nephrolithiasis. Gross hematuria (A) associated with severe colicky pain was the presenting complaint of this patient with primary hyperoxaluria. Secondary hyperoxaluria may occur with increased absorption of oxalate (eg, inflammatory bowel disease, extensive bowel resection). Calcium oxalate stone that was passed by the patient is shown (B). (Photo contributor: Shella Mongia, MD.)

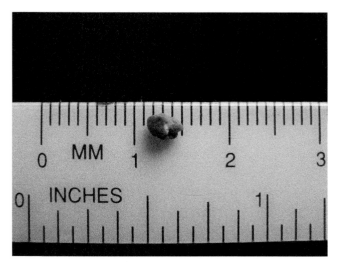

FIGURE 16.29 ■ Nephrolithiasis. This 4-mm renal stone was "easily" passed by the patient. This is typical for stones <5 mm. Notice its irregular shape and jagged contours, explaining presence of red blood cells in the urine as these stones move down the ureters. (Photo contributor: Mark Silverberg, MD.)

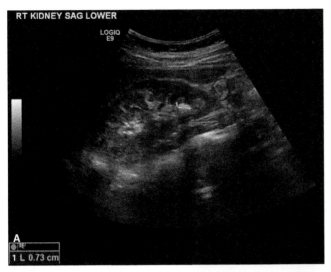
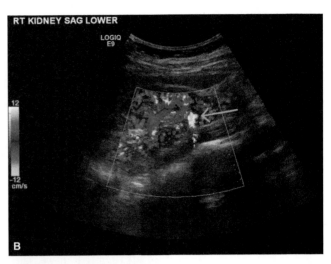
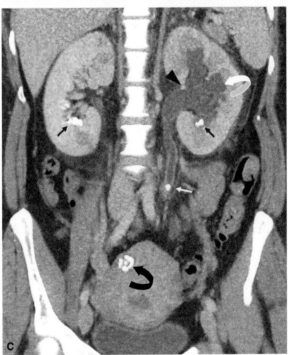

FIGURE 16.30 ▪ Nephrolithiasis. (**A**) Sagittal view of the right kidney in an adolescent demonstrates a 7-mm stone in the lower pole (calipers). There is posterior acoustic shadowing effect indicative of stone (red arrow) that is useful for distinguishing between stone and echogenic renal sinus fat. (**B**) Color flow image demonstrates apparent strong color flow within the stone (green arrow), a counterintuitive artifact known as "twinkle." (**C**) Obstructive uropathy. Oblique coronal CT view of the abdomen in a different patient presenting with left flank pain and hematuria. The left kidney displays perinephric fat stranding and moderate hydroureteronephrosis (curved white arrow). There is an obstructing calculus located at the left mid ureter (white arrow) with associated urothelial enhancement. There are also multiple nonobstructive calyceal calculi in both kidneys (black arrows), and incidentally noted calcified uterine fibroid (curved black arrow). (Photo contributors: Ryan Logan Webb, MD [A, B], and Dan Portal, MD, and Josh Greenstein, MD [C].)

may present with flank pain, whereas a stone obstructing the ureterovesical junction may result in urinary urgency and frequency mimicking bacterial cystitis. A stone in the renal calyces may cause pain during jumping and running.

Patients with kidney stones may present with recurrent gross hematuria or incidental finding of microscopic hematuria. Gross or microscopic hematuria is found in 33% to 90% of children with nephrolithiasis. UTI may be the presenting

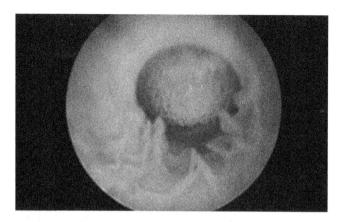

FIGURE 16.31 ■ Nephrolithiasis. A cystoscopic image shows a stone in the urethra that was pushed in the bladder and subsequently fragmented with laser. This 8-year-old child presented with decreased force of stream and dysuria. His urinalysis showed microscopic hematuria. He was seen a year earlier with similar symptoms and had a negative CT scan and US of kidneys and bladder. (Photo contributor: Mark Horowitz, MD.)

sign of nephrolithiasis in preschoolers and infants. The differential diagnosis of acute severe abdominal pain from an obstructive stone includes acute appendicitis, pyelonephritis, ectopic pregnancy, ovarian torsion, bowel obstruction, Henoch-Schönlein purpura, and biliary colic.

Emergency Department Treatment and Disposition

In patients suspected to have acute abdominal pain from urinary tract stones, obtain urinalysis, serum electrolytes, BUN, creatinine, carbon dioxide, calcium, and in postmenarchal girls, a urine pregnancy test. Evaluate urine microscopy for presence of RBCs, bacteria, abnormal crystals, and microcrystalline casts. Presence of positive leukocyte esterase and nitrite in urine dipstick suggests UTI. Send any "passed" stones for analysis, and instruct patients to keep any stones they pass at home (use urine strainers or paper coffee filters to strain urine). Renal US is a valuable imaging technique for detecting hydronephrosis from obstructive stone and usually allows visualization of calculi ≥3 mm. A noncontrast CT scan is the gold standard imaging modality for the diagnosis of nephrolithiasis because it can show the size and location of the calculus and level of obstruction and rule out other conditions that may mimic symptoms of nephrolithiasis. CT scanning,

however, exposes the patient to large amount of radiation and should be reserved for situations where invasive intervention is planned. In an average-sized adult, kidney stones <5 mm in diameter can easily pass down the ureters, whereas stones >10 mm are generally unable to do so. Stones of intermediate size can get stuck in the ureter and cause renal colic.

For a patient with renal colic or obstructive renal stone, consult pediatric nephrologist and urologist. Encourage oral water intake ad lib. In patients unable to tolerate oral fluids, infuse D5 half-normal saline IV to help flush the stone down the ureter. Use tamsulosin, an α-adrenergic blocker, 0.4 mg orally once daily to dilate the ureter. Other helpful drugs include oral nifedipine to dilate the ureter, IV steroids to decrease ureteral mucosal edema, and progesterone intramuscular to decrease ureteral spasm. Make it a priority to control pain with NSAIDs or opioids. Admit patients with an obstructive stone and intractable vomiting, severe pain, single functional kidney, history of renal transplantation, or evidence of infection. Up to 50% of children will pass obstructive stones with increased fluid intake and tamsulosin within 2 weeks of diagnosis. In those with persistent hydronephrosis, obstruction can be relieved using shock wave lithotripsy to fragment the stone(s), percutaneous nephrolithotomy, or cystoscopic and ureteroscopic retrieval of stones. Long-term preventive measures for idiopathic calcium oxalate stones include increased water intake, low salt intake (to decrease calcium excretion), increased intake of fruits and vegetables (increases urinary citrate), lower intake of animal proteins, and in certain cases, supplemental potassium citrate.

Pearls

1. Calcium oxalate is the most common constituent of human renal stones.
2. The 2 most common abnormalities associated with idiopathic calcium oxalate stones in children are hypercalciuria and hypocitraturia.
3. Calcium phosphate stones occur with distal renal tubular acidosis and hyperparathyroidism.
4. Hexagonal crystals in the urine suggest cystinuria. Both cystine and uric acid stones are radiolucent.
5. Medications used to dilate the ureters to facilitate the passage of stones in patients with renal colic include an α-adrenergic blocker such as tamsulosin and calcium channel blocker such as nifedipine.

Clinical Summary

Hypocalcemia refers to a reduction in the concentration of ionized calcium in serum or whole blood. Hypocalcemia may be asymptomatic if mild or manifest with jitteriness, tetany, and carpopedal spasm if moderate. If acute and severe, hypocalcemia may also present with life-threatening complications including seizures, refractory heart failure, hypotension, and laryngospasm. Hypocalcemia can cause psychological symptoms, particularly emotional instability, anxiety, and depression. Less common psychological symptoms are confusional states, hallucinations, and frank psychosis.

Hypocalcemia characteristically causes prolongation of the QT interval in the ECG. Torsades de pointes (polymorphic ventricular tachycardia associated with a prolonged QT interval) can potentially be triggered by hypocalcemia but is much less common than with hypokalemia or hypomagnesemia.

Papilledema can occur in patients with severe hypocalcemia. Rarely, optic neuritis (distinguished by decreased visual acuity) may be present.

Emergency Department Treatment and Disposition

The initial goal of the laboratory evaluation is to determine if true hypocalcemia is present. Factitious hypocalcemia can occur in the face of hypoalbuminemia and is corrected by the following formula: Corrected Ca = 0.8 × (4 g/dL - patient's albumin [g/dL]) + measured serum Ca level. Low ionic blood calcium can result from various causes including hypoparathyroidism, vitamin D deficiency, vitamin D resistance, magnesium deficiency, and hyperphosphatemia, as shown in Figure 16.32. If low ionized calcium is confirmed, obtain detailed personal and family

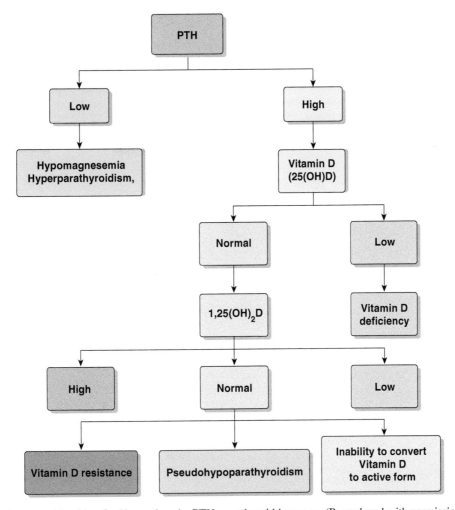

FIGURE 16.32 ■ Laboratory Algorithm for Hypocalcemia. PTH, parathyroid hormone. (Reproduced with permission from Tenenbein M, Macias CG, Sharieff GQ, et al. *Strange and Schafermeyer's Pediatric Emergency Medicine*. 5th ed. McGraw-Hill Education; New York, NY, 2019.)

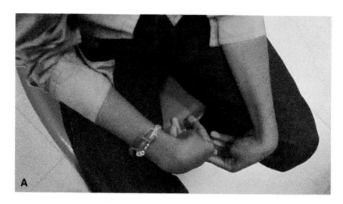

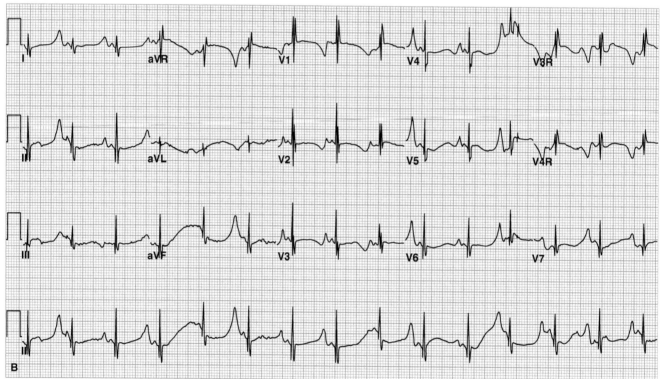

FIGURE 16.33 ■ Hypocalcemia. (**A**) A 9-year-old girl with chronic renal disease presented with carpopedal spasm due to hypocalcemia. She was treated with IV calcium gluconate reversing her symptoms. (**B**) A 12-lead ECG shows a sinus rhythm with prolonged QT interval (QTc >500 milliseconds). Torsades de pointes is unusual with hypocalcemia. (Photo contributors: Rajpal Singh, MD [A], and Shyam Sathanandam, MD [B].)

history for aforementioned causes and symptoms. A family history of hypocalcemia suggests a genetic cause. A history of head and neck surgery or the presence of a neck scar suggests postsurgical hypoparathyroidism. Latent tetany can be elicited by various maneuvers. Carpopedal spasm of the forearms and hand can be elicited by inflating the BP cuff in the arm 20 mm Hg above systolic pressure for >3 minutes (Trousseau sign). Twitching of the muscle at the margin of the lips can be elicited by tapping the facial nerve anterior to external auditory

meatus (Chvostek sign). Obtain blood for total and ionized serum calcium, magnesium, electrolytes, glucose, phosphorus, parathyroid hormone (PTH) levels, vitamin D metabolites (25-hydroxyvitamin D and 1,25-dihydroxyvitamin D), alkaline phosphatase, and obtain ECG.

IV calcium is indicated for symptomatic patients (carpopedal spasm, tetany, seizures) and for patients with a prolonged QT interval. IV calcium is also indicated for asymptomatic patients with serum calcium of ≤7.5 mg/dL who may develop serious complications if untreated. IV calcium should be given as a 10-mg/kg dose of elemental calcium over 5 to 10 minutes under ECG monitoring as 10% calcium gluconate or 10% calcium chloride. Calcium gluconate is usually preferred because it is less likely to cause tissue necrosis if extravasated. IV calcium should be continued until patient is receiving an effective regimen of oral calcium and vitamin D. Symptoms of hypocalcemia refractory to calcium supplementation may be caused by hypomagnesemia. This can be managed with IV magnesium sulphate salt. For patients with milder acute hypocalcemia (serum corrected calcium concentration of 7.5–8.0 mg/dL) or a serum ionized calcium concentration >3.0 to 3.2 mg/dL who are asymptomatic or patients with chronic hypocalcemia, oral calcium supplementation is preferred.

Pearls

1. Hypomagnesemia may cause hypocalcemia, both by inducing resistance to PTH action and by diminishing its secretion. In patients with hypomagnesemia, hypocalcemia is difficult to correct without first normalizing the serum magnesium concentration.

2. Hypoparathyroidism, a major cause of pediatric hypocalcemia, is caused by impaired secretion or production of PTH or a defect in the calcium-sensing receptor that regulates PTH secretion.

3. Hypocalcemia with high levels of PTH may be caused by vitamin D deficiency or defects in its metabolism or action and genetic mutations causing deficiency of 1-α-hydroxylase.

Clinical Summary

Hypercalcemia and high ionized serum calcium can result from increased calcium absorption from the gut, increased calcium release from the bones, and decreased urinary excretion of calcium. Increased intestinal calcium absorption occurs under the influence of high 1,25-dihydroxyvitamin D (calcitriol; >150 ng/mL) as in vitamin D toxicity, impaired degradation of calcitriol, or nonrenal calcitriol production by activated macrophages in granulomatous disease and subcutaneous fat necrosis. Hypercalcemia due to ingestion of a large dose of calcitriol usually lasts only 1 to 2 days because of its relatively short biologic half-life, whereas hypercalcemia caused by excess vitamin D ingestion lasts longer. Increased calcium release from bone resorption can result from several causes, including primary hyperparathyroidism, production of PTH-related peptide (PTHrp) by malignant cells, bone metastasis, thyrotoxicosis, immobilization, and vitamin A toxicity.

Decreased renal calcium excretion (eg, thiazide diuretics or stage 4 or 5 chronic kidney disease) generally does not result in significant hypercalcemia but can exacerbate hypercalcemia from other causes.

The severity of hypercalcemia has diagnostic implications. Primary hyperparathyroidism is often associated with borderline or mild hypercalcemia (serum calcium often <11 mg/dL); values >13 mg/dL are unusual in primary hyperparathyroidism. Patients with hypercalcemia of malignancy often have a higher serum concentration and a more rapid increase in serum calcium and are more symptomatic.

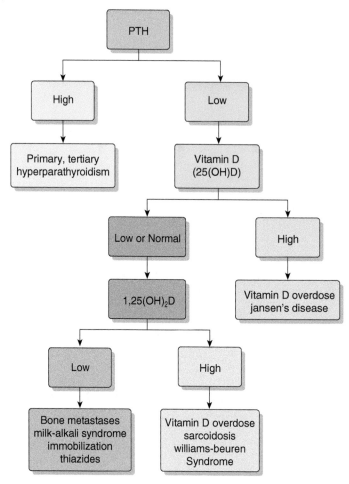

FIGURE 16.34 ■ Laboratory Algorithm for Hypercalcemia. PTH, parathyroid hormone. (Reproduced with permission from Tenenbein M, Macias CG, Sharieff GQ, et al. *Strange and Schafermeyer's Pediatric Emergency Medicine*. 5th ed. McGraw-Hill Education; New York, NY, 2019.)

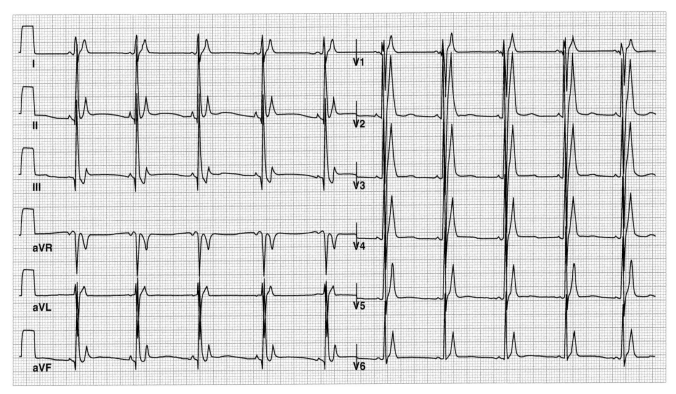

FIGURE 16.35 ■ Hypercalcemia. A 12-lead ECG shows sinus rhythm with a short QT interval (QTc <330 milliseconds), with tall, symmetrical, peaked T waves in a patient with hypercalcemia from vitamin D toxicity. (Photo contributor: Shyam Sathanandam, MD.)

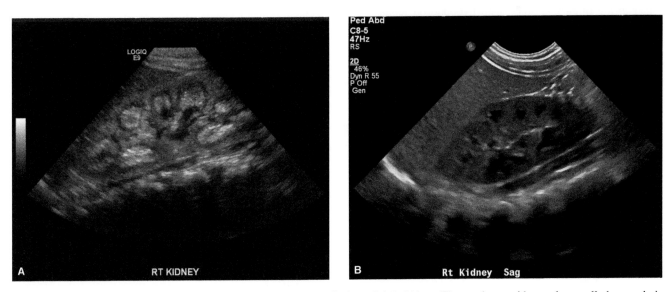

FIGURE 16.36 ■ Medullary Nephrocalcinosis. (**A**) Longitudinal US view of right kidney. The renal pyramids are abnormally hyperechoic (red asterisk) representing the fine calcifications of medullary nephrocalcinosis. (**B**) Longitudinal US view of the normal right kidney of a different patient for comparison. Note the normal dark appearance of the renal pyramids. (Photo contributors: Ryan Logan Webb, MD, and Josh Greenstein, MD.)

The signs and symptoms of hypercalcemia depend on its chronicity and severity. Typical signs of hypercalcemia include constipation, urinary concentrating defect, lethargy, hypotonia, and nephrocalcinosis.

Emergency Department Treatment and Disposition

A review of diet and medications including calcium and vitamin supplements is important to assess for drug-induced hypercalcemia and milk-alkali syndrome. The initial goal of the laboratory evaluation is to differentiate hypercalcemia mediated by PTH from other causes such as vitamin D toxicity, malignancy, and granulomatous disease. An elevated or high-normal value of serum intact PTH in the presence of hypercalcemia indicates primary hyperparathyroidism, whereas a low or low-normal serum intact PTH level (<20 pg/mL) is most consistent with non–PTH-mediated hypercalcemia. Such patients should be referred to an endocrinologist for further evaluation and tests (eg, measurements of PTHrp, 25-hydroxyvitamin D, and calcitriol levels to assess for hypercalcemia of malignancy and vitamin D toxicity).

Evaluation of serum phosphate concentration also may be helpful in selected cases of hypercalcemia. Hyperparathyroidism and humoral hypercalcemia of malignancy due to PTHrp are often associated with hypophosphatemia due to inhibition of renal proximal tubular phosphate reabsorption. In comparison, the serum phosphate concentration is normal or elevated in patients with hypercalcemia due to vitamin D toxicity, granulomatous diseases, immobilization, thyrotoxicosis, milk-alkali syndrome, and metastatic bone disease.

Patients with asymptomatic or mildly symptomatic hypercalcemia with serum calcium <12 mg/dL do not require immediate treatment. Serum calcium levels of 12 to 14 mg/dL may be well tolerated chronically and may not require immediate treatment. However, acute rise may cause symptoms and require more aggressive measures. In general, patients with a serum calcium concentration >14 mg/dL require treatment, regardless of symptoms.

Initial therapy of severe hypercalcemia includes IV administration of isotonic saline to correct volume depletion due to hypercalcemia-induced urinary salt wasting and also because hypovolemia exacerbates hypercalcemia by impairing the renal clearance of calcium. The rate of administration of saline should be based on the extent of dehydration and the tolerance of the cardiovascular system for volume expansion.

A loop diuretic, such as furosemide 1 to 2 mg/kg every 2 to 4 hours, is indicated as adjunct to saline infusion in patients with renal disease and heart failure to prevent fluid overload as well as to facilitate urinary calcium excretion by inhibiting calcium reabsorption in the thick ascending limb of the loop of Henle. Glucocorticoids are helpful in treating hypercalcemia caused by vitamin D intoxication or endogenous overproduction of calcitriol since they counteract the effects of vitamin D in mediating increased absorption of dietary calcium. Additional therapies to inhibit osteoclast-mediated bone resorption (eg, salmon calcitonin) may be indicated in patients who have severe symptoms of hypercalcemia or whose serum calcium concentrations remain moderately or markedly elevated even after volume expansion. All such patients would require hospitalization and endocrinology and nephrology consultations. Hemodialysis may be indicated in patients with severe malignancy-associated hypercalcemia and chronic kidney disease or heart failure in whom hydration cannot be safely instituted.

Pearls

1. Symptoms and signs of hypercalcemia depend on its chronicity and severity.
2. Serum calcium levels >13 mg/dL are likely to be associated with malignancy or vitamin D toxicity and are rare with primary hyperparathyroidism.
3. Inducing saline diuresis is the first-line treatment for symptomatic hypercalcemia.

Clinical Summary

Hypokalemia is generally defined as a serum potassium level of <3.5 mmol/L, whereas severe hypokalemia is defined as a level of <2.5 mmol/L. Chronic hypokalemia is most commonly related to excessive potassium loss in the urine or gut. Renal potassium loss can be mediated by excess aldosterone or other mineralocorticoids or use of diuretics or can result from intrinsic renal tubular disorders such as Bartter syndrome, Gitelman syndrome, and distal renal tubular acidosis. Gastrointestinal losses result from diarrhea, vomiting, and laxative abuse.

Approximately 98% of total body potassium is intracellular. Cellular potassium uptake is stimulated by insulin and catecholamines. Relatively small changes in potassium distribution can cause clinically significant changes in the potassium level in the extracellular fluid. Sudden onset of hypokalemia from transcellular potassium shift is noted in patients with abuse of adrenergic drugs, rapid correction of diabetic ketoacidosis, refeeding of patients with anorexia nervosa, familial periodic hypokalemic paralysis, and thyrotoxicosis periodic

paralysis; the acute hypokalemia in the latter 2 conditions occurs after carbohydrate-rich meals or strenuous exercise.

The manifestations of hypokalemia are related to the severity and acuity of the reduction in serum potassium. Patients with chronic mild hypokalemia are often asymptomatic; if present, symptoms are often from the underlying cause of the hypokalemia. The symptoms of severe acute hypokalemia are predominantly related to muscle weakness and cardiac arrhythmias. These include fatigue, constipation, ileus, and muscle cramps. The cramps usually begin in the lower extremities, progress to the trunk and upper extremities, and can worsen to the point of rhabdomyolysis and paralysis. Other symptoms include palpitations from cardiac arrhythmias and psychological symptoms such as psychosis. Severe hypokalemia may manifest as life-threatening complications of cardiovascular collapse and acute respiratory failure from respiratory muscle paralysis.

ECG findings of hypokalemia include depression of the ST segment, decrease in the amplitude of the T wave, and an increase in the amplitude of U waves, which occur at the end of the T wave. Hypokalemia also results in prolonged

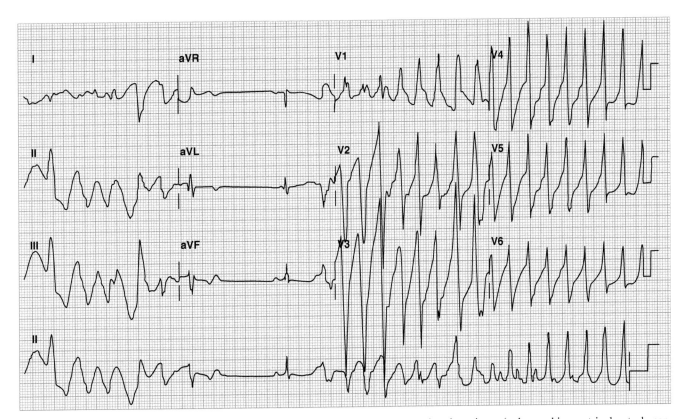

FIGURE 16.37 ■ Hypokalemia. Severely prolonged QT interval leading to torsades de pointes (polymorphic ventricular tachycardia) is seen in a patient with acute diarrheal illness and excessive vomiting with serum potassium value of <2 mEq/L. (Photo contributor: Shyam Sathanandam, MD.)

QT interval, wide P waves, prolonged PR interval, prolonged QRS duration, depressed ST segment, and inverted T waves. These conduction abnormalities predispose to sinus bradycardia, premature atrial and ventricular beats, paroxysmal atrial or junctional tachycardia, atrioventricular block, and ventricular tachycardia or fibrillation.

In most cases, the cause of hypokalemia is apparent from the history and physical examination. Evaluating patients for associated metabolic alkalosis, metabolic acidosis, or hypomagnesemia is important. In the absence of known diuretic use, assessment of urine potassium excretion is critical for establishing renal versus nonrenal potassium wasting from the gastrointestinal tract (ie, a spot urine potassium level of <20 mmol/L indicates nonrenal potassium loss, and urine potassium loss of >20 mmol/L in a patient with hypokalemia indicates ongoing, excessive renal potassium secretion). Associated metabolic alkalosis would suggest vomiting, Bartter syndrome, Gitelman syndrome, or mineralocorticoid excess.

Emergency Department Treatment and Disposition

Obtain arterial or venous blood gas, ECG, serum creatinine, BUN, calcium, and electrolytes.

The urgency of treatment of hypokalemia depends on the acuity and severity of hypokalemia as well as associated comorbid conditions. Therapy should address preventing and treating life-threatening complications, minimizing potassium losses by removing offending drugs, treating the underlying condition, and replenishing potassium stores. The goals of potassium replacement are to raise the serum potassium concentration to a safe level and then replace the remaining deficit at a slower rate over days to weeks to allow for equilibration of potassium between plasma and intracellular stores. Patients with hypokalemia due to potassium redistribution (eg, hypokalemic periodic paralysis) have no potassium deficit and need very low rates of potassium administration because they

are at risk of hyperkalemia once the redistributed potassium returns to the extracellular fluid.

If the potassium level is <2.5 mmol/L, the patient requires hospitalization and IV potassium at a concentration of 30 to 40 mEq/L. Patients needing potassium concentrations of >40 mEq/L should be closely monitored with ECG and serum potassium levels. Sodium chloride 0.9% is the preferred initial infusion fluid because 5% glucose may cause transcellular shift of potassium into cells. Potassium can be administered as potassium chloride, potassium phosphate, potassium bicarbonate, or bicarbonate precursors such as potassium citrate, acetate, or gluconate. Oral potassium bicarbonate or IV potassium acetate is preferred in patients with hypokalemia associated with metabolic acidosis (eg, renal tubular acidosis or diarrhea). Potassium phosphate is used in patients with hypokalemia and hypophosphatemia, as might occur with diabetic ketoacidosis. Potassium chloride is preferred in patients with alkalosis as well as all other patients because it raises the serum potassium concentration at a faster rate than potassium acetate. Magnesium replacement is necessary if concurrent hypomagnesemia is present either from chronic diarrhea or renal magnesium losses from Gitelman syndrome or nephrotoxic drugs; it is hard to correct hypokalemia without magnesium replacement.

Patients with a potassium level of 2.5 to 3.5 mmol/L may need only oral potassium replacement. Potassium chloride salt is used in patients with metabolic alkalosis, and potassium citrate is used in patients with metabolic acidosis. Oral potassium should be taken with plenty of fluid, either with or after meals.

Pearls

1. Administer IV potassium replacement under close supervision since high concentration or rapid infusion can result in life-threatening hyperkalemia.

2. For potassium replacement, use potassium chloride, potassium acetate, or potassium phosphate depending on associated alkalosis, acidosis, or hypophosphatemia.

Clinical Summary

Hyperkalemia is usually defined as a serum or plasma potassium level >5.5 mEq/L. Signs and symptoms of hyperkalemia are affected by the rate of rise of serum potassium level and the underlying cause. Mild (<6 mEq/L) to moderate (6.0–7.0 mEq/L) elevations of potassium concentrations may not produce symptoms in many children. However, significant acute hyperkalemia may be associated with potentially life-threatening disturbances in cardiac conduction including palpitations, syncope, or asystole. ECG changes that generally occur at a concentration >7 mEq/L in children with chronic hyperkalemia may occur at lower levels with an acute rapid increase in potassium concentration, as with tumor lysis or significant crush injury. In infants, the average serum potassium level is higher than in children; therefore, ECG changes are usually seen at higher levels of serum potassium. The following is the general range of serum potassium levels and the corresponding ECG changes:

- Serum potassium = 5.5 to 6.5 mEq/L: tall peaked T waves with a narrow base and shortening of the QT interval
- Serum potassium = 6.5 to 8.0 mEq/L: peaked T waves, prolonged PR interval, decreased or disappearing P wave, widening QRS complex, and amplified R wave

- Serum potassium >8.0 mEq/L: absent P wave, bundle branch block, progressive widening of QRS complex that eventually merges with the T wave to form a sinusoidal pattern followed by ventricular fibrillation or asystole

Severe acute hyperkalemia (potassium level >7 mEq/L) can cause muscle weakness or paralysis that is usually ascending, beginning in the legs and progressing to the trunk and arms, and can progress to flaccid paralysis. These findings may mimic those seen in patients with Guillain-Barré syndrome.

Emergency Department Treatment and Disposition

Obtain detailed history including history of acute or chronic renal disease, such as edema, oliguria, brown urine, or proteinuria; HTN (suggestive of acute glomerulonephritis); recent hemorrhagic colitis (suggestive of HUS); arthralgia, abdominal pain, or purpura (suggestive of HSP); or systemic symptoms of systemic lupus erythematosus, trauma, or chemotherapy for tumors. Assess patient for intravascular volume status, signs of shock, heart failure, muscle weakness, and neurologic signs. Obtain arterial or venous blood gas, ECG, serum creatinine, BUN, calcium, and electrolytes.

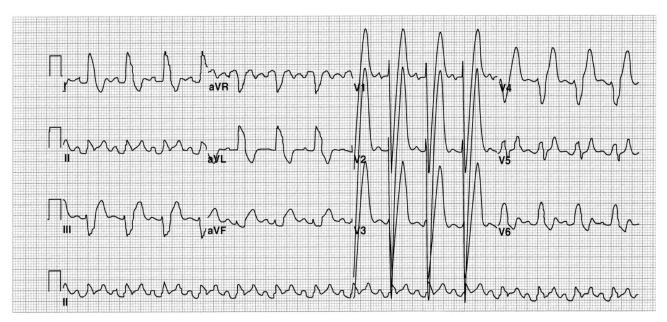

FIGURE 16.38 ■ Hyperkalemia. A 12-lead ECG in a 17-year-old adolescent with renal failure shows sinus rhythm, first-degree atrioventricular block, broad notched P waves, left bundle branch block, QRS duration of 0.16 seconds, marked QT prolongation (QTc = 0.52 seconds), tall, broadened T waves, and diffuse ST segment abnormalities. (Photo contributor: Shyam Sathanandam, MD.)

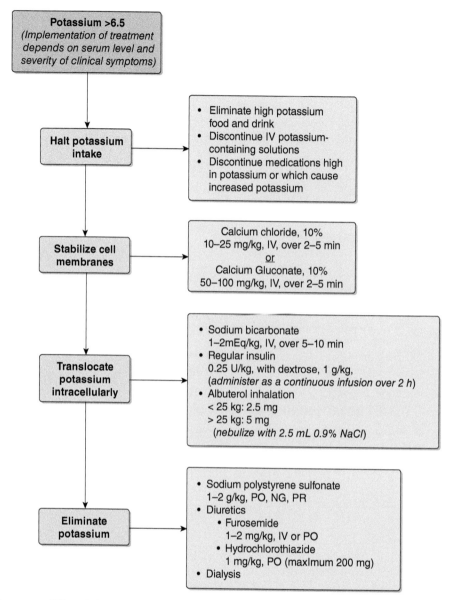

FIGURE 16.39. ▪ Treatment of Hyperkalemia. (Reproduced with permission from Tenenbein M, Macias CG, Sharieff GQ, et al. *Strange and Schafermeyer's Pediatric Emergency Medicine.* 5th ed. McGraw-Hill Education; New York, NY, 2019.)

The therapy should address prevention and treatment of life-threatening complications, minimizing potassium entry into circulation by removing offending drugs, debriding damaged tissue, and enhancing potassium excretion out of the body. For patients with severe hyperkalemia, those with signs or symptoms of hyperkalemia (ECG changes or muscular weakness or paralysis), or patients with potassium levels between 6 and 7 mEq/L who are at risk for further increases in potassium, initial emergent therapeutic interventions are directed toward counteracting the adverse cardiac effects and

moving the potassium from the extracellular to the intracellular fluid compartment. These measures, which are transient in effect, are shown in Figure 16.39.

Loop diuretics and intestinal cation exchange resins such as sodium polystyrene sulfonate are used in patients with persistent, moderate hyperkalemia (5.5–6.5 mEq/L) and as adjuncts for those with more severe hyperkalemia. Kayexalate can be given as retention enema in those with impaired intestinal motility. Dialysis is initiated in patients with persistent hyperkalemia who are unresponsive to diuretic or cation exchange therapy. Generally, hemodialysis is more effective than peritoneal dialysis in providing a sufficiently rapid decrease in serum potassium concentration.

After initial emergent management of the child with potentially life-threatening hyperkalemia or asymptomatic patients who present with more modest hyperkalemia (potassium levels <7 mEq/L), further management consists of hospitalization, nephrology consultation, identification and treatment of reversible causes of hyperkalemia, minimizing intake of potassium, and removal of drugs that may induce or worsen hyperkalemia, such as angiotensin-converting enzyme inhibitors, angiotensin receptor blockers, aldosterone antagonists, and nonselective β-blockers.

Pearls

1. Physical findings of hyperkalemia may be absent if the potassium level is mildly elevated.
2. Physical findings of hyperkalemia include ascending muscle weakness and paralysis.
3. Cardiac arrhythmias can occur with hyperkalemia.

Chapter 17

TOXICOLOGY

Mark K. Su
Madeline H. Renny

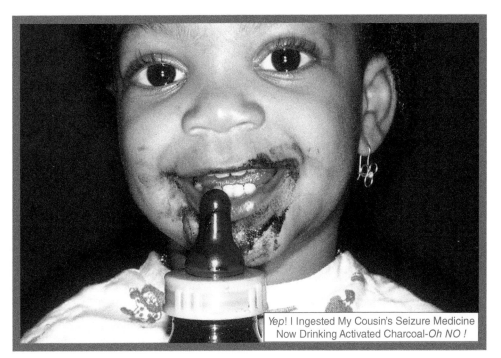

Yep! I Ingested My Cousin's Seizure Medicine Now Drinking Activated Charcoal-*Oh NO !*

(Photo contributor: Binita R. Shah, MD)

The authors acknowledge the special contributions of Ronak R. Shah, MD, Mae De La Calzada-Jeanlouie, MD and Rachel S. Weiselberg, MD to the prior edition.

THE EVALUATION AND MANAGEMENT OF POISONING IN CHILDREN: GENERAL APPROACH AND GI DECONTAMINATION

Clinical Summary

The incidence of pediatric poisoning follows a biphasic curve, with about 90% of cases occurring in children age 1 to 6 years and a second smaller peak of 10% to 15% of cases occurring in adolescents. Most ingestions in children are of a single agent (frequently nontoxic household products) and unintentional/accidental. The most frequently reported pharmaceutical exposures in children <6 years of age include analgesics, cough and cold preparations, cardiovascular agents, topical preparations, sedative hypnotic agents, and antidepressants. Adolescent toxic ingestions are more likely to be multiple pharmaceutical agents and intentional.

The most important factor in successfully treating a patient with a toxicologic exposure is to recognize a toxicologic etiology in the patient who presents with undifferentiated symptoms. Poisoning must be considered in the differential diagnosis of multiple conditions, especially when a patient presents with cyanosis, shock, vomiting, diarrhea, hypothermia or hyperthermia, abnormal behavior, or altered mental status. A thorough history must be obtained with a focus on the identification of the toxin, timing, dosage, route, intent of ingestion, and symptom development since ingestion.

The patient and/or care providers may be able to directly identify the involved toxin because of a known exposure (eg, medications taken, intentional overdose attempt, substance abuse, exposure to occupational chemicals). Determining whether the exposure was intentional or not may aid in

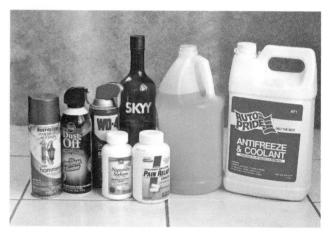

FIGURE 17.2 ■ Medications and Poisons Frequently Ingested by Adolescents. Pharmaceutical agents and other substances that are intentionally ingested in the context of a suicide attempt by adolescents include analgesics, sedative-hypnotics, cyclic antidepressants, antihistamines, ethylene glycol, and windshield washer fluid (methanol). (Photo contributor: Ronak R. Shah, MD.)

assessing the reliability of the history given by the patient. Regardless of intent, patients may or may not report accurate amounts, and it may be necessary to search through medication containers and count the number of remaining pills or measure approximate quantities of liquid.

Prehospital health care workers may aid in identification of the toxin and information about dosage/route at the time of arrival in the ED with findings of containers or other evidence of possible toxins and can provide information on any treatment and attempts at decontamination prior to hospital arrival.

Coingestions or multiple agents should be suspected, especially in adolescent patients; in addition, the potential for nonoral routes of exposure (dermal, rectal, ocular, parenteral, or transplacental) should be considered because the route of exposure affects the severity and evolution of the patient's condition.

Determination of symptoms since ingestion will aid in recognition of *toxidromes* (see below) as well as determination of degree of toxicity. Attention must be paid to past medical history and comorbidities with a focus on the patient's medications, including herbal supplements, dietary supplements, over-the-counter medications, and alternative medical therapies.

Samples of the substance may be available (eg, plants, mushrooms). For potential carbon monoxide (CO) poisoning, the local fire department may also be notified to quantify the amount of CO in a building. A poison control center or

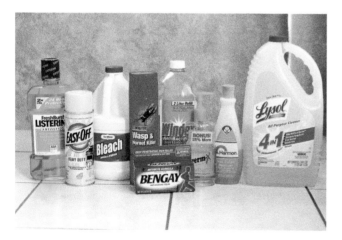

FIGURE 17.1 ■ Household Products Frequently Ingested by Young Children. Household cleaners, cosmetics, and plants are among the leading nonpharmaceutical agents ingested by children. Some of these products contain potential toxic substances including sodium hydroxide, alcohol, methyl salicylate (eg, Listerine), and sodium hypochlorite (eg, bleach). (Photo contributor: Ronak R. Shah, MD.)

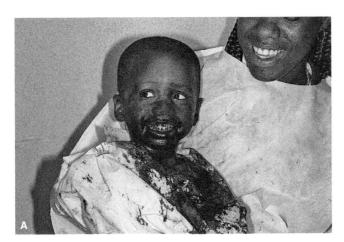

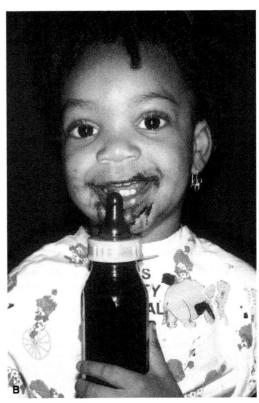

FIGURE 17.3 ■ Activated Charcoal (AC) Administration. A 3-year-old child presented after unintentionally drinking 4 ounces of Dimetapp liquid (grape flavor) 1 hour prior to arrival in the ED. He was completely asymptomatic. (**A**) As seen here, AC is poorly accepted by young children, and often, there is a battle between the hospital staff and the child over its administration. AC should *not* be routinely administered in the management of all poisoned patients. (**B**) A smiling face with a bottle full of AC given to this girl who accidentally ingested carbamazepine (sibling's seizure medication). (Photo contributor: Binita R. Shah, MD.)

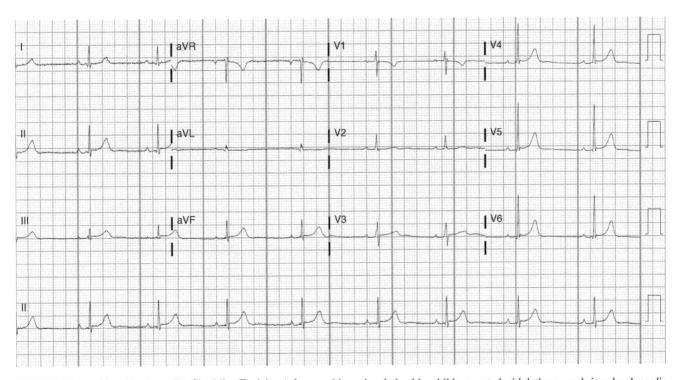

FIGURE 17.4 ■ Sinus Bradycardia; Clonidine Toxicity. A 3-year-old previously healthy child presented with lethargy and sinus bradycardia following unintentional ingestion of his grandmother's clonidine. His heart rate would increase to 120 bpm when stimulated but would drop to 50 bpm when stimulation was withdrawn. (Photo contributor: Sushitha Surendran, MD.)

TABLE 17.1 ▪ THE POISONED PATIENT: TOXICOLOGIC CLUES AND TESTS TO PERFORM AT THE BEDSIDE

- Cyanosis unresponsive to supplemental O_2 administration = methemoglobinemia
- "Chocolate brown" blood = methemoglobinemia
- Therapeutic response to glucose = hypoglycemic agents, alcohols, salicylates
- Therapeutic response to naloxone = opioids (possibly other agents, angiotensin-converting enzyme inhibitors [ACEIs], clonidine, valproic acid)
- Coma: alcohol, sedative hypnotics, opioids, cyclic antidepressants, anticholinergics, CO, salicylates, isoniazid, organophosphates, anticonvulsants, antihistamines, clonidine, phencyclidine (PCP), phenothiazines (see mnemonic COMATOSE PATIENT, Table 13.5)
- Respiration
  1. Bradypnea: opioids, alcohols, benzodiazepines, clonidine, barbiturates, γ-hydroxybutyrate (GHB)
  2. Tachypnea: salicylates, sympathomimetics, methanol, ethylene glycol, theophylline, caffeine, cocaine
  3. Wheezing: organophosphates
  4. Kussmaul: salicylates, methanol, ethylene glycol
- Pulse
  1. Bradycardia: β-blockers, calcium channel blockers, clonidine, digoxin, sedative hypnotics, opioids, organophosphates, phenylpropanolamine
  2. Tachycardia: anticholinergics, sympathomimetics (cocaine, amphetamines, over-the-counter [OTC] cold remedies), theophylline, caffeine, iron, salicylate, cyclic antidepressants (CAs)
  3. Dysrhythmias: anticholinergics, CAs, phenothiazines, β-blockers, calcium channel blockers, organophosphates, CO, cyanide (CN)
- BP
  1. Hypotension: β-blockers, calcium channel blockers, clonidine, opioids, iron, CAs, phenothiazines, CO, CN
  2. Hypertension: phenylpropanolamine (OTC cold remedies), sympathomimetics, PCP, cocaine, amphetamines, anticholinergics, antihistamines
- Temperature
  1. Hypothermia: alcohols, opioids, benzodiazepines, clonidine, barbiturates, phenothiazines, CAs, CO, antidepressants, hypoglycemic agents
  2. Hyperthermia: sympathomimetics, anticholinergics, salicylates, cyclic antidepressants, cocaine, amphetamines, theophylline, phenothiazines
- Bedside Glucose Analysis
  1. Hyperglycemia: salicylates, iron, isoniazid
  2 Hypoglycemia: hypoglycemic agents, alcohols, salicylates
- Arterial Blood Gas
  1. CO: normal PO_2, normal hemoglobin saturation and normal pulse oximetry, elevated lactate
  2. Methemoglobinemia: normal or increased PO_2, decreased hemoglobin saturation and decreased pulse oximetry, elevated lactate
  3. Carboxyhemoglobin and methemoglobin levels
- ECG: terminal 40-ms frontal plane QRS vector, prolonged QRS = CAs (sodium channel–blocking agents)
- Urine ferric chloride assay (1 mL of urine + few drops of 10% ferric chloride): purple = salicylates, phenothiazines
- Urine:
  1. Calcium oxalate crystals = ethylene glycol
  2. Ketones = acetone, isopropyl alcohol, salicylates
- Fluorescence under Wood's lamp: ethylene glycol from antifreeze (fluorescein additive)
- Gastric contents deferoxamine test: (deferoxamine + hydrogen peroxide added to gastric contents yields a rose color) = iron

(Continued)

- Skin
  1. Cherry red = CO, CN
  2. Blue/cyanosis = methemoglobinemia
  3. Flushing = anticholinergics, sympathomimetics, ethanol, antihistamines, niacin
  4. Hot, dry skin = anticholinergics
  5. Diaphoresis = sympathomimetics, salicylates, cocaine, PCP, organophosphates
  6. Jaundice = acetaminophen, mothballs (naphthalene-induced hemolysis), toxic mushrooms (eg, amanita phalloides)
- Odor
  1. Acetone = isopropanol, methanol, chloroform, salicylate
  2. Wintergreen = methyl salicylate
  3. Alcohol = mixed ethanol (pure ethanol is odorless), isopropyl alcohol, methanol
  4. Garlic = organophosphates, arsenic, thallium, phosphorus
  5. Coal gas = CO
  6. Bitter almond = CN
  7. Rotten eggs = hydrogen sulfide
  8. Fruity = isopropanol, ethanol, amyl nitrite
  9. Mothballs = camphor, naphthalene
  10. Petroleum = petroleum distillate
  11. Pears = chloral hydrate
- Extrapyramidal signs (rigidity, dysphonia, torticollis, oculogyric crisis) = phenothiazines
- Myoclonus/rigidity = phenothiazines, anticholinergics, haloperidol
- Nystagmus = phenytoin, PCP, alcohol, barbiturates, sedative-hypnotics, carbamazepine, CO, lithium
- Psychosis/delirium = PCP, anticholinergics, phenothiazines, cocaine, heroin, sympathomimetics, lysergic acid diethylamide (LSD), marijuana, ethanol, antihistamines
- Ataxia = alcohols, phenytoin, barbiturates, benzodiazepines, CO
- Fasciculations = organophosphates
- Paralysis = organophosphates, botulinum toxin, carbamates, heavy metals
- Blindness = methanol, quinine

TABLE 17.2 ▪ MNEMONICS FOR POISONINGS AND TOXIDROMES

A. *Increased anion gap metabolic acidosis:*

MUD PILES
*M*ethanol
*U*remia
*D*iabetic ketoacidosis
*P*henformin, *P*araldehyde
*I*ron, *I*soniazid
*L*actic acidosis (caused by CO, CN, seizure, shock)
*E*thylene glycol
*S*alicylates

B. *Anticholinergics:*
Hot as a hare (elevated temperature)
Red as a beet (flushed skin)
Blind as a bat (mydriasis)
Mad as a hatter (delirium)
Dry as a bone (decreased secretions)

ACIDOSIS
*A*lcohols (methanol, ethylene glycol)
*C*arbon monoxide (CO) or *C*yanide (CN)
*I*ron
*D*iabetic ketoacidosis
*O*ther (uremia, paraldehyde)
*S*eizures or shock (lactic acidosis)
*I*soniazid
*S*alicylates

(Continued)

TABLE 17.2 ■ MNEMONICS FOR POISONINGS AND TOXIDROMES (*CONTINUED*)

C. *Cholinergics: DUMBELS*
   Diarrhea
   Urination
   Miosis
   Bronchorrhea/Bronchospasm
   Emesis
   Lacrimation
   Salivation
D. *Miosis: COPS*
   Clonidine, Cholinergics
   Opioids (except meperidine and diphenoxylate/atropine sulfate), Organophosphates
   Phenothiazines, Phencyclidine
   Sedative-hypnotic coma (barbiturates, benzodiazepines, ethanol)
E. *Mydriasis: WASH*
   Withdrawal (sedative-hypnotic, opioid, ethanol)
   Anticholinergics (atropine)
   Sympathomimetics
   Hallucinogens
F. *Radiopaque substances*: *COCAINE*
   Cocaine packets
   Opioids packets
   Chloral hydrate
   Arsenic (heavy metals, lead, mercury)
   Iron
   Neuroleptics (phenothiazines, cyclic antidepressants)
   Enteric-coated preparations (eg, aspirin)
G. *Drugs or chemicals producing seizures: CAMPHOR BALLS*
   Camphor, Cocaine, Carbon monoxide, Cyanide, Caffeine, Carbamazepine
   Amphetamines, Anticholinergics (cyclic antidepressants, antihistamines)
   Methylxanthines (theophylline), caffeine
   Phenothiazines or Phencyclidine
   Hypoglycemic agents (sulfonylureas, insulin), Heavy metals (eg, lead)
   Opioids (tramadol, meperidine), Organophosphates
   Rodenticides (strychnine, thallium, arsenic)
   Barbiturates, Benzodiazepines (withdrawal seizures)
   Alcohols (methanol, ethylene glycol), ethanol (withdrawal seizures)
   Lidocaine
   Lithium
   Salicylates

TOXIDROMES (Examples of compounds categorized by their associated toxidromes):
1. Anticholinergics: atropine, cyclic antidepressants (CAs), antipsychotics, antihistamines, phenothiazines, and antispasmodics
2. Sympathomimetics: amphetamines (phenylpropanolamine, ephedrine, methamphetamine), cocaine, methyl xanthines (eg, caffeine, theophylline)
3. Opioids: heroin, methadone, morphine, codeine, meperidine
4. Sedative-hypnotics: barbiturates, benzodiazepines, ethanol
5. Cholinergics: organophosphates and carbamate insecticides
6. Hypermetabolics: salicylates
7. Withdrawal: opioids, benzodiazepines, ethanol

Modified with permission from Finberg L, Kleinman RE. *Saunders Manual of Pediatric Practice.* WB Saunders; Philadelphia, PA, 2002.

TABLE 17.3 ■ MEDICATIONS AND TOXINS FOR WHICH QUANTITATIVE SERUM CONCENTRATIONS AID IN THE MANAGEMENT OF A POISONED PATIENT

- Medications
  1. Acetaminophen
  2. Salicylates
  3. Iron
  4. Carbamazepine
  5. Phenobarbital
  6. Phenytoin
  7. Valproic acid
  8. Theophylline
  9. Digoxin
  10. Lithium
- Toxins
  1. Carboxyhemoglobin
  2. Methemoglobin
  3. Ethanol
  4. Methanol
  5. Ethylene glycol

product manufacturer should be contacted if the ingredients of a product are unknown. Review of drug and chemical databases (eg, Poisindex®) is also useful.

Consider child abuse in very young infants in the setting of repeated ingestions, or if the child's developmental level and skills preclude performance of the described events (eg, a child too young to open child-resistant containers).

Perform a thorough physical examination beginning with vital signs. Possible *toxidromes* (toxicologic syndromes that are characteristic signs and symptoms seen with certain poisons or classes of poisons) should be identified as these aid diagnosis and management of acutely ill patients, especially when a history of poisoning is lacking (see Table 17.2).

Laboratory studies should be performed, *if clinically indicated*, for diagnosis or to guide therapy (see specific chapters for agents and laboratory studies that may prove useful in management). These should include serum electrolytes, including glucose, BUN, and creatinine to determine renal function and calculation of anion gap. Obtaining serum osmolality will determine if substances causing an increased osmolal gap were ingested. These include ethanol, methanol, isopropyl alcohol, and ethylene glycol (osmolal gap = measured serum osmolality – calculated osmolality). Toxicology screens (either urine or serum) may occasionally help

in determining occult coingestions; however, they are rarely helpful in the acute management of patients. Many laboratory tests are used by consultants (eg, psychiatry) or admitting providers for management and disposition decisions.

All patients with an intentional suicidal overdose should have serum acetaminophen and salicylate levels determined. All female patients of childbearing age should have a pregnancy test performed. If there is any gastric aspirate/vomitus, note appearance, pills, and possible odors.

Radiographic studies may be useful for management or confirmation of a diagnosis with a high index of suspicion, for example, ingestion of iron tablets. Chest radiographs may show pulmonary edema or aspiration pneumonitis consistent with hydrocarbon exposure. Abdominal radiographs may show other radiopaque substances. However, it is important to note that absence of toxins generally considered to be radiopaque does not exclude ingestion.

Emergency Department Treatment and Disposition

Proper external decontamination before entry into the ED is necessary to protect health care personnel and prevent contamination of the ED. This may involve removal of all clothing and washing the skin.

All patients should have airway, breathing, and circulation (ABCs) stabilized based on abnormal vital signs *before* any diagnostic tests are performed. Focus on *treating the patient, not the poison*. Patients may have more than 1 type of exposure or ingestion, complicating the identification of distinct toxidromes. Consultations with the local medical toxicologist or regional poison control center may also be helpful.

Unresponsive patients may empirically be given IV dextrose (1 g/kg) and IV naloxone (1–2 mg, may be repeated several times) followed by IV thiamine and be observed for a response. Patients with altered mental status should be evaluated for all causes of altered sensorium including nontoxicologic causes (see mnemonic COMATOSE PATIENT; Table 13.5).

Motor seizures are generally well controlled by benzodiazepines. Anticonvulsant medications, such as phenytoin, are not recommended in the treatment of most toxin-induced seizures. If the toxic agent is known, seizures may be controlled with specific therapy (eg, pyridoxine for acute isoniazid toxicity).

Gastrointestinal (GI) decontamination by syrup of ipecac is no longer recommended, and use of orogastric lavage is also of limited value. Orogastric lavage is indicated when there is a potentially life-threatening ingestion of a toxin with no definitive antidote. The greatest benefit is most likely to be seen in a patient who presents within 60 minutes of ingestion. Patients presenting after 60 minutes may also benefit if the suspected agent is known to delay GI motility. Contraindications include ingestion of caustics, hydrocarbons, and foreign bodies (FBs); bleeding diathesis; and an unprotected airway. Complications include aspiration pneumonia, GI perforation, laryngospasm, and emesis.

Decontamination with activated charcoal (AC) is indicated if a patient has ingested a potentially toxic amount of a poison that is known to be adsorbed by AC. AC does *not* adsorb acids, alkalis, lithium, iron (most metals), alcohols, or hydrocarbons. AC administration is likely to be most effective if begun within 60 minutes of ingestion, but may also be given after 60 minutes, especially if there is delayed gastric emptying, bezoar formation, and enterohepatic or enteroenteric circulation of the toxin. AC is given orally as a slurry in water or fruit juice (also by nasogastric or orogastric tube), and the usual single dose (children/adults) is 1 to 2 g/kg up to 50 g, and a 10:1 ratio of AC to drug is considered ideal. Multiple-dose AC (0.5–1 g/kg every 4–6 hours) should be performed if a patient has ingested a large quantity of agents that decrease gastric motility (eg, anticholinergics, enteric-coated preparations), theophylline, phenobarbital, carbamazepine, quinine, or dapsone. Patients should have good GI motility as evidenced by normal bowel sounds and passage of stool (ie, no evidence of GI obstruction). Contraindications include intestinal obstruction or perforation, altered sensorium (absent gag reflex/unprotected airway), and caustics (may obscure endoscopic visualization of gastroesophageal injury). Complications include pulmonary aspiration, intestinal obstruction, constipation, and development of charcoal bezoars. If desorption of ingestant from AC is a possibility, a single dose of cathartic may be given to an adolescent who has ingested a large amount of drugs. Administration of a cathartic alone has *no* role as a method of gut decontamination. Routine use of a cathartic with AC is *not* recommended. Complications of cathartics include nausea, vomiting, diarrhea, abdominal pain, and dehydration with electrolyte disturbances (following multiple doses, which should not be repeatedly given for >24 hours). Contraindications include absent bowel sounds, ingestion of caustics, or GI irritants.

Whole bowel irrigation (WBI) should be performed in patients who have ingested FBs, packets containing toxins, iron, and sustained-release or enteric-coated tablets. *WBI should not be routinely used in the management of the poisoned patient.* WBI is commonly performed by the continuous administration of a bowel-cleansing solution containing polyethylene glycol electrolyte solution (PEG ELS) via an oral or nasogastric tube. It is given at a rate of 0.5 L/h until the rectal effluent is clear. In older children and adolescents, it should be given at a rate of 1 to 2 L/h. There is no systemic absorption of PEG ELS, and no significant adverse effects of prolonged WBI with PEG ELS have been demonstrated.

Certain toxins can be managed with the administration of toxin-specific antidotes. Prophylactic use of antidotes is not recommended because of potentially serious side effects with inappropriate administration. Life-threatening poisonings such as opioids, cholinergics, cyclic antidepressants, methemoglobinemia, CO, and cyanide require simultaneous use of an antidote with the initial stabilization of vital signs.

Inpatient hospitalization and/or observation in a monitored bed is indicated if the patient manifests significant toxicity or has suicidal intent, identification of poison is unclear, ingested substance has delayed toxicity, or if the patient will require further management such as urinary alkalinization (eg, salicylates, phenobarbital), hemodialysis (eg, methanol, ethylene glycol, salicylates, lithium), or WBI (eg, iron). Consider ICU admission for patients who manifest significant toxicity or those in whom management will require rigorous nursing care.

Patients can be discharged home if the ingestion was unintentional, if the patient (and/or guardians) has received appropriate counseling and social service intervention, the product or drug has been determined to be benign, the amount ingested is less than the smallest amount known to produce toxicity (*note that the history is often unreliable*), the patient has no signs of toxicity since the time of ingestion, the time elapsed since the ingestion is greater than the longest interval known between ingestion and peak toxicity, and child abuse or neglect is not considered likely.

Pearls

1. The most important factor in successfully treating a patient with a toxicologic exposure is to recognize that there is a toxicologic etiology of the patient's condition.

2. GI decontamination has not been shown to improve patient outcome; however, removal of toxin by GI decontamination before adsorption may prevent or mitigate toxicity. It is critical to ask, "Has the child ingested a potentially toxic dose?" and "What is the time since ingestion?"

3. Gastric lavage should *not* be performed unless the patient has ingested a potentially life-threatening amount of a poison and toxin is expected to be remaining in the stomach.

4. AC should only be administered if a patient has ingested a potentially toxic amount of a poison that is known to be adsorbed by AC. A nasogastric tube should not be placed for the sole purpose of AC administration.

5. WBI should be performed in patients presenting with potentially toxic ingestion of iron, lead, packets of illicit drugs, or sustained-release or enteric-coated tablets.

Clinical Summary

Acetaminophen (APAP) overdose can lead to hepatic necrosis, fulminant hepatic failure, and death. The therapeutic dose is 10 to 15 mg/kg with maximum dosage of 80 mg/kg/day. Acute toxicity usually occurs at doses above >150 mg/kg taken as a single dose.

Clinical presentation is dependent on amount of time since ingestion, and patients may be completely asymptomatic initially. After 24 hours, patients may also present with GI symptoms of nausea, vomiting, and malaise. After 24 to 72 hours, GI symptoms may lessen, during which time hepatic damage is occurring. Patients may have right upper quadrant pain or tenderness. After 72 to 96 hours, anorexia, nausea, and vomiting worsen. Progression to fulminant hepatic failure may occur by 4 to 5 days after ingestion.

The differential diagnosis of hepatotoxicity includes viral hepatitis, other drug- or toxin-induced hepatitis (eg, isoniazid, carbamazepine, *Amanita phalloides* mushroom, phenytoin), alcoholic hepatitis, hepatobiliary disease, Reye syndrome, and ischemic hepatitis (usually following a prolonged period of hypotension).

Evaluation should include a careful history with particular attention to comorbidities that may predispose the patient to development of hepatotoxicity and formulations that decrease GI motility (eg, combination preparations containing anticholinergic agents such as diphenhydramine or opioids). Laboratory tests should include serum APAP concentration, CBC, glucose, electrolytes, BUN, creatinine, phosphate, prothrombin time (PT), international normalized ratio (INR), serum

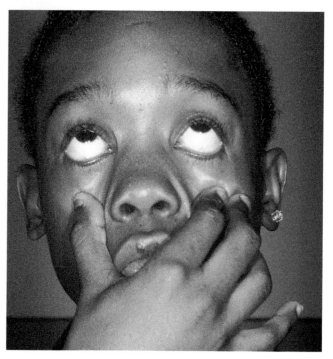

FIGURE 17.6 ■ Hepatotoxicity; Acetaminophen (APAP) Overdose. This 15-year-old girl presented to ED 16 hours after ingestion of 32.5 g of APAP (100 tablets of 325 mg each). Her serum APAP value of 62 µg/mL (plotted on nomogram; see Figure 17.7) was above the line and in the "potentially toxic" area of the figure. Therapy with oral N-acetylcysteine (NAC) was initiated. Her serum aspartate aminotransferase (AST) level was initially mildly elevated to 368 IU/L, and rose to a peak of 7600 IU/L with development of jaundice and coagulopathy (international normalized ratio, 2.5) over the next 72 hours. Her AST level and hepatic function normalized after day 5 with a full recovery. (Photo contributor: Ronak R. Shah, MD.)

transaminases (alanine and aspartate aminotransferase), and serum bilirubin. A venous or arterial blood gas (ABG) with lactate should also be obtained for patients who are acutely ill on ED presentation. A high anion gap with high lactate metabolic acidosis is reported following large APAP overdoses. The Kings College criteria of poor prognostic indicators following APAP overdose include a serum pH <7.3, INR >6.5, serum creatinine >3.4 mg/dL, and grade III or IV hepatic encephalopathy. It has also been suggested that elevated serum lactate and phosphate values, in combination with the Kings College criteria, are prognostic markers of severe APAP-induced hepatotoxicity. Once a serum APAP concentration has been obtained 4 hours after ingestion, the Rumack-Matthew nomogram should be applied to determine necessity for antidotal treatment.

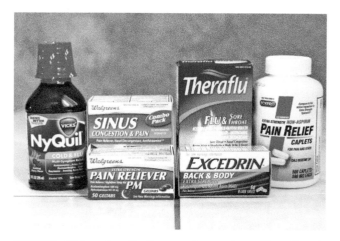

FIGURE 17.5 ■ Over-the-Counter Preparations That Contain Acetaminophen. (Photo contributor: Ronak R. Shah, MD.)

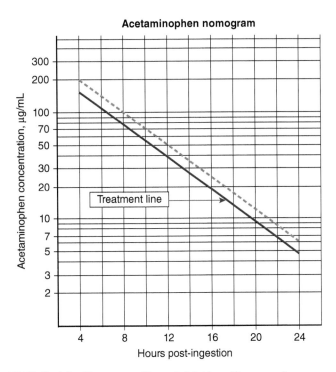

Acetaminophen nomogram

FIGURE 17.7 ■ Acetaminophen (APAP) Toxicity Nomogram (Rumack-Matthew Nomogram).

1. Risk of toxicity is best evaluated by comparing serum APAP concentration to the time of ingestion.

2. Measure serum APAP concentrations after a single, acute overdose of an immediate-release preparation between 4 and 24 hours after ingestion, and plot results on the nomogram to determine the need for antidotal therapy.

3. Serum levels drawn before 4 hours may not represent peak concentrations and still should be checked at 4 hours after ingestion. The optimal level is drawn at 4 hours after ingestion or as soon after 4 hours as possible. (The 4-hour level is not necessarily the peak. In fact, many people who overdose probably have much higher APAP concentrations prior to 4 hours.)

4. Values that fall above the "upper line or original line" are considered to be "potentially toxic" and represent an approximately 60% incidence of severe hepatotoxicity and 5% mortality, if untreated.

5. "Lower line" that runs parallel to the upper line has been arbitrarily lowered by 25% (in order to add greater sensitivity and additional safety margin) and represents APAP acetaminophen concentration considered to be toxic in the United States. (Historically, the "upper line" was still used in the United Kingdom until 2012, but their guidelines have since been changed and they no longer use this nomogram.) Values that fall below the "lower line" are considered to have decreased potential for toxicity and are associated with a significantly lower risk of hepatotoxicity and fatalities are not expected to occur.

6. The nomogram may be used for sustained-release preparations of APAP, and treatment should be instituted if the 4-hour level is in the "Potential for Toxicity" area. Also, this is a rare setting in which a second APAP level may be drawn 4 to 6 hours later, if the initial level is in the "Toxicity Unlikely" area. If the second level is in the "Potential for Toxicity" area, treatment should be implemented.

7. The nomogram is also not applicable if the time of ingestion is uncertain, if ingestion occurred >24 hours before presentation, or if repeated ingestion has occurred.

(Reproduced with permission from Hoffman RS, Howland M, Lewin NA, et al. *Goldfrank's Toxicologic Emergencies.* 10th ed. McGraw-Hill Education; New York, NY, 2015.)

Emergency Department Treatment and Disposition

GI decontamination is primarily achieved through the administration of AC (1–2 g/kg orally). Antidotal therapy with *N*-acetylcysteine (NAC) can be empirically administered if >150 mg/kg of APAP has been ingested and the patient presents soon after ingestion via IV as 3 doses over 21 hours. The initial loading dose is 150 mg/kg diluted in 3 mL/kg of D5 ½ normal saline (NS), infused over 60 minutes. The second dose is 50 mg/kg diluted in 7 mL of D5 ½ NS infused over the subsequent 4 hours. The third dose of 100 mg/kg diluted in 14 mL of D5 ½ NS is then infused over 16 hours. NAC dosing needs to be adjusted for children weighing

<40 kg because of adverse effects associated with hyperosmolarity and hyponatremia due to excessive fluid administration.

All patients who have a toxic APAP level require a full course of NAC therapy and should be admitted. Patients with signs and/or symptoms of significant hepatotoxicity or other end organ toxicity should be admitted to the ICU. Patients presenting after 24 hours following an overdose and with clinical evidence of hepatotoxicity (eg, altered mental status, jaundice) should be started on IV NAC immediately. Patients should be hospitalized for supportive care.

Contact the poison control center for all patients with APAP toxicity, patients who have developed signs and symptoms of hepatotoxicity, patients presenting with ingestion of extended-release preparations, or those presenting more than 24 hours after ingestion. Indications for transfer to a liver transplantation center in patients who develop hepatotoxicity include assessment of the Kings College criteria: if a patient has an arterial pH <7.3 after fluid resuscitation or grade III or IV encephalopathy, creatinine >3.3 mg/dL, and INR >6.5. Psychiatry should be consulted for all cases of self-harm.

Pearls

1. APAP is the most widely used analgesic-antipyretic in the United States and accounts for more overdoses and overdose fatalities per year than any other pharmaceutical agent.

2. All patients presenting with an intentional overdose of medication should have a serum APAP concentration checked.

3. Severe APAP toxicity may produce fulminant hepatic failure 3 to 5 days after ingestion.

Clinical Summary

The most common salicylate therapeutically used is acetyl-salicylic acid (ASA; aspirin). Many over-the-counter products contain salicylates, including Ben-Gay® and Pepto-Bismol®, as well as the highly concentrated salicylate product, oil of wintergreen. Toxicity generally occurs at doses of >150 mg/kg, with >300 mg/kg considered as potentially lethal. Ingested ASA tablets may occasionally form concretions (bezoars) or cause pylorospasm, resulting in delayed and prolonged absorption. Enteric-coated preparations may also result in delayed or prolonged absorption.

Clinical findings of salicylate toxicity include nausea, vomiting, epigastric pain, and possible hematemesis. Hyperpnea and tachypnea may lead to respiratory alkalosis and acute lung injury. Patients with salicylate toxicity present to the ED with tinnitus, deafness, delirium, seizures, or coma. A high anion gap metabolic acidosis develops after significant ingestions of salicylate. Increased sweating, vomiting, and tachypnea lead to dehydration and electrolyte disturbances, and hypoglycemia occurs due to energy failure.

Differential diagnosis of other causes of increased anion gap metabolic acidosis should be considered (see Table 17.2). Other etiologies must also be considered for hypoglycemia, gastroenteritis, and acute respiratory distress syndrome (ARDS).

Take a careful history with attention to amount, time of ingestion, intent, possibility of coingestions, and type of

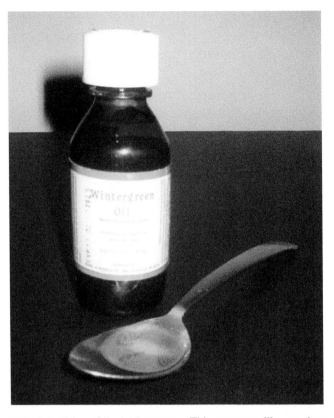

FIGURE 17.9 ■ Oil of Wintergreen. This sweet-smelling product contains 100% methyl salicylate. One teaspoon contains 7000 mg of methyl salicylate (equivalent to 21.5 tablets of aspirin, each containing 325 mg). In a 10-kg child, the minimum toxic salicylate dose of about 150 mg/kg body weight can almost be achieved with ingestion of 1 mL (1 mL = 1400 mg of methyl salicylate = 140 mg/kg for a 10-kg child). As little as 1.5 mL (2100 mg) can kill a small child; thus, ingestion of this preparation is potentially very dangerous. (Photo contributor: Robert J. Hoffman, MD.)

preparation (ie, immediate-release vs enteric-coated). Laboratory tests should include CBC, serum electrolytes, glucose, BUN, creatinine, venous blood gases (VBG), liver transaminases, coagulation studies, serum calcium, and ketone concentrations.

A serum salicylate concentration should be obtained on presentation and every 2 hours thereafter for the first 4 to 8 hours. If the salicylate level is >30 mg/dL, obtain serial concentrations hourly until a consistent decrease is noted. Determine urinary pH in all patients and obtain a urine pregnancy test in girls of reproductive age. Abdominal radiographs may demonstrate enteric-coated tablets, concretions, or bezoars. A CXR may show acute lung injury.

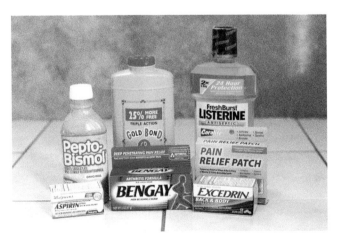

FIGURE 17.8 ■ Household Agents That Contain Salicylates. (Photo contributor: Ronak R. Shah, MD.)

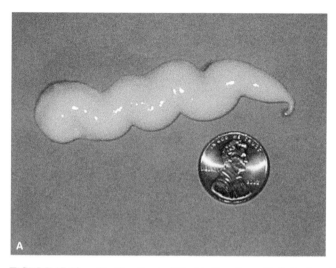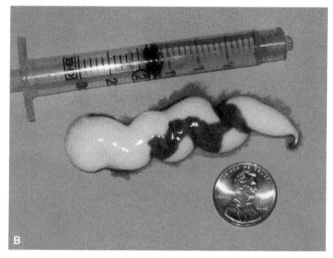

FIGURE 17.10 ■ Positive Ferric Chloride Reaction with Salicylate-Containing Topical Cream. (**A**) A 14-month-old Chinese boy was found unconscious with vomitus on floor of his grandmother's bedroom. An open tube of a topical rubefacient was also in the room, and the parents reported that the vomitus smelled like the rubefacient (a very strong, pleasant smell of wintergreen or mint). A sample of the rubefacient balm was available (most of the package label was worn off, and the remaining label, printed in Chinese, did not identify the ingredients). (**B**) Positive ferric chloride reaction. Application of ferric chloride to the product yielded a purple color (positive ferric chloride test). In its natural state, ferric chloride is translucent brown, and upon reaction with salicylate it produces a purple hue. (Photo contributor: Robert J. Hoffman, MD.)

Emergency Department Treatment and Disposition

All patients should be fluid resuscitated with IV crystalloid solution and electrolyte abnormalities corrected (eg, add potassium supplementation to IV fluids after urine output is established). In the case of GI bleeding, administer blood products such as packed RBCs.

Treat patients with large ingestions, metabolic acidosis, symptoms of severe toxicity, or serum salicylate level >70 mg/dL with an initial sodium bicarbonate bolus of 1 to 2 mEq/kg followed by a continuous infusion made from 3 ampules (44–50 mEq each) of $NaHCO_3$ in 1 L D5W and infused at 1.5 to 2 times maintenance fluid rate to alkalinize the urine (goal of urinary pH of 7.5–8.0) unless there is encephalopathy, cerebral edema, pulmonary edema, blood pH >7.55, renal failure, or serum sodium >150 mEq/L. Measure urinary pH hourly and titrate the $NaHCO_3$ infusion accordingly. Serum potassium must be closely monitored and replaced as necessary. Hypokalemia limits the ability to properly alkalinize the urine.

A nephrology consultation should be obtained, and hemodialysis is indicated for patients who are severely poisoned,

hemodynamically unstable, comatose, or seizing; who have pulmonary edema, cerebral edema, or oliguric renal failure; or who have rising salicylate levels despite GI decontamination, aggressive medical management, and proper urinary alkalinization.

In most cases, AC should be given after an acute overdose of salicylate. Multiple-dose AC (0.5–1 g/kg) may be given for an additional 1 to 2 doses. WBI should be performed if concretions are seen on abdominal x-ray or there is a history of ingestion of enteric-coated preparations. Gastric endoscopy may rarely be required for bezoar removal.

Asymptomatic patients observed for a minimum of 4 to 6 hours, with nontoxic serum salicylate levels and no significant acid-base abnormalities, should be medically cleared. Consult the local medical toxicologist, regional poison control center, psychiatry (suicidal intent), and rarely gastroenterology (possible endoscopic removal of aspirin bezoars), as indicated.

Hospitalize symptomatic patients for repeat doses of AC, urinary alkalinization, observation, hemodialysis, and supportive care.

Pearls

1. Treat patients based on clinical and metabolic abnormalities not absolute serum salicylate concentration (unless very high [>100 mg/dL]).

2. Salicylate toxicity initially causes a respiratory alkalosis that progresses to a metabolic acidosis with increased anion gap.

3. In contrast to adolescents and adults, young children present without apparent respiratory alkalosis.

4. Endotracheal intubation in salicylate-poisoned patients is harmful because of transient apnea and respiratory acidosis. If a patient is intubated, adjust ventilator settings to account for the patient's increased minute ventilation prior to intubation. Failure to manage this aspect of a patient's care may result in abrupt and rapid demise due to acute respiratory acidosis.

Clinical Summary

Iron supplements are commonly available as ferrous fumarate, ferrous gluconate, and ferrous sulfate, each containing 33%, 12%, and 20% elemental iron, respectively. Children's multivitamin tablets contain 10 to 18 mg of elemental iron per tablet; adult multivitamins contain up to 65 mg of elemental iron per tablet. To risk stratify patients following ingestion of an iron supplement, determine the amount of *elemental* iron ingested. Signs of toxicity usually begin with ingestions of >20 mg/kg.

There are 5 stages of iron toxicity commonly described. In stage I, the first 12 hours after exposure, profuse GI symptoms occur including abdominal pain, nausea, vomiting, and diarrhea (occasionally bloody). In stage II, 6 to 24 hours after ingestion, GI symptoms improve, although patients may still be ill and develop metabolic acidosis and/or hypovolemia. In stage III, 1 to 3 days after ingestion, multiorgan failure develops. Patients may develop altered mental status, renal failure, respiratory failure, and cardiovascular collapse. During stage IV, 2 to 5 days after ingestion, hepatic failure is characterized by coagulopathy and elevations in serum transaminases, ammonia, and bilirubin, as well as hypoglycemia. In stage V, some patients develop gastric outlet and small bowel obstruction 1 to 2 weeks after overdose.

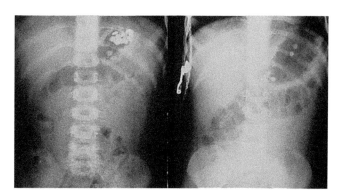

FIGURE 17.11 ■ Radiopaque Tablets in Iron Poisoning. A flat plate of abdomen shows presence of radiopaque tablets (left panel) in a 2-year-old child presenting about 1 hour after ingestion of a number of ferrous sulfate tablets. Gastric lavage was performed (whole bowel irrigation was not routinely used for GI decontamination of such cases in the past). The right panel radiograph, which was taken shortly after lavage, shows removal of almost all of the tablets. Currently, whole bowel irrigation would be the method of choice for GI decontamination in such patients. Identification of radiopaque tablets confirms diagnosis in a patient with a suspected iron overdose and helps guide gastric decontamination. (Photo contributor: James G. Linakis, PhD, MD.)

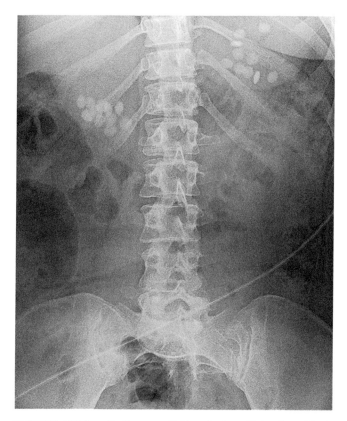

FIGURE 17.12 ■ Radiopaque Tablets in Iron Poisoning. Single frontal view of the abdomen shows multiple ingested radiopaque iron pills. This 17-year-old girl with altered mental status was found by her family with a bottle of vodka and mumbling "pills." The patient was prescribed iron supplements after a spontaneous miscarriage 2 months ago. The patient was obtunded and intubated for airway protection. After this kidney, ureters, and bladder (KUB) radiograph, whole bowel irrigation was initiated via nasogastric tube. The patient's serum iron rose as high as 350 μg/dL, but chelation therapy was initiated with deferoxamine because of an anion gap of 24, with a serum pH of 7.1, and her altered mental status. (Photo contributor: Ronak R. Shah, MD.)

Differential diagnosis includes acute GI injury (eg, poisoning by APAP, salicylates, mushrooms, heavy metals, theophylline, and NSAIDs) and acute gastroenteritis (eg, *Salmonella, Shigella,* viral). Increased anion gap metabolic acidosis from other etiologies should be considered (see Table 17.2). Consider other causes of acute hepatitis or acute surgical abdomen.

Obtain a thorough history with careful attention to amount, time of ingestion, intent, possibility of coingestants, and specific type of preparation (eg, ferrous sulfate, fumarate). Laboratory analysis should include CBC (may show anemia or leukocytosis), VBG (metabolic acidosis), electrolytes

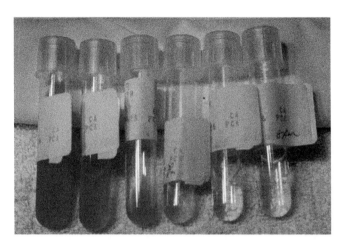

FIGURE 17.13 ■ Vin Rose Urine; Iron Poisoning. An example of the progression of coloration of vin rose urine (from excreted ferrioxamine complex) over 15 hours of chelation with deferoxamine is shown. Deferoxamine chelates only free iron (but not iron present in transferrin, hemoglobin, hemosiderin, or ferritin). (Reproduced with permission from Strange GR, Ahrens WR, Schafermeyer RW, et al. *Pediatric Emergency Medicine.* 3rd ed. McGraw-Hill Education; New York, NY, 2009.)

(increased anion gap, hyperglycemia or hypoglycemia), PT/partial thromboplastin time (PTT) (coagulopathy), transaminases, serum lactate, and a type and screen. Obtain serum iron concentrations and abdominal x-rays to check for presence of radiopaque pills and GI perforation.

Emergency Department Treatment and Disposition

If pill fragments are visualized on the kidney, ureters, and bladder (KUB) radiograph, WBI with GoLYTELY® (25 mL/kg/h up to maximum 1–2 L/h) should be initiated. AC does not adsorb iron and should not be used. Endoscopy should be used to remove adherent particles or bezoars.

For severely ill patients, initiate chelation therapy with deferoxamine mesylate as soon as possible. Indications for chelation therapy include severe GI symptoms, hypotension, shock, metabolic acidosis, or serum iron concentration >500 µg/dL. Deferoxamine should be infused slowly over 20 minutes at a dose of up to 15 mg/kg/h via continuous infusion. Infusion should be started at lower doses and titrated up if patient's clinical course does not improve or titrated down if patient develops hypotension or ARDS. Monitor BP; if hypotension occurs, decrease the infusion rate or temporarily stop the infusion.

Consult with the local medical toxicologist or regional poison control center, psychiatry, and gastroenterology as needed.

Asymptomatic patients should be discharged 6 hours after ingestion provided there is no clinical evidence of iron toxicity (eg, vomiting), the serum iron level is <500 µg/mL, and psychiatry consultation has been provided for patients with intentional self-harm.

All other patients should be admitted to the hospital. Patients with persistent vomiting, shock, lethargy, GI bleed, or metabolic acidosis should be admitted to the ICU.

Pearls

1. Do not use declining serum iron concentrations as a sign of clinical improvement or response to therapy as this may reflect iron uptake into cells.

2. Serum iron measurement is unreliable in patients receiving deferoxamine.

3. Antidotal treatment should *not* be delayed while awaiting serum iron concentrations or other laboratory tests in patients who are severely ill; iron poisoning is classically a clinical diagnosis.

Clinical Summary

Opioids are found in many forms including morphine, meperidine, codeine, oxycodone, methadone, hydromorphone, buprenorphine, and fentanyl as well as street drugs such as heroin. Opioid use is ubiquitous and has increased to epidemic proportions; thus, opioid toxicity is a common occurrence in the ED. Less common scenarios are "body packing" and "body stuffing." "Body packing" is intentional transport of opioids inside a body cavity and is accomplished via ingestion of drug packets wrapped in condoms, latex, or tape. Generally, packets have multiple layers to prevent leakage. "Body stuffing" implies haphazard ingestion of contraband and is usually without layers or intent to prevent leakage.

Therapeutic and toxic doses of opioids vary, as does individual tolerance. Toxicity is affected by coingestants, especially those that cause CNS depression (eg, alcohol, benzodiazepines).

Opioid toxicity is characterized by CNS depression, miosis, and respiratory depression. Other CNS signs may include seizures due to hypoxia and coma. GI involvement typically

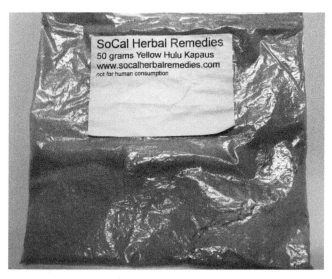

FIGURE 17.15 ■ Kratom Powder. Kratom powder purchased from the Internet. Kratom is a tropical tree (*Mitragyna speciosa*) native to Southeast Asia that possesses both opioid-like and stimulant effects. Kratom is being used for abuse purposes as well as to self-treat opioid withdrawal. Currently, it is legal for purchase in some states in the United States, whereas others have banned its sale. (Photo contributor: Mark K. Su, MD, MPH.)

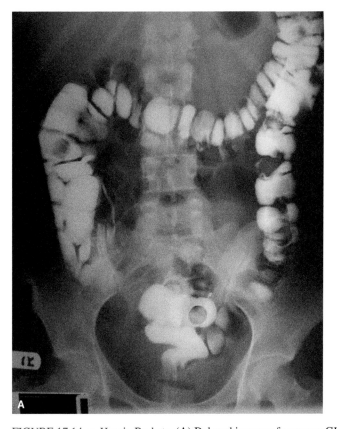

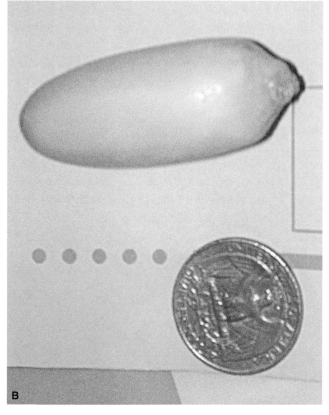

FIGURE 17.14 ■ Heroin Packets. (**A**) Delayed images of an upper GI series showing multiple filling defects within contrast-filled loops of large bowel (seen in the rectum and just below the hepatic flexure). Subsequently, these packets were found to contain heroin. (**B**) Heroin packet recovered from a "mule" or "body packer." (Photo contributor: Mark K. Su, MD, MPH.)

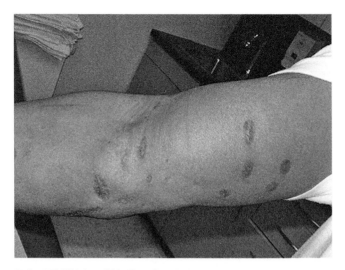

FIGURE 17.16 ■ Skin Popping. This habitual drug user bears the scars of his addiction. The large erosions in his arm are due to "skin popping," which is typically done using cocaine or heroin. It is when the user injects the drug directly under the skin instead of into a vein. This route of administration may result in prolonged duration of effect and the user does not have to find a vein, which often is difficult. (Photo contributor: Mark Silverberg, MD.)

is associated with decreased motility and constipation with chronic use. Following overdose, patients typically have hypotension or bradycardia and, in some cases, hypoxia due to the development of acute lung injury.

TABLE 17.4 ■ COMPARISON OF OPIOID AND SEDATIVE-HYPNOTIC TOXICITY

	Opioids	Sedative-Hypnotics
Vital signs	Bradypnea, bradycardia, hypotension, hypothermia	Bradypnea, bradycardia, hypotension, hypothermia
Pupils	Miosis (except meperidine)	Mydriasis, miosis (early)
CNS	Lethargy to coma	Coma, nystagmus, ataxia
Other	Acute lung injury, track marks	Bullae
Antidote	Naloxone	Flumazenil (for benzodiazepines only)

Reproduced with permission from Finberg L, Kleinman RE. *Saunders Manual of Pediatric Practice.* WB Saunders; Philadelphia, PA, 2002.

Differential diagnosis includes altered mental status (see mnemonic COMATOSE PATIENT, Table 13.5) and miosis from other etiologies.

Obtain a thorough history with careful attention to amount, time of ingestion, intent, and possibility of coingestions. Laboratory analysis is not typically needed unless there is concern for coingestions. An ABG may be useful in patients with hypoxia or hypoventilation. CXR may be performed to evaluate for aspiration or acute lung injury.

Emergency Department Treatment and Disposition

AC adsorbs orally ingested opioids and can be used for GI decontamination. Consider multiple-dose AC for body packers. Use WBI with polyethylene glycol (25 mL/kg/h up to maximum 1–2 L/h) for asymptomatic body packers and extended-release preparations.

Airway and respiratory support are essential. Naloxone causes immediate reversal of CNS and respiratory depression and is given IV, intramuscularly (IM), subcutaneously, and sublingually. In children, the initial dose of naloxone is 0.01 mg/kg IV, and the dose may be repeated up to a total of 10 mg. Failure to respond to 10 mg of naloxone reliably excludes opioids as the cause of respiratory depression. Judicious use of naloxone is not associated with significant side effects except acute opioid withdrawal, which is generally not acutely life threatening. However, in opioid-dependent neonates, acute opioid withdrawal may be associated with significant toxicity including seizures.

Patients with prolonged duration of opioid toxicity should be admitted. Admission to the ICU for continuous monitoring is indicated for patients with persistent altered mental status, recurrent respiratory depression, or hypoxia, or if additional naloxone is necessary. Older patients may be discharged from the ED if they are asymptomatic after 6 hours of observation and have been evaluated by psychiatry (if indicated). All body packers should be admitted to the hospital until all packets are eliminated from the body.

Consult medical toxicology, poison control center, psychiatry (intentional ingestion), and, for body packers, gastroenterologist and/or surgery.

Pearls

1. Naloxone is generally effective for 30 to 60 minutes; many opioids exert their effects for a longer time. Patients should be observed for more than 90 minutes; in case of reoccurrence of CNS or respiratory depression, naloxone should be readministered.
2. Children may have unusual sensitivity to opioids and can display signs of toxicity at therapeutic doses.
3. Maintain a high index of suspicion for aspirin and APAP, which are often present in combination with opioids.
4. For chronic opioid users, start with small doses of naloxone for diagnostic and therapeutic purposes to decrease the likelihood of acute withdrawal. Excessive naloxone administration may result in withdrawal symptoms refractory to supportive care.
5. Body packers may place packets containing contraband in the ears, vagina, or rectum. Careful inspection of all body cavities is warranted.
6. Opioid toxicity due to synthetic opioids (eg, fentanyl) may require higher doses of naloxone.

Clinical Summary

Cocaine is most often used via nasal insufflation and intra-venously or, in its "freebase" or "crack" form, smoked and inhaled through the lungs. Inhalational and IV routes have peak effect within 5 minutes, whereas insufflation produces a peak in 20 minutes. Although short lived, rapid, intense euphoria is the usual impetus for recreational cocaine use.

Cocaine causes multisystem symptoms including tachy-cardia, hyperthermia, and hypertension. Head/neck examina-tion may reveal mydriasis or nasal septal perforation. Cardiac effects include acute myocardial ischemia, aortic dissection, fatal dysrhythmias, and cardiac arrest. Chronic use may lead to congestive heart failure, myocarditis, or dilated cardiomy-opathy. Pulmonary signs include wheezing pneumothorax, pneumomediastinum, or pulmonary edema. Bowel ischemia and infarction are caused by splanchnic vasospasm. Patients may develop acute kidney injury because of renal infarction or rhabdomyolysis. Neurologic effects include agitation, seizures, intracerebral hemorrhage, or infarction. Acute cocaine toxicity can be indistinguishable from acute psychiatric disease.

Cocaine washout syndrome refers to persistent lethargy and altered mental status following repeated use over a short period caused by depletion of CNS catecholamines. This con-dition manifests as a depressed mental status or coma. The patient's condition usually improves over several hours with supportive care.

The differential diagnosis includes toxicity from other stimulants (eg, amphetamines, synthetic cathinones), oral decongestants, thyroid hormone, and β-adrenergic agents (eg, clenbuterol), neuroleptic malignant syndrome, malignant hyperthermia, and serotonin syndrome present similarly to acute cocaine toxicity but are typically noted to have muscu-lar rigidity, hyperthermia, and altered mental status. Nontoxi-cologic etiologies in the differential include hypoglycemia, pheochromocytoma, hyperthyroidism, alcohol or sedative-hypnotic withdrawal, and acute psychosis.

Obtain a thorough history with careful attention to amount, time of ingestion, intent, and possibility of coingestants. Use serum chemistries, BUN, creatinine, and glucose to evaluate for alternative causes of altered mental status or seizures and to assess for dehydration and renal function. Obtain an ECG and CXR in patients with chest pain. Abdominal radiographs may help evaluate for body packing/stuffing. Brain CT is use-ful to assess for intracerebral hemorrhage or infarction. If

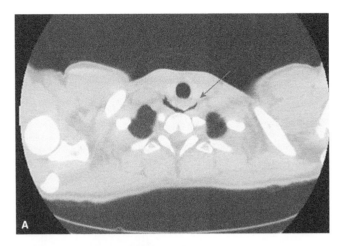

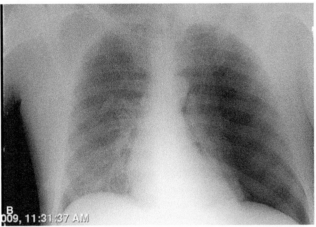

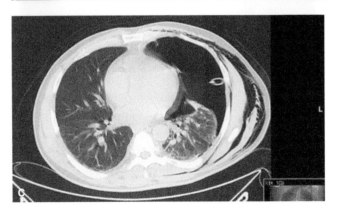

FIGURE 17.17 ■ Pulmonary Complications Related to Crack Cocaine Inhalation. (**A**) Forceful inhalation may be associated with complications including acute respiratory distress syndrome, pneu-monitis, pneumothorax, or pneumomediastinum. A chest CT shows pneumomediastinum (arrow) in a 17-year-old boy who presented with severe chest pain after smoking crack cocaine. (**B, C**) Left pneu-mothorax is seen in a different patient on chest radiograph and CT after smoking crack cocaine. (Photo/legend contributors: Mark K. Su, MD, MPH [A], Anika Backster, MD [B, C], and John Amodio, MD.)

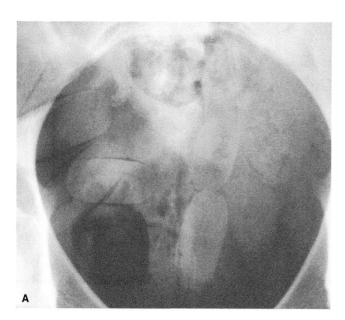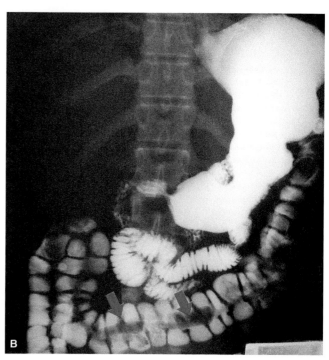

FIGURE 17.18 ■ Body Packing. (**A**) Radiopaque packets seen with body packing. Magnified frontal projection of pelvis reveals multiple well-defined radiopaque densities within the pelvic bowel loops. Note the air around some of the packets implying that packets were not tightly sealed. There is a risk of spontaneous perforation of such packets. This asymptomatic adolescent male was arrested at the airport as a suspected mule and brought to the ED. Whole bowel irrigation was performed, and analysis of these packets showed cocaine. (**B**) Cocaine packets. Single frontal view of abdomen after barium ingestion demonstrates tubular filling defects (arrows) in mid transverse colon compatible with ingested packets. Severe toxicity may result if packet ruptures. (Photo contributors: Mark K. Su, MD, MPH [A], and Mark Silverberg, MD [B].)

there is suspicion for subarachnoid hemorrhage and the brain CT is negative, lumbar puncture should be performed. Creatine kinase will be elevated in the setting of rhabdomyolysis. In patients with severe hyperthermia, elevated serum transaminases and coagulopathy may occur. Serum troponin may be elevated if patient develops myocardial ischemia or infarction. Obtain serum aspirin, APAP, and urine drug screens to evaluate for coingestants if there is a suspicion of intentional self-harm.

Emergency Department Treatment and Disposition

Stabilize ABCs. GI decontamination is not recommended because ingestion is rare except in the case of body packing/stuffing. Management is primarily supportive and includes management of hypertension, psychomotor agitation, hyperthermia, seizures, pneumothorax, cardiac dysrhythmias, cerebral infarction, intracerebral hemorrhage, pulmonary edema, and rhabdomyolysis. Aggressive IV hydration may help prevent renal impairment due to rhabdomyolysis. Treat myocardial ischemia or infarction with oxygen, nitrates, and aspirin, and avoid β-blockers. Use phentolamine or IV nitrates to manage acute severe hypertension and sodium bicarbonate and lidocaine for cardiac dysrhythmias. Admit patients with symptoms that do not resolve quickly, severe toxicity, or serious sequelae of cocaine intoxication. All patients presenting with myocardial ischemia, hyperthermia, intracranial hemorrhage, or severe agitation should be admitted to the ICU for monitoring and management. Patients with mild toxicity may be discharged on clinical improvement and referred for drug counseling.

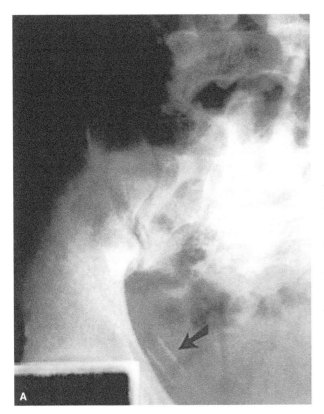 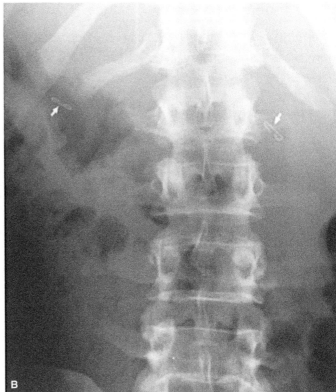

FIGURE 17.19 ▪ Two "Body Stuffers." Radiography infrequently helps with the diagnosis. (**A**) An ingested glass crack vial is seen in the distal bowel (arrow). The patient had ingested his contraband several hours earlier at the time of a police raid. Only the tubular-shaped container, and not the xenobiotic, is visible radiographically. The patient did not develop signs of cocaine intoxication during 24 hours of observation. (**B**) Another patient in police custody was brought to the ED for allegedly ingesting his drugs. The patient repeatedly denied this. The radiographs revealed "nonsurgical" staples in his abdomen (arrows). When questioned again, the patient admitted that he had swallowed several plastic bags that were stapled closed. (Reproduced with permission from Nelson LS, Hoffman RS, Howland MA, et al. *Goldfrank's Toxicologic Emergencies*. 11th ed. McGraw-Hill Education; New York, NY, 2019. Photo contributor: The Fellowship in Medical Toxicology, New York University School of Medicine, New York City Poison Center.)

Pearls

1. β-Blockers used alone to control heart rate or elevated BP due to cocaine intoxication should be avoided, if possible; these agents could exacerbate cocaine-induced coronary vasospasm and result in severely elevated BP.

2. Do not use haloperidol to control agitation of suspected cocaine intoxication because it can impair heat dissipation and may cause extrapyramidal side effects.

3. Benzodiazepines are the treatment of choice for psychomotor agitation, hyperthermia, seizures, tachycardia, and hypertension.

4. Asymptomatic cocaine body packers may be treated with WBI. Symptomatic body packers who have signs of cocaine leakage (eg, abdominal pain, tachycardia) require immediate surgical intervention. Body stuffers usually do well with administration of activated charcoal and supportive care.

METHEMOGLOBINEMIA

Clinical Summary

Methemoglobin (MetHb) is hemoglobin in which the normally reduced ferrous ion (Fe^{2+}) is oxidized to the ferric form (Fe^{3+}), preventing binding of oxygen (O_2) to the abnormal hemoglobin (Hgb) and impairing O_2 unloading by normal Hgb. Thus, symptoms of methemoglobinemia are related to decreased O_2 delivery to the tissues. Serum MetHb concentration >3% is termed *methemoglobinemia* and usually occurs in the setting of oxidative stress (eg, sepsis, toxins, or drugs such as nitrates, topical anesthetics, aniline dyes, quinine, sulfonamides, hydrocarbons, and food additives containing nitrites or nitrates).

Clinically, patients present with signs and symptoms of tissue hypoxia, including tachycardia, tachypnea, hypotension, cardiac dysrhythmias, cardiac arrest, dyspnea, nausea, vomiting, lethargy, confusion, coma, seizures, and persistent cyanosis despite supplemental O_2 therapy. Phlebotomy may show the pathognomonic sign of *chocolate brown blood*. Pulse oximetry readings are usually decreased, with O_2 saturation readings characteristically around 85%.

Differential diagnosis includes CO poisoning (although patients are not typically cyanotic), sulfhemoglobinemia, and cardiac/pulmonary causes of cyanosis.

Obtain a thorough history with careful attention to amount, time of ingestion, intent, and possibility of coingestants. Consider underlying conditions that increase risk for methemoglobinemia. Obtain ABG with co-oximetry. ABG will give disparate O_2 saturation compared to the pulse oximeter because the ABG O_2 saturation is based on the amount of dissolved O_2 in blood, whereas co-oximetry quantifies alternative Hgbs such as MetHb and carboxyhemoglobin. Pulse oximetry assesses the ratio of oxyhemoglobin to deoxyhemoglobin only and will usually be decreased. The difference in O_2 saturation between ABG and pulse oximetry is referred to as the *saturation gap*. A CBC should be obtained to evaluate for anemia, especially if hemolysis is suspected. (Occasionally, agents that are associated with methemoglobinemia may cause hemolysis) Serum chemistry aids in evaluating acid-base status because patients may have an increased anion gap metabolic acidosis.

Emergency Department Treatment and Disposition

Stabilize ABCs and begin decontamination immediately. GI decontamination remains controversial, but most children can be administered 1 dose of AC (dose: 1–2 g/kg) if there are no contraindications.

Severity of symptoms correlates with serum MetHb concentrations. A MetHb concentration >50% is considered severe, and a concentration >70% is potentially fatal. Treat all symptomatic patients and any with a MetHb concentration

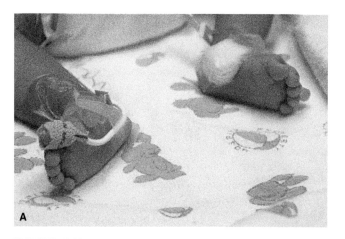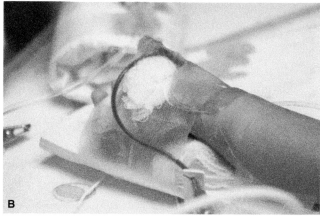

FIGURE 17.20 ■ Methemoglobinemia. (**A**) An infant presenting with dusky discoloration of the entire body. He presented with hypovolemic shock due to acute gastroenteritis and methemoglobinemia. Infants with diarrhea may develop methemoglobinemia without any exogenous toxic exposures. His arterial blood gases while receiving 100% oxygen by nasal cannula showed the following: pH 7.176, PaO_2 271.4 mmHg, PCO_2 19.7 mm Hg, O_2 saturation 100%, HCO_3 7 mmol/L, and BE 20 mmol/L, and the MetHb value was 27.6%. (**B**) Blood containing MetHb has a distinct chocolate-brown color and provides an important clue to the diagnosis. Arterial blood from the patient is shown. (Photo contributor: Irma Fiordalisi, MD.)

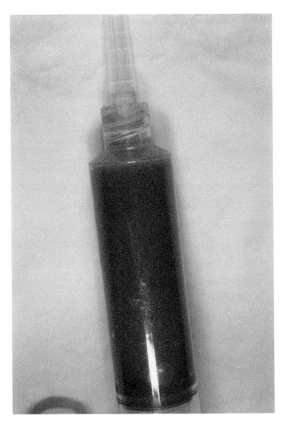

FIGURE 17.21 ■ Chocolate-Colored Blood in Methemoglobinemia. A 23-day-old neonate presenting with hypovolemic shock with methemoglobinemia also had chocolate-brown blood as shown here. His MetHb value was 40.2%, and arterial blood gases showed pH of 7.02 with severe metabolic acidosis (HCO₃ of 2.8 mmol/L and BE 26.7 mmol/L). He was resuscitated with IV fluids followed by IV methylene blue. This was followed by an immediate marked improvement in cyanosis, metabolic acidosis, and peripheral perfusion. (Photo contributor: Ronak Shah, MD.)

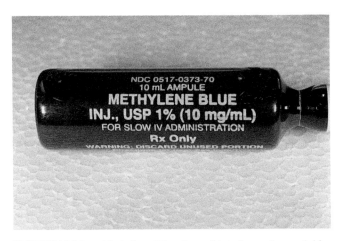

FIGURE 17.22 ■ Methylene Blue. An antidote for methemoglobinemia is available as 1% methylene blue (10 mg/mL) for IV administration. (Photo contributor: Ronak R. Shah, MD.)

of >20% with an initial dose of methylene blue 1 to 2 mg/kg IV over 5 minutes. If clinical improvement is not seen within 1 hour, repeat serum MetHb measurement and repeat dose of methylene blue to a maximum of 7 mg/kg over 3 hours. In patients with glucose-6-phosphate dehydrogenase (G6PD) deficiency or known NADPH-MetHb reductase deficiency, methylene blue may not be effective or may precipitate hemolysis. Although it has been effectively used in these patients, it should be used with caution and awareness of possible adverse effects. Consider hyperbaric O_2 or exchange transfusion in patients who do not respond to methylene blue or have MetHb concentration >70%. Use caution when administering repeated doses because methylene blue is a weak oxidant that may induce methemoglobinemia at higher concentrations.

All patients (especially infants and young children) who receive therapy with methylene blue should be admitted to an ICU for continuous monitoring and supportive care. Consult medical toxicology, poison control center, and hematology for evaluation of underlying conditions that may predispose to development of methemoglobinemia.

Pearls

1. Methemoglobinemia may present with profound cyanosis with minimal symptoms.
2. Methemoglobinemia should be suspected in patients *with cyanosis despite a normal Po_2 determination from ABG or cyanosis unresponsive to supplemental O_2 therapy.*
3. Pulse oximetry and standard ABG analysis give disparate O_2 saturation. A blood gas with co-oximetry must be obtained to determine the presence of MetHb.
4. Neonates are at risk of developing methemoglobinemia because of lower levels of NADPH-MetHb reductase and the presence of fetal Hgb, which is more readily oxidized than adult Hgb.
5. Methylene blue may cause hemolysis, methemoglobinemia, and a significant decrease in O_2 saturation on pulse oximetry, especially in patients predisposed to methemoglobinemia (eg, G6PD deficiency, NADPH-MetHb reductase deficiency).
6. Sulfhemoglobinemia results in falsely elevated MetHb levels. Suspect sulfhemoglobinemia in cyanotic patients who do not respond to O_2 therapy or who fail to improve after treatment with methylene blue.

ORGANOPHOSPHATE AND CARBAMATE INSECTICIDE TOXICITY

Clinical Summary

Organophosphate and carbamate exposures usually occur as unsupervised ingestion of pesticides, malathion (used to treat head lice), or medications such pyridostigmine or neostigmine (used to treat myasthenia gravis). The highly toxic nerve agents sarin, soman, and tabun are organophosphates.

Organophosphates bind to the active site of acetylcholinesterase and inactivate it, leading to postsynaptic excitation. Carbamate toxicity is similar to that of organophosphate toxicity, but it is generally reversible and of shorter duration and usually less severe than organophosphate toxicity. However, there are exceptions, including medicinal carbamates such as physostigmine (antidote for anticholinergic toxicity) and the cyclic antidepressant donepezil (treatment for Alzheimer disease). These agents readily cross the blood–brain barrier and have a long half-life.

The severity and extent of toxicity are dependent on the specific agent, dose, and route of exposure. Inhalation leads to rapid symptomatology (within as little as 5 minutes), whereas effects after skin absorption may be prolonged or delayed. Agents with higher lipid solubility are likely to produce delayed, prolonged, or cyclical toxicity.

The major clinical presentation of these agents occurs from hyperactivity of the parasympathetic nervous system, leading to the classic DUMBELS symptoms (see mnemonic; Table 17.2). Nicotinic receptor activation will result in autonomic instability, and neuromuscular junction hyperactivity manifests as twitching, weakness, ineffectual muscle contraction, and ultimately, paralysis. The CNS effects are confusion, coma, seizures, ataxia, and respiratory depression.

An *intermediate syndrome* is reported to develop 1 to 4 days following acute organophosphate poisoning despite therapy with atropine and oximes (eg, pralidoxime). Signs and symptoms include cranial nerve palsies, nuchal weakness, acute respiratory paralysis, proximal limb weakness, and depressed reflexes. This occurs more commonly with organophosphates that are highly fat soluble and may last up to 15 days; most patients have a full recovery. Delayed peripheral neuropathy may develop 1 to 3 weeks after organophosphate exposure and causes a distal flaccid paralysis with variable recovery (months to years) but that may be permanent.

Differential diagnosis includes other direct-acting cholinergic agents (eg, pilocarpine producing identical symptomatology), nicotine poisoning (symptoms of nicotinic receptor hyperactivity), opioid toxicity, muscarine-containing mushrooms, and bradycardia from other drugs (eg, digitalis). Nontoxicologic causes of acute neuromuscular weakness include Eaton-Lambert syndrome and myasthenia gravis.

History should focus on the agent, amount, time, and route of exposure. Physical examination should focus on vital signs, with careful attention to cardiovascular and neuromuscular status, respiratory effort, and motor strength. Note the amount of respiratory secretions, presence of garlic odor, fever, tenesmus, blurry vision, heart block, or cardiac dysrhythmias. CBC findings include leukocytosis with a normal differential and hemoconcentration due to fluid loss. Serum

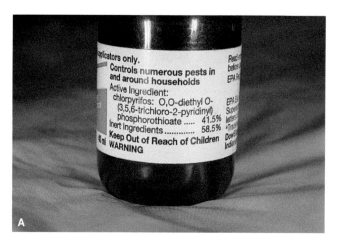

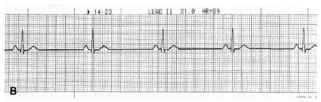

FIGURE 17.23 ■ Organophosphate Insecticide Toxicity. (**A**) A 10-year-old boy presented with lethargy and numerous episodes of vomiting that started shortly after receiving a liquid preparation thought to be cough syrup (given by grandmother). Actually what he received was a commercial pesticide containing chlorpyrifos and "inert" ingredients (pesticides contain hydrocarbon solvent carriers such as petroleum distillates and aromatic hydrocarbons as "inert" ingredients. The hydrocarbon diluent may contribute to the overall picture of toxicity). (**B**) The patient had bradycardia, increased salivation, and bilateral diffuse rales with wheezing and miosis. Gastric lavage contents gave a petroleum-like odor. A total of 16 doses of atropine within the first 6 hours were required to remain free of respiratory secretions. Two hours after arrival to ED, he also became disoriented and developed tongue fasciculations. He was started on pralidoxime. Both atropine and pralidoxime were continued for the next 36 hours until he was fully oriented with an absence of any respiratory secretions. (Photo contributor: Ronak R. Shah, MD.)

electrolytes may show an increased anion gap, hyperglycemia, hypokalemia, hypomagnesemia, and prerenal azotemia. A blood gas may show metabolic acidosis. If the exposure is intentional, serum APAP and salicylate levels should also be obtained on presentation.

Emergency Department Treatment and Disposition

Decontamination is of the utmost importance to prevent further toxicity and protect the health care providers. Remove the patient's clothes, and wash all exposed surfaces thoroughly. Universal precautions to prevent transdermal absorption of toxins by health care providers are essential.

Stabilize ABCs and treat pulmonary edema, respiratory distress, altered mental status, and hypotension as indicated. If a patient presents soon after an overdose and has not vomited yet, gastric lavage should be performed for large overdoses.

Atropine and pralidoxime are specific antidotes. For all patients with signs of muscarinic excess (eg, bronchorrhea, bronchospasm, or bradycardia), give atropine 0.05 mg/kg IV (adult dose is 2–5 mg; minimum dose of 0.1 mg in children), and repeat as needed every 5 to 15 minutes until pulmonary and oral secretions are controlled. After atropine administration, pralidoxime (treats both muscarinic and nicotine toxicity) may be given as an IV bolus of 25 mg/kg (up to 1 g) over 30 minutes. If fasciculations continue, repeat the dose of pralidoxime after 1 hour, and then every 6 to 12 hours over the subsequent 48 hours as needed. Alternatively, after initial bolus, pralidoxime may be given as a continuous IV infusion at 10 to 20 mg/kg/h. Effects are usually seen within the first 10 minutes of administration.

Admit all patients with significant symptoms or with evolving toxicity. Most patients should be admitted to the ICU for close observation and monitoring of CNS and cardiopulmonary status. Asymptomatic patients with unintentional exposures may be discharged home after a 6-hour observation period. However, some organophosphates may present with delayed toxicity, especially if the route of exposure was dermal.

Pearls

1. Paralytic agents administered therapeutically for intubation may have an increased duration of action when combined with organophosphates and carbamates.
2. When death occurs, it is usually from respiratory failure; endotracheal intubation and mechanical ventilation may be necessary early in the course of treatment if there are significant respiratory symptoms.
3. Atropine should be given until the drying of secretions is noted and should *not* be titrated to tachycardia or mydriasis.
4. Symptoms vary greatly; nerve agents may present with predominant nicotinic and CNS effects rather than muscarinic effects.
5. Atropine and pralidoxime given together have synergistic effects against signs and symptoms of cholinesterase inhibition, thus decreasing atropine requirements.
6. Although atropine alone is usually adequate for carbamate toxicity, pralidoxime should also be given when there is uncertainty about the agent involved (organophosphate and carbamate toxicity may be indistinguishable) and the patient's symptoms are severe.
7. Give pralidoxime only after atropine (faster onset of action).

CASTOR BEAN AND ROSARY PEA INGESTION

Clinical Summary

Castor beans are found in the fruit of *Ricinus communis*, a large, leafy plant that may be green or red, and are hard and shiny with grey and brown streaks. Rosary peas (also called jequirity pea, crab's eye, Buddhist's rosary bead, and prayer bead) are found in the fruit of *Abrus precatorius*, a high-climbing, woody, green vine found in India, Florida, and the Caribbean. Rosary peas are hard and may be bright red with a black center, black with a white center, or white with a black center. Castor beans and rosary peas are used in jewelry and toys. *R communis* is also the source of castor oil, used as a purgative and as a lubricant for engines. Ricin and abrin are found within the seeds and are extremely potent toxins. Toxicity occurs when the seed casing is broken via chewing or digestion and there is subsequent GI absorption. Fortunately, toxicity is usually limited by poor GI absorption of the seed if it isn't chewed or broken into smaller pieces.

Although toxicity via ingestion is rare, if toxicity does occur, patients usually present 2 to 48 hours after ingestion with abdominal pain with bloody vomiting and diarrhea. Acutely poisoned patients have tachycardia, hypotension, cardiac dysrhythmias, CNS depression, seizures, and sometimes, cerebral edema. Multiorgan injury typically occurs after 24 hours, and hepatic failure, acute kidney injury, lethargy, stupor, and death can occur.

Differential diagnosis includes organophosphates and other cholinergic agents, toxins that cause seizures (see CAMPHOR BALLS; Table 17.2) or CNS depression, and infectious gastroenteritis.

Obtain a careful history, including identification and number of seeds ingested if observed and the timing of ingestion. Ask patients if they chewed the seed and analyze symptoms occurring after ingestion. Physical examination should focus on vital signs, mental status, and proper evaluation of the abdomen. Obtain CBC and type and screen in any patient with GI hemorrhage and to assess for possible hemolytic anemia. Coagulation studies may be abnormal, and serum chemistries may show elevated BUN and creatinine suggestive of dehydration or renal injury.

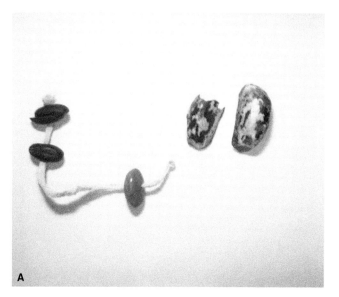 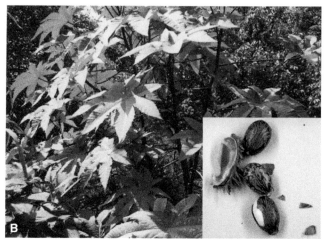

FIGURE 17.24 ■ Bracelet Made with Castor Bean Seeds. (**A**) One of the seeds from this bracelet was chewed and eaten by an infant presenting with lip swelling and new onset of wheezing shortly after chewing the seed. He was readmitted with anaphylaxis (hypotension, angioedema, and wheezing) about 2 weeks after the first admission, again after chewing the seeds from a necklace that was also made of castor beans (purchased with this bracelet as a matching set). Allergic reactions are well recognized and reproducible with patch testing. The castor plant flourishes in warm climates, including the southwestern United States and Mexico. It produces clusters of pods containing seeds. Castor bean seeds are almond-sized and glossy with a mottled black, dark brown, gray, and white coating. (**B**) The castor bean plant. The seedpods come in bunches, 2 of which appear near the center of the image. Each seedpod typically contains 3 seeds. Inset: Castor beans (*Ricinus communis*), which contain the toxalbumin ricin. By interfering with protein synthesis, ricin may cause multiorgan system failure when administered parenterally. However, its oral absorption is poor, and most oral ingestions cause gastroenteritis. (Photo contributor: Ronak R. Shah, MD [A], and [B] Reproduced with permission from Hoffman RS, Howland M, Lewin NA, et al. *Goldfrank's Toxicologic Emergencies*. 10th ed. McGraw-Hill Education; New York, NY, 2015.)

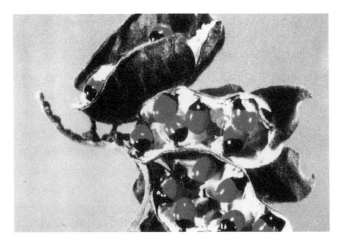

FIGURE 17.25 ■ Rosary Pea (*Abrus precatorius*). The fruit is a pea-shaped pod approximately 4 cm in length. When opened and dried, 3 to 5 scarlet pea-sized seeds with a small black spot at the point of attachment are found. As shown, these seeds are glossy and colored bright red and black. The rosary pea contains the toxalbumin abrin. *A precatorius* has many common names including jequirity pea, rosary pea, Indian bean, Buddhist's rosary bead, prayer bead, and crab's eye. It thrives in the tropical climates of South and Central America, the Caribbean, and Florida. (Reproduced with permission from Goldfrank LR, Lewin NA, Flomenbam NE, et al. In: *Goldfrank's Toxicologic Emergencies*. 6th ed. McGraw-Hill Education; New York, NY, 1998.)

Emergency Department Treatment and Disposition

Stabilize ABCs, and treat hypovolemic shock, seizures, CNS depression, and cerebral edema. No antidote exists; treatment is supportive. Initiate aggressive fluid resuscitation in all hypovolemic patients. GI decontamination is accomplished with AC for most patients; if symptomatic, gastric lavage and/or WBI should be performed to decrease the gut burden.

Admit all symptomatic patients for observation and supportive care. Asymptomatic patients may be safely discharged after a period of observation of at least 6 hours.

Pearls

1. Toxicity occurs when seeds are chewed rather than when ingested whole.
2. All patients who have ingested rosary peas or castor beans should be observed for the possible development of toxicity.

Clinical Summary

Phenothiazines (eg, prochlorperazine, chlorpromazine, thioridazine), historically called *neuroleptics,* are commonly prescribed as antiemetics, antipsychotics, and anxiolytics.

Extrapyramidal side effects such as dystonia, akathisia, parkinsonism, or tardive dyskinesia result from these agents in both acute and chronic ingestions. Symptoms may be delayed up to 24 hours after ingestion, and patients are usually awake, alert, and aware of their symptoms. Dystonic reactions manifest as oculogyric crisis, torticollis, opisthotonos, trismus, difficulty speaking, facial grimacing, or chorea-like movements. In akathisia, typically seen 5 to 60 days after starting neuroleptic therapy, there is extreme restlessness or the feeling that the "body wants to jump out of its skin." Parkinsonism, typically seen 2 to 3 months after starting neuroleptic therapy, includes resting tremor, bradykinesia, a shuffling gait, or mask-like facies. Tardive dyskinesia develops months to years following initiation of antipsychotic therapy and is the only extrapyramidal symptom that is associated with long-term use of these agents It involves involuntary bucco-linguo-masticatory movements and choreo-athetoid movements. In neuroleptic malignant syndrome, an idiosyncratic and potentially life-threatening reaction to antipsychotic therapy, there is hyperthermia, muscular rigidity, autonomic instability, and altered mental status ranging from extreme confusion to catatonia. Altered mental status is almost always seen. In large overdoses (specifically with thioridazine and mesoridazine), seizures and cardiac dysrhythmias are reported to occur.

Phenothiazines also have anticholinergic properties, so tachycardia, hypertension, and hyperthermia may occur (the classic toxidrome is described as "Red as a Beet, Dry as a Bone, Mad as a Hatter, Hot as a Hare, and Blind as a Bat"). Urinary retention may also occur (anticholinergic effects). Cardiac conduction effects, including QT prolongation, QRS widening, atrioventricular (AV) block, or fatal dysrhythmias, are reported with thioridazine and mesoridazine. Adverse GI effects associated with chronic uses include constipation, ileus, and cholestatic or hepatocellular jaundice. Rarely, hematologic effects of anemia or agranulocytosis are seen.

Differential diagnosis of phenothiazine toxicity includes medical causes of altered mental status such as meningitis, intracranial hemorrhage, and cerebral ischemia. Other causes of cardiac conduction abnormalities include electrolyte disturbances, myocardial ischemia, cyclic antidepressants, and toxicity from other type Ia antidysrhythmics (eg, diphenhydramine).

Obtain a focused history on agent involved, dose, time of ingestion, chronicity of ingestion, and intent. Perform a physical

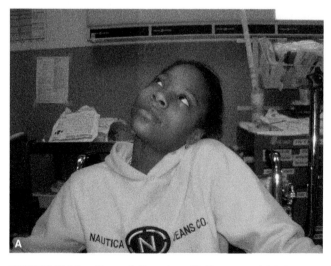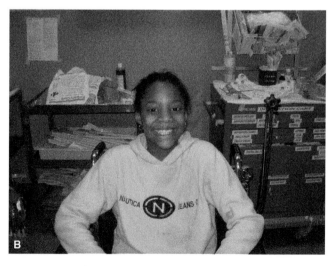

FIGURE 17.26 ■ Dystonic Reaction. (**A**) Extrapyramidal signs seen here such as torticollis, inability to speak, and trismus were the presenting complaints in this girl who was brought to the ED from the school, and there was no history available. Based on her clinical findings, phenothiazine toxicity was suspected. (**B**) Dramatic improvement after IV diphenhydramine. Extrapyramidal signs are very frightening to caregivers (especially in a previously healthy child without any history of ingestion), and following the dramatic improvement, treating physicians are often lauded as heroes. Subsequently, we learned that this patient's uncle was receiving mesoridazine for anxiety, and the patient confessed to taking her uncle's medication. (Photo contributor: Mark Silverberg, MD.)

examination focusing on vital signs, including orthostatic BP and cardiovascular and neurologic status. Order serum chemistries, liver function tests (may show transaminitis or increased bilirubin), creatine kinase (elevated in rhabdomyolysis), and urinalysis (red, pink, purple, orange, or rust colored). Abdominal radiographs may show radiopaque phenothiazine tablets.

Consult medical toxicology or regional poison control center as needed. Consult psychiatry in cases of intentional overdose or for patients taking phenothiazines for psychiatric disorders.

Emergency Department Treatment and Disposition

Treatment begins with stabilization of ABCs. Treat cardiac dysrhythmias such as QRS widening >100 milliseconds with IV bolus of NaHCO$_3$ (1–2 mEq/kg) until QRS interval narrows; this may be repeated once. NaHCO$_3$ may exacerbate QT prolongation by causing hypokalemia. Acid-base status should be assessed by frequent blood gases to monitor serum pH; it should not exceed 7.55. Continuous cardiac monitoring should be done. Treat seizures with benzodiazepines. Accomplish GI decontamination with gastric lavage and AC for large or recent ingestions.

Treat acute dystonic reactions with diphenhydramine 1 mg/kg IV or IM or benztropine 0.5 to 2.0 mg IV or IM. Treat akathisia and drug-induced parkinsonism with anticholinergic agents (diphenhydramine or benztropine) and benzodiazepines. Tardive dyskinesia is usually irreversible but may respond to changing the dose of the antipsychotic agent or discontinuation. Treatment of neuroleptic malignant syndrome includes rapid cooling and pharmacologic agents such as benzodiazepines and dopamine agonists such as bromocriptine and amantadine.

Admit all symptomatic patients presenting with acute overdose unless symptoms are minor and last <6 hours. Admit patients with cardiovascular instability or CNS depression to the ICU. Even though patients with acute dystonic reactions may respond to therapy (eg, diphenhydramine), extended-release products may require admission for extended observation. Patients may be discharged from the ED after appropriate GI decontamination if they do not develop seizures, hypotension, or ECG changes after a 6-hour observation period.

Pearls

1. Response to parenteral diphenhydramine or benztropine mesylate can be diagnostic as well as therapeutic in patients presenting with acute extrapyramidal signs such as a dystonic reaction.

2. Patients may develop signs of toxicity while receiving therapeutic doses of phenothiazines or with an acute overdose. Signs and symptoms of toxicity or adverse drug effects may also develop unpredictably after chronic therapy.

3. A previous history of extrapyramidal signs is strongly associated with recurrence on repeat challenge of the drug.

4. Phenothiazines may cross-react with urine drug assays for cyclic antidepressants resulting in a false-positive test result.

Clinical Summary

Many drugs (eg, antihistamines, cyclic antidepressants) and plants (eg, jimson weed, nutmeg, potatoes) possess anticholinergic properties, and exposure occurs through ingestion, intraophthalmic use, or inhalation, or even transdermally. The classic symptoms of anticholinergic toxicity are described

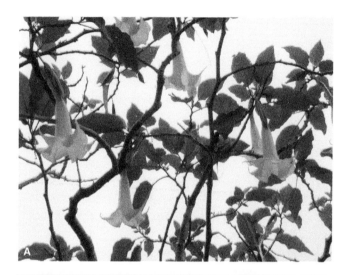

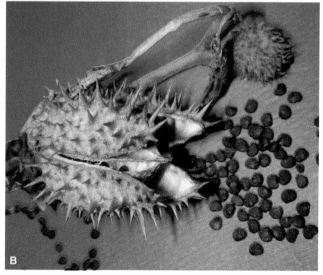

FIGURE 17.27 ■ Jimson Weed. Jimson weed plant initially has white trumpet-shaped flowers (**A**) that become a prickly fruit (pod) following maturation (**B**). The pod of Jimsonweed holds multiple small seeds that contain atropine, hyoscyamine, and scopolamine. These plants are often used as hallucinogens or as asthma remedies. Other plants with anticholinergic properties include henbane and mandrake. (Photo contributors: Angela Anderson, MD [A], and Reproduced with permission from Knoop KJ, Stack LB, Storrow AB, et al. *The Atlas of Emergency Medicine,* 4th ed. McGraw-Hill Education; New York, NY, 2016. Photo contributors: Matthew D. Sztajnkrycer, MD [B].)

by the mnemonic "Red as a Beet (flushing), Hot as a Hare (hyperthermia), Dry as a Bone (skin and mucus membrane dry), Blind as a Bat (mydriasis with blurry vision), and Mad as a Hatter (agitation and hallucinations)." Vital signs abnormalities include tachycardia and hyperthermia. GI examination shows decreased bowel sounds, constipation, or ileus. Patients may have urinary retention, psychomotor agitation, CNS agitation or depression, seizures, or coma. Patients are at risk of rhabdomyolysis from psychomotor agitation and from specific anticholinergic agents (ie, doxylamine). Differential diagnosis includes ingestion of sympathomimetic agents and other organic causes of altered mental status (see phenothiazines).

Obtain a history focused on the agent involved, dose, and timing of exposure including both prescription and over-the-counter medications and possible plant ingestion. Physical examination should focus on vital signs, pupillary reactivity, skin characteristics, bowel and bladder function, and neurologic status. ECG may show sinus tachycardia or cardiac dysrhythmias such as QRS widening or an R wave in aVR suggesting cyclic antidepressants or other sodium channel blockers. Order serum electrolytes, salicylates, and APAP levels if there is suspicion of coingestion of if the exposure was intended for self-harm. Serum BUN and creatinine may be elevated because of dehydration or renal failure from rhabdomyolysis. Urine may be concentrated as suggested by an elevated urine specific gravity.

Emergency Department Treatment and Disposition

Stabilize ABCs, and treat altered mental status, agitation, CNS depression, cardiac dysrhythmias, or seizures. Treat intraocular exposure by irrigation with normal saline. Accomplish GI decontamination with gastric lavage if patient presents within 1 hour of ingestion, or decontaminate with AC. Decreased GI motility seen with anticholinergics may allow both gastric lavage and AC to have an increased efficacy despite delay in presentation.

Physostigmine is a specific antidote and should be used if there is severe agitation, recurrent or refractory seizures, or severe hallucinations and/or delirium. Physostigmine administration can be diagnostic to determine if altered mental status is due to anticholinergic toxicity. Care must be taken during administration because excessive physostigmine can cause harmful cholinergic side effects. Continuous cardiac

TABLE 17.5 ▪ COMPARISON OF SYMPATHOMIMETICS AND ANTICHOLINERGICS

	Sympathomimetics	Anticholinergics
Vital signs	Tachyarrhythmias, hypertension/ tachycardia, hyperthermia	Tachyarrhythmias, hypertension, hyperthermia
Pupils	Mydriasis	Mydriasis
CNS	Hyperalert/agitation, hallucinations, delirium/psychosis	Coma/agitation/delirium, hallucinations, extrapyramidal movements
Skin	Severe sweating	Dry, hot, flushed
Urine	Normal	Retention
GI	Increased bowel sounds	Decreased bowel sounds (ileus)

Reproduced with permission from Finberg L, Kleinman RE. *Saunders Manual of Pediatric Practice.* WB Saunders; Philadelphia, PA, 2002.

monitoring, atropine, and an airway tray must be available at the bedside. Give physostigmine slowly as an IV push (over 2–5 minutes) at a dose of 0.02 mg/kg (up to 2 mg) and repeat every 5 to 10 minutes until anticholinergic symptoms improve. If cholinergic toxicity develops, administer atropine (dose is typically half of total amount of physostigmine given).

Admit all patients with signs of significant toxicity. Admit those with significant tachycardia, altered mental status, seizures, or hyperthermia to an ICU. Discharge patients if they are asymptomatic following a 6- to 12-hour observation period (or 4–6 hours after their last dose of benzodiazepine), and if they have received appropriate GI decontamination and

psychiatric evaluation. Check for coingestants such as APAP or aspirin if the ingestion was intended for self-harm.

Pearls

1. A careful history is of utmost importance as many diverse agents and plants contain anticholinergic substances.
2. Refer patients attempting "to get high" to substance abuse counseling to help prevent future repetition of events.
3. Physostigmine is contraindicated in patients with suspected cyclic antidepressant ingestion.

Clinical Summary

Isoniazid (INH) is an antimicrobial commonly prescribed to treat or prevent tuberculosis. Ingestion of 80 to 150 mg/kg of INH typically produces seizures, although seizures may occur with ingestion of as little as 40 mg/kg. Acute ingestion of 2 to 3 g causes acute toxicity in most patients, and ingestion of 10 to 15 g frequently causes death if untreated. The classic triad of symptoms is refractory seizures, coma, and increased anion gap metabolic acidosis. Seizures are typically generalized tonic-clonic and occur 1 to 2 hours after ingestion. Patients with severe INH toxicity present with hyperthermia, tachycardia, and hypotension. Patients may present with Kussmaul respirations due to metabolic acidosis or respiratory depression due to seizures. Patients may initially complain of nausea, vomiting, and dizziness. Patients may also develop anuric or oliguric renal failure secondary to prolonged seizures and rhabdomyolysis.

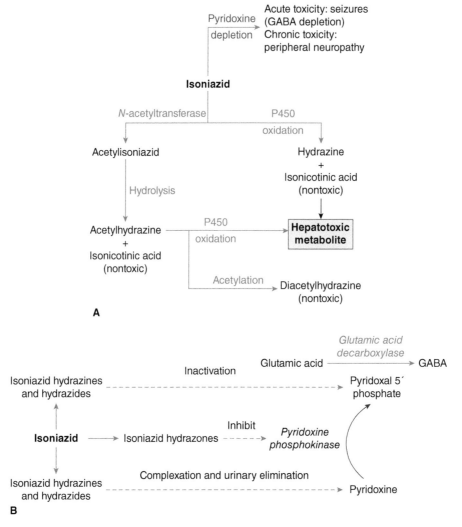

FIGURE 17.28 ■ Mechanisms of Acute Isoniazid Neurotoxicity. (**A**) The effect of isoniazid on pyridoxine, leading to reduced activation and a diminished supply of pyridoxine. (**B**) The mechanism of the inactivation of pyridoxal 5′-phosphate resulting in the reduction of the synthesis of GABA. GABA is the main inhibitory neurotransmitter of the CNS, and a decrease in the availability of GABA (with resultant loss of its vital inhibitory influence) is the presumed etiology of isoniazid-induced seizures. Isoniazid also enhances inactivation of GABA via transamination. (Reproduced with permission from Nelson LS, Lewin NA, Howland MA, et al. *Goldfrank's Toxicologic Emergencies.* 9th ed. McGraw-Hill Education; New York, NY, 2011.)

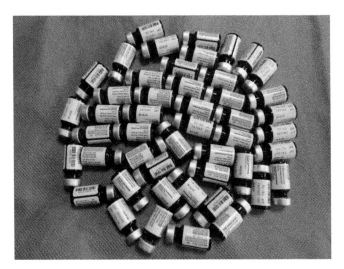

FIGURE 17.29 ▪ Pyridoxine, an Antidote for Isoniazid-Induced Seizures. Dose for pyridoxine is 1 g per gram of isoniazid ingested, or 5 g if the quantity is unknown. Shown here are 50 vials of pyridoxine (100-mg/mL vial) that were used to provide 5 g of pyridoxine to an adolescent female patient who presented in status epilepticus with an unknown amount of isoniazid ingestion for a suicide attempt. Do not lose your patience while opening 50 vials (or 100 vials if the only available concentration is 50 mg of pyridoxine per 1-mL vial) while the patient is in status epilepticus! Ask for additional help! (Photo contributor: Ambreen Kahn, MD.)

Differential diagnosis includes other causes of increased anion gap metabolic acidosis and other causes of seizures with anion gap acidosis (primarily because of *lactic acidosis*; see CAMPHOR BALL mnemonic; Table 17.2).

Obtain a history focused on preparation involved, dose, timing, and symptoms. Physical examination should focus on vital signs, cardiopulmonary assessment, abdominal pain, and neurologic status. Consider CXR, head CT, and lumbar puncture to evaluate for other causes of altered mental status and seizures.

Order serum chemistries (increased anion gap metabolic acidosis, hyperglycemia), serum ketones (elevated), serum lactate (increased), urinalysis (glycosuria, ketonuria, myoglobinuria), transaminases (increased), creatine kinase (elevated from rhabdomyolysis), and serum creatinine (elevated from rhabdomyolysis and acute kidney injury).

Emergency Department Treatment and Disposition

Stabilize ABCs and treat seizures, hypotension, and altered mental status. Accomplish GI decontamination with gastric lavage in the case of a large ingestion if the patient presents early and is not yet symptomatic. AC may also be given early if the patient has not developed seizures or altered mental status.

Pyridoxine (vitamin B_6) is the antidote for INH-induced seizures and also may be used in patients presenting with seizures of unknown origin who are refractory to conventional anticonvulsants. If the amount of INH ingested is known, give pyridoxine on a *gram-for-gram* basis up to a maximum of 5 g. If the INH amount ingested is unknown, give 70 mg/kg to a maximum of 5 g and repeat once if there is no improvement in the patient's status. If active seizures persist despite 2 adequate doses of pyridoxine, question diagnosis of INH toxicity and administer other GABAergic agents (eg, benzodiazepines or barbiturates). If IV pyridoxine is not available, give a slurry of crushed vitamin B_6 tablets orally, at the same dose. Adverse neurologic effects of excess pyridoxine can occur with chronic use but are uncommon with acute administration in the setting of most INH overdoses. Admit patients with altered mental status, seizures, or other signs of serious INH toxicity to an ICU for continuous monitoring and supportive care. Consult medical toxicology, the regional poison control center, and psychiatry as needed.

Pearls

1. Classic clinical presentation is the triad of refractory seizures, coma, and increased anion gap metabolic acidosis.
2. *Consider acute INH toxicity in any patient with status epilepticus* and no prior history of seizures.
3. The dose of pyridoxine is 1 g for every 1 g of INH ingested and may deplete hospital stores. A 5-g empiric dose may require up to *100 vials* of medication.
4. Prolonged coma may occur after INH overdoses for unclear reasons.

CAMPHOR TOXICITY

Clinical Summary

Camphor is an ingredient found in over-the-counter liniments (eg, Ben-Gay, Children's Vaporizing Rub, Vicks VapoRub, Deep Down Rub), antipruritics, cold remedies, antiseptics, topical anesthetics, and aphrodisiacs. Typically, the concentration of camphor is limited to 11% in the United States; however, higher concentrations can be found in non-US products. Camphor is also found in moth repellents, lacquers, varnishes, explosives, embalming fluid, and cosmetics. Camphor toxicity can occur through inhalation, ingestion, or dermal absorption. Although significant toxicity is rare, death has been reported.

Clinical symptoms include tachycardia, burning sensation in oropharynx, visual disturbances (veiling, darkening, or flickering), and an aromatic odor on the breath. Patients often present with nausea and vomiting; clinically, patients may have headache, fasciculations, confusion, delirium, coma, tremors, and seizures (typically seen as early as 5 minutes and as late as 2 hours after ingestion). Severe toxicity can result in cardiovascular collapse.

Obtain a careful history with attention to dosage, time, route, intent of exposure, and symptoms since exposure, and assess neurologic status. Serum camphor levels are not readily available or clinically useful. Serum chemistries with liver function tests may reveal a toxic hepatitis.

Emergency Department Treatment and Disposition

Treatment is primarily supportive, and there is no specific antidote. Decontamination must be performed to prevent further exposure. Gastric lavage may be beneficial if the patient presents shortly after exposure to a large amount of liquid product. AC is not indicated because of inefficacy of adsorption.

Patients who are asymptomatic 6 hours after exposure may be discharged home after appropriate decontamination and psychiatric evaluation (if indicated). Admit any patient who presents with significant signs of toxicity (eg, seizures, altered mental status, hepatotoxicity) from camphor exposure for continued monitoring and supportive care.

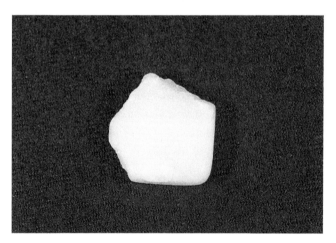

FIGURE 17.30 ■ Camphor Cube. A previously healthy toddler presented with afebrile status epilepticus. An odor of camphor was noted in his vomitus. His mother found the infant chewing on this camphor cube (shown here with a portion eaten away). Camphor cubes were used at home as moth repellent. It should be noted that camphor mothballs are illegal in the United States, but these mothballs were obtained from abroad. (Photo contributor: Ronak R. Shah, MD.)

Pearls

1. In liquid form, camphor has potential morbidity with ingestion of as little as 50 mg/kg and is potentially fatal at a dose of 100 mg/kg.
2. Consider camphor toxicity in all cases of toxin-induced seizures (especially in patients who have access to over-the-counter preparations containing camphor).
3. Patients with camphor toxicity may seize abruptly without antecedent signs or symptoms. Seizures are rare following dermal contact or inhalation exposure. Seizures may be recurrent or develop into status epilepticus with respiratory depression, a common cause of morbidity and mortality in camphor toxicity.

Clinical Summary

Many common household products contain hydrocarbons (HCs) including solvents, polishes, felt-tipped markers, glues, paints, car waxes, stain removers, and paint thinners. Exposure to HCs commonly occurs through inhalation, ingestion, or dermal routes. Several terms are used to describe intentional inhalation for the purpose of abuse including "sniffing," "bagging," and "huffing," and each technique differs in its exact method of inhalation.

The HCs naphthalene and paradichlorobenzene (PDB) are commonly found in moth repellent products. However, unlike camphor-containing mothballs, PDB ingestions are usually nontoxic. Naphthalene ingestion may precipitate methemoglobinemia, especially in patients with decreased ability to handle oxidative stress (ie, patients with G6PD deficiency).

Pulmonary aspiration is the most common serious side effect of ingesting liquid HCs, and risk increases with decreased viscosity and increased volatility of the HC. Patients who aspirate HCs present with dyspnea, cough, chest tightness, or hypoxia and may develop bronchitis, interstitial pneumonitis, pulmonary edema, or aspiration pneumonia.

Lower-molecular-weight HCs are more readily absorbed systemically, and rapid CNS distribution to the brain occurs with some agents, leading to CNS depression or excitation. Myocardial irritation and depression from halogenated HCs predispose patients to cardiac dysrhythmias and sudden death from ventricular fibrillation. This has been described as *sudden sniffing death*. Significant hepatic toxicity may result from exposure to halogenated HCs. Patients may complain of nausea, vomiting, or abdominal pain. Hematologic effects include disseminated intravascular coagulation. Certain HCs lead to the development of renal tubular acidosis (eg, toluene). Ocular complaints include eye irritation, pain, lacrimation, and blurring of vision. Vital sign abnormalities include tachycardia, bradycardia, tachypnea, bradypnea, hypoxia, and fever.

Differential diagnosis includes other causes of CNS depression such as ethanol, opioids, benzodiazepines, and hypoglycemic agents and other causes of altered mental status such as infection, trauma, and cerebral ischemia.

Obtain a thorough history focused on the agent involved, route of exposure, timing, intent, dose, and symptoms. Physical examination should focus on vital signs and neurologic

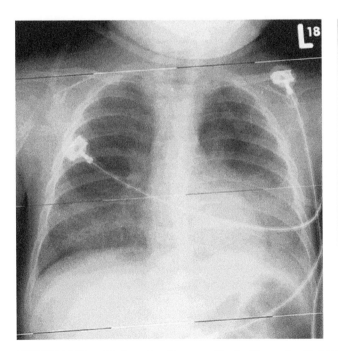
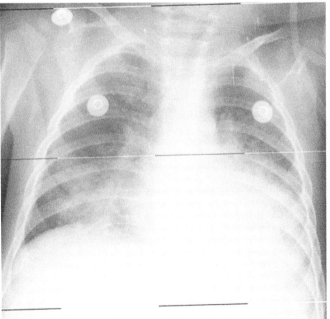

FIGURE 17.31 ■ Hydrocarbon Pneumonitis. An 18-month-old child was found by his parents coughing with an open bottle of paraffin lamp oil next to him and paraffin oil spillage on his clothing. He presented with several episodes of vomiting, persistent coughing, and tachypnea, with O$_2$ saturation of 90% on room air requiring hospitalization to the pediatric ICU. He experienced progressive respiratory distress and hypoxia. These serial CXRs demonstrate pneumonitis that progressed over a 4-day period (pulmonary damage reaches its peak about 3 days after aspiration). (Photo contributor: Mark K. Su, MD, MPH.)

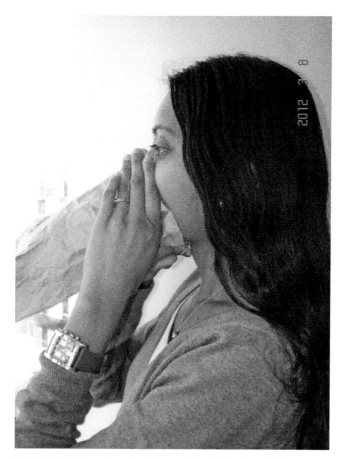

FIGURE 17.32 ■ Bagging Hydrocarbon (HC) Abuse. This is common among adolescents because of the ease of acquisition of products such as paints, model glue, and various solvents. Two methods of HC abuse include huffing and bagging, as demonstrated in the photo. (Photo contributor: Toral R. Shah, BS, PA-C.)

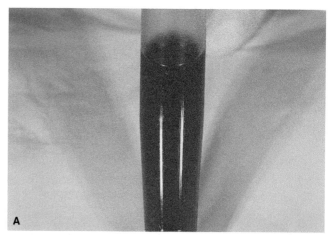

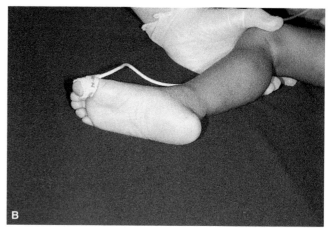

FIGURE 17.33 ■ Acute Hemolytic Anemia in a Child with G6PD Deficiency Following Exposure to Naphthalene Mothballs. Reddish urine (hemoglobinuria; **A**) and extreme pallor (**B**) were seen in a 2-year-old African American male child with sickle cell anemia presenting with lethargy, poor feeding, and a HgB value of 5 g/dL with signs of hemolysis on the peripheral smear. Two days prior to his presentation to the ED, he was found playing with naphthalene mothballs that his mother was using as moth repellent. Ingestion of <1 naphthalene mothball by a patient with G6PD deficiency can result in significant toxicity. (Photo contributor: Ronak R. Shah, MD.)

and cardiopulmonary assessment. A CXR may show pulmonary edema, aspiration pneumonia, or pneumonitis. In chronic exposure, CBC may demonstrate aplastic anemia or leukemia. Serum electrolytes may demonstrate acute renal failure. Elevated serum transaminases are evidence of hepatic injury. ABG analysis confirms hypoxia, hypercarbia, and assessment of pulmonary status.

Emergency Department Treatment and Disposition

Management is primarily supportive, and external decontamination and adequate skin and respiratory protection of health care professionals are essential. Stabilize ABCs and treat respiratory distress, seizures, coma, and cardiac dysrhythmias. Reserve gastric lavage only for those with large, recent ingestions or coingestions because it may result in increased risk of aspiration. AC should not be used; it does not adsorb HC and may increase risk of emesis and aspiration. Prophylactic antibiotics and steroids are not recommended even for patients who have confirmed aspiration on CXR.

Patients believed to have ingested small amounts and who are asymptomatic require only observation with no intervention. Discharge patients who remain asymptomatic over a 6-hour observation period. A CXR should be obtained 6 hours

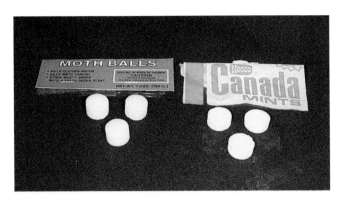

FIGURE 17.34 ▪ Candy Look-Alikes. As seen here, a naphthalene mothball could easily be mistaken for candy and be unintentionally ingested. (Reproduced with permission from Shah BR, Laude TL. *Atlas of Pediatric Clinical Diagnosis.* WB Saunders; Philadelphia, PA, 2000.)

after ingestion to asses for aspiration in asymptomatic children. Radiographic evidence of aspiration in the absence of symptoms requires prolonged observation and possible admission. Order labs for symptomatic patients to evaluate and monitor respiratory status. Admit anyone with altered mental status, cardiac dysrhythmias, or respiratory insufficiency to the ICU for continuous monitoring and supportive care.

Admit patients exposed to naphthalene mothballs if signs of acute hemolytic anemia or methemoglobinemia are present. Perform packed RBC transfusion in hemodynamically unstable or symptomatic patients with Hgb value of ≤6 g/dL or Hgb of 6 to 9 g/dL with ongoing hemolysis. Use parenteral hydration to maintain adequate urine output and urinary alkalinization to prevent renal damage from precipitation of Hgb in renal tubules. Follow asymptomatic patients with G6PD deficiency closely as outpatients. Hemolysis and methemoglobinemia usually occur 1 to 2 days after exposure; patients should be monitored with serial CBCs, and parents should be told to bring the child to the ED immediately if dark urine, pallor, jaundice, or any symptoms of anemia occur. Asymptomatic patients who are not G6PD deficient can be sent home with close outpatient follow-up.

Pearls

1. Less than 1 naphthalene mothball in a patient with G6PD deficiency can cause significant toxicity.
2. Neonates without G6PD deficiency may develop hemolytic anemia or methemoglobinemia on exposure to naphthalene mothballs because fetal Hgb is more susceptible to oxidant stress.
3. Parents should be advised not to use naphthalene or camphor mothballs; cedar mothballs are a safe alternative.
4. Perform GI decontamination with great care because it may result in increased risk of aspiration pneumonitis.
5. CXR may be unreliable because radiographic findings often lag physical examination findings by 4 to 6 hours.

ECSTASY/MOLLY TOXICITY

Clinical Summary

3,4-Methylenedioxymethamphetamine (MDMA), also known as "Ecstasy" or "Molly," is an entactogen known for its euphoric and stimulant effects. Commonly used street slang names for MDMA include "E," "X," or "Adam." Popular in the club and rave scene, users describe feelings of inner peace, empathy, self-confidence, and a heightened sense of awareness. Once ingested, the onset of action is approximately 20 minutes, but the duration of action can last hours or even days. Although not fully elucidated, the effects of MDMA appear to be mediated by the enhanced secretion of serotonin, inhibition of its reuptake mechanism in the synapse, and release of dopamine.

MDMA is available as a tablet and is frequently adulterated with other drugs such as ketamine or caffeine. As a recreational drug, it is associated with a wide range of effects, including mydriasis, tachycardia, hypertension, bruxism, hyperthermia, psychosis, seizures, and coma.

Individuals abusing MDMA may present to the ED with agitation or exhibiting signs of acute psychosis. It is of utmost importance to control agitation with the use of benzodiazepines and assess for other untoward effects (eg, rhabdomyolysis, acute kidney injury, hepatotoxicity, and hyperthermia).

Emergency Department Evaluation and Management

Treatment is supportive; there is no specific antidote. Monitor vital signs, mental status, and oxygen saturation continually. Hyponatremia may develop as a result of the inappropriate secretion of antidiuretic hormone. Increased free water intake from exertion may exacerbate and contribute to hyponatremia. Laboratory evaluation should include measurement of electrolytes, serum transaminases, renal function, and creatine phosphokinase. Assess for cerebral edema with a head CT if altered mental status is present, and obtain an ECG to look for other potential coingestants and potential dysrhythmias. Consider endotracheal intubation to protect the airway. Treat hyperthermia with active cooling.

Observe individuals with mild toxicity for 6 to 8 hours. Moderate to severe cases of MDMA toxicity associated with persistent CNS involvement should be admitted to the ICU. Consult psychiatry in self-harm attempts and for substance abuse counseling.

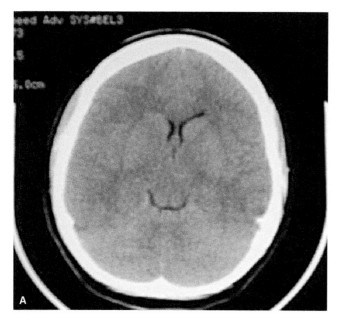

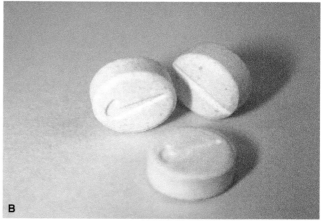

FIGURE 17.35 ■ Ecstasy (Methylenedioxymethamphetamine [MDMA]) Toxicity. (**A**) Head CT scan of a young woman who experienced MDMA-induced syndrome of inappropriate antidiuretic hormone secretion (SIADH) shows effacement of the brain with disappearance of gyri and sulci as well as slit ventricles. Her serum sodium was 119 mmol/L. She had taken the drug at a party the previous evening and was brought to the ED by college roommates, who noticed her to be delirious the following morning. (**B**) Ecstasy tablets seized in New York City. (Photo contributor: Robert J. Hoffman, MD.)

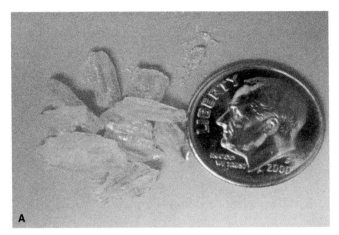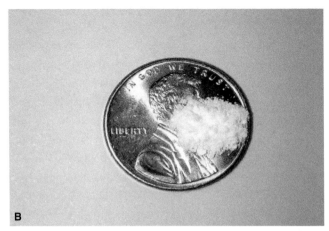

FIGURE 17.36 ■ Methamphetamine Toxicity. Differential Diagnosis of Ecstasy (MDMA) Toxicity. Methamphetamine and MDMA are both substituted amphetamines with sympathomimetic properties. MDMA has more serotonergic properties; methamphetamine is mostly sympathomimetic and causes large amounts of dopamine to be released into the brain. Methamphetamine may be found in various forms including powder, pills, or crystal form. Here is methamphetamine in crystalline form (**A**). Methamphetamine on a penny (**B**). Methamphetamine is highly potent. This small quantity approximates that typically used to maintain euphoria or a "high" over a 24-hour period. (Photo contributor: Robert J. Hoffman, MD.)

Pearls

1. Always assess for other causes for altered mental status (eg, infection, intracranial hemorrhage).
2. Control agitation and seizure activity with benzodiazepines.
3. Treat significant hyponatremia with hypertonic saline (3% NaCl) in patients with altered mental status and/or seizures.
4. In young children with unintentional suspected MDMA ingestion, notify child protective services and social worker.

Clinical Summary

Ketamine is a nonopioid anesthetic known for its dissociative effects. Ketamine usage as a recreational drug is associated with a wide range of effects, including inebriation, anxiety, slurred speech, sedation, hallucinations, nystagmus, mydriasis, chest pain, complete dissociation, and coma. It is available as a clear liquid or white/off-white powder, which can be injected IM or IV, insufflated (snorted), or ingested. Individuals may also exhibit an emergence reaction during the recovery phase, which is characterized by confusion, delirium, hallucinations, irrational behavior, and vivid dreams. This reaction is more commonly seen in adults. Monikers commonly used include "Special K" or simply "K."

Emergency Department Treatment and Disposition

Treatment for ketamine toxicity is supportive; there is no specific antidote. Monitor vital signs, mental status, and oxygen saturation continually. If there is altered mental status, obtain blood glucose and electrolyte measurements, ECG, and cardiac monitoring. Endotracheal intubation should be considered in cases of prolonged CNS or respiratory depression. Patients should be observed until they are asymptomatic or admitted to the hospital depending on the severity of symptoms.

Pearls

1. GI decontamination with AC is not indicated, especially in the obtunded patient without a protected airway.
2. Control agitation and seizure activity with benzodiazepines.
3. Always consider the possibility of a coingestion.
4. Consider other causes of altered mental status, despite drug history.
5. Supportive care is the mainstay of treatment, with supplemental oxygen, symptomatic therapy, and IV hydration.

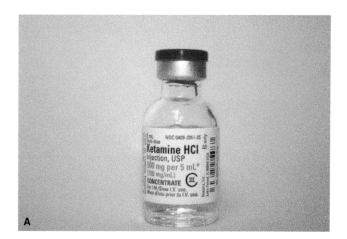 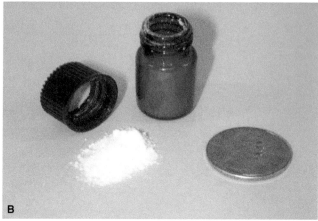

FIGURE 17.37 ■ Ketamine. (**A**) Pharmaceutical ketamine. (**B**) "Cooked" ketamine. Ketamine that was heated to precipitate the active ingredient from the liquid solution. (Photo contributors: Mae De La Calzada-Jean Louie, DO [A], and Robert J. Hoffman, MD [B].)

Clinical Summary

Dextromethorphan (DXM) is an antitussive medication commonly found in formulations containing antihistamines, analgesics, cough suppressants, decongestants, and expectorants. Its availability without a prescription makes it susceptible to abuse, especially in the adolescent population. Its allure as a drug of abuse is associated with a heightened sense of perceptual awareness, euphoria, and visual hallucinations. DXM exhibits effects similar to other well-known *N*-methyl D-aspartate (NMDA) antagonists (eg, phencyclidine [PCP] and ketamine) and is also known to cross-react with urine drug screens for PCP, resulting in a false-positive test.

Use as a recreational drug is associated with a wide range of effects including nausea, vomiting, tachycardia, respiratory depression, seizure activity, stupor, ataxia, hyperexcitability, dystonia, psychosis, and coma. When taken in combination with other serotonergic agents, individuals can develop *serotonin toxicity (or syndrome)* (altered mental status, autonomic hyperactivity, and neuromuscular abnormalities). Street names for DXM include "Robo," "Skittles," or "Triple C."

Emergency Department Treatment and Disposition

Treatment is supportive; there is no specific antidote. GI decontamination with AC is not necessary; seizures and CNS depression have been observed within 30 minutes of ingestion. Continually monitor vital signs, mental status, and oxygen saturation. Observe patients for 3 to 6 hours until they are asymptomatic. Admit patients with persistent respiratory and CNS depression. Consult social services in cases involving young children and psychiatry in self-harm attempts.

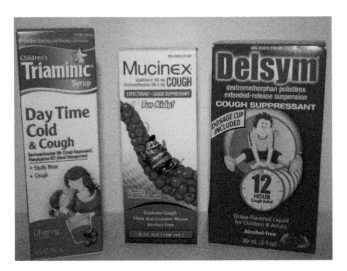

FIGURE 17.38 ■ Various Formulations Containing Dextromethorphan. (Photo contributor: Mae De La Calzada-Jeanlouie, DO.)

Pearls

1. Always consider the possibility of toxicity from ingestion of DXM products due to the presence of other toxins (eg, APAP).
2. Use AC only in the awake and alert patient with a protected airway.
3. Control agitation and seizures with benzodiazepines.
4. Supportive care is the mainstay of treatment, with supplemental oxygen, symptomatic therapy, and IV hydration.

MARIJUANA TOXICITY

Clinical Summary

Derived from the *Cannabis* plant, the use of "medicinal" marijuana in history dates back to 400 BC. The active ingredient of marijuana is Δ^9-*tetrahydrocannabinol* (THC). THC binds to the cannabinoid receptor (CB_1), which results in inhibition of neurotransmitter release through various intracellular mechanisms. Marijuana use is associated with alteration of perception and euphoria. Monikers commonly used include "Dope," "Ganja," "Mary Jane," and "Hashish."

With recreational usage of marijuana, individuals can experience euphoria, short-term memory impairment, disinhibition, impaired motor coordination, lethargy, slurred speech, and ataxia. In cases involving young children, the agent is commonly ingested; these patients can present with drowsiness, mydriasis, hypotonia, or particulate matter in the mouth. Ingestion of cannabis has become increasingly prevalent due to the use of medicinal cannabis and legalization of recreational marijuana.

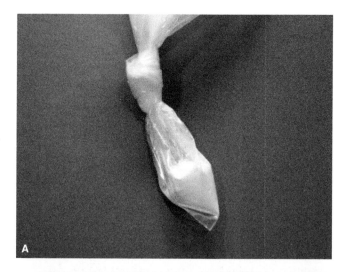

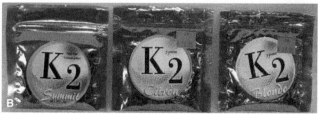

FIGURE 17.40 ■ Examples of K2 Spice or JWH-018. (**A**) Suspected synthetic cannabinoid K2 Spice (JWH-018) used by an individual who complained of difficulty breathing and chest pain after smoking it. (**B**) K2 is a synthetic psychoactive agent resembling marijuana but varying in clinical effects and is undetected by routine urine toxicology testing for marijuana. (Photo contributors: Mae De La Calzada-Jeanlouie, DO [A], and Cindy Moran BS; Arkansas State Crime Laboratory [B].)

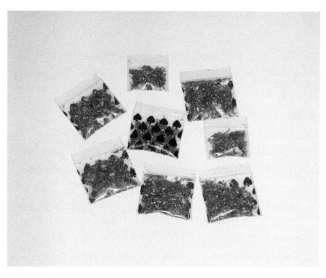

FIGURE 17.39 ■ Marijuana. Marijuana leaves in small plastic bags (a total of 8 bags) were found on an adolescent male who was brought to the ED with a stab wound to the chest. Marijuana refers to material obtained from the leaves and flowers of the Indian hemp plant, *Cannabis sativa*. A few examples of other names by which it is known include pot, weed, smoke tea, joint, hashish, Colombian ganja, ace, bush, rope, Jamaican, and Panama red. Marijuana is the most commonly used drug in the Unites States, and with the advent of medical cannabis and legalization of recreational marijuana, childhood exposures have significantly increased. Reported cases of cannabis toxicity include altered mental status and lethargy. After nicotine, alcohol, and caffeine, marijuana is probably the most commonly abused substance in the world. (Photo contributor: Binita R. Shah, MD.)

Recently, newer designer drugs known as synthetic cannabinoids or synthetic cannabinoid receptor agonists have emerged as an alternative to marijuana. These drugs were initially marketed as herbal incense, but since these products have been associated with significant toxicity, many compounds have been identified and banned by the US Food and Drug Administration. Slang terms used for these agents include "Spice" and "K2." These variations of marijuana are modified chemical structures of THC that bind to the cannabinoid receptors (CB_1 and CB_2). Originally synthesized for laboratory animal research, short- and long-term effects in humans have yet to be determined from these synthetic agents. Acute symptoms are variable and can resemble those of THC but with greater potency. Toxicity associated with these synthetic compounds includes seizures, cerebrovascular accidents, myocardial infarction, acute kidney injury, rhabdomyolysis, and death.

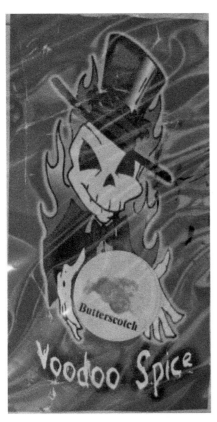

FIGURE 17.41 ■ Incense. A combination of herbal products, marketed as incense, containing synthetic cannabinoids. (Photo contributor: Cindy Moran BS; Arkansas State Crime Laboratory.)

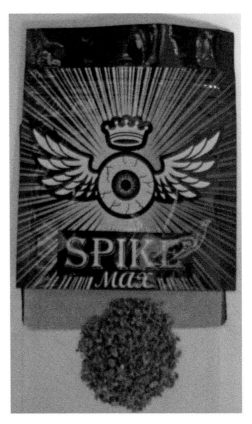

FIGURE 17.42 ■ Organic Material Resembling Marijuana, Laced with a Synthetic Cannabinoid. This product marketed as "fragrant potpourri/incense" contains organic material resembling marijuana that is laced with the synthetic cannabinoid. (Photo contributor: Cindy Moran BS; Arkansas State Crime Laboratory.)

Emergency Department Treatment and Disposition

Treatment for these patients is focused on supportive care; there is no specific antidote. AC can be used to decrease absorption from ingestion of cannabis but may be difficult to administer in the young child. While in the ED, continuously monitor patient's vital signs, mental status, and oxygen saturation. Patients presenting with altered mental status will need a blood glucose and electrolyte measurement, ECG, and cardiac monitoring. These individuals can often be observed in the ED for 4 to 6 hours until asymptomatic. Incorporate social services in cases involving young children or psychiatry in self-harm attempts.

Pearls

1. AC is indicated for use in patients who have ingested marijuana products, except in the obtunded patient without a protected airway.
2. Place agitated or hallucinating individuals in a quiet room.
3. Extreme agitation and seizure activity should be controlled with benzodiazepines.
4. Consider other causes of altered mental status.
5. Do not rely on urine toxicology testing for synthetic cannabinoids because they will not be detected by routine THC testing.

ETHYLENE GLYCOL TOXICITY

Clinical Summary

Ethylene glycol (EG) is a highly toxic alcohol. Antifreeze is the major source of exposure. It has a sweet taste, which makes it appealing to young children and animals. Some antifreeze formulations introduce bitter agents in an attempt to counteract this appeal and mitigate potential toxicity.

EG is rapidly absorbed following ingestion. It undergoes metabolism by alcohol dehydrogenase to glycoaldehyde, which is then metabolized by aldehyde dehydrogenase to glycolic acid. EG has a half-life of about 4 hours when metabolized by alcohol dehydrogenase. EG, itself, is eliminated by the kidneys, with a half-life of 11 to 18 hours.

Signs and symptoms of toxicity include tachycardia, tachypnea, nausea/vomiting, CNS depression, and seizures. Hypocalcemia, high anion gap metabolic acidosis, acute kidney injury, increased osmolal gap, and urinary calcium oxalate crystals are all findings of EG toxicity. Differential diagnosis includes other types of toxic alcohols (eg, methanol) and ethanol or sedative-hypnotic ingestion; other causes of increased anion gap metabolic acidosis (see Table 17.2) and seizures are also considerations.

Emergency Department Treatment and Disposition

Obtain serum electrolytes with calcium, measured serum osmolality, BUN, creatinine, lactate, and blood gas. Calculate the anion gap and osmolal gap (ie, the difference between measured osmolality and calculated osmolality). Check urine for calcium oxalate crystals. Order serum EG and methanol levels; however, because of their turnaround times, these results might not be obtained in a clinically relevant manner. If the child is believed to have ingested a trivial amount of EG, he or she can be observed for 12 hours in the ED with serial laboratory testing to assess for acidosis. Consult the regional poison control center or medical toxicologist for any questions and management recommendations. Psychiatry should be notified for intentional suicidal ingestions. Prior to ED discharge, consider social work consult. If the child becomes symptomatic during observation or develops any laboratory abnormalities (eg, anion gap metabolic acidosis, lethargy), he or she should be treated with antidotal therapy and admitted to the ICU.

Because this is a liquid toxin that is rapidly absorbed and distributed, no gastric decontamination is advised. Antidotal therapy for EG toxicity first consists of pharmacologic blockade of EG metabolism by inhibition of alcohol dehydrogenase. Although IV ethanol has been used historically and is effective at blocking alcohol dehydrogenase, it is complicated to administer and is associated with complications such as hypoglycemia. The current treatment of choice is fomepizole. Thiamine and pyridoxine are also recommended to enhance formation of nontoxic metabolites.

If the patient has altered mental status, acute kidney injury, and worsening acidosis or electrolyte abnormalities that are not responding to conventional medical treatment, emergent hemodialysis should be performed. Occasionally, more than 1 course of hemodialysis will be necessary for large ingestions.

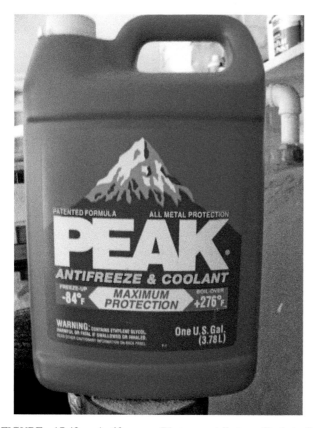

FIGURE 17.43 ■ Antifreeze. (Photo contributor: Rachel S. Weiselberg, MD.)

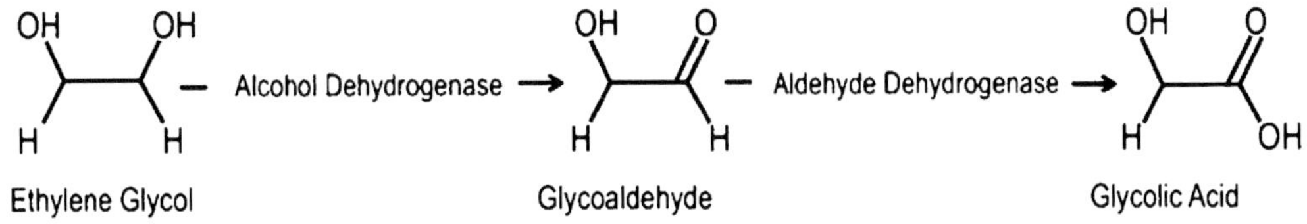

OH   OH   OH   O   OH   O

— Alcohol Dehydrogenase →   — Aldehyde Dehydrogenase →

H   H   H   H   H   OH

Ethylene Glycol   Glycoaldehyde   Glycolic Acid

FIGURE 17.44 ■ Metabolism of Ethylene Glycol. (Photo contributor: Rachel S. Weiselberg, MD.)

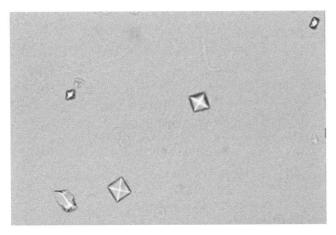

FIGURE 17.45 ■ Calcium Oxalate Crystals. (Photo contributor: Loring Bjornson, PhD, DABCC, FACB.)

Pearls

1. Osmolal gap = measured osmolality – (2Na + BUN/2.8 + glucose/18 + ethanol/4.6). Normal osmolal gap range is between 14 and +10. A normal osmolal gap *does not* exclude toxicity.

2. If ethanol has also been ingested, it will be preferentially metabolized by alcohol dehydrogenase, delaying metabolism and onset of toxicity of EG.

3. Consult the renal service early to ensure timely hemodialysis when indicated.

4. Fomepizole is a blocking agent that only prevents EG metabolism and is dosed every 12 hours.

5. Endogenous clearance of EG does occur after fomepizole administration, but the EG half-life is approximately 18 hours with normal kidney function. Therefore, the need for hemodialysis will necessitate consideration of clinical and laboratory status of the patient.

Clinical Summary

Methanol is a toxic alcohol that can be found in windshield wiper fluid, antifreeze, solvents, and homemade ethanol (eg, moonshine).

Signs and symptoms of toxicity include tachycardia, tachypnea, nausea/vomiting, occasional hepatitis or pancreatitis, visual impairment (from blurry vision to blindness), ataxia, CNS depression, and seizures. Methanol is osmotically active, creating an osmolal gap. As it is metabolized to formic acid, it causes a high anion gap metabolic acidosis. Differential diagnosis includes ingestion of other types of toxic alcohols or ethanol and other causes of elevated anion gap metabolic acidosis (see Table 17.2).

Methanol is rapidly absorbed and distributed following ingestion. It undergoes metabolism by alcohol dehydrogenase (like ethanol) to formaldehyde, which is then metabolized by aldehyde dehydrogenase to formic acid. Methanol has a half-life of up to 28 hours when metabolized by alcohol dehydrogenase. The parent compound appears to be slowly eliminated by the lungs, with a half-life of 30 to 54 hours.

Emergency Department Treatment and Disposition

Obtain serum electrolytes, measured serum osmolality, BUN, creatinine, liver enzymes, and blood gas. Calculate the anion gap and the osmolal gap. Order a serum methanol concentration (and EG concentration if unknown ingestion); however, because of turnaround time, these results might not be obtained in a clinically relevant manner.

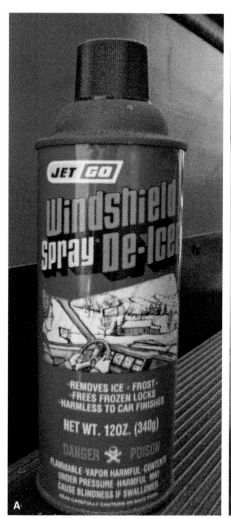
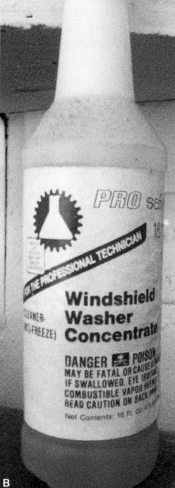
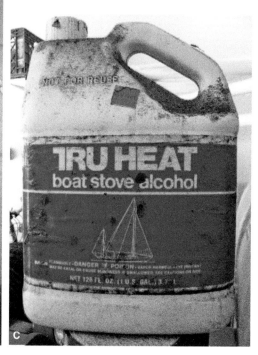

FIGURE 17.46 ■ Methanol-Containing Household Products. (Photo contributor: Rachel S. Weiselberg, MD.)

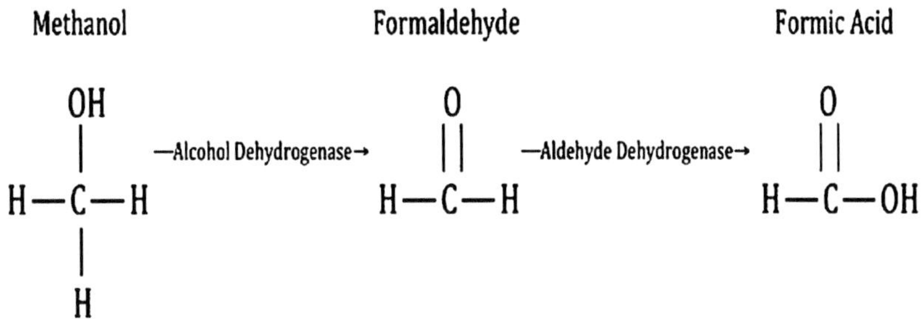

Methanol   Formaldehyde   Formic Acid

OH   O   O
| —Alcohol Dehydrogenase→ || —Aldehyde Dehydrogenase→ ||
H—C—H   H—C—H   H—C—OH
|
H

FIGURE 17.47 ■ Metabolism of Methanol. (Photo contributor: Rachel S. Weiselberg, MD.)

If methanol ingestion is suspected, the child will need a minimum period of 12 hours of observation and serial blood work in the ED. Consult the regional poison center or medical toxicologist for management recommendations and psychiatry for intentional suicidal ingestions. Consider social work consult prior to discharge. If the child becomes symptomatic during observation or develops any laboratory abnormalities (eg, anion gap metabolic acidosis, lethargy), he or she should be treated and admitted.

Because this is a liquid toxin (very similar to EG) that is rapidly absorbed and distributed, no gastric decontamination is advised. Antidotal therapy for methanol toxicity first consists of pharmacologic blockade of alcohol dehydrogenase. Although IV ethanol has been successfully used historically, it is complicated to administer and is associated with complications such as hypoglycemia. The current initial treatment of choice is fomepizole. Folic acid may also provide benefit in the detoxification of formic acid.

If the patient has altered mental status, vision changes, acute kidney injury, and worsening acidosis or electrolyte abnormalities that are not responding to conventional medical treatment, consult the renal service for emergent hemodialysis.

Pearls

1. As methanol is metabolized, the osmolal gap will get smaller while the anion gap will grow larger.
2. Osmolal gap = measured osmolality − (2Na + BUN/2.8 + glucose/18 + ethanol/4.6). Normal osmolal gap is −14 to +10. A normal osmolal gap *does not* exclude toxicity.
3. Delayed onset of toxicity can occur, and patients should be observed for prolonged periods and possibly admitted.
4. After fomepizole administration, endogenous clearance of methanol is extremely slow. The vast majority of patients with methanol ingestions will require hemodialysis.

ETHANOL TOXICITY

Clinical Features

Ethanol, more commonly referred to as alcohol, is one of the most frequently used and socially accepted drugs in the world. Ethanol abuse is a significant social disease that afflicts many adults. Ethanol is responsible for the greatest number of yearly deaths in the 15- to 45-year-old age group. In young children, ethanol exposures are usually unintentional, and significant toxicity occasionally occurs. Common household products containing ethanol include mouthwashes, antitussive medications, and perfumes and colognes.

In adolescents, intentional abuse of ethanol-containing beverages is extremely common and much more likely to be dangerous. Ethanol concentration is expressed usually as *proof* or *percent*. In the United States, percent refers to one-half of the proof. Among the general public, "proof" is commonly used, but in science, percent (or mg/dL) is used as the unit of concentration.

Important considerations in the patient history include amount, time of ingestion, intent, possibility of coingestants, and awareness of possible factors delaying absorption. In general, increasing concentrations of ethanol will result in CNS depression and, occasionally, respiratory depression.

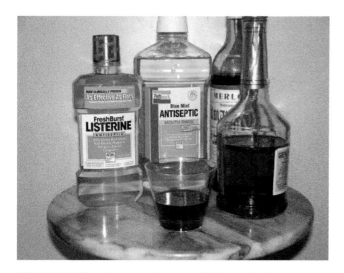

FIGURE 17.48 ■ Common Sources of Ethanol for Young Infants and Children. Common household products containing ethanol that are unintentionally ingested by infants and young children include mouthwashes, antitussive medications, perfumes, and colognes. Alcohol content of these preparations varies significantly (eg, the alcohol content in mouthwash varies from 5% to almost 30%). Accidental ingestion of wine from leftover wine glasses after parties (especially New Year's or Christmas Eve) is a common cause of a toddler presenting with hypoglycemic seizures. (Photo contributor: Binita R. Shah, MD.)

Depending on the age of the patient, the quantity ingested, and the individual, the clinical manifestations can be markedly different. Occasionally, paradoxical CNS stimulation may occur from CNS disinhibition. In cases of massive ingestions, respiratory depression, loss of protective reflexes, coma, and death may occur.

Ethanol metabolism interferes with gluconeogenesis, and significant hypoglycemia may occur, especially in young children with low glycogen stores. The acute neuroglycopenia can cause generalized tonic-clonic seizures. Symptomatic hypoglycemia in adolescents and healthy adults is less frequent. Other effects of ethanol include myocardial depression, vasodilatation, dysrhythmias (eg, atrial fibrillation), hypotension and tachycardia, gastritis, pancreatitis, skin flushing, urticaria, and hypothermia.

Differential diagnosis includes overdose of other sedative-hypnotic agents (eg, benzodiazepines), hypoglycemia from other etiology (eg, oral hypoglycemia agents), infection (eg, meningitis), head trauma, and ingestion of toxic alcohols (eg, methanol, EG).

Emergency Department Treatment and Disposition

History should focus on determining the agent involved, amount, time of ingestion, and intent. The patient's mental status may impede obtaining a thorough history. Initial stabilization of ABCs is necessary, especially in patients with a depressed mental status. Hypotension and reflex tachycardia may be prominent. Obtain an ECG to detect any cardiac dysrhythmias and electrolyte disturbances and a bedside fingerstick glucose test on all patients with altered mental status. If unavailable, give empiric treatment with IV dextrose.

GI decontamination will rarely be necessary for isolated ethanol ingestions but should be considered in patients presenting with a recent massive ingestion of significant quantity of coingestants. In patients with persistent altered mental status, consider other etiologies besides ethanol intoxication (see COMATOSE; Table 13.5).

Obtain serum chemistry (including calcium, magnesium, and phosphate), ketones, CBC, and ethanol concentration. Coingestants (eg, APAP) and subsequent toxidromes should be sought in patients who present with intentional ingestion. Although individual variation exists, ethanol intoxication in non–alcohol-dependent individuals is usually apparent at a blood ethanol concentration of 50 mg/dL.

Supportive care (eg, IV fluids, warm blankets) is the mainstay of therapy. In cases of massive overdose with respiratory depression, hemodialysis is effective at removing ethanol from the body. Patients with simple intoxication may be discharged home after a period of observation. Admit patients with hemodynamic instability, persistent altered mental status, hypoglycemia, and coingestants. Consult medical toxicologist, regional poison control center, psychiatry (if intentional), or social services (for suspected abuse) as necessary.

Pearls

1. Consider ethanol intoxication in the differential diagnosis of altered mental status and/or hypoglycemia.
2. Significant head or neck trauma may be overlooked in trauma patients who are intoxicated. Have a low threshold to perform a head CT to look for intracranial hemorrhage.
3. No measures of enhanced elimination of ethanol aside from hemodialysis are effective at removing ethanol from the body.
4. Parents should be educated on proper storage of ethanol-containing beverages. Older children may need to be referred for substance abuse counseling.
5. Patients who have ingested toxic alcohols (ie, methanol and ethylene glycol) may present in a similar clinical manner to ethanol intoxication, but these patients can develop a high anion gap metabolic acidosis that does not improve with standard supportive measures. Suspicion of these agents must be high to prevent missing the diagnosis.

Clinical Summary

Opioids: Opioids (eg, OxyContin®, Percocet®, Vicodin®, fentanyl) are a class of medications known for their analgesic effects. They are derived from naturally occurring opiates, such as morphine. Although indicated for moderate to severe pain, prescription opioids have become an increasing source of drug abuse. Users not only experience a euphoric effect but also develop tolerance and physical dependence, thus resulting in fortified behavior. There are a number of opioid receptors in the CNS; however, opioids primarily exert their analgesic effects through the μ (mu) opioid receptor. The μ receptors are present in the peripheral and central nervous systems and modulate pain perception by inhibition of the presynaptic release of neurotransmitters, hyperpolarization of the postsynaptic membrane, and activation of a descending inhibitory system.

Benzodiazepines: Benzodiazepines (eg, Xanax®, Valium®, Ativan®, Klonopin®) are members of a family known as sedative hypnotics. They are commonly prescribed to treat anxiety, agitation, sleep disturbances, and seizure disorders. In a controlled setting, benzodiazepines are frequently administered for sedation. Benzodiazepines exert their effect by binding to $GABA_A$ receptors, resulting in GABAergic neurotransmission potentiation. These drugs are frequently abused in combination with other drugs and are sought after for their calming and relaxing effects. Like opioids, individuals can develop tolerance and physical dependence.

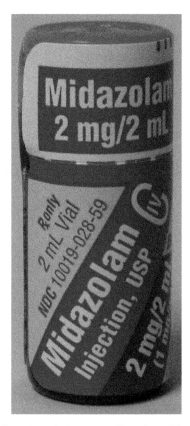

FIGURE 17.50 ■ Prescription Benzodiazepines. (Photo contributor: Mae De La Calzada-Jeanlouie, DO.)

Emergency Department Treatment and Disposition

For Opioid Toxicity: Treatment for these patients is focused on supportive care and airway maintenance. Individuals who present to the ED with respiratory or CNS depression secondary to opioid overdose can be given naloxone, an opioid receptor antagonist. When administering the antidote, always begin with a low dose and titrate to arousal or improvement of respiration; rapid reversal may result in withdrawal symptoms in opioid-tolerant patients. Individuals should be closely monitored because naloxone is relatively short acting compared to some opioids and patients can have recurrence of opioid toxicity.

Some oral opioid preparations are available in combination with APAP or aspirin. APAP or salicylate toxicity may result from these combination preparations. Serum levels for these "coingestants" should be obtained in conjunction with renal and hepatic function tests, especially in overdose cases, and toxicity must be treated appropriately (see earlier sections on acetaminophen and salicylate toxicity).

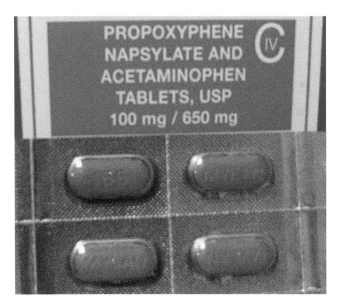

FIGURE 17.49 ■ Propoxyphene. (Photo contributor: Mae De La Calzada-Jeanlouie, DO.)

For Benzodiazepine Toxicity: Flumazenil is a benzodiazepine receptor antagonist; however, its use is rarely indicated except in iatrogenic oversedation. Extreme caution should be used when giving this antidote to patients with long-standing benzodiazepine use because patients can develop withdrawal seizures that may be difficult to treat. While in the ED, patients should have their vital signs (including cardiac monitor), mental status, and oxygen saturation continually checked. An ECG should be performed to look for other potential coingestants. Laboratory evaluation should include measurement of electrolytes, renal function, hepatic function, APAP, and salicylate concentrations.

For Opioid and Benzodiazepine Toxicity: With mild toxicity, these individuals can often be observed in the ED for 6 to 8 hours. In moderate to severe cases, designated by persistent CNS involvement, admit these patients to the ICU. Consult social services in cases involving young children or psychiatry in self-harm attempts.

Pearls

1. In acute overdoses, impending respiratory depression should be taken into consideration before entertaining the utility of AC; risk of aspiration is high.
2. Naloxone is a short-acting antidote; a continuous infusion may be necessary in patients with ingestion of long-acting opioids.
3. Always consider the possibility of a coingestion.
4. Consider other causes of altered mental status, despite drug history.

β-BLOCKER AND CALCIUM CHANNEL BLOCKER TOXICITY

Clinical Summary

β-Blockers (BBs) and calcium channel blockers (CCBs) are antihypertensive medications that can be toxic in young children after ingesting as little as 1 tablet. β-Blockade of $β_1$ receptors in the heart slows cardiac conduction at the sino-atrial (SA) and AV nodes and decreases inotropy, thereby decreasing BP. Blockade of $β_2$ receptors causes constriction of the peripheral vasculature, bronchospasm, hyperkalemia, and hypoglycemia.

Diltiazem and verapamil are CCBs that exert their primary effect on the heart, slowing cardiac conduction at the SA and AV nodes, decreasing inotropy, and thus lowering BP. The dihydropyridine CCBs act more peripherally, causing dilata-tion of the vasculature to lower BP, which may result in a *reflex tachycardia*. Calcium channel blockade of pancreatic β islet cells inhibits insulin release, resulting in hyperglycemia.

The differential diagnosis for toxicity from these agents includes cardioactive steroid (eg, digoxin), imidazoline (eg, clonidine), opioid, sedative-hypnotic, and cholinergic toxicity.

The pharmacokinetics vary widely based on the drug and formulation taken. Most of the immediate-release preparations

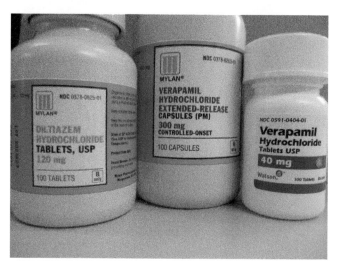

FIGURE 17.52 ■ Commonly Prescribed Calcium Channel Blockers. (Photo contributor: Rachel S. Weiselberg, MD.)

usually have an effect within 1 to 2 hours and not later than 6 hours. The extended-/controlled-/sustained-release products have later onset and peak effects and are more likely to be associated with delayed toxicity.

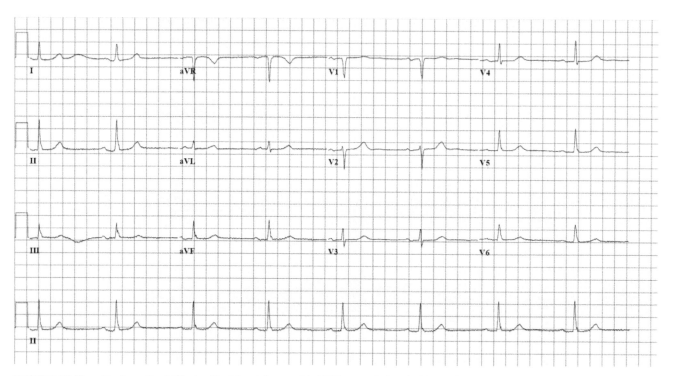

FIGURE 17.51 ■ Bradycardia; β-Blocker Toxicity. A 5-year-old child became lethargic 1 hour after mother found him playing with grandma's propranolol bottle, and his presenting ECG showed sinus bradycardia. (Photo contributor: Rachel S. Weiselberg, MD.)

Emergency Department Treatment and Disposition

Because there are a wide variety of BBs and CCBs, it is important to determine the name of the drug, the strength, the formulation, the maximum number of tablets that may have been ingested, and the time of ingestion. Consider social work and psychiatry consults as needed.

Obtain vital signs, including BP. Obtain an ECG, and place child on a cardiac monitor. Send for serum electrolytes, BUN, and creatinine, and check a bedside glucose.

Gastric decontamination may be indicated, depending on the timing of the ingestion and specific preparation (ie, immediate vs sustained release), with orogastric lavage, AC, and WBI all potential options. The choice of decontamination technique will vary depending on the severity of the overdose; orogastric lavage and WBI are generally reserved for patients with large overdoses.

The ability to observe the asymptomatic patient in the ED and discharge home will vary based on the drug and formulation. For some immediate-release preparations, if the child is completely asymptomatic and with normal vital signs at 6 to 8 hours, it may be safe to discharge home.

For any child with signs or symptoms of toxicity or overdose of a sustained-release preparation, admission to an ICU is advised.

Treatment is similar for both BBs and CCBs. IV fluids and atropine can be given initially. There is no true order in which to administer treatment, but glucagon and calcium salts are often the next step. Vasopressors, such as norepinephrine, may be necessary in severe cases of hemodynamic instability. High-dose insulin–euglycemia therapy has been shown to improve cardiac function. When these treatments are insufficient, an intra-aortic balloon pump or extracorporeal membrane oxygenation may be required. Extracorporeal removal (eg, hemodialysis) is generally ineffective for most lipophilic BBs and CCBs.

Pearls

1. BBs and CCBs can be highly toxic in young children, with significant toxicity occurring from only a single pill. Early consultation with the regional poison control center or medical toxicologist is advised.
2. Aggressive early decontamination and treatment are important.
3. High-dose insulin is given as a 1 unit/kg bolus with a dextrose bolus of 0.5 g/kg, followed by an insulin drip of 0.5 unit/kg/h, titrated to effect, with dextrose infusion of 0.5 g/kg/h.
4. Standard Pediatric Advanced Life Support (PALS) measures are generally ineffective for toxicity of these agents.

Clinical Summary

Clonidine is an imidazole derivative that acts via central α_2 agonism to produce its antihypertensive effect. In addition to being used to treat hypertension, it may be used therapeutically for attention-deficit/hyperactivity disorder, Tourette syndrome, neuropathic pain, and opioid withdrawal.

Following overdose, vital sign abnormalities may include an initial period of hypertension and tachycardia, followed by hypotension and bradycardia, respiratory depression,

hypoxia, and hypothermia. Lethargy, coma, miosis, and decreased deep tendon reflexes can be seen. A clonidine withdrawal syndrome has also been described that is manifested by hypertension, anxiety, agitation, headache, and confusion.

The toxicologic differential diagnosis of clonidine overdose includes BB, CCB, digoxin, and opioid toxicity.

Clonidine is available as tablets and patches. Ingestion of a single 0.1-mg tablet or a patch may cause toxicity in a small child. The onset of action for tablets is 30 to 90 minutes, with a half-life of 12 to 16 hours. Toxicokinetics are delayed for

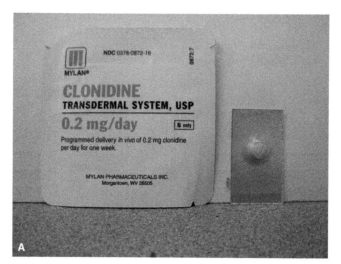

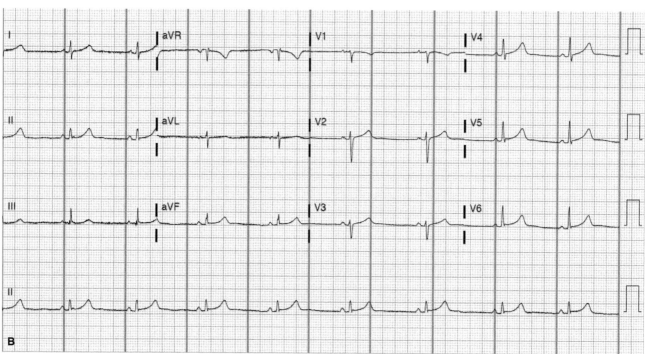

FIGURE 17.53 ■ Clonidine Toxicity. (**A**) Clonidine in 2 Formulations. (**B**) An 18-year-old woman with bradycardia (HR of 54 bpm). She intentionally took her grandmother's clonidine tablets. (Photo contributors: Rachel S. Weiselberg, MD [A], and Sushitha Surendran, MD [B].)

patch ingestion, and symptom onset may be delayed. The drug is mainly eliminated by the kidneys, but a considerable portion is also excreted in the bile.

Emergency Department Treatment and Disposition

GI decontamination with AC is advised if the airway is protected. There is a role for WBI in the case of an ingested patch.

All patients should have an ECG and cardiac monitoring. Send for serum electrolytes, BUN, and creatinine.

If the child ingests the tablet form of clonidine and is asymptomatic after 4 hours of observation, the child can be discharged home from the ED. If the child ingests a patch or if the child is symptomatic, admission to the ICU is advised.

There is no antidote for clonidine; treatment is supportive. Perform endotracheal intubation if airway protection is necessary. Naloxone may reverse some of the CNS and respiratory depression in some patients, but the therapeutic response is inconsistent. Atropine, pacing, and vasopressors can be used as needed for bradycardia and hypotension, but use of these is rarely needed.

Consultation with the regional poison control center or medical toxicologist for management recommendations is advised. Consult social services in cases involving young children or psychiatry in self-harm attempts.

Pearls

1. As little as 1 dose of clonidine can be toxic in a child.
2. AC should be given if the airway is protected.
3. Supportive care is the mainstay of therapy for most symptomatic patients.
4. Naloxone may be attempted to reverse CNS depression. The dose of naloxone for infants and children up to age 5 years or weighing 20 kg is 0.1 mg/kg. Children >5 years or weighing >20 kg should be given 2 mg. Naloxone can be given up to a maximum of 10 mg in a single dose.

CYCLIC ANTIDEPRESSANT TOXICITY

Clinical Summary

Cyclic antidepressants (CAs; eg, imipramine, amitriptyline, desipramine, nortriptyline) are commonly used medications for the treatment of various disorders including depression, nocturnal enuresis, anxiety disorders, attention-deficit/hyperactivity disorder, and migraine headaches. They are one of the most common causes of reported deaths from pharmaceutical products in the United States.

CAs inhibit CNS reuptake of norepinephrine, serotonin, and dopamine. Not all CAs have 3 rings; hence, the term *cyclic antidepressants* is a better classification than the more often used term *cyclic antidepressants*.

Toxicity from CAs is mostly attributed to cardiovascular and CNS effects. Toxicity may occur with therapeutic doses as well but is usually less clinically significant. Anticholinergic effects (central and peripheral) may be prominent. Central effects include lethargy, delirium, hallucinations, seizures,

and coma. Peripheral effects include dry skin, tachycardia, mydriasis, decreased bowel sounds, and urinary retention. Neurologic effects include depressed or altered mental status, seizures secondary to anticholinergic toxicity, and GABA antagonism. Cardiovascular effects include type Ia sodium channel blockade ("quinidine-like") leading to conduction delays and myocardial depression. On the ECG, this manifests as a prolonged QRS interval and possibly wide complex ventricular dysrhythmias and negative inotropy, and hypotension occurs secondary to vasodilation from α-adrenergic blockade. Tachycardia usually occurs secondary to anticholinergic effect and the normal reflexive physiologic response to hypotension.

The differential diagnosis includes agents causing CNS depression, especially those that impair cardiac conduction (eg, type Ia antidysrhythmics, phenothiazines) and other medical etiologies of CNS depression (eg, meningitis, intracranial hemorrhage, cerebral ischemia). Electrolyte imbalances

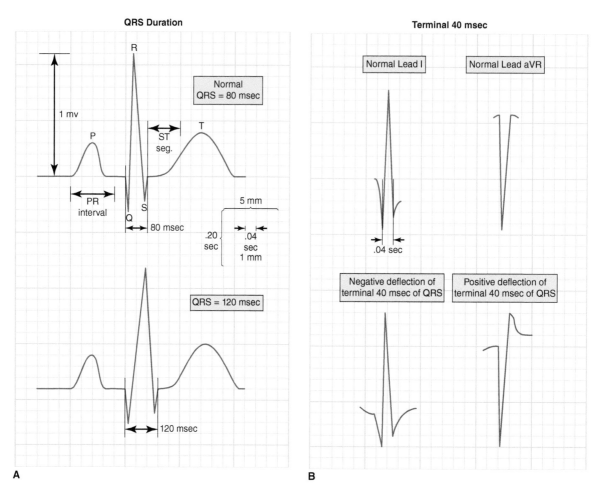

FIGURE 17.54 ■ QRS Duration and Terminal 40 Milliseconds in Cyclic Antidepressant Toxicity. (**A**) Example of QRS widening on ECG. (**B**) Right axis deviation of the terminal 40 milliseconds of the QRS complex.

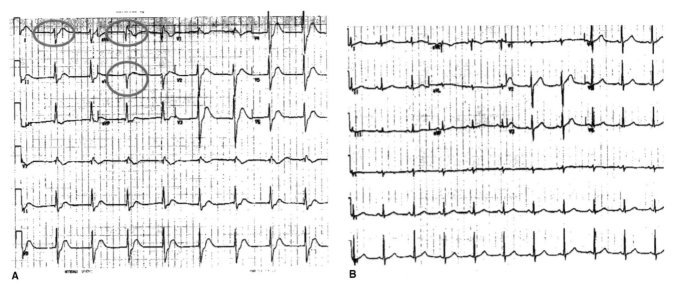

FIGURE 17.55 ▪ Cyclic Antidepressant Toxicity. (**A**) ECG of patient after overdose of amitriptyline. QRS duration of 160 milliseconds and terminal 40-millisecond axis changes in leads I, aVL, and aVR (circled in red) are seen. (**B**) ECG of the same patient after treatment with sodium bicarbonate, demonstrating narrowing of QRS complex (QRS duration 80 milliseconds). (Photo contributor: Mark K Su, MD, MPH.)

leading to cardiac conduction abnormalities are also a consideration.

Emergency Department Treatment and Disposition

History should focus on determining agent involved, dose, time of ingestion, and intent. Patient's mental status may impede obtaining a thorough history. Physical examination should focus on vital signs, including evaluation for anticholinergic effects and observation of mental status. Obtain a 12-lead ECG as soon as possible. The QRS interval is highly predictive of toxicity. This is based on a previous landmark study where approximately 30% of patients with a QRS duration >100 milliseconds had seizures; there was a 50% prevalence of ventricular dysrhythmias in patients with a QRS duration >160 milliseconds. In addition, in the setting of an acute overdose, the terminal 40-millisecond right axis changes (S waves in leads I and aVL and R in aVR) had a positive predictive value of 66% and a negative predictive value of 99%. Obtain serum APAP levels to evaluate for occult ingestion. Consult medical toxicologist, regional poison control center, psychiatry, and social services as needed.

Consider GI decontamination with AC if no contraindications; perform gastric lavage if patients have life-threatening toxicity or a history of a large recent ingestion. AC should be administered with caution because patients may have a rapid deterioration in mental status.

Sodium bicarbonate should be administered to patients with signs of significant cardiac toxicity (ie, prolonged QRS duration on the 12-lead ECG). Hypotension is managed initially with IV fluids and/or NaHCO₃ and then vasopressors if hypotension persists. Patients may be discharged from ED if they do not develop seizures, hypotension, or ECG changes after a 6-hour observation period and evaluation by a psychiatrist (if indicated) is completed. Admit patients with seizures, cardiac dysrhythmias, or CNS depression to an ICU for monitoring.

Pearls

1. CA toxicity presents with cardiovascular and CNS effects.
2. A 12-lead ECG is the best diagnostic test to determine if a patient has significant CA toxicity.
3. A QRS duration >100 milliseconds is concerning for CA (and other sodium channel blocker) toxicity.
4. CAs have a narrow therapeutic window, and ingestion of small amounts may be toxic in young children.
5. Physostigmine should not be given to reverse anticholinergic toxicity from CAs because of potential deleterious cardiovascular consequences.

LEAD TOXICITY

Clinical Summary

Lead is a heavy metal that can be found in paint, food/liquids cooked or stored in ceramic vessels, fishing weights, bullets, and many other items. Pediatric lead screening is based on risk of exposure generally at 12 and 24 months of age. Symptoms are usually seen once blood lead levels (BLLs) are >50 μg/dL. BLLs of >70 μg/dL are usually associated with severe toxicity.

GI symptoms (abdominal pain, vomiting, anorexia) are common in acute lead toxicity, but these are nonspecific. CNS findings correlate with lead levels. As levels exceed 70 μg/dL, children are at risk for encephalopathy and may exhibit change in mental status, incoordination, seizures, and coma. Early symptoms of lead poisoning can be misdiagnosed as gastroenteritis or a behavioral disorder.

Lead is best absorbed when ingested or inhaled and is transported by RBC throughout the body. The majority of lead is stored in bone. Other areas of deposition are the liver, kidney, and brain. The kidneys are the primary site of excretion, followed by the liver. The half-life of lead in children is approximately 10 months in the blood, 40 days in soft tissue, and up to 20 years in bone.

Important information that should be obtained regarding lead exposures includes the following: take a medical history, determine the age of the patient's home, recent remodeling, family history including pica, and patient's country of origin. Perform a full neurologic exam, including fundoscopy.

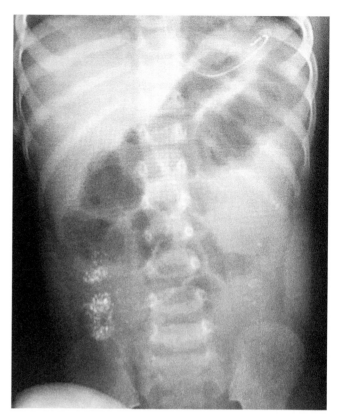

FIGURE 17.57 ■ Lead Intoxication. Single frontal view of the abdomen demonstrates multiple radiopaque densities consistent with ingested leaded material in a child with a history of pica. (Photo contributor: Darien Sutton-Ramsey, MD.)

Emergency Department Treatment and Disposition

Discharge asymptomatic patients with serum lead level of <45 μg/dL home if return to safe lead-free environment is possible. Arrange follow-up with primary care and notify local health department (or lead bureau). Asymptomatic children with BLLs between 45 and 70 μg/dL may undergo outpatient chelation, but admission may be necessary, especially if adequate follow-up cannot be arranged.

Check CBC with peripheral smear for basophilic stippling, the whole BLL, basic chemistry panel with renal function, and urinalysis. Obtain an abdominal radiograph to look for ingested FBs and radiographs of long bones to look for lead lines. Perform WBI if radiographs show lead FBs in the GI tract and there is no contraindication. Children should be admitted to the hospital for chelation therapy if there are severe symptoms or the BLL is >70 μg/dL. Admit patients with lead encephalopathy to the pediatric ICU. Consult local

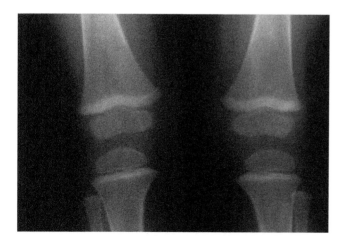

FIGURE 17.56 ■ Lead Toxicity. Single anteroposterior view of the knees shows dense metaphyseal bands involving the femora, bilateral tibias, and bilateral fibulas, compatible with chronic lead toxicity. (Photo contributor: John Amodio, MD.)

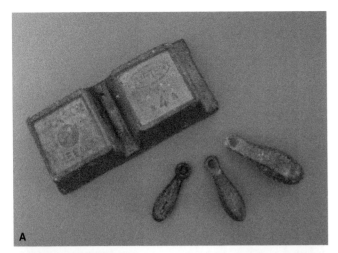

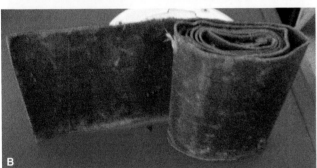

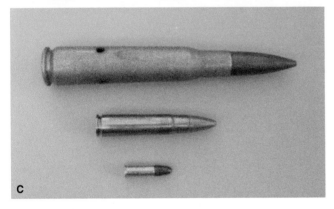

FIGURE 17.58 ■ Potential Household Sources of Lead. Lead fishing weights (**A**), lead ballast (**B**) and lead bullets (**C**). These sources of lead may cause significant toxicity if ingested by children. (Photo contributor: Rachel S. Weiselberg, MD.)

medical toxicologist or regional poison control center for management recommendations.

Depending on the case, chelation may be performed with oral succimer, intramuscular dimercaprol (BAL), and IV edetate calcium disodium (CaNa$_2$EDTA). Succimer therapy alone is given for asymptomatic or minimally symptomatic patients; for children with acute encephalopathy, administer both BAL and CaNa$_2$EDTA. Benzodiazepines are first-line therapy for seizures.

Pearls

1. With mild symptoms, lead toxicity can be missed.
2. Most asymptomatic children with mildly elevated BLLs can be managed safely in the outpatient setting.
3. For acute lead encephalopathy, start BAL at 75 mg/m^2 IM (every 4 hours for 5 days) as soon as possible. If the patient is still in the ED 4 hours later, give the second IM dose and then start the CaNa$_2$EDTA at 1500 mg/m^2/day (can be divided or given continuously).
4. Check siblings of affected children for lead poisoning.
5. Patients who are discharged home from the ED must be sent to a safe, lead-free environment.

Clinical Summary

Caustics are agents that cause both functional and histologic damage on contact with body surfaces. Caustic substances are commonly associated with agents with extremes of pH such as acids and alkalis (bases). However, they are a diverse group of agents, and other factors besides pH (eg, concentration, amount, and intrinsic characteristics of a particular substance) can determine the potential for tissue injury. Examples of various caustic agents include hydrochloric acid, sodium hydroxide, hydrofluoric acid, mercuric chloride, and phenol. A significant number of cases occur in the pediatric population, especially in children <5 years old.

Direct contact of any external or internal tissue surface by a caustic agent can result in injury.

Pain is usually the first symptom. Because most caustic agents are ingested, localization of pain to the oropharynx, chest, and abdomen is most common. GI effects such as nausea, vomiting, drooling, and inability to swallow are often present. Upper airway injury may result in the development of stridor, and rapid deterioration of respiratory status may occur.

Although signs of physical injury around the mouth and oropharynx may be visualized, significant esophageal injury may still be present in the absence of physical examination findings. Burns on the face and upper chest (ie, "dribble burns") may be apparent. Ocular injury may occur, and examination of the eyes for pH, abrasions, and ulcers is very important. Examination of the chest may reveal subcutaneous emphysema, abnormal breath sounds, or pericardial friction rub (Hamman crunch). Examination of the abdomen may reveal tenderness and peritoneal signs; however, peritoneal signs may be absent even with significant intestinal perforation.

For some patients, long-term or delayed complications of caustic ingestion may be particularly troublesome, especially when GI strictures develop. The patient may suffer from repeated hospitalizations and nutritional deficiencies and may require multiple esophageal dilatations. Other laryngotracheal and pharyngeal injuries, such as stenosis or reflux, can further contribute to morbidity and patient discomfort. Pyloric obstruction and impaired gastric function may also occur.

History should focus on determining agent involved, amount, time of ingestion, and intent. The patient's mental status may impede obtaining a thorough history.

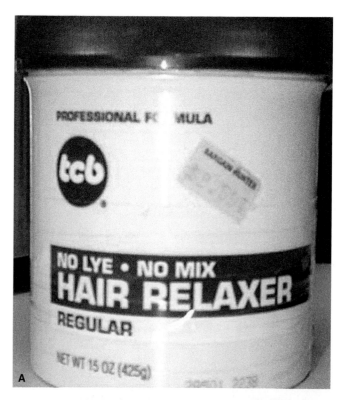

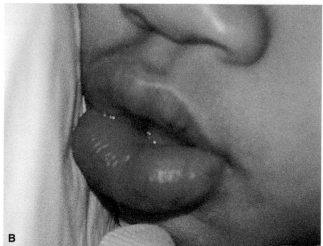

FIGURE 17.59 ■ Caustic Injury. (**A**) A toddler was found with a substance on his mouth and hands from the container that contained lithium hydroxide (strong base) as one of the major ingredients. (**B**) He was brought to the ED about 4 hours after the exposure with drooling and 2 episodes of emesis. Oropharyngeal burns with erythema and swelling of the lips were noted. Fiberoptic laryngoscopy showed no evidence of edema of vocal cords or hypopharynx. Endoscopy revealed no evidence of injury. One day later, he was able to eat and drink without difficulty. (Photo contributor: Howard Greller, MD.)

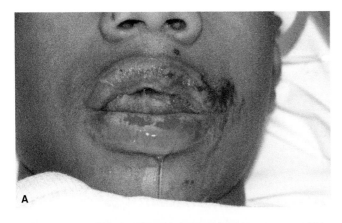

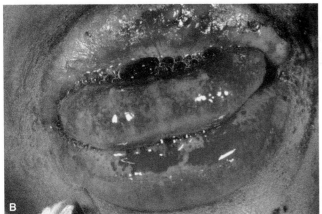

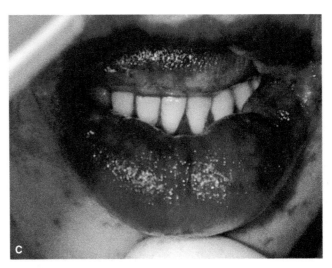

FIGURE 17.60 ▪ Caustic Burns. (**A, B**) Adolescent male who drank lye for a suicide attempt is shown presenting with drooling and burns on the lip and tongue, which is also edematous. Endoscopy revealed evidence of submucosal lesions, ulcerations, and exudates. (**C**) Photograph demonstrating burns to the lips and tongue of a 20-year-old boy following ingestion of sodium hydroxide. (Photo contributor: Binita R. Shah, MD [A, B], and [C] reproduced with permission from Nelson LS, Hoffman RS, Howland MA, et al. *Goldfrank's Toxicologic Emergencies,* 11th ed. McGraw-Hill Education; New York, NY, 2019. Photo contributor: The Fellowship in Medical Toxicology, New York University School of Medicine, New York City Poison Center.)

Emergency Department Treatment and Disposition

Initial stabilization of ABCs is crucial because injury occurs so rapidly. Establish 2 large-bore IVs to administer fluids. Order serum chemistry, CBC, PT/PTT (INR), and blood gas with serum lactate concentration. Coingestants (eg, APAP) and subsequent toxidromes should be sought for in patients who present with intentional ingestion. Order type and screen for blood products. Plain radiographs of the chest and abdomen may be useful to assess for perforation. As clinically indicated, consult with medical toxicologist, regional poison control center, gastroenterology, surgery, otolaryngology, and psychiatry (if intentional).

Emesis should never be induced because tissue injury may be exacerbated by reexposing potentially damaged areas. AC should *not* be given. If a solid substance has been ingested, a small quantity of water may be given to dissolve the agent. This will also be effective if the caustic material becomes lodged at an area of anatomic narrowing.

Imaging studies such as contrast studies with gastrograffin or barium and CT are not useful in the acute setting. Emergent endoscopy should be performed in patients with intentional suicidal ingestions and in children with unintentional ingestions if they have 2 of the following 3 signs: vomiting (inability to drink), drooling, or stridor. The optimal time to perform endoscopy is controversial, but ideally, it should be performed within 24 to 48 hours of injury. Critically ill patients may benefit from surgical intervention to remove necrotic tissue. Indications for surgical intervention include obvious perforation, presence of peritoneal signs, and persistent hypotension. Coagulopathy and acidosis are also poor prognostic findings. Various endoscopic grading systems of GI burns exist. In general, burns can be classified as follows:

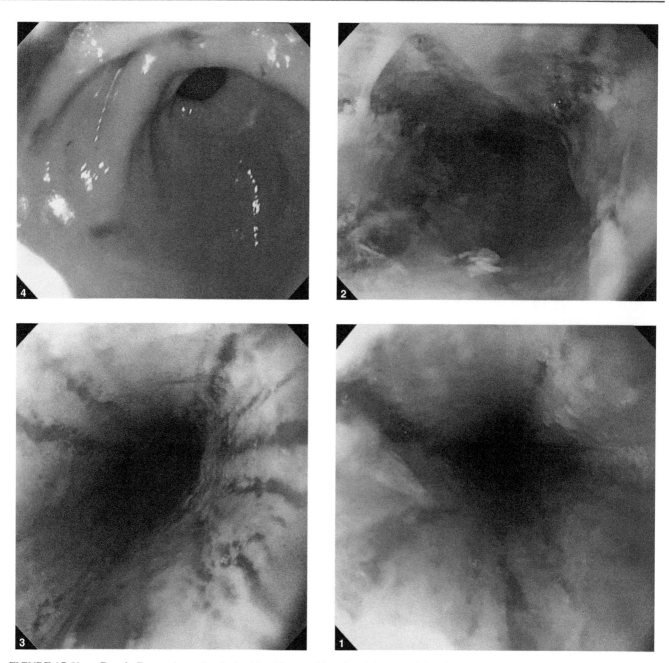

FIGURE 17.61 ■ Caustic Burns. A previously healthy 14-year-old male adolescent with unintentional ingestion of heavy-duty degreaser (he thought he was drinking wine!) presented with chest pain and drooling. His endoscopy showed grade IIb (circumferential) lesions (Photo contributor: Mark K. Su, MD, MPH.)

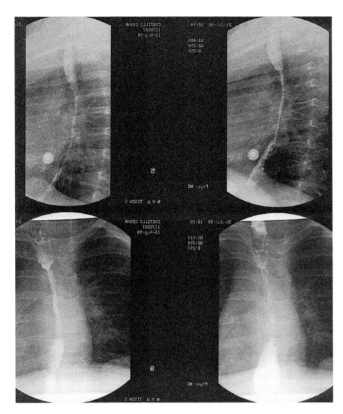

FIGURE 17.62 ■ Lye Stricture. Several projections of the esophagus from a barium swallow demonstrate a long mid esophageal stricture. The patient had swallowed lye several months prior and complained of dysphagia. (Photo contributor: Dr. John Amodio.)

Grade	Findings/Prognosis	Implications
Grade 0	No injury	No stricture formation
Grade I	Hyperemia or edema of mucosa	No stricture formation
Grade IIA	Submucosal lesions, ulcerations and exudates	Usually no stricture formation
Grade IIB	Circumferential	Often develop strictures
Grade III	Deep ulcers; necrosis	Almost always develop strictures; other complications

Pearls

1. Dilution or neutralization is *not* recommended in the ED.
2. Absence of obvious burns on physical examination does not exclude significant GI tract injury.
3. Suspect child abuse with exposures in very small infants and children.
4. If grade IIB lesions are visualized on endoscopy, administration of corticosteroids is associated with decreased development of esophageal strictures.
5. Patients with significant caustic injuries to the GI tract require long-term follow-up for many years to monitor for development of complications, including malignancy.

NICOTINE

Clinical Summary

Nicotine is primarily derived from the tobacco plant, most often from the species *Nicotiana tabacum*. Most nicotine exposures and poisonings that occur in children are from ingestion of tobacco cigarettes or other nicotine-containing products, nicotine pesticides, and more recently, nicotine liquid in electronic cigarettes (e-cigarettes). Nicotine is highly addictive, leading to dependency, and its long-term use is associated with many chronic diseases. Nicotine is well absorbed via inhalation, ingestion, or dermal exposure. Overall, nicotine is a rare cause of acute poisoning, but severe toxicity and death can occur.

The lethal dose of nicotine is approximately 0.5 to 1 mg/kg in adults. Severe toxicity can occur in children at even lower doses. One tobacco cigarette contains approximately 10 to 30 mg of nicotine and, when smoked, delivers 0.5 to 3 mg of absorbed nicotine. E-cigarettes contain varying but substantial concentrations of liquid nicotine in a reservoir or cartridge (0–59 mg/mL). These liquid nicotine products can be flavored and brightly colored and may be sold in large-volume replacement bottles with attractive packaging, making them particularly appealing to young children.

Nicotine binds to nicotinic receptors (nAChR) in the brain, sympathetic and parasympathetic ganglia, and neuromuscular junction, and stimulates acetylcholine release. Severe toxicity presents in 2 phases. Early signs and symptoms of nicotine toxicity present within the first hour and are related to cholinergic excess; these include diaphoresis, salivation, bronchorrhea, vomiting, and diarrhea. Hypertension and tachycardia may occur, as well as neurologic symptoms, such as headache, dizziness, tremor, fasciculations, ataxia, agitation, confusion, and seizures. One to 4 hours after ingestion, the late manifestations occur, including bradycardia, hypotension, dysrhythmias, coma, and neuromuscular blockade with respiratory muscle paralysis and apnea.

Differential diagnosis includes exposure to cholinergic agents, such as pesticides, nerve agents, malathion, and neostigmine, as well as other life-threatening toxins that cause acute GI symptoms, including heavy metals, ricin, and colchicine.

Obtain a history focused on type of product, route, dosage, timing, and symptoms. Physical examination should focus on vital signs, cardiopulmonary assessment, and neurologic status. Obtain IV access and basic laboratory studies. Consider CXR, ECG, head CT, and lumbar puncture for further evaluation. Serum or urine nicotine concentrations are not useful in acute management of nicotine toxicity.

Emergency Department Treatment and Disposition

Mild symptoms (vomiting, agitation) should resolve within 12 hours. Patients who are asymptomatic or with only mild symptoms can be observed for several hours and then discharged home if there are no significant comorbidities or suicidal intent.

Treatment of severe toxicity is primarily supportive. Decontamination with AC is indicated but may be limited by the risk of pulmonary aspiration from vomiting, seizure, or depressed level of consciousness. Ensure airway protection and respiratory support. Atropine can be used to treat excess secretions, wheezing, or bradycardia. Treat hypotension with IV fluids and vasopressors if necessary. Treat seizures with benzodiazepines. Consult the regional poison control center or medical toxicologist for any questions and management recommendations. Patients with signs or symptoms of severe toxicity should be admitted to an ICU for continuous monitoring and supportive care.

Pearls

1. Nicotine poisoning usually occurs after ingestion of nicotine-containing products, with liquid nicotine from e-cigarettes becoming a more frequent source of exposure.
2. Nicotine toxicity presents with signs and symptoms of cholinergic excess early (vomiting, diarrhea, salivation, bronchorrhea, diaphoresis) and, in severe toxicity, progresses to seizures, dysrhythmias, hypotension, bradycardia, and neuromuscular blockade with respiratory paralysis.
3. Treatment is symptomatic and supportive.

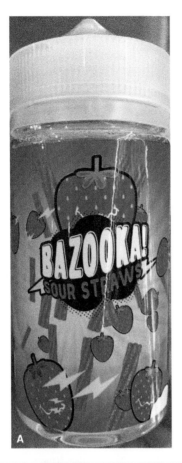
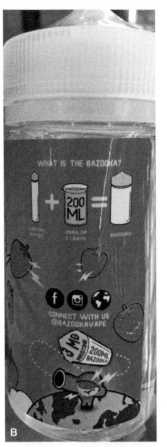
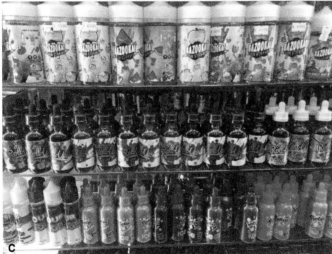
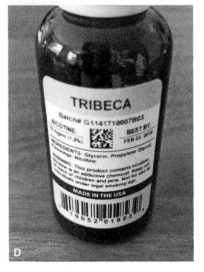

FIGURE 17.63 ■ Various Liquid Nicotine Products for Use with E-Cigarettes. (**A–D**) Many liquid nicotine products are brightly colored and multiflavored with decorative packaging, making them particularly attractive to young children. Nicotine content varies among products, and many are sold in large-volume bottles. (Photo contributors: Madeline H. Renny, MD [A–C], and Daniel J Repplinger, MD [D].)

Clinical Summary

Caffeine-containing beverages are ubiquitous throughout the world and often imbibed for their stimulant effects. Caffeine is also found in over-the-counter supplements in both tablet and powdered form. It is aggressively marketed for alertness or dieting and has become increasingly popular in energy drinks. Powdered caffeine has caused multiple deaths in recent years, so its sale is limited or prohibited in many parts of the United States. Medically, caffeine is used to treat neonatal apnea and as an analgesic adjuvant.

Caffeine is a methylxanthine, causing the release of endogenous catecholamines and also functioning as an adenosine antagonist. Acute ingestions >20 mg/kg are potentially toxic, and those >150 to 200 mg/kg may be lethal.

Clinical manifestations of caffeine toxicity include severe nausea and vomiting, tachycardia, atrial and ventricular dysrhythmias (including supraventricular tachycardia [SVT]), myocardial infarction, headache, agitation, and seizures.

Differential diagnosis includes sympathomimetic toxicity, from substances such as amphetamines and cocaine, and other substances or syndromes that can cause seizures and status epilepticus, such as cyclic antidepressants, camphor, bupropion, INH, and withdrawal syndromes.

Obtain a history focused on type of product, dosage, timing, and symptoms. Physical examination should focus on vital signs (look for a widened pulse pressure due to enhanced inotropy and peripheral vasodilation), cardiopulmonary assessment, and neurologic status. Obtain an ECG and basic laboratory studies, including serum chemistries to assess for electrolyte disturbances (most often hypokalemia, but can also see hypomagnesemia and hypophosphatemia) and anion gap (high anion gap metabolic acidosis), blood gas and lactate, creatinine kinase (assess for rhabdomyolysis), and serum caffeine level, which may correlate with acute toxicity.

Emergency Department Treatment and Disposition

Address ABCs. Multiple-dose AC is indicated to limit absorption and enhance elimination. Orogastric lavage should be considered in patients who present early after potentially life-threatening ingestions. Antiemetics (eg, ondansetron, metoclopramide) may be used.

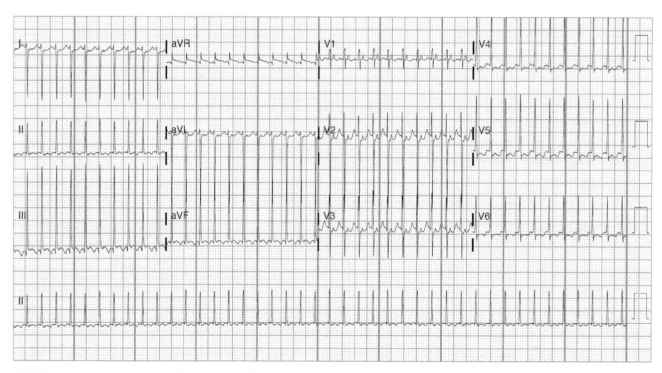

FIGURE 17.64 ■ Supraventricular Tachycardia (SVT) from Caffeine Toxicity. A 12 lead ECG shows regular narrow complex tachycardia (HR of 250 bpm) with retrograde P waves. Caffeine toxicity can present with atrial and ventricular dysrhythmias, including SVT. The primary treatment for caffeine-induced SVT is the administration of benzodiazepines or a calcium channel blocker, such as diltiazem. (Photo contributor: Sushitha Surendran, MD.)

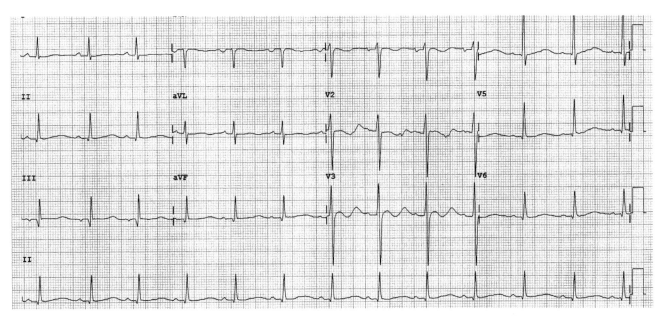

FIGURE 17.65 ■ Hypokalemia from Caffeine Toxicity. Caffeine toxicity can lead to electrolyte disturbances, most often hypokalemia. In severe hypokalemia, U waves may be noted on an ECG, as seen here. Patients with symptomatic hypokalemia with ECG changes should be treated with supplemental potassium. (Photo contributor: Robert S. Hoffman, MD.)

IV fluids should be given for hypotension, followed by vasopressor therapy if hypotension persists after fluid resuscitation. Phenylephrine is the first-line pressor of choice, followed by norepinephrine. Esmolol can be used for refractory hypotension (to reverse β_2-adrenergic–mediated vasodilation). If a patient has SVT, then adenosine is unlikely to be successful in converting the rhythm. The primary treatment for caffeine-induced SVT is the administration of benzodiazepines or a CCB, such as diltiazem. Intractable seizures may occur and should be treated aggressively with benzodiazepines and then barbiturates or another sedative-hypnotic (eg, propofol) if these are unsuccessful. Patients with symptomatic hypokalemia with ECG changes should treated with supplemental potassium.

Extracorporeal removal with hemodialysis is indicated for patients with an acute serum caffeine concentration >90 μg/mL or a serum caffeine concentration >40 μg/mL and seizures, hypotension unresponsive to IV fluid, or ventricular dysrhythmias.

Consult the regional poison control center or medical toxicologist for any questions and management recommendations. Patients with caffeine toxicity should be admitted to an ICU for continuous monitoring.

Pearls

1. Caffeine is ubiquitously used throughout the world, but its excessive consumption in supplements and energy drinks can lead to severe poisoning and even death.
2. Caffeine toxicity presents with vomiting, tachycardia, dysrhythmias, intractable seizures, and electrolyte abnormalities.
3. Treatment includes multiple-dose AC, specific therapies for hypotension and dysrhythmias, electrolyte repletion, aggressive treatment of seizures, and hemodialysis in severe poisoning.

Chapter 18

ENVIRONMENTAL EMERGENCIES

Jeanine E. Hall
Christine S. Cho

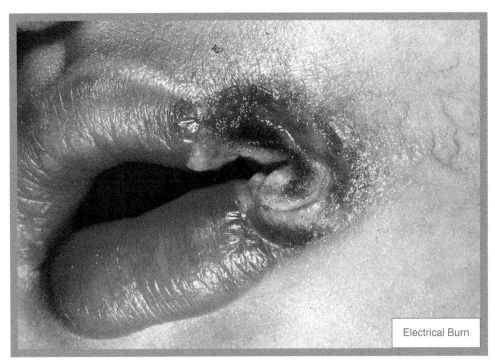

Electrical Burn

(Photo contributor: Binita R. Shah, MD)

The authors acknowledge the special contributions of Mark Silverberg, Teresa Bowen Spinelli, and Chaiya Laoteppitaks to prior edition.

807

THERMAL BURNS

Clinical Summary

The extent of burn-related injury depends on the amount of heat, the delivery medium (gas, liquid, solid, or vapor), and the duration of contact. Scald burns are most common in children. The majority of thermal injuries occur within the home, and approximately 60% of pediatric burn patients are male. In the United States, burn-related injuries in children result in approximately 300 ED visits and 2 deaths daily. Burns can be graded by depth and amount of damage.

Emergency Department Treatment and Disposition

Most thermal burns can be treated in the outpatient setting with appropriate follow-up with a burn specialist as clinically indicated. Pain should be managed as soon as possible in all patients presenting for burn management. Extent of the burn should be estimated using 1 of the following methods: Lund-Browder chart (most accurate), rule of nines (adults only; pediatric version available), or palmar surface (palm + finger tips = 1% burn surface area). Minor burns involve <10% body surface area (BSA) and do not involve the airway, hands, face, or genitalia. Minor burn management requires local wound management consisting of cooling methods (tepid water 55–65°F or 13–18°C) to reduce extension of burn, cleaning, debridement, topical antimicrobial application, and dressing. Controversy exists regarding unroofing intact blisters. The wound should be irrigated with cool saline, and necrotic skin should be debrided. A topical antimicrobial ointment such as a triple-antibiotic ointment and/or an advanced burn dressing should be applied. Silver sulfadiazine has been commonly used in the past but may lead to a delay in wound healing. A sterile dressing should then be applied and the patient should be provided adequate analgesics and close follow-up.

For significant (>10% BSA) and major (>20% BSA) thermal injuries in patients with preexisting medical conditions, the possibility of multiorgan failure needs to be anticipated, and screening labs such as a CBC, electrolytes, glucose, BUN, creatinine, creatine phosphokinase, and urinalysis should be ordered. Any history or signs of significant smoke inhalation (carbonaceous sputum, hoarse voice, singed nasal hair, or evidence of hypoxia) should prompt a CXR. All patients who were in a fire should have carboxyhemoglobin

TABLE 18.1 ■ CLASSIFICATION OF THERMAL BURNS

Depth	Former Classification	Tissue Affected	Clinical Manifestations	Treatment/Outcome
Superficial or epidermal	First degree	Epidermis	Redness, warm or hot to touch, painful	Local burn first aid No scarring Heals within 3–5 days
Partial-thickness (superficial)	Second degree	Epidermis/upper layer of dermis	Redness, painful, fluid-filled blisters	Heals spontaneously within 3 weeks without functional impairment or hypertrophic scarring
Partial-thickness (deep)	Second degree	Epidermis/lower layer of dermis	Blisters, red or waxy dry skin	Heals within 3–9 weeks; scarring is likely to occur Hypertrophic scarring treated with excision and grafting
Full-thickness	Third degree	Epidermis/dermis, hair follicles, sweat glands, other adnexal skin structures	Paresthesia (loss of tactile sensation) Dry or leathery skin texture Charred, blackened, or white in appearance	Excision and grafting
Fourth degree (deep full-thickness)	Fourth degree[a]	Cutaneous and subcutaneous structures, including muscle, fascia, bone	Paresthesia (loss of tactile sensation)	Excision and grafting Amputation may be required in some cases

[a]Not universally used.

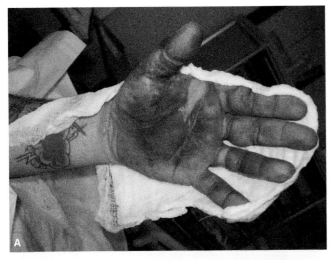

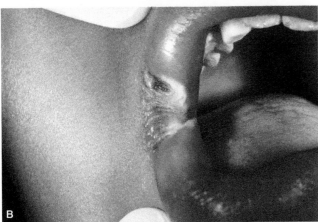

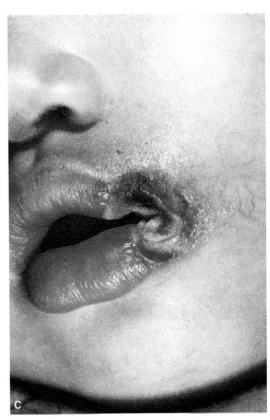

FIGURE 18.1 ■ Electrical Burns. (**A**) These burns to the hand were sustained by an electrician who was working on a high-voltage wire while constructing our new ED. (**B, C**) Third-degree burns to the commissure of the mouth after chewing on an electrical cord are seen in 2 different toddlers. These patients need to be followed very closely as they are prone to delayed bleeding because tissue necrosis can erode to the labial artery 5 to 10 days after the initial injury. (Photo contributors: Mark Silverberg, MD [A], and Binita R. Shah, MD [B, C].)

(CO-Hgb) concentration determined from a venous blood sample. A pulse oximetry level (>96%) without visual signs of oral burns *and* a normal venous CO-Hgb level (<5%) virtually rules out the possibility of inhalation injury. Patients with CO-Hgb levels above baseline should be placed on high-flow oxygen to help dissociate the carbon monoxide (CO) from their hemoglobin. Patients with significant CO-Hgb levels require transfer to a hyperbaric chamber. Hyperbaric oxygen has been shown to decrease the long-term neurologic sequelae associated with CO poisoning and should be employed even if the CO-Hgb level has been returned back to normal with simple high-flow oxygen. Cyanide poisoning should also be considered in fire victims. Laboratory findings will include an elevated anion gap and lactate level. Significantly, burned

patients should be resuscitated in the ED and transferred to a burn center when possible. Patients with burns that meet the following American Burn Association criteria should be transferred to a burn center: partial-thickness burns >10% total BSA; burns involving face, feet, genitalia, perineum, or major joints; third-degree burns; electrical burns; chemical burns; inhalational injury; burn injury in patients with preexisting medical disorders that could complicate management, prolong recovery, or affect mortality; any patient with burns and concomitant trauma in which the burn injury poses the greatest risk of morbidity or mortality; burned children in hospitals without qualified personnel or equipment for the care of children; and burn injury in patients who will require special social, emotional, or rehabilitative intervention.

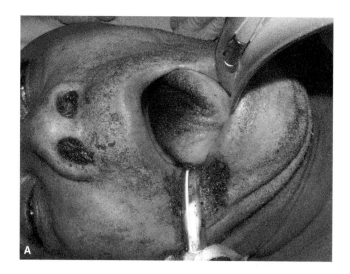

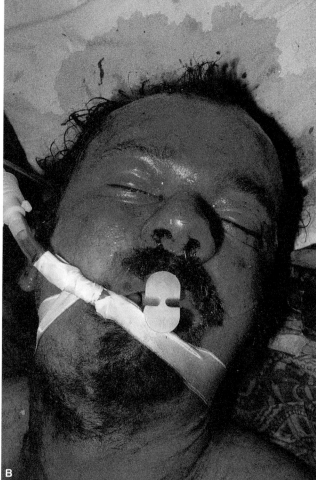

FIGURE 18.2 ■ Inhalation Injuries Following Fire. (**A**) Soot in the oral cavity is a clinical cue that a patient may have sustained a lung injury while in a fire. (**B**) Picture of a young man with second- and third-degree burns to the face and a CO-Hgb level of 32%. His oropharyngeal burns and carbonaceous sputum necessitated intubation on arrival in the ED. After resuscitation and stabilization, he was transported to a hyperbaric chamber. (Photo contributors: Mark Silverberg, MD [A], and Michael Lucchesi, MD [B].)

The Parkland formula (4 mL/kg × body weight in kilograms × percentage of BSA burned) is used for calculating the amount of Ringer's lactate needed for initial resuscitation for burn shock. Half of this volume should be given in the first 8 hours after the burn occurred and half in the following 16 hours. Treating physicians should remember that this volume is in addition to regular maintenance fluids. Fluid resuscitation is deemed adequate if urine output is maintained at 0.5 mL/kg/h for adults and 0.5 to 1.0 mL/kg/h for children <30 kg. Burns are considered traumatic injuries, so any patient with a significant burn should be evaluated by a trauma team. Circumferential burns of an extremity need to be monitored closely and should prompt urgent surgical evaluation should symptoms of compartment syndrome develop.

Electrical burns to the corner of the mouth caused by chewing on an electrified wire deserve special mention. They need to be followed closely because they are prone to delayed bleeding as tissue necrosis can erode into the labial artery 5 to 10 days after the initial injury.

Clinicians should inquire about the patient's tetanus status and give a tetanus booster in patients who have not had a booster in the past 5 years. In addition, tetanus immunoglobulin should be given to patients who have not completed the tetanus immunizations schedule.

Pearls

1. All burn patients should initially receive supplemental oxygen until it is determined that they do not need it.
2. Pain should be addressed as early as possible in clinical course and treated appropriately.
3. Children with large percentage of BSA burns are at risk for developing hypothermia.
4. Children with significant burns need comprehensive fluid management with the use of aids such as the Parkland formula for calculating maintenance plus ongoing deficits for burn shock.
5. Burns as a manifestation of non-accidental trauma is seen in 10% of children with abuse.

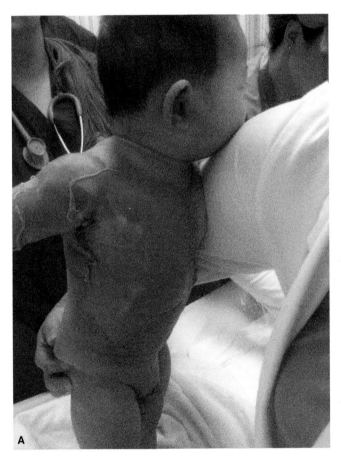
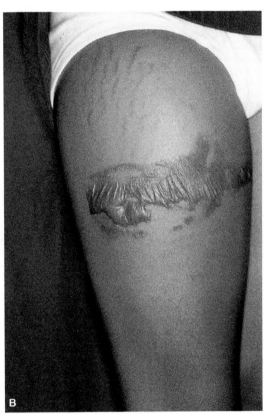

FIGURE 18.3 ▪ Second-Degree Burns. **(A)** This child sustained second-degree burns to his trunk and upper arm after accidentally pulling down a cup of hot soup from the table and required a transfer to a burn center. **(B)** An image of a 10-year-old boy who sustained a second-degree burn with blistering to the anterior surface of the upper thigh from an accidental spilling of hot cooking oil from a frying pan.

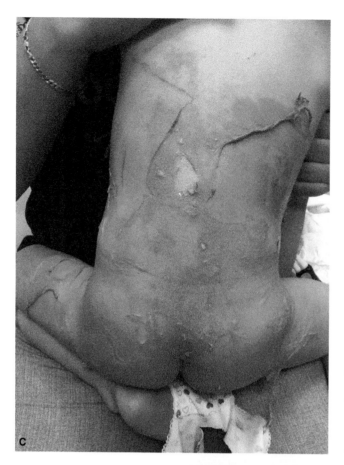

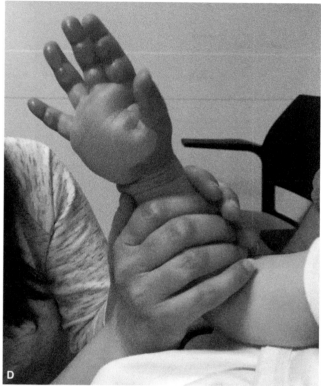

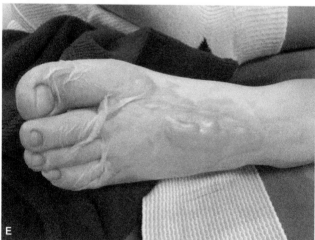

FIGURE 18.3 ■ (*Continued*) (**C**) A 4-year-old girl who sustained a second-degree burn to her torso, buttocks, and upper thighs after falling into a very large pot of soup that a relative had left on the floor. (**D**) The hand of a 16-month-old toddler who sustained a second-degree burn to the palmar surfaces of his bilateral hands after touching the inside of an open oven door. (**E**) An image of the left foot of a child who sustained a second-degree burn after spilling a cup of noodles on his foot. (Photo contributors: Barry Hahn, MD [A], Binita R. Shah, MD [B], Jeanine E. Hall, MD [C, D], and Kathryn Pade, MD [E].)

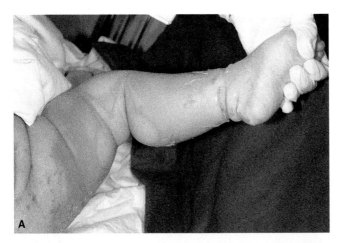

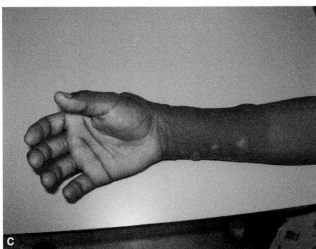

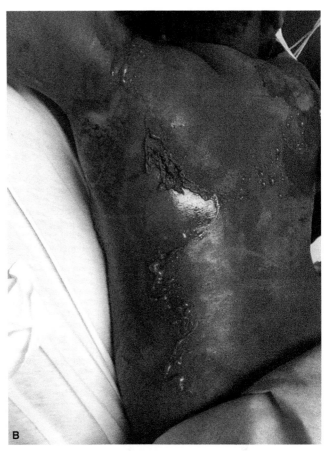

FIGURE 18.4 ■ Circumferential Burns. (**A**) A 9-month-old infant sustained circumferential burns to the ankle, calf, and thigh after accidentally pulling hot soup from the table while in grandmother's lap. Inflicted burns from child abuse need to be considered in such cases. The pattern of the burn seen here is consistent with a splash injury and not an immersion injury (see Figure 1.20). (**B**) Superficial partial-thickness burns are seen in this child with autism and seizure disorder presenting to the ED after a possible seizure in the bathtub, when he fell into the tub partly filled with warm water. Given the concerning history, child protective services was called. Circumferential burns to an extremity (**C**) or chest (**B**) put the patient at risk for a compartment syndrome and may require a fasciotomy should contracture of the eschar develop. (Photo contributors: Binita R. Shah, MD [A], Virteeka Sinha, MD [B], and Mark Silverberg, MD [C].)

Clinical Summary

Cold injuries range from frostnip to frostbite (see Table 18.2). Frostbite classification was historically based on degrees (ie, first, second, or third degree), but this does not accurately predict long-term outcome; therefore, classifying burns as superficial or deep is preferred. Prognostic classification symptoms are being developed. History should focus on exposure temperature, duration of exposure, wind velocity, clothing, freeze-thaw-freeze events, in-field treatment, and underlying comorbidities. Distal areas are always affected first, which usually include fingers, toes, extremities, nose, and ears and even the cornea. Note that swelling and blistering may not be present until after rewarming has taken place. Caretakers should focus on vital signs, assessment of the degree of hypothermia, and resuscitation. Retained sensation, normal skin color, and clear fluid within blisters (if present) indicate positive prognosis. Nonblanching, cyanotic, firm skin and dark fluid-filled blisters indicate poor prognosis. Risk factors include extremes of age, homelessness, altered mental status (drug/alcohol use, head trauma), nicotine or other vasoconstrictive drug use, preexistence of peripheral vascular disease, and diabetes.

Emergency Department Treatment and Disposition

Rewarming begins in the field after it is assured that frozen regions will not be reexposed. Refreezing causes considerably

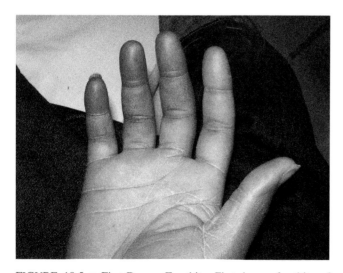

FIGURE 18.5 ■ First-Degree Frostbite. First-degree frostbite of the third, fourth, and fifth digits on a homeless teenage drug abuser taken on a very cold day in January. Demarcation has already begun. (Photo contributor: Mark Silverberg, MD.)

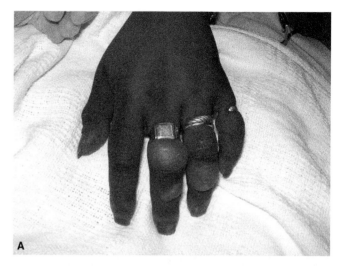

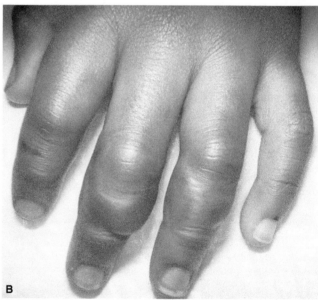

FIGURE 18.6 ■ Second-Degree Frostbite. (A) Clear fluid-filled blisters are the hallmark of second-degree frostbite. This patient's rings also needed to be cut off immediately. (B) A 5-year-old child who was playing in the snow for several hours sustained frostbites to the second, third (with clear fluid blister), and fourth digits. The picture was taken several hours after the injury occurred. (Photo contributors: Mark Silverberg, MD [A], and Binita R. Shah, MD [B].)

more tissue damage than if the limb was left cold and rewarmed later. Upon ED arrival, stabilize airway, breathing, and circulation (ABCs) including management of hypothermia, cardiac dysrhythmias, intoxication, head injury, and hypoglycemia—all of which could have caused the cold exposure. Remove all wet garments, which can cause continued heat loss. Also remove any constrictive items such as rings and other jewelry

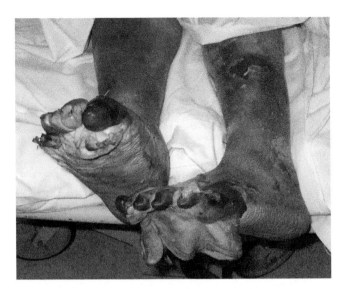

FIGURE 18.7 ■ Third-Degree Frostbite. Severe third-degree frostbite in a schizophrenic homeless 20-year-old boy, who chronically wore wet socks and shoes. The hemorrhagic fluid-filled blisters have been rubbed off by walking. (Photo contributor: Mark Silverberg, MD.)

as swelling is expected upon rewarming. Initiate rapid active rewarming of affected areas with immersion in 37°C to 39°C water for 10 to 30 minutes. Rewarming should be continued until the skin tissue is red/purple and pliable. Analgesia should be provided for reperfusion pain. Clear blisters may be aspirated to remove inflammatory mediators that can worsen tissue destruction, but hemorrhagic blisters should be left intact. The affected extremity should be elevated, splinted, and dressed with a dry sterile dressing.

Laboratory studies such as a CBC, electrolytes, creatine phosphokinase, and serum myoglobin values should initially be obtained to identify a baseline and evaluate for rhabdomyolysis. Surgery may be consulted, but debridement should never take place until definite demarcation has occurred. Patients should be admitted for observation and supportive care unless frostbite is very superficial and painless.

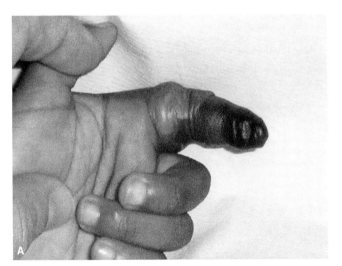

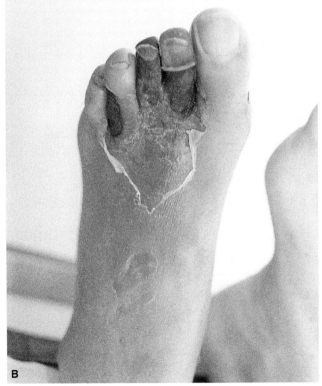

FIGURE 18.8 ■ Fourth-Degree Frostbite. (**A**) An image of the index finger of a 6-year-old boy with frostbite several weeks after the injury. He had gone sleigh riding wearing a torn glove on that hand and had gone unsupervised for several hours with his family at night. (**B**) An image of the foot of 17-year-old boy several weeks after he sustained frostbite to his second, third, fourth, and fifth toes. Note the irregular pattern of demarcation, which required eventual surgical debridement. (Photo contributors: Michael Stracher, MD [A], and Michael Lucchesi, MD [B].)

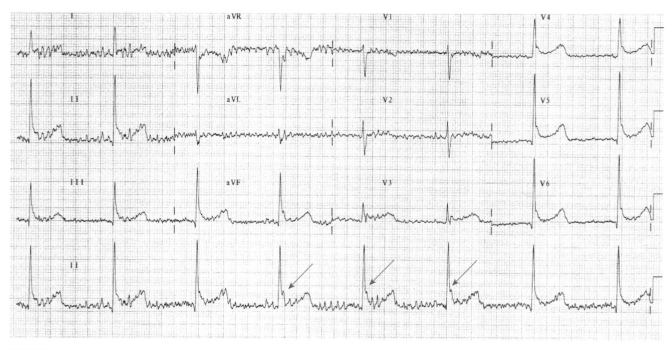

FIGURE 18.9 ■ ECG in Hypothermia. This ECG of a patient with a core temperature of 91°F depicts the classic J-waves (Osborn waves or camel-hump sign, arrows) of hypothermia as described by J.J. Osborn in 1953. Note also the jagged baseline caused by shivering. (Photo contributor: Mark Silverberg, MD.)

Pearls

1. Treat hypothermia aggressively as it can lead to malignant arrhythmias.
2. Management of frostbite cannot begin until core temperature is >35°C.
3. Rewarming should not be initiated if there is a possibility of refreezing.
4. Dry rewarming (such as near an open fire) is uneven, dangerous, and should be avoided if possible.
5. Active rewarming should take place in 37°C to 39°C water for 10 to 30 minutes or until thawing is complete.
6. The true extent of frostbite may take up to 6 months to demarcate. Escharotomy/fasciotomy may be indicated in the acute setting.

TABLE 18.2 ■ CLASSIFICATION OF COLD INJURIES

	Thickness	Clinical Manifestations
Frostnip	Superficial	Reversible ice crystal formation resolves with warming
Frostbite: first degree	Superficial	Irreversible ice crystal formation
		Insensate central wide region surrounded by ring of hyperemia
Frostbite: second degree	Superficial	Irreversible ice crystal formation
		Clear or milky blisters with surrounding erythema
Frostbite: third degree	Deep	Irreversible ice crystal formation
		Hemorrhagic blisters
Frostbite: fourth degree	Deep	Irreversible ice crystal formation
		Initial appearance: Mottled, red or cyanotic
		Final appearance: Dry, black, focal necrosis

Clinical Summary

Anaphylaxis is a type I IgE-mediated hypersensitivity reaction caused by mast cell degranulation following antigen exposure *in a previously sensitized individual.* Anaphylactoid reactions are indistinguishable from true anaphylaxis except that no prior sensitization exists. Clinical criteria for the diagnosis of anaphylaxis are defined by National Institute of Allergy and Infectious Diseases (https://www.niaid.nih.gov). The most frequent triggers include medications, food, and insect envenomation. Diffuse pruritus, sweating, urticaria, and lip, face, and mouth swelling are often the first signs of anaphylaxis, with hypotension or even total cardiovascular collapse occurring if not addressed rapidly. Excessive pulmonary secretions and bronchospasm result in wheezing and difficulty breathing. Diarrhea, nausea, and gastrointestinal (GI) upset are also common. About 80% of patients present with a predictable uniphasic course, in which signs and symptoms occur early and respond to therapy. A biphasic pattern can also be seen with a second episode of anaphylaxis occurring up to 8 hours after apparent recovery. Rarely, symptoms persist for days to weeks.

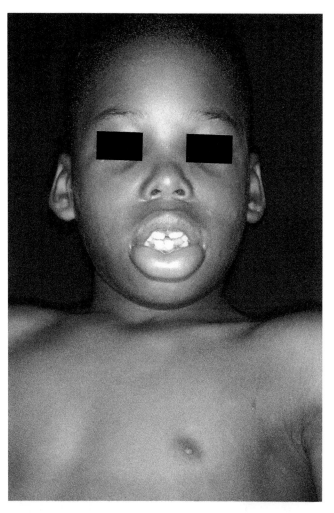

FIGURE 18.11 ■ Anaphylaxis. This child developed swelling of lips, difficulty breathing, and hypotension requiring epinephrine fluid boluses after eating eggs. (Photo contributor: Binita R. Shah, MD.)

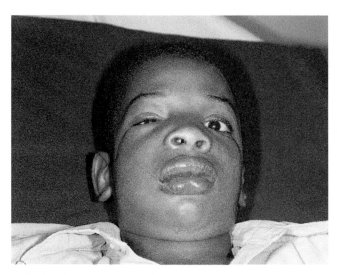

FIGURE 18.10 ■ Anaphylaxis. Right-sided periorbital and facial swelling and lip swelling (angioedema), wheezing, hoarseness of the voice, and urticaria were the presenting complaints in this child after eating peanuts. Angioedema usually involves the loose connective tissues of the ear or the periorbital or perioral areas, but may involve the oropharynx or extremities. (Photo contributor: Binita R. Shah, MD.)

Emergency Department Treatment and Disposition

Parenteral epinephrine (0.01 mg/kg of a 1:1000 solution, 1 mg/mL; maximum pediatric dose: 0.3 mg; maximum adult dose: 0.5 mg) is the drug of choice for anaphylaxis; it is given intramuscularly (IM) and can be repeated every 5 to 15 minutes as needed for persistent symptoms. The administration of epinephrine should not be delayed if anaphylaxis is suspected. Patients undergoing previous treatment with β-blocking agents may not respond to epinephrine and may require glucagon to bypass the adrenergic receptor complex. Second-line therapy for the management of anaphylaxis include

817

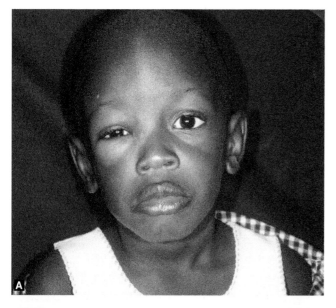

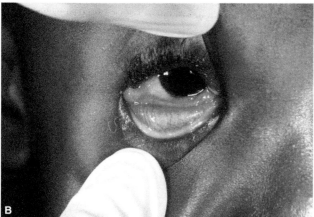

FIGURE 18.12 ■ Anaphylaxis. (**A, B**) Swelling of the lower eye-lid and chemosis (swelling of conjunctiva) associated with urticaria and wheezing were the presenting complaints of this child after an "insect" bite. (Photo contributor: Binita R. Shah, MD.)

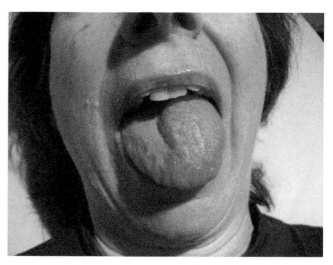

FIGURE 18.13 ■ Unilateral Angioedema of the Tongue. This young adult developed angioedema in the left side of her tongue after eating a kiwi. She had a known strawberry allergy but had never had kiwi before. (Photo contributor: Mark Silverberg, MD.)

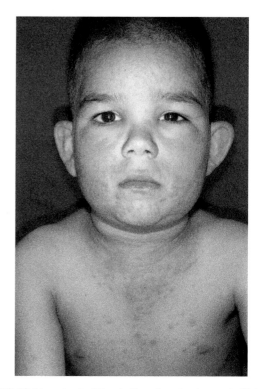

FIGURE 18.14 ■ Acute Allergic Reaction. Acute onset of intensely pruritic, erythematous maculopapular rash, bilateral periorbital edema, and swelling of the left ear were the presenting complaints of this child. The etiology of this acute allergic reaction was unclear. (Photo contributor: Binita R. Shah, MD.)

antihistamines, β₂-adrenergic agonists, and glucocorticoids and should only be administered after epinephrine. The antigen must be removed whenever possible (eg, discontinuation of medication infusion or removal of an insect's stinger). Of note, a credit card can be used to "flick" the stinger out as tweezers or forceps may actually instill more antigen if the venom sac is compressed. A tourniquet may be applied to delay systemic absorption of the allergen in the case of injection or sting.

All patients should receive an immediate assessment of their ABCs. If there is tongue or pharyngeal edema, establish a secure airway and administer 100% oxygen. Supplemental oxygen should also be provided via face mask to patients showing signs of respiratory distress. Inhaled β_2-agonist and anticholinergics (nebulized albuterol and ipratropium, respectively) aid breathing by reversing bronchospasm and decreasing pulmonary secretions. Hypotension should be treated initially with an IV crystalloid bolus (20 mL/kg), but pressors may become necessary in the setting of refractory hypotension. Repeat fluid boluses may be administered to compensate for the marked peripheral vasodilation and third spacing that may accompany anaphylaxis. IV aminophylline may also be used in very severe cases, although very few patients progress this far. Antihistamines do not reverse end-organ effects or hypotension in patients with anaphylaxis. They block further release of histamine and vasoactive mediators and provide symptomatic relief in anaphylactic reactions accompanied by urticaria and angioedema. A combination of H_1- and H_2-receptor–blocking agents such as diphenhydramine and famotidine, respectively, can be synergistic in effect and should be used. Corticosteroids do not play a role in the immediate reversal of anaphylaxis because their onset of action is delayed for 4 to 6 hours. However, they may inhibit or lessen biphasic (usually occurring within 8–10 hours after resolution of initial symptoms) and protracted anaphylactic reactions, including bronchospasm, with their anti-inflammatory properties and should be given in the ED. All patients with moderate to severe reactions requiring resuscitation must be hospitalized and observed for 24 to 48 hours, even in the absence of persistent symptoms.

Patients with milder reactions can be sent home after 6 to 8 hours of observation. Antihistamines and steroids should be prescribed to these patients orally for the next 72 hours. Upon discharge, patients should be referred to an allergist for potential identification of anaphylaxis trigger and desensitization immunotherapy. Patient and/or parent education regarding possible future recurrences is important. They must be prepared for severe reactions because a mild reaction at the hospital visit does not guarantee that future episodes will not be life threatening. Patient with severe reactions should wear a medical alert bracelet that indicates precipitating agents, if known. Insect exposure should be avoided, and patients should be instructed to avoid wearing things that attract insects such as perfumes or bright-colored clothing. Latex-free gloves and catheters should be used with patients who are allergic to latex. Parents and older children should be educated about the risk of recurrence of anaphylaxis, provided a prescription, and educated about epinephrine autoinjectors (eg, Auvi-Q, EpiPen, EpiPen JR).

Pearls

1. Anaphylaxis is a potentially life-threatening manifestation of an IgE-mediated hypersensitivity reaction involving *2 or more* organ systems.
2. Life-threatening features include upper airway obstruction (laryngeal, pharyngeal, and lingual edema) and hypotensive shock due to profound vasodilation and increased vascular permeability.
3. Epinephrine IM (0.01 mg/kg of a 1:1000 solution, 1 mg/mL; maximum pediatric dose: 0.3 mg; maximum adult dose: 0.5 mg) should be given to all patient with a diagnosis of or high clinical suspicion for anaphylaxis.

Clinical Summary

The brown recluse spider (violin or fiddle back spider; *Loxosceles reclusa*) is a small orange to reddish brown spider measuring 6 to 12 mm in length that is found in the midwestern and southeastern United States. It can be identified by the classic brown, violin-shaped mark on its dorsal surface. These spiders are not usually aggressive and bite only when threatened.

Initially, bites are red and may be pain free. Most become firm and heal with little scarring over days or weeks. However, severe and/or systemic envenomations occasionally occur. In these patients, there is localized pain and tissue destruction with systemic symptoms. The bite can cause pain, pruritus, and erythema to the affected skin. Within 24 hours, an erythematous halo may form around the bite. Depending on the amount of venom delivered, bites may progress over days (as early as 48–72 hours) to weeks to large necrotic defects that may require reconstructive cosmetic surgery to repair. Systemic signs and symptoms include fever and chills, nausea, morbilliform rash formation, arthralgias, and myalgias. Renal failure, hemolysis, thrombocytopenia, disseminated intravascular coagulopathy, and seizures may all occasionally be seen and very rarely may progress to coma or death in small children. The constellation of symptoms classically known as loxoscelism includes necrosis at the bite site, nausea, malaise, fever, hemolysis, and thrombocytopenia.

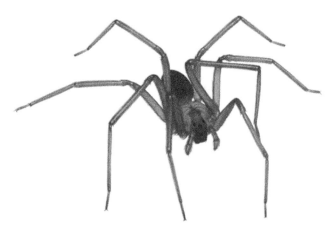

FIGURE 18.15 ■ Brown Recluse Spider (*Loxosceles reclusa*). This venomous arachnid can be identified by its brown color and the typical violin-shaped pattern on the dorsal cephalothorax. (Reproduced with permission from Klaassen CD, Watkins III JB. *Casarett & Doull's Essentials of Toxicology.* 3rd ed. McGraw-Hill Education; New York, NY, 2015.)

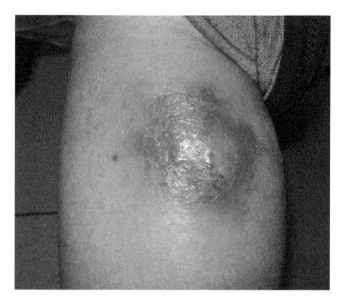

FIGURE 18.16 ■ Brown Recluse Spider Bite. This patient stated that she was bitten by a 1-inch-long brown spider with a dark brown marking on its back that "looked violin-shaped." The bite rapidly progressed to form this lesion only 2 days after the event, making the brown recluse spider the likely culprit, although the offending arachnid was never captured or definitively identified. (Photo contributor: Mark Silverberg, MD.)

Emergency Department Treatment and Disposition

ED care can vary from local wound care to ICU hospitalization. There are no specific tests to diagnose brown recluse spider envenomation, so definitive diagnosis depends on identifying the offending arachnid. Patients with systemic symptoms should receive a CBC including platelet count, coagulation profile, serum electrolytes, creatinine, BUN, and urinalysis. A local poison center may be helpful in identifying the species of spider when available.

Brown recluse spider bites typically require local wound cleansing, splinting (for immobilization), tetanus prophylaxis, and pain management. Long-term cosmetic reconstruction may be necessary because the toxin in recluse venom can cause massive local tissue destruction. Surgery should not be performed until 6 to 8 weeks after initial bite as early surgery may increase inflammatory response and effects of venom. Some advocate early use of dapsone (leukocyte inhibitor) for these bites to limit the local inflammatory response, but no scientific study has ever proven its efficacy. Dapsone use is not advocated in children. It also should not be used in

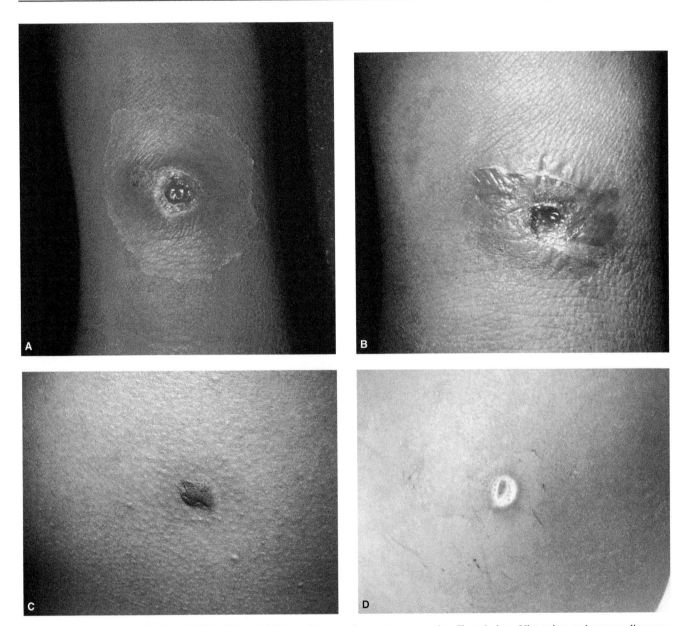

FIGURE 18.17 ▪ Brown Recluse Spider Bites. (A) Extremities are the most commonly affected sites. Ulceration and surrounding erythema on the forearm at the bite site are seen. (B) Local intense erythema, induration, and bullous lesion followed by eschar and a deep ulcer on the hand of a different child following a spider bite. (C) Halo of erythema surrounding an area of tissue destruction on the arm of a patient as a result of a spider bite. (D) Same lesion as in (C) after 11 days of bite. (Photo contributors: Binita R. Shah, MD [A, B], and David B. Liss, MD [C, D].)

patients with glucose-6-dehydrogenase deficiency due to risk of hemolysis. Patients with systemic manifestations or evidence of a rapidly expanding necrotic lesion should be admitted for observation. If hemolysis is present, maintenance of urine output, urine alkalinization with IV sodium bicarbonate to keep the urine pH >7, and close monitoring of renal function and hematocrit are required. Heat can accelerate tissue destruction and should not be applied. Steroid creams usually do not help, and overcutting to extract the venom with a suction device should never be attempted. Hyperbaric oxygen use in patients with brown recluse spider bites remains controversial. High-voltage electrotherapy from stun guns has been reported but has never been shown to be effective in scientific studies. Other home remedies have not been proven useful.

Pearls

1. Monitor patients for evidence of hemolysis, renal failure, or coagulopathy. Smaller children are more likely to develop these systemic manifestations.

2. The shorter the time to the onset of symptoms following a spider bite, the more severe is the envenomation.

3. Dapsone use is not advocated in children for brown recluse spider bites. Furthermore, its use is contraindicated in patients with glucose-6-dehydrogenase deficiency because it can cause hemolysis.

Clinical Summary

Widow spiders (hourglass spiders; *Latrodectus mactans, Latrodectus bishop, Lactrodectus geometricus, Latrodectus hesperus, Latrodectus variolus*) range in size from 2.5 to 3.5 cm and have large fangs and a distinct red hourglass-shaped mark on their ventral surface. These arthropods are found in outdoor areas throughout the world, with *L mactans* found most commonly in the East, *L hesperus* in the West, and *L variolus* in the North.

The bite of a black widow spider causes a pinprick sensation. Envenomations tend to cause local erythema and pain but considerably more systemic effects known as latrodectism. Muscle spasms of the back, abdomen, and chest are classic and may become severe enough to require narcotic analgesics. Pain associated with this bite usually resolves within 48 to 72 hours. Hemodynamic instability and coagulopathy are also common. Systemic symptoms include nausea and vomiting, weakness, hypertension, tachycardia, diaphoresis, and facial edema. Classic "facies latrodectismica" is characterized by sweating, contortion, and grimacing. Black widow envenomations are graded based on symptoms. Grade 1 envenomations cause minimal or no symptoms at the bite site and have normal vitals. Grade 2 envenomations cause diaphoresis at the bite site and muscle spasms at the bite site and trunk; the patient otherwise has normal vitals. Grade 3 envenomations cause more generalized diaphoresis, more severe muscle spasms, nausea, vomiting, and headache. Tachycardia and elevated BP are also present.

Emergency Department Treatment and Disposition

ED care can range from simple local wound care to hospitalization and antivenom administration. There are no specific tests to diagnose *Latrodectus* envenomation, so definitive diagnosis requires identification of the spider. A local poison center may be helpful in identifying the arachnid and locating the appropriate antivenom.

CBC including platelet count, coagulation profile, serum electrolytes, creatinine, BUN, and urinalysis should be obtained. Therapy can be guided by using the envenomation grading symptoms. Patient with grade 1 envenomation may only require NSAIDs for pain control. Patients with grade 2 and 3 envenomations make require opioids and benzodiazepine to manage the muscle cramps. IV benzodiazepines are used for treatment of muscle spasms, replacing the use of calcium gluconate for this indication. Antivenin is indicated in small children for severe envenomations with systemic symptoms and is available as a hyperimmune horse serum, which can be given IM or IV. Indications for antivenin include life-threatening hypertensive crisis, muscle spasms not controlled by IV opioids and IV benzodiazepines, priapism, tachycardia, and respiratory difficulty. Antivenom usually relieves symptoms rapidly, although it may precipitate anaphylaxis or serum sickness. Hospitalization is recommended for all *Latrodectus*-envenomated pediatric patients. Tetanus status should be elicited and vaccine given if not up to date.

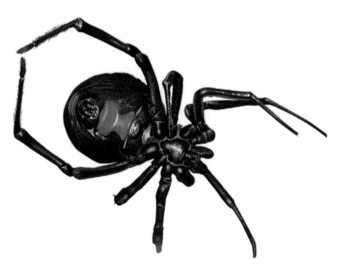

FIGURE 18.18 ■ Black Widow Spider (*Latrodectus mactans*). The classic deep red-orange hourglass marking on the black abdomen of the black widow spider is very recognizable. (Reproduced with permission from Klaassen CD, Watkins III JB. *Casarett & Doull's Essentials of Toxicology*. 3rd ed. McGraw-Hill Education; New York, NY, 2015.)

Pearls

1. The classic red hourglass-shaped mark on their abdomen makes widow spiders easier to identify.

2. The hallmark of black widow spider envenomation is muscle cramping, usually affecting the abdomen, back, and chest.

3. Abdominal pain and rigidity associated with nausea and vomiting can mimic acute abdomen.

Clinical Summary

Scorpions, like spiders, are members of the class Arachnida. Of the approximately 1500 venomous species of scorpion found throughout the world, 50 are potentially dangerous to humans, with only 1 species, *Centruroides exilicauda* (the bark scorpion), residing in North America. All scorpions have hard exoskeletons with flat and elongated bodies armed with claws in the front and a whip-like tail in the back. Their tail ends in a bulbous segment known as the telson that contains 2 venom glands and the stinger. Scorpion venom is usually a heterogeneous mixture containing multiple proteins, many of which are neurotoxins that typically activate ion channels such as fast sodium channels. Humans are often stung on the hands or feet as they try to pick up or step on a scorpion. Children frequently manifest worse toxicity because of their small size. Envenomated individuals immediately complain of severe pain at the sting site (worsened by tapping on the area) progressing to local erythema and edema. Systemic symptoms are rare but include nausea, vomiting, hypersalivation, sweating, hyperthermia, anxiety, autonomic instability, myoclonus, and cardiac dysrhythmias. "Roving" eye movement is common in children as well as agitation, weakness, muscle fasciculations, and opisthotonos. Symptoms typically last 24 to 48 hours, although when fatal, death is usually due to cardiogenic shock or pulmonary edema. Pancreatitis is seen in up to 80% of victims of *Tityus trinitatis* scorpion stings.

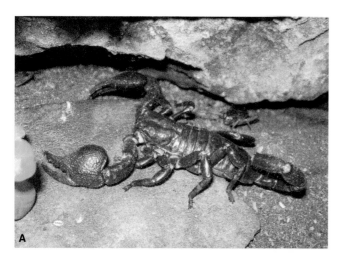

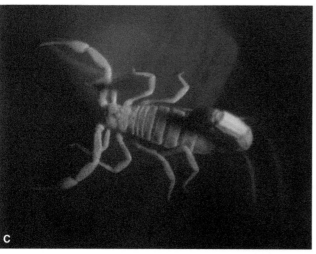

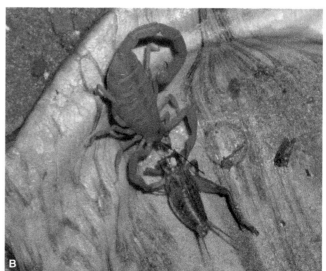

FIGURE 18.19 ■ Scorpions. (**A**) Emperor scorpion (*Pandinus imperator*). Because of their impressive size and the relatively low toxicity of their venom, emperor scorpions are often kept as pets. Found in the wild only in Africa, they can grow to 8 inches in length. (**B**) Arizona hairy scorpion (*Hadrurus arizonesis pallidus*) eating its prey. (**C**) Fluorescing under a Wood's lamp. (Photo contributors: Mark Silverberg, MD [A], and Michael D. Levine, MD [B, C].)

Emergency Department Treatment and Disposition

It is important to get a thorough history surrounding the sting and a description of the scorpion if no specimen is available. Initial first aid involves cleaning the wound with soap and water and applying ice to the sting site. ED care is supportive with analgesics plus benzodiazepines for myoclonus, muscle spasms, and agitation. Tetanus prophylaxis should be checked and updated when indicated. Atropine is typically not needed for excessive oral secretions, although it can be used if necessary. Esmolol or labetalol can be used to treat hypertension and tachydysrhythmia. Barbiturates should be avoided as they may potentially increase the toxic effects of the venom by an unknown mechanism. Administration of antivenin is recommended in all cases of severe envenomation when available. Benzodiazepine use should be avoided or limited if antivenom will be given due to potential of oversedation, leading to possible intubation once the excitatory effects of the scorpion venom have been reversed. Observation for 24 hours is prudent for closer monitoring of all envenomated children. Contact the American Association of Poison Control Centers to be connected to a local poison control center to help take care of a patient envenomated by a scorpion.

Pearls

1. "Roving" eye movements, muscle fasciculations, and opisthotonos are some of the signs seen in children with scorpion stings.
2. Antivenom may exist for some scorpion species.
3. All scorpions fluoresce in the dark when exposed to a Wood lamp.

DOG BITES

Clinical Summary

Dog bites in children occur disproportionately to the head and face, which is typically closer to a dog's mouth than the heads of adults. Male children are twice as likely to suffer dog bites. School-aged children are at higher risk of sustaining a dog bite, with children <5 years old sustaining the highest rate of serious injury. Most bites occur from an animal owned by the family, a family friend, or a neighbor. Soft tissue injury as a result of a dog bite can be classified as a laceration, puncture wound, or avulsion. Facial fractures can also occur but are rare. Approximately 10% to 15% of dog bites become significantly infected, and these are usually polymicrobial in nature. Larger wounds can be easily cleansed and debrided and are paradoxically less likely to become infected than are minor lacerations or puncture wounds, which quickly close over the bacterial inoculum.

Emergency Department Treatment and Disposition

The basic principles of general wound care apply to all dog bites. Radiographs of the injury should be obtained to rule out the presence of foreign bodies or fracture. Revision of the wound edges may be necessary after injuries are thoroughly cleansed. Because almost all animal bites are contaminated, meticulous wound toilet and copious irrigation are essential. Suturing is controversial. In recent years, the consensus has changed from never suturing such wounds to one of loosely approximating them to obtain the best possible cosmetic

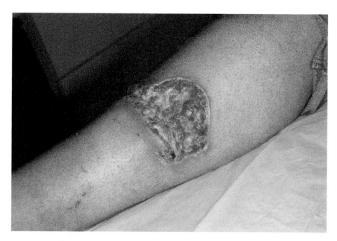

FIGURE 18.21 ■ Dog Bite by a Pit Bull. This picture was taken in a patient 2 weeks after a bite on the leg. (Photo contributor: Binita R. Shah, MD.)

appearance without actually closing the wound. Close observation for wound infections is essential in these cases. Puncture wounds should not be sutured due to increased risk of infection. Tissue adhesives should never be used because they trap bacteria and help create an anaerobic environment where bacteria can flourish. After wound care, the limb should be immobilized and elevated to reduce swelling. Tetanus should always be updated when indicated, and tetanus immune globulin may be needed in unimmunized individuals. Rabies prophylaxis should be considered in an unprovoked attack by a suspicious animal. The patient should be instructed to see a physician in 24 to 48 hours to have his or her wounds reevaluated for signs of infection.

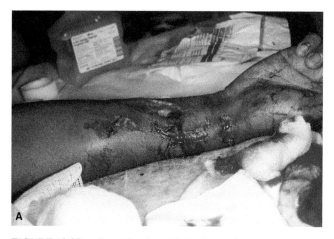

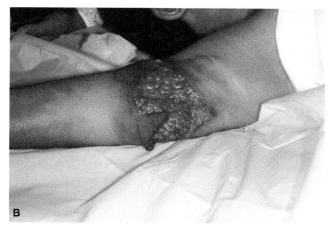

FIGURE 18.20 ■ Dog Bites by a Pitt Bull. Multiple bites are seen on the forearm (**A**) and upper arm (**B**). Dog bite wounds cause a spectrum of tissue injuries that vary from scratches and abrasions to contusions and lacerations. Dog bites occur in the head and neck area in 60% to 70% of victims age 5 years or younger and in 50% of those who are age 10 years or younger. (Photo contributor: Binita R. Shah, MD.)

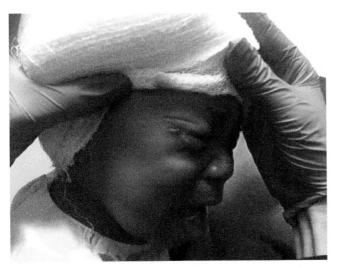

FIGURE 18.22 ■ Dog Bite to Face. This child sustained a dog bite to the face involving the right upper and lower eyelid. (Photo contributor: Kathryn Pade, MD.)

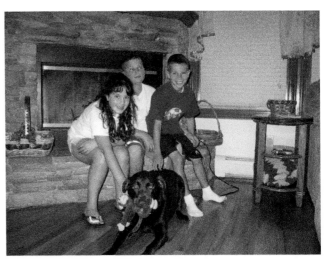

FIGURE 18.24 ■ The "Bear." Sometimes a teddy and sometimes a grisly, but always a "Bear." The Lucchesi family children with their dog (who is biting a stuffed monkey but not the children!). The dogs that most often bite people are not strays or wild dogs, but rather pets well known to the victim and owned by the family (15%) or neighbors (75%). Many injuries could be avoided by proper parental education of children regarding their behavior in the presence of animals. When impartially investigated, most instances of animal bites turn out to be the fault of the child, not the animal. (Photo contributor: Michael Lucchesi, MD.)

There is no advantage in giving antibiotics to patients who present >24 hours after injury with an uninfected dog bite. Conversely, individuals who present with an already infected wound should always receive antibiotics. Amoxicillin plus clavulanic acid is a good single-drug regimen to start until cultures can identify a causative organism(s). Common organisms isolated from cultures include both aerobic (*Pasteurella, Streptococcus, Staphylococcus,* and *Neisseria*) and anaerobic (*Fusobacterium, Porphyromonas, Prevotella*) organisms. A combination of an extended-spectrum cephalosporin or trimethoprim-sulfamethoxazole plus clindamycin is suitable to cover most offending organisms in penicillin-allergic patients.

The effectiveness of antibiotic prophylaxis in fresh bites is less well established. The location of the bite may play a

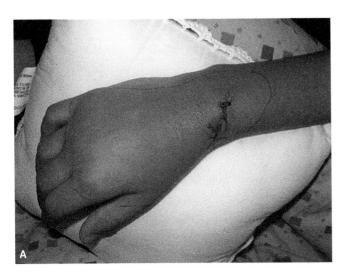

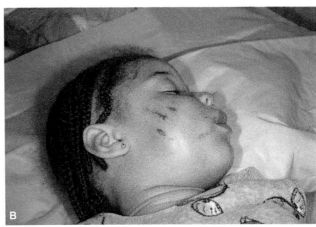

FIGURE 18.23 ■ Cellulitis; Dog Bite. (**A**) This dog bite to the hand became infected despite being only loosely closed and the patient being started on oral antibiotics 2 days earlier. (**B**) Severe local tenderness and rapidly spreading erythema were seen in this febrile patient who came back 12 hours after being discharged from the ED following a bite by a German shepherd that was owned by the family. (Photo contributors: Mark Silverberg, MD [A], and Binita R. Shah, MD [B].)

role in choosing to initiate prophylactic antibiotics. Wounds at high risk of becoming infected are those located on the hand, foot, below knee, and scalp or face (in infants). Wounds >12 hours old, contaminated wounds, puncture-type wounds, and extensive crush injuries are also at high risk of developing infection. Antibiotic prophylaxis should be given to individuals who meet high-risk criteria as well as immunocompromised and asplenic patients.

Pearls

1. Dog bites usually have a significant amount of devitalized tissue because of the nature of dog's flat, crushing teeth, and strong muscles of mastication.
2. Dog bites present a significant potential for morbidity in childhood. Most injuries are minor, although fatalities do occur and infections may be common.
3. Bite wound infections are usually polymicrobial in nature.

Clinical Summary

Rabies is an RNA virus transmitted primarily through saliva present in animal bites, although it may be transmitted via direct mucosal exposure, airborne laboratory accidents, and transplantation of tissues harboring undiagnosed rabies. Depending on the inoculum site, rabies virus may take an average of 4 to 12 weeks to become symptomatic, but this period can range from days to years. Transmission by airborne virus in bat-filled caves or by human bite has been theorized but never documented.

Initial peripheral infection produces an acute illness with malaise, fever, and headache and progresses to more central symptoms, including anxiety, seizures, dysphagia, and eventually coma, which is invariably fatal within days. The primary cause of death is respiratory arrest. Only a handful of cases are published in the medical literature describing survivors of rabies once neurologic symptoms are present.

Emergency Department Treatment and Disposition

Guidelines for postexposure prophylaxis (PEP) are given in Table 18.3. Rabies PEP requires administration of 2 agents unless there has been previous immunization and a documented adequate rabies antibody titer, in which case rabies immune globulin (RIG) is not required. All others should receive 1 dose of RIG (20 IU/kg) to provide temporary passive immunity. The Centers for Disease Control and Prevention (CDC) recommends the entire dose be infiltrated into the soft tissues surrounding the bite. If that is impractical, the amount unable to be infiltrated should be injected into a large muscle distant from the injection site of the active vaccine. Active immunization agents such as human diploid cell vaccine (HDCV) or RabAvert produce longer lasting active immunity to the virus. The development of newer vaccines has markedly reduced the incidence of reactions previously associated with PEP.

The CDC recommends active immunization of previously unvaccinated immunocompetent individuals with 4 doses of HDCV or purified chick embryo cell vaccine (PCECV). Individuals who have already received a full series of PEP or who previously had a documented adequate rabies virus–neutralizing antibody titer should receive 2 doses. Immunocompromised hosts should receive 5 doses. Regardless of weight or age, the dose is 1 mL injected into a large muscle group. Single doses should be administered on days 0, 3, 7,

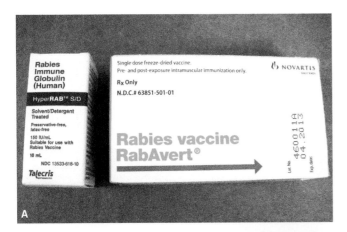

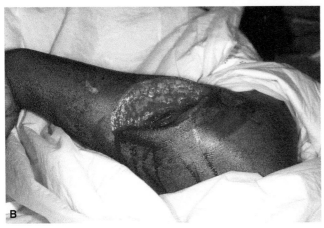

FIGURE 18.25 ■ Rabies Vaccine and Rabies Immune Globulin for Postexposure Prophylaxis. (**A**) RabAvert and rabies immune globulin are the typical medications given to any patient attacked by a rabid animal to induce both active and passive immunity respectively. (**B**) Bites by a pit bull on the extensor surface of the forearm following an "unprovoked" attack by a stray dog in a child. Rabies immunoglobulin and rabies vaccine were given to this child. (Photo contributors: Mark Silverberg, MD [A], and Binita R. Shah, MD [B].)

TABLE 18.3 ■ GUIDELINES FOR POSTEXPOSURE PROPHYLAXIS (PEP)	
Domestic animal found fully vaccinated	PEP not needed
Domestic animal, vaccination status unknown; or wild animal, captured and appearing healthy	Observe animal for 10 days; if symptoms occur in animal, initiate PEP until animal is euthanized and tested
Wild animal, unavailable for observation	Initiate PEP

and 14, with day 0 being the day of initial presentation. Immunosuppressed patients should receive a fifth and final dose on day 28.

PCECV (RabAvert) has been developed for use in patients who develop sensitivity to 1 of the other vaccines. The entire series must be completed. If there is any patient-related deviation from the schedule, the manufacturer or local poison control center should be contacted for advice on timing of series completion.

Bat exposures deserve special mention, with most human rabies cases diagnosed in the United States being bat variants. Because bat teeth are so small, such bites can go virtually unnoticed. If a patient believes that he or she *could have been* bitten by a bat, regardless of the findings on physical examination, rabies PEP should be initiated. Rabies prophylaxis should also be administered to anyone who has an open wound or mucous membrane that could have become contaminated with bat saliva or other potentially infectious material or who has occupied the same closed space with a bat during a time of altered perception (eg, asleep, intoxicated, developmentally immature, mentally impaired), regardless of the findings on physical examination.

Pearls

1. Always consider PEP after animal bites because rabies is almost always fatal after symptoms develop. Exposure to an animal that even *might be* rabid should lead to consideration of rabies PEP.
2. Postexposure treatment consists of passive immunization with RIG in addition to active immunization.
3. Local health authorities should be consulted when there is doubt about the local rabies status of a particular species of biting animal.

Clinical Summary

It is estimated that 5% to 15% of all animal bite injuries are inflicted by cats, and girls are twice as likely as boys to be bitten. Cat bites are typically puncture wounds and have a high chance of becoming infected and causing osteomyelitis. Approximately 15% to 50% of cat bites become significantly infected, so excellent wound care and close follow-up is essential. Cat bites are usually polymicrobial in nature.

Emergency Department Treatment and Disposition

Basic principles of general wound care apply to cat bites. Radiographs of the site of injury should be obtained to rule out the presence of foreign bodies or fracture. Revision of the wound edges may be necessary after the injuries are thoroughly cleansed. Cat bites should almost never be sutured or glued closed because they are often narrow, deep puncture wounds that are difficult to irrigate. After wound care, the limb should be immobilized and elevated to prevent swelling. Tetanus should always be updated when indicated and tetanus immune globulin may be administered in unimmunized individuals. Rabies prophylaxis may be considered in an unprovoked attack by a suspicious animal. The patient should be instructed to see a physician in 24 to 48 hours to have his or her wounds reevaluated for infection.

There is no advantage in giving antibiotics to patients who present >24 hours after injury with uninfected cat bite

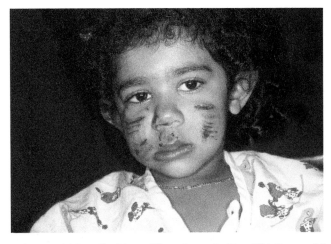

FIGURE 18.27 ■ Cat Bite and Scratches to the Face. This 3-year-old girl presented with bilateral scratches and puncture wounds (around the lips) inflicted by the cat owned by her family. Cat scratches are most commonly seen on the upper extremities or periorbital region. Cat bites are located on upper extremities in two-thirds of cases and usually consist of puncture wounds rather than lacerations or contusions. (Photo contributor: Binita Shah, MD.)

wounds. Conversely, individuals who present with an already infected cat bite should always receive antibiotics. A combination of an extended-spectrum cephalosporin or trimethoprim-sulfamethoxazole plus clindamycin is suitable to cover most offending organisms in penicillin-allergic patients. Prophylactic antibiotics for fresh cat bites are probably indicated. Hand wounds present a special problem with cat bites because 30% or more become infected. Cats have much smaller jaw parts than dogs, so many cat bites occur on the hands and fingers because that is all they can fit in their mouth. Because of the complexity of the tissue planes of the hand and the presence of avascular tendon sheath spaces, there is a high propensity for spread of infection and potential for significant morbidity.

Pearls

1. Cat bite wound infections are usually polymicrobial in nature.
2. Hand wounds tend to become infected more often than those located elsewhere. Considering the complexity of the hand's structure and the ease with which infection spreads along contaminated tissue planes, function can be easily compromised or destroyed. Thus, every bite of the hand should be considered potentially serious.

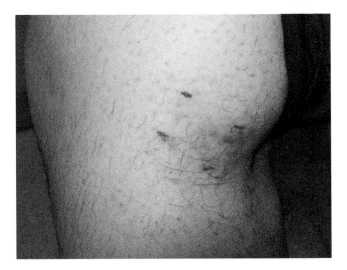

FIGURE 18.26 ■ Cat Bite. Four fang puncture wounds are seen on this teenage fireman's leg who attempted to remove a dozen cats from a house after a fire. (Photo contributor: Mark Silverberg, MD.)

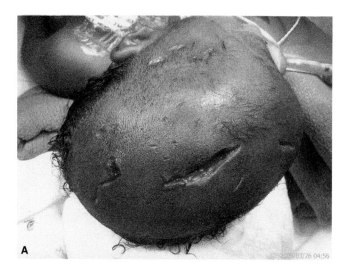

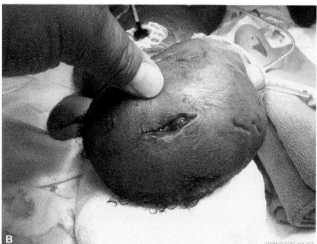

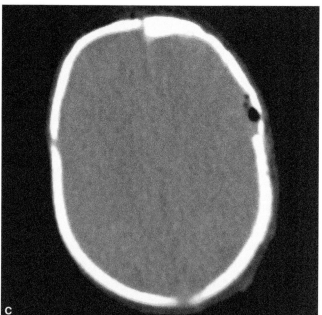

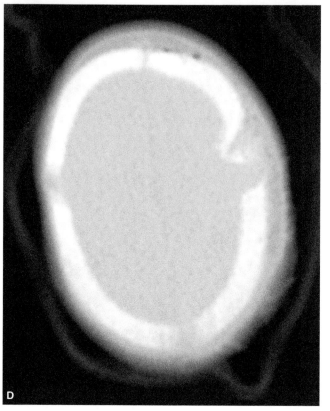

FIGURE 18.28 ■ Newborn Attacked by a Family Cat. (**A, B**) This 47-day-old ex-29-week preemie was brought home from the hospital only hours prior to being attacked in the crib by a cat. Baby had multiple lacerations of the scalp and eyelids. The largest laceration (**B**) revealed an open depressed skull fracture and dural laceration with exudation of the brain. Craniectomy with wound exploration, debridement, elevation of the depressed skull fracture, and dural repair were done in the operating room (OR). Brain cortical injury with local necrosis was also noted. (**C, D**) CT scan axial images demonstrate a complex depressed skull fracture with intracranial air. A small left frontal subdural hemorrhage is also present. Baby was not sedated (very young age) to get "perfect quality" CT images, but it provided enough information on the extent of injuries prior to bringing the baby to OR. (Photo contributors: Mark Thompson, MD [A, B], and John Amodio, MD [C, D].)

Clinical Summary

Human bites are common occurrences in childhood, and of these, 5% require suturing and 5% to 30% will become infected. In children younger than 10 years old, boys are more commonly bitten, whereas in older children, girls are bitten more often. Human bites are classified as occlusional bites or clenched fist injuries. Occlusional bites occur when the teeth close directly onto the skin tissue, whereas clenched fist injuries occur when the closed hand comes into contact with teeth upon impact (typically during an altercation). Abrasions account for 66% to 75% of bite injuries. The remainder is evenly distributed between punctures and lacerations. Human bites in children are commonly located on the face, upper extremities, or trunk.

Infections of human bites are typically polymicrobial. Risk factors for infection include delay in initial care >20 hours, concomitant crush injuries, punctures or deep lacerations, complete wound closure of deep wounds, and larger intraoral bites. Viral infections such as hepatitis B and C, HIV, and herpes may also be transmitted, and PEP should be considered when appropriate.

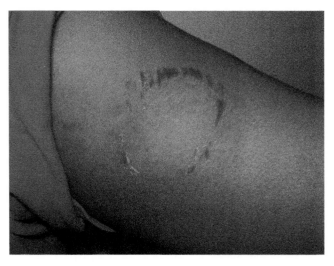

FIGURE 18.30 ■ Human Bite. This teenager was bitten on the upper arm during a fight at school over a new boyfriend. Because the bite does not break the skin, she does not need to be placed on antibiotics. (Photo contributor: Mark Silverberg, MD.)

Emergency Department Treatment and Disposition

The general principles of wound management apply. All human bites that break the skin must be considered contaminated, and meticulous wound toilet and copious high-pressure irrigation are essential. Suturing is somewhat controversial because some studies suggest sutured wounds may be more susceptible to infection. A thorough examination should be performed on all patients with bite wounds to the hand with special attention in evaluating for joint involvement or tendon injury.

The repair of intraoral bite wounds deserves special mention. The intraoral portion of a through-and-through bite wound to the cheek or lip should be tightly approximated with absorbable sutures. Once closed, a new suture tray should be opened, and the external layers of the face can be irrigated and sterilely prepared and then closed in the regular fashion as if the intraoral rent was not present. Never use saliva-contaminated instruments to suture extraorally.

Contusions and abrasions resulting from human bites generally do not become infected. There also seems to be no advantage in administering antibiotics to patients who present

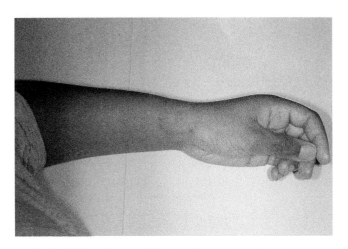

FIGURE 18.29 ■ Human Bite. An 11-year-old girl with a human bite sustained during a fight at school. Most human bite injuries in children are minor. Abrasions (as seen here) account for two-thirds to three-quarters of bite injuries in children. Bites are most commonly seen on the upper extremities. (Photo contributor: Binita R. Shah, MD.)

>24 hours after injury with uninfected wounds. The utilization of prophylactic antibiotics for fresh human bite wounds is more controversial. Antibiotic prophylaxis should be administered to all deep puncture wounds, sutured full-thickness wounds, full-thickness wounds of the hand, and high-impact wounds such as sports- or fight-related wounds that likely contain crushed tissue. Amoxicillin and clavulanic acid are effective first-line treatments until antibiotic cultures are obtained. Extended-spectrum cephalosporin or trimethoprim-sulfamethoxazole plus clindamycin are effective alternatives for patients who are allergic to penicillin. Tetanus prophylaxis should be considered in all bite wounds and updated as needed. After wound care, an affected limb should be sterilely dressed, immobilized, and elevated. Appropriate follow-up care (within 36 hours) should also be arranged for these patients.

Pearls

1. All human bites must be managed as contaminated wounds.
2. Infection is the most common type of morbidity associated with human bites. If not aggressively treated, human bite infections can lead to serious permanent dysfunction of the injured area.
3. Always rule out child abuse when a small child presents with a human bite.
4. Joint involvement and tendon injuries should be considered when a patient has a clenched fist hand injury.

Clinical Summary

The corals, sea anemones, and hydroids all have thousands of specialized cells along their tentacles called nematocysts. Each contains a toxin-filled coiled poison dart called a cnidocil. When triggered, the nematocyst rapidly discharges the cnidocil into the target, releasing toxin into the victim.

Coral can be soft or hard. Both can sting, but hard corals can also cause abrasions or lacerations. With the exception of fire coral, nematocysts of most corals cannot penetrate human skin. Fire coral and hydroids can cause pain and urticaria, which subsides by 90 minutes. Symptoms can progress to produce hemorrhagic or ulcerative lesions. Inflammation can take up to 1 week to resolve. Most sea anemones (class Actiniaria) cannot penetrate human skin, although there are more poisonous Indo-Pacific varieties that can cause painful stings, rashes, and itching on contact. Systemic envenomations are rare, but in severe cases, evidence of organ damage may be seen. Complications include long-term skin changes such as hyperpigmentation and hypopigmentation and eschar formation. Local reactions to these organisms are common, but allergy to their venom is also a possibility. Full anaphylaxis can be seen in some envenomations by this class of animals.

Emergency Department Treatment and Disposition

Treatment should begin in the field with removal of macroscopic pieces of tentacle. This will prevent further

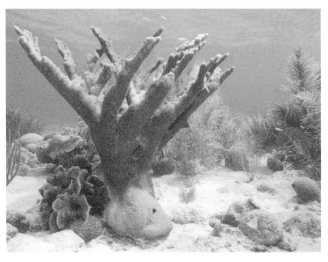

FIGURE 18.32 ■ Hard Coral. Hard corals come in all shapes, colors, and sizes. This hard coral appears in the shape of an underwater tree. Multiple soft corals can also be seen in the background. (Photo taken in Bonaire, the Netherlands Antilles. Photo contributor: Mark Silverberg, MD.)

envenomation because nematocysts remain active despite the tentacles being severed from the organism body. No specific antivenom exists against these species, so symptomatic relief is the goal of ED treatment. Rinsing the wound immediately with vinegar may prevent further discharge of nematocysts, but its effectiveness in this group is less clear than with the box jellyfish. Baking soda has been advocated by some to reduce wound pain when applied shortly after the sting. Tetanus status should be assessed and updated as needed. Antihistamines

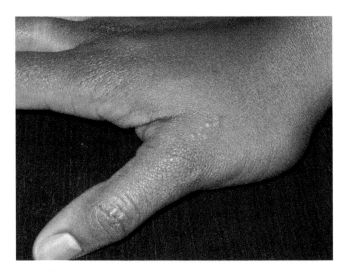

FIGURE 18.31 ■ Hydroid Injury. The typical sting pattern on the hand of a teenager after contacting a hydroid while scuba diving. (Photo taken in Speyside, Tobago. Photo contributor: Allysia Guy, MD.)

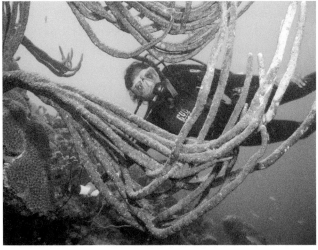

FIGURE 18.33 ■ Soft Coral. A relaxed diver poses among soft corals with long, flowing branches. (Photo taken in Bonaire, the Netherlands Antilles. Photo contributor: Donita Dyalram, MD, DDS.)

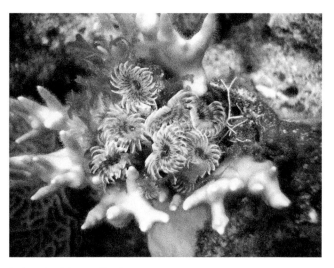

FIGURE 18.34 ■ Fire Coral. A bunch of tan-colored fire coral is seen here surrounding a cluster of feather duster worms. Notice the white hair-like projections so typical of fire coral. (Photo taken in Bonaire, the Netherlands Antilles. Photo contributor: Mark Silverberg, MD.)

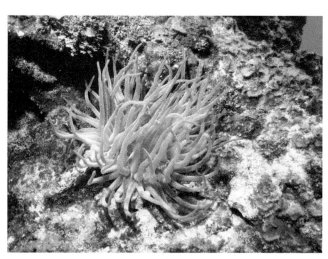

FIGURE 18.35 ■ Sea Anemone. A large purple sea anemone is pictured here, although they come in many other colors, shapes, and sizes. (Photo taken at the barrier reef in Belize. Photo contributor: Mark Silverberg, MD.)

may be used to alleviate itching; topical corticosteroids may also alleviate itching. More severe skin reactions may require systemic corticosteroids. A 5- to 10-day course of prednisolone is typically adequate. Patients without evidence of a systemic reaction 4 to 6 hours after being stung may be safely discharged home. When evidence of systemic illness exists, the patient should be admitted for 24 hours of observation to follow the progression of the symptoms. The treating physician may want to contact experts in marine envenomation at the Divers Alert Network (phone: 919-684-9111, 800-446-2671) for any additional information.

Lacerations and abrasions from hard corals should be x-rayed for foreign bodies and cleansed well using high-pressure saline irrigation to remove all foreign material. Devitalized tissue can be excised to further prevent infection. Lacerations should not undergo tight primary closure as they are prone to infection; approximation with adhesive strips or

delayed closure may be preferred. Antibiotic prophylaxis is not indicated for immunocompetent patients with stings or minor wounds. Dermatology follow-up may be indicated for more severe skin reactions.

Pearls

1. As with all aquatic animals that "sting" you, vinegar may be beneficial to prevent further coral, hydroid, and anemone nematocyst envenomation, and it may also denature the venom proteins, thus alleviating symptoms.

2. Treatment is primarily supportive, with antihistamines for itching and analgesics for contusions and painful stings.

3. Simple skin reactions can be treated with topical steroid preparations, whereas worse reactions should receive oral steroids.

Clinical Summary

Although it appears to be a jellyfish, the Portuguese man-of-war is a collection of hydroids in a colony with a float at the top. The long trailing tentacles can measure 10 m in length, and broken tentacles that have washed ashore days later can still sting beachgoers. Box jellyfish (cubozoan jellyfish) are the world's most dangerous jellyfish. *Chironex fleckeri*, the Australian box jellyfish, has been linked to at least 70 deaths (mostly in children) that are usually due to cardiovascular collapse. Children are at particular risk, with smaller individuals more likely to suffer a significant envenomation. True jellyfish (scyphozoans) are found worldwide, ranging in size from a few millimeters to 2 m across.

Jellyfish tentacles contain thousands or even millions of nematocysts that fire toxin-laden cnidocils at high velocity into flesh. Toxins released are a combination of neurotoxins, cardiotoxins, and dermonecrotic substances. Symptoms vary from mild skin irritation to localized pain with redness and itching to life-threatening circulatory collapse. Long-term skin changes, such as hyperpigmentation and hypopigmentation, lichenification, and keloid or eschar formation, are common. Portuguese man-of-war envenomations cause acute-onset severe pain with linear rashes, vesiculation, and necrosis. Pain can improve within hours, whereas skin findings may take up to 72 hours to improve. Severe envenomations, especially by box jellyfish, can lead to full-thickness dermal necrosis and even multiorgan system failure in some cases that may prove fatal.

Emergency Department Treatment and Disposition

Treatment begins in the field with the removal of all tentacles, which may be scraped off with a credit card or paper plate; some recommend covering the area with clean beach sand first. Immediately rinse the wounds with seawater (if the water is known to be free of tentacles). Rinsing the wound with 5% acetic acid (vinegar) prevents further discharge of nematocysts and may inactivate the venom. For box jellyfish envenomation, soak the area for at least 30 minutes in vinegar or place a vinegar-soaked cloth on the wound after tentacle parts have been removed with thick gloves or some

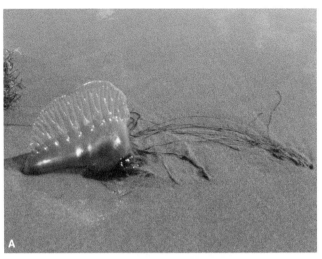

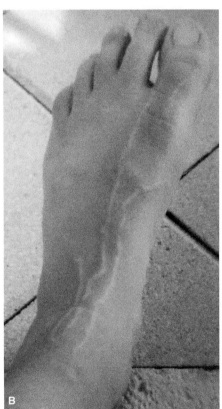

FIGURE 18.36 ■ The Portuguese Man-of-War or Bluebottle (*Physalia physalis*). (**A**) Although not a true jellyfish, envenomation by this organism is similar. This hydroid colony trails long stinging tentacles off of its float that can measure up to 10 m in length. Photo taken in Miami, Florida. (**B**). An adolescent presenting to the ED with pain, swelling, and erythema to her left foot after envenomation by Portuguese man-of-war off the coast of Florida. (Photo contributors: Matthew T. Timberger, MD [A], and Madeline H. Renny, MD [B].)

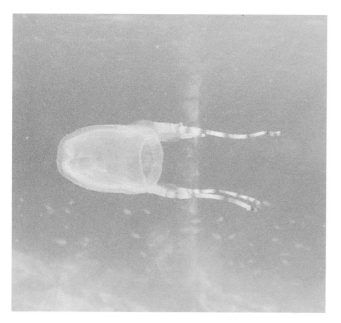

FIGURE 18.37 ▪ Jellyfish. The sting from this 5-inch jellyfish swimming in shallow water can be quite painful. True jellyfish like this one are always radially symmetrical. (Photo taken in Bonaire, the Netherlands Antilles. Photo contributor: Mark Silverberg, MD.)

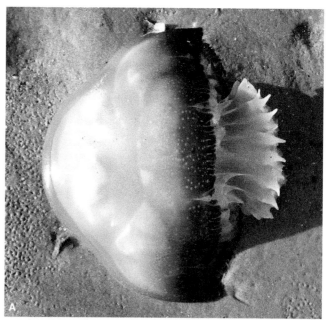

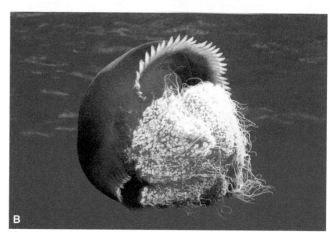

FIGURE 18.38 ▪ Jellyfish. (Photos taken in Myrtle Beach, South Carolina, and Andaman Sea in Thailand. Photo contributors: Mark Silverberg, MD [A], and Matthew T. Timberger, MD [B].)

sort of tool. The use of 5% acetic acid in Portuguese man-of-war envenomations is controversial because this has been shown to worsen cnidocyst discharge in vitro. Lidocaine may be effective in preventing further nematocyst firing and may help with topical pain control. For Portuguese man-of-war and jellyfish envenomations, place the affected extremity into hot water (45°C). Of note, hot water immersion should be avoided in box jellyfish envenomations. Alcohol, papain, urine, and ammonia have not been proven effective. A box jellyfish antivenin may be available for IV or IM use (sheep-derived immunoglobulin). If antivenin is not available, pressure and immobilization should be used until definitive care is available.

In the ED, monitor cardiovascular status. Treat nonfacial dermonecrotic injuries (essentially chemical burns) with silver sulfadiazine. Cleanse wounds with normal saline after treatment with acetic acid. Tetanus status should be assessed and updated as needed. Mild local reactions may be treated with antihistamines and topical corticosteroids. More severe skin reactions may require systemic corticosteroids. Patients without evidence of systemic reaction 6 hours after being stung may be discharged with good follow-up instructions. Patients with any evidence of systemic illness must be observed closely for at least 8 hours. In the setting of clinical improvement after treatment, discharge may be safe, although rebound illness has been reported. Patients with unrelenting signs of systemic envenomation should be admitted for observation. Prophylactic antibiotics are not normally indicated for immunocompetent patients. Dermatology follow-up may prove helpful for more severe skin reactions. Experts in marine envenomation may be sought through local poison control centers or through the Divers Alert Network (919-684-9111, 800-446-2671). Burn specialists may be required for management of severe dermal necrosis.

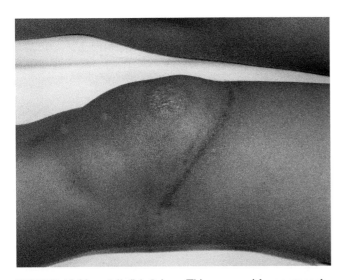

FIGURE 18.39 ■ Jellyfish Injury. This young girl was stung by a jellyfish on her left leg 3 to 4 days earlier while playing in the surf off the coast of the Dominican Republic. Hyperpigmentation is typical of such injuries after the pain subsides. (Photo contributor: Mark Silverberg, MD.)

Pearls

1. As with all animals that "sting" you, vinegar should be effective in treating most jellyfish envenomations, although lidocaine can be mixed with it for added benefit.
2. Most jellyfish envenomations do not have an antivenom, except the Australian box jellyfish, *C fleckeri*.
3. Hot water (45°C) immersion can be used in Portuguese man-of-war and jellyfish envenomations but should be avoided in box jellyfish envenomations.

Clinical Summary

Sponges have a matrix-like skeleton of silicon dioxide or calcium carbonate and can cause injuries in 1 of 3 ways. Their silicate or calcite spicules can penetrate the skin and may be coated with toxin. This can lead to a spicule or irritant dermatitis that may progress to abscess formation around difficult-to-remove foreign material. They can cause contact dermatitis very much like that from poison ivy. Symptoms from this reaction are similar to those of poison ivy with itching and redness. Desquamation may also occur, and erythema multiforme has been reported after such an injury. Finally, they may harbor venomous cnidarians, particularly hydroids. Most symptoms caused by sponges are brief in duration, but resolution may

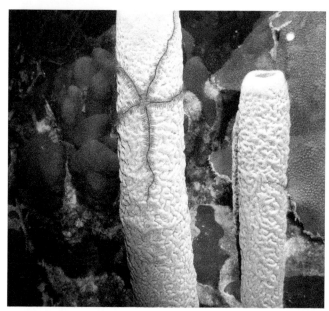

FIGURE 18.41 ■ Starfish on a Purple Tube Sponge. Echinoderms like this starfish have sharp toxin-covered spines projecting out from their legs that can easily become imbedded in human skin. (Photo taken in Bonaire, the Netherlands Antilles. Photo contributor: Mark Silverberg, MD.)

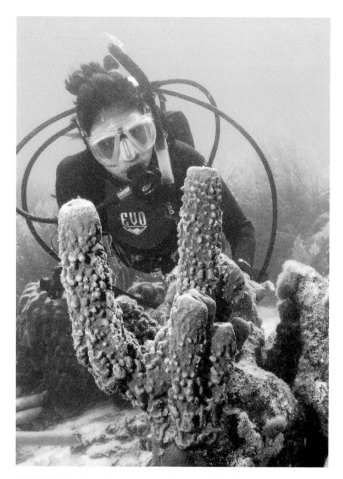

FIGURE 18.40 ■ Brown Tube Sponge. This diver is investigating a brown tube sponge, although she is keeping a good safe distance from it to avoid injury. (Photo taken in Cozumel, Mexico. Photo contributor: Donita Dyalram, MD, DDS.)

take up to a week or more in rare cases. Allergy to sponges has also occasionally been described, causing vesiculation, edema, and even urticaria or anaphylaxis.

Emergency Department Treatment and Disposition

Because it impossible to distinguish which of the 3 mechanisms of injury occurred, treat for all 3, beginning in the field. Rinse the affected area with vinegar, if available. Gently pat the wound dry and apply adhesive tape over the area and slowly remove the tape to remove much of the exposed spicular material. Soak the area again in vinegar for 20 to 30 minutes.

In the ED, wounds should be well irrigated with normal saline. For mild reactions, topical steroids may prevent or reduce secondary inflammation. Tetanus status should be evaluated and updated if necessary. Severe skin reactions may require treatment with a tapering course of oral steroids. Antibiotics should rarely be needed, except where deep tissue penetration or injury has occurred. Urticaria and itching should respond to antihistamine therapy. Dermatologist follow-up is indicated for more severe skin reactions. Experts in marine envenomation may be sought through local poison control centers or through the Divers Alert Network (919-684-9111, 800-446-2671).

Pearls

1. Exposed sea sponge spicules can be removed with adhesive tape.
2. Vinegar may help alleviate symptoms caused by sponge envenomation.

STABBING MARINE ANIMALS: STARFISH, SEA URCHINS, AND CROWN-OF-THORNS STARFISH

Clinical Summary

Echinoderms (starfish and sea urchins) stab with spines that cause penetrating trauma as well as envenomation. Species vary in toxicity, although, as with most other toxic marine animals, the most dangerous varieties are found in the Indo-Pacific region.

Injuries from these animals occur when their sharp spines pierce the skin or a joint. When stabbed, venom coating the spines along with the integumentary sheath, seawater, particulate matter, and microorganisms enter the tissues. These spines are quite brittle and often crumble when one tries to remove them, resulting in chronic pain, tattooing, granuloma, or abscess formation around retained foreign material. Besides the physical injury, envenomation from the poisonous species of echinoderms may occur, leading to severe local pain or nonspecific generalized symptoms such as malaise, body aches, neuromuscular weakness, and hypotension. Deaths have been attributed to severe envenomations due to respiratory failure or from overwhelming sepsis if infected retained spines are not removed or treated adequately. The crown-of-thorns starfish has toxin-coated spines. Its venom is hemolytic, hepatotoxic, myonecrotic, and an anticoagulant. Pain from a crown-of-thorns starfish puncture wound can resolve within 30 minutes to 3 hours. Sea urchin puncture wounds can cause pain and muscle aches lasting up to 24 hours. Tenosynovitis can develop if a spine enters the joint space.

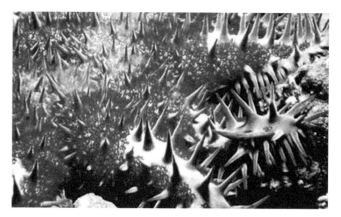

FIGURE 18.43 ■ Spines on the Crown-of-Thorns Sea Star (*Acanthaster planci*). This beautiful starfish is surrounded on all exposed sides by sharp spines, making it look quite menacing, and produces venom in glandular tissue underneath the epidermis, which is released via its spiny surfaces. (Reproduced with permission from Kasper DL, Fauci AS. *Harrison's Infectious Diseases,* 3rd ed. McGraw-Hill Education; New York, NY, 2017. Photo contributor: Paul Auerbach, MD.)

Emergency Department Treatment and Disposition

Treatment should begin in the field. Visible spines should be carefully removed as they fracture easily. Because the toxins from these creatures are usually heat labile, immersion in hot water (114°F/45.6°C) for 30 to 90 minutes may relieve the pain by denaturing the venom proteins. Foreign bodies must be sought with radiographs and/or sonography. An x-ray, US, CT scan, or MRI may be necessary to find all foreign material embedded in the tissues. All puncture wounds should be aggressively cleansed, although it is usually hard to reach the bottom of the tract. Most echinoderm spines crumble easily, and the clinician should try to avoid crushing them during extraction. All foreign material must be removed including the integument sheath when possible. Penetrated joints should be evaluated in an operating room setting. Tetanus vaccination should be updated if necessary. Antibiotics such as a quinolone that have activity against marine organisms such as *Vibrio* species are indicated for deep wounds, especially in the hand or foot. Treatment for the envenomation is generally supportive because no antivenin exists for these creatures. Experts in marine envenomation may be sought through local poison control centers or through the Divers Alert Network (919-684-9111, 800-446-2671).

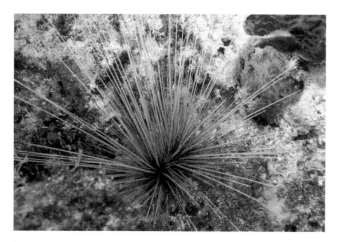

FIGURE 18.42 ■ Sea Urchin. This spiny sea urchin uses its long thin spines to protect its soft central body. The integument-covered spines are capable of delivering venom to an individual who is unlucky enough to be impaled while swimming or stepping on it. (Photo taken in Grand Cayman. Photo contributor: Mark Silverberg, MD.)

Pearls

1. Venom from starfish and sea urchins is usually heat labile, so soak affected body parts in the warmest water that the patient can tolerate to denature the proteins and help alleviate symptoms.

2. Seek (and expect) foreign bodies in the skin when a patient has been stabbed by these creatures because their spines are quite brittle and break easily.

3. No antivenom exists, so treatment is supportive.

Clinical Summary

The Scorpaenidae family includes the venomous lionfish, frogfish, scorpionfish, stonefish, and devilfish. Common to this diverse group are the venomous integument-covered spines on their dorsal and ventral fins. The stonefish (*Synanceia* species) is by far the most dangerous of these creatures, with venom that induces severe localized pain in addition to multiple nonspecific systemic symptoms. Lionfish are frequently kept in aquaria and thus are a more common source of envenomation than might be expected.

Clinically, patients envenomated by any of these fish will complain of intense pain at the injury site surrounded by erythema and swelling. Pain symptoms peak at 60 to 90 minutes and can last for hours to days in patient envenomated by the scorpionfish or stonefish, respectively. The associated wounds can have a cyanotic appearance. The affected site may develop cellulitis or become necrotic. Systemic effects such as nausea and vomiting may be present along with hemolysis, hypotension, and neuromuscular weakness. Death can occur (within 6–8 hours) rarely with severe envenomations due to respiratory failure or overwhelming sepsis.

Emergency Department Treatment and Disposition

Treatment should begin in the field. Immersion in hot water (114°F/45.6°C) for 30 to 90 minutes may relieve some of the

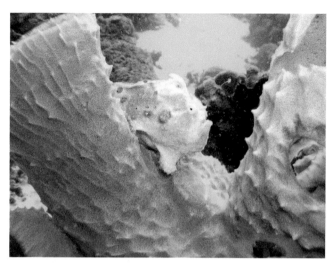

FIGURE 18.45 ■ Frogfish (*Antennarius multiocellatus*). The long lure frogfish blend in with their surroundings amazingly well, making them difficult to spot. They dangle a small projection off of their head as "bait" while they "fish." When a small fish investigates the moving lure, they end up becoming the meal. (Photo taken in Bonaire, the Netherlands Antilles. Photo contributor: Mark Silverberg, MD.)

pain, but narcotic analgesics in liberal doses will likely be required for stonefish injury. Tetanus status should be ascertained and updated when necessary. Foreign bodies must be sought with plain radiography, sonography, CT scan, or even MRI because spines can break off easily. Wounds should be cleansed and debrided aggressively. Penetrated joints should

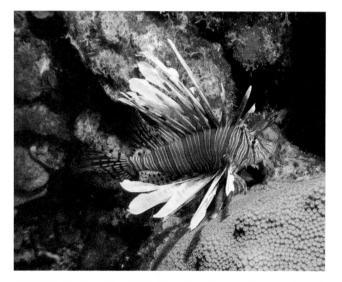

FIGURE 18.44 ■ Lion Fish (*Pterois volitans*). Although beautiful, the lion fish sports many dangerous poison-covered spines on its dorsal fin that induce an extremely painful envenomation. (Photo taken in Bonaire, the Netherlands Antilles. Photo contributor: Mark Silverberg, MD.)

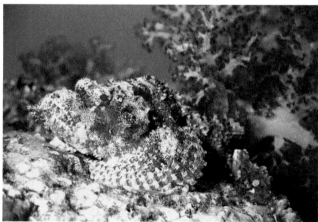

FIGURE 18.46 ■ Scorpionfish (Scorpaenidae Species). The amazing camouflage of these fish make them very difficult to spot, which also makes them quite easy to accidentally put your hand down on when diving. (Photo taken in Andaman Sea, Thailand. Photo contributor: Matthew T. Timberger, MD.)

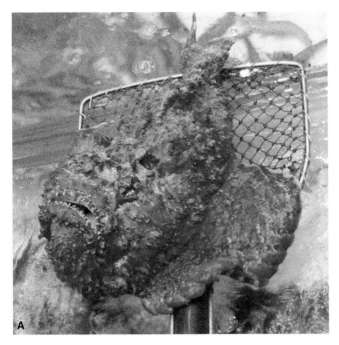
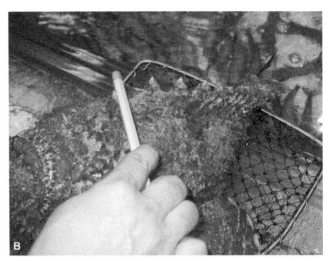

FIGURE 18.47 ■ Stonefish (*Synanceia* Species). (**A**) Of all the fish in the scorpionfish family, the venom of the stonefish is the most potent and induces an extremely painful envenomation. (**B**) Note the stinging spines on the close-up. (Reproduced with permission from Nelson LS, Hoffman RS, Howland MA, et al. *Goldfrank's Toxicologic Emergencies,* 11th ed. McGraw-Hill Education; New York, NY, 2019. Photo contributor: The Fellowship in Medical Toxicology, New York University School of Medicine, New York City Poison Center.)

be addressed in an operating room setting. An antibiotic such as a quinolone that has activity against marine organisms is indicated for deep penetrations and wounds that occurred more than 6 to 12 hours before presentation.

ED care is supportive, except in the case of severe stonefish envenomation. Stonefish antivenom is produced by CSL, Ltd., of Australia, from the venom of *Synanceia trachynis* and may be available for use in the Indo-Pacific region to treat systemic envenomation. Experts in marine envenomation may be sought through local poison control centers or through the Divers Alert Network (919-684-9111, 800-446-2671).

Pearls

1. Toxin components of these fish are usually heat labile, so soak them in the warmest water that the patient can tolerate (without burning the patient) to denature the proteins and help alleviate symptoms.

2. Antivenom is available for stonefish envenomation.

Clinical Summary

Stingrays are cartilaginous fish with a long, sharp barb on their tail used for defense, which is often deployed when they are stepped on or frightened. The barb is coated with venom and covered by an integumentary sheath. Venom contains phosphodiesterase, serotonin, and 5′-nucleotidase. As the venom-coated barb is forcefully driven into the tissues, seawater, particulate matter, and microorganisms are also dragged in with it. Case reports have documented all kinds of visceral injuries in addition to pneumothoraces and hemothoraces. Most ED visits for stingray injuries are for physical trauma of the lower extremities in the form of lacerations, although envenomation can lead to systemic symptoms such as nausea, vomiting, diaphoresis, diarrhea, hypotension, syncope, muscle cramps, neuromuscular weakness, headaches, seizure, cardiac dysrhythmias, and even respiratory failure in rare cases of severe envenomation. Deaths do occur from stingray injuries but are usually due to penetrating trauma to the chest, neck, or abdomen or from overwhelming sepsis originating from an untreated or undertreated barb wound.

Emergency Department Treatment and Disposition

Treatment should begin in the field. Immersion in hot water (114°F/45.6°C) for 30 to 90 minutes may relieve some pain, although any retained barb should be left in place just in case it is tamponading a vascular injury. Because the barb can easily be broken off and left inside the body, radiographs, sonography, or even CT scans or MRI should be used to rule out retained barb fragments.

All stingray barb injuries must be treated as if they are life-threatening penetrating stab wounds even when in the lower extremities. Abdominal injuries should be worked up for evidence of visceral injury, and chest trauma should be treated following Advanced Trauma Life Support (ATLS) protocol. Impaled stingray barbs are often difficult to remove if found lodged in the tissues because of their serrated nature

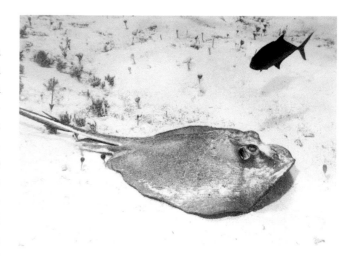

FIGURE 18.48 ■ Stingray. Stingrays such as this one sport a long, sharp barb on their tail (arrow) that is used defensively when the stingray is disturbed or even stepped on. (Photo taken in Grand Cayman. Photo contributor: Mark Silverberg, MD.)

and may require a trip to the operating room if more than shallowly embedded. Tetanus status should be updated when indicated. Wounds must be cleansed and debrided aggressively to remove all foreign material and bits of integument. Penetrated joints should also be addressed in an operating room setting. An antibiotic such as a quinolone that has activity against marine organisms is indicated for deep wounds. Patients should be observed for 6 hours after injury, after which neurologic involvement is unlikely to occur. Care for envenomation is supportive because no antivenin is available.

Pearls

1. Toxin components are usually heat labile, so soak them in the warmest water that the patient can tolerate to denature the proteins and help alleviate symptoms.
2. Treat stingray injuries like any other penetrating trauma before dealing with the envenomation.
3. Retained foreign bodies are likely with stingray injuries. Any number of radiologic modalities can be used to rule them out.

STABBING MARINE ANIMALS: CONE SHELLS (FAMILY CONIDAE)

Clinical Summary

Cone shells are small, snail-like mollusks that usually inhabit tropical waters, with the species found in the Indo-Pacific region being the most toxic. They are carnivorous animals that can deliver a highly venomous bite. Cone shell venom is an extremely toxic set of neurotoxins that paralyze its prey. Neurologic impairment may persist for days to weeks, making mechanical ventilation the only bridge to survival in those bitten. Clinically, the patient may initially be asymptomatic, but stinging or sharp pain usually develops at the site. Numbness, pallor, or cyanosis surrounding the wound often follows, with paresthesias spreading up the extremity. Perioral numbness, nausea, and vomiting are common early signs of systemic toxicity progressing to cranial nerve dysfunction, muscle paralysis, hypotension, and coma in severe envenomations. Respiratory failure is the usual cause of death in these patients (can occur within 1 hour), although cardiac failure and cerebral edema have also been reported. Peak activity of venom is within the first 12 hours, but neurologic deficits may persist for days.

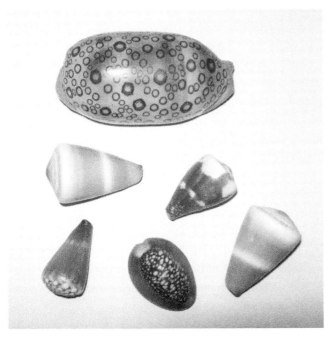

FIGURE 18.49 ■ Cone Shell Variety. Cone shells come in many shapes, colors, and sizes and make lovely room decorations. However, a shell collector must make sure that the animal has evacuated its home before picking it up to avoid injury from envenomation. A Cowrie shell is seen at the top with multiple different cones below it. (Photo contributor: Matthew T. Timberger, MD.)

Emergency Department Treatment and Disposition

Field management is essential and includes pressure and immobilization, which should begin as soon as possible to prevent the lymphatic spread of toxins. Apply a stack of gauze pads (sterile if available) over the bite and wrap with modest pressure using an elastic bandage. The dressing should be snug, as when wrapping a sprained ankle, but circulation should not be compromised and should be checked frequently. Immobilize the extremity if possible and do not remove the dressing until resuscitative equipment or definitive care is available. Submersion of the wrapped area in hot water (114°F/45.6°C) for 30 to 90 minutes has been suggested.

Treatment in the ED is supportive, and a ventilator and intubation equipment must be available in case of respiratory failure. Patients without respiratory weakness should be observed for 8 to 12 hours. Tetanus status should be assessed and updated as needed. The wound must be carefully cleansed and explored for foreign bodies; plain films or sonography may reveal a retained object, but CT or MRI is more accurate. Antibiotics should be considered for deep injuries, for wounds over joints, and in patients with immune impairment or with significant comorbidities such as diabetes mellitus. Experts in marine envenomation may be sought through local poison control centers or through the Divers Alert Network (919-684-9111, 800-446-2671).

Pearls

1. Toxin components of cone shells are usually heat labile, so soak them in the warmest water that the patient can tolerate to denature the proteins and help alleviate symptoms.
2. Cone shell venom is neurotoxic.
3. The pressure/immobilization technique may help stop the spread of venom through the lymphatic system.

Clinical Summary

Blue-ringed octopuses are small (<25 cm) and found throughout the Indo-Pacific living in tide pools and among coral heads and rocks. The octopus produces a highly potent venom that is transmitted through a chitinous beak during a bite. Some believe that other body parts may contain low levels of venom, making these creatures poisonous as well as venomous. The chief component of the venom is a tetrodotoxin-like agent that blocks cellular sodium channels and produces neuromuscular paralysis. Initially the bite may be asymptomatic, but numbness or pain at the bite site usually occurs within 15 minutes, along with pruritus, erythema, and, occasionally, urticaria. By 30 minutes, facial numbness and weakness typically ensue. Cranial nerve dysfunction is common, and voluntary or involuntary muscle paralysis soon follows, culminating in respiratory failure. Hypotension may occur but is not a consistent feature. Peak activity of blue-ringed octopus venom is within the first 12 hours, but neurologic effects may persist for 3 to 4 days.

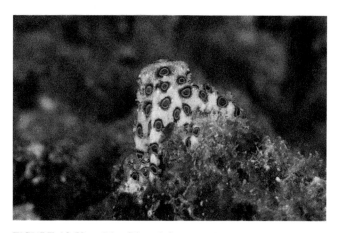

FIGURE 18.50 ■ Blue-Ringed Octopus. The blue-ringed octopus demonstrates its iridescent blue colorations, seen when the animal is threatened. (Reproduced with permission from Knoop KJ, Stack LB, Storrow AB, et al. *The Atlas of Emergency Medicine,* 4th ed; McGraw-Hill Education; New York, NY, 2016. Photo contributor: Kevin J. Knoop, MD.)

Emergency Department Treatment and Disposition

Field management is essential. Place a stack of gauze pads over the bite and wrap with a pressure bandage as snugly as possible without compromising circulation. The extremity involved should be immobilized and the dressing kept in place until resuscitative equipment or definitive care is available. The wrapped limb may be submerged in hot water for 30 to 90 minutes.

In the ED, provide cardiovascular and respiratory support, and draw baseline labs. Because respiratory paralysis is common, ventilator support may become necessary, so intubation equipment should be available. Patients without respiratory weakness should be observed for 8 to 12 hours and are unlikely to deteriorate after this period. Laboratory findings are nonspecific, although coagulation studies should be performed, as other components of the venom may have anticoagulant properties. Itching and urticaria can be relieved with histamine blockade with an agent such as diphenhydramine, and pain can be addressed with NSAIDs or narcotics if severe. Basic local wound care using an antiseptic preparation followed by copious irrigation should be provided in an effort to remove all marine life and bacteria. Tetanus status should be checked and updated as needed. Antibiotics may be considered for deep injuries, for bites over joints, and in patients with immune impairment or with significant comorbidities such as diabetes mellitus. Experts in marine envenomation may be sought through local poison control centers or through the Divers Alert Network (919-684-9111, 800-446-2671).

Pearls

1. Respiratory support is the hallmark of treatment.
2. The pressure/immobilization technique should be used prior to hospital arrival.
3. A paralyzed victim may be fully alert.

Clinical Summary

Lightning can injure patients by a direct strike, spread of ground current after a strike, or blunt trauma produced by the explosive force of current discharged to a nearby object. Lightning injuries vary widely from cuts and scrapes, to mild mental disorientation without physical effect, to asystole or cardiac arrest. Classification of lightning injuries into organ systems affected is common.

Cardiovascular manifestations tend to directly affect the myocardial conduction pathway, and cardiac arrest is the only direct cause of death due to lightning. When lightning strikes cause asystole, spontaneous circulation often returns after early and only brief cardiopulmonary resuscitation (CPR). Other arrhythmias may also occur (most commonly ventricular fibrillation). QT prolongation is most common and generally resolves spontaneously within a few weeks to months.

Neurologic effects are among the most frequent nontraumatic sequelae. Altered mental status, which may include confusion or amnesia, is often seen and may compromise the reliability of the history. Patients may also develop acute

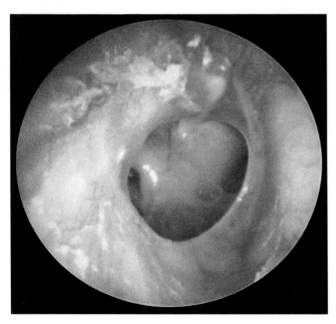

FIGURE 18.51 ■ Perforated Tympanic Membrane Following a Lightning Strike. Tympanic membrane perforation is one of many injuries that commonly result after being struck by lightning. An otoscopic examination, therefore, must be performed on every lightning-injured patient to avoid missing this injury. Near-total perforation of the tympanic membrane is seen in this image. Such perforation can also result from acute or chronic otitis media. (Photo contributor: Neil Sperling, MD; see also Figure 9.5.)

pain syndromes, paresthesias, temporary paralysis, vertigo, cataracts, and tinnitus. In the most severe cases, anoxic brain injury may occur because of cardiovascular collapse or neurologic respiratory failure.

Dermatologic consequences are generally obvious. Entrance and exit wounds appear similar to traditional electrocution burns and can be quite serious. Diffuse skin burns may also occur because of sweat or rain water being vaporized into steam when a large lightning current passes over the body. Deeper internal burns occur rarely. The phenomenon called Lichtenberg figures or lines are fernlike patterns created on the skin and are considered a pathognomic finding of lightning strikes.

Emergency Department Treatment and Disposition

Evaluate and stabilize the ABCs, and then perform a thorough history and physical examination, after which patients should be observed in a monitored setting. Cervical spine precautions are especially important if there is altered mental status or other signs of neurologic dysfunction. Remove wet clothing to avoid hypothermia, and complete a thorough secondary survey. Order plain films of the extremities if there is tenderness or deformity. If the patient's sensorium is altered or the patient has suffered a loss of consciousness, obtain a noncontrast head CT scan to rule out intracranial bleeding or cerebral contusion. Although no specific laboratory tests are diagnostic of a lightning-injured patient, creatine kinase and myoglobin levels may help to identify complications such as rhabdomyolysis. The remainder of the workup should follow ATLS guidelines for trauma patients. If cardiac irregularity is present on a screening ECG, admission is warranted for telemetry monitoring.

Pearls

1. Injuries occur either from a direct strike itself or indirectly from the energy released by the conduction of current to a ground surface.
2. Early CPR is often associated with successful return of spontaneous circulation when lightning causes asystole.
3. No set guidelines exist for the workup of a lightning-injured patient, and clinicians should maintain a high index of suspicion for rhabdomyolysis.

Clinical Presentation

Snake bites are uncommon and have a wide spectrum of presentations depending on the timing of the bite, amount of venom delivered, and species and type of venom. Most snake bites are harmless and are caused by nonpoisonous snakes. The 2 most common classes of venomous snakes are the Elapidae and Viperidae families. Elapids include cobras, mambas, sea snakes and kraits, and the coral snake. In North America, coral snakes have red, yellow, and black bands and bear a close resemblance to king snakes, which are not venomous. Coral and king snakes have a different sequence of colored bands, so that they may be distinguished from one another with the mnemonic "Red on Yellow, Kill a Fellow; Red on Black, Friend of Jack (or Venom Lack)."

Snakes in the Viperidae family such as rattlesnakes, true vipers, and lanceheads cause bites that often bear *typical* double puncture marks made by mobile fangs that swing out when biting. These snakes usually have narrow, slit-like pupils and large poison glands located behind their powerful jaws, causing them to exhibit triangular heads that are distinctly separate from their bodies.

Elapid venoms are neurotoxins that cause systemic symptoms including lethargy, weakness, ptosis, aphasia, and, in severe cases, respiratory depression or arrest. Snakes of the Elapidae family have short, fixed fangs and must chew the victim to inject enough venom to be harmful, and thus, these bites do not display "typical" double fang marks. Elapid bites may also manifest symptoms in a delayed fashion (up to hours later) when only small amounts of venom penetrate the skin.

Effects of Viperidae venom are usually rapid and more localized to the bite site, with erythema, swelling, and ecchymosis being common. Systemic symptoms may occasionally arise, which can include paresthesias of the tongue, a metallic

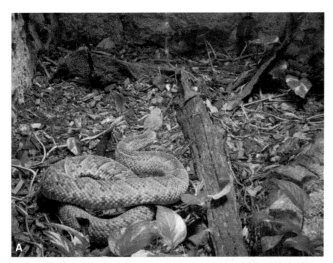

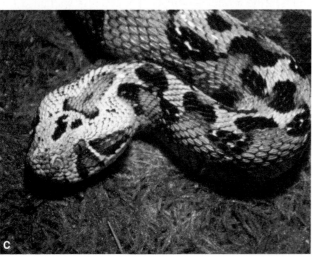

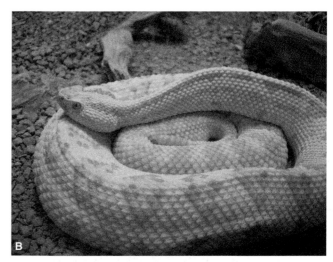

FIGURE 18.52 ■ Snakes of the Viperidae Family. (**A**) The rattlesnake is typical for snakes of the Viperidae family. Notice the triangular-shaped head, which Elapidae do not possess. The rattle at the tip of its tail sets these snakes apart from all of the others in its family. (**B**) South American rattlesnake (*Crotalus durissus*). This is the "xanthic" phase of the South American rattlesnake, which is a rare, special form of albinism. Notice the diamond-shaped head and the rattle at the tip of the tail, setting these snakes apart from the other vipers. (**C**) Ethiopian mountain viper (*Bitis parviocula*). This viper species is found only in southwest Ethiopia and bears the typical diamond-shaped head that all vipers display. They hiss when teased but do not possess a rattle. ([A] Photo taken in Playa Del Carmen, Mexico; photo contributor: Lawrence Silverberg, DPM; and [B, C] photos taken at the San Diego Zoo; photo contributor: Mark Silverberg, MD.)

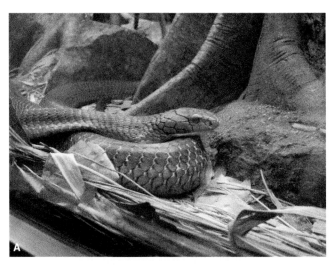
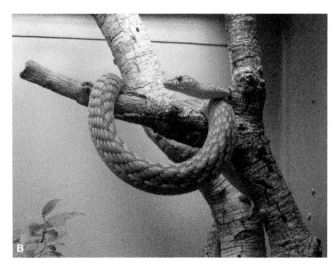

FIGURE 18.53 ■ Snakes of the Elapidae Family. (**A**) The king cobra (*Ophiophagus hannah*) is the world's longest venomous snake and can measure up to 5.5 m. When undisturbed, they have cylindrical bodies that taper slightly at the head. However, when confronted or agitated, they rear up and display the typical cobra "hood." (**B**) West African green mamba (*Dendroaspis viridis*). The green mamba is an arboreal (tree climbing) snake in the Elapidae family that possesses potent neurotoxins that can easily kill the birds and lizards on which it preys. (Photos taken at the San Diego Zoo. Photo contributor: Mark Silverberg, MD.)

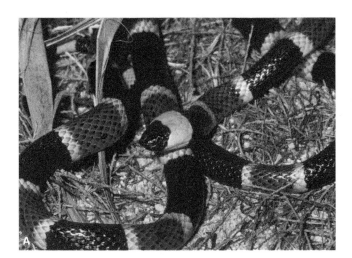

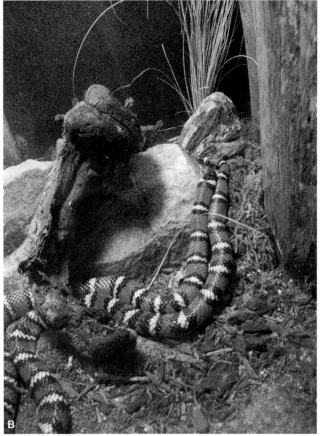

FIGURE 18.54 ■ Coral Snake ("Red on Yellow, Kill a Fellow") versus king snake ("Red on Black, Friend of Jack or Venom Lack"). (**A**) A close-up view of the striking and distinctive markings of the highly venomous coral snake. The coral snake can be identified by the yellow and red bands that touch, whereas the red and black bands do not. The coral snake is a member of the Elapidae family and is venomous. (**B**) This king snake appears similar to the coral snake but has a different band pattern with adjacent red and black bands. It is only a mimic of the coral snake and is harmless. (Photo contributor: Mike Cardwell, MS; reproduced with permission from Knoop KJ, Stack LB, Storrow AB, et al. *The Atlas of Emergency Medicine,* 4th ed. McGraw-Hill Education; New York, NY, 2016 [A]; and Mark Silverberg, MD [B].)

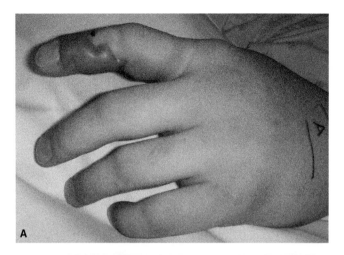

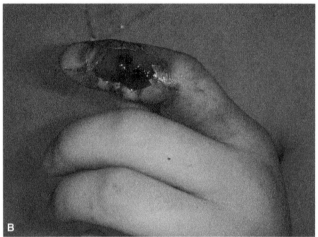

FIGURE 18.55 ■ Snake Bite. (**A**) Left index finger of patient who sustained a snake bite. (**B**) Evolution of snake bite wound during hospitalization. (Photo contributor: Michael D. Levine, MD.)

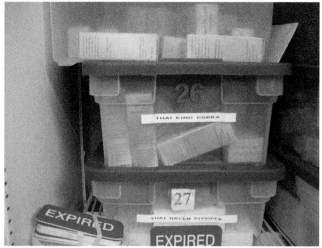

FIGURE 18.56 ■ Antivenom. Large zoos keep most of the world's stock of antivenom for dangerous snakes. Because the supply is so small, even expired vials are kept on hand. (Photo taken at the San Diego Zoo. Photo contributor: Mark Silverberg, MD.)

taste in the mouth, generalized pain, hypotension, and even shock. Up to 30% of venomous snake bites seen are "dry bites" where no toxin was instilled. The volume of venom depends on time since the snake's last bite, degree of threat perceived by the snake, size of the snake, and size of the victim. Early development of systemic manifestations may signal a significant envenomation, especially if the venom was directly introduced into a vessel.

Emergency Department Treatment and Disposition

Assess and stabilize ABC status first, with special attention to airway compromise or vascular collapse. Perform a complete physical with a full visual examination with the patient wholly undressed. Bulla formation, ecchymosis, petechiae,

or muscle fasciculations indicate increased severity of envenomation. Use caution in unconscious patients, ensuring that snake bites are not presumed to be merely puncture wounds.

Obtain plain radiographs of the bite site to rule out fracture or retained foreign bodies such as broken fangs. Cleanse the affected area with high-pressure irrigation and address pain control. Evaluate for compartment syndrome, which may necessitate fasciotomy. Rarely, snake bite coagulopathy can develop; therefore, baseline coagulation studies should be obtained. Follow CBC closely as thrombocytopenia may also ensue. Check creatine kinase levels and electrolytes as rhabdomyolysis may develop.

If the snake can be confirmed to belong to the Crotalinae subfamily (rattlesnakes, water moccasins, and copperheads) of the Viperidae, use Crotalidae polyvalent immune fab (CroFab) to arrest or reverse symptom progression. The initial dose of CroFab is 4 to 6 vials delivered via IV. If symptoms resolve, give an additional 2 vials every 6 hours for 3 more doses. If the symptoms continue to progress despite being sure that the patient was bitten by a snake of the Crotalinae subfamily, give 4 to 6 more vials every hour until symptoms begin to resolve. As with all animal bites, tetanus immunization should be updated when indicated. Antibiotics are often given, although no study has every proven them to be beneficial in preventing wound infections. Any patient discharged must be given close follow-up within 24 to 48 hours for reevaluation of the wound and given detailed discharge instructions describing potential complications.

Pearls

1. Contact the local poison center to assist with snake identification and attempt to determine the type of venom delivered to anticipate its effects and look for an antivenom.

2. Certain venoms can have delayed manifestations, such as compartment syndrome, thrombocytopenia, rhabdomyolysis, and electrolyte disturbances.

3. Offer close follow-up to discharged patients for reevaluation of wounds.

Clinical Summary

High-altitude illness (HAI) is a term used to describe the continuum of symptoms an individual can develop as a result of ascending to a higher altitude. Acute mountain sickness (AMS), high-altitude cerebral edema (HACE), and high-altitude pulmonary edema (HAPE) represent various presentations of HAI. HAI varies depending on speed of ascent and the individual's own innate ability to adapt to elevation. Reduced ambient pressure and low oxygen tension at high altitudes are thought to be the cause of tissue injury. Children with respiratory illnesses, otitis media, congenital cardiopulmonary disease, sickle cell disease, asthma, and Down syndrome have an increased risk of developing HAI.

AMS usually begins at altitudes >2000 m (6560 ft) as early as 1 hour after ascent, but may develop as late as 2 days after beginning climbing. Patients with AMS appear ill but will have no distinct physical findings. Headache is the most common complaint, along with GI symptoms such as nausea and vomiting. Constitutional complaints such as weakness, dizziness, and lightheadedness may also be present.

HAPE presents as a cough with thin, clear to yellowish sputum. Other common symptoms include chest tightness or dull pain, but frank shortness of breath with tachypnea may also be present. In severe cases, patients can develop hypoxia.

HACE is considered the most serious and life threatening of high-altitude diseases. It is usually seen in individuals who continue ascent despite early signs of AMS and HAPE. Ataxia is often the first sign and is typically followed by altered mental status. In rare cases, patients can have focal neurologic deficits, such as nerve palsy. Without prompt treatment, further neurologic deterioration to coma and death can occur.

Emergency Department Treatment and Disposition

Descent, even by a small amount, is the treatment for any high-altitude illness; if descent is not an option due to weather or injury, rest at the current altitude may allow acclimatization. Typically, climbers recognize the symptoms and return down to a medical facility. Most will no longer have symptoms, and further treatment is rarely indicated.

Regardless of presentation, climbers should be thoroughly evaluated for HAI as well as dehydration or hypothermia. Climbers may take acetazolamide to prevent altitude illness. The recommended prophylactic dosage is 125 mg taken twice daily beginning 2 to 3 days prior to ascent, but it can be started as late as 8 to 24 hours before ascent. Side effects of this drug include paresthesias, urinary frequency, and blurry vision, which can be mistaken for AMS itself. Benzolamide may have less CNS effects compared to acetazolamide. Slow ascent may be more effective in preventing symptom development.

If medical prophylaxis fails and descent is not an option, a portable hyperbaric chamber called a Gamow bag (pronounced gam-off) can be used. Such a device serves as a descent simulator and is composed of a nylon bag forming a sealed chamber and a manual foot pump to pressurize it. Oxygen can also be concentrated in the chamber for an added benefit. Deployment of this device can simulate a descent of up to 2000 m (65,000 ft) and can be accomplished within minutes. Because acclimatization may take up to 24 hours and the device is totally portable, the patient can be transported down to a lower altitude within the Gamow bag where symptoms should not recur when the patient emerges. Dexamethasone is used to treat both AMS and HACE. Dexamethasone is dosed 4 mg every 6 hours for both AMS and HACE, but requires a loading dose of 8 mg for patients with HACE and should be given via the IM route. In patients with AMS, dexamethasone can be given enterally, parenterally, or IM. Nifedipine and phosphodiesterase inhibitors have been used in the treatment of HAPE.

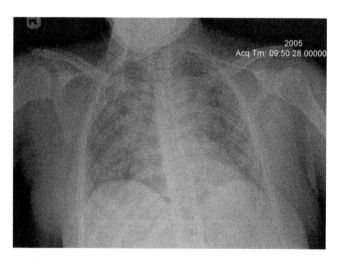

FIGURE 18.57 ■ High-Altitude Pulmonary Edema. It is not uncommon for climbers to experience shortness of breath and cough as they top altitudes of 2500 meters (8200 ft). This climber had to be air lifted off of Mt. Kilimanjaro due to respiratory distress. (Photo taken at base camp of Mt. Kilimanjaro, Northeastern Tanzania. Photo contributor: Mark Silverberg, MD.)

Pearls

1. Prophylactic use of acetazolamide can help with acclimatization and avoidance of the development of altitude sickness.

2. HAI can present with a spectrum of severity, most often affecting the respiratory and neurologic systems.

3. Development of signs or symptoms of altitude sickness should prompt individuals to descend, which is the only definitive treatment for altitude illness.

Chapter 19

ORTHOPEDICS

Konstantinos Agoritsas
Ameer Hassoun
Jennifer H. Chao
Sathyaseelan Subramaniam
Andrea T. Cruz
Ryan Logan Webb
Josh Greenstein

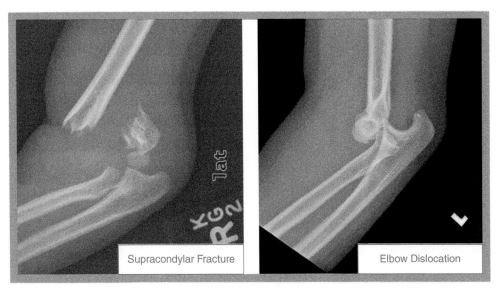

Supracondylar Fracture

Elbow Dislocation

(Photo contributors: John Amodio, MD, and Ryan Logan Webb, MD)

The author acknowledges the special contributions of Michael Lucchesi, MD, Rita Nathawad, MD, and Diana E. Weaver, MD, to prior editions.

Clinical Summary

Fractures are caused by high-energy forces on bones and may result from blunt or penetrating trauma. Fracture size and shape are determined by the amount of energy absorbed, the focus of energy, and mass and resistance of the affected bone. Obvious deformities may or may not be present, depending on the degree of fracture angulation and the presence of associated joint dislocation. Patients present with swelling and tenderness. If mental status is intact and there is no associated nerve damage, patients will complain of pain on palpation. Ecchymosis may not be present for minutes to hours and is dependent on associated tissue damage, thickness and integrity of overlying skin, and the degree of vascular injury.

Emergency Department Treatment and Disposition

Obtain plain films that ensure the entire injured area is evaluated at various angles, as fractures are often present on one view but not another. Provide analgesia, elevate the fractured bone, and apply cold compresses after more serious, associated injuries have been ruled out. Provide IV antibiotics for

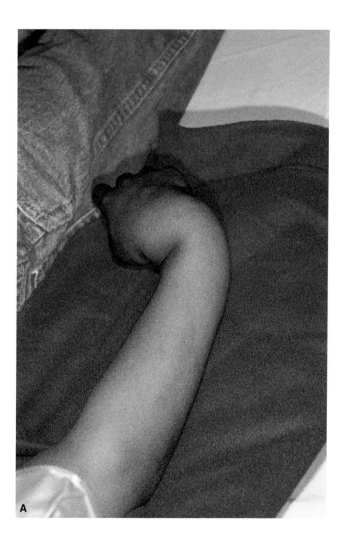

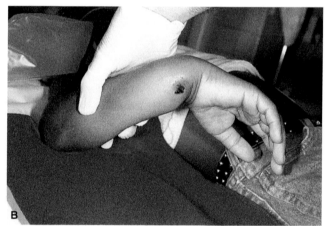

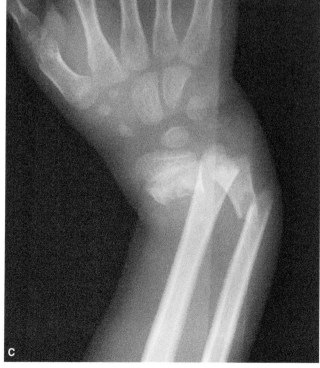

FIGURE 19.1 ■ Open Fractures. (**A**) A picture of a wrist showing obvious severe deformity. (**B**) A puncture wound at the site of the deformity is diagnostic for an open fracture. (**C**) X-ray demonstrating a markedly displaced fracture of the distal radius and ulna. There is also a dislocation of the distal radioulnar joint. (Photo contributor: Binita R. Shah, MD.)

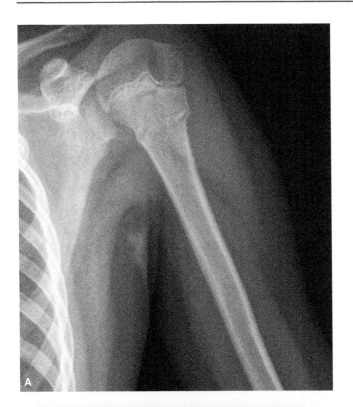

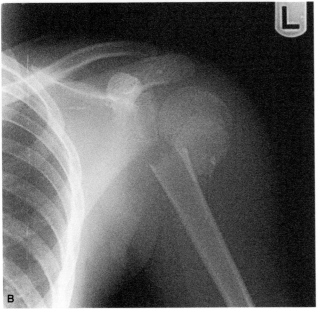

FIGURE 19.2 ■ Complete Fractures. (**A**) Frontal view of the humerus demonstrates a complete, nondisplaced fracture of the diametaphysis. (**B**) Frontal view of the humerus in a different patient shows complete fracture of the diametaphysis with medial displacement of the distal fragment by 1 bone shaft's width. (Photo/legend contributors: Carlos Barahona, MD, and John Amodio, MD.)

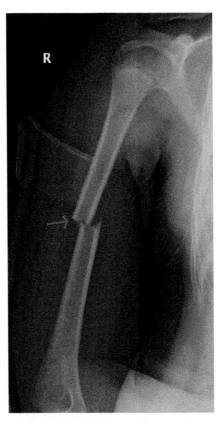

FIGURE 19.3 ■ Transverse Fracture. A complete transverse fracture of the humerus. The distal segment is displaced one-half shaft width medially. (Photo contributors: Ryan Logan Webb, MD, and Josh Greenstein, MD.)

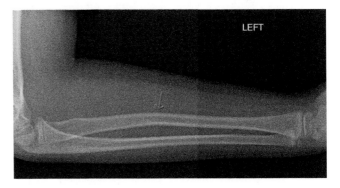

FIGURE 19.4 ■ Bowing Fracture. A 9-year-old girl with left forearm injury. Lateral view of the left forearm reveals no discrete cortical break or dislocation; however, the radius demonstrates a mildly abnormal dorsal bend consistent with bowing fracture (red arrow). Compare with the normal physiologic gentle curve of the ulna. Bowing fracture is a subtype of incomplete fracture. (Photo contributors: Ryan Logan Webb, MD, and Josh Greenstein, MD.)

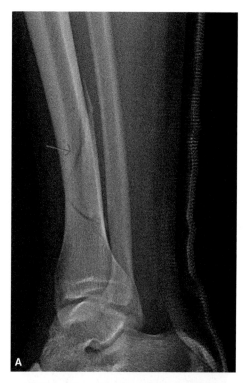

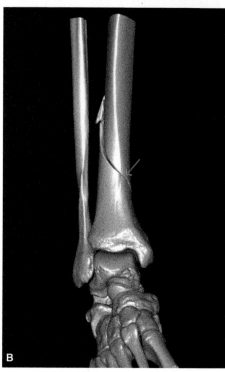

FIGURE 19.5 ■ Spiral Fracture. (**A**) Lateral view of the right lower leg shows the spiraling course of a tibial diaphyseal fracture (red arrow) in an adolescent male with ankle injury. (**B**) Three-dimensional reconstruction from CT scan, with AP view showing the spiral fracture (red arrow). Spiral fractures occur within long bones as a sequela of rotating-force injury. (Photo contributors: Ryan Logan Webb, MD, and Josh Greenstein, MD.)

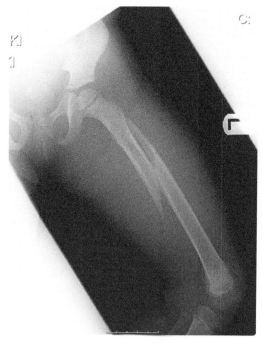

FIGURE 19.6 ■ Oblique Fracture. An oblique fracture through the mid left femoral shaft is seen in a young child. In the absence of a significant dependable mechanism, child abuse should be strongly considered. (Photo contributor: Michael Lucchesi, MD.)

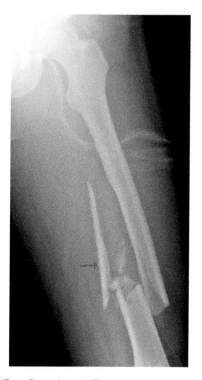

FIGURE 19.7 ■ Comminuted Fracture. Comminuted fracture of the femoral midshaft is seen in a 25-year-old man after a motorcycle accident. A large "butterfly fragment" is medially displaced (red arrow). (Photo contributors: Ryan Logan Webb, MD, and Josh Greenstein, MD.)

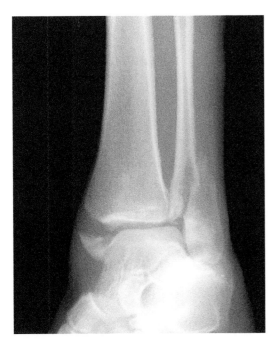

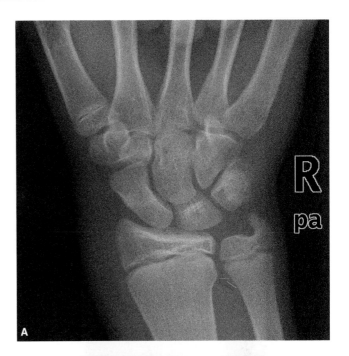

FIGURE 19.8 ■ Avulsion Fracture and Oblique Fracture. Oblique view of ankle demonstrates an avulsion fracture of the medial malleolus and an oblique fracture of the lateral malleolus (Weber B bimalleolar fracture). (Photo contributor: Michael Lucchesi, MD.)

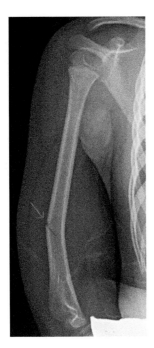

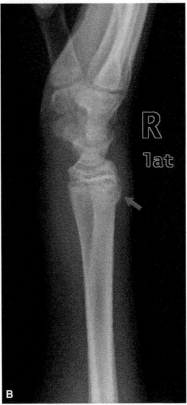

FIGURE 19.9 ■ Greenstick Fracture. Internally rotated view of the right humerus shows an oblique incomplete fracture of the right humerus. There is a clear cortical break on the posterolateral aspect of the bone (red arrow); however, no break is seen on the anteromedial aspect, consistent with a greenstick fracture. This 4-year-old girl's arm was caught against her bed post and was injured as she fell while trying to remove it. The mechanism of injury was felt to be consistent with the fracture. (Photo contributors: Ryan Logan Webb, MD, and Josh Greenstein, MD.)

FIGURE 19.10 ■ Torus Fracture (Buckle Fracture). (**A, B**) Frontal and lateral views of the wrist show torus fracture of distal radius. (Photo contributor: Tian Liang, MD.)

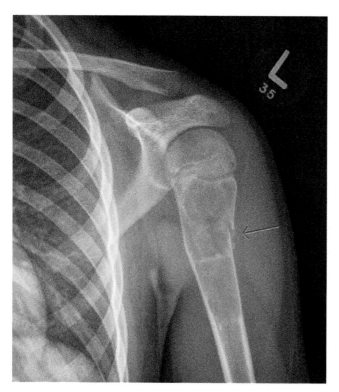

FIGURE 19.11 ■ Pathologic Fracture. Pathologic fracture of unicameral bone cyst. AP view of the left shoulder shows a lucent, mildly expansile lesion within the left proximal humeral metadiaphysis in a 11-year-old boy after a fall. A pathologic fracture is seen with obvious cortical break at the lateral aspect (red arrow). The lesion demonstrates a narrow zone of transition with no periosteal reaction or aggressive features. (Photo contributors: Ryan Logan Webb, MD, and Josh Greenstein, MD.)

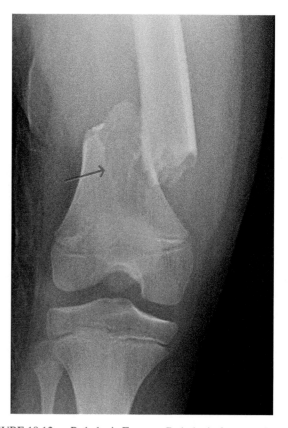

FIGURE 19.12 ■ Pathologic Fracture. Pathologic fracture of nonossifying fibroma (common lesion in adolescence). A displaced distal femoral shaft fracture is seen in this 12-year-old girl who fell off a pedal scooter. An associated well-defined, "bubbly" lucency is seen within the femoral metaphysis (red arrow). Lesion shows thin sclerotic borders with no periosteal reaction, soft tissue mass, or aggressive features. Fractures in this location normally occur only following high-energy trauma such as motor vehicle accident. Be suspicious of injuries that seem discordant with their mechanism. (Photo contributors: Ryan Logan Webb, MD, and Josh Greenstein, MD.)

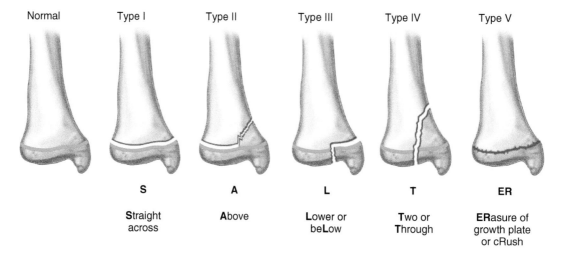

FIGURE 19.13 ■ Schematic Drawings of Salter-Harris Classification of Growth Plate Fractures. (Reproduced with permission from Moore EE, Feliciano DV, Mattox KL. *Trauma*. 8th ed. McGraw-Hill Education; New York, NY, 2017.)

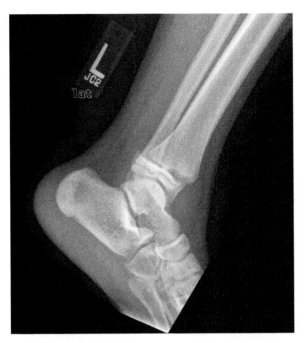

FIGURE 19.14 ■ Salter-Harris Type I Fracture. Lateral view of the ankle shows Salter-Harris I fracture of the distal tibia. Note widening of the physeal plate and anterior displacement of the distal tibia. (Photo/legend contributors: Tian Liang, MD, and John Amodio, MD.)

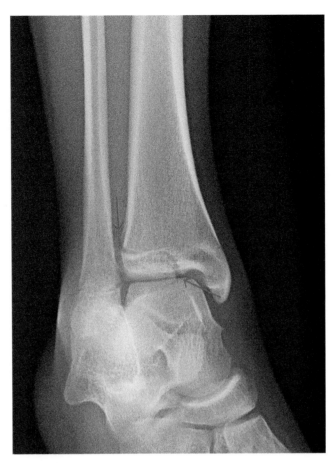

FIGURE 19.16 ■ Salter-Harris Type III Fracture. An oblique view of the right ankle reveals a sagittally oriented fracture of the epiphysis (red arrow) and disruption and widening of the lateral physis (blue arrow) consistent with Salter-Harris type III fracture. Such fractures involve the epiphysis and physis while sparing the metaphysis. (Photo contributors: Ryan Logan Webb, MD, and Josh Greenstein, MD.)

patients with open fractures to prevent osteomyelitis. Orthopedic consultation is recommended for many types of fractures but specifically for open fractures as they need wound irrigation often in the operating room. After adequate immobilization and consultation, most patients with isolated closed extremity fracture can be discharged with expeditious follow-up. Admit all patients with open fractures for observation and continued parenteral antibiotics or patients with complicated fractures for operative management.

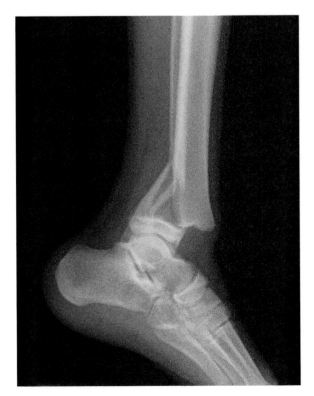

FIGURE 19.15 ■ Salter-Harris Type II Fracture. Lateral view of the ankle demonstrates comminuted and displaced Salter-Harris II fracture of the distal tibia. (Photo/legend contributors: Tian Liang, MD, and John Amodio, MD.)

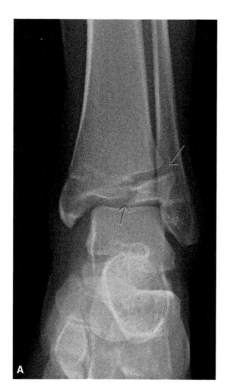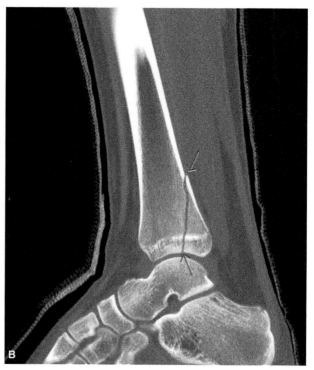

FIGURE 19.17 ■ Salter-Harris Type IV Fracture. (A) AP view of left ankle shows sagittally oriented fracture of the epiphysis (red arrow) and horizontally oriented disruption/widening of the lateral physis (blue arrow). (B) A follow-up CT scan sagittal image also shows fracture of posterior tibial metaphysis (red arrow) and epiphysis (blue arrow) representing Salter-Harris type IV fracture. When combined with the fractures seen on AP view, this injury pattern is termed triplane fracture. (Photo contributors: Ryan Logan Webb, MD, and Josh Greenstein, MD.)

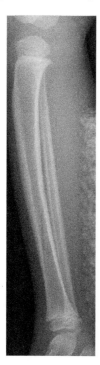

Pearls

1. Treat any fracture with an open wound as an open fracture until proven otherwise.
2. Use a radiologic marker in the area of the laceration or puncture to aid in identifying possible foreign bodies when obtaining radiologic images.
3. Exploration and irrigation should be done by someone with expertise in open-wound care.
4. Maintain a high suspicion for child abuse when mechanisms of injury do not fit the injury pattern, particularly spiral long bone fractures.
5. Immobilize occult fractures, and if they are in the area of the physis, treat these as Salter-Harris type I fractures.

FIGURE 19.18 ■ Toddler's Fracture. Lateral view of the leg shows a spiral fracture of the midshaft of the tibia. A spiral fracture in a nonambulatory infant is highly suspicious of nonaccidental trauma. (Photo/legend contributors: Tian Liang, MD, and Ryan Logan Webb, MD.)

TABLE 19.1 ■ TYPES OF FRACTURES

Fracture Type	Defining Features
Open fracture	Perforation or avulsion of skin and soft tissue overlying fracture site, often caused by sharp bony fragments forcing their way through skin A high propensity toward infection
Closed fractures	Skin and soft tissue overlying fracture intact
Complete fractures	Complete separation or discontinuity of bone
Incomplete fractures	Do not extend completely through bone; leaves portion of cortex intact (eg, Greenstick, Bowing fracture)
Occult fractures	Fracture not immediately apparent on x-ray, but clinically has a high index of suspicion because of physical findings; often detected on follow-up radiologic studies
Transverse fractures	Perpendicular to long axis of bone
Oblique fractures	Not perpendicular to long axis of bone
Comminuted fractures	More than 2 fragments of bone present and has typical shattered appearance (often pieces are large and form typical Y or T shape)
Avulsion fractures	Bone fragment pulled away from cortex at the site of tendon insertion, which may be extremely small and appears as a chip or flake in proximity to a bony tuberosity
Impacted fractures	Fragmented segments driven into each other; these may be complete or incomplete, and the fracture line may not appear as a lucency but as a more dense area
Torus (Buckle) fracture	An incomplete fracture in which 1 side of long bone cortex buckles outward and typically occurs at the base of long bones (fracture named from Greek architecture in which a *torus* is typically a bump at base of a column); these fractures are often subtle on x-ray

TABLE 19.2 ■ FRACTURES WITH SPECIAL CONSIDERATIONS

Fracture Type	Defining Features
Epiphyseal fractures	(See Table 19.3)
Spiral fractures	Occurs down shaft of long bone in a circumferential manner and caused by a twisting around long axis of bone. Often seen in child abuse.
Greenstick fractures	Limited to infancy and early childhood, these occur along the shaft of long bone transversely through 1 side of the cortex and then abruptly along the longitudinal axis of bone without disrupting the opposite cortex. Similar to the pattern of breaking a green stick.
Stress fractures	Seen in healthy people, usually athletes, in response to a repeated stress, and often not radiologically apparent until weeks after symptoms appear. Eventually fractures manifest as thin line of radiolucency or periosteal callus without an underlying fracture.
Pathologic fractures	Occur in diseased bone with characteristically minor injury and are often transverse and surrounded by areas of demineralized bone. Often seen in metastatic bony disease, areas with bone cysts, or in patients with osteogenesis imperfecta.

TABLE 19.3 ■ SALTER-HARRIS CLASSIFICATION OF EPIPHYSEAL FRACTURES

The Salter-Harris classification is the most widely used classification for epiphyseal fractures and gives a general prognosis for risk of premature closure of physes, as well as generalized treatment guidelines. There are 5 types differentiated by location and involvement of physeal growth plate.

Type	Features	Management
Type I	Fracture line goes through physis, not involving epiphysis or metaphysis.	Usually managed by closed reduction (joint space not involved and perfect alignment not required).
Type II	Fracture line through a portion of physis and extends through metaphysis on either side of bone.	Closed reduction except for type II fracture of distal femur, which requires anatomical alignment by either open or closed technique.
Type III	Fracture line goes through portion of physis and extends through epiphysis into joint space on either side of bone.	Fractures usually require open alignment of physis and articular surface.
Type IV	Fracture line goes through portion of metaphysis, extends through physis, involves portion of epiphysis, and thus enters joint space.	Fractures require open alignment of physis and articular surface.
Type V	Fracture is a crush injury, compressing physis, and is not always initially recognized. Often diagnosed retrospectively with premature physeal closure.	

TABLE 19.4 ■ FRACTURE COMPLICATIONS

Fracture Type	Complication	Features
All	Ligament injury	Common with fractures near joints or in areas with known ligamentous insertions.
	Neurovascular compromise	Caused by direct damage to or pressure on vessel/nerve and progresses with time. Manifests as loss of sensation, tingling, diminished pulses.
	Direct nerve injury	Immediate loss of function/sensation distal to injury and usually permanent without surgical repair.
	Compartment syndrome (especially with crush injures)	Edema and swelling cause increased pressure in closed fascial compartments impairing oxygenation to the tissue and initiating a vicious cycle of necrosis, edema, and swelling.
		Occurs most frequently in anterior/posterior compartments of thigh/calf, followed by peroneal compartments of legs, volar and dorsal compartments of forearm; less commonly with interossei of hands or gluteus medius.
		Manifests as the "5 P's": pain, paresthesia (occur first), pallor, pulseless, paralysis (irreversible damage, if all signs present).
	Fat embolism	Occurs frequently with trauma (clinically significant in about 30% of cases); manifests with signs of pulmonary embolism.
	Volkman ischemic contracture	End result of ischemic injury to muscle or nerve (synonymous with irreversible damage). Rare without preceding compartment syndrome.
	Nonunion of fracture	Occurs when fractured parts not placed in close proximity and more frequent in bones with tenuous blood supply (eg, femoral neck, scaphoid wrist).
	Posttraumatic reflex dystrophy	Manifests weeks to months after injury as weakness or pain in the affected extremity.
Open fractures	Contamination	Dirt, sand, glass.
		Bacterial (self-inoculation from normal skin flora or infection from mammalian bite that caused fracture, boxer's fracture).
	Foreign body	May or may not be seen on x-ray (glass dependent on size/lead content).
	Osteomyelitis	Frequently from contiguous focus of infection or hematogenous.

Clinical Summary

Tuft fractures result from crush injuries or falls. The tuft or the distal portion of the distal phalange is located directly beneath the nail bed, and fractures to this area are most often caused by a crush injury. Most tuft fractures do not involve the distal interphalangeal (DIP) joint space. Patients present with swelling, pain, and erythema, and there is often a subungual hematoma (see Figure 19.21).

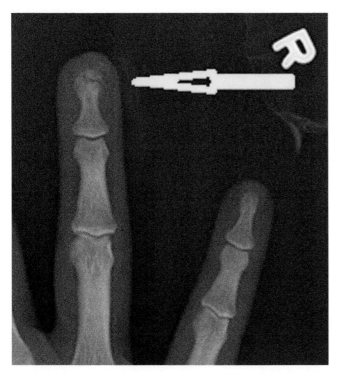

FIGURE 19.19 ■ Tuft Fracture. Frontal view of the right hand showing a tuft fracture (arrow) at the distal portion of the fourth digit. (Photo contributor: David Sarkany, MD.)

Emergency Department Treatment and Disposition

Obtain x-rays of the digit and consider x-rays of the hand and wrist if there is tenderness in those areas. Subungual hematomas are extremely painful and may act as a distracting injury. Refer all patients for orthopedic follow-up and consult orthopedics emergently for open fractures and phalanx fractures with extension into the joint space and extensor or flexor tendon rupture. Fractures involving the joint space should have orthopedic follow-up in 48 to 72 hours. Perform cautery drainage for subungual hematoma of ≥50% of the nail bed or as necessary for pain control.

Pearls

1. Apply hairpin aluminum splints without putting pressure on the distal phalanx to provide protection against inadvertent contact.
2. Axial loading of the finger will always elicit pain.
3. Always evaluate the other digits and the wrist, with attention to scaphoid tenderness.

Clinical Summary

Phalangeal fractures often occur from a fall on an outstretched hand, although they can also occur from a crush injury. Distal phalangeal fractures are most often secondary to crush injuries. Osteomyelitis is often associated with open fractures, including nail plate lacerations and fractures associated with drained subungual hematomas. Swan-neck deformity results from an intra-articular avulsion fracture or tendon tear of the dorsal surface of the distal phalanx. If not treated properly, hyperextension deformity of the proximal interphalangeal (PIP) joint with simultaneous flexion of the DIP joint may occur. The resultant swan-neck appearance of the finger is the reason for its name.

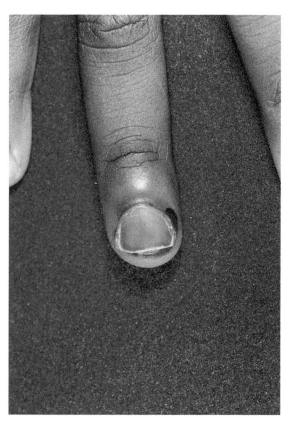

FIGURE 19.21 ■ Subungual Hematoma. A picture of a 100% subungual hematoma, which was sustained from a crush injury to the distal phalanx. There was no underlying tuft fracture. This was drained using cautery. (Photo contributor: Binita R. Shah, MD.)

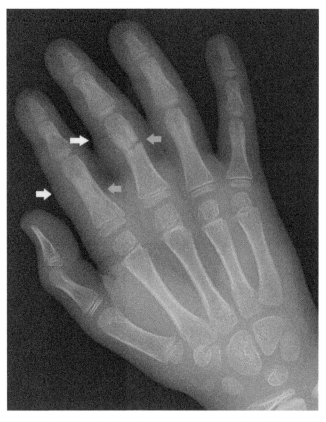

FIGURE 19.20 ■ Phalanx Fracture. Anteroposterior radiograph of the hand showing an acute vertical fracture of the proximal phalanx of the second digit and an acute transverse fracture of the proximal phalanx of the third digit (blue arrows) in this 7-year-old child after having a door closed on his hand. There is overlying soft tissue swelling (yellow arrows). (Photo contributors: Jonathan Stern, MD, and Josh Greenstein, MD.)

Emergency Department Treatment and Disposition

Obtain x-rays with special attention to chip or avulsion fractures that do not produce a great degree of swelling and may go undetected. If subungual hematoma is present, it may be drained for pain control, especially if >50% of the nail is involved. Use cautery through the nail or careful drilling with an 18-gauge needle. Repair any nail bed lacerations with removal of the entire nail after digital block. Consult orthopedics or a hand specialist for all open fractures, comminuted fractures, fractures involving the joint space, and fractures with any degree of digit rotation or any significant degree of angulation. In general, because of the increased mobility from the second to the third to the fourth to the fifth metacarpal bones, a higher degree of angulation is tolerated. Angulation

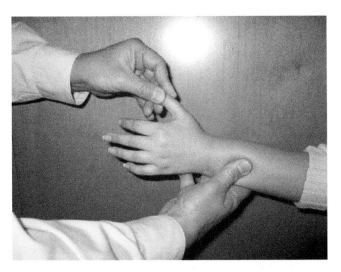

FIGURE 19.22 ▪ Axial Loading of a Digit. An image demonstrating the proper technique of axial loading of the thumb. (Photo contributor: Michael Lucchesi, MD.)

of 30 to 40 degrees can be tolerated for the fifth metacarpal, 30 degrees for the fourth metacarpal, 20 degrees for the third metacarpal, and 10 degrees for the second metacarpal.

Pearls

1. Bony tenderness can often be elicited by applying axial loading with the finger in the extended position.
2. Although degrees of angulation deformities can be tolerated, a rotational deformity of the digit, however slight, is not acceptable.
3. Detect rotational deformities by having the patient flex all 5 digits as in making a fist. All digits should point toward or just pass the scaphoid. Any deviation from this can indicate malrotation and thus require urgent evaluation by a hand specialist.
4. Thoroughly scrutinize lacerations over any joints on the dorsum of the hand to ensure the dorsal hood is not violated, not violated suggesting an open joint that would necessitate emergent consultation.

Clinical Summary

Mallet finger result from dorsal avulsion fracture in which the extensor mechanism of the DIP joint is destroyed, leaving the DIP joint in partial flexion. Mallet finger may occur

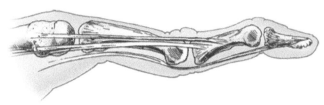

FIGURE 19.24 ■ Swan-Neck Deformity. If a mallet fracture is treated improperly, a hyperextension deformity will occur at the PIP joint. This is secondary to an imbalance between the ruptured extensor tendon and the unopposed distal flexor tendon. (Reproduced with permission from Sherman SC. *Simon's Emergency Orthopedics.* 7th ed. McGraw-Hill Education; New York, NY, 2014.)

if there is forced flexion of the distal phalanx when the finger is in taut extension. This is often seen after playing basketball or baseball when the ball hits and creates axial loading of an outstretched finger. Patients present with the inability to fully extend the DIP joint.

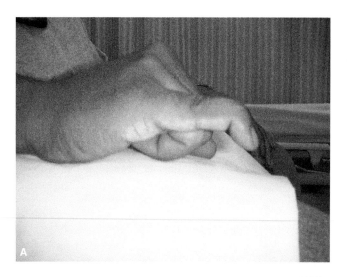

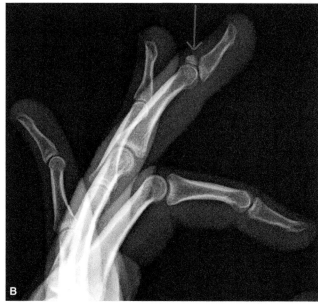

FIGURE 19.23 ■ Mallet Finger. (**A**) An image of the fifth digit of an adolescent who sustained a direct blow to the tip of his finger while playing basketball. The youth was unable to extend the DIP joint. (**B**) Lateral view of the hand in a different patient shows a fracture at the dorsal base of the third distal phalanx (red arrow). This type of injury results from forced flexion of the digit, causing either avulsion fracture at the site of extensor ligament attachment or ligamentous injury in which no fracture is seen. (Photo contributors: Mark Silverberg, MD [A], Ryan Logan Webb, MD, and Josh Greenstein, MD [B].)

Emergency Department Treatment and Disposition

Obtain standard x-rays of the digit. Avulsion fracture may not be apparent on x-ray. The DIP joint should be immobilized in full extension so that the finger is straight. If the finger has laxity at the PIP as well, then splint the digit with the DIP in extension and the PIP in partial flexion with an aluminum splint on the dorsal aspect of the digit. This will keep the avulsed tendon in contact with its area of origin. If not properly treated, a swan-neck deformity may occur. Discharge patients with orthopedic or hand specialist follow-up in 72 to 96 hours.

Pearls

1. The injury is relatively painless unless there is an associated phalanx fracture.
2. Mallet finger is a clinical diagnosis, with the inability to fully extend the DIP joint being pathognomonic.

Clinical Summary

Bennett fracture is a transverse fracture of the first metacarpal base extending into the joint and is associated with metacarpal dislocation. In Rolando fracture, the metacarpal fracture is comminuted. These are usually seen with a fall on an outstretched hand and are often associated with high-impact sports such as skiing. Patients present with a swelling and significant tenderness at the base of the thumb.

Emergency Department Treatment and Disposition

Obtain standard x-rays of the hand, thumb, and wrist and consider scaphoid x-rays. Missed fractures are associated with a significant amount of morbidity. Nonunion is a common complication if not treated in a timely and proper manner.

Pearls

1. Closed treatment with cast immobilization and short period of splinting is possible with Bennett fractures characterized by small avulsion fractures and minimal articular involvement, but most of these fractures often require operative repair.

2. Often these injuries will require a CT scan to reveal the full extent of the articular comminution and to facilitate repair.

3. Arthritis, limited range of motion, and decreased grip strength are fairly common complications.

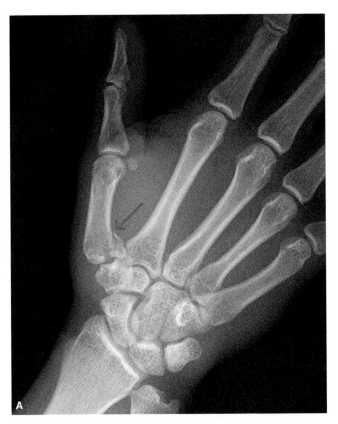 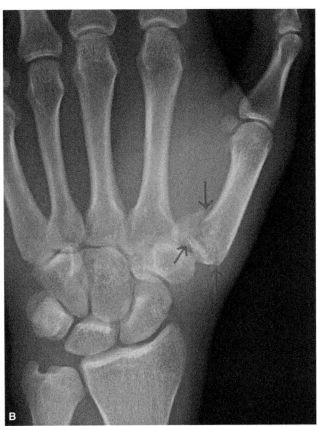

FIGURE 19.25 ■ Bennett and Rolando Fractures. (**A**) Bennett fracture in a 25-year-old male. Acute slightly displaced fracture of the medial base of the first metacarpal (red arrow), which contacts the first carpometacarpal joint. No comminution is seen. (**B**) Rolando fracture in a 20-year-old male. Acute comminuted fracture of the base of the first metacarpal (red arrows), with a fracture line contacting the first carpometacarpal joint. (Photo contributors: Ryan Logan Webb, MD, and Josh Greenstein, MD.)

BOXER'S FRACTURE

Clinical Summary

Fracture of the fourth or the fifth metacarpal neck is called a boxer's fracture and is the most common metacarpal fracture. Volar angulation of the distal bone is almost always present. Most commonly, this results from hitting a wall with the fist rather than from boxing injuries. Patients present with swelling, tenderness, and sometimes ecchymosis over the dorsal aspect of the involved metacarpal. Comminution of the anterior cortex is common, resulting in volar angulation of the metacarpal head. Fractures isolated to the metacarpal neck have few complications. Because of the mobility of the fifth metacarpal-carpal joint, angulation up to 40 degrees, and some report up to 60 degrees, is well tolerated. Angulation of >40 degrees or any rotational deformity if not reduced will result in an inability to maintain the normal tucked-in position of a clenched hand. This will lead to further vulnerability to injury of the fifth digit. Up to 50 degrees of angulation of the fifth metacarpal can be accepted before operative management is warranted, but these cases require urgent hand specialist consultation.

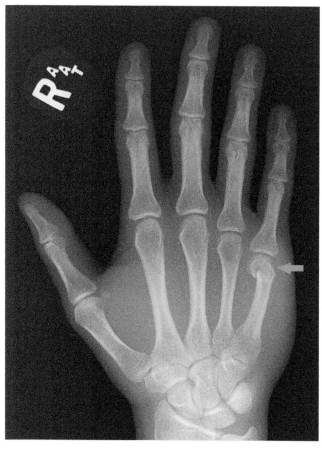

FIGURE 19.26 ■ Boxer's Fracture. Anteroposterior radiograph of the hand showing an acute displaced fracture of the fifth metacarpal neck (blue arrow) compatible with a boxer's fracture in a 22-year-old man who presented to the ED after punching a refrigerator. (Photo contributors: Jonathan Stern, MD, and Josh Greenstein, MD.)

Emergency Department Treatment and Disposition

Obtain standard x-rays of the hand, including anteroposterior (AP) and lateral views. The lateral view is essential to determine the amount of volar angulation. Splint closed fractures with an ulna gutter splint and discharge with instructions for orthopedic or hand specialist follow-up. Urgent orthopedic referral is indicated for intra-articular fractures, unstable fractures, displaced fractures of the metacarpal shaft, and fractures with significant angulation >40 degrees.

Pearls

1. Consult orthopedics for evaluation in the ED if there is angulation >40 degrees for the fifth or >30 degrees for the fourth digit or any rotational deformity.
2. Clinched fist-to-mouth injuries resulting in a puncture or laceration over the fourth or fifth metacarpophalangeal (MCP) joints need antibiotics (broad spectrum antibiotics that cover aerobes and anaerobes) in the ED, scrutiny for involvement of the MCP joint, and admission when associated with a fracture.

Clinical Summary

Scaphoid fractures are the most common carpal fractures and occur by falling on an outstretched hand or after seemingly minor trauma.

Emergency Department Treatment and Disposition

Physical examination reveals pain and swelling of the radial wrist. The classic presentation is snuffbox tenderness, although this is not specific to scaphoid fractures. To assess snuffbox tenderness, have the patient fully flex the thumb into the palm with the second through fifth digits flexed over it, and actively flex the wrist medially into ulnar deviation and palpate the snuffbox. Another useful sign may be pain with axial loading to the first metacarpal. This is assessed by keeping the thumb in the extended position while the examiner holds it by the distal phalanx and gently pushes into its origin. Patients may present with diminished grip strength when compared to contralateral wrist. If any of these tests elicit pain, scaphoid fracture should be suspected. Obtain standard x-rays of the wrist, including scaphoid views (ulna deviation views of the wrist). Consult orthopedics for all radiologically apparent injuries of the carpal bone or dislocations.

Pearls

1. Nonunion is the most common complication of a scaphoid/navicular fracture, and this requires open pinning with subsequent decreased mobility.

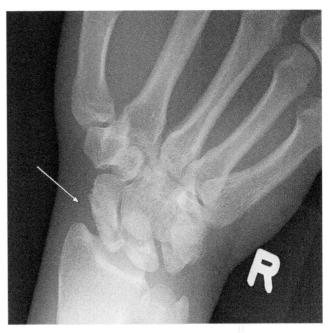

FIGURE 19.27 ■ Scaphoid Fracture. Scaphoid view of the right wrist demonstrating a nondisplaced scaphoid fracture (arrow). (Photo contributor: David Sarkany, MD.)

2. Blood is primarily supplied to the distal scaphoid, so fractures of the proximal scaphoid have severed blood supply and a high incidence of avascular necrosis of the proximal pole.

3. When images are negative and history or exam is concerning for scaphoid fracture, conservative management with thumb spica splint and follow-up in 2 weeks with repeat radiography is recommended.

FOREARM FRACTURES

Clinical Summary

Distal radius fractures are often referred to as a "dinner fork" deformity and result from a fall onto outstretched hand (FOOSH injury). They are common in school-aged children after a FOOSH injury, where the child braces a fall with their wrist, leading to a fracture. In some cases, the force bends the distal radius and causes a buckle (torus) fracture. In other cases, the force causes only 1 cortex to break, leaving the other side intact, which is known as a greenstick fracture. In more severe cases, a Colles fracture occurs when the distal segment is angulated posteriorly and Smith fracture occurs when the distal segment is angulated anteriorly. Simultaneous ulnar styloid fracture is often present with a distal radius fracture. On examination, patients with distal radius fractures demonstrate swelling and tenderness.

Emergency Department Treatment and Disposition

Standard 2-view radiographs of the forearm should suffice. Obtain radiographs of humerus, elbow, or wrist if examination reveals swelling or tenderness and thus concern for injury there as well. Nonangulated or minimally angulated buckle or greenstick fractures of the forearm have excellent healing potential, and thus traditional casting may not be required. Recent studies support management of buckle fractures with

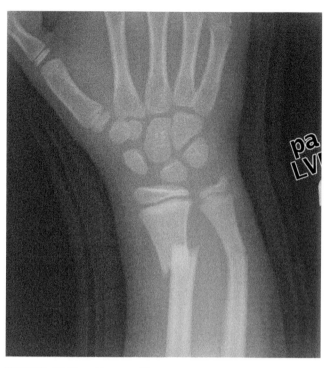

FIGURE 19.29 ■ Forearm Fracture. Posteroanterior view of the wrist shows complete fracture of the distal radius with overriding of fracture fragments. There is a greenstick fracture of the distal ulna. (Photo contributor: Tian Liang, MD.)

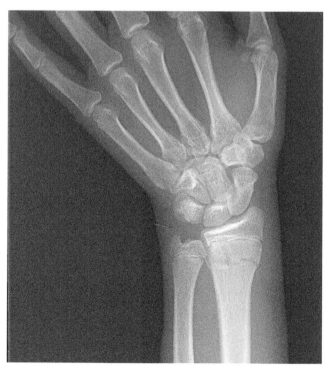

FIGURE 19.30 ■ Forearm Fracture. Frontal view of the wrist shows complete fracture of the distal radius and avulsion of the ulna styloid (Photo/legend contributors: Shashidhar Rao Marneni, MD, and John Amodio, MD.)

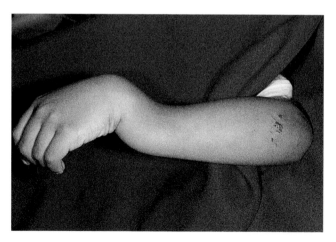

FIGURE 19.28 ■ Forearm Fracture. A photograph of the wrist of a child who fell from a fence, showing an obvious "dinner fork" deformity. Radiograph showed transverse fracture of the distal shaft of the radius and ulna. (Photo contributor: Binita R. Shah, MD.)

874

minimal or no angulation with a removable splint. Consult orthopedics for more significant distal radius fractures at risk for subsequent angulation, including mildly angulated fractures, unstable fractures, and fractures of both the radius and ulna.

Pearls

1. Definitive treatment for all displaced distal radius fractures is closed reduction.
2. It is essential to test for median nerve injury.
3. The younger the child and the more distal the fracture, the more angulation is acceptable without reduction.

GALEAZZI FRACTURE DISLOCATION AND MONTEGGIA FRACTURE DISLOCATION

Clinical Summary

Galeazzi fracture dislocation is fracture of the distal radial shaft associated with a distal radioulnar disruption. Monteggia fracture dislocation is fracture of the proximal third of the ulna with a radial head dislocation. The most common mechanism of injury is a fall on the arm. Tenderness on palpation is always present, but swelling and deformity may be minimal.

Emergency Department Treatment and Disposition

Obtain complete x-rays of the radius and ulna as well as the wrist. Consult orthopedics for evaluation and treatment in the ED, and immobilize, elevate, and ice the injury while awaiting consultation.

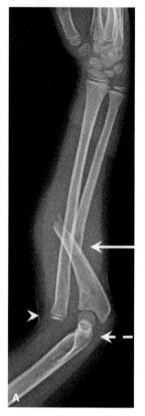
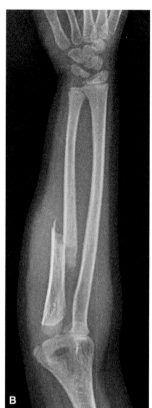

FIGURE 19.32 ■ Monteggia Fracture. (**A**) Right Monteggia fracture in a 6-year-old girl. Lateral radiograph of the forearm demonstrates the 2 components of the Monteggia fracture: fracture of the ulnar shaft (solid arrow) and dislocation of the proximal head of the radius (arrowhead) from the humerus (dashed arrow). Anterior dislocation of the radial head makes this case a Bado class I Monteggia fracture, which is the most common type. (**B**) The ulnar fracture is well visualized on the AP view, but the radial head dislocation is not as apparent. (Photo contributors: Brandon Z. Lei, MD, and Josh Greenstein, MD.)

Pearls

1. Both Galeazzi fracture dislocation and Monteggia fracture dislocation require open reduction and internal fixation in the operating room.
2. Neurovascular complications with Galeazzi fracture dislocations are uncommon.
3. Monteggia fracture dislocations are associated with radial nerve injury.

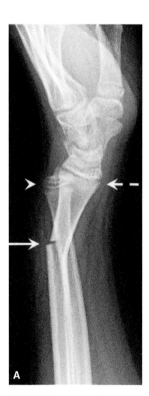
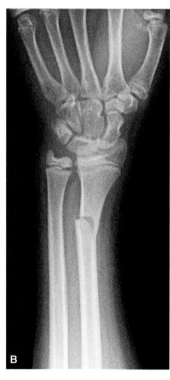

FIGURE 19.31 ■ Galeazzi Fracture. (**A**) Left Galeazzi fracture in a 13-year-old girl. Lateral radiograph of the forearm readily demonstrates the 2 components of a Galeazzi fracture: distal radial fracture (solid arrow) and dislocation of the joint between the distal radius (dashed arrow) and the head of the ulna (arrowhead), which are normally in alignment and fully overlapping. (**B**) The radial fracture is also well visualized on the AP view, but the radioulnar joint dislocation is not as apparent. (Photo contributors: Brandon Z. Lei, MD, and Josh Greenstein, MD.)

Clinical Summary

Olecranon fractures are usually due to a direct blow to the elbow. Patients present with tenderness and swelling over the posterior elbow and pain on flexion and extension.

Emergency Department Treatment and Disposition

Obtain x-rays of the elbow including AP and lateral views. Splint nondisplaced fractures with the elbow in 90 degrees of flexion and orthopedic referral as an outpatient in the next several days.

Pearls

1. Olecranon fracture is associated with ulnar nerve injury.
2. Consult orthopedics for evaluation and treatment in the ED for fractures with >2 mm of displacement.
3. When caused by a direct blow, consider child abuse.

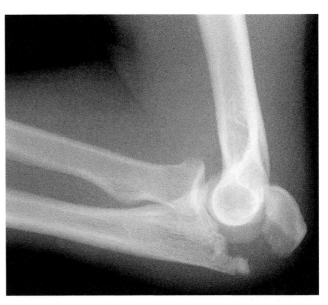

FIGURE 19.33 ■ Olecranon Fracture. Lateral view of the elbow shows a comminuted fracture of the olecranon with posterior displacement of the major fragment. (Photo/legend contributors: Mark Silverberg, MD, and John Amodio, MD.)

Clinical Summary

Radial head fractures occur in adults and adolescents, and radial neck fractures typically occur in children. These fractures are typically associated with other fractures including those of the medical epicondyle, olecranon, proximal ulna, and lateral condyle. The mechanism is usually from a FOOSH injury, and the patient presents with tenderness over the radial head or neck and pain with supination and pronation.

Emergency Department Treatment and Disposition

Evaluate for point tenderness of the lateral distal elbow over the radial head. Obtain standard x-rays of the elbow, although fractures may not be apparent on x-ray and fat pad signs are often the only evidence of a fracture. A small anterior fat pad may be normal. A "sail sign" or a large anterior fat pad is

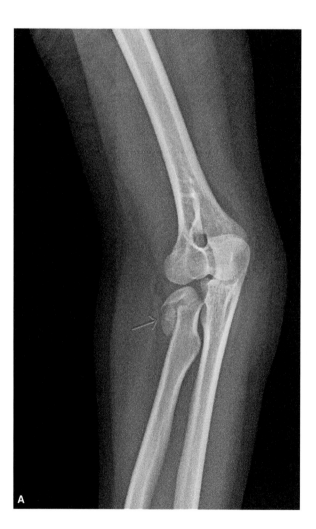

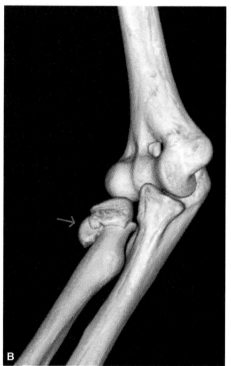

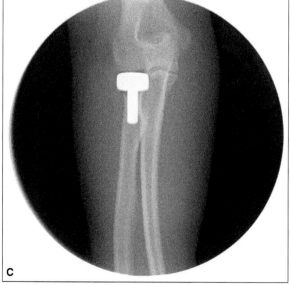

FIGURE 19.34 ■ Radial Head Fracture. Radial head fractures have a variety of appearances, from barely noticeable hairline fracture to displaced and obvious deformities. Shown here is one such example in a 22-year-old woman after trauma. (**A**) Obvious deformity of the radial head. The radial head is comminuted and displaced (red arrow). (**B**) CT 3-dimensional reconstruction showing the displaced radial head fracture (red arrow). (**C**) Interoperative fluoroscopic image showing placement of radial head prosthesis. (Photo contributors: Ryan Logan Webb, MD, and Josh Greenstein, MD.)

abnormal. A posterior fat pad suggests a fracture. Treat with a sling for comfort and early mobilization for occult radial head fractures and those with minimal displacement. Fractures with >2 mm of displacement require reduction in the ED and may require operative intervention if unstable.

Pearls

1. Neurovascular complications are rare in minimally displaced radial head fractures.
2. Radial neck fractures, which are also common in children, are usually buckle fractures that can easily be overlooked on x-rays.

Clinical Summary

Supracondylar fractures are caused by FOOSH injuries, typically in children age 3 to 10 years old. Patients present with a swollen elbow and tenderness over both the lateral and medial epicondyles and limited range of motion. The injury is a result of elbow hyperextension with a FOOSH injury.

Emergency Department Treatment and Disposition

Obtain 3 views of the elbow, including AP, lateral, and oblique views. X-rays may show the fracture line, an anterior fat pad sign (displaced anterior fat pad), a posterior fat pad, or an abnormal anterior humeral line. The anterior humeral line is drawn down the anterior cortex of the humerus on the lateral x-ray of the elbow and should pass through the center of the ossification center of the capitellum. The radiocapitellar line draws down the center of the radius and should bisect the capitellum. Management is based on the Gartland classification. Type 1 fractures are nondisplaced or minimally displaced and are managed with long arm posterior splint with the elbow at 90 degrees of flexion and the forearm in a neutral position and outpatient referral to orthopedics within 7 days. Casting should be avoided because it can lead to compartment syndrome. Type 2 fractures are displaced with posterior cortex attached and are managed with attempted reduction and immobilization after orthopedic consultation. Type 3 fractures involve complete displacement and require operative management. Every patient with a supracondylar fracture must have a complete neurovascular examination prior to and after reduction and immobilization.

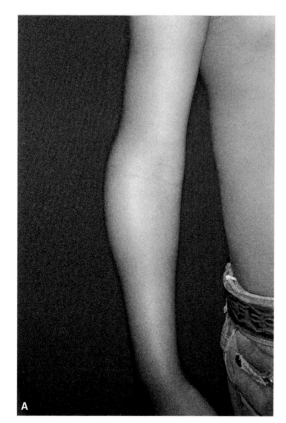

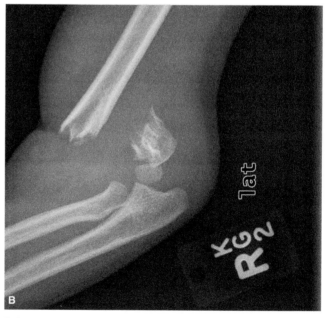

FIGURE 19.35 ■ Supracondylar Fracture. (**A**) Clinical picture of a supracondylar fracture with marked soft tissue swelling in a child with a history of falling on an outstretched arm. (**B**) Lateral projection of the right elbow shows a supracondylar fracture of the humerus with severe anterior displacement of humerus. The capitellum is in normal anatomic alignment with the radial head. (Photo contributors: Binita R. Shah, MD, and John Amodio, MD.)

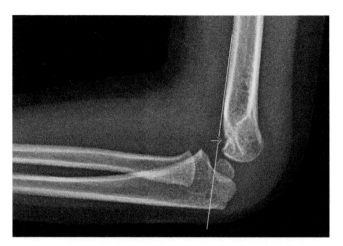

FIGURE 19.36 ■ Supracondylar Fracture. Gartland type 2 supracondylar fracture. Lateral view of the elbow demonstrates elbow effusion with posterior fat pad sign and anterior fat pad sail sign. A break is seen in the anterior cortex (red arrow). The anterior humeral line (blue line) passes just anterior to the capitellum, indicative of posterior angulation of the distal humerus. (Photo contributors: Ryan Logan Webb, MD, and Josh Greenstein, MD.)

Pearls

1. Incidence of nerve injuries associated with supracondylar fractures is reported to be 10 to 20%. The median nerve and the radial nerve are most often injured.

2. A positive "OK" sign indicates injury to anterior interosseous nerve. There is loss of strength of the thumb interphalangeal joint in flexion as well as the index DIP joint in flexion. This injury renders the patient unable to perform the "OK" sign, with the thumb and index finger apposed against resistance.

3. Brachial artery compromise can lead to Volkmann contracture (compartment syndrome of the forearm), which will lead to muscle and nerve fibrosis and drastic loss of function.

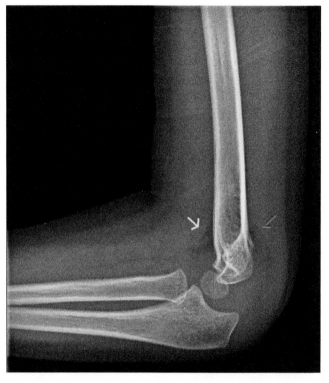

FIGURE 19.37 ■ Anterior and Posterior Fat Pads. Lateral view of left elbow demonstrates posterior fat pad (red arrow) as well as anterior fat pad sail sign (yellow arrow) in a 5-year-old boy who fell. The anterior humeral line (red line) is not displaced, bisecting the middle third of the capitellum. AP and oblique views demonstrated no clear fracture line, thus representing a nondisplaced supracondylar humeral fracture. Many of these fractures are bowing-type fractures, and a clear fracture line will not be seen. A small anterior fat pad can be seen normally; however, visualization of an enlarged anterior fat pad or a posterior fat pad indicates joint effusion/hemorrhage. (Photo contributors: Ryan Logan Webb, MD, and Josh Greenstein, MD.)

HUMERUS FRACTURE

Clinical Summary

Humerus fractures may be due to a fall (FOOSH injury) or a direct blow, the latter of which should alert the clinician to the possibility of abuse. Patients present with decreased movement of the extremity, localized swelling, and difficulty raising the affected arm.

Emergency Department Treatment and Disposition

Obtain perpendicular AP and lateral views of the entire humerus. Most fractures are minimally displaced and can be treated with a sling for 3 to 4 weeks with good results. Closed reduction is preferred for severely displaced fractures of the

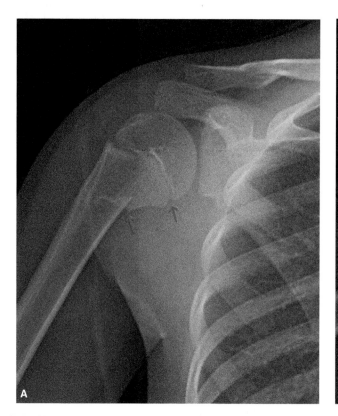
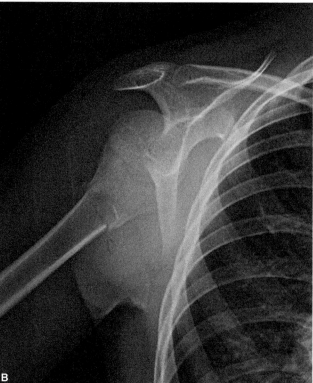

FIGURE 19.38 ■ Humeral Neck Fracture. (**A**) A frontal view of the humerus in external rotation in an 8-year-old boy showing a minimally angulated fracture of the humeral neck, with a clear cortical break seen medially (red arrow). This is not to be confused with the normal humeral physis (blue arrow). (**B**) Humerus in internal rotation is showing a nondisplaced fracture of the humeral neck (red arrow). (Photo contributors: Ryan Logan Webb, MD, and Josh Greenstein, MD.)

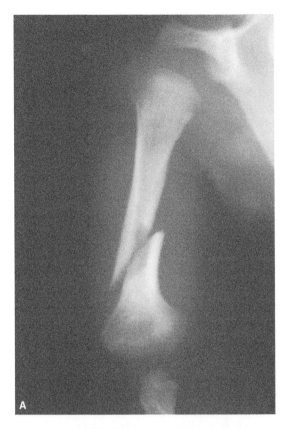

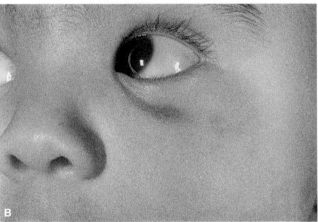

FIGURE 19.39 ■ Nonaccidental Trauma. (**A**) An oblique fracture of the humerus is seen in this 3-month-old infant presenting with inconsolable crying. (**B**) A small bruise is seen in the periorbital region. The humerus and femur are among the most frequently fractured long bones in abusive injuries. Most common types of abusive fractures are spiral (oblique) or transverse. (Photo contributor: Binita R. Shah, MD.)

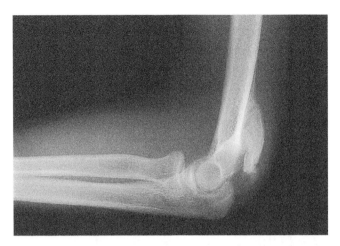

FIGURE 19.40 ■ Myositis Ossificans. Lateral view of the elbow demonstrates a dense calcification/ossification of the posterior aspect of the elbow joint extending from the distal humeral shaft to the olecranon process. The posttraumatic myositis ossificans was related to a subperiosteal hematoma sustained from a stab wound, which occurred 3 months previously. This 16-year-old presented with a frozen elbow after months of immobilization. (Photo contributor: Michael Lucchesi, MD.)

metaphysis with a goal of <15 degrees. In patients younger than 10 years old, up to 20 degrees of angulation can be treated nonoperatively because of the significant remodeling potential.

Pearls

1. Adhesive capsulitis (frozen shoulder) can occur with proximal fracture and raises the possibility of neglect.
2. Brachial plexus injuries and axillary nerve and artery injuries are associated.
3. Young children have open epiphyses and usually suffer epiphyseal separation rather than fractures.
4. Humeral shaft fractures typically involve the middle third, and 10% to 20% have radial nerve injury. The brachial artery can also be injured.
5. Displacement is significant if there is separation of >1 cm or angulation of >45 degrees.
6. Myositis ossificans can be avoided by active routine exercise rather than just simple passive stretching in the recuperatory phase.

CLAVICLE FRACTURE

Clinical Summary

Clavicle fractures are the most common fracture in children and are commonly caused by a direct blow or fall on the shoulder. The majority of clavicle fractures occur in the middle of the clavicle. Most children present with refusal to use or raise the injured arm. Older children and adolescents may hold their arm against their body to help support the arm and to limit motion. Patients present with pain on clavicular palpation, swelling, or gross deformity. Thorough neurovascular testing is imperative given the proximity of the clavicle to the brachial plexus and subclavian veins.

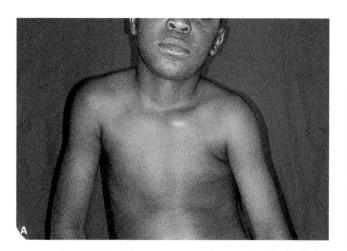

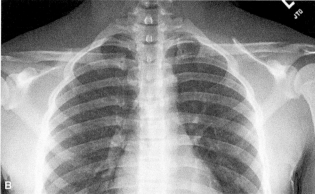

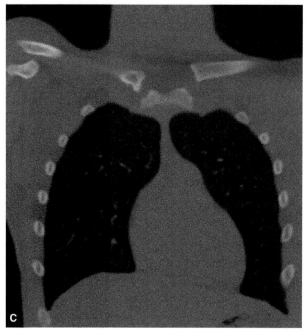

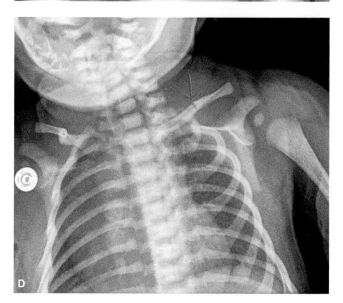

FIGURE 19.41 ■ Clavicular Fracture/Dislocation. (**A**) A picture of a 9-year-old boy who suffered a fall, sustaining a clavicular dislocation. (**B**) Angled AP view of the clavicles showing the left clavicular head is elevated compared with the right (red asterisks) in a 16-year-old boy with clavicular injury during wresting. (**C**) Coronal CT slice confirming the left-sided sternoclavicular dislocation with left clavicular head elevated compared with the right (red asterisks). Superior dislocations are usually anterior, in contradistinction with inferior dislocations, which are often posterior and more serious injuries, potentially damaging mediastinal or vascular structures. (**D**) A neonate with asymmetric Moro reflex on exam. AP view demonstrates nondisplaced fracture of the left mid clavicle (red arrow), consistent with birth trauma. Clavicular fractures may be displaced and obvious or nondisplaced and subtle. Sometimes they are greenstick fractures, and the single cortical break may not be visible on frontal view, necessitating angulated AP cephalic view for the diagnosis. (Photo contributors: Mark Silverberg, MD [A], Ryan Logan Webb, MD, and Josh Greenstein, MD [B, C, D].)

Emergency Department Treatment and Disposition

Fractures can be identified with AP shoulder view or with a 30-degree cephalad tilt for better visualization. Nonoperative management with a sling aimed at limited range of motion initially is the mainstay treatment for midshaft fractures with up to 2 cm of displacement or shortening. Simple nondisplaced clavicle fractures can be followed up by a general pediatrician, and those that are completely displaced should be seen by orthopedics as an outpatient. Discharge the patient and educate the caregivers that fractures heal with the formation of a lump that may take months to resolve. Athletes should be advised to use a sling for the first 2 days and thereafter as needed for comfort. They should also be advised to avoid contact sports for at least 8 to 10 weeks to avoid repeat fractures.

Pearls

1. Eighty percent of clavicle fractures involve the middle third of the clavicle.
2. Significant bone remodeling in children allows for better cosmetic outcomes and lower rates of nonunion compared with adults.
3. In children, nonoperative clavicle fractures heal within 3 to 6 weeks but take longer to heal in skeletally mature adolescents.

Clinical Summary

Scapular fractures are most often caused by a high-energy direct blow to the scapular area and rarely by an indirect force. Patients present with local pain, swelling, and decreased and painful abduction of the arm. Associated injuries such as rib fractures, pulmonary injury, splenic injury, and humeral fractures are common and may delay the diagnosis.

Emergency Department Treatment and Disposition

Obtain plain radiographs for the shoulder, including axillary views of the shoulder/scapula. If a displaced scapula is suspected, obtain CT imaging, especially if operative intervention is planned. Complications are always related to

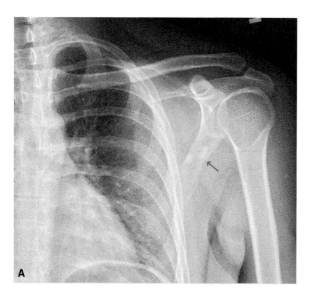

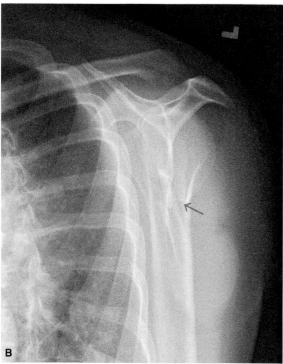

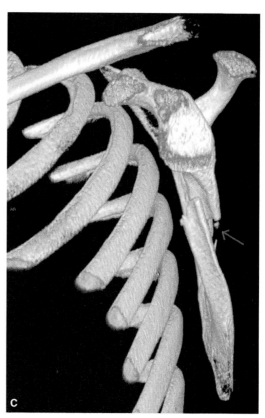

FIGURE 19.42 ■ Scapular Fracture. (**A**) AP view of left shoulder shows acute fracture of the body of the scapula (red arrow) in a 22-year-old man after trauma. (**B**) Y view of the scapula shows displacement of the scapular body fracture (red arrow). (**C**) CT 3-dimensional reconstruction, Y view better shows the comminution of the fracture (red arrow). (Photo contributors: Ryan Logan Webb, MD, and Josh Greenstein, MD.)

associated injuries, and thus identification and treatment of those injuries is paramount. Consult orthopedics as needed for those injuries. In rare cases when the mechanism of injury is localized and other injuries are ruled out, immobilize the shoulder with a sling and discharge the patient with instructions for early progressive range-of-motion exercises and use of shoulder out of the sling as pain subsides.

Pearls

1. Scapular fractures are rare in childhood.
2. Scapular fractures necessitate investigation for other injuries (rib fractures, pneumothoraces, and vertebral fractures).
3. Fifty percent of scapular fractures involve the scapular body and spine.

Clinical Summary

Femur fractures are most commonly associated with high-energy force injuries (motor vehicle accidents and falls from significant heights). There is a bimodal age distribution that correlates directly with type of injury. In infants and toddlers, child abuse should always be suspected (especially in infants who are not ambulatory). Patients usually present with swelling and tenderness on palpation, although deformity may or

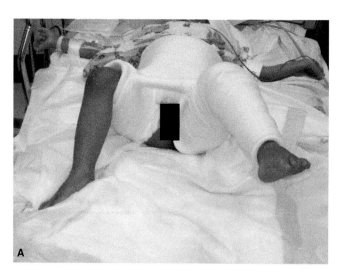

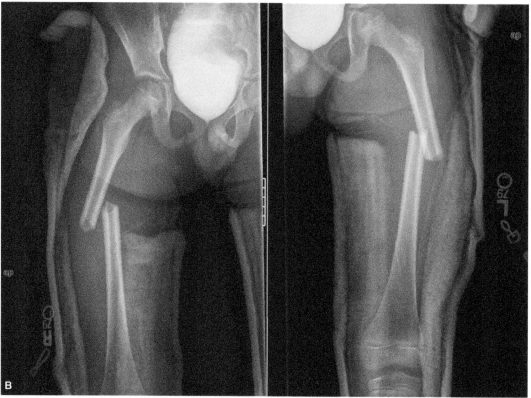

FIGURE 19.43 ■ Femur Fractures. (**A**) A 2-year-old boy fell while jumping on the bed and sustained a left midshaft femur fracture. A hip spica cast was used for immobilization. (**B**) Anteroposterior view of bilateral femora (different patient) demonstrates bilateral femoral fractures of the proximal femoral shafts with medial displacement of the distal fracture fragments in a child involved in a motor vehicle accident. The fracture fragments are overriding and are displaced medially >1 shaft width. There is an overlying cast. Contrast is seen in the bladder from the patient's prior CT scan with IV contrast. (Photo contributors: Jessica Stetz, MD [A], and Rachelle Goldfisher, MD [B].)

may not be present. Other concomitant and life-threatening injuries should also be identified (eg, Waddell triad: femur fracture secondary to pedestrian accidents in young children can be associated with severe head injury and thoracoabdominal injury).

Emergency Department Treatment and Disposition

Early immobilization and analgesia are the top priorities in management. Early reduction of obvious deformity is also indicated. Meticulous examination of the skin is an important step in identifying open fractures and need for treatment with parenteral antibiotics.

Femur x-rays should be obtained after appropriate pain control. Consider obtaining hip and knee views as well because there is a high incidence of associated injuries.

Consult orthopedics emergently. Immobilize the hip, and assess and document neurovascular status and admit patients expeditiously. Ultimate treatment in children <6 years old is more complex. Depending on the fracture, definitive treatment may be external splinting, open reduction, or internal fixation.

Pearls

1. Hemorrhage is the most serious complication. Overweight adolescents can extravasate 1.5 L of blood into the thigh after a femur fracture.

2. Neurovascular injury and avascular necrosis of the femoral head is likely especially with fractures of the base of the femoral neck.

3. Midshaft femur fractures, especially spiral fractures in infants, should alert the clinician to the possibility of child abuse (see Figure 1.32).

PATELLA FRACTURES

Clinical Summary

Patellar fractures usually result from a direct injury to the patella (fall on a flexed knee or direct impact on the dashboard during automobile accidents) or from a sudden forceful contraction of the quadriceps. Patients present with a tender swollen prepatellar area, and if there is a complete transverse fracture, they are unable to maintain the leg extended against gravity.

Emergency Department Treatment and Disposition

Early immobilization and pain control are indicated. Obtain patella x-rays including a sunrise view, which are diagnostic.

Operative management is indicated for displaced or complex fractures and for fractures that disrupt the extensor function. Consult orthopedics emergently for evaluation in the ED. For all other fractures, knee immobilization and outpatient orthopedic follow-up are indicated. Without treatment, nonunion of the patella can occur, especially in displaced fractures.

Pearl

1. Complete transverse fractures, especially if displaced, need surgical open reduction and internal fixation.

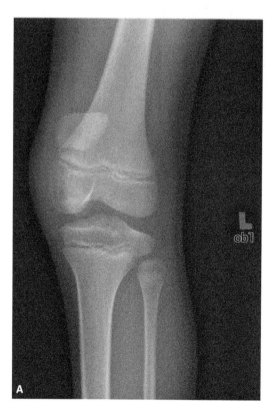 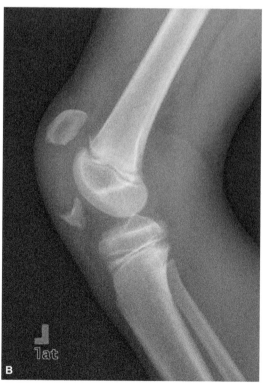

FIGURE 19.44 ■ Patella Fracture. (**A, B**) Oblique and lateral views of the left knee demonstrate an avulsion fracture of the lower third of the patella. The proximal portion has been retracted by the quadriceps. There is an overlying soft tissue deformity. (Photo/legend contributors: Shashidhar Rao Marneni, MD, and Rachelle Goldfisher, MD.)

Clinical Summary

Maisonneuve fracture is a proximal fibular spiral fracture with an unstable disruption of the tibiofibular syndesmosis. External rotation of the ankle is a common mechanism. Patients present with an obvious ankle fracture, although the ankle may appear to be without deformity and pain on palpitation of the proximal calf (proximal fibular tenderness).

Emergency Department Treatment and Disposition

Splinting and non–weight bearing should be the initial ED management. Ankle radiographs might show a widened mortise. When x-rays include the proximal fibula, fractures are usually obvious. Complications include significant arthritic changes and future difficulty in ambulation if left untreated. Nonunion of the tibiofibular syndesmosis can also occur. Although most patients with these injuries can eventually be discharged from the ED, they should not be discharged without orthopedic consultation.

Pearls

1. When evaluating an injured ankle, always palpate the calf and anterior lower extremity for tenderness.
2. Maisonneuve fracture is usually associated with deltoid ligament rupture and ankle fractures; evaluate the proximal lower leg when these are diagnosed.

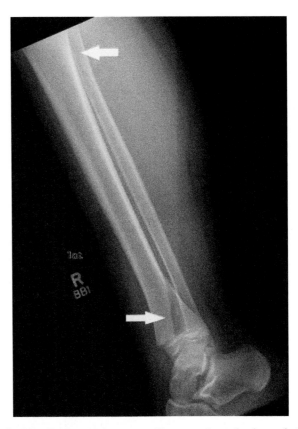

FIGURE 19.45 ■ Maisonneuve Fracture. Lateral view of the leg demonstrates a Salter-Harris II fracture of the distal tibia and a nondisplaced fracture of the proximal fibula, compatible with a Maisonneuve fracture in an adolescent male. (Photo/legend contributors: Tian Liang, MD, and John Amodio, MD.)

ANKLE FRACTURE AND SPRAIN

Clinical Summary

Ankle fractures are one of the most common fractures in children and skeletally immature athletes. Distal fibular physical fractures are the most common, with low potential for long-term complications. Patients present with swelling that is most pronounced over the lateral malleolus. Joint stability is recognized by isolated pain to medial or lateral malleolus; there is no marked swelling, deformity, or malalignment, and there is no associated injury to ligaments.

Epiphyseal injuries that are usually caused by sheering and avulsion forces have no adult counterpart, because they occur at the epiphyseal growth plates. The medial malleolus is shorter than the lateral malleolus, which allows the talus to invert more than evert. The deltoid ligament stabilizes the medial aspect of the ankle joint and offers stronger support than the thinner lateral ligaments. As a result, the ankle is more stable and resistant to eversion injury than it is to inversion injury. Differential diagnosis includes Maisonneuve fracture and proximal metatarsal fracture. Complications include

arthritis and chronic pain with undiagnosed proximal metatarsal fractures.

Emergency Department Treatment and Disposition

Obtain 3-view ankle radiographs (AP, lateral, and mortise) because up to 20% of fractures are seen only in 1 view. Isolated soft tissue swelling on radiographs points to the diagnosis of sprain even in skeletally immature children. Avulsion off the distal fibula in anterior talofibular tears is occasionally seen. If there is no documented fracture, joint instability, or neurovascular deficit, treat such patients with ice, elevation, and splinting and arrange for follow-up with orthopedics. Nonfractures with clinical ligamentous injury (or sprains in which ligamentous injury is indeterminate) need telephone orthopedic consultation and urgent orthopedic follow-up (within 1 week) after adequate immobilization in the ED. Consult orthopedics emergently in the ED for any gross

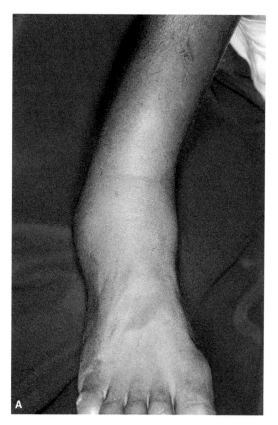 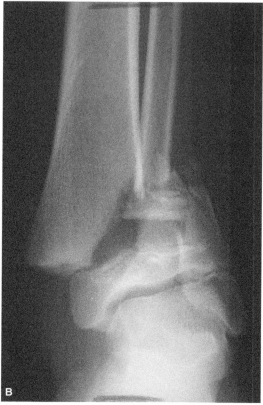

FIGURE 19.46 ■ Ankle Fracture. (A) Image of a grossly deformed ankle with surrounding soft tissue swelling. (B) Radiograph shows a comminuted fracture of the distal fibula and a Salter-Harris type II fracture of the distal tibia with medial displacement of the tibial and fibula fragment. The ankle mortise appears to be intact. (Photo/legend contributors: Binita R. Shah, MD, and John Amodio, MD.)

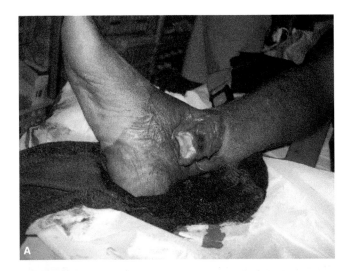

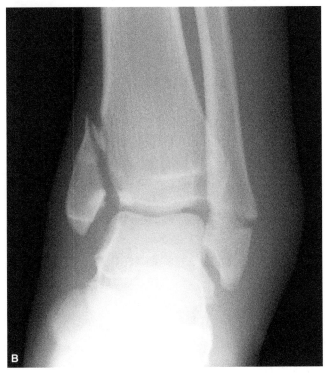

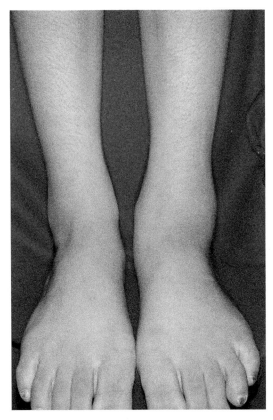

FIGURE 19.48 ■ Ankle Sprain. Image of a left ankle sprain with soft tissue swelling in an adolescent who presented after an inversion injury. Ankle radiographs were negative. (Photo contributor: Binita R. Shah, MD.)

FIGURE 19.47 ■ Ankle Fractures. (**A**) In this type II open ankle fracture (type II is >1 cm but <10 cm, open), the tibia is seen protruding through the skin and the articular cartilage is visible. (**B**) Radiograph from a different patient shows a bimalleolar fracture with a comminuted fracture of the medial malleolus and a distal fibular fracture. (Photo contributor: Mark Silverberg, MD.)

ligamentous deformities (laxity on examination), any neurovascular deficits, or any ankle fracture or open ankle fracture. CT evaluation for complex ankle fractures (triplane, displaced Salter-Harris III, Salter-Harris IV) can provide key information for later operative management but is not indicated emergently in the ED.

Pearls

1. Twisting injuries that cause fractures in children are usually minimally displaced, but with involvement of the articular surface, they may require open reduction and internal fixation.

2. The ankle joint usually adheres to the ring or pretzel axiom. A fracture in one part of the ring is often associated with a second injury. Always look for an associated medial malleolar fracture when a spiral fracture of the fibula proximal to the ankle mortise is seen.

3. A vertical fracture of the medial malleolus is also associated with either a lateral malleolar fracture or a fracture of the lateral ligaments.

4. Ninety percent of ankle sprains involve the lateral ligaments.

5. Ligamentous injuries occur in the following order of frequency: anterior talofibular, calcaneofibular, and posterior talofibular.

CALCANEAL FRACTURE

Clinical Summary

Calcaneal fractures can occur from significant high-energy trauma (fall or jump from a height). The axial loading on the foot can lead to compression. These patients usually present with severe heel pain associated with inability to bear weight. Swelling and tenderness are usually evident, and deformity may also be observed. Contralateral calcaneal fracture, thoracolumbar compression fractures, and lower extremity fractures can occur concomitantly.

Emergency Department Treatment and Disposition

Obtain standard foot x-rays (PA, lateral, and axial) with the addition of a calcaneal view. Böhler angle (normally 20 to 40 degrees) may be decreased. Böhler angle is formed by the intersection of the 2 lines between the superior margin of the posterior tuberosity of the calcaneus through the superior tip of the posterior facet, and the superior margin of the posterior tuberosity through the superior tip of the anterior process. CT scan is indicated for displaced or suspected occult fractures with a nondefinitive radiograph. Consult orthopedics or podiatry emergently for displaced, open, or intra-articular fractures or fractures with neurovascular involvement or skin tinting because these entities require meticulous surgical care. Nondisplaced body fractures that do not involve articular surfaces might benefit from immobilization in a compression dressing. Instruct these patients to ice and elevate the ankle and avoid weight bearing. Refer patients with calcaneal injuries to orthopedics within few days. Evaluate the need to admit these patients for pain control and monitoring because early complications are common. Complications include, acutely, compartment syndrome and disruption of the subtalar joint. Chronic complications include arthritis, heel spurs, plantar fasciitis, complex regional pain syndrome, and malunion.

Pearls

1. Tarsal bone fracture is the most common accompanying fracture to a calcaneal injury.
2. Injury of the calcaneus should warrant evaluation of the lumbar sacral spine, which has a high rate of associated injury.
3. Calcaneal fractures are bilateral in 10% of calcaneal injuries.

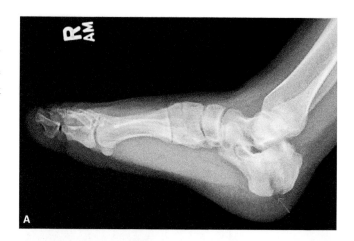

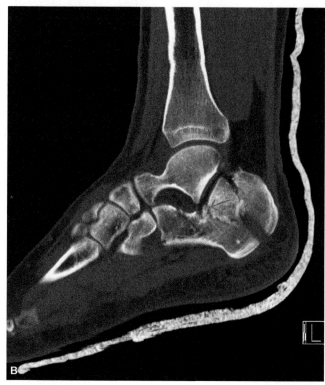

FIGURE 19.49 ■ Calcaneal Fracture. Acute comminuted fracture of the calcaneus in a 19-year-old boy. (**A**) Multiple fracture lines traversing the calcaneus, the most obvious seen on the posteroinferior surface (red arrow). (**B**) CT sagittal image depicting the comminuted fracture, with fracture line contacting the posterior subtalar joint (red arrow). (Photo contributors: Ryan Logan Webb, MD, and Josh Greenstein, MD.)

Clinical Summary

An acute fracture of the proximal diaphysis or the junction between the metaphysis and diaphysis is usually caused when a forceful load is placed on the ball of the foot or there is forced oblique lateral plantar flexion. Patients present with mild swelling and point tenderness over the base of the fifth metatarsal. This fracture carries with it the risk of painful nonunion.

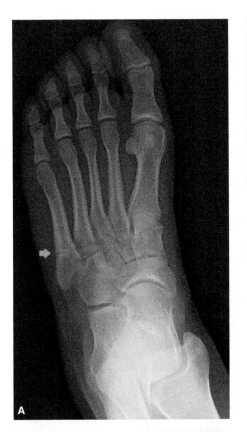

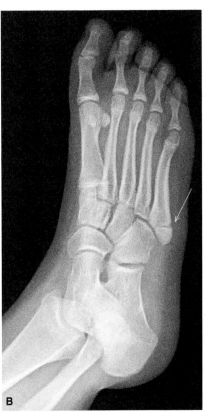

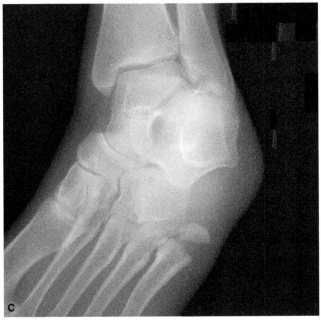

FIGURE 19.50 ■ Jones and Pseudo-Jones Fractures. (**A**) An oblique view of the foot demonstrates a nondisplaced transverse fracture of the fifth metatarsal extending to the intermetatarsal joint compatible with a Jones fracture. (**B**) An oblique view of the foot demonstrates a nondisplaced fracture through the base of the fifth metatarsal (arrow) extending to the tarsometatarsal joint, representing a pseudo-Jones fracture. Fracture line extends to the tarsometatarsal joint but not the intermetatarsal joint, ruling out Jones fracture. (**C**) Oblique view of the foot demonstrates a displaced avulsion fracture of the fifth metatarsal tuberosity, compatible with a pseudo-Jones fracture, and this injury may require fixation. (Photo contributors: Mark Raden, MD [A], Daniel Eisman, MD, Ryan Logan Webb, MD [B], and Mark Silverberg, MD [C].)

Emergency Department Treatment and Disposition

Obtain standard x-rays of the foot. Initial treatment includes pain control and below-the-knee non–weight bearing cast or splint with orthopedic follow up within 1 week. Surgical repair depends on fracture location. The closer the fracture is to the mid-shaft, the more likely it will need surgery. Surgery has been shown to improve healing and recovery in adolescent athletes.

Pearl

1. Transverse proximal fifth metatarsal fractures have a completely different prognosis, require urgent/emergent orthopedic or podiatric consultation, and have a high incidence of delayed union or nonunion.

Clinical Summary

Lisfranc fractures are tarsometatarsal dislocations or fractures and are most commonly seen with strong, blunt compression force (motor vehicle accident) or severe rotational stress. Patients present with significant midfoot swelling and tenderness and inability to bear weight. Degenerative arthritis and decreased circulation to the distal foot are occasional complications.

Emergency Department Treatment and Disposition

Obtain AP, lateral, and oblique views of the foot and consider ordering a foot CT, which is useful in identifying occult injuries. Consult orthopedics emergently, as these cases most commonly require open reduction and internal fixation. Provide ice, immobilization, elevation, and analgesics, and admit patients for open reduction and internal fixation.

Pearls

1. Lisfranc fracture is the most common midfoot fracture.
2. Fracture of the base (proximal) of the second metatarsal is nearly pathognomonic.
3. Dislocations may involve 1 or several tarsometatarsal joints.
4. Separation of the base of the first and second metatarsals is highly suggestive of Lisfranc fracture.

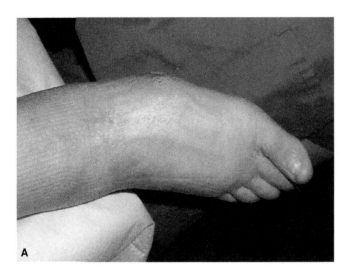
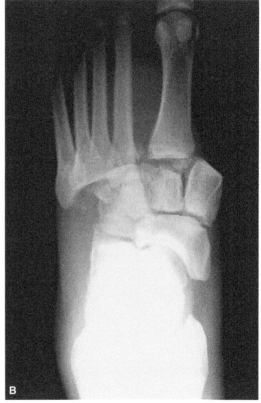

FIGURE 19.51 ■ Lisfranc Fracture. (**A**) Picture of a developmentally delayed adolescent whose foot was caught in a metal door, resulting in tenderness and deformity of the midfoot. (**B**) Frontal view of the midfoot in a different patient shows fractures of the middle and lateral cuneiforms and fractures of the metatarsal bases, with lateral displacement of metatarsals, compatible with the homolateral type of Lisfranc fracture. (Photo/legend contributors: Mark Silverberg, MD, and John Amodio, MD.)

Clinical Summary

Stress fractures of the metatarsals are almost always secondary to repetitive overuse of the forefoot. Anatomic (pes planus and long second metatarsal bone), physiologic (obesity and osteopenia), or external factors (poorly fitted shoes) are common risk factors. Patients present with pain on ambulation and, in particular, exertion. Erythema, swelling, and pain on palpation are all rare. Arthritis and chronic pain may occur if the stress fractures are not treated appropriately.

Emergency Department Treatment and Disposition

Order x-rays, although these are usually negative (x-ray changes usually appear 2–6 weeks after injury). No laboratory tests are needed because stress fractures are mechanical problems and do not cause laboratory abnormalities. Consider a bone scan, which may be positive. Instruct patients on appropriate rest and use of NSAIDs as needed. Immobilization (with a boot or a cast) is more often used in children when compared to adults due to failures in compliance. Refer athletes to an orthopedic sports medicine specialist.

Pearls

1. Metatarsal stress fractures are the second most common fracture after tibial stress fractures.
2. The main differential diagnosis is shin splints, which are usually bilateral; stress fractures are usually unilateral.

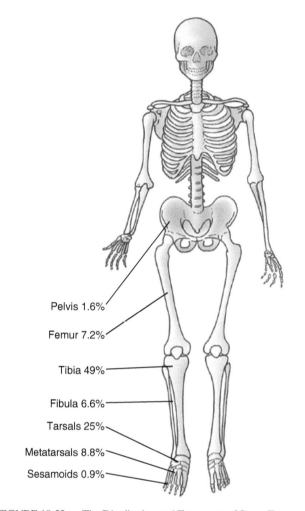

Pelvis 1.6%

Femur 7.2%

Tibia 49%

Fibula 6.6%

Tarsals 25%

Metatarsals 8.8%

Sesamoids 0.9%

FIGURE 19.52 ■ The Distribution and Frequency of Stress Fractures. (Reproduced with permission from Sherman SC. *Simon's Emergency Orthopedics.* 7th ed. McGraw-Hill Education; New York, NY, 2014.)

Clinical Summary

Interphalangeal joint dislocation usually results from a pull and twist of an isolated finger or a fall on a hand with the fingers locked in extension. The mechanism is often a hyperextension of the proximal (PIP) or distal (DIP) joint. Patients present with obvious angulation of PIP or DIP joint and inability to flex the affected joint.

Emergency Department Treatment and Disposition

Obtain x-rays of the digit in at least 2 views and look for articular surface fractures as well as avulsion fractures. If there is

an overlying laceration, after applying a digital nerve block, examine the wound carefully for the possibility of an open joint or tendon laceration. Consult a hand or orthopedic specialist for any suspicion of an open joint or in dislocations associated with fractures or tendon laceration. Initiate antibiotics for patients with open joints or fractures. They will likely require further wound irrigation in the operating room and continued IV antibiotics. Reduce isolated dislocations without an associated fracture or open joint with axial traction. If there is dorsal displacement of the DIP or PIP joint and there is difficulty with reduction, the volar plate may be entrapped and require hyperextension prior to relocation. If this does not work, consult orthopedics or a hand specialist because it may require operative reduction. If successful, for the DIP joint, the finger should

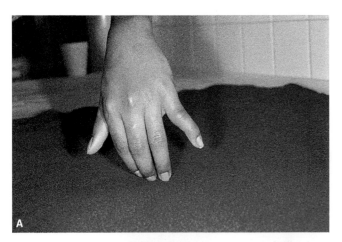

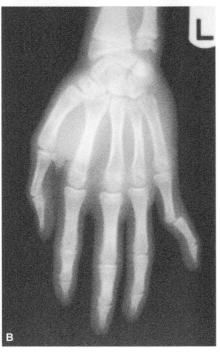

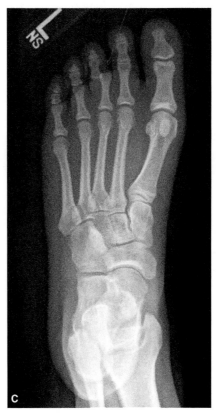

FIGURE 19.53 ■ Interphalangeal Joint Dislocation. (**A**) Picture of obvious proximal interphalangeal (PIP) joint deformity of the fifth digit. (**B**) Frontal radiograph (intentionally shown upside down for correlating with clinical photograph) of the finger demonstrates PIP dislocation, which was easily reduced with axial traction after digital block. (**C**) A frontal view of the foot in a different child shows a lateral dislocation of the third middle phalanx. (Photo contributors: Binita R. Shah, MD [A, B], and Tian Liang, MD [C].)

be splinted in mild flexion for 2 weeks; for the PIP joint, the fingers may be buddy taped for 3 to 6 weeks. Volar dislocations of the PIP joint should be similarly reduced but splinted in extension for 6 to 8 weeks, because there is damage to the central slip and collateral ligament. Obtain a postreduction x-ray to ensure proper alignment. Discharge patients with expeditious follow-up by orthopedics or a hand specialist.

Pearl

1. Proper immobilization after reduction of a volar PIP joint dislocation is important to prevent a boutonnière deformity.

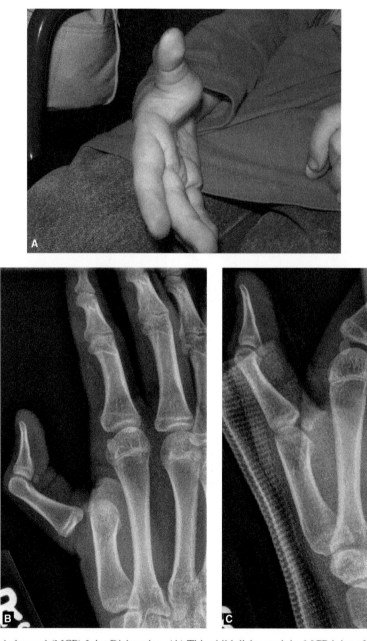

FIGURE 19.54 ■ Metacarpophalangeal (MCP) Joint Dislocation. (**A**) This child dislocated the MCP joint of his thumb as a result of hyperextension force while falling on an outstretched hand. Gentle traction along with a good analgesic was used to put it back in place. MCP joint dislocation is sometimes seen in pediatrics, with thumb MCP dislocation being the most common type. (**B**) First MCP dislocation. The first phalanx is shown dislocated dorsally from the MCP joint in this 14-year-old boy. (**C**) Postreduction images show restoration of anatomic alignment. (Photo contributors: Mark Silverberg, MD [A], and Ryan Logan Webb, MD [B, C].)

Clinical Summary

Lunate and perilunate dislocations are usually caused by extreme hyperextension of the wrist with ulnar deviation, and perilunate dislocation is the most common wrist dislocation. Patients present with pain and swelling to the wrist. There may be a protruding deformity on the dorsum of the wrist (dorsal dislocations) or a concavity over the dorsum of the wrist (volar dislocations). With a perilunate dislocation, the lunate remains in anatomic position. The remainder of the hand is displaced either volar or dorsally. With lunate dislocation, x-rays show that the capitate is aligned and the lunate is displaced, resembling a spilled tea cup. High suspicion must be maintained for this injury because it is commonly missed on primary presentation and results in significant morbidity.

Emergency Department Treatment and Disposition

Obtain standard x-rays; the lateral view will show misalignment of the distal radius, the proximal border of the lunate, and the proximal border of the capitate. Consult orthopedics emergently for all wrist dislocations for treatment in the ED. Almost all dislocations will require surgery, either after reduction in a delayed fashion or immediately.

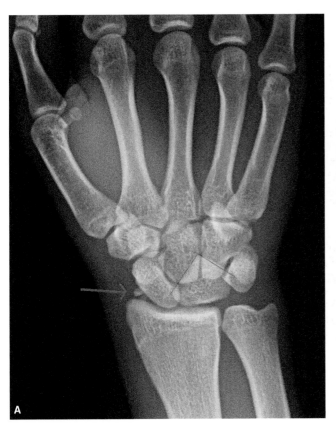
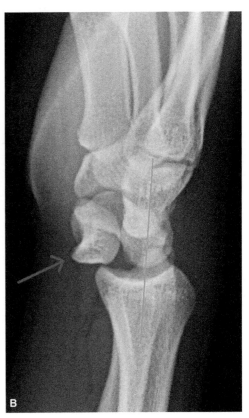

FIGURE 19.55 ■ Lunate Dislocation. (**A**) AP view of the wrist in a 17-year-old boy with lunate dislocation. Lunate bone takes on an unusual "piece of pie" shape, which is characteristic of the diagnosis (red lines). Also noted is a small fracture fragment (red arrow) presumably off the scaphoid bone. (**B**) Lateral view confirms the diagnosis. The crescent moon–shaped lunate bone is rotated volarly (red arrow). The radiocapitate alignment is normal (blue line). (Photo contributors: Ryan Logan Webb, MD, and Josh Greenstein, MD.)

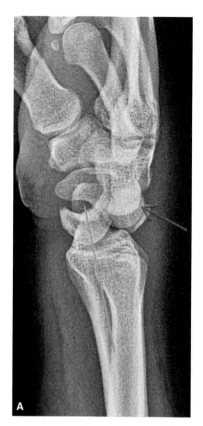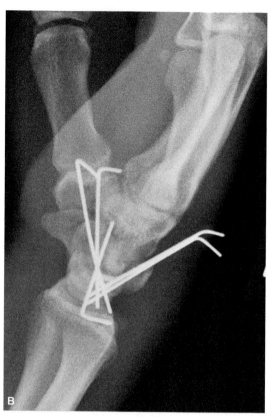

FIGURE 19.56 ■ Perilunate Dislocation. Lateral view of the wrist in a patient with perilunate dislocation. (**A**) The capitate bone (red arrow) is displaced posteriorly from its normal articulation from the lunate bone. The radiolunate alignment is normal (blue line). (**B**) Postreduction with restoration of radial-lunate-capitate alignment and percutaneous fixation with multiple K-wires. (Photo contributors: Ryan Logan Webb, MD, and Josh Greenstein, MD.)

Pearls

1. Undiagnosed wrist dislocations could result in neurologic or vascular compromise as well as severe mobility limitations. Median nerve injury and scaphoid fractures are also common complications.
2. The lunate usually dislocates volarly.

Clinical Summary

Elbow dislocations are relatively rare in pediatrics because fracture is more common. The incidence of dislocation increases in patients over the age of 10 years. When dislocation occurs, a fracture and/or neurovascular injury is often associated. They are most commonly associated with a fall on an extended, abducted arm. Patients present with the elbow held in flexion. The olecranon process may be palpated at a more posterior position than normal.

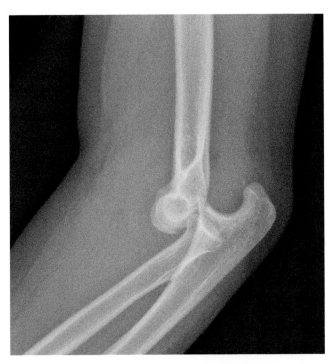

FIGURE 19.57 ■ Elbow Dislocation. Lateral view of left elbow is shown in a 12-year-old girl with elbow dislocation. The radius and ulna are dislocated posteriorly relative to the humerus. Posterior dislocation is the most common type of elbow dislocation. (Photo contributors: Ryan Logan Webb, MD, and Josh Greenstein, MD.)

Emergency Department Treatment and Disposition

First, perform a neurovascular exam. If there are absent or weak pulses, immediate reduction with appropriate pain control is indicated. Reduction of a posterior dislocation is performed using traction and flexion. Obtain an AP and lateral x-ray of the elbow before and after reduction. An oblique view may be helpful to discern fractures. If there is associated fracture or the reduction is not successful as demonstrated on the postreduction lateral elbow x-ray, have orthopedics see the patient in the ED.

Pearls

1. Medial epicondyle fractures are often associated with elbow dislocations, at a rate that may be as high as 30% to 40%.
2. Ulnar nerve injuries are associated with elbow dislocation.
3. Brachial artery injuries are associated with elbow dislocation.

Clinical Summary

Shoulder dislocations are very common in adolescents and young adults and are rare in children younger than age 10 years. Anterior shoulder dislocations are the most common (95%), and usually, the humeral head is in the subcoracoid position. Anterior force placed on the arm while in abduction with external rotation is a common mechanism resulting in an anterior dislocation. Patients present with the arm held in abduction with internal rotation, unable to abduct or externally rotate the shoulder; the normal contour of the shoulder is lost. Physical examination reveals a loss of shoulder contour in comparison to the opposite side. Axillary nerve injury is common. Hill-Sachs lesions (compression fracture of the posterolateral humeral head) and Bankart lesions (fracture of the glenoid rim) are associated with anterior dislocations, and detachment or tear of the rotator cuff may occur.

Posterior dislocations account for 2% to 4% of injuries and are rarely seen in sports; however, the diagnosis can be missed. Mechanisms associated with posterior shoulder dislocation

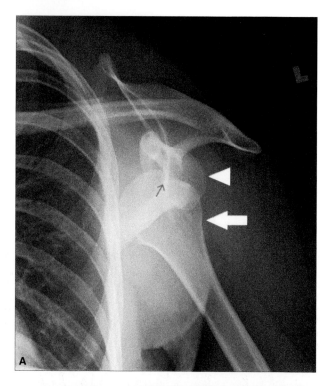

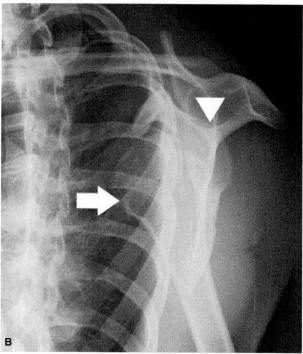

FIGURE 19.59 ■ Anterior Glenohumeral Joint Dislocation. (**A**) Frontal radiograph of the left shoulder in a patient with an anterior shoulder dislocation. Note that the humeral head (arrow) is dislocated anterior to the glenoid as well as inferior to its normal position. There is a Hill-Sachs fracture impaction deformity on the humeral head (red arrow). (**B**) Y view. The humeral head (arrow) is dislocated anterior to the glenoid (arrowhead), resting underneath the coracoid process. (Photo contributors: Berenice Lopez Leal, MD, and Ryan Logan Webb, MD.)

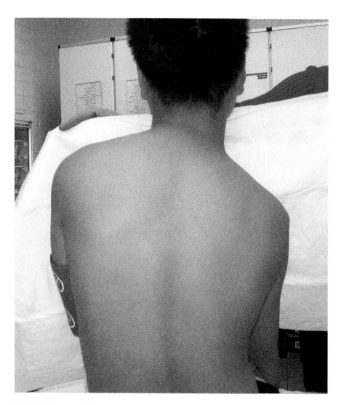

FIGURE 19.58 ■ Anterior Glenohumeral Joint Dislocation. Loss of normal contour of the right shoulder is seen in an adolescent with shoulder dislocation following a fall. (Photo contributor: Binita R. Shah, MD.)

904

include trauma to the arm when it is flexed, adducted, and internally rotated; seizures; and electric shock.

Emergency Department Treatment and Disposition

Obtain radiographs including AP, lateral, and axillary views. The axillary view is difficult to obtain in a patient with a posterior dislocation, but it is diagnostic and helpful in differentiating anterior and posterior dislocations. One of the several techniques to reduce a shoulder dislocation is the traction–countertraction technique, where the patient lays supine and an assistant loops a sheet under the axilla of the affected arm. A practitioner applies traction to the affected arm at 45 degrees of abduction, sometimes for up to 20 minutes to overcome muscle forces. Once the head of the humerus slips into the joint, a clunk is usually felt. Another method is the Stimson technique. Postreduction imaging should evaluate for the congruity of the joint and to identify any associated fractures. The ED physician should attempt reduction with analgesia and, if

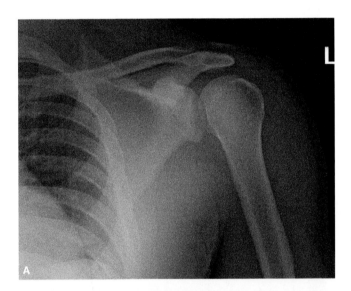

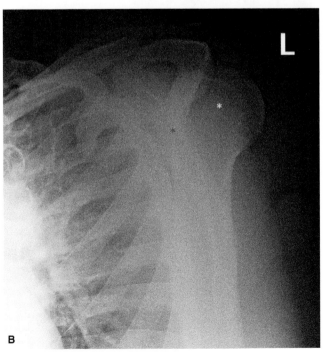

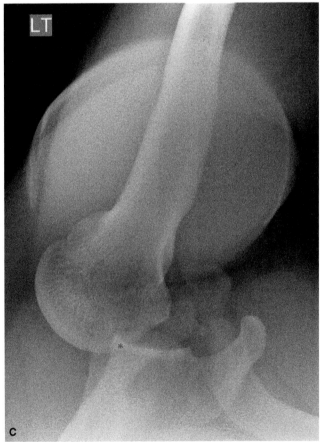

FIGURE 19.60 ■ Posterior Glenohumeral Joint Dislocation. (**A**) An essentially unremarkable AP view of the left shoulder is shown in a 24-year-old man presenting with posterior glenohumeral joint dislocation. (**B**) Y view shows the humeral head (yellow asterisk) positioned posteriorly relative to the glenoid (red asterisk). (**C**) Axillary view confirms the diagnosis, with obvious posterior dislocation and the humeral head impacted on the posterior glenoid (red asterisk). There is an impaction fracture deformity on the anteromedial humeral head, the "reverse Hill-Sachs" lesion. (Photo contributors: Ryan Logan Webb, MD, and Josh Greenstein, MD.)

needed, sedation. Always check for axillary nerve injury over the deltoid area, immobilize the limb with a sling and swathe, and discharge the patient with instructions for follow-up by orthopedics in a few days. If reduction attempts are not successful, consult orthopedics emergently.

Pearls

1. Anterior shoulder dislocations usually displace the humeral head inferiorly, which when minimal is easily missed on x-ray, including the "Y" view. Thus, the axillary view is important for ruling out a shoulder dislocation.

2. Up to 35% of first-time dislocations are associated with axillary nerve neuropraxia and decreased sensation over the deltoid.

3. If there is an isolated fracture of the lesser tuberosity of the humerus, maintain a high suspicion of index for posterior dislocation, which may not be immediately radiologically apparent.

4. Hill-Sachs lesions are cortical depression fractures of the humeral head and occur with 90% to 100% of dislocations.

Clinical Summary

Posterior hip dislocations result from a direct blow along the femoral axis and most commonly occur in front-end motor vehicle accidents when the patient is thrown forward and hits the dashboard with the knee. Anterior dislocations result from forced abduction, as with external blunt trauma such as when an automobile strikes a pedestrian. In posterior dislocations, patients present with the leg adducted, flexed, and internally rotated. In anterior dislocations, the leg is abducted, flexed, and externally rotated at the hip.

Emergency Department Treatment and Disposition

Obtain routine hip and pelvic x-rays and consult orthopedics emergently. Assess and document neurovascular status on arrival and before and after reduction attempts. All dislocations require significant sedation and analgesia for reduction. For the posterior dislocation, place the patient in the supine position and have 1 caretaker apply steady pressure on both superior iliac crests to stabilize the pelvis. Straddle the patient, flex the knee to 90 degrees, and pull the leg toward the

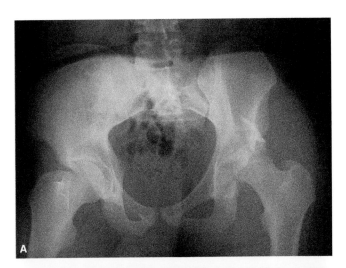

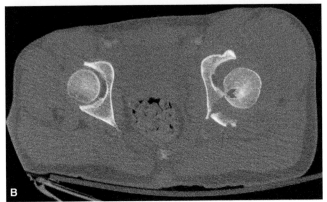

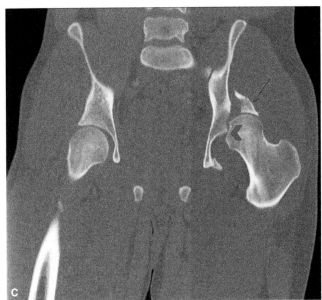

FIGURE 19.61 ■ Hip Dislocation and Posterior Acetabular Wall Fracture. (**A**) AP view of the pelvis demonstrates posterosuperior dislocation of the left hip in a 16-year-old male adolescent following a blunt trauma to the left hip. (**B, C**) Axial and coronal CT reconstructions of the pelvis demonstrate a displaced posterior wall left acetabular fracture (arrows) and subsequent posterosuperior dislocation of the left femoral head in respect to the left acetabulum. The femoral head is impacted on the remaining posterior acetabular wall (arrowheads). (Photo contributors: Caitlin Feeks, DO, and Cheryl H. Lin, MD.)

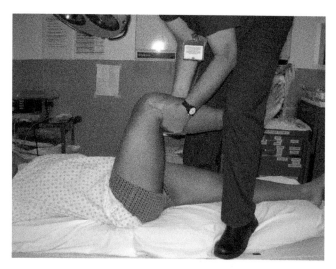

FIGURE 19.62 ■ Proper Technique for Reduction of Posterior Hip Dislocation. With the patient lying on the back and the hip and knee flexed to 90 degrees, reduction is performed by applying traction perpendicular to the bed, toward the ceiling. (Photo contributor: Mark Silverberg, MD.)

ceiling. For anterior dislocation reduction, place the patient supine and flex the hip to convert the anterior dislocation to a posterior dislocation. Then reduce the posterior dislocation as described above. Assess and document neurovascular status after each reduction attempt. A CT scan of the hip is needed to evaluate for fractures after reduction.

Pearls

1. Posterior dislocations account for 90% of hip dislocations.
2. Acetabular and femoral head fractures can be difficult to diagnose and often require CT for diagnosis.
3. Twenty-five percent of hip dislocations are associated with knee injuries, and almost 5% are associated with ipsilateral femur fractures.
4. Avascular necrosis of the femoral head is a common complication associated with significant morbidity.
5. Sciatic nerve injury may occur with posterior hip dislocations.

Clinical Summary

Knee dislocation results from a direct blow to the knee as in a motor vehicle accident or significant fall. Dislocations are classified by tibial displacement relative to the femur. Anterior and posterior dislocations are most common, but medial, lateral, and rotary dislocations can occur. Patients present with an obvious deformity and tenderness on palpation. Some may spontaneously reduce, but a high suspicion for neurovascular injury must be maintained. Dislocations are often associated with fractures. Distal pulses may be diminished.

Emergency Department Treatment and Disposition

If pulses are present, obtain standard x-rays of the knee including AP and lateral views and a sunrise view of the

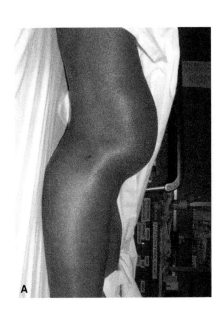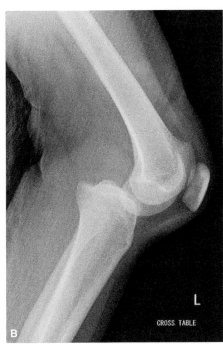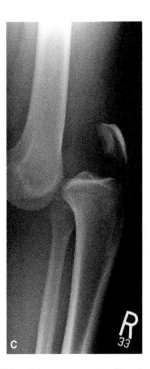

FIGURE 19.63 ■ Knee Dislocations. (**A**) Posterior knee dislocation. This patient slipped down a flight of icy steps and suffered a knee dislocation. The anterior surface of the tibia is no place near the anterior surface of the femur and knee. (**B**) Posterior knee dislocation is seen in 15-year-old girl presenting after a fall from a trampoline with awkward landing on her left leg. She immediately felt a "pop," felt pain, and was unable to ambulate. No neurovascular symptoms or signs were appreciated. Lateral radiograph of the knee demonstrates a posterior dislocation. Her knee was successfully reduced; however, a follow-up knee MRI showed extensive ligament and tendon injury requiring reconstruction. (**C**) Anterior dislocation of the tibia, fibula, and patella relative to the femur is seen in a 21-year-old man kicked by a horse. (Photo contributors: Mark Silverberg [A], Gregory Emmanuel, MD, Ryan Logan Webb, MD, and Josh Greenstein, MD [B, C].)

patella. If pulses are absent, immediate reduction is indicated. In all cases of knee dislocation, emergent orthopedics consult should be obtained because there is a high incidence of neurovascular injury and reduction should take place promptly in the ED. If orthopedic consultation is not immediately available, provide sedation analgesia and reduce the dislocation with longitudinal traction and pressure toward the normal knee position. The decision regarding whether a patient needs a CT angiogram can be based on clinical signs and the ankle-brachial index (ABI). Without other evidence of popliteal artery injury, patients with an ABI of >0.90 can be monitored

without CT angiography. Admit any patient with a suspicion of popliteal artery injury.

Pearls

1. Complications are very common and include popliteal artery injury (up to 40%) and peroneal nerve injury (25%–35%).

2. Peroneal nerve injury will produce paresthesias over the dorsum of the foot, diminished dorsiflexion of the foot, and/or decreased sensation between the first and second toes.

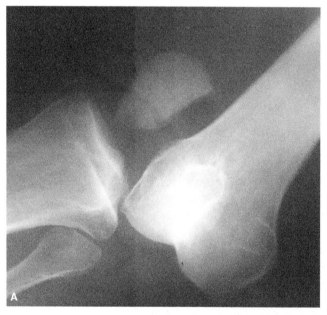

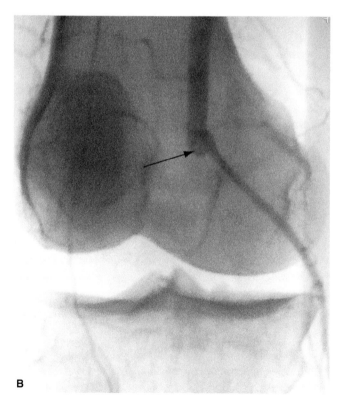

FIGURE 19.64 ■ Anterior Knee Dislocation (Tibiofemoral Dislocation). (**A**) The tibia is displaced far anterior to the femoral condyles with both translational and a rotational component to dislocation. This is the most common form of knee dislocation and results from forceful hyperextension. (**B**) Despite immediate reduction of the dislocation, the popliteal artery was torn and completely thrombosed (arrow). (Photo contributor: Michael H. Siegel, MD.)

Clinical Summary

Ankle dislocation may be caused by forced inversion or eversion. Patients usually present with obvious deformity. The most frequent ankle dislocation is a lateral dislocation. With lateral dislocation, the foot is usually obviously displaced laterally and the skin on the medial side will be tense. Avascular necrosis and reflex sympathetic dystrophy are known complications after dislocation.

Emergency Department Treatment and Disposition

Obtain standard 3-view x-rays, including the AP, lateral, and mortise views and consult orthopedics emergently. If consultation is not immediately available, check vascular integrity, provide sedation and analgesia, and then perform reduction with inline traction by grasping the calcaneus and the forefoot. Check vascular integrity after reduction. Open ankle dislocations require urgent surgery. Approximately 30% of dislocations cannot be reduced in the ED and require operative reduction. Postreduction CT is indicated to evaluate for associated injuries including fractures and talonavicular dislocation.

Pearls

1. Fifty percent of ankle dislocations are open.
2. Ankle dislocations are often associated with malleolar fractures.
3. If pulses are not present, reduce the dislocation prior to x-ray evaluation; otherwise, x-rays should always be taken before reduction.
4. Lateral dislocations are almost always associated with fractures of the malleolus or distal fibula.

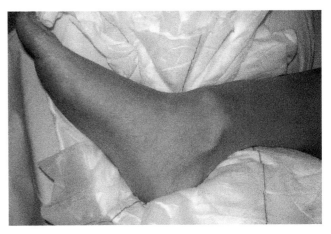

FIGURE 19.65 ■ Ankle Dislocation. This teenager tripped over a soccer ball while trying to kick it. The underlying ankle dislocation is obvious as it tents the skin. (Photo contributor: Mark Silverberg, MD.)

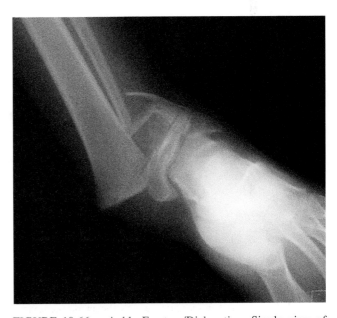

FIGURE 19.66 ■ Ankle Fracture/Dislocation. Single view of the ankle shows a Salter-Harris II fracture of the tibia with lateral dislocation of the of the distal fragment. There is a comminuted fracture of the fibula with lateral displacement of the distal fibula as well. (Photo/legend contributors: Rachael George, MD, and Rachelle Goldfisher, MD.)

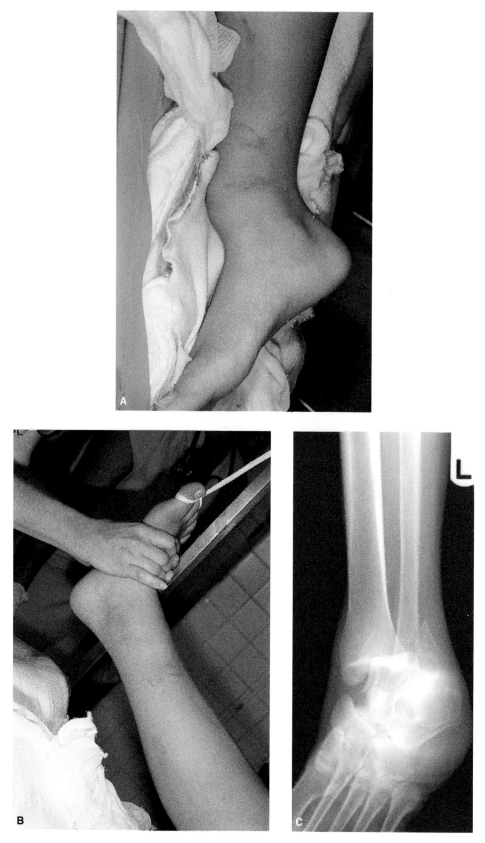

FIGURE 19.67 ■ Ankle Fracture/Dislocation. (**A, B**) Image of ankle dislocation with a gross deformity prior to and after reduction. (**C**) Posteriorly displaced oblique fracture of the distal fibula. Posterior dislocation of the talus is also noted (it is preferred to name the direction of dislocation based on the movement of the distal fragment). (Photo contributor: Binita R. Shah, MD.)

Clinical Summary

Patellar twisting injury to an extended knee is a frequent mechanism of dislocation. Females or patients with an increased Q angle (measured between the line made by connecting the anterior superior iliac spine to the midpoint of the patella and the line connecting the midpoint of the patella to the tibial tubercle) are at increased risk for patellar dislocation. Patients generally present with the patella displaced laterally and limited movement of the knee secondary to pain and tenderness on palpation. Differential diagnosis of patella dislocation includes anterior cruciate or other ligamentous tear, patella fracture, femoral condyle fracture, contusion, or sprain.

Emergency Department Treatment and Disposition

Most patellar dislocations are lateral. They are usually immediately apparent and may be reduced prior to x-rays. If there is concern for other pathology or significant fracture, obtain radiographs prior to any reduction attempts. Reduce the dislocation by having the patient flex at the hips while you apply pressure medially on the patella and extend the knee. If the first attempt is not successful, provide sedation analgesia for subsequent attempts. After successful reduction, obtain standard x-rays including AP and lateral of the knee and sunrise view of the patella to assess for osteochondral fractures. Immobilize the knee and refer the patient for orthopedic consultation. Few complications are associated with a patella dislocation. Orthopedic consultation is rarely emergent and can be made in several days to a week after successful reduction.

Pearls

1. More than 90% of patellar dislocations are lateral.
2. If the patella has self-relocated prior to presentation, the patient will likely have a positive "apprehension test," or tense up or grab the examiner's hand when the patella is pushed laterally and the knee is flexed to 30 degrees.
3. It is important to refer patients for quadriceps strengthening and rehabilitation after dislocation to prevent chronic dislocations.

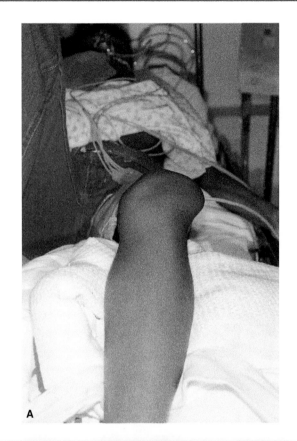

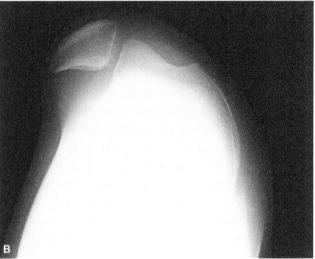

FIGURE 19.68 ■ Lateral Patella Dislocation. (**A**) Image of a 12-year-old girl after a fall, with blunt trauma to the knee and obvious deformity. (**B**) Sunrise view radiograph of the patella demonstrating a patella dislocation. (Photo contributor: Binita R. Shah, MD.)

Clinical Summary

Pelvic avulsion fractures are commonly seen in boys during late adolescence when the muscles and tendons are stronger than the physis. They present with the history of a "pop" and sudden pain to the area avulsed after maximal muscle contraction, such as with sprinting or jumping. There are a number of sites around the pelvis that may be avulsed, with the most common being the ischial tuberosity (attachment of hamstrings) and the anterior inferior iliac spine (attachment of rectus femoris).

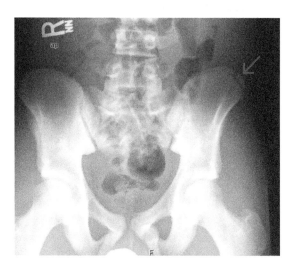

FIGURE 19.69 ■ Pelvic Brim Avulsion. AP view of the pelvis shows avulsion of the left iliac apophysis (arrow). Soft tissue density projects over the left inferior pubic ramus synchrondrosis. (Photo contributor: Jennifer H. Chao, MD.)

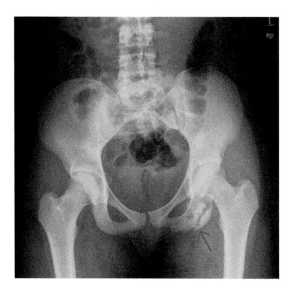

FIGURE 19.70 ■ Ischial Tuberosity Avulsion. AP view of the pelvis demonstrates chronic avulsion fracture of the left ischial tuberosity (arrow), the hamstring origin site. (Photo/legend contributors: Jennifer H. Chao, MD, and Ryan Logan Webb, MD.)

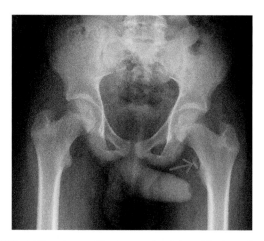

FIGURE 19.71 ■ Lesser Trochanter Avulsion. AP view of the pelvis demonstrates avulsion of the left inferior trochanteric apophysis (arrow). (Photo contributor: Jennifer H. Chao, MD.)

Emergency Department Treatment and Disposition

Pelvic and hip x-rays are needed to confirm the diagnosis of an avulsion fracture. Most avulsions will heal well with 4 to 6 weeks of rest. Patients should be made non–weight bearing and should follow up with orthopedics or a sports physician to assess for the unlikely need for surgical repair.

Pearl

1. Indications for surgical repair include painful nonunion and significant (>3 cm) displacement of the fragment.

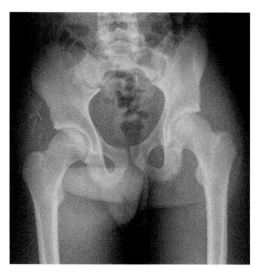

FIGURE 19.72 ■ Anterior Superior Iliac Spine Avulsion. AP view of the pelvis demonstrates avulsion of the right anterior superior iliac spine (arrow). (Photo contributor: Jennifer H. Chao, MD.)

Clinical Summary

Tibial tubercle avulsion fractures are seen primarily in boys during late adolescence, when the quadriceps muscle and tendon are stronger than the proximal tibial physis. Patients present with a history of a "pop" and sudden pain and deformity to the proximal tibia after significant muscle contraction, such as with sprinting or jumping. On physical examination, they are often unable to extend the knee against resistance.

This finding will help differentiate Osgood-Schlatter disease (no physeal involvement) from a true avulsion fracture.

Emergency Department Treatment and Disposition

Knee x-rays are needed to confirm the diagnosis of an avulsion fracture. There may be a finding of patella alta on the lateral x-ray. Orthopedics consult is necessary to determine operative management versus conservative management with reduction and a cylindrical cast. Compartment syndrome is a known complication.

Pearls

1. Keep in mind that compartment syndrome may occur with this type of injury.
2. Osgood-Schlatter disease or a fragmented tibial tuberosity on x-ray may be confused with an avulsion fracture. The ability to extend the knee against resistance and lack of physeal involvement on x-ray helps to differentiate the 2 conditions.

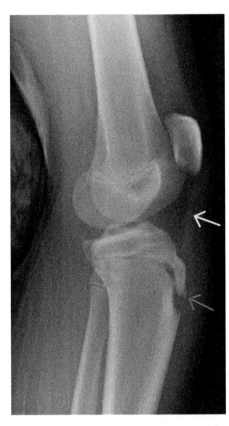

FIGURE 19.73 ■ Tibial Tubercle Avulsion. Lateral view of the knee shows avulsion of the physis of the tibial tubercle (red arrow). Note the superior displacement of the patella (patella alta). There is marked soft tissue swelling anteriorly and poor definition of the patella tendon (yellow arrow). (Photo contributor: Jennifer H. Chao, MD.)

Clinical Summary

Gamekeeper's thumb is a tear of the ulnar collateral ligament of the MCP thumb joint. The name is derived from gamekeepers who were prone to the injury, because they killed fowl by snapping the birds' necks with their hands. Today, this injury is more often associated with falling on an outstretched hand (forced abduction of the thumb) and is referred to as skier's thumb, because skiing accidents represent the most common cause. Patients present with pain on abduction and extension of the thumb associated with swelling at the ulnar aspect of thumb's MCP joint. There is also a laxity of >20 degrees of the ulnar collateral ligament with the thumb in full extension. There is decreased range of motion of the thumb and functionality of the hand with a decreased strength of the pincer grip.

Emergency Department Treatment and Disposition

Obtain x-rays and provide analgesia with 2% lidocaine without epinephrine before checking laxity of the ligament with the thumb in full extension. The injury may not be apparent on x-ray or may appear as an avulsion fracture of the proximal phalanx base on the medial side. Apply ice acutely to reduce swelling. Immobilize the injury with thumb spica splinting with the MCP joint flexed to about 20 degrees. After immobilization, patients with closed injuries can be sent home with orthopedic or hand specialist follow-up in 48 to 72 hours.

Pearl

1. The inability to hold the pincer grip (ie, make the "OK" sign) with the thumb and index finger is key to diagnosing this injury.

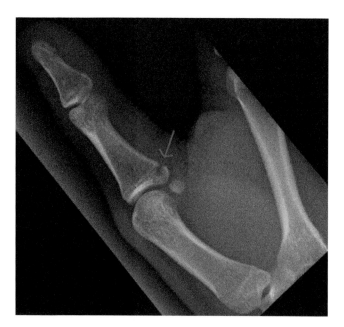

FIGURE 19.74 ■ Gamekeeper's Thumb. A 16-year-old boy presented with a history of a fall landing on his thumb in full extension. Acute oblique fracture of the medial base of first proximal phalanx (red arrow), consistent with an avulsion fracture at the site of ulnar collateral ligament attachment (gamekeeper's thumb), is seen. (Photo contributors: Ryan Logan Webb, MD, and Josh Greenstein, MD.)

Clinical Summary

When a caretaker pulls a child by the arm to safety, sudden traction of the pronated extended forearm results in the displacement of the annular ligament over the radial head, with the ligament becoming trapped between the radial head and the capitellum. This is also known as radial head subluxation or "temper-tantrum elbow" or "pulled elbow." Patients usually refuse to move the arm, holding it in pronation at the side and flexed at the elbow. Supination elicits pain. Occasionally, a deformity is seen with prominence and displacement of the radial head. Complications are extremely rare with simple subluxation of the radial head or its reduction procedure.

Emergency Department Treatment and Disposition

Radiographs are often unnecessary and may not be helpful, because the radial head and lateral humeral condyle may not be ossified in a young child. If radiographs are obtained, the radiology technician will supinate and flex the elbow to 90 degrees to obtain a proper lateral x-ray of the elbow; such manipulations can result in joint reduction. Reduce the subluxation unless there are external signs of trauma (eg, swelling, extreme tenderness, ecchymosis), suspicion of elbow or forearm fracture or dislocation, or known mechanism of injury unlikely to result in radial head subluxation. Reduction is done by supination and flexion (traditional reduction technique) or using the hyperpronation technique (pronation and flexion). The latter requires fewer attempts and has greater success. In supination and flexion, grasp the palm of the involved hand as if to shake it, and encircle the elbow with the other hand with the thumb placed over the radial head. Fully supinate the arm in one quick deliberate motion while applying gentle longitudinal traction, and in a continuous motion, flex the elbow to the shoulder. For hyperpronation, apply gentle longitudinal traction, and place the forearm in hyperpronation and then flex the elbow. Most often, an audible or palpable pop or click is felt by the thumb lying over the radial head as the annular ligament is freed from the joint,

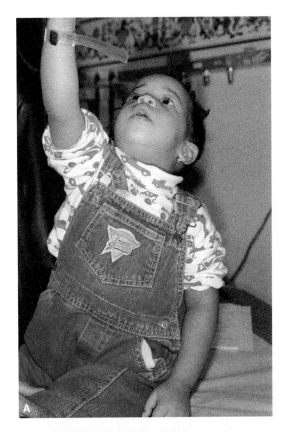

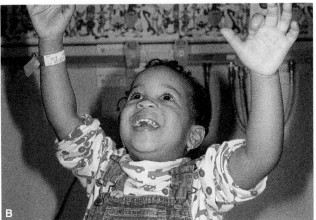

FIGURE 19.75 ■ Nursemaid's Elbow (Radial Head Subluxation). (**A**) Image of a child with nursemaid's elbow on the left side, which is the more common side because the adult who pulled on the arm is more likely to be right handed. The child refuses to use the left arm. (**B**) Within 15 minutes after reduction, the child freely uses the arm. (Photo contributor: Binita R. Shah, MD.)

and this signals successful reduction. If no click is heard or felt, attempt reduction again in 15 minutes. After a successful reduction, no treatment, radiographs, or immobilization is required.

Pearls

1. Indications for radiography include either unsuccessful attempts at reduction or the presence of swelling or significant tenderness, suggesting another diagnosis, or when there is question or doubt about the mechanism of injury.

2. Let the child sit comfortably in the caregiver's lap for reduction. Gentle examination of the uninvolved arm first may make the examination of the injured arm easier. Exclude any point tenderness before attempting reduction.

3. With successful reduction, movement usually returns in 5 to 15 minutes, although it may take longer if subluxation has been present for several hours.

4. If there are recurrent subluxations, consider posterior immobilization with the elbow flexed to 90 degrees and the forearm in supination.

5. The strength of the annular ligament and the size of the radial head increase with age, making this subluxation uncommon after the age of 5 years.

Clinical Summary

Acromioclavicular (AC) injuries are caused by direct blow to the superior or lateral aspect of the shoulder or to the acromion itself. These injuries are common in contact sports (hockey, American football, and rugby). Shoulder appearance is usually normal, and patients present with pain on gravity traction of the arm. These injuries are classified into the following: First-degree injuries have incomplete tear of the AC ligament, with no subluxation. Second-degree injuries have subluxation of the AC joint and distal clavicular separation <50% of the clavicular diameter in relation to the acromion. In third-degree injuries, the clavicular separation is >50% of its diameter in relation to the acromion. Fourth-degree injury represents complete dislocation and posterior displacement of the distal head of the clavicle into the trapezius muscle. Fifth-degree injury is defined by superior dislocation of the joint of 1 to 3 times the normal spacing with increased coracoclavicular ligament distance and disruption of deltotrapezial fascia. Sixth-degree injury is complete dislocation with inferior displacement of distal clavicular head.

Emergency Department Treatment and Disposition

Obtain AC x-rays including weight-bearing views. In first-degree injuries, x-rays including stress views are negative. In second- and third-degree injures, subluxation may be seen with stress views. For third- to sixth-degree injuries, consult orthopedics for evaluation in the ED, as surgical repair is indicated. For first- and second-degree injuries, immobilize the limb with a sling and swathe, and discharge the patient with a referral for orthopedic follow-up. The sling should be worn for 4 to 6 weeks. Future contact sport activity is limited. Neurovascular complications are extremely rare.

Pearls

1. AC injuries are fairly common among athletes in contact sports.
2. AC stress test is performed by bringing the arm across the body, approximating the elbow with the contralateral shoulder. A positive test produces pain in the area.

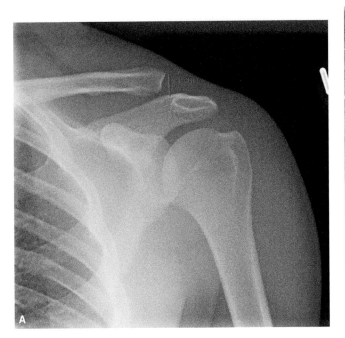
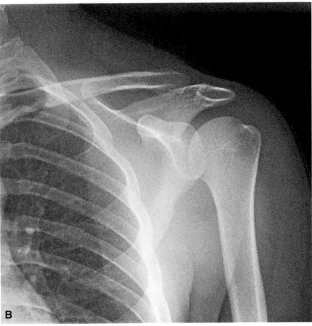

FIGURE 19.76 ■ Acromioclavicular (AC) Injury. A 22-year-old man presented with AC joint tenderness after a fall. (**A**) AP view of the shoulder shows 1-cm separation of the distal clavicle from the acromion (red line) consistent with AC joint injury. (**B**) A follow-up radiograph a few years later shows healing of the injury and restored alignment. (Photo contributors: Ryan Logan Webb, MD, and Josh Greenstein, MD.)

Clinical Summary

Slipped capital femoral epiphysis occurs when the femoral epiphysis becomes displaced from the femoral neck. Classically, the patient is an obese adolescent, complaining of dull aching pain at the hip, groin, thigh, or knee, without any history of injury. Over time, a classic limp becomes apparent. Because of the rapid bone growth and activity level in prepubescent children, the femoral epiphysis is displaced.

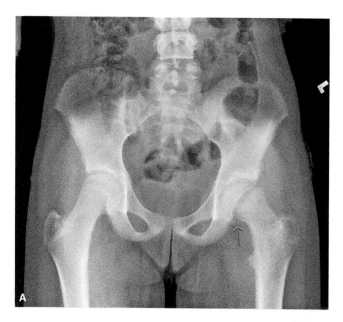

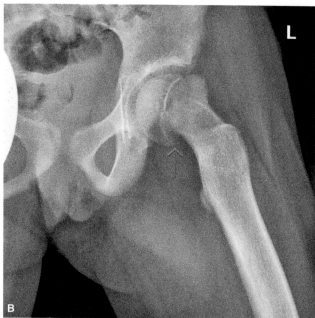

FIGURE 19.77 ■ Slipped Capital Femoral Epiphysis. An 11-year-old obese girl presented with hip pain. (**A**) Widening of the physis is seen (earliest radiographic sign), with anterolateral displacement of the femoral metaphysis from the epiphysis (red arrow), which moves posteromedially. (**B**) Frog-leg lateral view better depicts the slippage (red arrow) and may be positive in cases with apparently normal AP view. (Photo contributors: Ryan Logan Webb, MD, and Josh Greenstein, MD.)

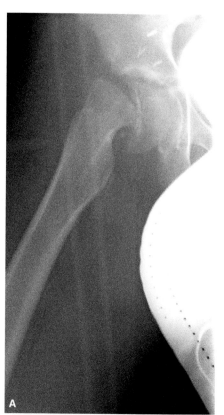

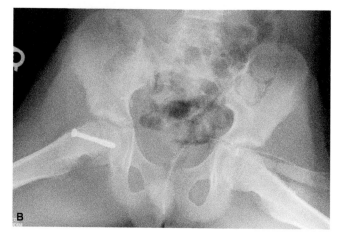

FIGURE 19.78 ■ Slipped Capital Femoral Epiphysis (SCFE). A 12-year-old boy suffered a traumatic SCFE after being tossed by tornado and thrown against a fence. (**A**) AP radiograph of the right hip demonstrates a grade 2 SCFE. (**B**) AP radiograph of the pelvis shows postreduction of the SCFE in normal anatomic alignment. In this case, the slippage has been reduced; however, often the malaligned epiphysis is left in place, referred to as "in situ pinning." (Photo contributor: Stuart A. Bradin, DO.)

This entity can be classified according to presentation (pre-slip, acute, acute-on-chronic, or chronic), stability (stable or unstable), or severity when it is compared to the unaffected side (mild, <30 degrees; moderate, 30–50 degrees; or severe, >50 degrees). Differential diagnosis of slipped capital femoral epiphysis includes transient synovitis of the hip, septic arthritis, degenerative arthritis, and bursitis.

Emergency Department Treatment and Disposition

Obtain AP and lateral views of both hips; frog-leg or cross-table lateral views should be obtained to visualize lateral projections. These views will show a widened and displaced capital epiphysis that is also displaced posteriorly and inferiorly. Evaluate for kidney or endocrine diseases when the presentation is atypical (age <10 years or >16 years or weight <50th percentile) Complications include avascular necrosis, chondrolysis, further slippage, and degenerative arthritis of the hip. Consult orthopedics emergently. Depending on the degree of slippage, treatment may be conservative or may require internal fixation with application of screws.

Pearls

1. Slipped capital femoral epiphysis occurs in children from ages 10 to 16 years (years of rapid bone growth) and in boys more often than girls.
2. There is a higher association with children who are overweight.
3. In 20% to 40% of cases, both hips are involved.
4. There is a peak incidence in the summer months, when there is increased outdoor physical activity.
5. The history may include minor trauma, but it usually has an insidious onset of symptoms.

LEGG-CALVÉ-PERTHES DISEASE

Clinical Summary

Legg-Calvé-Perthes disease, or avascular necrosis of the femoral head, results from an ill-defined etiology, is not secondary to any injury, and is also known as osteochondrosis of the femoral head. Onset is usually insidious and may progress from months to years. The problem is seen in children aged 3 to 12 years, and it peaks around 5 to 7 years of age. It is usually a self-limiting disorder. Eighty percent of cases are seen in boys, and it is usually unilateral (10%–20% are bilateral). Patients usually present with a limp and a vague complaint of pain in the groin, inner thigh, or hip and have limited abduction of the hip and internal rotation on flexion or extension. Symptoms are exaggerated during times of excessive activity or exertion (summer months). Acute complications are unusual, and long-term complications include arthritis and limited mobility.

Emergency Department Treatment and Disposition

Obtain x-rays (a pelvic view), which early on may be normal or demonstrate only joint space widening. Later findings include a flattening of the femoral head known as coxa plana. Refer patients for orthopedic consultation, which does not need to take place in the ED.

Pearls

1. Legg-Calvé-Perthes disease is fairly rare in African Americans.
2. Ten percent of cases are familial.

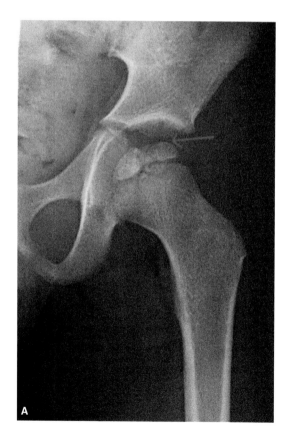

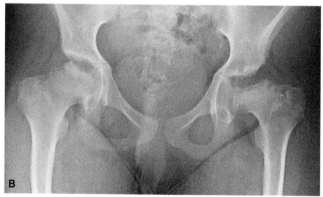

FIGURE 19.79 ■ Legg-Calvé-Perthes Disease (LCPD). (**A**) Left femoral epiphysis height loss and mild fragmentation (red arrow) consistent with LCPD is shown in a 4-year-old boy presenting with bilateral leg pain. Radiograph of his right hip was unremarkable. (**B**) A more advanced case of LCPD in an 11-year-old girl is shown with fragmentation and flattening of both femoral heads. (Photo contributors: Ryan Logan Webb, MD, and Josh Greenstein, MD.)

Clinical Summary

Anterior cruciate ligament (ACL) tears are the most common ligamentous injury of the knee in children and skeletally immature adolescents. It is classically caused by noncontact injuries during sports, yet a direct blow to the knee can also be culprit. Patients present with history of a pop at the time of injury followed by a swollen, diffusely tender knee within 1 hour. Clinicians should perform various standardized tests such as drawer test, Lachman test etc. in order to establish the diagnosis. The anterior drawer sign and positive Lachman test are fairly sensitive for diagnosis. ACL tears are often associated with fractures (eg, tibial eminence fracture) or medial meniscus tear. Complications include arthritis, chronic pain, and limited range of motion.

Emergency Department Treatment and Disposition

Obtain standard x-rays including AP and lateral films of the knee, which usually demonstrate joint effusion and soft tissue swelling but no bony abnormalities. Acute management includes rest, ice, compression, elevation, and pain medications (RICED). Refer patients with stable knee joints for outpatient orthopedic follow-up within 48 hours. Immobilize the knee, and provide crutches for avoidance of weight bearing. Definitive treatment is surgical repair by orthopedics.

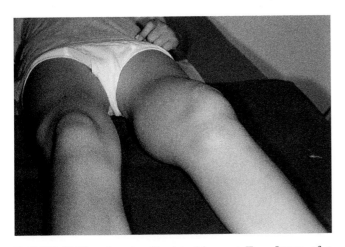

FIGURE 19.80 ■ Anterior Cruciate Ligament Tear. Image of a 10-year-old boy who sustained an anterior cruciate ligament tear while playing football. Note the marked diffuse swelling of the left knee in comparison to the normal right knee. (Photo contributor: Binita R. Shah, MD.)

Pearls

1. ACL tears are the most common serious ligament injury of the knee.
2. Seventy-five percent of ACL tears will present with hemarthrosis.
3. A tense hemarthrosis may decrease the sensitivity of the anterior drawer sign and Lachman test.
4. All tender, swollen knees should be immobilized, and weight bearing should be avoided until orthopedic follow-up.

Clinical Summary

Osgood-Schlatter disease is a traction apophysitis of the proximal tibial tubercle and occurs during a normal or slightly advanced activity level for children aged 9 to 14 years. It affects 20% of adolescents participating in sports activities. It is usually unilateral, but it can asymmetrically affect both knees in up to half of cases. Patients present with a tender swollen tibial tuberosity and pain. Erythema over the tibial tuberosity may be present. There is usually no history of direct injury. The only complication is a lack of participation in the routine activities of an adolescent. There are no significant long-term complications of diagnosed Osgood-Schlatter disease.

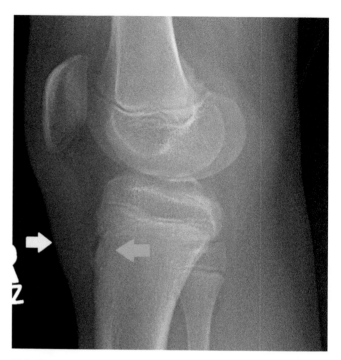

FIGURE 19.82 ■ Osgood-Schlatter Disease. A lateral view of the knee demonstrates fragmentation of the tibial tuberosity (blue arrow) and associated patellar tendon thickening and Hoffa's fat pad inflammation (yellow arrow) in a 14-year-old boy presenting with knee pain. (Photo contributors: Jonathan Stern, MD, and Josh Greenstein, MD.)

Emergency Department Treatment and Disposition

Osgood-Schlatter disease is not an acute infectious/inflammatory process; thus, no laboratory values or imaging studies contribute to the diagnosis. Consultations are not necessary unless the patient is a high-functioning individual. When the diagnosis is made, only rarely is there a reason for a consultant to see the patient in the ED. Treatment is rest and NSAIDs.

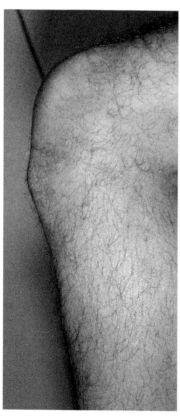

FIGURE 19.81 ■ Osgood-Schlatter Disease. A lateral picture of the knee demonstrates a protuberance over the tibial tuberosity (exquisitely tender on direct palpation) in this young basketball player. (Photo contributor: Raffi S. Kapitanyan, MD.)

Pearls

1. Osgood-Schlatter disease is extremely common. The activity level of the patient and point tenderness are key to its diagnosis.

2. If systemic signs or symptoms are present, another diagnosis is likely.

Clinical Summary

Achilles tendon rupture is a rare entity in children and young adolescents. It usually results from forced dorsiflexion of the ankle, usually related to strenuous athletic activity. Direct trauma to a taut tendon is a secondary cause. Most patients present with severe pain at the posterior part of the ankle with inability to bear weight, yet the absence of pain does not rule out tendon rupture. On examination, there is tenderness at distal calf, with or without a palpable defect in the tendon 1.5 to 2 inches (narrowest point) proximal to the calcaneus (hematoma might mask tendon defects). On squeezing the calf (Thompson test), there is no plantar flexion, and when the patient is laying prone, feet misalignment will be observed (Matles sign). Complete tears are rarely undiagnosed but lead to a difficult surgical repair. Partial tears that are undiagnosed could lead to complete tears.

Emergency Department Treatment and Disposition

Obtain tibia/fibula and ankle films, although these are usually negative. Bedside US can provide a quick diagnostic confirmation and further details on injury type (partial-thickness vs full-thickness tear). Apply a posterior splint in a neutral position and instruct the patient to avoid weight bearing with crutches. Ice and NSAIDs can help with pain and swelling. Consult orthopedics for definitive treatment and follow-up. Partial tears should also have orthopedic referral for extended immobilization.

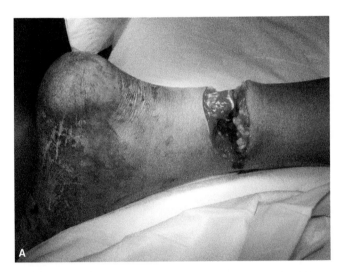

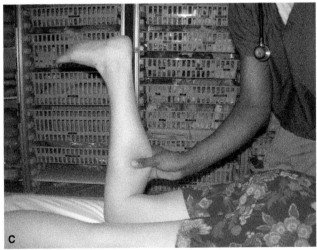

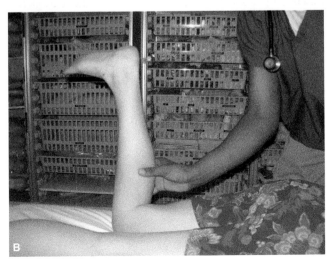

FIGURE 19.83 ■ Achilles Tendon Laceration and Positive Thompson Test Seen in Achilles Tendon Rupture. (**A**) This skateboarder fell on a chain link fence while jumping over it and transected his Achilles tendon. (**B**) Image of a patient in the proper position for a Thompson test prior to squeezing the calf. (**C**) Image of a positive Thompson test, demonstrating no plantar flexion of the foot after the calf is squeezed. This test is positive with complete tears of the Achilles tendon. (Photo contributor: Mark Silverberg, MD.)

Pearls

1. Although Achilles tendon rupture is rare, it is most commonly seen in adolescent athletes in the pediatric population.

2. Normally the posterior splints are applied with the ankle at 90 degrees, but in this case, the ankle should be splinted in gravity equinus position, which is the position of the ankle when the foot is hanging off the bed.

3. The Achilles tendon is able to regenerate when partially sectioned and heals well with immobilization.

4. Partial tears can be missed in 25% of cases.

5. Surgical repair of complete rupture of Achilles tendon can help prevent repeat tendon rupture in the future.

FOREIGN BODIES AND PENETRATING INJURIES

Clinical Summary

Foreign bodies and penetrating injuries are most often seen on the plantar aspect of the foot or the palmar surface of the hand. Less commonly, these result from falling objects or projectiles. Patients present with a puncture wound, which may be subtle when on the plantar aspect of the foot. Pain is usually present, especially if there is associated bony involvement. Complications may include cellulitis, retained foreign body, fibrosis, and chronic pain. Osteomyelitis is common

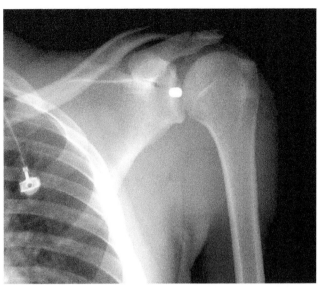

FIGURE 19.85 ■ Intra-articular Foreign Body (Bullet). AP view of the glenohumeral joint shows an intra-articular bullet lodged within the glenoid fossa. There was no fracture or dislocation confirmed also on other views. The bullet required urgent removal in the operating room. (Photo contributor: Michael Lucchesi, MD.)

after inoculation into the bony matrix. Septic arthritis, either from direct penetration of the joint capsule or via direct spread from a focus of osteomyelitis, may occur.

Emergency Department Treatment and Disposition

Obtain x-rays of the involved area whenever there is suspicion of a penetrating injury with foreign bodies that are radiopaque. Note that the ability to see glass on x-ray is dependent on its lead content. Order US to detect subcutaneous foreign bodies. Whether a foreign body is seen on imaging or not, if there is a high suspicion, consult orthopedics and provide parenteral antibiotics in the ED. Admit patients with penetrating foreign bodies for definitive removal when indicated or for an initial course of parenteral antibiotics when removal is not indicated.

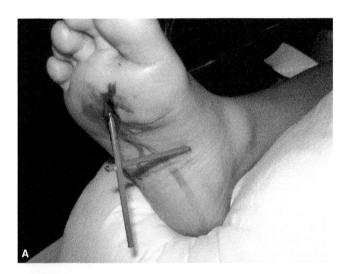

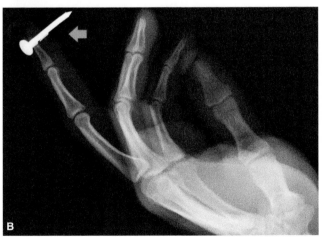

FIGURE 19.84 ■ Foreign Bodies and Penetrating Injuries. (**A**) This child was playing at a construction site and stepped on a wire mesh. He was cut away from the larger piece and subsequently taken to the operating room to have this part removed. (**B**) Lateral view of the hand in a different patient shows a nail embedded in the patient's distal third digit (blue arrow). Follow-up radiograph after removal showed no osseous abnormalities. (Photo contributors: Mark Silberberg, MD [A], Jonathan Stern, MD, and Josh Greenstein, MD [B]. (See also Figure 20.97.)

Pearl

1. Of particular concern is a plantar puncture wound of the foot through sneakers, which are often colonized by *Pseudomonas*. Often a small piece of material from the sneaker is left in the puncture cavity and is very difficult to locate. Infection is inevitable if it is not found and removed.

927

Clinical Summary

Paronychia is an infection involving the nail fold of the nail, and patients present with swelling, tenderness, and fluctuance at the nail base. Paronychia is associated with nail biting but can also be caused by any penetrating injury at the base of the

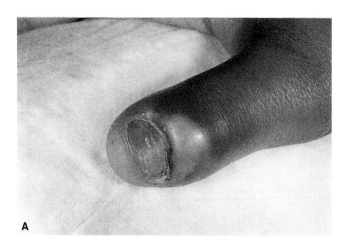

A

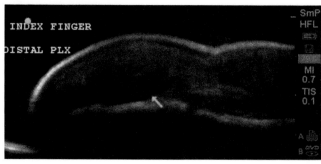

FIGURE 19.87 ■ Digital US. Point-of-care US by an emergency physician demonstrating pus collection (arrow) on the volar aspect of the distal index finger in a 6-year-old patient complaining of index finger tip pain and swelling. (Photo contributor: Sathyaseelan Subramaniam, MD.)

nail. Spread of infection can occur proximally. A felon (infection of the volar surface of the distal phalanx pulp space) is also a complication of an untreated paronychia. Differential diagnosis of a paronychia includes contusion, retained foreign body, tuft fracture, and hair tourniquet syndrome.

Emergency Department Treatment and Disposition

Radiographic evaluation is not necessary unless there is a recent history of significant trauma. Provide adequate anesthesia with a digital block, and incise and drain with a no. 11 blade scalpel sliding up the nail proximally underneath the cuticle and eponychium. Depending on the location of the paronychia, the incision can extend toward a lateral nail fold if needed. Incision will usually produce purulent material that can be cultured. In severe cases, antibiotics covering *Staphylococcus aureus* and *Streptococcus pyogenes* should be given.

Pearls

1. Place a gauze wick to allow for additional drainage in large wounds.
2. Administer tetanus vaccination as indicated; antibiotics can be prescribed in severe cases after obtaining a wound culture.

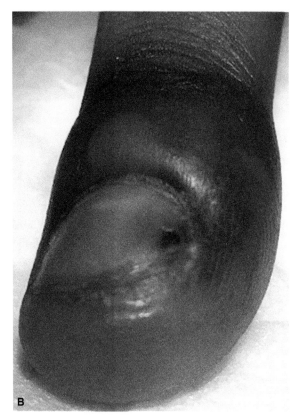

B

FIGURE 19.86 ■ Paronychia. (**A**) Paronychia of the thumb with localized cellulitis, which was drained after digital block. (**B**) Paronychia in a 10-year-old girl with a history of biting her fingers regularly presented with new complaints of swelling and pain in her right hand third digit. (Photo contributors: Binita R. Shah, MD [A], and Sathyaseelan Subramaniam, MD [B].)

Clinical Summary

Flexor tenosynovitis usually results from puncture wounds along the volar aspect of the digit. Patients present with Kanavel signs:

1. Symmetric or fusiform swelling of the finger
2. Tenderness over the flexor tendon sheath
3. Pain with passive extension
4. Finger held in a flexed position

The most common pathogens causing tenosynovitis include *S aureus* and *Streptococcus* species, followed by *Pseudomonas* species.

Emergency Department Treatment and Disposition

Obtain x-rays of the digit to rule out occult fracture or foreign body and investigate for osteomyelitis. Septic arthritis, ascending cellulitis, joint fibrosis, and limited mobility are complications of tenosynovitis. Consult orthopedics emergently and admit patients for continuous elevation of the infected limb and IV antibiotics (eg, oxacillin or clindamycin for patients who are allergic to penicillin). Severe cases and cases that do not respond to antibiotic therapy may require incision and drainage, irrigation, and debridement in the operating room.

Pearls

1. Not all cases of tenosynovitis are dramatic on presentation. When there is a question, consult a hand surgeon.
2. With no barriers to the spread of infection, the entire tendon sheath usually becomes involved.

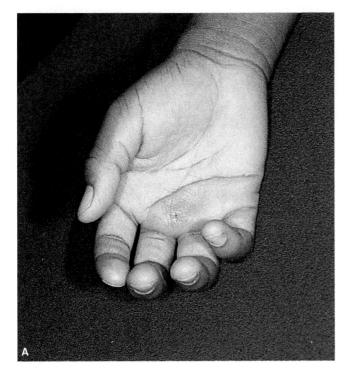

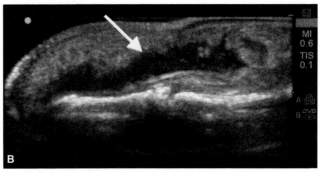

FIGURE 19.88 ■ Flexor Tenosynovitis. (**A**) Palmer view of a child shows fusiform swelling of the third and fourth digits caused by a puncture wound to the palm over the MCP joint resulting in tenosynovitis. (**B**) Point-of-care US image by emergency physician demonstrating collection (arrow) tracking along flexor tendon of second digit confirming diagnosis of flexor tenosynovitis in a 16-year-old girl. (Photo contributors: Binita Shah, MD, and Sathyaseelan Subramaniam, MD.)

Clinical Features

Osteomyelitis is an infection of the bone more often seen at the junction of metaphysis and epiphysis. Half of all cases occur in children <5 years of age, and one-quarter occur by 2 years of age. Clinical presentation varies with age. Younger children are more likely to have external findings of edema, tenderness, erythema, and warmth at the involved site. Toddlers will present with refusal to use the affected limb and tenderness on examination. Older children may only report mild symptoms with point tenderness. The most common sites are long bones such as the tibia, femur, and humerus. Fever and a history of other nonspecific symptoms such as irritability and poor appetite are helpful clues but are not always present.

Acute osteomyelitis usually occurs by hematogenous seeding from a prior bacteremia, and thus, there is typically a single offending organism (Table 19.5). Vaccination has dramatically decreased the incidence of *Haemophilus influenzae* type b–associated osteomyelitis; however, it should be considered in underimmunized populations. Infection of the bone can also occur as a result of direct inoculation of pathogens, as in penetrating injury or extension from local infection.

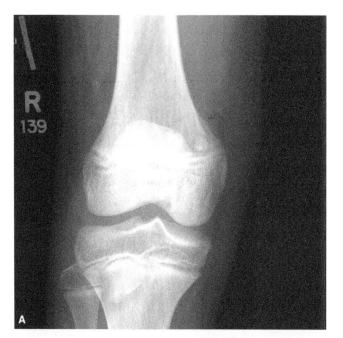

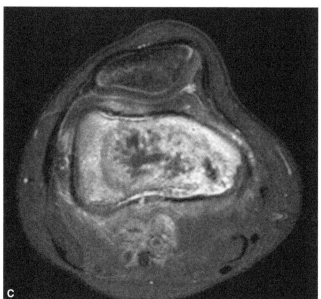

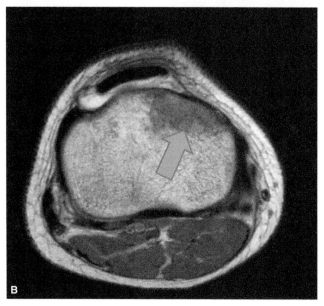

FIGURE 19.89 ■ Acute Osteomyelitis. (**A**) Frontal projection of the right knee shows area of cortical destruction along the medial aspect of the right knee (arrow). (**B**) Axial T1-weighted image of the right knee shows area of decreased bone marrow signal in the medial aspect of the knee (arrow) corresponding to the area of bone destruction seen on the radiograph. (**C**) Axial T1-weighted image with fat suppression, after gadolinium administration, shows marked enhancement of the bone marrow with enhancing surrounding inflammatory reaction (arrows). (Photo/legend contributors: Rita Nathawad, MD, and John Amodio, MD.)

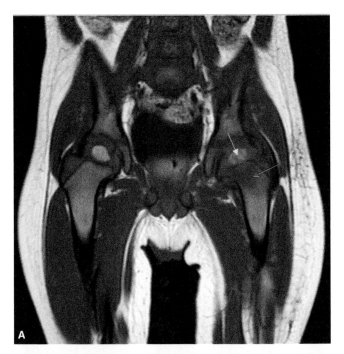

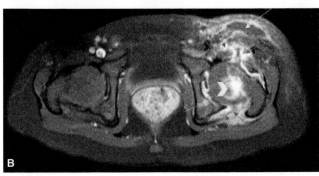

FIGURE 19.90 ■ Acute Septic Arthritis of the Left Hip and Osteomyelitis of the Left Proximal Femur. A 2-year-old girl presented crying with pain and not moving her left leg. (**A**) Coronal T1 sequence showing abnormal T1 hypointense signal within the left femoral metaphysis (red arrow) as well as heterogeneous signal within the epiphysis (yellow arrow). Compare with the contralateral normal side. (**B**) Axial fat-saturation postgadolinium T1 sequence demonstrating complex left hip joint effusion with thickened enhancement of the left hip joint capsule (red arrows) with a contiguous anterior thigh soft tissue rim-enhancing abscess (yellow arrow). Enhancement within the femoral head (yellow arrowhead) is consistent with osteomyelitis, when paired with the T1 heterogeneous signal on image A. Enhancement within the left posterior acetabular wall (blue arrow) is most likely reactive, given normal corresponding T1 signal. (Photo/legend contributors: Sathyaseelan Subramaniam, MD, and Cheryl H. Lin, MD.)

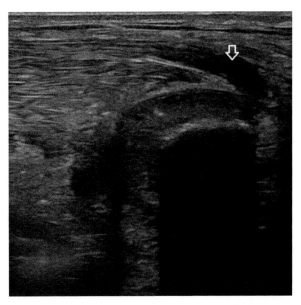

FIGURE 19.91 ■ Acute Osteomyelitis. Clavicular osteomyelitis in an 18-year-old boy with right anterior neck pain and fever. Swelling over the neck was revealed by point-of care US to be due to collection of pus along medial clavicle (arrow). Emergency physician performed bedside aspiration of the purulent material, which grew *Staphylococcus aureus*. Hyperechoic point is demonstrated within the collection as the needle tip in short axis during the procedural aspiration. (Photo contributor: Sathyaseelan Subramaniam, MD.)

Differential diagnosis includes septic arthritis, bony tumors (eg, osteogenic sarcoma), metastatic bony lesions (eg, leukemia, neuroblastoma), cellulitis, hemoglobinopathies (bone infarction), and fracture.

Emergency Department Treatment and Disposition

Evaluate any healthy child presenting with focal skeletal pain or decreased limb function for osteomyelitis. Analgesia should be provided for pain control. Although not diagnostic, a CBC with differential and inflammatory markers (eg, erythrocyte sedimentation rate [ESR] and C-reactive protein [CRP]) should be obtained. Blood culture (positive in 36%–74% of cases) may be useful for antimicrobial agent choice. Order x-rays, noting that these will not show evidence

TABLE 19.5 ■ PATHOGENS CAUSING OSTEOMYELITIS IN SPECIFIC CLINICAL SETTINGS

Clinical Setting	Pathogen
All osteomyelitis	*Staphylococcus aureus* (most common)
	Streptococcus pyogenes (second most common)
	Staphylococcus pneumoniae, other gram negatives (*Haemophilus influenzae, Kingella kingae, Salmonella* spp)
Nosocomial infection	Enterobacteriaceae, *Pseudomonas aeruginosa, Candida* spp
Diabetes mellitus	Streptococci and anaerobic bacteria
Bites (human and animal)	Streptococci, anaerobic mouth flora (ie, *Eikenella corrodens*), *Pasteurella multocida*
Immunocompromised patients	*Aspergillus* spp, *Candida* spp, *Mycobacteria* spp
Puncture wound to foot	*P aeruginosa*
Sickle cell disease	*Salmonella* spp, *S aureus, S pneumoniae*
Exposure to tuberculosis	*Mycobacterium tuberculosis*
Neonate	*S aureus, Streptococcus agalactiae*, enteric gram negatives (ie, *Escherichia coli*), coagulase-negative *Staphylococcus*

of bone destruction until 10 to 14 days after the onset of infection but can be used to exclude trauma. In consultation with pediatric orthopedics and infectious diseases, an MRI or bone scan should be considered. Both have high sensitivity (>95%) for diagnosis. MRI is preferable as it better outlines the inflammatory changes, is more useful for drainage of purulent material, and does not expose the child to ionizing radiation. If multifocal disease is a possibility, then a bone scan is preferred.

Unless in overt sepsis, prescribe empiric antibiotics after culture of bone specimens if possible. Anti-staphylococcal β-lactam antibiotics such as oxacillin or ceftriaxone are adequate. However, clindamycin or vancomycin should be strongly considered if local antibiograms suggest a high prevalence of methicillin-resistant *S aureus*. Different antibiotic regimens may be necessary if the clinical history points toward an atypical pathogen (Table 19.5). Drainage of bone collections, if present, may be both diagnostic and therapeutic.

Pearls

1. Consider acute osteomyelitis in any child with fever and decreased use of an extremity.
2. Osteomyelitis may be associated with septic arthritis in young children.
3. Radiographic findings will be delayed; MRI or bone scan is preferred for making the diagnosis.
4. Obtain cultures prior to initiation of antibiotics (if possible).

Clinical Summary

Although there is some debate over the definition of chronic osteomyelitis, most patients have symptoms for >2 to 3 weeks. Typically, patients have waxing and waning symptoms for months. Often there is a prior history of inadequately treated or untreated acute osteomyelitis, a surgical procedure, or major trauma. Fever and other nonspecific signs of infection may be present intermittently or not at all. A painful and poorly functioning extremity and the presence of draining sinuses and necrotic tissue are important clues to diagnosis. Chronic osteomyelitis is often seen in children with peripheral neuropathy when a lesion on the extremity is not noticed and subsequently becomes infected. Lesions are most commonly polymicrobial (eg, *S aureus, Pseudomonas aeruginosa*, coagulase-negative *Staphylococcus*, anaerobes, fungi) but occasionally are due to a single organism. Children without adequate access to health care may present late in the course of illness with chronic osteomyelitis.

Emergency Department Treatment and Disposition

Obtain CBC, ESR, and CRP, which may be elevated but are often normal. Consult orthopedics and infectious disease for appropriate workup, management including hospitalization,

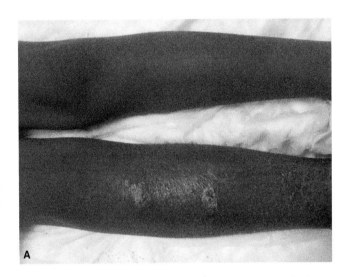

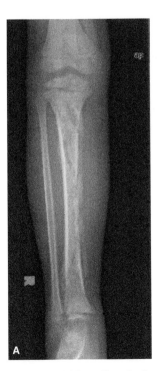
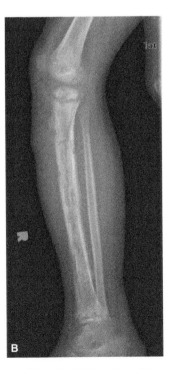

FIGURE 19.92 ■ Chronic Osteomyelitis. (**A, B**) Frontal and lateral projections of the right leg demonstrate extensive osteolytic and osteosclerotic areas, in both tibia and fibula, with periosteal reaction compatible with chronic osteomyelitis. (Photo contributor: John Amodio, MD.)

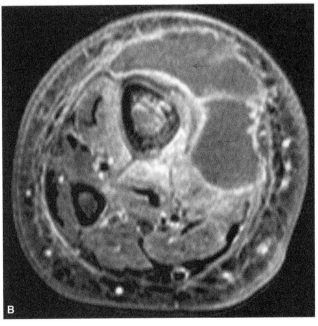

FIGURE 19.93 ■ Chronic Osteomyelitis. (**A**) This 6-year-old boy (same patient as in Figure 19.92) presented with a swollen, crythematous right leg with 2 draining sinuses following an injury he suffered 2 months earlier. Bone culture was positive for *S aureus*. (**B**) Axial T1-weighted image, after gadolinium administration, through the right leg shows diffuse heterogeneous enhancement of the bone marrow with soft tissue abscess (arrows). Diffuse inflammatory reaction surrounding the bones is also seen. (Photo contributors: Haamid Chamdawala, MD [A], and John Amodio, MD [B].)

933

and choice and duration of antibiotics. Order radiographs and CT with contrast and MRI to delineate the extent of disease and find sinus tracts. Obtain blood and/or bone cultures (preferable) before initiating antibiotic therapy. Do not use surface cultures from draining sinuses or skin ulcers because these are not representative of the causative pathogen organism. Diagnosis is ultimately made from biopsy histopathology and culture. The primary treatment is adequate debridement of dead tissue and removal of sinus tracts by a specialist trained in such procedures. Antibiotics are a supplement to these procedures and will be continued for at least 3 months and often longer depending on the clinical presentation.

Pearls

1. Patients with chronic osteomyelitis often are symptomatic for weeks to several months.
2. Draining sinuses are a hallmark of this disease.
3. Debridement of dead tissue is crucial to treatment.

Clinical Features

Osteomyelitis is the second most common infection (after pneumonia) in patients with sickle cell disease (SCD). Patients present with fever and pain of the affected area. Signs and symptoms are similar to those described in acute osteomyelitis (see page 930); however, patients with SCD may be ill appearing with a more acute onset and may have multiple boney foci. The most common pathogen is *Salmonella* species followed by *S aureus, Streptococcus pyogenes, Streptococcus pneumoniae*, and other gram-negative organisms (eg, *Shigella* species, *Escherichia coli*). It is difficult to differentiate osteomyelitis from vaso-occlusive crisis in these patients. Both diagnoses can present with fever, leukocytosis, and elevation of inflammatory markers. The persistence of symptoms despite adequate hydration and pain control should prompt further workup for osteomyelitis.

Emergency Department Treatment and Disposition

Obtain CBC, blood culture, ESR, and CRP. Order imaging studies including plain radiographs, bone scan, and/or MRI, which may show more extensive lesions with osteomyelitis versus simple infarction. Consult orthopedic, infectious disease, and hematology for additional diagnostic workup and management including hospitalization. Gadolinium-67 or bone marrow scan of lesions with technetium-99m sulfur colloid will show increased uptake of radionuclide with infection as compared to infarction. Diagnosis often requires biopsy for

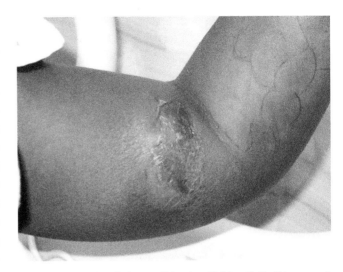

FIGURE 19.94 ■ Osteomyelitis in Sickle Cell Disease. A 15-year-old girl with sickle cell anemia presented with left arm pain for 6 weeks followed by swelling that was associated with discoloration of the skin, tenderness, and warmth. (Photo contributor: Haamid Chamdawala, MD.)

histopathology and culture. Time and clinical condition of the patient permitting, all appropriate cultures (blood and bone) are obtained prior to a presumptive antibiotic regimen (eg, high-dose ceftriaxone and vancomycin).

Pearl

1. Differentiation from vaso-occlusive crisis often requires bone biopsy and culture.

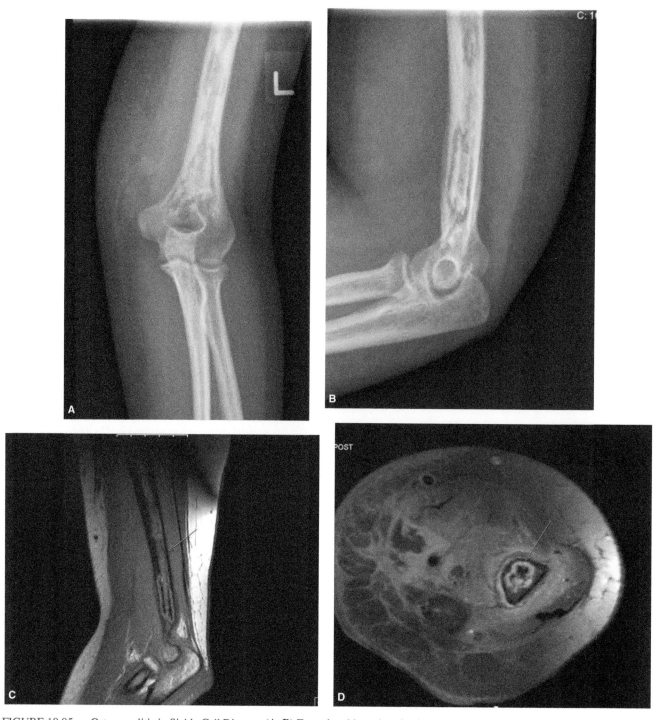

FIGURE 19.95 ■ Osteomyelitis in Sickle Cell Disease. (**A, B**) Frontal and lateral projections of the left humerus and elbow show extensive areas of lysis and sclerosis in the distal humerus with periosteal reaction. (**C**) Sagittal T1-weighted image of humerus demonstrates extensive replacement of the normal bone marrow signal (arrow). (**D**) Axial image of the distal humerus demonstrates enhancing bone marrow signal (arrow) with extensive enhancing, surrounding inflammatory response. Biopsy of the humerus revealed osteomyelitis and culture grew *Salmonella*. (Photo contributor: John Amodio, MD.)

Clinical Summary

Septic arthritis results from microbial invasion of the joint space, and clinical presentation varies with age and pathogen type. Infants present with a swollen and painful extremity held in a fixed position. Children present with a limp or refusal to use the limb, and adolescents report pain and have limited use of a specific joint. Most patients have signs of edema, redness, warmth, and tenderness, although the younger the patient, the more difficult it is to localize the affected joint because these signs involve the entire limb. Fever is more common in younger patients. Large joints of the lower extremity such as the hip and knee are most commonly affected. Pediatric emergency physicians commonly employ Kocher's criteria to evaluate the likelihood of a septic joint. This clinical prediction rule confers a point to each of the following factors: non–weight-bearing joint, fever >38.5°C, WBC >12,000/mm³, and

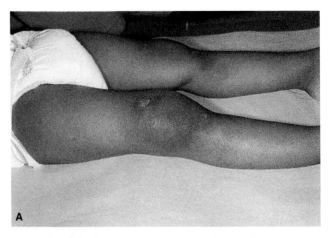

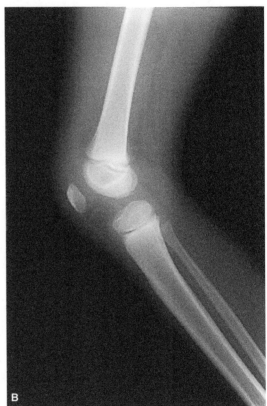

FIGURE 19.96 ■ Septic Arthritis. (**A**) A picture of a young child with septic arthritis of the right knee. (**B**) The x-ray demonstrates an opacification of the suprapatellar bursa indicative of a joint effusion. (Photo contributor: Binita R. Shah, MD.)

TABLE 19.6 ■ ETIOLOGIES AND DIAGNOSIS OF SEPTIC ARTHRITIS BY AGE

Age	Pathogen
Neonate	*Staphylococcus aureus*
	Streptococcus agalactiae
	Enteric gram negatives
	Salmonella spp
	Coagulase-negative *Staphylococcus*
Child	*S aureus* (most common)
	Streptococcus pyogenes (second most common)
	Streptococcus pneumoniae
	Other gram negatives (*Haemophilus influenzae, Kingella kingae, Salmonella* spp)
Adolescent	*S aureus*
	S pyogenes
	Neisseria gonorrhoeae

Diagnosis of Septic Arthritis

1. Suggested by a positive culture from a synovial aspirate or direct visualization of bacteria on Gram stain.
2. WBC count of the synovial fluid is essential; following WBC counts assists in diagnosis
   - <50,000/high-power field (HPF): likely inflammatory
   - 50,000–75,000/HPF: possibly infectious; differential of the WBC should be done; presence of immature neutrophils (bands) suggests infection
   - 75,000–100,000/HPF: likely infectious; strongly consider septic arthritis if the differential shows any immature neutrophils (bands)
   - >100,000/HPF: diagnosis of septic arthritis very likely

ESR >40 mm/h. The cumulative score and the corresponding predicted probability of septic arthritis are often used. However, *Kingella kingae* is a gram-negative bacterium that can present similarly to transient synovitis, with lack of fever or rise in inflammatory markers, resulting in delayed diagnosis and devastating consequences to the infected joint.

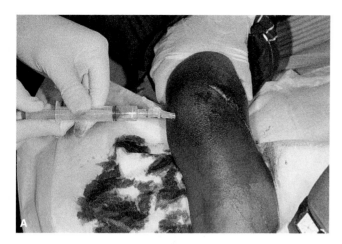
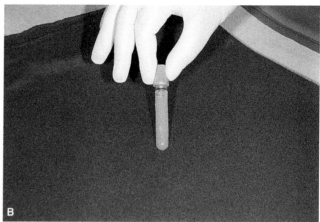

FIGURE 19.97 ■ Septic Arthritis. (**A**) A diagnostic arthrocentesis was performed in the ED in a child with septic arthritis following a laceration repair 1 week earlier. (**B**) The arthrocentesis yielded 15 mL of purulent straw-colored fluid, which on analysis had a WBC count of 110,000/high-power field. Subsequently it grew *Streptococcus pyogenes*. (Photo contributor: Binita R. Shah, MD.)

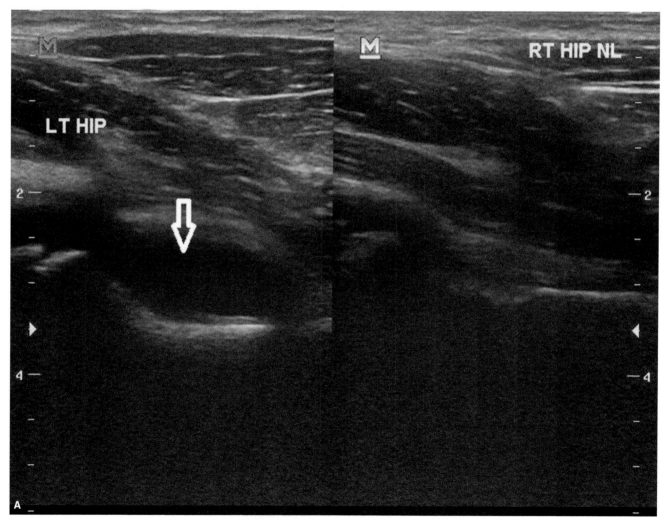

FIGURE 19.98 ■ Septic Arthritis; Point-of-Care US (POCUS). (**A**) 4-year-old child presented with limp of left lower extremity and fever for 2 days. POCUS demonstrates a left hip effusion (arrow) compared to right hip.

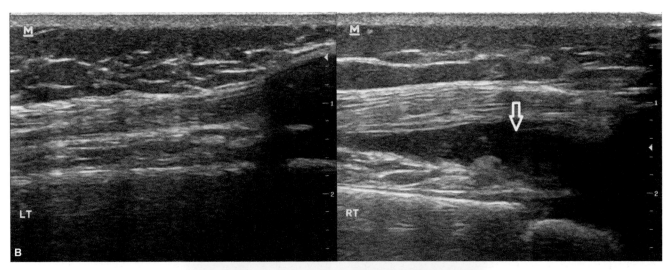

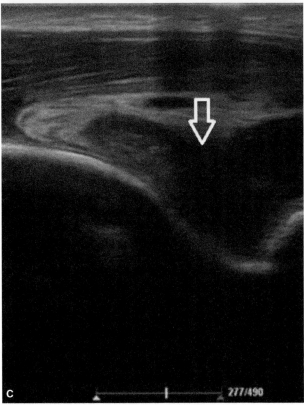

FIGURE 19.98 ■ (*Continued*) (**B**) Afebrile 2-year-old girl presented with right knee swelling and limp. Knee POCUS demonstrates a right knee effusion (arrow) compared to the left. Joint aspiration revealed WBC of 90,000 cells/mm³, concerning for septic arthritis. (**C**) A 14-year-old boy presented with 2 weeks of increasing right elbow swelling. POCUS demonstrates an echogenic elbow effusion (arrow). Aspiration at bedside revealed purulent material with a WBC of 180,000 cells/mm³ and *S aureus* growth from joint fluid culture. (Photo contributor: Sathyaseelan Subramaniam, MD.)

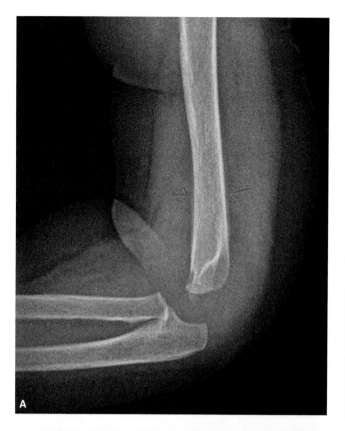

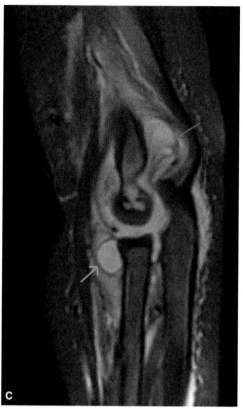

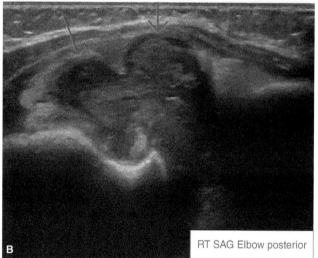

FIGURE 19.99 ■ Septic Arthritis. (**A**) Lateral view of the elbow in a 10-month-old infant presenting with elbow swelling. It reveals an elbow effusion as well as slight periosteal reaction (red arrows) along the anterior and posterior humerus, indicating a subacute process. (**B**) US of the elbow from a posterior approach shows thickened hyperemic synovium and heterogeneous material distending the joint capsule (red arrows), concerning for septic arthritis. Olecranon fossa of the distal posterior humerus (red asterisk) for anatomic reference. (**C**) Sagittal short tau inversion recovery sequence confirms the thickened synovium and joint fluid posteriorly (red arrow) and anteriorly (blue arrow). There is also abnormal T2-hyperintense signal within the distal humerus (red asterisk). Correlating with additional MRI sequences, findings were consistent with osteomyelitis of the distal humerus with septic arthritis. (Photo contributor: Ryan Logan Webb, MD.)

The differential includes Legg-Calvé-Perthes disease, slipped capital femoral epiphysis, trauma, rheumatologic conditions (eg, rheumatic fever, Lyme arthritis, juvenile rheumatoid arthritis), other infections such as osteomyelitis or pyomyositis, and arthritis due to viruses (eg, rubella, parvovirus). Transient synovitis and postinfectious reactive arthritis should be considered as diagnoses of exclusion only.

Emergency Department Treatment and Disposition

Order WBC count (may be elevated with a neutrophil predominance) and ESR and CRP. Obtain blood culture. Order radiographs of the involved joint, which will show capsular widening, soft tissue edema, and displacement of normal fat lines. If a septic hip is suspected, obtain hip films in a frog-leg position, which may show medial displacement of the obturator muscle into the pelvis (obturator sign). US and MRI may also be useful. Consult orthopedics and infectious disease for immediate additional diagnostic workup and therapy, including hospitalization. Septic joints must be drained immediately as delay may lead to permanent physical disability. Collect joint fluid for cell count and differential, glucose, Gram stain, and culture. Collect specimens in a heparinized syringe, as an inflamed joint may contain fibrinogen, clotting factors, and protein, which can cause the specimen to clot and make cell count and differential determinations difficult. Synovial fluid cell count will be elevated with a predominance of neutrophils, glucose will be low, and Gram stain and culture may be positive. Some fastidious organisms such as *K kingae* will grow more readily if joint fluid is inoculated directly into a blood culture bottle. Administer antibiotics after obtaining Gram stain and cultures; presumptive therapy should cover common etiologies (Table 19.6). Injection of antibiotics into the joint space is unnecessary as the vascular nature of these spaces allows for high levels of parenteral antibiotic concentrations in the joint. Total duration of therapy is typically 3 weeks.

Pearls

1. Septic arthritis is a surgical emergency, and immediate drainage is vital to preserve joint function.
2. Gram stain of the joint aspirate *must* be done; it may show the presence of bacteria, which may not grow in culture (culture specimens are often sterilized by the bacteriostatic properties of the synovial fluid).

Clinical Summary

Neonatal osteomyelitis is an uncommon infection, but when it occurs, diagnosis is often delayed because the initial symptoms are nonspecific. Patients present anywhere along the spectrum of well appearing with no fever and decreased movement of an extremity to toxic appearing with signs of septic shock. The affected area is swollen, discolored, painful to touch, and held in a fixed position. Newborns with septic arthritis of the hip will present with the leg in abduction with external rotation. There may be multiple foci of infection because infection spreads readily in this age. The thin bone cortex and loose periosteum in neonates allow infection to spread easily into adjacent joints and muscles. Risk factors include prematurity, heel lancet punctures, scalp electrode, venous or arterial lines, or a history of prior skin and soft tissue infection. *S aureus* is the most common pathogen, but other organisms include *Streptococcus agalactiae,* enteric gram-negative organisms such as *E coli,* and vaginal pathogens such as *Neisseria gonorrhoeae.* Consider coagulase-negative *Staphylococcus* and *Candida* if there is a history of central venous catheters. The differential diagnosis for a neonate presenting with limited use of an extremity should also include trauma (eg, child abuse), congenital malformation, malignancy, and femoral vein thrombosis.

Emergency Department Treatment and Disposition

Order WBC count, ESR, and CRP, which are typically elevated with infection. Obtain blood culture and urine culture and consider lumbar puncture (depending on the clinical scenario) preferably before initiation of antibiotics. Order plain radiographs because lesions in the neonate are detected earlier and more easily because neonatal bone is less ossified. Bone scan is not useful because the bone is not well mineralized. Consult orthopedics and infectious disease for additional workup and therapy, including hospitalization. Needle aspiration of soft tissue or incision and drainage of bone should be performed for Gram stain and culture. Lesions should be drained and sent for culture in a timely manner to facilitate prompt initiation of broad-spectrum antimicrobials (eg, vancomycin and cefotaxime). If a nosocomial source of infection is considered, broader gram-negative coverage with a carbapenem or antipseudomonal drug instead of a cephalosporin may be indicated. Consider fungal coverage with amphotericin if the infection is related to an indwelling catheter.

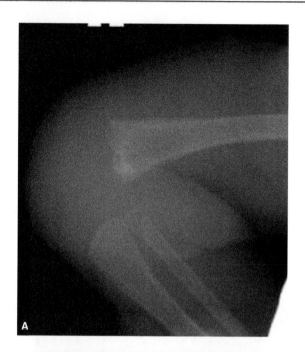

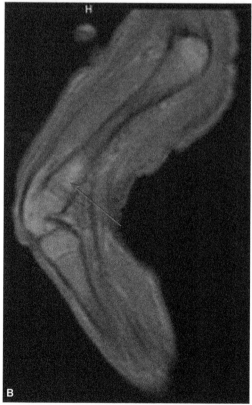

FIGURE 19.100 ■ Neonatal Osteomyelitis. (**A**) Lateral view of the distal femur demonstrates moth-eaten appearance of the metaphysis with periosteal reaction. (**B**) Sagittal T2-weighted images show abnormal bone marrow signal in the distal femoral metaphysis (red arrow) with increased signal in the surrounding soft tissue. The area of abnormal bone marrow signal corresponds to the area of plain film abnormality. (Photo contributor: John Amodio, MD.)

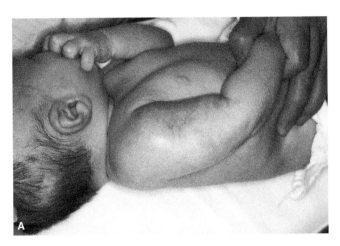

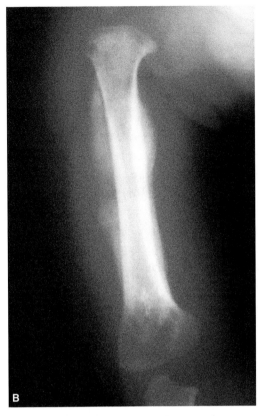

FIGURE 19.101 ■ Neonatal Osteomyelitis (OM). (**A**) Acute osteomyelitis of the humerus in a 3-week-old neonate. In acute OM, soft tissue swelling, local warmth, and tenderness are seen secondary to pus dissecting through the periosteum and soft tissues. (**B**) Frontal view of the right humerus shows cortical thickening, sclerosis, and diffuse periosteal reaction 10 days after the initial presentation. (Reproduced with permission from Shah BR, Laude TL. *Atlas of Pediatric Clinical Diagnosis*. WB Saunders; Philadelphia, PA, 2000.)

Pearl

1. Inappropriately managed osteomyelitis and/or septic arthritis in the neonate can lead to devastating consequences such as permanent bone or joint deformity, arthritis, gait abnormality, and growth disturbances.

Clinical Summary

Osteoarticular tuberculosis (TB) composes <5% of all TB cases. The causative organisms can be either *Mycobacterium tuberculosis* or *Mycobacterium bovis*. The latter species, transmitted via ingestion of dairy products, often occurs in the absence of pulmonary involvement. The most common site of osteoarticular TB is the spine, where the spondylitis is referred to as Pott disease. The thoracic and lumbar spines are equally affected, and the cervical spine is least often involved. Destruction of the anterior vertebral bodies results in the classic kyphotic gibbus deformities characteristic of spinal TB. Multiple vertebral bodies may be affected by contiguous spread; skip lesions in the spine can be seen with hematogenous dissemination. Intervertebral disk spaces are spared until late in the illness course.

The most common symptoms are back pain. In preverbal children, the first symptom parents may notice is limp or reluctance to walk. Spasming of the paraspinal muscles can cause apparent spinal rigidity. Because TB causes cold abscesses, lesions are typically not tender to the touch. Progressive kyphotic deformities and epidural abscesses can result in cord compression and paraplegia. Constitutional symptoms such as fever, malaise, and weight loss are not uniformly seen. Pott disease of the cervical spine should be on the differential diagnosis of chronic torticollis and hoarseness (from both compression on the airway and because osteoarticular TB can be seen in association with laryngeal TB). Pus can track through tissue planes and emerge at distant sites, often in the absence of other signs of inflammation.

Emergency Department Treatment and Disposition

Frontal and lateral radiographs of the entire spine are the first step in the evaluation process for children with suspected Pott disease. Radiographic findings may include destruction of multiple vertebral bodies, with the anterior aspect of the bodies more affected than the posterior. Abnormal calcification of the surrounding ligamentous structures is common. CT is more sensitive than MRI for the early detection of small vertebral lesions and paravertebral abscesses. However, evaluation for epidural abscesses is best done via MRI. MRI is also far more sensitive for detecting cord involvement and intravertebral abscesses.

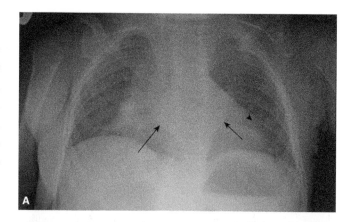

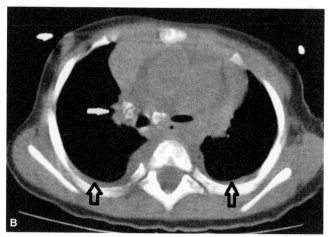

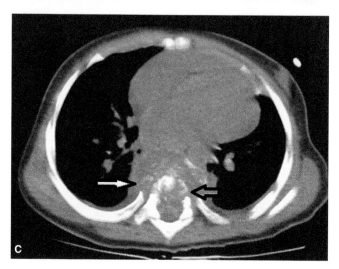

FIGURE 19.102 ■ Pott Disease. (**A**) AP view of the chest shows a paraspinal mass (arrows). (**B, C**) CT scan of the chest demonstrates enlarged calcified mediastinal and right hilar lymph nodes (yellow arrow), small bilateral pleural effusions (black arrows), a paraspinal mass (white arrow) and destruction of the adjacent vertebral body (orange arrow). (Photo/legend contributors: Diana Weaver, MD, and John Amodio, MD.)

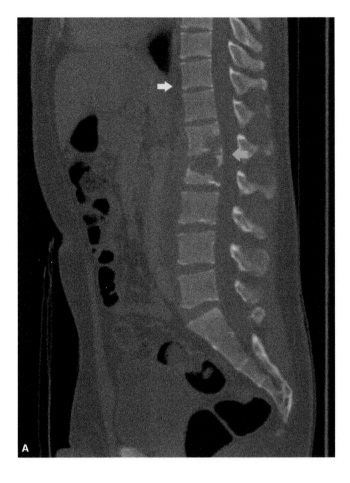

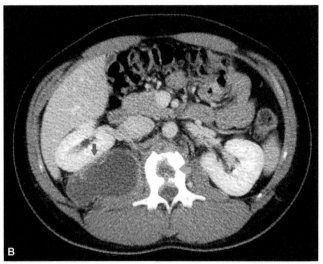

FIGURE 19.103 ■ Pott Disease. A 22-year-old man with a history of Pott disease and retroperitoneal tuberculosis presented with back pain. (**A**) Sagittal CT image of the abdomen demonstrates osseous destruction of the L1 and L2 vertebral bodies with involvement and narrowing of the L1-L2 disk space compatible with diskitis/osteomyelitis (blue arrow). There is also the beginning of kyphosis of the thoracic spine, which is classic in Pott disease (yellow arrow). (**B**) Axial CT of the same patient again shows the osseous destruction of the L2 vertebral body (blue arrow) with a right psoas abscess (red arrow). (Photo contributors: Jonathan Stern, MD, and Jeremy Neuman, MD.)

A CXR should be obtained in all children with suspected Pott disease. Although positive in only 50% of children, this can be the first indication that a child has TB, given the duration of time it takes for cultures and other TB testing to return. Also, recognition of pulmonary TB allows for isolation of the child to prevent nosocomial spread. Children with suspected Pott disease and abnormal CXRs should be placed in negative-pressure rooms, and all providers should use N95 respirators. Although Pott disease with a normal CXR does not require isolation, all providers in the operating room, if a child were to require stabilization or biopsy, should also wear N95 respirators.

Absolute indications for surgical intervention from the ED include marked neurologic deficits potentially correctable by surgery; progressive spinal instability or kyphosis (including respiratory distress from restrictive lung disease); and worsening neurologic deficits despite optimal medical therapy.

Surgeons may be consulted after the child is admitted to obtain material for biopsy or to drain abscesses.

All children in whom Pott disease is suspected should be tested for HIV. Additionally, children should have CBCs obtained because malignancy is also on the differential diagnosis, and hepatic transaminases should be obtained because almost all TB drugs are hepatically metabolized.

Pearls

1. Pott disease should be on the differential diagnosis of the child presenting with kyphosis or with vertebral body destruction of subacute/chronic onset.

2. CXRs are abnormal in 50% of children with Pott disease, and these children may have contagious forms of TB.

3. Neurosurgical or orthopedic intervention is needed for children with marked neurologic deficits.

Chapter 20

TRAUMA

Joshua Nagler
Caitlin A. Farrell
Marc Auerbach
Sydney C. Butts

Roman Shinder
Ilaaf Darrat
Lamont R. Jones

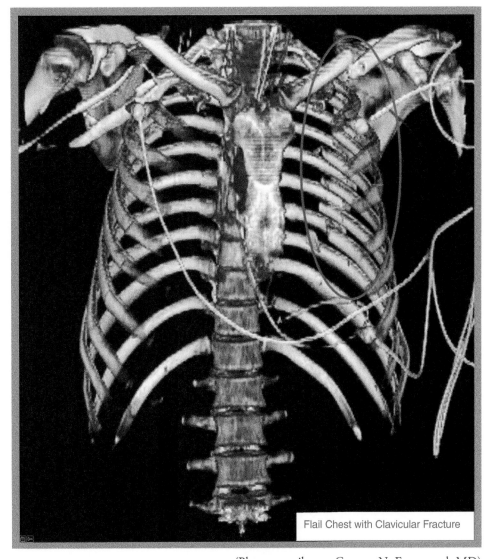

Flail Chest with Clavicular Fracture

(Photo contributor: Gregory N. Emmanuel, MD)

The authors acknowledge the special contributions of Karen Santucci, Bonny J. Baron, Audrey J. Tan, Behrad Aynehchi, Baljeet Kaur Purewal, Christopher I. Doty, Chaiya Laoteppitaks, Cynthia L. Benson, Ee Tein Tay, and Michael Lucchesi to prior edition.

Clinical Summary

Pediatric head trauma occurs commonly, with most injuries being minor; however, seemingly low-risk presentations may have intracranial injuries, and thus it is important to maintain a high index of suspicion.

Emergency Department Treatment and Disposition

The initial diagnosis and treatment of a head-injured infant or child involves evaluation in a standardized and algorithmic manner performed by a multidisciplinary and interprofessional team of providers. Selected head injury outcomes can worsen when there are delays in the time to definitive care (eg, epidural hematomas). This necessitates a prompt approach to diagnosis and treatment of all head-injured patients. First, providers should assess the airway, breathing, and circulation during a primary trauma survey. During this evaluation, providers may need to implement interventions informed by their assessment (eg, providing oxygen, inserting endotracheal tubes, beginning fluid resuscitations, immobilizing the cervical spine, raising the head of the bed).

This is followed by a more comprehensive and detailed head-to-toe secondary survey. This survey involves a thorough neurologic assessment. Pertinent positive findings on this assessment such as neurologic deficits or pupillary defects provide objective evidence of intracranial injury. The Glasgow Coma Scale (GCS) quantifies neurologic findings and allows uniformity in description and communication among team members involved in taking care of the patient. A GCS score of 14 to 15 is categorized as mild head injury; a GCS score of 9 to 13 as moderate head injury; and a GCS score <9 as severe head injury. Modified versions of this scale for children and infants have been created, such as the AVPU (alert, verbal, painful, unresponsive). Concurrent with the primary and secondary survey, additional point-of-care diagnostic tests, such as laboratories (type and cross-match, coagulation profiles, CBC, complete metabolic panel, toxicology screening) and imaging studies (x-rays and US, especially focused assessment

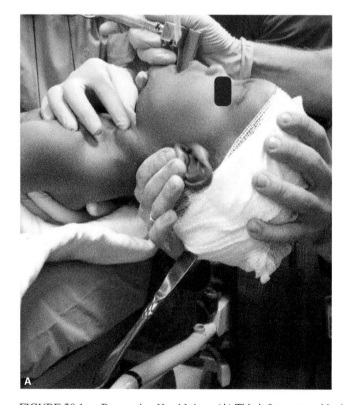
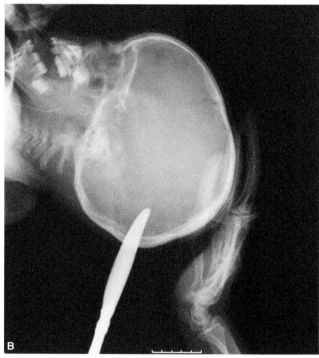

FIGURE 20.1 ■ Penetrating Head Injury. (**A**) This infant was stabbed in the head with a butter knife during a domestic dispute between his mother and angry father. He suffered no neurologic deficits after the knife was removed by neurosurgery in the operating room. (**B**) A lateral projection of the skull demonstrates the butter knife embedded within the occipital-parietal region of the skull. (Photo/legend contributors: Mark Silverberg, MD, and John Amodio, MD.)

948

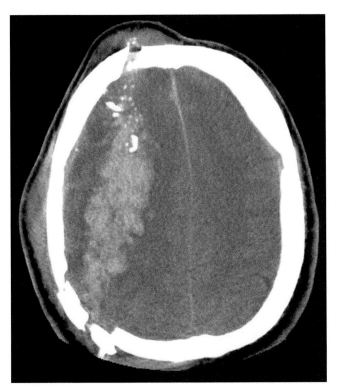

FIGURE 20.2 ▪ Penetrating Head Injury. An axial slice from a non-contrast head CT shows a penetrating gunshot wound with fracture of the frontal and parietal bones and large hemorrhagic contusion along the tract of the bullet. High-density bullet fragments are also noted in the frontal region of the brain. (Photo/legend contributors: Mark Silverberg, MD, and John Amodio, MD.)

with sonography in trauma [FAST]), are obtained. The definitive test for severely head-injured patients is a noncontrast CT of the head. This test should be obtained in patients with penetrating injury, a high-risk mechanism of blunt injury, clinical signs of basilar or depressed skull fracture, a posttraumatic seizure, a large scalp hematoma (especially parietal/temporal), repetitive vomiting, prolonged lethargy, amnesia, past history of bleeding diathesis (eg, hemophilia), significant past medical history (eg, shunts), or suspected abusive head injury (<1 year of age). Any patients with intracranial injury should be promptly evaluated by a neurosurgeon to determine the need for medical or surgical interventions. Patients with foreign bodies should only be manipulated during operative removal by a neurosurgeon.

In patients with cervical spine tenderness, with neurologic deficits, and/or who are unable to be evaluated based on their mental status, lateral neck radiographs and/or CT of the neck should be obtained. When signs of herniation are present, such as Cushing triad (bradycardia, hypertension, and irregular

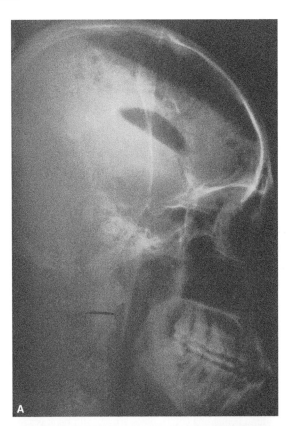

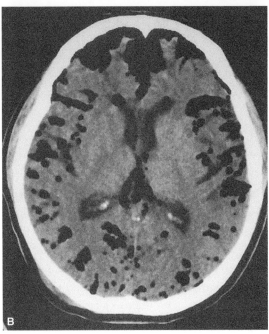

FIGURE 20.3 ▪ Pneumocephalus. (A) Lateral skull film of a 19-year-old man who sustained multiple stab wounds to the head, demonstrating extensive pneumocephalus. The bony matrix could not be conclusively evaluated because of the pneumocephalus. (B) A CT scan of the head of the same patient demonstrates numerous pockets of air in the sulci with marked subarachnoid pneumocephalus. (Photo/legend contributors: Binita R. Shah, MD, and John Amodio, MD.)

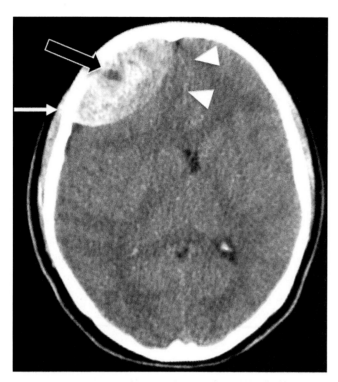

FIGURE 20.4 ■ Epidural Hematoma. Axial noncontrast CT scan in a patient following head trauma demonstrates a right frontal acute epidural hematoma (EDH, black arrow) with biconvex shape. Note the posterior border of the EDH is limited by the coronal suture (white arrow). Mass effect is present with compression of the right frontal lobe and leftward midline shift (arrowheads). Following craniotomy and evacuation of EDH, mass effect and midline shift had resolved. (Photo contributors: Rabia Malik, MD, and Vinodkumar Velayudhan, DO.)

respirations), neuroprotective measures such as elevation of the head of the bed and mild hyperventilation (targeting end-tidal carbon dioxide to 30 to 35 mm Hg) must be initiated prior to imaging. Recent large-cohort studies on children with minor head injury have been published that give clinicians access to clinical decision rules that help guide the need for CT scan, observation, or discharge from the ED without any imaging. These minor head injury rules, such as the Pediatric Emergency Care Applied Research Network (PECARN) head injury prediction rule, have been validated and successfully applied worldwide and have led to the reduction in unnecessary CT scans in children. Patients who meet low-risk criteria should be observed for a period of time as part of a tertiary survey because injuries such as epidural and subdural hematomas can progress over time after the initial injury.

The tertiary survey can involve a period of observation, including assessment after oral intake as well as adequacy of age-appropriate ambulation. Children with low-risk injuries can be identified using validated head injury decision tools, which provide the ED clinician tools to safely avoid exposing the child to ionizing radiation from CT scans.

Patients with elevated intracranial pressure identified by signs of herniation should be managed with neuroprotective agents. Treatment with 3% normal saline or mannitol should be administered to temporarily reduce intracranial pressure when there is clinical evidence of raised intracranial pressure with worsening vital signs. Pain should be managed with narcotic analgesics as appropriate. Endotracheal intubation should be performed with medications to paralyze and sedate the patient in order to blunt the spike in intracranial pressure. Short-acting paralytics are preferred in order to obtain a neurologic examination. Prophylaxis for seizure in head-injured patients can be initiated if severe intracranial hemorrhage is present and/or the patient requires paralysis for their interventions, which has a potential to mask overt seizure activity.

Patients may require admission for observation, neurosurgical consultation, or transfer to a higher level of care. Patients who are discharged require written instructions for the family and communication with the patient's medical home or pediatrician related to follow-up. Communication with the caretaker should include the directive to return to the ED immediately if the patient develops any of the following: (1) excessive sleepiness or difficulty in awakening; (2) confusion or abnormal behavior; (3) severe progression of headache; (4) intractable vomiting or nausea; (5) abnormal gait; (6) ataxia; (7) unequal pupils, double vision, or any visual disturbance; (8) seizures; or (9) bleeding or watery drainage from the nose or ear. Patients and care providers should be provided clear instructions regarding activities and returning to sport. Resources have been developed by the CDC to support providers and families in this process. "Heads Up" program link (https://www.cdc.gov/headsup/youthsports/index.html).

Pearls

1. Diffuse brain injury (concussion or diffuse axonal injury) is the most common type of head injury.

2. Prevent secondary brain injury in patients presenting with head trauma or multiple trauma with timely and age-appropriate management.

3. Patients with epidural hematoma may present with the classic lucid interval and acutely deteriorate ("talk and die").

Clinical Summary

Skull fractures occur because of a direct impact to the calvarium. The parietal bone is involved most frequently. Linear fractures are most common (about 75%), followed by depressed and basilar fractures. Approximately 30% of children with depressed skull fractures have an associated intracranial injury. Typical head injury mechanisms include falls, sports injuries, and motor vehicle collisions. The morbidity and mortality from closed head injuries increase when there are associated extracranial injuries. Skull fractures are classified by appearance, location, degree of depression, and whether there is an associated scalp laceration. Comminuted skull fractures are multiple linear fractures. Open skull fractures are rare but increase the risk of CNS infection. Physical examination findings for skull fractures vary and include hematoma, a palpable step-off or skull defect, and crepitus.

Most linear skull fractures heal without complications and do not require surgical interventions.

Emergency Department Treatment and Disposition

For a detailed approach to head trauma, see page 948. CT of the head is the ideal test for diagnosis. Although radiographs may rule in a fracture, they cannot exclude intracranial injury. Clinical assessment is more difficult in children <2 years of age and especially those <3 months old, although these children are more susceptible to injury from even minor trauma. Children of this age are also at greater risk of being victims of physical abuse, developing a growing fracture, and having associated intracranial injuries. ED providers must maintain a high index of suspicion and a lower threshold for obtaining

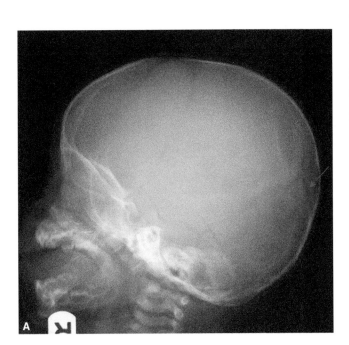
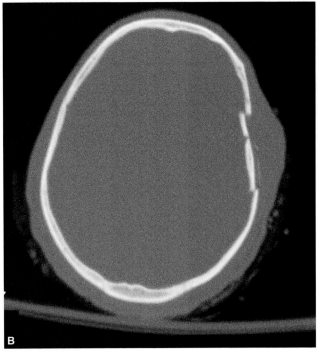

FIGURE 20.5 ■ Skull Fractures. (**A**) A lateral projection of the skull shows a fracture of the parietal region (arrow). (**B**) An axial CT slice shows a comminuted depressed fracture of the left parietal bone in a different patient. (Photo/legend contributors: Mark Silverberg, MD, and John Amodio, MD.)

radiographic imaging, typically CT, in this age group. Additionally, in nonverbal patients, a further diagnostic evaluation for physical abuse should be obtained, which may include skeletal survey and other laboratory testing. All patients in whom child abuse is suspected should be reported to child protective services, and some may need to be hospitalized.

ED providers must consult neurosurgery for patients with depressed, basilar, or widely diastatic skull fractures, and these patients often need to be hospitalized for observation to an ICU for frequent neurologic checks. All patients with persistent neurologic deficits, persistent vomiting, suspected nonaccidental injury, or unreliable guardians should also be hospitalized.

Pearls

1. Consider hospitalization for children with skull fracture if the patient is <6 months old, the patient has a large scalp swelling over the fracture, injury follows a known high-energy mechanism of injury, or the fracture location is concerning (eg, crossing a suture, extending into posterior fossa, or in a dural venous sinus or a vascular groove).

2. Normal variants, such as vascular grooves, open metopic sutures, posterior fossa sutures, and accessory sutures, may mimic skull fractures on plain radiographs.

Clinical Summary

Basilar skull fractures (BSFs) are injuries that involve the base of the skull, typically involving the petrous portion of the temporal bone (but can involve any skull base). Patients present with distinct clinical findings (80% of cases) that include Battle sign (postauricular ecchymosis suggesting a mastoid fracture), raccoon eyes or periorbital ecchymosis (intraorbital bleeding from orbital roof fractures), hemotympanum, CSF rhinorrhea or otorrhea or cranial nerve palsies, tinnitus, hearing loss, anosmia, nausea, vomiting vertigo, or nystagmus. BSFs with underlying dural tears have an increased association with CSF leaks and thus an increased risk of intracranial infection (eg, *Streptococcus pneumoniae, Streptococcus pyogenes, Haemophilus influenzae*). Other complications include hearing loss (conductive or sensorineural in up to half of the children).

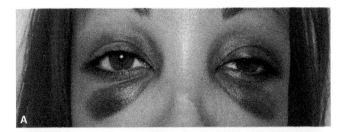
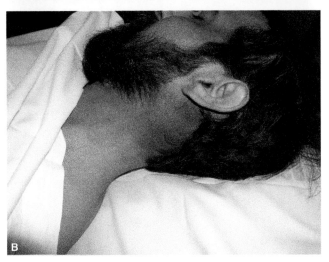

FIGURE 20.7 ■ Basilar Skull Fracture. (**A**) "Raccoon eyes" are pictured here in this teenager with a 4-day-old basilar skull fracture. (**B**) Battle sign occurs when blood from a skull fracture tracks down to the neck and is visible there as a blue/purple discoloration seen under the skin. In this case, there are some green hues as well, signifying that the blood has been around for a while and is starting to break down. (Photo contributor: Mark Silverberg, MD.)

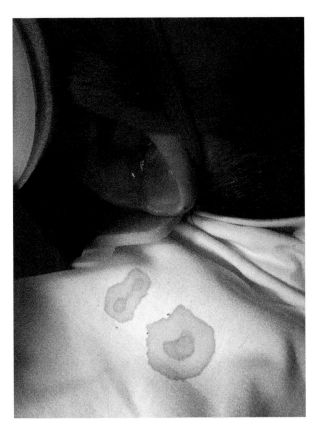

FIGURE 20.6 ■ Otorrhea; Basilar Skull Fracture. Otorrhea is seen here coming from the ear of this patient with a basilar skull fracture. When CSF is dripped onto filter paper or fabric, it forms these classic "rings." (Photo contributor: Cynthia Benson, MD.)

Emergency Department Treatment and Disposition

For a detailed approach to head trauma, see page 948. In addition, when performing CT of the head, these patients need dedicated temporal bone tomography cuts that require a specific protocol (up to 40% of BSFs are missed by CT scan). Children may need to be hospitalized to the ICU for neurologic monitoring and neurosurgical management.

Pearls

1. BSF usually results from a considerable force.
2. Do not insert a nasogastric tube because it may lead to inadvertent passage through an injured cribriform plate.
3. Cranial nerve palsies (eg, I, VII, VIII, X) may be seen immediately or a few days after the injury as intracranial swelling increases.

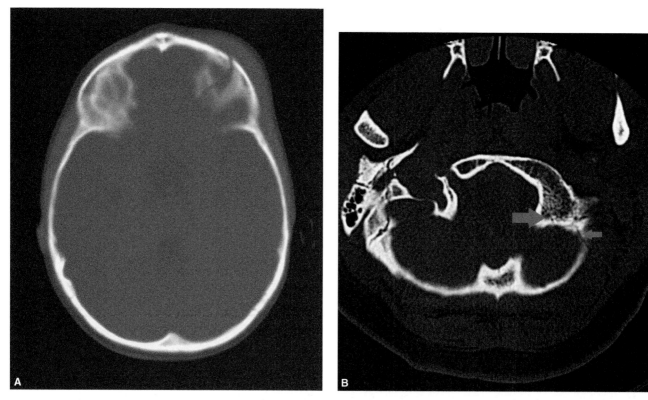

FIGURE 20.8 ■ Basilar Skull Fracture. (**A**) An axial CT slice through the roof of the orbits shows a nondisplaced fracture of the roof of the left orbit. (**B**) An axial CT slice of the cervical spine demonstrates an acute nondisplaced fracture of the left skull base/occipital bone extending into the left occipital condyle (red arrows) in a patient presenting to the ED with headache, vomiting, and dizziness after falling off a ladder from 8 feet and hitting the back of her head on the floor. (Photo contributors: Mark Silverberg, MD [A], Danielle Del Re, MD, and Dan Klein, MD [B].)

Clinical Summary

Subdural hematoma (SDH) occurs when the bridging veins between the dura and the arachnoid membranes are disrupted. SDHs are seen with significant mechanisms of injury and are often associated with underlying brain injury (eg, intracerebral hematomas, contusions). SDH may be bilateral and occur more commonly than epidural hematoma. Nonaccidental trauma is a common etiology, especially when the child is <2 years of age, and infants may present without any history of trauma with symptoms of irritability, a full fontanelle, vomiting, altered mental status, seizures, and/or focal neurologic signs. Predisposing factors for development of SDHs with minor or no history of injury include osteogenesis imperfecta, glutaric aciduria type I, arachnoid cysts, cerebral atrophy, history of hydrocephalus, or bleeding disorders.

Emergency Department Treatment and Disposition

For a detailed approach to head trauma, see page 948. As above, when there is suspicion of child abuse, patients need additional testing. All patients with an SDH should be hospitalized in an ICU for close monitoring. When necessary to operate, a craniotomy or craniectomy will effectively evacuate subdural hemorrhage in roughly 80% of patients. Many of these patients will have associated intraparenchymal injuries. Even in the most critically injured children, surgical intervention may not be helpful.

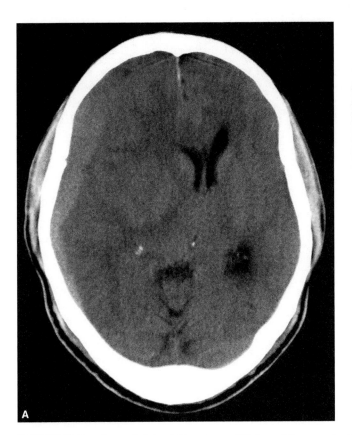
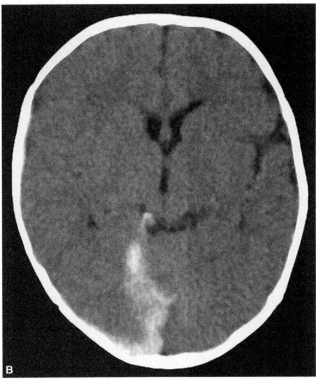

FIGURE 20.9 ■ Acute Subdural Hematoma. (**A**) An axial noncontrast head CT slice shows acute right subdural hematoma with a midline shift from significant mass effect. (**B**) An axial noncontrast CT scan demonstrates posterior interhemispheric subdural hematoma with dissection into quadrigeminal plate cistern. (Photo/legend contributors: Mark Silverberg, MD, and John Amodio, MD.)

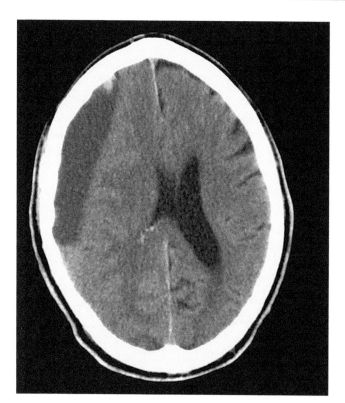

FIGURE 20.10 ■ Subdural Hematoma. An axial noncontrast head CT slice shows a large right subdural hematoma with a "hematocrit effect" indicating acute and chronic hemorrhage (hematocrit effect with fluid-fluid levels is the result by layering of heavier cellular elements of blood located dependent to a liquid supernatant and can be seen on CT or MRI). There is significant mass effect present, with a midline shift. Also note effacement of the right cerebral gyri from cerebral edema. (Photo/legend contributors: Mark Silverberg, MD, and John Amodio, MD.)

Pearls

1. The majority of SDHs in infants and children <2 years old are caused by inflicted head injuries, and children may present with very nonspecific clinical signs.

2. SDHs are seen as areas of increased density that appear concave (or crescent shaped), covering and compressing the gyri and sulci over an entire hemisphere.

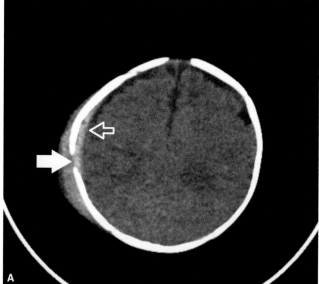

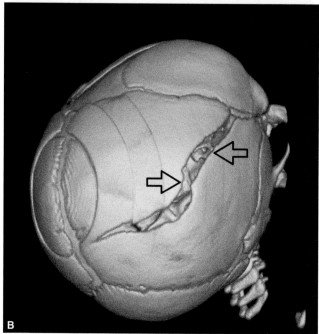

FIGURE 20.11 ■ Acute Subdural Hematoma. (**A**) Axial CT image demonstrates an acute displaced right parietal bone fracture (solid arrow) with underlying acute subdural hematoma (hollow arrow) in a 1-month-old infant presenting with right scalp swelling following "trauma." This is nonaccidental trauma (abusive head injuries/ shaken impact syndrome) unless and until proven otherwise. A multidisciplinary team including child abuse specialist, social worker, and child protective services will need to be consulted during evaluation of such injuries. (**B**) A 3-dimensional reformatted CT image better illustrates the acute displaced parietal bone fracture and can be useful for identifying nondisplaced fractures. (Photo contributors: Gregory N. Emmanuel, MD, and Dan Klein, MD.)

Clinical Summary

Epidural or extradural hematoma (EDH) is collection of blood between the dura and overlying calvarium. Common causes include low-velocity impact (falls) and nonaccidental injury, motor vehicle collisions (adolescents), and occasionally forceps delivery in neonates. Delayed EDH may occur in polytrauma patient. EDHs may be of arterial or venous origin. Temporal EDHs are often due to injury to the middle meningeal artery (about 80%) or injury to the middle meningeal vein and dural sinus. In children, there are fewer temporal EDHs, and the most common sites are frontal, parietooccipital, and posterior fossa. A patient with EDH may present with an asymptomatic period (lucid period) followed by headache, vomiting, and altered mental status that may progress to signs and symptoms of uncal herniation (ipsilateral fixed or dilated pupil with contralateral hemiparesis).

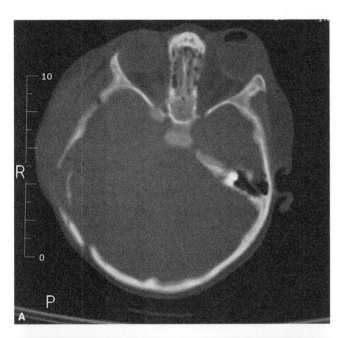

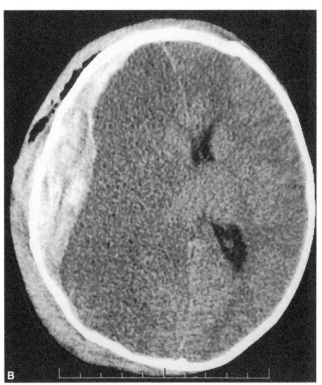

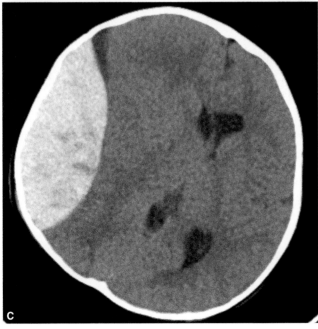

FIGURE 20.12 ■ Epidural Hematoma. The head CT scan of a 12-month-old boy who had a 27-inch television fall onto his head. (**A**) Multiple skull fractures of the right frontal, temporal, and occipital bones are seen in this bone window. (**B**) A large area of hyperdensity extending from the right frontal to the right parietal region, representing a large epidural hematoma, is seen. Extensive hypodensity involving the right cerebral hemisphere and left frontal lobe, compatible with cerebral edema, and significant mass effect compressing the right lateral ventricles and causing a midline shift to the left are also seen. Diffuse soft tissue swelling and air overlying the right side of the skull are also seen. (**C**) Axial CT image in an 11-month-old infant following "blunt trauma" demonstrates large epidural hematoma with significant mass effect. Nonaccidental trauma needs to be excluded when there is lack of plausible explanation in evaluating such injuries. (Photo contributors: Binita R. Shah, MD [A, B], Gregory N. Emmanuel, MD, and Dan Klein, MD [C].)

Emergency Department Treatment and Disposition

For a detailed approach to head trauma, see page 948. Prompt evaluation and timely diagnosis are critical for successful management of an EDH. Imaging will reveal a biconvex or lenticular increased density of fresh blood. EDH is usually unilateral and localized and does not cross suture lines (because the outer layer of dura attaches to the skull there, preventing blood from expanding past it). Consult neurosurgery emergently because the evacuation of EDH is necessary if there is any evidence of worsening mental status, an expanding bleed, or midline shift. Hospitalize all patients with EDH in an ICU (even if EDH is small and patient is asymptomatic) for close monitoring and serial head CT scans.

Pearls

1. Expanding EDHs are potentially life threatening and often lead to herniation if not recognized promptly.
2. Infants and young children have a higher frequency of venous EDHs.
3. Younger children with open sutures may not be symptomatic until their condition is critical.
4. EDHs may occur without evidence of an overlying fracture, making the diagnosis challenging.

Clinical Summary

Brain contusions (intracerebral hematomas) result from direct external contact forces or from the brain striking the inner surface of the skull during an acceleration/deceleration type of trauma. A classic coup injury will occur at the site of impact, and a contrecoup injury will occur at a site remote to the impact site. Most contusions occur in the frontal and temporal lobes (may occur anywhere in the brain). These areas of bruising are associated with localized edema, ischemia, and mass effect.

Emergency Department Treatment and Disposition

For a detailed approach to head trauma, see page 948. In addition to a CT, an MRI should be obtained because it is more sensitive in discovering cerebral contusions since CT may not reveal nonhemorrhagic contusions or small petechial

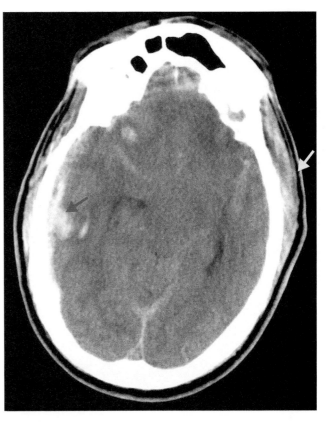

FIGURE 20.14 ■ Coup and Contrecoup Injury. The head CT scan of a young male patient who after becoming intoxicated fell to the ground, striking the left side of his head. Note the large left-sided scalp contusion (coup injury, yellow arrow). Also note the right-sided cerebral contusion (contrecoup injury, red arrow). (Photo contributor: Mark Silverberg, MD.)

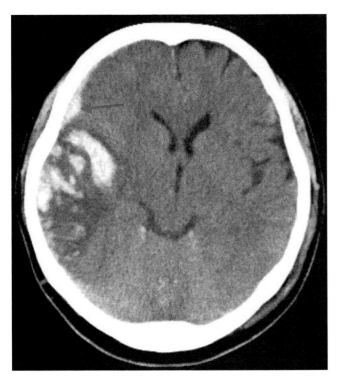

FIGURE 20.13 ■ Cerebral Contusion. An axial noncontrast head CT slice shows blood within the gyri and brain parenchyma compatible with cerebral hemorrhagic contusion. A small subdural hematoma is also present (arrow). There is a slight shift of the midline from mass effect. (Photo/legend contributors: Mark Silverberg, MD, and John Amodio, MD.)

hemorrhages. Consult neurosurgery, and admit to ICU patients with CT evidence of cerebral contusion or neurologic signs or symptoms or patients who have unreliable caretakers. Patients with simple concussions or nonhemorrhagic contusions with no neurologic symptoms can be discharged home with detailed instructions explaining what to watch for in case of cerebral injury.

Pearls

1. Patients with brain contusions may present with focal neurologic signs and/or confusion and an impaired level of consciousness.
2. MRI is the modality of choice to diagnose nonhemorrhagic cerebral contusions.
3. Brain contusions may delay the recovery process of a concussion.

CEREBRAL CONCUSSION

Clinical Summary

Mild traumatic brain injury (TBI) is a fairly common and important public health problem. It is usually benign but can have serious short- and long-term sequelae. A concussion is defined as a complex pathophysiologic process affecting the brain, induced by traumatic biomechanical forces. The hallmarks of concussion are headache and confusion with or without amnesia, often without a history of loss of consciousness. Frequently observed signs/symptoms of a concussion are vacant stare, unrelenting headache, memory deficits, incoordination, inability to focus, perseveration, slurred or incoherent speech, emotional extremes, and disorientation. Early posttraumatic seizures (within the first week after a head injury) occur in <5% of mild or moderate TBIs and are associated with a higher risk of posttraumatic epilepsy. It should be noted that a substantial number of children with concussion can have minor symptoms or be asymptomatic at initial presentation.

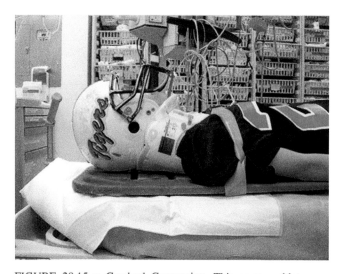

FIGURE 20.15 ■ Cerebral Concussion. This young athlete sustained a cerebral concussion during a football game. It is important to leave the helmet on until it can be properly removed by a person who is trained to do so without risking further injury. (Photo contributor: Randi Ozaki, MD.)

Emergency Department Treatment and Disposition

For a detailed approach to head trauma, see page 948. As stated earlier, not all patients with mild head injury require a CT scan, and clinical decision tools have been developed that can assist providers in risk stratifying patients to determine the need for a CT. Lower risk patients should be observed over a period of time with imaging performed when there are signs of deterioration. Patients with a GCS score <15, any abnormality on CT scan, history of a seizure, not tolerating fluids, any abnormal bleeding parameters, or a home environment where the patient cannot be checked on regularly require admission to the hospital. If a patient is discharged, instruct the caregiver to seek medical care if there is difficulty waking the child, vomiting, a worsening headache, deteriorating vision, restlessness or confusion, weakness or numbness, or any evidence of urinary or bowel incontinence.

Guidelines for return to play are available through the CDC website. With severe concussions, it is best to recommend that the child have a follow-up with their primary doctor and not play contact sports for at least 1 week after all symptoms have resolved. Consult neurology and/or a sports medicine specialist for patient and caregiver counseling to help avoid second-impact syndrome—a phenomenon where patients develop permanent neurologic symptoms after a second concussion soon after the first event.

Pearls

1. A mild TBI/concussion is an injury to the brain that results from acceleration/deceleration or a blunt force and generally does not show up on any radiologic imaging modality.
2. Patients who suffer a TBI need to be evaluated by a professional, and evidence based advice to guide return to play is recommended.

Clinical Summary

Nasal septal hematomas are collections of blood between the avascular septal cartilage and perichondrium and are almost always associated with facial trauma such as from motor vehicle collisions, sporting injuries, or assault. Intranasal surgery may also cause such an injury. Buckling forces result in tearing of the submucosal vessels underlying the perichondrium. Because the perichondrium is the sole blood supply to the cartilage, hematomas result in avascular necrosis of the cartilage if not drained promptly. Stagnant blood may promote bacterial proliferation and abscess formation as well. Accompanying fracture of the 2- to 4-mm-thick septal cartilage may lead to the formation of bilateral hematomas. Common complaints include nasal obstruction, pain, and epistaxis. Fever is less frequent in the acute phase but may mark the progression of a hematoma to an abscess. Associated physical findings include external nasal deformity and significant tenderness to palpation. Early diagnosis and drainage are critical to prevent consequences of cartilaginous ischemia, including septal perforation and saddle-nose deformity. Failure to manage these collections may result in more serious complications, including intracranial extension of any infection that develops as a result of the hematoma.

Emergency Department Treatment and Disposition

Perform a physical examination with a nasal speculum and a headlight. An asymmetric septum with a blue or red hue confirms the diagnosis, and direct palpation along the septum with a gloved finger or cotton-tipped applicator will reveal swelling or fluctuance. Use endoscopic nasal examination with a fiberoptic scope to better visualize the hematoma and better determine its extent.

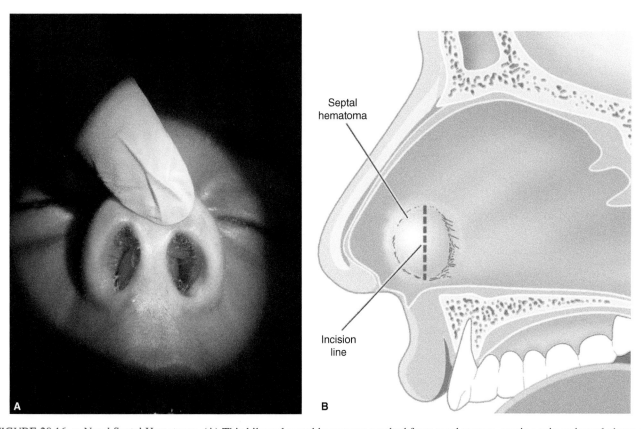

FIGURE 20.16 ■ Nasal Septal Hematoma. (**A**) This bilateral septal hematoma resulted from nasal trauma, causing pain and nasal obstruction. Rapid drainage of the hematoma is required to prevent the development of a septal necrosis or septal abscess. (**B**) Nasal septal hematoma evacuation. Nasal septal hematoma with markings for a vertical incision through the mucoperichondrium. (Photo contributors: Jessyka Lighthall, MD [A], and [B] reproduced with permission from Reichman EF. *Emergency Medicine Procedures*. 3rd ed. McGraw-Hill Education; New York, NY, 2019.)

Perform incision and drainage as soon as possible; this may require ENT consultation and may need to be done in an operating room, especially in young children. Incise the mucosa over the area of greatest fluctuance without involving the cartilage. If bilateral hematomas are present, stagger the incisions to avoid iatrogenic perforation. Suction clots and purulent fluid and collect cultures. Place a small passive drain, such as a cut Penrose or large vessel loop, under the septal flap to prevent reaccumulation and suture it to the edge of the incision. Small bilateral anterior packs or septal splints are placed in the nostrils to prevent recollection. Antibiotics that cover gram-positive organisms and β-lactamase–producing organisms are prescribed. Patients with a septal abscess are recommended to receive a course of IV antibiotics due to the risk of septic thrombophlebitis of nasal veins, which are valveless and allow potential intracranial spread of infection.

Obtain a CT scan of the brain and sinuses in any patient with signs of systemic infection to rule out septal abscess.

Refer patients for follow-up with an otolaryngologist to remove packing and drains within 5 days. Patients will also need annual follow-up for monitoring of septal developmental abnormalities due to potential septal cartilage destruction.

Pearls

1. Septal hematomas in children can occur with minor trauma, including simple falls or altercations. Younger children, including infants and toddlers, presenting with septal hematomas without concomitant injuries should raise the suspicion of child abuse.
2. Abscess formation is the most common complication of septal hematomas; failure to manage this collection may result in serious complications, including intracranial abscesses, orbital cellulitis, meningitis, and cavernous sinus thrombosis.

Clinical Summary

Nasal fractures are the most common facial fractures in children and must not be confused with nasoorbitoethmoid (NOE)-type injuries, which are far less frequent (Table 20.1). Typical etiologies of nasal trauma include falls, sports injuries, motor vehicle collisions, and physical confrontations. The nasal bones articulate with the nasal septum, which can also be fractured. Patients may complain of pain and nasal obstruction. Significant obstruction may result in mouth breathing and new-onset snoring. Fracture/dislocations of the nasal bones are typically associated with swelling and ecchymosis in the region and occasionally an overlying laceration. Many patients will also present with epistaxis.

Emergency Department Treatment and Disposition

Manage immediate life-threatening injuries first and stabilize airway, breathing, and circulation. Perform a complete physical examination, including a nasal speculum examination to exclude septal hematoma. Control epistaxis with cold packs

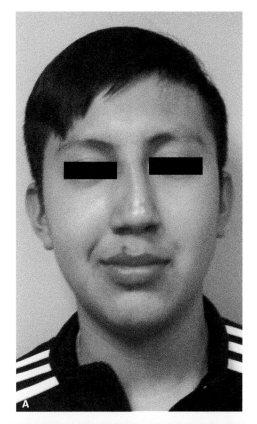

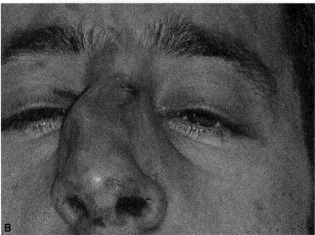

FIGURE 20.17 ■ Nasal Fracture. (**A**) A 15-year-old boy with a moderately displaced nasal fracture from an elbow to the nose while playing basketball. (**B**) This gentleman was assaulted with the butt of a gun. His severely displaced nasal fracture is obvious. (Photo contributors: Sydney C. Butts, MD [A], and Mark Silverberg, MD [B].)

TABLE 20.1 ■ EXPECTED CLINICAL FINDINGS IN PATIENTS PRESENTING WITH SIMPLE NASAL FRACTURES COMPARED TO NASOORBITOETHMOID (NOE) FRACTURES

Clinical Finding	Isolated Nasal Fracture	NOE Complex Fracture
Mucosal lacerations	+/−	+/−
Bony step-offs or deviations	+/−	+
Swelling or edema	++	+++
Septal disruption	+	+
Septal hematoma	+/−	+/−
CSF rhinorrhea	−	+/−
Double vision or decreased visual acuity	−	+/−
Localized facial numbness	−	+/−
Telecanthus	−	++
Enophthalmos	−	+/−
Nasal telescoping	−	++
Flattened nasal dorsum	−	++
Periorbital ecchymosis	+/−	++

and light pressure and consider use of topical decongestants to help control bleeding and aid visualization as well. If these methods do not stop the bleeding, use nasal packing. Document mucosal lacerations, septal deviation, or septal hematoma.

963

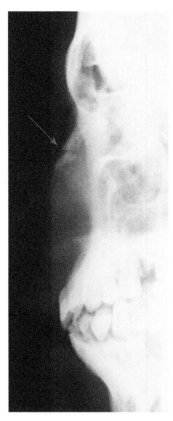

FIGURE 20.18 ■ Nasal Fracture. This lateral view of the nasal bones shows a depressed nasal bone fracture. The anterior maxillary spine is intact (arrow). (Photo/legend contributors: Mark Silverberg, MD, and John Amodio, MD.)

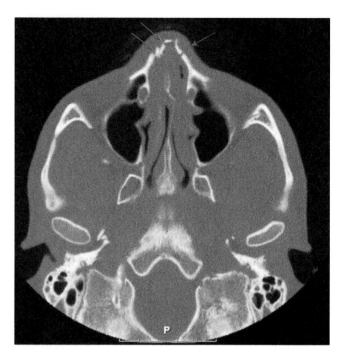

FIGURE 20.19 ■ Nasal Fracture. An axial CT slice demonstrates bilateral comminuted nasal bone fractures (arrows) that were sustained when an unrestrained driver hit his face on the steering wheel in a motor vehicle accident. There is also nasal septal deviation. (Photo/legend contributors: Mark Silverberg, MD, and John Amodio, MD.)

Plain films of the nasal bones are not routinely needed to diagnose an isolated nasal fracture. Nasal fractures can often be diagnosed based on history and physical examination (Table 20.1). Imaging is useful in the diagnosis when patients have severe swelling associated with the injury that obscures assessment of the deformity of the nasal bones. Imaging should also be ordered when additional facial fractures are suspected. It should be noted that the sensitivity of plain films of the nasal bones is not high (reported at 50%), and this should be considered when interpreting the findings. A noncontrast maxillofacial CT scan is the most sensitive imaging modality, especially in cases where the history and physical exam findings suggest more complex injuries of the nose or midface.

Refer patients with nasal pyramid deformity or obstruction to a facial trauma surgeon for closed nasal reduction under general anesthesia within 3 days. Because healing in children is faster than in adults, closed nasal reduction should be planned 4 to 7 days after the injury to be effective and avoid sequelae.

Patients may be discharged with analgesics such as acetaminophen or NSAIDs and discharge instructions to avoid nose blowing and heavy lifting or physical exertion. Instruct patients to use cold packs to decrease swelling. Prescribe prophylactic antibiotics that cover gram-positive bacteria to prevent toxic shock syndrome to all patients with nasal packing.

Pearls

1. Effective management of nasal fractures prevents secondary deformity and the need for additional reconstructive procedures.
2. Manage simple nondisplaced nasal fractures conservatively with ice packs to reduce swelling and analgesics. Early follow-up within 3 to 5 days is essential. Delayed follow-up results in treatment delays and potential complications.
3. Imaging should only be ordered in patients if the history and physical examination do not support the diagnosis of nasal fracture. Imaging should be ordered immediately and should not delayed until swelling has resolved.

Clinical Summary

The mandible is one of the most frequently fractured bones in children, and falls and motor vehicle collisions are the most common causes. In older children, mandible fractures may also result from sports injuries and interpersonal violence. The condyle is the most common fracture site, representing up to 50% of all mandible fractures. In 20% of patients, both condyles will be fractured. Older children are potentially exposed to higher velocity/higher impact injuries, with greater degrees of displacement and comminution. There is a significant rate of associated injuries among these patients.

Jaw pain is a common complaint among patients. Lip or tooth numbness may be present secondary to injury to the inferior alveolar nerve, and there may be associated dental injuries or tooth avulsions that must be documented. Physical examination may reveal trismus, malocclusion and pain with jaw opening, floor of mouth swelling, or hematoma. Some fractures may result in retrognathia and tongue collapse with airway obstruction. Intraoral lacerations may also be seen. Deviation of the jaw with opening can suggest the presence of a condylar fracture with occlusion shifted as well. Ecchymosis over the chin or lacerations of the ear canal are external signs associated with some mandibular fractures.

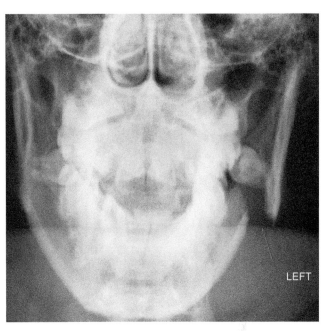

FIGURE 20.21 ■ Mandible Fracture. This frontal projection of the mandible demonstrates a displaced fracture of the left mandibular ramus (arrow). (Photo/legend contributors: Mark Silverberg, MD, and John Amodio, MD.)

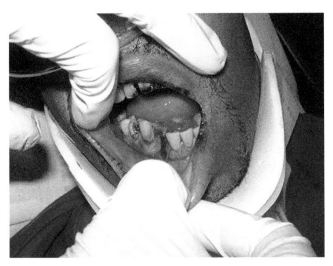

FIGURE 20.20 ■ Mandible Fracture. The occlusal surface of this patient's lower incisors is at a different level from the surrounding teeth with a bleeding gap between them. The underlying mandible fracture is obvious. (Photo contributor: Mark Silverberg, MD.)

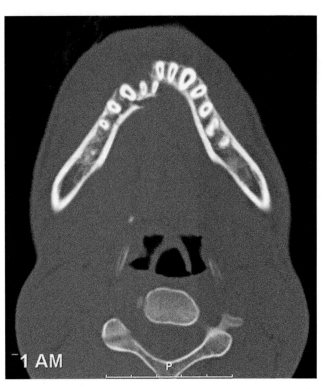

FIGURE 20.22 ■ Mandible Fracture. This axial CT shows a displaced mandible fracture with a "free-floating" section. (Photo/legend contributors: Ambreen Kahn, MD, and John Amodio, MD.)

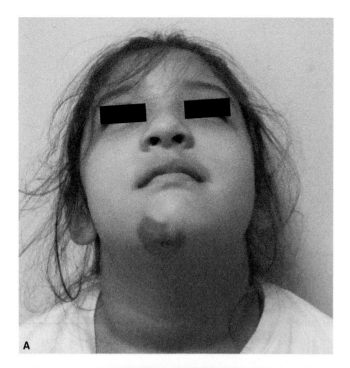

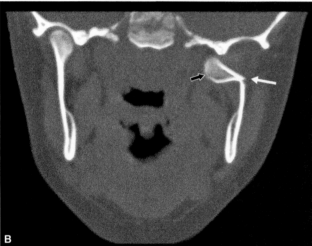

FIGURE 20.23 ■ Mandible Fracture. (**A**) A 5-year-old girl was playing and tripped, landing on her chin, resulting in ecchymosis, pain, and deviation of the chin to the left with mouth opening. The condyle—the weakest region of the mandible—is the most frequently fractured site in the pediatric mandible. The chin will deviate toward the side of the fracture. Nonsurgical treatment is often effective even with severe dislocation. (**B**) Subcondylar mandibular fracture. Coronal noncontrast CT demonstrates a displaced fracture through the left mandibular neck (white arrow). The left mandibular condyle is dislocated medially (black arrow). Note the normal right temporomandibular joint with the condyle positioned in the condylar fossa. (Photo/legend contributors: Sydney Butts, MD, and Vinodkumar Velayudhan, DO.)

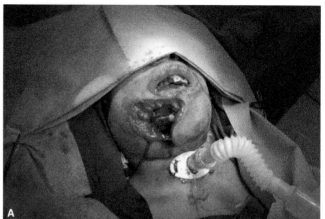

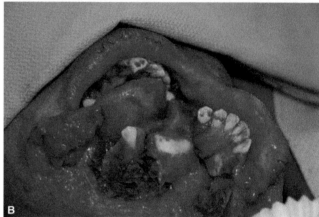

FIGURE 20.24 ■ Mandible Fracture. (**A, B**) This 17-year-old patient was hit by a bus and sustained a comminuted mandible fracture and severe lower lip and cheek lacerations. Significant mandibular comminution can result from high-velocity injuries. The patient also had a maxillary dental alveolar fracture and multiple avulsed maxillary teeth. (Photo contributor: Sydney C. Butts, MD.)

Emergency Department Treatment and Disposition

As a first priority, stabilize the patient and perform a complete physical examination, including a facial trauma survey with palpation of the bony craniofacial skeleton for step-offs, mobile bony segments, or crepitus, and a neurosensory assessment with attention to cranial nerve function, particularly the trigeminal nerve. Assess for other facial fractures and rule out cervical spine injuries. Obtain a panoramic radiograph or panorex if the patient is able to sit upright. If the patient cannot sit or cervical spine immobilization is needed, a plain film mandible series may be shot, which also allows imaging of any dental injuries. In general, a maxillofacial CT scan (with axial and coronal reconstruction) is frequently ordered in patients with suspected facial fractures. Multiplane protocols allow better visualization of fracture fragments or dislocations. If other facial fractures are present, a CT scan is mandatory.

Consult facial trauma surgery for all mandible fractures and dentistry if associated dental trauma is present. Obtain a CXR in patients with avulsed teeth that cannot be accounted for to rule out tooth aspiration. Provide temporary stabilization of fractured mandibular segments with circumdental wires, such as a bridle wire, until definitive management is planned. In young children, this requires sedation and is most easily accomplished in a procedure suite or the operating room.

Admit patients with floor of mouth swelling, associated severe midfacial fractures, pain resulting in poor oral intake, severe associated soft tissue injury requiring operative repair, or pain that is not well controlled with oral analgesia. All other patients may be discharged with appropriate follow-up and adequate analgesia. Acetaminophen or NSAIDs are appropriate initial choices. Mandibular fractures in children heal more quickly than in adults, so a follow-up appointment should be scheduled within 24 to 72 hours if open reduction is being considered. Provide antibiotics that cover oral flora and instruct patients to adhere to a soft diet.

Pearls

1. Mandible fractures can occur in predictable patterns (eg, combination of a symphyseal fracture with bilateral condylar fractures, a body fracture with a contralateral condylar fracture, parasymphyseal fractures with unilateral or bilateral condylar fractures). Exclude a possibility of a second fracture with appropriate imaging and clinical examination.

2. Exclude condylar fracture in a patient with chin ecchymosis, chin laceration, or a history of a blow to the chin from a punch, a fall, or the chin hitting the dashboard of an automobile.

MIDFACIAL FRACTURES (MAXILLARY/LE FORT, FRONTAL SINUS, NASOORBITOETHMOID)

Clinical Summary

Fractures of the midface and upper face with various degrees of bony disruption are usually caused by motor vehicle accidents, falls, or interpersonal violence. There are several important anatomic features of the pediatric craniofacial skeleton. The paranasal sinuses are not fully formed at birth. Before the development of the maxillary sinuses, pure Le Fort pattern fractures are rare. Similarly, frontal sinus fractures are rare until at least school age as postnatal development of the frontal sinus is not significant until the adult size is attained in adolescence. The lack of frontal sinuses and prominence of the calvaria in infants and toddlers result in a higher proportion of frontal skull and skull base fractures.

Maxilla/Le Fort Fractures

The Le Fort fracture patterns describe fracture lines that occur with some reproducibility after impact forces delivered to the maxilla. Varying degrees of midfacial retrusion and elongation are the hallmarks of these bony disruptions. The Le Fort I fracture line runs just above the maxillary alveolus from the rim of the pyriform aperture laterally ending at the pterygoid plates posteriorly. Patients will present with malocclusion—often an anterior open bite—and the alveolus will be mobile

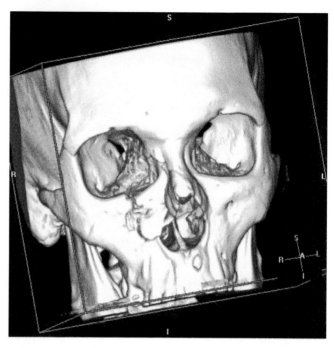

FIGURE 20.26 ■ Le Fort Fracture. Nasoorbitoethmoid fracture. This 3-dimensional CT reconstruction shows fracture involving the bone at the junction of the orbital rim, ethmoids, maxilla, nasal bone, and skull base. Patients can have many symptoms including diplopia, tearing, nasal deformity, telecanthus, and facial numbness. A combination of all of these findings suggests a serious injury best evaluated with CT scan imaging. (Photo contributor: Sydney C. Butts, MD.)

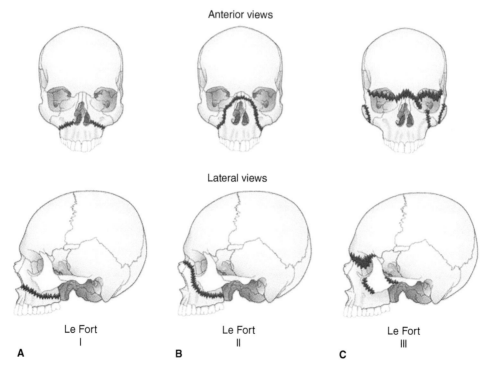

FIGURE 20.25 ■ Schematic Drawing of Le Fort Fractures. Le Fort fracture classification system. (Reproduced with permission from Stone CK, Humphries RL. *Current Diagnosis and Treatment Emergency Medicine*. 8th ed. McGraw-Hill Education; New York, NY, 2017.)

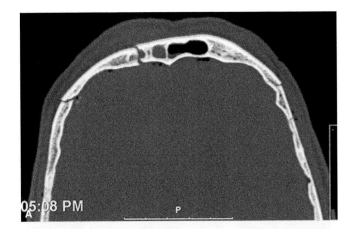

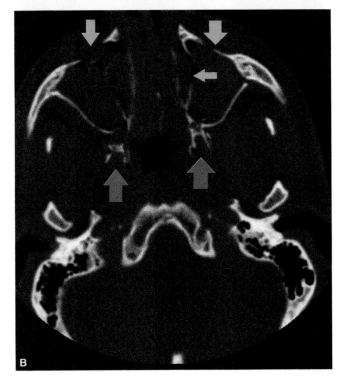

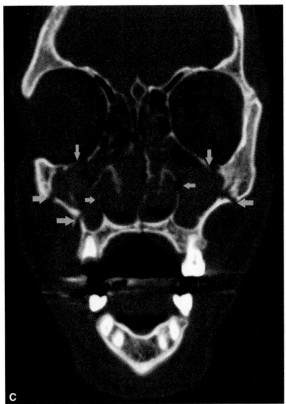

FIGURE 20.27 ■ Midfacial Fractures. (**A**) This axial CT shows a comminuted right frontal bone fracture with intracranial air. A small amount of fluid is noted within the frontal sinuses. (**B, C**) Axial and coronal CT scans of the maxillofacial region demonstrate multiple fractures including bilateral maxillary sinus anterior, medial, and posterolateral wall fractures (blue arrows), bilateral orbital floor fractures traversing the infraorbital foramen (green arrows), and comminuted fractures of the bilateral pterygoid plates (purple arrows) in a patient presenting to the ED postassault after sustaining blunt trauma to the face by a baseball bat. (Photo contributors: Mark Silverberg, MD [A], Danielle Del Re, MD, and Dan Klein, MD [B].)

when manipulated. The Le Fort II fracture is also known as a pyramidal fracture. These fracture lines begin at the root of the nose where the nasal bones articulate with the frontal bones and run inferolaterally across the medial orbital walls to the lateral maxilla. The Le Fort III fracture is also referred to as craniofacial separation. This high fracture line results in maxillary separation from the cranial base. Step-offs and bony mobility will be palpable at the fracture sites. Hypesthesia of the second division of the trigeminal nerve (V2) is a common finding. Significant epistaxis may be a presenting feature in Le Fort II/III fractures. CSF rhinorrhea from a concomitant skull base injury may also be present. Many patients

have marked midfacial edema and periorbital ecchymosis. Patients may also complain of visual acuity change, diplopia, or other ocular symptoms related to the fracture's disruption of the bony orbit.

Nasoorbitoethmoid Fractures

Several physical findings distinguish NOE fractures from other midface fractures. The fractured segment of bone that results from an NOE fracture is demarcated medially by the nasal cavity, laterally by the orbit, and superiorly by the anterior skull base. This segment of bone is the site of attachment of the medial canthal tendon. The 3 types of fractures, as described by

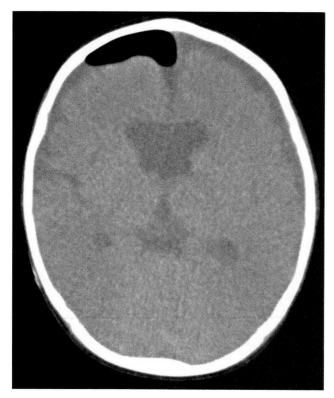

FIGURE 20.28 ■ Pneumocephalus. A large amount of pneumocephalus is noted in this axial CT in a patient who blew his nose after sustaining multiple facial fractures. (Photo contributor: Mark Silverberg, MD.)

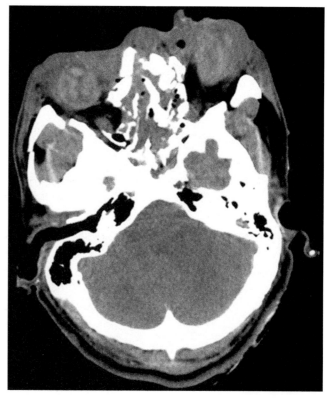

FIGURE 20.29 ■ Nasoorbitoethmoid Fracture (NOE). Single axial view at the level of the orbits in soft tissue algorithm demonstrates multiple fractures of the medial orbital walls and nasal septum. There is bilateral preseptal periorbital soft tissue edema. Hyperdensity in the right choroidal space of the right globe is compatible with choroidal hemorrhage. The left globe is deformed and not completely imaged; globe rupture and vitreous hemorrhage cannot be excluded. A characteristic V shape of the posterior globe may represent an orbital hematocyst (tented globe). (Photo/legend contributors: Barry Hahn, MD, and Steven Pulitzer, MD.)

Markowitz, are defined by worsening severity of comminution of this central region, with the most severe resulting in marked comminution and avulsion of the medial canthal tendon from the bone. Physical findings include extraocular muscle restriction resulting in diplopia, nasal obstruction (lateral nasal wall impingement), epiphora, telecanthus (lateral displacement of the medial canthus), and loss of nasal dorsal support with telescoping. The proximity of the skull base and frontal sinus results in frequent simultaneous injuries of these regions.

Frontal Sinus Fractures

Frontal sinus fractures are rare under the age of 6 years, as pneumatization of the frontal bone is not significant until then. Forehead lacerations, deformity, and hypesthesia of the first division of the trigeminal nerve (V) are physical findings associated with fractures of the anterior table of the frontal sinus. Fractures of the posterior table of the frontal sinus can result in dural lacerations and leakage of the CSF from the nose. CSF rhinorrhea is a presenting feature in 18% to 30% of frontal sinus fractures and should be actively sought by holding the patient's head in a dependent position and looking for

clear fluid leakage. A significant percentage of children with frontal sinus fractures will have an additional craniofacial fracture or intracranial injury.

Emergency Department Treatment and Disposition

Provide hemodynamic resuscitation and secure the airway first. Order CT imaging of the head and facial bones (axial and coronal planes). Request ophthalmologic consultation for any midfacial fractures that involve the orbit or in any patient with a change in visual acuity or positive findings on the initial ocular assessment. Document visual acuity, pupillary reflexes, and extraocular muscle motility.

Consult otolaryngology for all patients with unresolving epistaxis. Approach patients with skull base fractures who require intranasal packing to control bleeding with extreme caution to avoid worsening of the cranial base injury. Obtain otolaryngology and neurosurgery evaluations for all patients with CSF rhinorrhea. If possible, collect the fluid and send for glucose and β_2-transferrin to confirm its origin.

Debride, clean, and repair minor facial lacerations in the ED. Repair more extensive lacerations in the operating room where better anesthesia and hemostasis can be achieved. It may be possible to use lacerations to access underlying fractures, obviating the need to make additional incisions. In these cases, irrigate the wound and dress it with sterile gauze. Admit patients with midfacial trauma because there is a high incidence of associated neurologic injuries or other injuries distant to the head and neck. Discharge only those with the mildest injuries after evaluation by the facial trauma team with arrangements made for close follow-up. Prophylactic antibiotics for midfacial fractures are not routinely recommended (in contrast to mandibular fractures). Factors that would prompt use of antibiotics would be contaminated wounds, significant soft tissue loss, or frank signs of infection upon presentation.

Pearls

1. NOE fractures can be misdiagnosed as simple nasal bone fractures. Overlying edema and inability to examine anxious or uncooperative patients are obstacles to diagnosis.
2. High-impact forces, massive midfacial swelling, V2 sensory disturbance, and ocular signs and symptoms raise suspicion of a midfacial fracture rather than an isolated nasal fracture.
3. Involve facial trauma surgeons early to avoid complications of facial growth restriction, subsequent procedures, and suboptimal function.

Clinical Summary

Orbital blowout fractures involve the thin bones of the floor and medial wall of the orbit while the orbital rim remains intact. These typically result from impact by a projectile larger than the orbit, such as a ball or fist. Because of the high incidence of concomitant intraocular injury, an ocular examination must always be performed on patients who have sustained orbital trauma. Common signs and symptoms include lid edema and ecchymosis, diplopia, enophthalmos, and infraorbital nerve hypesthesia. Air leakage from the sinuses may manifest as orbital emphysema, which will demonstrate crepitus on palpation of the lids or globe proptosis if severe. Binocular diplopia can occur if there is gaze restriction due to extraocular muscle or orbital edema or tissue entrapment.

Emergency Department Treatment and Disposition

Obtain a CT scan of the orbits with axial and coronal reconstruction in all cases of suspected orbital fracture. Coronal sections offer the best view of the orbital floor. Examine the CT carefully for a trapdoor fracture with entrapment of the inferior orbital tissues. There is usually minimal loss of the floor integrity and a lack of blood in the maxillary sinus. However, on clinical examination, there is significant limitation on vertical globe excursion associated with pain, nausea, vomiting, bradycardia, or syncope. Immediate repair, usually within 24 hours, is indicated; consult a facial trauma surgeon urgently. If trapdoor fractures and entrapment are not present, discharge the patient with instructions not to blow his or her nose, to keep the mouth open during sneezing, and to apply ice packs to the orbit for the first 24 to 72 hours. Nose blowing and closed mouth sneezing can cause intraorbital air entry from the paranasal sinuses that can lead to compressive optic neuropathy visual loss, especially in the setting of medial wall fractures. Provide nasal decongestants and as-needed analgesics for 7 days. A short course of oral steroids can aid in decreasing periorbital edema and orbital scar formation, facilitating a more detailed postinjury exam and surgical assessment earlier in the postinjury timeline.

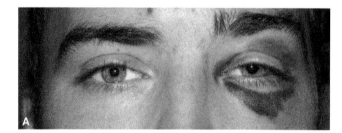
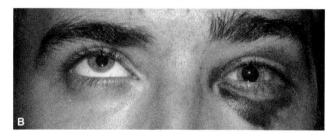
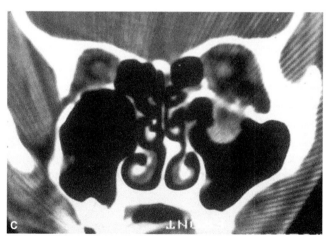

FIGURE 20.30 ■ Orbital Floor Blowout Fracture. (**A**) An adolescent patient after blunt trauma to left orbit with an elbow. (**B**) Same patient with severe limitation on superior excursion (the "hallmark sign"). His dilated left pupil is due to eye drops to facilitate the posterior eye examination and not due to traumatic injury. (**C**) A coronal CT scan shows entrapment of the inferior rectus muscle and soft tissue attachments. Because the fracture size is small and the tissue is minimally incarcerated, radiologic diagnosis can be missed. Urgent surgical repair is advised when signs of entrapment of the inferior rectus muscle or nearby attachments exist clinically and on the CT scan. (Photo contributor: Roman Shinder, MD.)

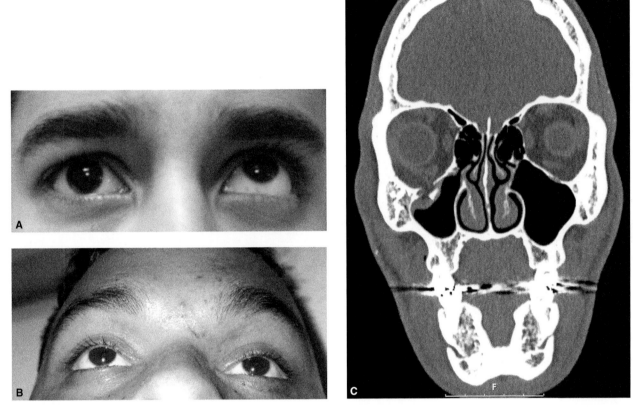

FIGURE 20.31 ▪ Orbital Floor Blowout Fracture. (A) An adolescent patient after blunt trauma to right orbit during basketball showing decreased right eye elevation during upgaze. (B) Left eye enophthalmos is appreciated 1 week after the injury in a different patient with orbital floor blowout fracture. It is useful to determine the presence of enophthalmos by viewing the globe position after the periorbital edema subsides. The larger the fracture, the greater is the likelihood of an enophthalmos. (C) A coronal CT in a different patient demonstrates right orbital floor fracture with inferior displacement of fracture fragment into right maxillary sinus. (Photo contributors: Roman Shinder, MD [A, B], and Mark Silverberg, MD [C].)

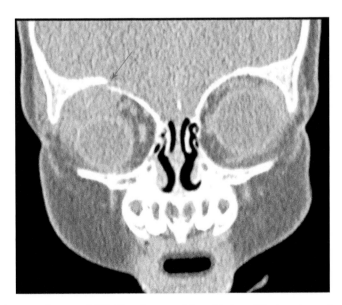

FIGURE 20.32 ▪ Orbital Roof Fracture. A coronal CT slice shows a right orbital roof fracture (arrow) with a large orbital hematoma in a 3-year-old boy who had a television fall on his head. Such fractures are more common in young children, and most do not require repair. (Photo contributor: Sydney C. Butts, MD.)

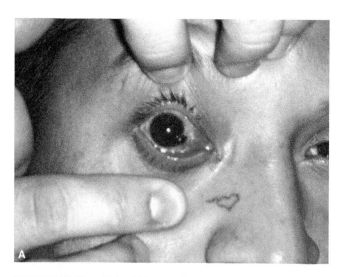
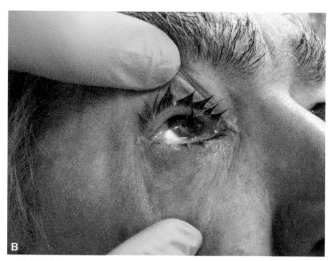

FIGURE 20.33 ■ Orbital Trauma, Ruptured Globe. (**A**) Digital retraction of the right eyelids discloses a full-thickness corneal laceration (open globe) at the 4 o'clock peripheral cornea with iris prolapse through the wound. Conjunctival injection and subconjunctival hemorrhage are also noted. (**B**) This patient fell face first onto his shoe rack, perforating his cornea. The dark-colored iris can be seen here protruding from the defect (arrow). (Photo contributors: Barry Hahn, MD [A], and Mark Silverberg, MD [B].)

Pearls

1. Double vision is the most common complaint of patients with orbital blowout fractures.
2. Decreased motility due to entrapment is most commonly seen on superior excursion with patients classically unable to elevate past the midline.
3. As the swelling and hemorrhage within the orbit subside, eye movements will improve and the double vision will improve or resolve.
4. Consult surgery for open reduction of large fractures, nonresolving double vision, enophthalmos of ≥2 mm, or clinical entrapment.
5. In cases of extraocular muscle entrapment, urgent surgical consultation is necessary to prevent muscle ischemia, chronic motility disturbance, and diplopia.

Clinical Summary

Facial fractures are less common in children than in adults and are more likely to occur in children >6 years old. Midface fractures, which include the zygomas, are rare in children because of the elastic properties of the pediatric skeleton. The paired zygomas compose the malar (cheek) regions of the face, providing midfacial width and cheek projection, and with their 4 suture attachments, they compose the zygomatico-maxillary complexes (ZMCs). A ZMC fracture is a quadripod

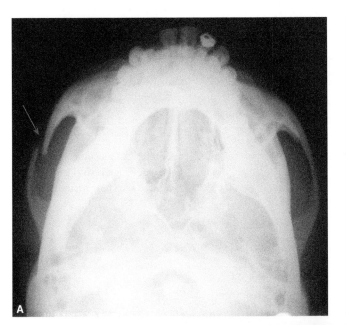

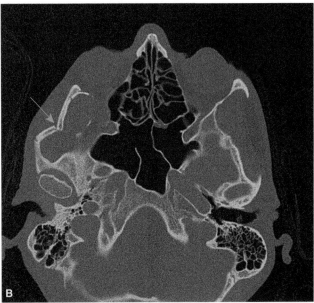

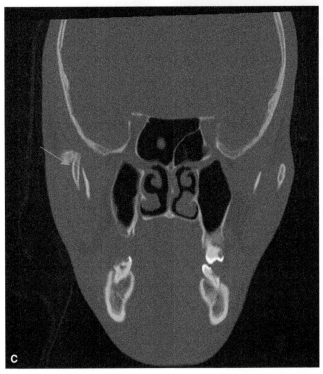

FIGURE 20.34 ■ Zygomatic Arch Fractures. (**A**) This "jug handle" view of the skull shows a mildly displaced right zygomatic arch fracture (arrow). (**B**) An axial CT view shows a comminuted fracture of the right zygomatic arch (arrow). (**C**) Coronal CT view of right arch fracture impinging on the coronoid process. (Photo contributors: Mark Silverberg, MD [A], and Ilaaf Darrat, MD [B, C].)

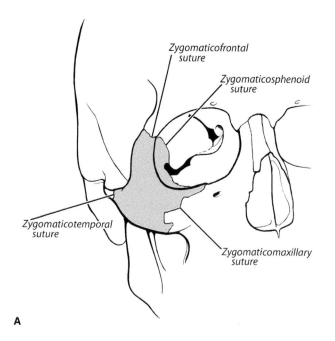

A

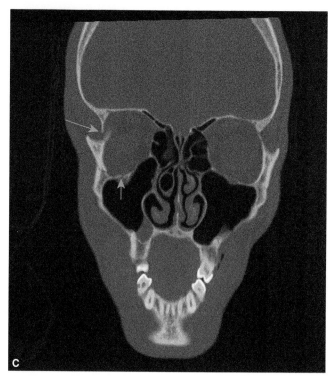

C

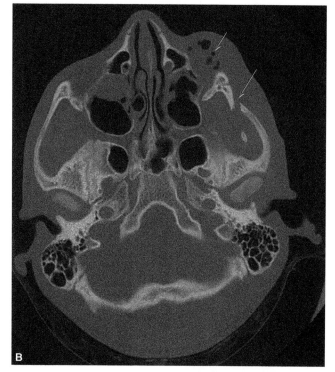

B

FIGURE 20.35 ▪ Tripod Fracture. (**A**) Drawing illustrating the quadripod nature of the zygoma. (**B**) A maxillofacial axial CT scan view in an adolescent after an assault shows a displaced left zygomaticomaxillary complex (ZMC) fracture. The malar process has been pushed backward, resulting in a typical ZMC fracture (long arrow). Also notice the subcutaneous air (short arrow) that probably escaped from the maxillary sinus at the time of the trauma. (**C**) A maxillofacial coronal CT scan view in a different patient shows a right displaced ZMC fracture with a lateral orbital wall fracture (long arrow) and an orbital floor fracture (short arrow). (Photo contributors: Lamont R. Jones [A], Sydney C. Butts, MD [B], and Ilaaf Darrat, MD [C].)

fracture because fractures of the zygoma involve 4 sutures—the term *tripod fracture* is not the most accurate description of this complex fracture.

Patients with zygomatic fractures present with a loss of malar projection (which can be seen from a bird's-eye or worm's-eye view) and bony step-offs at the orbital rim and the lateral orbital rim. Possible ocular findings include enophthalmos, exophthalmos, restricted gaze, and diplopia. Other associated findings include cheek numbness due to hypesthesia of maxillary division of the trigeminal nerve and trismus (difficulty opening the mouth because of impingement of the coronoid process from a posteriorly displaced ZMC fracture).

Emergency Department Treatment and Disposition

Stabilize airway, breathing, and circulation and the cervical spine, and perform a full head and neck examination. Plain radiographs are of limited value. Order a high-resolution (at most 1.5-mm thickness) maxillofacial CT scan with axial and either true coronal or reconstructed coronal view as this is the best imaging modality to evaluate midfacial fractures. Three-dimensional reformats may also be helpful when available. If the patient has a mobile or displaced ZMC or zygomatic arch fracture with a cosmetic or functional deformity, consult a facial trauma surgeon. Manage patients with isolated nondisplaced or minimally displaced zygomatic arch or ZMC fractures with supportive care, observation, and instructions to follow up in 7 to 10 days. Because ZMC fractures involve the orbital rim and usually the orbital floor, all of these patients should be evaluated by an ophthalmologist prior to discharge from the ED to rule out vision loss or retinal, anterior chamber, or other globe injury.

Pearls

1. The ZMC provides facial width and cheek bone shape.
2. The ZMC is a quadripod complex and not a tripod structure because of its articulation with the temporal, maxillary, frontal, and sphenoid bones.
3. ZMC or zygomatic arch fractures that cause cosmetic or functional deformities will likely require surgical intervention.

Clinical Summary

Facial injuries that involve the soft tissue can result from either blunt or penetrating trauma and may occur in isolation or with associated facial skeletal fractures. Soft tissue injuries can range from simple lacerations to avulsion injuries with significant tissue loss. Animal bites can also be a cause of soft tissue injuries of the face in children. Interpersonal violence resulting in stabbing or human bites is an additional causative factor in adolescents. Several specific subsites have unique presentations that must be recognized and managed appropriately.

Penetrating injury to the cheek can result in transection of the parotid or Stensen duct that runs horizontally, just inferior to the zygomatic arch, and parallel to the buccal branch of the facial nerve, explaining the concurrence of facial nerve injuries in a significant number of duct injuries. Wound exploration may reveal pooling of saliva, especially on parotid massage, suggesting injury. Confirm the diagnosis by cannulating the duct from its intraoral opening with a lacrimal probe. The tip of the probe will be visualized within the wound.

Injuries of the lateral cheek/preauricular region, especially near the tragus of the ear, can result in the main trunk of the facial nerve being severed. The temporal branch of the facial nerve, which is responsible for forehead movement, is vulnerable along a path from the tragus to the lateral brow. The marginal mandibular branch may be transected when the injury occurs in the region of the lower border of the mandible. Paralysis of this branch results in elevation of the corner of the mouth. The zygomatic and buccal branches are vulnerable

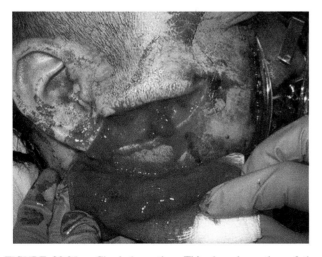

FIGURE 20.36 ■ Cheek laceration. This deep laceration of the cheek was made by a boxcutter. With injuries in this region, the examining provider must look for injuries to the parotid gland, duct, and facial nerve. (Photo contributor: Mark Silverberg, MD.)

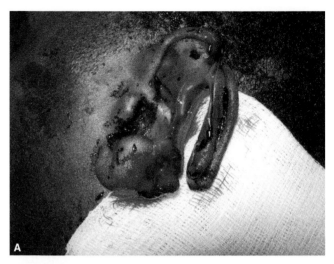

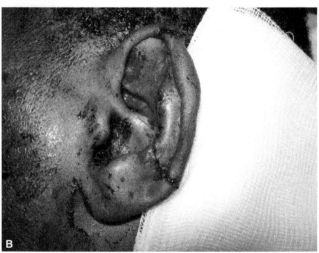

FIGURE 20.37 ■ Auricular Trauma. (**A**) Composite injuries to the ear involve multiple tissue types such as cartilage, connective tissue, and skin. Each must be approximated in the appropriate manner. (**B**) The same patient after his multiple layer closure. This wound should be examined by a physician in 24 to 48 hours to make sure the tissue is viable. (Photo contributor: Mark Silverberg, MD.)

in the midcheek region. Inability to close the eye and drooping of the upper lip are the sequelae, respectively. It is imperative that all facial nerve branches are evaluated prior to any manipulation of the wound. Penetrating injuries of the lateral cheek may also result in trauma to the external carotid artery with acute hemorrhage.

Injury to the ear is complicated by the involvement of cartilage or soft tissue loss. Composite tissues losses (eg, skin and cartilage) require special attention if successful reimplantation or partial salvage of the tissue is to be achieved.

Eyelid lacerations, periocular trauma, and injury to the nasal lacrimal system constitute several possible soft tissue

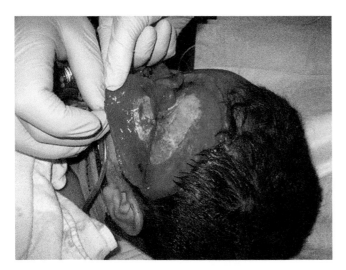

FIGURE 20.38 ▪ Scalp Laceration. The scalp is an extremely vascular region of the body. Lacerations of this region have been known to bleed an excessive amount from transected veins and arteries if direct pressure is not applied. (Photo contributor: Mark Silverberg, MD.)

injuries. Excessive tearing (epiphora) is a cardinal sign that the nasal lacrimal ductal system is not functioning.

Scalp trauma ranges from simple lacerations to complex avulsions with exposed calvarial bone. Scalp avulsions often occur between the galea aponeurosis layer and the periosteum of the skull; however, the entire scalp layer may be missing, leaving exposed bare bone. Scalp injuries can be associated with massive hemorrhage (5 arterial branches that provide blood supply to the scalp emanate from both internal and external carotid arteries).

Emergency Department Treatment and Disposition

First stabilize airway, breathing, and circulation following Advanced Trauma Life Support (ATLS) protocols. Next begin evaluation of the facial trauma and provide tetanus and antibiotic prophylaxis with coverage of gram-positive organisms and anaerobes if the injury involves the nasal, pharyngeal, or oral cavities. For dog bites, obtain information about the rabies immunization status of the dog and administer rabies prophylaxis and immunoglobulin. Amoxicillin/sulbactam will cover *Pasturella multocida*, which is present in the saliva of dogs. Use simple pressure, gauze packing, hemostatic agents, or vessel ligation for hemostasis at the wound site. If there is massive hemorrhage from a significant arterial bleed, perform vessel exploration and ligation in the operating room. In some severe instances, obtain interventional radiology consultation for embolization.

Explore all wounds under sterile conditions after copious irrigation with sterile normal saline and close all wounds that can be safely repaired in the ED, optimally in a separate treatment area for privacy, minimization of patient/caregiver anxiety, and proper lighting and instrumentation. Facial wounds heal very well given their excellent blood supply; primary closure up to 24 hours after the injury is acceptable. Consider the use of conscious sedation to facilitate the repair. Otherwise, a low threshold for intraoperative repair should be adopted in the pediatric population.

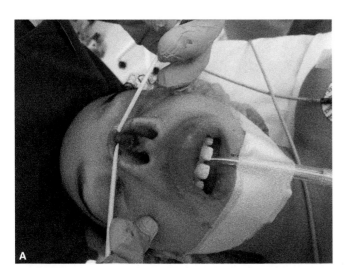
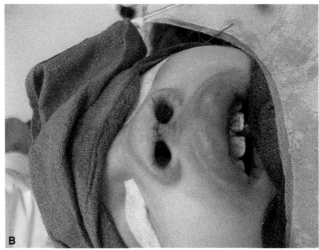

FIGURE 20.39 ▪ Nose Laceration. (**A**) This toddler tripped and fell against a table at home, resulting in a laceration of the columella down to the level of the cartilage of the nasal tip. Given the patient's age and deep soft tissue involvement, the repair was performed in the operating room. (**B**) After repair in the operating room. (Photo contributor: Sydney C. Butts, MD.)

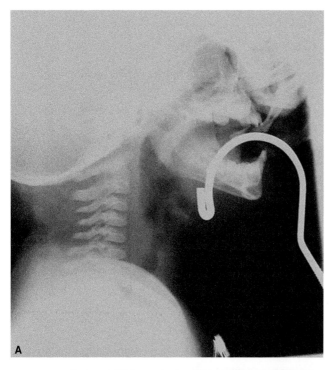

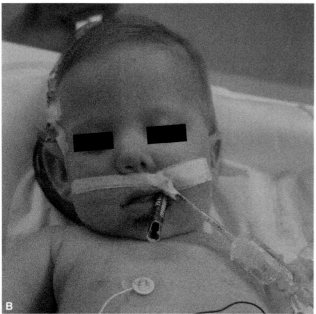

FIGURE 20.40 ■ Oropharyngeal Penetrating Trauma. (**A**) Lateral projection of the neck in a toddler shows a wire hanger impaled through child's mouth, into submental soft tissues. (**B**) A toddler presented to the ED after tripping and falling while chewing on a pen, which lodged into the posterolateral oropharyngeal wall. The potential for vascular injury to the internal carotid artery dictates that extraction be performed in the operating room, and vascular imaging is also recommended to assess for any vessel injury. The pen was successfully removed with no associated vascular injury. (Photo contributors: Ernesto Jose Jule, MD [A], and Sydney C. Butts, MD [B].)

If parotid duct injury is suspected, consult otolaryngology or plastic surgery. If a duct injury is confirmed, send the patient to the operating room for repair.

Diagnosis of a facial nerve injury is easiest when the patient is conscious and can follow commands. Consult the facial trauma team if there is a mechanism that may have resulted in facial nerve injury in an unconscious or unresponsive patient to coordinate the timing of wound exploration. It is possible for a seemingly minor penetrating trauma to be underestimated in the light of more serious injuries. Intraoperative exploration and repair of nerve transections should occur within 3 days of the injury.

Repair lacerations of the ear that extend through the skin to the cartilage without tissues loss by reapproximating the cartilage followed by soft tissue repair. If skin is absent and cartilage is exposed, daily wound care with antibiotic ointment and sterile dressing may be required until more definitive repair can be performed. If ear tissue is avulsed, reattach it primarily, noting that avulsed ear tissue longer than 1.5 cm is not likely to survive. Other options include delayed reconstruction or banking the cartilage (removing the outer layer of skin) underneath the temporal scalp so that it can be used in the future secondary repair as a structural graft. For large, near-total ear avulsion injuries, consult otolaryngology or plastic surgery for microvascular techniques of reattachment.

Similar tenets of repair apply to the nose as to the ear, particularly if there is a composite injury. Use layered closure of wounds (nasal lining, cartilage, deep soft tissue, and skin).

Consult ophthalmology for all periocular trauma for a comprehensive examination of the globe. If possible, consult oculoplastic surgery for evaluation and management of patients with these delicate injuries to avoid secondary complications.

Repair extensive scalp injuries in the operating room and consult neurosurgery for concomitant skull or intracranial injury. Even seemingly minor degrees of tissue loss are challenging wounds to close as scalp tissue is quite inelastic. If repair can be accomplished in the ED, use layered closure with attention to repair of the galea aponeurosis and then the skin to prevent soft tissue depressions. Use pressure dressings or passive drains as needed.

Pearls

1. Salivary duct injuries require surgical subspecialist consultation to repair.
2. Auricular avulsions are injuries where initial intervention makes a significant impact on outcome. If the avulsed ear can be salvaged, it should be put on ice immediately.

LIP LACERATION INVOLVING THE VERMILION BORDER

Clinical Summary

Emergency physicians frequently care for children with lip lacerations. Common causes of lip trauma include falls, sports-related injuries, assaults, motor vehicle collisions, and animal or human bites. Careful assessment is required because lip laceration may be associated with other oral maxillofacial findings depending on the mechanism of injury. When planning repair of lip lacerations, it is important to appreciate the anatomic boundaries of the lip. The vermilion border marks the transition between the dry mucosa of the lip and the facial skin. Meticulous evaluation and achieving accurate anatomical repair are important in lip lacerations involving the vermilion border in order to have acceptable cosmetic outcomes.

Emergency Department Treatment and Disposition

Lip lacerations that result in disruption of the vermilion border require careful management in order to avoid cosmetic deformity. Wound repairs with even small degrees of malalignment at the vermilion border will have an unacceptable cosmetic result. Thorough wound evaluation and preservation of the anatomic alignment of the vermilion border are the key elements in achieving optimal wound closure and long-term cosmetic outcomes.

Carefully evaluate the laceration and the intraoral cavity for underlying alveolar fractures or loose, missing, or damaged teeth. After appropriate analgesia, irrigate the wound and place the first suture to approximate the edges of the vermilion border. If the injury extends to the orbicularis oris muscle, first repair the musculature with buried absorbable sutures, taking care to maintain good alignment. Use 5.0 or 6.0 absorbable sutures to close the defect inside the vermilion border. Next, approximate the skin edges. In young children, use absorbable sutures on all tissues to avoid the additional challenge of suture removal. In older children, monofilament nonabsorbable sutures may be used on skin beyond the vermilion border, which should be removed in 3 to 5 days. Patients requiring multiple layered repair may benefit from

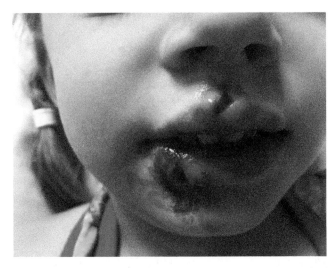

FIGURE 20.41 ■ Lip Lacerations. Lip lacerations must be repaired very carefully. Even slight misalignment of the vermilion border will be noticeable. Proper alignment at the vermillion cutaneous border is a key step of proper repair. (Photo contributor: Joshua Nagler, MD.)

consultation with a plastic or oral surgeon, depending on the comfort and skill set of the emergency medicine provider.

Pearls

1. Marking the wound edges with a surgical skin marker or methylene blue can aid with proper alignment of the vermilion border.
2. Injected local anesthesia may distort anatomy and interfere with wound margin approximation. Use of epinephrine may also blanch tissue locally, reducing contrast across the vermillion border and making alignment more difficult. An infraorbital nerve block can be used for the upper lip, and a mental nerve block will anesthetize the lower lip to provide adequate analgesia without local tissue distortion. Ultimately, decisions regarding approach to analgesia need to be customized based on patient factors (eg, cooperation and complexity of the wound) as well as provider experience and comfort with regional and local analgesia in children.

TONGUE LACERATION

Clinical Summary

Pediatric tongue lacerations often occur after a fall or a collision with another person or an object. Sports-related injuries are common in older children. Injury commonly results from the tongue being trapped between the teeth. The tongue is a highly vascular, muscular organ, and bleeding following injury can be profuse. Tongue injuries associated with significant lingual edema and large hematomas must be monitored closely, as they have potential to cause upper airway compromise and respiratory distress.

Emergency Department Treatment and Disposition

First, stabilize the airway and control bleeding. Inspect the wound for embedded teeth or foreign bodies including food. Irrigate the wound, taking care to prevent airway compromise. Lingual lacerations tend to heal rapidly because of the rich vascular supply. Small, superficial, linear lacerations generally heal without intervention. Primary closure of tongue lacerations is indicated in select cases to avoid functional or cosmetic deformity. Indications for primary closure include: deeper lacerations that involve the muscular layer or bisect the whole tongue and remain gaping, lateral tongue lacerations, lacerations with persistent bleeding, large avulsion-type injuries, and lacerations with a high potential for cosmetic deformity if not repaired (ie, "anterior split tongue").

Provide topical anesthesia by applying lidocaine (4%)–soaked gauze for 5 minutes, or for larger lacerations, use local infiltration or a regional nerve block. Regional anesthesia is less painful than local infiltration. An inferior alveolar block will include the lingual nerve, providing anesthesia to the anterior two-thirds of the tongue. Some patients may require procedural sedation or general anesthesia prior to local or regional analgesia and for wound repair. Use a gauze sponge to better grasp the tongue during the procedure. Alternatively, if the tip of the tongue is anesthetized, use of a towel clamp or placement of a temporary suture can be used to help stabilize the tongue.

Use absorbable sutures for wound repair, burying the knots when possible. Edema of the tongue can be severe in the first 48 hours, and tight sutures may increase lingual edema or produce local tissue necrosis. Therefore, place stitches wide and tie loosely. All 3 layers (inferior mucosa, muscle, and superior mucosa) of the tongue can be closed. Alternatively, some recommend closing only the muscular layer and allowing the mucosa to heal on its own. Approximating the muscle generally provides adequate hemostasis. The use of routine antibiotic prophylaxis for tongue injuries is controversial. Consider antibiotic treatment for complex, contaminated wounds. Instruct patients to eat a soft diet for 2 to 3 days and rinse their mouths after each meal to prevent food entrapment in the defect.

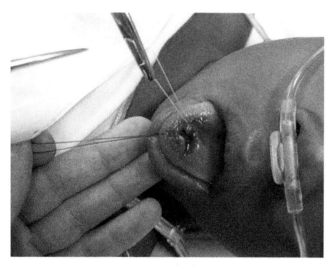

FIGURE 20.42 ■ Tongue laceration. By putting a large suture through the anterior one-third of the tongue, it may make it easier to withdraw the tongue from the mouth to suture. (Reproduced with permission from Greenberg MI. *Greenberg's Text-Atlas of Emergency Medicine*. Lippincott Williams & Wilkins; Philadelphia, PA, 2005.)

Pearls

1. Bury knots whenever possible as the constant motion of the tongue easily unties sutures in the oral cavity. Alternatively, each suture should be tied with at least 4 locking square knots.
2. A bite block can be used during laceration repair to protect both the patient and the physician. Procedural sedation may be required in young or uncooperative children.
3. A majority of tongue lacerations do not need surgical repair and can be managed conservatively.

Clinical Summary

The temporomandibular joint (TMJ) is formed by the articulation of the condyle of the mandible and the temporal bone. The TMJ may dislocate anteriorly (most common), posteriorly, laterally, or superiorly. The direction of TMJ dislocation refers to the position of the condyle in relation to the temporal fossa. Unilateral or bilateral TMJ dislocations may occur. TMJ dislocation results in stretching of the ligaments and severe spasm of the muscles that control jaw movement. Trismus prevents the condyle from returning to the temporal fossa. Unilateral dislocation is most common, but symmetric bilateral dislocation may occur.

TMJ dislocations typically occur after extreme jaw opening following yawning or lengthy dental procedures. Anterior traumatic TMJ dislocations can occur following blunt trauma. The patient presents with jaw or mouth pain, trismus, drooling, difficulty speaking, and malocclusion. Traumatic posterior and superior dislocations are usually due to a direct blow to the chin and can be associated with injury to the mandibular fossa, external auditory canal, or the skull base. Lateral dislocations are secondary to trauma to the side of the face and are associated with mandibular fractures.

Emergency Department Treatment and Disposition

Begin with a thorough head and neck examination to evaluate for associated injuries and any facial asymmetry. In unilateral dislocation, the jaw deviates to the side opposite the dislocation. Inspect the mouth for intraoral lacerations, which may indicate open fractures. CT scans or panoramic radiographs are useful for traumatic dislocations to evaluate for mandibular fractures.

Manual reduction can be performed by placing the patient in a seated position in a chair with his or her head against a wall. With gloved hands, place the clinician's thumbs on the patient's inferior molars and exert bilateral, steady force. For anterior dislocation, direct the force inferiorly and posteriorly. Procedural sedation may be needed in uncooperative patients or excessive masseter spasm.

Consultation with oral maxillofacial surgeons is recommended if the TMJ dislocation is posterior or superior; associated with mandibular fracture, recurrent, difficult, or failed reductions, or open dislocations; or presents with associated cranial nerve injuries. Refer patients with uncomplicated dislocations for outpatient follow-up with oral maxillofacial surgery within a few days.

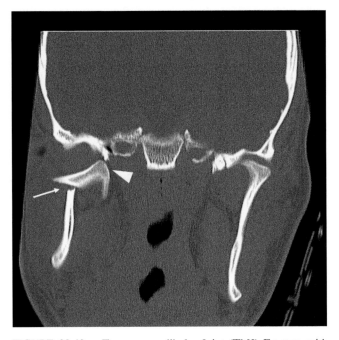

FIGURE 20.43 ■ Temporomandibular Joint (TMJ) Fracture with Dislocation. Coronal CT shows a displaced fracture through the right mandibular neck (arrow). The mandibular condyle is dislocated medially from the right TMJ (arrowhead). This was managed operatively. (Photo/legend contributors: Joshua Nagler, MD, and Vinodkumar Velayudhan, DO.)

Pearls

1. Traumatic TMJ injuries in children may have an impact on growth of the facial bones.
2. Patients with prior TMJ dislocations are prone to recurrence.
3. When performing closed reduction, care must be taken to avoid injury to the clinician's thumbs, which may occur when the patient's jaw snaps closed following reduction. This can be accomplished by wrapping the clinician's thumbs with gauze (with or without incorporation of tongue blades) and with use of a bite block. Gauze should have a trailing end for retrieval should it become dislodged during reduction.

PENETRATING NECK INJURY

Clinical Summary

Penetrating anterior neck injuries are a diagnostic and management challenge. The high density of vital structures in a confined area makes the neck vulnerable to significant vascular, aerodigestive, and neurologic injuries. Mechanisms of injury include gunshots, stabbing, and injuries secondary to miscellaneous sharp objects. The degree of blast effect from gunshot wounds is related to mass, velocity, and range of the bullet. Traditionally, the anterior neck has been subdivided into 3 anatomic zones based on the accessibility of underlying structures. Zone I lies between the clavicles and the cricoid cartilage. Zone II injuries involve the midportion of the neck between the cricoid and angle of the mandible, making it the most surgically accessible, because both proximal and distal vascular control can be easily obtained. Zone III injuries are contiguous with the cranium and are found below the skull but above the angle of the mandible. Classifying an external wound to a particular zone does not ensure that the trajectory of the penetrating implement and injuries to underlying structures are confined to that anatomic zone.

Emergency Department Treatment and Disposition

Stabilize the airway, evaluate ventilation, and rapidly achieve hemostasis of vascular injuries. Early airway management is vital, because blood or air dissecting through the deep fascial layers of the neck can quickly distort the anatomy and cause airway compromise. Perform tube thoracostomy expeditiously to relieve hemothoraces and pneumothoraces. Control active bleeding with direct pressure and avoid clamping bleeding vessels, because this may result in unintended injury to neurologic or other vascular structures. If the patient is hemodynamically unstable or has obvious signs of airway injury, immediate surgical repair is indicated.

On initial physical examination, determine whether or not the penetrating injury has violated the platysma muscle. All wounds deep to the platysma are significant injuries that require diagnostic evaluation and surgical consultation. Identify clinical signs and symptoms suggestive of vascular, aerodigestive, and neurologic injuries. Clinical signs indicative of significant injury include active arterial bleeding, expanding hematomas, diminished or absent pulses, air or bubbling in the wound, bruits or thrills, ED hypotension, massive hemothorax, lateralizing signs, hemoptysis, hematemesis, and tracheal deviation.

Management decisions in hemodynamically stable patients not requiring immediate surgery are guided by mechanism of injury, wound location, signs and symptoms, and preferences based on availability of specialized personnel. Imaging studies may provide further data affecting decisions regarding nonoperative management or the need for surgical exploration.

Pearls

1. Transcervical gunshot wounds are twice as likely to cause significant injuries as those that do not cross the midline.
2. Shotgun wounds usually involve multiple zones of the neck.
3. A benign physical examination may not be adequate to exclude the presence of injuries. Use diagnostic imaging or surgical exploration for wounds that have violated the platysma.
4. Penetrating esophageal injuries are often initially asymptomatic. Delayed recognition of these injuries can result in severe neck space infections or mediastinitis.

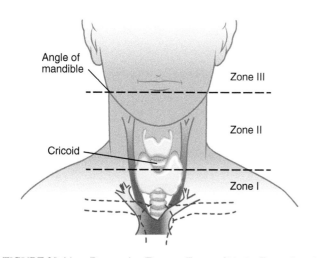

FIGURE 20.44 ■ Penetrating Trauma: Zones of Neck. (Reproduced with permission from Doherty GM. *Current Surgical Diagnosis and Treatment.* 14th ed. McGraw-Hill Education; New York, NY, 2015.)

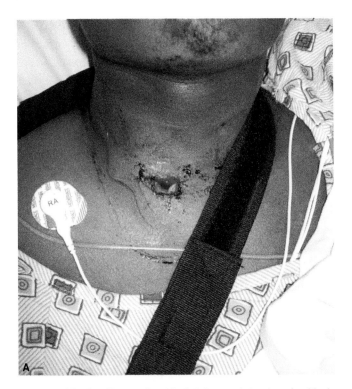

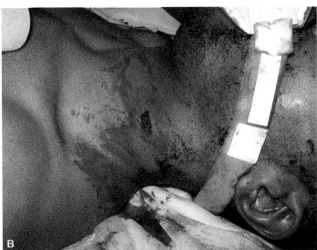

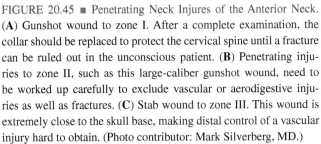

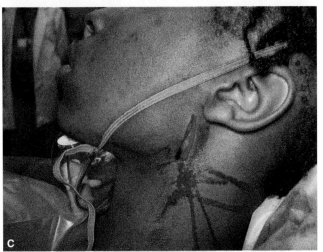

FIGURE 20.45 ▪ Penetrating Neck Injures of the Anterior Neck. (A) Gunshot wound to zone I. After a complete examination, the collar should be replaced to protect the cervical spine until a fracture can be ruled out in the unconscious patient. (B) Penetrating injuries to zone II, such as this large-caliber gunshot wound, need to be worked up carefully to exclude vascular or aerodigestive injuries as well as fractures. (C) Stab wound to zone III. This wound is extremely close to the skull base, making distal control of a vascular injury hard to obtain. (Photo contributor: Mark Silverberg, MD.)

Clinical Summary

Cervical spine injury (CSI) occurs in only 1% to 2% of blunt pediatric trauma patients. Motor vehicle collisions and falls are the most common mechanisms of injury. Injuries related to sports and recreational activities (eg, diving) are also common in adolescents, whereas inflicted injuries (eg, non-accidental trauma) may occur in infants and younger children. The incidence of CSI secondary to penetrating injury is very low in young children but increases during adolescence and approaches the adult incidence in the late teenage years.

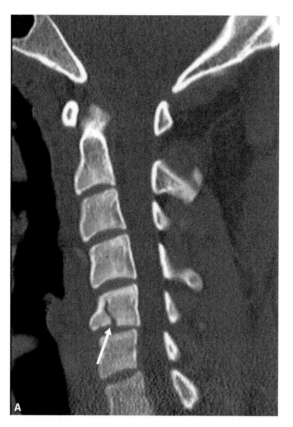

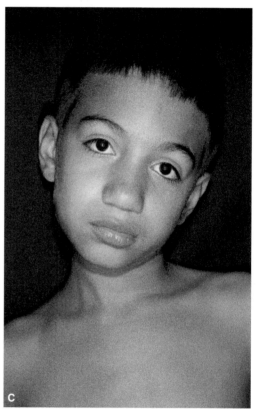

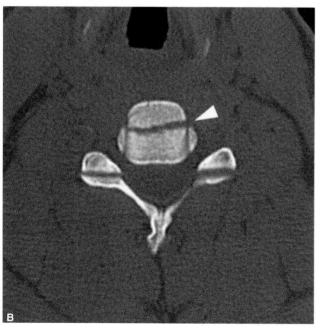

FIGURE 20.46 ■ Cervical Spine Injuries. Vertical compression fracture of C5. (**A**) Sagittal CT demonstrates compression of the C5 vertebral body with a fracture extending through the anterior body (white arrow). (**B**) Axial CT shows the coronally oriented fracture (arrowhead). (**C**) Torticollis. Neck pain, torticollis, limitation of neck movements, and muscle spasm are some of the findings seen with cervical spine injury. However, torticollis can result from many etiologies, as seen in this child presenting with acute onset of torticollis not related to trauma. He woke up with muscle spasm and neck stiffness ("wry neck"). (Photo/legend contributors: Caitlin A. Farrell, MD, Vinodkumar Velayudhan, DO [A, B], and Binita R. Shah, MD [C].)

There is a 2:1 predominance in boys to girls. This injury has significant morbidity, and a high index of suspicion for these injuries is appropriate in all trauma patients.

Although anatomic features may predispose to upper CSI in younger children, epidemiologic data suggest that higher cervical injury occurs equally in all pediatric age groups. Hyperflexion, hyperextension, and axial loading are associated with different types of injuries. Certain conditions may also predispose to CSI, including Down syndrome, Klippel-Feil syndrome, achondrodysplasia, mucopolysaccharidosis, Ehlers-Danlos syndrome, Marfan syndrome, osteogenesis imperfecta, Larsen syndrome, juvenile rheumatoid arthritis, juvenile ankylosing spondylitis, renal osteodystrophy, rickets, and previous history of CSI or cervical spine surgery. Pediatric trauma patients with predisposing conditions or high-risk mechanism should undergo appropriate radiologic imaging. Recent data suggest that imaging should be obtained if any of the following are present: neck pain, midline posterior neck tenderness, decreased range of motion, torticollis, depressed mental status, focal neurologic findings, or other significant injuries (eg, to the torso).

The cervical spine is commonly considered as 2 columns: anterior and posterior. The anterior column is composed of the vertebral bodies and interposed annulus fibrosus and vertebral disks, which are held in alignment by the anterior and posterior longitudinal ligaments. The posterior column contains the spinal canal as well as the bony elements formed by the pedicles, the transverse processes, the articulating facets, the laminae, and the spinous processes. Any injury or combination of injuries that affects both of these columns is unstable.

Emergency Department Treatment and Disposition

All trauma patients should be evaluated as though they might have a spinal injury until it has been excluded. Plain radiographs are often the primary imaging modality to evaluate for potential spine injuries in most cases of pediatric trauma and should consist of a supine lateral view, an anteroposterior (AP) view, and an open-mouth odontoid view in children who are old enough to cooperate. An adequate lateral spine radiograph must reveal all 7 cervical vertebrae and include the C7/T1 junction. CT imaging of the cervical spine should be obtained in pediatric patients with any of the following: neurologic findings, a GCS score <8, a highly concerning mechanism of injury, abnormal radiographs, or when plain films are inadequate for complete cervical spine assessment. If a head CT is ordered to rule out intracranial injury, particularly in younger children, extension of the study to include the upper cervical spine may be used, given the challenges of imaging this area in children using plain radiographs. Radiation exposure is significantly greater when using CT imaging rather than conventional radiography, and children are particularly susceptible. Patient, provider, and institutional factors should be considered when determining the optimal imaging strategy for injured children with possible CSI. Absence of fracture on CT or plain radiographs does not rule out traumatic injury to the spinal cord. Spinal cord injury without radiographic evidence of fracture or dislocation (ie, SCIWORA) can result from the elastic nature of the pediatric cervical spine. Up to 50% of children with spinal cord injury found on MRI have no fractures on primary radiologic survey.

Pearls

1. Assess all children for CSI emergently if they have neurologic symptoms (eg, focal neurologic deficit, signs of neurogenic shock, altered mental status, urinary retention, or priapism), significant associated injuries, or a palpable step-off in the cervical spine.

2. Obtain MRI for all patients with neurologic deficits but no initial radiographic abnormalities to diagnose ligamentous injury or changes in injury to the spinal cord.

Clinical Summary

Fractures of the first cervical vertebra, also known as Jefferson fractures or fracture of the "atlas," result in disruption of the C1 ring, typically into 4 parts and less commonly into 2 or 3 parts. The mechanism of injury is an axial load, commonly associated with diving accidents or roll-over motor vehicle collisions. C1 is compressed between the occipital condyles of the cranium and the body of C2. This is an unstable fracture due to a loss of bony connection and interrelation from the cranium and the lower spine. A high index of suspicion is warranted for associated C2 fractures as these are often seen with Jefferson fractures. Other fractures of the C1 ring have little clinical significance.

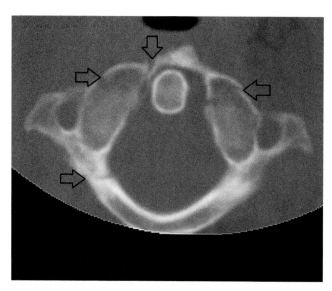

FIGURE 20.47 ■ Jefferson Fracture. Axial CT image of C1 demonstrates 4 C1 fractures (arrows) compatible with a 4-part Jefferson burst fracture. (Photo/legend contributors: Gregory N. Emmanuel, MD, and Marlena Jbara, MD.)

Emergency Department Treatment and Disposition

Immobilize the cervical spine and obtain cervical spine series and odontoid view plain radiographs. Findings of a C1 burst fracture include 1 or both of the lateral masses of C1 laterally displaced over the body of C2. In addition, the predental space is often widened (>5 mm in children). Order a CT for fracture visualization and to rule out other fractures of the cervical spine. Consult neurosurgery emergently for patients with Jefferson fractures. Carefully observe spinal cord precautions. Provide adequate analgesia while maintaining the ability to monitor the patient's mental status and neurologic status. Carefully assess the patient's airway and breathing, as C1 spinal cord injuries are often associated with respiratory failure.

All patients with Jefferson fractures require hospitalization, usually to intensive care. Treatment should include appropriate analgesia if the patient is not already sedated and intubated and continued spinal immobilization. Decisions regarding surgical management of the fracture should be made in conjunction with neurosurgery.

Pearls

1. Patients with spinal cord injury at the C1 level will have normal sensation and motor control of the face from cranial nerve innervation, with concomitant loss of sensation and motor function of the rest of the body.
2. Burst fractures of C1 are often associated with vertebral artery injury and subsequent neurovascular deficits.
3. Respiratory failure requires careful but emergent endotracheal intubation, with many patients requiring tracheostomy and dependence on mechanical ventilatory support.

Clinical Summary

The odontoid process of C2 (also known as the dens) is a bony projection off the superior aspect of the C2 body that articulates with the anterior ring of C1. These 2 bones are kept in tight approximation by the thick transverse ligament (also known as the cruciate ligament) that stabilizes the C1/C2 articulation. Fractures that disrupt the transverse ligament lead to C1/C2 instability with subsequent risk of cord injury.

Odontoid fractures are categorized into 3 types based on the involvement of the transverse ligament and the body of C2. Type I odontoid fractures are avulsions of the tip of the dens at the insertion site of the alar ligament. These fractures are mechanically stable but are sometimes associated with atlantooccipital dislocation, which is a life-threatening injury. Type II odontoid fractures consist of a horizontal fracture at the base of the dens separating the dens (and the transverse ligament) from the rest of C2. This is the most common type of odontoid fracture. It is considered an unstable fracture because the transverse ligament, along with the dens and C1, is separated from the body of C2 and the rest of the spine. Type III odontoid fractures exhibit a fracture plane extending down into the body of the axis (C2) and are unstable.

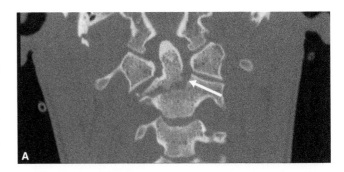

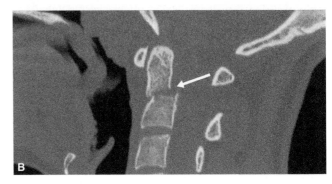

FIGURE 20.48 ■ Dens Fracture. Type III Dens Fracture. Coronal (**A**) and sagittal (**B**) CT images demonstrate a displaced fracture extending through the body of C2 inferior to the dens (white arrows). (Photo/legend contributors: Caitlin A. Farrell, MD, and Vinodkumar Velayudhan, DO.)

Emergency Department Treatment and Disposition

Immobilize the cervical spine and consult neurosurgery emergently for patients with type II or III odontoid fractures. Instability at the C1–C2 junction can lead to cord trauma, which may be associated with paralysis of respiratory muscles and respiratory failure.

As with Jefferson fractures, all of these patients require admission to the hospital usually in an ICU. Treatment should include appropriate analgesia if the patient is not already sedated and intubated along with spinal immobilization. Type I odontoid fractures are usually managed conservatively with outpatient immobilization in a cervical collar. Type II and III dens fractures are at risk for nonunion in patients with >10 degrees of angulation or >5 mm of translation; therefore, surgical arthrodesis is preferred over external fixation devices such as a halo.

Pearls

1. Type I odontoid fractures are commonly stable, although may be associated with atlantooccipital dislocation, which can be devastating.

2. The odontoid, or open-mouth, view will often reveal odontoid fractures in children able to cooperate with such imaging; however, CT allows for coronal and sagittal reconstructions, which can better detect and delineate these injuries.

3. Type II odontoid fractures may be missed on axial CT images because the fracture plane is often parallel to the image acquisition plane. Such fractures are often identified using reconstructed coronal images.

Clinical Summary

Traumatic spondylolisthesis of C2 is also known as "hangman's fracture" and occurs most commonly as a result of high-speed motor vehicle collisions. The mechanism of injury commonly results in axial loading and lateral flexion. Traumatic spondylolisthesis of C2 always results in bilateral pedicle fractures. The degree of disruption of the associated disc and anterior and posterior ligaments varies depending on the severity of the lateral flexing forces and the amount of distraction of the fracture fragments. Increased distraction of C2 on C3 increases the likelihood of spinal cord injury.

Emergency Department Treatment and Disposition

Stabilize the cervical spine and obtain emergent neurosurgical consultation. Carefully assess the patient's airway and breathing because upper cervical spinal cord injuries are often associated with respiratory failure. Patients with C2 fractures require MRI to evaluate for possible spinal cord involvement. In patients without spinal cord injury, fractures can often be managed on an outpatient basis with cervical traction.

Pearls

1. Hangman's fractures affect both the anterior and posterior columns of the spine and therefore are considered to be unstable.

2. Due to a relatively larger AP diameter of the spinal canal at this level, nondisplaced C2 fractures commonly occur without associated spinal cord injury.

3. When associated with unilateral or bilateral facet dislocation at the level of C2, this injury is unstable and has a high rate of neurologic complications.

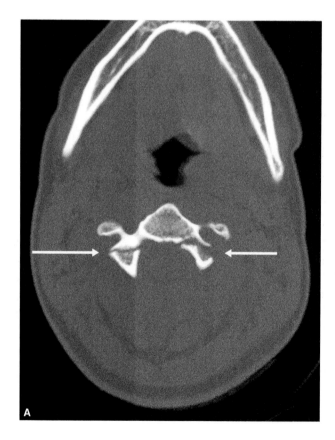

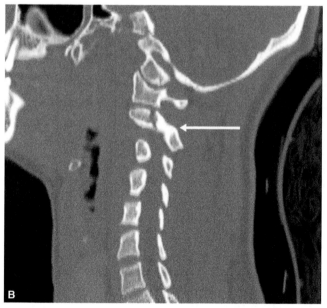

FIGURE 20.49 ■ Hangman's Fracture. (**A**) Axial CT image demonstrates fractures through the pars interarticularis of C2 bilaterally (arrows). (**B**) Sagittal CT image to the right of midline demonstrates C2 pars interarticularis fracture (arrow). (Photo contributors: Marlena Jbara, MD, and Ami Gokli, MD.)

Clinical Summary

Extension teardrop fractures result from sudden hyperextension, which commonly results from blunt trauma to the forehead or rear-impact motor vehicle collisions. With this mechanism of injury, the anterior longitudinal ligament is stretched to the point of disruption and avulses off a small fragment of bone, creating the typical fracture pattern. This most commonly occurs at the lower cervical levels and is stable provided the neck remains in flexion. The injury is highly unstable when the neck is in extension due to disruption of the anterior stabilizing ligaments of the spine.

Emergency Department Treatment and Disposition

Immobilize the cervical spine and order radiographs. Findings of an extension teardrop fracture include a small avulsion of the inferior aspect of the anterior surface of the vertebral body. Prevent extension of the neck and consult neurosurgery promptly. Perform a careful neurologic assessment to assess for evidence of spinal cord injury. Treatment of isolated teardrop fractures is cervical orthosis. Fixation may be required if there are other associated cervical injuries.

Pearls

1. Extension teardrop fractures may be associated with the central cord syndrome as a result of the ligamenta flava buckling into the spinal canal during hyperextension.

2. If endotracheal intubation is indicated, it is imperative that neck extension is avoided by performing 2-person intubation with 1 person maintaining manual in-line stabilization. If available, intubation should be performed with the use of indirect laryngoscopy (fiberoptic or video).

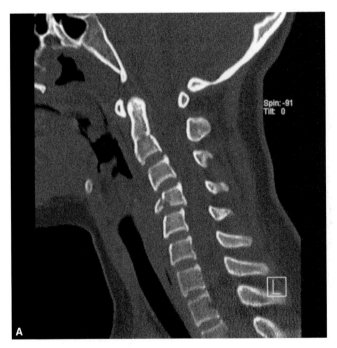 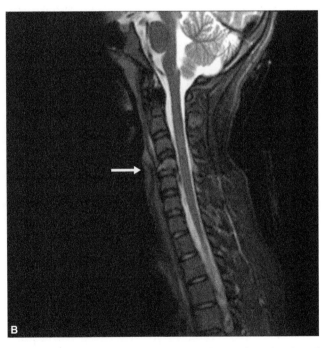

FIGURE 20.50 ■ Extension Teardrop Fracture. (**A**) Sagittal CT slice through midline with white arrow denoting a triangular-shaped anterior-inferior C4 corner fracture and minimal spondylolisthesis of C4–C5 consistent with hyperflexion teardrop mechanism of injury. (**B**) Sagittal MRI T2-weighted image demonstrates C4 anterior-inferior endplate fracture with bone marrow edema and prevertebral soft tissue swelling. (Photo contributors: Ami Gokli, MD, and Marlena Jbara, MD.)

ANTERIOR FLEXION FRACTURES (FLEXION TEARDROP)

Clinical Summary

Flexion teardrop fractures manifest with a displaced antero-inferior bony fragment. The mechanism of injury is forced flexion such as blunt trauma to the back of the head or deceleration motor vehicle collision. Severe flexion of the spine causes a compression-like fracture of the anterior aspect of the vertebral body, and a fragment resembling a teardrop is displaced anteriorly. The anterior longitudinal ligament may be disrupted and the anterior vertebral body crushed. In addition, as flexion continues, the posterior ligamentous complex and bony articulations may become disrupted and open up or "fan" out, potentially stretching or injuring the cord. With this mechanism, both anterior and posterior columns are disrupted, making this innocuous-appearing teardrop fracture one of the most unstable CSIs. Therefore, these patients are at significant risk for spinal cord injury.

Emergency Department Treatment and Disposition

Immobilize the cervical spine with mild traction. Obtain plain films and urgent neurosurgical consultation. A careful neurologic assessment is critical to assess for evidence of spinal cord injury. These fractures represent complete destabilization of spinal integrity and therefore require urgent neurosurgical evaluation for possible surgical fixation.

Pearls

1. Patients with flexion teardrop fractures above the C5 level are at high risk for respiratory compromise.
2. Intubate with minimal movement of the cervical spine and/or with indirect laryngoscopy (fiberoptic or video).

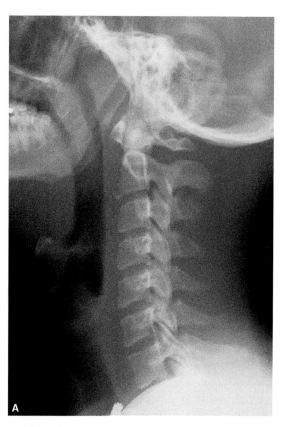 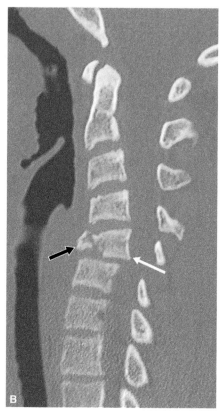

FIGURE 20.51 ■ Flexion Teardrop Fracture. (A) A triangular anteroinferior C2 endplate corner avulsion fracture consistent with hyperflexion teardrop mechanism of injury is seen on a lateral cervical spine radiograph obtained in a patient after motor vehicle trauma. (B, C) Sagittal CT and sagittal short tau inversion recovery (STIR) MRI in a different patient. (B) Sagittal CT demonstrates a burst fracture of the C5 vertebral body with a large "teardrop" fragment off its anteroinferior margin (black arrow). There is associated retrolisthesis of C5 on C6 into the spinal canal (white arrow).

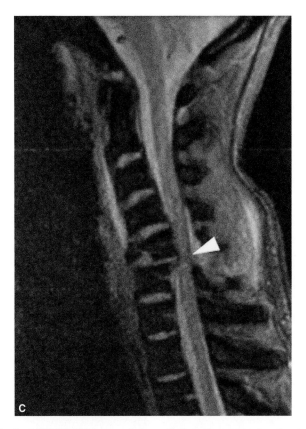

FIGURE 20.51 ■ (*Continued*) (**C**) Sagittal STIR MRI image shows spinal cord compression due to retrolisthesis (white arrow). (Photo/legend contributors: Daniel Luu, MD, Marlena Jbara, MD [A], and Caitlin A. Farrell, MD, Vinodkumar Velayudhan, DO [B, C].)

Clinical Summary

This is a rare but devastating, severely unstable spinal injury where the occipital condyles no longer articulate with the ring of C1. Very young children are at greatest risk given their large head relative to body size and weak spinal muscles.

The typical cause of injury is sudden deceleration in motor vehicle collisions, falls, or being struck in the head with a high-energy object. The mechanism of injury can be hyperextension, hyperflexion, distraction, or severe rotary forces. The complete disruption of ligamentous relationships between the spine and the cranium causes stretching of the brainstem and

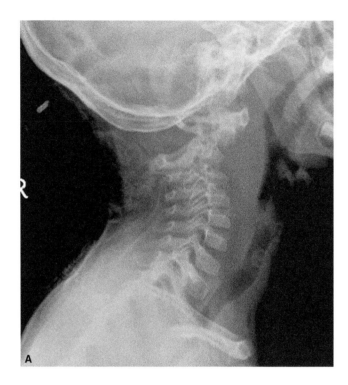

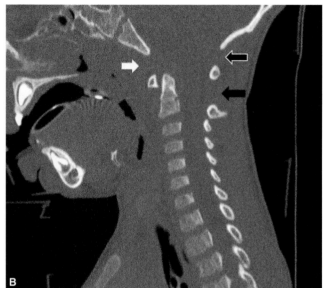

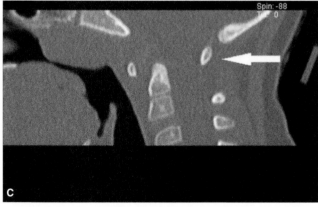

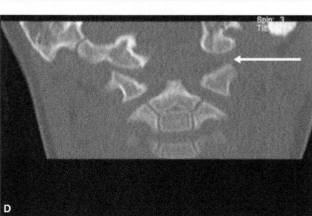

FIGURE 20.52 ■ Atlanto-occipital Dissociation. (**A**) Atlanto-occipital dislocation. Single lateral radiograph of the cervical spine demonstrates extensive prevertebral soft tissue swelling, anterior subluxation of C1, and the odontoid process with respect to the body of C2 due to a type II odontoid fracture and additional widening of the atlanto-occipital joint. (**B**) Atlanto-occiptal dislocation. Sagittal CT demonstrates marked widening of the distance from the tip of the clivus to the tip of the dens (white arrow), which should normally be 12 mm or less. Pronounced widening of the distance between the posterior arch of C1 and the occiput (black outlined arrow) and the C2 spinous process (black arrow) is also seen. (**C**) Atlanto-occipital subluxation. Sagittal CT through the midline demonstrates the anterior subluxation of the atlas relative to the occipital condyle with widening of the atlanto-dens interval (arrow). (**D**) Atlanto-occipital subluxation. Coronal CT slice demonstrates subluxation and asymmetric widening of the occipito-atlanto articulation (arrow). (Photo/ legend contributors: Konstantinos Agoritsas, MD, Steven Pulitzer, MD [A], Caitlin A. Farrell, MD, Vinodkumar Velayudhan, DO [B], and Ami Gokli MD, Marlena Jbara, MD [C, D].)

usually results in death secondary to respiratory arrest. If not immediately fatal, this dislocation is almost always associated with severe neurologic morbidity.

Emergency Department Treatment and Disposition

Immobilize the cervical spine and consult neurosurgery emergently. Order cervical spine plain films. Findings include increased space between the cranium and the ring of C1, best seen on the lateral view. Avoid traction, which may worsen neurologic injury. Assume these patients are in imminent respiratory failure and intubate with as little neck motion as possible. Prompt fixation is critical.

Pearl

1. Consider surgical airway management if video laryngoscopy or fiberoptic intubation is not possible.

SPINAL CORD INJURY WITHOUT RADIOGRAPHIC ABNORMALITY

Clinical Summary

Spinal cord injury without radiographic abnormality (SCIWORA) is a neurologic syndrome characterized by neurologic deficits without bony abnormality on plain radiographs or CT scan. The vast majority of patients with SCIWORA have myelopathy. SCIWORA is more common in younger children and can account for up to one-third of neurologic deficits in pediatric trauma victims. Such injury

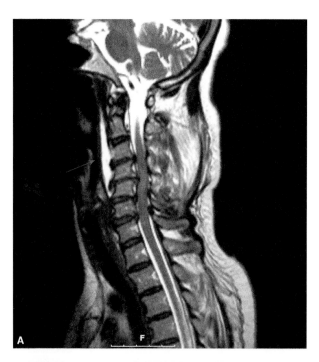

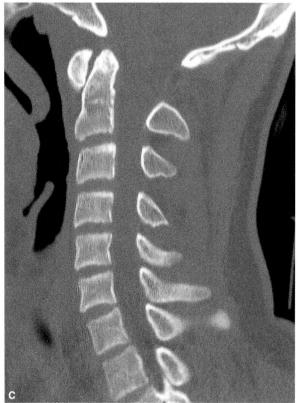

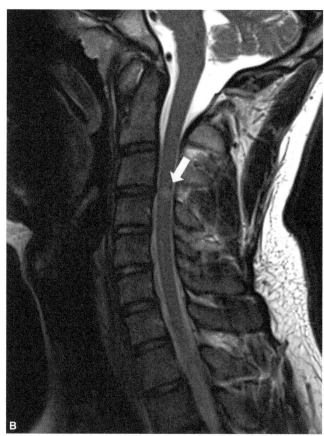

FIGURE 20.53 ■ Spinal Cord Injury without Radiologic Abnormality (SCIWORA). (**A**) Sagittal T2-weighted MRI of the cervical spine demonstrates prevertebral soft tissue swelling (arrow), reversal of the normal cervical lordosis, and disk herniations at C3–C4 and C4–C5. Hyperintense signal within the spinal cord at the C4–C5 level is compatible with spinal cord edema (hemorrhage not excluded in the setting of trauma). This patient was involved in a high-speed motor vehicle accident. (**B**) Sagittal T2-weighted MRI of the cervical spine in a different patient demonstrates high signal due to a spinal cord contusion at the C3–C4 level (arrow). (**C**) Corresponding sagittal CT image on the same patient shows no bony abnormality. Absence of findings on plain radiography and CT imaging in this patient with neurologic findings and spinal cord changes on MRI is consistent with SCIWORA. (Photo/legend contributors: Mark Silverberg, MD, Steven Pulitzer [A], and Caitlin A. Farrell, MD, Vinodkumar Velayudhan, DO [B, C].)

occurs because of the elastic nature of the pediatric spine. The mechanism of injury is usually hyperextension or flexion but can be rotational, lateral bending, or distraction as well. The degree of instability depends on which ligaments are torn or stressed. The severity of symptoms and neurologic findings can vary from minor to severe.

Emergency Department Treatment and Disposition

Immobilize the cervical spine and consult neurosurgery promptly. Monitor neurologic status closely. Most cases are treated with prolonged spinal immobilization.

Pearls

1. A normal CT or plain radiograph is not adequate to rule out a spinal cord injury in patients with altered mental status in whom a reliable neurologic assessment cannot be performed.

2. Monitoring of neurologic status is critical as these injuries may be caused by compression from spinal cord hemorrhage, which can progress.

BILATERAL FACET DISLOCATION

Clinical Summary

Bilateral facet dislocation is an extreme form of anterior subluxation caused by excessive cervical spine flexion. This hyperflexion results in ligamentous disruption and allows for marked anterior displacement of the spine at the level of injury, resulting in compromise of the spinal canal. The upper vertebrae's inferior articulating facets pass anterior to and above the superior articulating facets of the lower vertebrae and become "perched" there. There is often associated disk herniation, which further impinges on the spinal cord and can cause additional neurologic insult.

Emergency Department Treatment and Disposition

Immobilize the cervical spine and consult neurosurgery promptly. Order lateral plain films. Findings include anterior

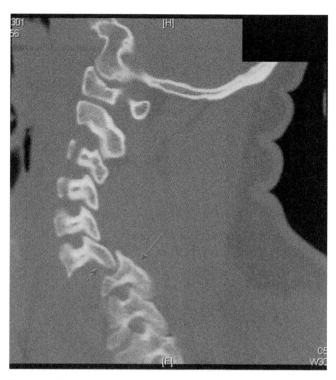

FIGURE 20.55 ■ Bilateral Facet Dislocations. Sagittal CT bone algorithm shows the inferior facet of C6 (short arrow) anterior to superior facet of C7 (long arrow) (jumped and locked facet). (Photo/legend contributors: Barry Hahn, MD, and Steven Pulitzer, MD.)

displacement that is more than half the AP diameter of the vertebral body and disarticulation of the facet joint. Treatment involves neurosurgical reduction of the dislocation to avoid further neurologic damage. Traction may increase the risk of injury if the injured disk retropulses into the canal. Perform a careful neurologic assessment for evidence of spinal cord injury before and after reduction.

Pearls

1. A significant number of bilateral facet dislocations are accompanied by disk herniation.
2. Any injury above C5 can be associated with respiratory compromise.

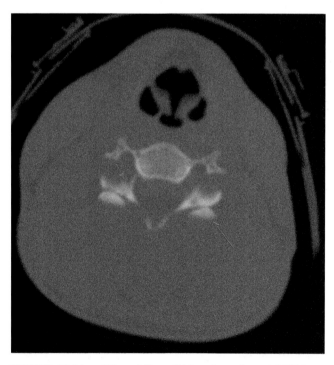

FIGURE 20.54 ■ Bilateral Facet Dislocations. An axial CT bone algorithm shows the inferior facet of C6 (short arrow) anterior to the superior facet of C7 (long arrow) (jumped and locked facet). Severe flexion is usually the mechanism that causes bilateral facet dislocations, as seen here. (Photo/legend contributors: Mark Silverberg, MD, and Steven Pulitzer, MD.)

998

Clinical Summary

Unilateral facet dislocation is a stable injury caused by simultaneous flexion and rotation. Patients often present with their head turned to one side with the inability to straighten it out. The inferior articular facet of a vertebra passes above and anterior to the superior articular facet of the vertebra below it and gets "locked" in the intervertebral foramen. Although the posterior ligament is usually torn, the "locking" of the facet into the intervertebral foramen makes this injury stable, and it is rarely associated with neurologic deficits.

Emergency Department Treatment and Disposition

Order plain films. Findings on the lateral radiograph include anterior displacement of the spine, less than one-half of the

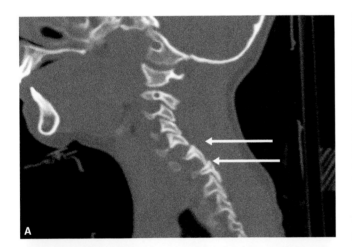

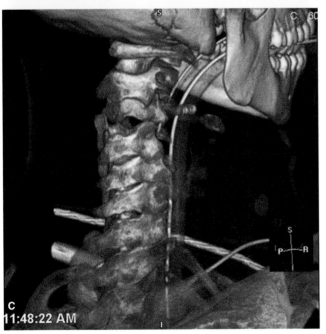

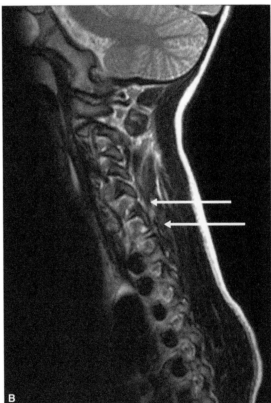

FIGURE 20.56 ■ Unilateral Facet Dislocation. (**A**) Sagittal CT to the right of the midline demonstrates perched facet at C5–C6 and jumped facet at C6–C7 (arrows). (**B**) Sagittal T2-weighted image to the right of the midline demonstrates perched facet at C5–C6 and jumped facet at C6–C7 (arrows). (**C**) This 3-dimensional; reconstruction of a posterior oblique view of the cervical spine in a different patient demonstrates a jumped and locked facet on the patient's left side at the C3 on C4 level. The right C3–C4 facet also seems to be at least partially disrupted. A rotational force is almost certainly responsible for this type of injury. (Photo/legend contributors: Ami Gokli, MD, Marlena Jbara, MD [A, B], and Mark Silverberg, MD, Steven Pulitzer, MD [C].)

diameter of a vertebral body. The AP view will show a discontinuity in the line connecting the spinous processes at the level of the dislocation. Provide analgesia and consult a spine surgeon (neurosurgery or orthopedics) promptly. These injuries may occasionally be reduced in the ED by a spine consultant under sedation with simple traction.

Pearls

1. Displacement of a vertebral body by more than one-half of its diameter should raise concern for bilateral facet dislocation. In such cases, immediate cervical immobilization should be performed.
2. This injury can be confused with torticollis but should be considered after acute neck trauma.

Clinical Summary

Anterior subluxation is an uncommon CSI that occurs when ligaments surrounding the posterior elements are disrupted but the anterior longitudinal ligament remains intact. Because both spinal columns are not affected, this injury pattern is considered mechanically stable. Isolated anterior subluxation is rarely associated with neurologic sequelae; however, cases with associated neurologic deficit have been reported.

Emergency Department Treatment and Disposition

Immobilize the cervical spine and order plain films. Findings include absence of fractures but widening (fanning) of interspinous processes and an offset of the anterior and posterior contour lines of the vertebral bodies on the lateral view. Avoid neck flexion because significant displacement can occur and impingement on the spinal cord can also occur. Consult neurosurgery promptly for evaluation in the ED.

Pearls

1. Anterior subluxation with a flexion mechanism is stable in extension but potentially unstable in flexion.
2. This injury can be confused with pseudosubluxation, which is a normal variant and usually occurs at the C2–C3 level in young children.
3. In true anterior subluxation, the spinolaminar line will be disrupted at the level of the injury, whereas in pseudosubluxation, this line will retain its smooth contour (within 2 mm).

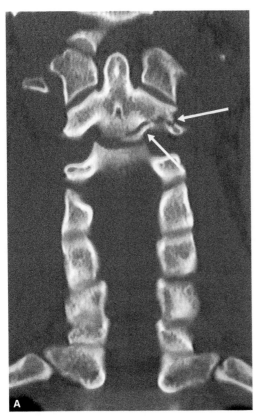
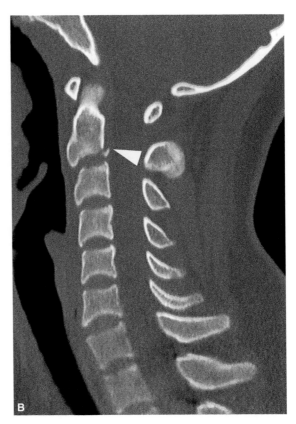

FIGURE 20.57 ■ Cervical Fracture with Subluxation. Fracture subluxation of C2. (**A**) Coronal CT demonstrates a fracture through the left lateral mass of C2 extending into the inferior vertebral body (arrows). (**B**) Sagittal CT again shows the fracture with minimal anterior subluxation (arrowhead) of C2 on C3. (Photo/legend contributors: Caitlin A. Farrell, MD, and Vinodkumar Velayudhan, DO.)

Clinical Summary

Clay shoveler's fracture is a stable injury that usually occurs after abrupt flexion of the neck combined with lower neck muscular contraction often from rapid torso/shoulder rotation. This violent muscular contraction results in avulsion of the longer spinal processes. C7 is most commonly affected, followed by T1 and then C6. This fracture can also be seen after direct blows to the spinous process or after forced flexion of the head and neck. Patients present with severe tenderness over the fractured spinous process, and a step-off may also be palpable. This fracture is always considered stable, and in isolation, it should not be associated with neurologic impairment. If neurologic deficits exist, other injuries should be sought.

Emergency Department Treatment and Disposition

Obtain plain films. Findings include an avulsed spinal process on the lateral view. Provide pain control and neurosurgical or orthopedic outpatient follow-up. Consider providing a cervical orthotic device for patient comfort. If significant trauma is also present, patients should be evaluated for additional injuries. This fracture can be caused by forced flexion, and flexion is a common mechanism for other, more severe CSIs.

Pearl

1. Plain films that do not adequately visualize the C7–T1 junction can miss this fracture, which most commonly occurs in this region of the cervical spine.

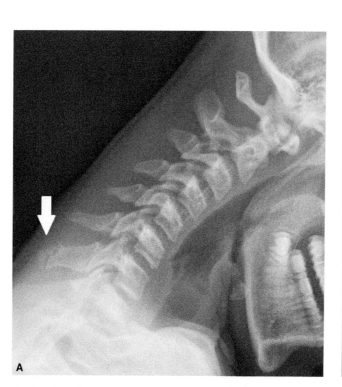
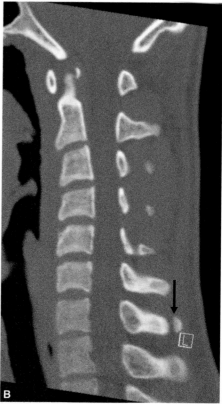

FIGURE 20.58 ■ Clay Shoveler's Fracture. (**A**) Lateral radiograph of the cervical spine in flexion demonstrates a displaced fracture (arrow) through the distal aspect of the C7 spinous process, consistent with a clay shoveler's fracture. (**B**) Sagittal CT image through the cervical spine demonstrates a displaced fracture (arrow) through the distal aspect of the C7 spinous process with a corticated edge. (Photo contributors: Ami Gokli, MD, and Marlena Jbara, MD.)

Clinical Summary

Tooth fractures are classified by the Ellis system. A class I Ellis fracture is through the enamel only, whereas a class II fracture is through enamel and dentin. Class III fractures involve the enamel, dentin, and pulp and lead to increased sensitivity and risk of infection.

A tooth concussion is consistent with minor traumatic injury to the supporting structures of the tooth, particularly the dentoalveolar ligament. There may be increased sensitivity to percussion, but there is no evidence of mobility or actual displacement of the tooth. Subluxation of a tooth is more severe than a concussion; there will be some mobility of the tooth without displacement. Luxation of a tooth implies displacement in the lateral plane. Caution must be taken not to miss a fracture of the tooth socket. Intrusion of a tooth is a traumatic impaction into the socket by an axial force. Such injuries may be associated with a dental root fracture. An extruded tooth is one that is outwardly displaced. An avulsed tooth is completely displaced out of its socket and is associated with periodontal ligament damage.

Emergency Department Treatment and Disposition

Manage class I Ellis fractures conservatively by referring to dentistry for potential filing or cosmetic repair. Treat patients who have class II Ellis fractures with antibiotics and consult

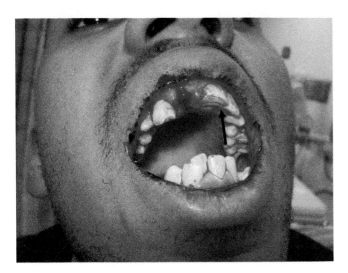

FIGURE 20.59 ■ Dental Trauma. After being struck in the mouth with a wrench, this patient avulsed tooth 8 and also suffered an Ellis class I fracture of tooth 7 (short arrow) and Ellis class III fracture of tooth 9 (long arrow). (Photo contributor: Mark Silverberg, MD.)

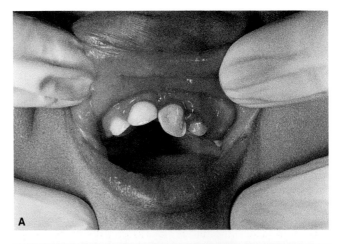

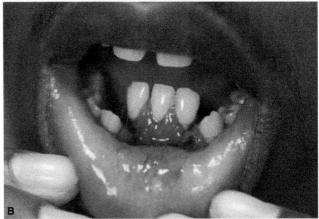

FIGURE 20.60 ■ Dental Trauma. (A) An image of a 2-year-old boy who sustained a subluxation of an upper anterior primary tooth after a fall. Management was conservative with frequent mouth rinsing and oral antibiotics. Had the tooth been completely avulsed, it would not have been reimplanted (primary teeth are never reimplanted). (B) An image of a mandibular alveolar ridge fracture with posterior displacement of the involved dentition. (Photo contributors: Binita R. Shah, MD [A], and Marc Baskin, MD [B].)

dentistry from the ED; cosmetic repair is usually indicated. Consult dentistry emergently for patients with class III Ellis fractures. Provide temporary coating, and initiate antibiotic therapy in the ED. Refer patients with concussed teeth for a nonemergent dental consultation. Advise these patients to avoid food or beverage with extremes of temperature.

Patients with subluxed teeth are at risk for pulpal necrosis. Consult dentistry for both primary and permanent subluxed teeth if there is >2 mm of mobility. Splinting reduces further damage and reduces the risk of avulsion with possible aspiration. With full luxation, there is increased risk of pulpal necrosis; consult dentistry for repositioning and bracing of the affected tooth in the ED.

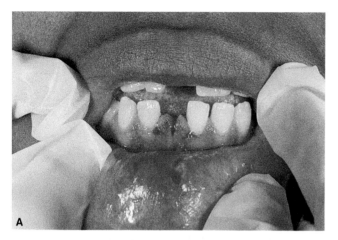

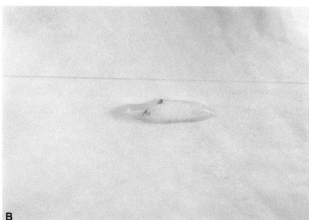

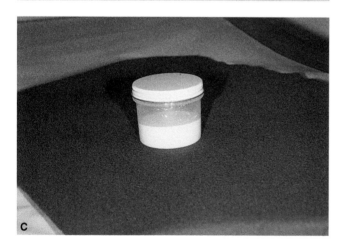

FIGURE 20.61 ■ Tooth Avulsion. (**A**) An image of an adolescent who was punched in the mouth and suffered an avulsion of her lower anterior incisor. The blow also caused subluxation of nos. 22, 23, and 24. The ideal scenario would have been to rinse the tooth with tap water and place it back into its socket and get to the ED as soon as possible. Other acceptable first-aid measures include placing the tooth in Hank solution, having the patient place the tooth under her tongue, or placing the tooth in a small container of milk. Unfortunately, the avulsed tooth (**B**) was left out to dry for over 2 hours before being placed in a container of milk (**C**). (Photo contributor: Binita R. Shah, MD.)

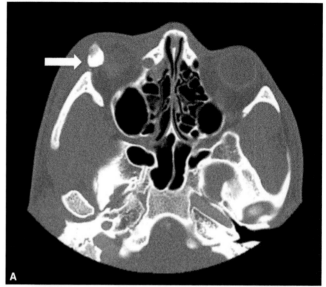

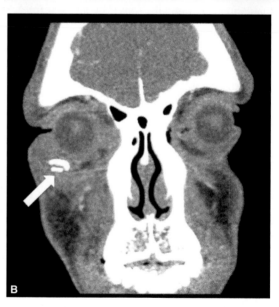

FIGURE 20.62 ■ Dental Trauma. An adolescent male who collided with his friend playing football was evaluated for facial trauma on the check and human bite (as he reported his friend's teeth hitting his face). His laceration was repaired, and he was sent home on antibiotics. He returned 2 days later for worsening pain and redness around the site. Axial (**A**) and coronal (**B**) CT images demonstrate a radiopaque foreign body (arrows, likely to be a tooth from his friend!), in the right check extending into the orbit inferior to globe. His wound was explored and irrigated, and a tooth was removed. (Photo contributors: Rabia Malik, MD, and Vinodkumar Velayudhan, DO.)

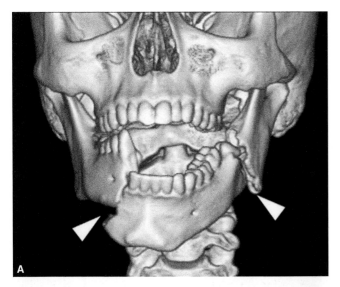

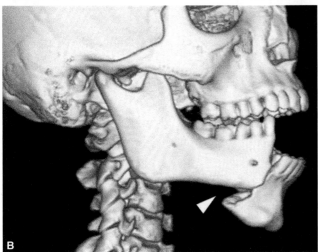

FIGURE 20.63 ▪ Mandibular and Dental Trauma. Bilateral mandibular fractures. Coronal (**A**) and oblique (**B**) 3-dimensional reconstructed CT images demonstrate displaced fractures (arrowheads) involving the right parasymphseal region of the mandible and the left mandibular angle with significant displacement and disruption of normal dental architecture and alignment. (Photo/legend contributors: Caitlin A. Farrell, MD, and Vinodkumar Velayudhan, DO.)

For intrusion of teeth, dental consultation is required to determine urgency of treatment. If a primary tooth is intruded on a permanent tooth, extraction of the intruded tooth is likely indicated. Caution parents that endodontic treatment or root canal may be necessary for the permanent tooth.

Consider extraction of severely extruded teeth in the ED to prevent aspiration. Either the ED provider or a dentist should reposition and splint the extruded tooth, and dental follow-up should be arranged.

Reimplant avulsed permanent teeth as quickly as possible (ideally within 30 minutes of avulsion) but do not reimplant primary teeth. Keep the tooth moist, preferably in Hank's balanced salt solution, but milk, water, or saliva also can also be used. Avoid touching the root and do not scrub the tooth; just rinse it gently. Consider local anesthesia or dental blocks to make this process more comfortable. Evacuation of any clot in the dental socket may also be warranted. Place the tooth in the socket and maintain firm pressure; then have the patient bite down firmly on folded gauze. The reimplanted tooth must then be splinted. Ensure dental follow-up because root canal is usually necessary.

Pearls

1. Provide broad-spectrum antibiotic coverage for any injury that leaves nerves or pulp exposed to saliva.
2. Primary teeth should never be reimplanted.

Clinical Summary

Pulmonary contusions are the most common thoracic injury in children. Most pulmonary contusions are secondary to blunt mechanisms, often motor vehicle–related injuries. The pulmonary capillaries are damaged, and this causes accumulation of blood in the alveoli, leading to progressive edema, atelectasis, consolidation, and ventilation-perfusion mismatch.

Patients with pulmonary contusions may have few external signs of injury. Bruising of the thoracic wall or fracture may often be absent. Clinical presentation depends on the degree of pulmonary injury. Initially, patients may be asymptomatic, or they may present with cough, chest pain, hemoptysis, tachypnea, or hypoxemia. Rarely respiratory failure is present from the start. Symptoms often progress over the next 48 hours because of continued bleeding and edema formation in the alveolar spaces.

Emergency Department Treatment and Disposition

Maintain a high index of suspicion for pulmonary contusion in all cases of pediatric blunt chest trauma. These injuries can be evaluated with CXR or CT scan. Plain films, although helpful in diagnosis, often lack sensitivity to detect small or

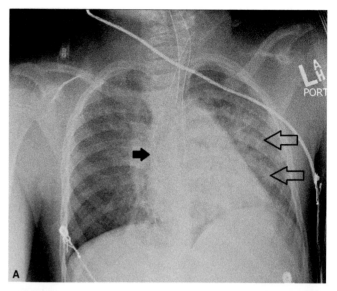

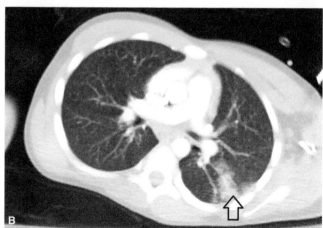

FIGURE 20.65 ■ Pulmonary Contusion. A 7-year-old child was found unresponsive outside on the ground with an open window seen on the second floor (child was presumed to have fallen from the second floor). (**A**) Trauma portable CXR demonstrates a diffuse patchy left-sided pulmonary contusion (hollow arrows). A malpositioned enteric tube is also present (solid arrow). The patient also had left-sided splenic and renal lacerations. (**B**) Axial CT view showing an arrow that denotes pulmonary contusion in the left posterior lung. (Photo contributors: Gregory N. Emmanuel, MD, and Josh Greenstein, MD.)

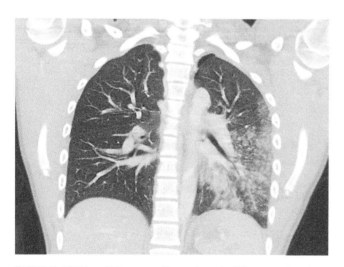

FIGURE 20.64 ■ Pulmonary Contusion. A CT scan using lung window algorithms demonstrates pulmonary contusion and apical pneumothorax on the left. This teenager was involved in a motor vehicle accident and sustained a rib fracture as well as solid organ injuries. (Photo/legend contributors: Caitlin A. Farrell, MD, and Ryan Logan Webb, MD.)

early contusions. Chest CT is more sensitive for detecting pulmonary contusions and can diagnose associated thoracic and abdominal injuries. Ventilation and oxygenation can be monitored with blood gas testing, capnography, and pulse oximetry measurement. Treatment is supportive for most pulmonary contusions and can include analgesia, supplemental oxygen, fluid restriction, incentive spirometry, and observation. Admission to an ICU is often warranted in patients with a high-risk mechanism of injury, an abnormal initial CXR, or a large contusion seen on CT due to the need for aggressive pulmonary toilet and close monitoring of respiratory status. Patients with large contusions that develop significant pulmonary shunting may require endotracheal intubation and mechanical ventilation.

Pearls

1. A normal initial CXR does not rule out a pulmonary contusion.
2. Pulmonary contusion in conjunction with rib fractures is associated with a high-energy injury.
3. Pneumonia is the most common complication of pulmonary contusion.

Clinical Summary

Isolated rib fractures are relatively rare in children. The compliant chest wall allows impacting forces to be transmitted directly to the underlying pulmonary parenchyma, without causing bony injury. When rib fractures are present, this indicates a high-energy mechanism, and severe underlying injuries should be suspected.

Flail chest occurs when a segment of the chest wall is separated from the rest of the thoracic cage. This is defined as at least 2 fractures per rib in 2 or more adjacent ribs. The flail segment paradoxically moves inward because of the normal negative intrapleural pressure of inspiration. Although this movement of the chest wall does increase the work of breathing, the major cause of hypoxemia is the underlying injury to the pulmonary parenchyma. Nearly all patients with flail chest have pulmonary contusions, which are the most common cause of respiratory failure following blunt chest wall trauma. Chest wall pain and inefficient ventilation further contribute to ventilatory failure.

Patients present with pain, dyspnea, tachypnea, hypoxia, chest wall tenderness/ecchymosis, and subcutaneous emphysema. Decreased breath sounds and dullness to percussion should raise suspicion of a hemopneumothorax. The diagnosis of flail chest is established most readily on CXR.

Emergency Department Treatment and Disposition

Stabilize the airway and provide ventilatory support with supplemental oxygen. Provide adequate analgesia and begin a complete diagnostic workup directed at evaluation and treatment of associated thoracic and abdominal injuries. Portable CXRs can help identify obvious pulmonary injuries that require immediate intervention. Chest and abdominal CT

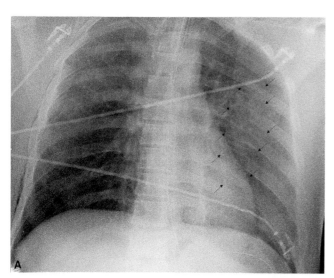

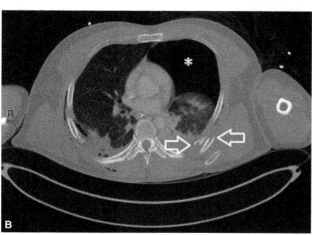

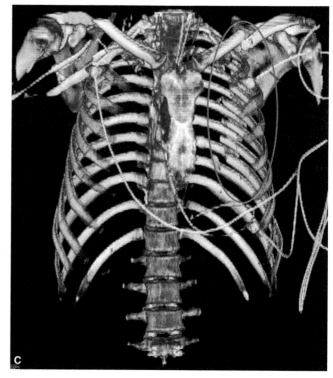

FIGURE 20.66 ■ Rib Fractures with Flail Chest. (**A**) Frontal CXR demonstrates multiple acute displaced rib fractures bilaterally. (**B**) Axial CT view of the chest demonstrates rib fractures (arrows) and large left pneumothorax (asterisk). (**C**) Three-dimensional reconstruction demonstrates contiguous left-sided rib fractures (circled) compatible with flail chest. A displaced left clavicular fracture is also seen. (Photo contributors: Sadie DeSilva, MS-4, Gregory N. Emmanuel, MD, and Josh Greenstein, MD.)

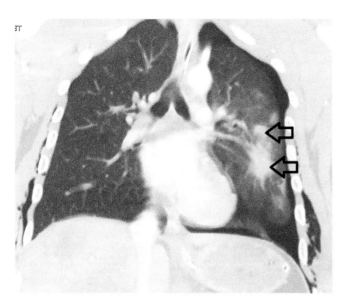

FIGURE 20.67 ■ Pulmonary Contusion. Coronal CT reformatted image shows left lung parenchyma opacification consistent with pulmonary contusion (arrows). (Photo contributors: Sadie DeSilva, MS-4, Gregory N. Emmanuel, MD, and Josh Greenstein, MD.)

scans are helpful to identify additional injuries. Consider an intercostal nerve block if systemic analgesics do not provide adequate pain control. If there is severe lung injury and ventilatory fatigue, consider mechanical ventilation in patients with concern for impending respiratory failure.

Patients with flail chest often require admission to an ICU for close monitoring of their respiratory status and observation for associated injuries. Provide adequate analgesia and chest physiotherapy to help prevent atelectasis and pneumonia.

Pearls

1. Unexplained rib fractures in children raise suspicion for child abuse. Multiple rib fractures, posterior rib fractures, or fractures in various stages of healing, especially in an infant, warrant an evaluation for child abuse.
2. The initial CXR may underestimate the degree of underlying pulmonary contusion.
3. Subtle flail segments are best appreciated by palpation of the chest during spontaneous ventilation.

Clinical Summary

Blunt or penetrating chest trauma can result in air accumulation in the pleural space. As the air volume continues to expand, normal ventilation becomes impaired and lung collapse progresses, leading to a ventilation-perfusion mismatch, resulting in hypoxia. In children with pneumothorax, the most common presenting complaints are chest pain and shortness of breath. Small pneumothoraces are often well tolerated, and children may manifest few if any symptoms. Children with larger pneumothoraces may show tachycardia, cyanosis, and decreased breath sounds on the affected side. Hyperresonance to percussion may also be noted. Subcutaneous emphysema is occasionally present when both pleural layers have been violated.

Tension pneumothorax occurs when there is a "1-way valve" air leak from the lung or through the chest wall. Progressive pleural air accumulation causes elevated intrathoracic pressure, leading to mediastinal shift and compression of the great vessels and contralateral lung, which results in

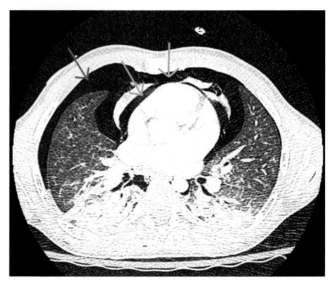

FIGURE 20.69 ■ Pneumothorax with Pneumomediastinum and Pneumopericardium. Midthoracic axial CT scan of the chest demonstrates bilateral pneumothoraces (red arrow), pneumomediastinum (green arrow), and pneumopericardium (blue arrow) in this adolescent with injuries from attempted hanging. (Photo/legend contributors: Caitlin A. Farrell, MD, and Ryan Logan Webb, MD.)

respiratory distress, tachycardia, and hypotension. Patients may present with ipsilateral decreased breath sounds and hyperresonance to percussion, jugular venous distention, and tracheal deviation to the opposite side. Pediatric patients with tension pneumothorax do not always manifest classic signs and symptoms, and the clinical presentation is often more subtle. The relatively short neck and increased soft tissue in children may make detection of jugular venous distention and tracheal deviation difficult. Consider tension pneumothorax in any pediatric patient with hypoxemia, tachycardia, and signs of shock.

Emergency Department Treatment and Disposition

When traumatic pneumothorax is diagnosed clinically, provide supplemental oxygen and prepare to place a thoracostomy tube emergently. If the patient is hypotensive, perform immediate needle decompression (midclavicular line in the second intercostal space), which converts the tension pneumothorax to a simple pneumothorax, and perform thoracostomy urgently for definitive treatment. Obtain an upright CXR or use US to confirm suspicion of a pneumothorax.

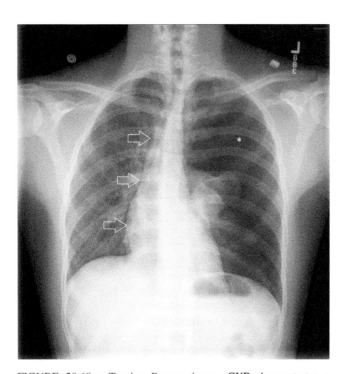

FIGURE 20.68 ■ Tension Pneumothorax. CXR demonstrates a large left pneumothorax (asterisk) with deviation of mediastinum to the right in this adolescent male (arrows) presenting with chest pain and diminished breath sounds on the left. (Photo contributors: Gregory N. Emmanuel, MD, and Josh Greenstein, MD.)

Pearls

1. Jugular venous distention may be absent in patients with tension pneumothorax and hypovolemia with active bleeding.
2. Young children are susceptible to tension pneumothorax because of their relatively mobile mediastinum.
3. Auscultate the lungs in the axilla because the more easily transmitted breath sounds in children across the chest and upper abdomen make clinical detection of a pneumothorax more difficult.
4. In the supine position, air in the pleural space tends to collect anteriorly and inferiorly, rather than in the apical location. The presence of a deep costophrenic angle (deep sulcus sign) on a supine film may be the only sign of pneumothorax.

Clinical Summary

Bleeding from the lung parenchyma, chest wall, or an intercostal vessel causing blood accumulation in the pleural space causes hemothorax. This is rare in infants and children because increased compliance of the ribs allows dissipation of traumatic forces. Hemothorax is most often associated with severe-impact blunt mechanisms such as high-velocity motor vehicle collisions or falls from moderate to extreme heights. Hemothorax secondary to penetrating injury is also rare in infants and young children, but the incidence increases dramatically in adolescents. As bleeding progresses, patients with hemothorax become hypoxic, tachycardic, and hypotensive. Physical examination often reveals decreased breath sounds and dullness to percussion on the affected side. A concomitant pneumothorax is often present with a hemothorax.

Emergency Department Treatment and Disposition

Obtain an immediate portable CXR in all patients with a significant mechanism of injury or clinical signs or symptoms of hemothorax. Use thoracostomy to decompress the pleura and drain blood from the pleural space. Place the chest tube laterally, in the midaxillary line at about nipple level, and directed posteriorly, and connect the chest tube to a water-seal apparatus. Obtain a repeat CXR to confirm proper positioning of the chest tube. Monitor the volume of blood drained and any ongoing blood loss, which usually stops spontaneously once the pneumothorax is evacuated. Operative intervention is indicated when the initial evacuation of blood is >10 to 15 mL/kg of body weight or there is persistent blood loss of >2 to 4 mL/kg per hour. Patients with hemothorax typically require ICU admission for close hemodynamic monitoring.

Pearls

1. Estimate appropriate chest tube size using either the patient's age plus 16 or 4 times the size of the appropriately sized endotracheal tube for intubation.
2. Hemothorax is often an indicator of multisystem injury. Perform a thorough diagnostic workup to avoid missed injuries.

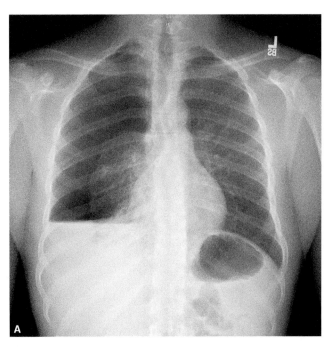

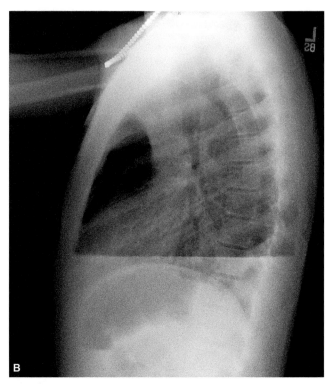

FIGURE 20.70 ■ Hemopneumothorax. (**A, B**) AP and lateral radiographs of the chest demonstrate a large right-sided pneumothorax with associated hemothorax. (Photo/legend contributor: Caitlin A. Farrell, MD.)

Clinical Summary

Traumatic airway obstruction is caused by penetrating or blunt trauma to the airway itself or from complications of other injuries. Relatively smaller airway diameter, less cartilaginous support, and a relatively large tongue and epiglottis make the pediatric airway more susceptible to obstruction. The airway may be occluded internally from secretions, blood, teeth, foreign bodies, or edema. External compression such as from hematoma formation in the neck with great vessel injury or from subcutaneous air can also lead to airway narrowing. Increased rate of respiration, nasal flaring, accessory muscle use, and presence of respiratory fatigue all indicate significant respiratory compromise. Cyanosis and hypoxemia are very late findings in upper airway obstruction. Stridor, gurgling, whistling, or grunting may indicate upper airway occlusion and should prompt rapid assessment and intervention.

Emergency Department Treatment and Disposition

Airway obstruction is immediately life threatening and must be recognized and corrected as part of the primary survey. If rapid removal of the obstruction is not possible, establishing a secure airway and initiating positive-pressure ventilation are required. Use suction to clear secretions and open the airway with the jaw thrust maneuver if CSI is suspected. High-flow

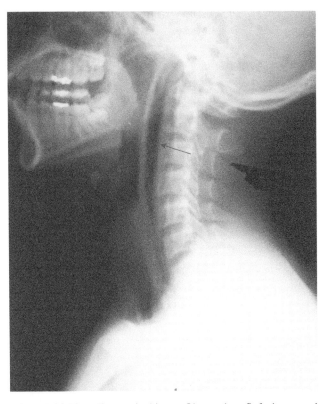

FIGURE 20.72 ■ Traumatic Airway Obstruction. Soft tissue neck x-ray of an adolescent who sustained a laryngeal fracture resulting in subcutaneous emphysema of the neck. Note the obvious soft tissue air tracking along the fascial planes (arrow). (Photo contributor: Michael H. Siegel, MD.)

oxygen should be provided. If signs of obstruction are still present, obtain plain films of the chest and neck to look for thoracic injuries or foreign bodies. Consider further evaluation with helical CT, laryngoscopy, or bronchoscopy. Consider rare but severe injuries, such as tracheobronchial tree injury. Consult pediatric trauma surgery and ENT as quickly as possible.

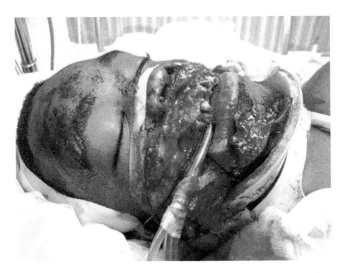

FIGURE 20.71 ■ Avulsion of Tissues of the Lower Face. After being struck by a city bus, this patient was dragged face down in the street. Multiple teeth have been avulsed out of their sockets and his upper lip has been torn off. Extensive injuries like these will require repair in the operating room. (Photo contributor: Mark Silverberg, MD.)

Pearls

1. The short length of an infant's trachea may easily result in intubation of the right mainstem bronchus.
2. Infants and young children have a large occiput, which results in passive flexion of the cervical spine when lying supine. Place a roll under the shoulders to anatomically align the airway and maintain maximal patency.
3. Young infants are preferential nose breathers. Trauma that results in nasal obstruction can lead to significant respiratory distress.

Clinical Summary

Blunt aortic injuries (BAIs) are rare in children and are usually associated with rapid deceleration mechanisms. Shearing forces and luminal compression occur against points of fixation, such as the ligamentum arteriosum. These injuries are most commonly caused by high-speed motor vehicle collisions and are less commonly due to falls from significant heights. Multisystem trauma is common, and nearly all patients have associated injuries. BAI has a high mortality rate, and most patients will die before reaching the ED.

Patient may complain of chest or back pain; however, patients often have no symptoms related to their BAI. There may be no external evidence of chest trauma. Physical findings associated with BAI include a "seatbelt sign," upper extremity hypertension or BP differential, decrease or loss of upper or lower extremity pulses, a new heart murmur, and

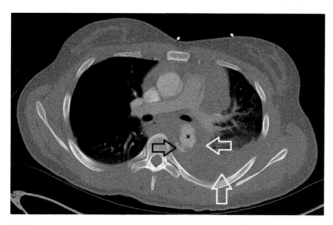

FIGURE 20.73 ■ Aortic Disruption. Axial post-contrast CT scan of the chest at the level of the pulmonary arteries. There is traumatic injury to the descending aorta (asterisk) with aortic rupture (black arrow) and surrounding mediastinal and thoracic hematoma (white arrows). The patient was successfully treated with an endovascular stent. (Photo contributors: Gregory N. Emmanuel, MD, and Ryan Logan Webb, MD.)

hypotension. Postoperative paraplegia is a significant complication of BAI.

Emergency Department Treatment and Disposition

Stabilize airway, breathing, and circulation and obtain a CXR. Radiographs are commonly normal or show only subtle changes. Mediastinal widening is the most consistent finding. Other findings may include loss of a defined aortic knob, deviation of the esophagus or main bronchus, an apical cap, hemothorax, or uncommonly, associated first or second rib fractures. In children, pulmonary contusion is more common than rib injury. If the patient has a high-risk trauma mechanism or the CXR is suggestive of aortic injury, order a CT scan of the chest, aortography, or transesophageal echocardiography (TEE). TEE is particularly useful in assessing small defects or when the diagnosis is in doubt after CT angiography or aortography.

Use IV short-acting β-blockers to control BP in patients without closed head injury. Decreasing the shear stress on the arterial wall may minimize the risk of rupture. Operative repair is required in BAI and may include endovascular stents in select situations for older children. Consult trauma surgery emergently.

Pearls

1. Maintain a high index of suspicion for BAI because the compliant chest wall in children may result in minimal or no external evidence of chest injury.
2. A normal CXR does not rule out BAI.
3. Thymic prominence in young children may make interpretation of the mediastinum difficult.

Clinical Summary

Traumatic diaphragm rupture (TDR) is rare in children and occurs most commonly in motor vehicle collisions in which the patient was restrained only by a lap belt. The sudden increase in intra-abdominal pressure may cause diaphragmatic tears, avulsions, or ruptures. Penetrating injuries may also involve the diaphragm. Any penetrating injury below the level of the nipple poses a risk of diaphragmatic injury.

The clinical presentation depends on the size and location of the rupture. Patients with small ruptures are usually asymptomatic. Those with larger ruptures and herniation of abdominal contents into the thoracic cavity may present with chest pain, decreased breath sounds on the side of the rupture, and respiratory distress. Bowel sounds may be heard on the affected side of the thorax. Displacement or compression of mediastinal structures can result in cardiovascular collapse.

Diaphragmatic herniation most commonly occurs on the left side because of the protective effects of the liver on the right side. The most common site of injury is the left posterolateral aspect, where the diaphragm is weakest. Missed diaphragmatic injuries may go undiagnosed for years. Long after the initial injury, patients may develop bowel obstruction or strangulation that is secondary to bowel herniation through a previously unrecognized diaphragmatic defect.

Emergency Department Treatment and Disposition

Timely diagnosis requires a high index of suspicion. Without visceral herniation, symptoms are minimal. Order a CXR and a CT scan of the chest and abdomen. Plain films may show only subtle abnormalities, such as an abnormal diaphragmatic contour. Note that a herniated liver may be easily mistaken for a raised hemidiaphragm. Larger defects may present with more obvious findings, such as intrathoracic visceral herniation or a nasogastric tube that remains in the thorax despite return of gastric contents. Diaphragmatic injuries are notoriously difficult to diagnose and may be missed even on CT. If TDR is strongly suspected, consider exploratory laparotomy, laparoscopy, or thoracoscopy to make the diagnosis.

Maintain adequate ventilation. Endotracheal intubation is warranted if the patient is in severe respiratory distress. Place a nasogastric tube for gastric decompression. Diaphragmatic tears do not heal spontaneously, and surgery is required for

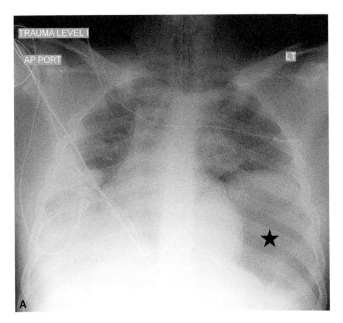
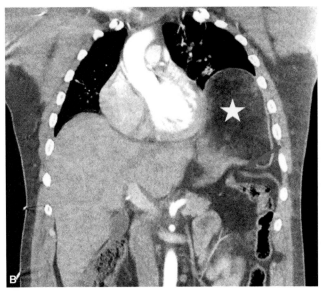

FIGURE 20.74 ■ Traumatic Diaphragmatic Injury. (**A**) Frontal CXR demonstrates an apparent elevated hemidiaphragm with the stomach bubble (star) overlying the left lower thorax in a 22-year-old man presenting after a motor vehicle accident. (**B**) Coronal CT of the chest and abdomen demonstrates a discontinuous left diaphragm (red arrow) with herniation of the stomach and surrounding mesenteric fat (star) into the thoracic cavity through the diaphragmatic defect. Many cases of traumatic diaphragmatic rupture are far more subtle and may be difficult to diagnose, even with the aid of CT. In these less obvious cases, simple elevation of the diaphragm or blurring of its contour could be a soft sign of injury. Where the diagnosis is missed, the patient is at risk for developing herniation of bowel through the defect weeks, months, or even years after the injury. (Photo contributors: Varun Mehta, MD, and Ryan Logan Webb, MD.)

definitive repair, regardless of the size of the defect. Consult surgery early, and admit all patients with diaphragmatic injuries.

Pearls

1. Children restrained only by lap belts are at higher risk for TDR than those who are fully restrained with lap and shoulder restraints or appropriate car seats.

2. Diaphragmatic rupture has been seen after minor blunt trauma. It is postulated that the timing of impact during the respiratory cycle may be more important than the magnitude of force.

3. Any impairment of diaphragmatic mobility can compromise ventilation.

4. The left side of the diaphragm is more prone to injury. However, right-sided injuries are less obvious and more easily missed.

Clinical Summary

Tracheobronchial tree injury (TBTI) is rare. It is most commonly caused by blunt trauma secondary to high-impact motor vehicle collisions. These injuries generally result from severe rapid deceleration or direct forces that occur when the child's elastic chest wall compresses the trachea and main bronchi against the vertebral bodies. In the majority of cases, TBTI is localized near the carina, or less frequently at the cricoid cartilage. In blunt trauma, rupture generally occurs in areas where the trachea is most fixed. TBTI from penetrating trauma is usually in the cervical region. TBTI frequently occurs in conjunction with other thoracic injuries. Overall mortality is high.

Children with TBTI often show only minimal symptoms initially and are less likely to have associated rib fractures, making TBTI a frequently missed or delayed diagnosis. Patients may complain of chest pain, dyspnea, or hemoptysis. Subcutaneous emphysema, stridor, decreased breath sounds, or cyanosis may be present.

Emergency Department Treatment and Disposition

Maintain a high index of suspicion in all patients with significant thoracic trauma. Order a CXR. Findings may include pneumothorax, pneumomediastinum, or subcutaneous emphysema. Treat any pneumothorax with tube thoracostomy. Consider large airway injury if the lung fails to reexpand, if there is a persistent air leak in the water seal, or if there is persistence of pneumomediastinum.

A high-resolution CT may confirm the diagnosis. Consider bronchoscopy to further assess the extent of the defect and aid in selective endotracheal intubation. Definitive management almost always involves surgical repair. Conservative treatment is reserved only for small lesions in patients without respiratory symptoms. Outcome is influenced by the extent of injury and the length of time delay in making the diagnosis. Consult surgery urgently and admit all patients with TBTI.

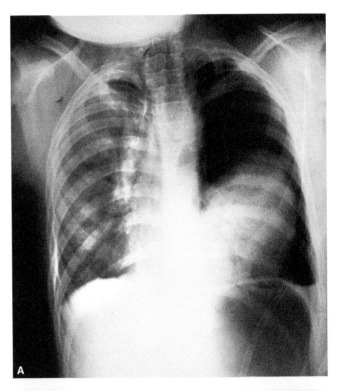

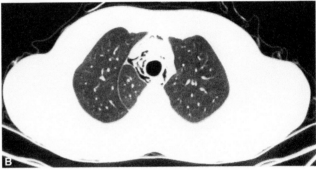

FIGURE 20.75 ■ Tracheobronchial Tree Injury. (**A**) Frontal CXR demonstrates left-sided pneumothorax with a peculiar position of the left lung. Rather than collapsing toward the hilum, the lung seems to have fallen to the dependent portion of the thorax ("fallen lung sign"). This is a rare finding on radiograph, but when present, the abnormal position of the lung and the left-sided pneumothorax are highly suggestive of rupture of the tracheobronchial tree. This was confirmed on a subsequent CT scan. (**B**) Pneumomediastinum. CT scan at level of the upper lobes demonstrates air within the mediastinum surrounding the trachea. Of incidental note, there is an azygous lobe and fissure, a normal anatomic variant. This patient was stabbed in the upper chest. A small hole was found in his trachea on bronchoscopy. (Photo/legend contributors: Michael H. Siegel, MD [A], and Mark Silverberg, MD, John Amodio, MD [B].)

Pearls

1. When possible, avoid positive-pressure ventilation in patients with concern for TBTI because it may worsen an injury by increasing air leakage from a tear, potentially resulting in tension pneumothorax.

2. Endotracheal intubation can convert a partial tracheal tear into a complete transection.

3. The "fallen lung" sign on plain film is rare but pathognomonic for TBTI. The involved lung drops to the dependent portion of the thoracic cavity as it hangs from only its vascular attachments at the hilum, indicative of complete bronchial transection.

Clinical Summary

Abdominal injuries account for approximately 22% of deaths in pediatric trauma. Up to 20% of children who present with a normal BP but a GCS score ≤10 have associated intra-abdominal injuries. Abdominal trauma is the leading cause of initially unrecognized fatal injuries in children. The most common causes of pediatric abdominal trauma are motor vehicle accidents and penetrating trauma. Falls account for a small number of abdominal injuries and typically lead to injury in children <2 years of age. Children's smaller bodies result in dissipation of traumatic forces over more organs, making multisystem trauma more likely. Solid abdominal organs are proportionately larger in children, leading to increased risk of direct injury. Young children have relatively less developed abdominal muscles and a more protuberant abdomen with less shock-dampening fat. The urinary bladder is an intra-abdominal organ in young children, making it more likely to be injured. Head injury is relatively more frequent in children with abdominal trauma, making the history and localization of pain and tenderness to palpation more difficult to determine. Physical examination also may be difficult or unreliable in infants aged <1 year, in children swallowing large amounts of air from excessive crying leading to abdominal distension, and with usage of illicit substances or spinal cord

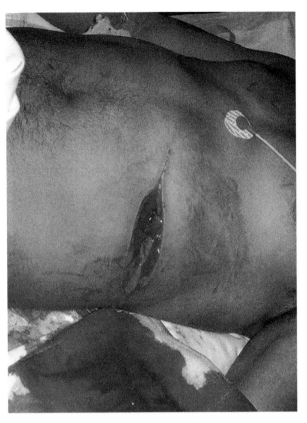

FIGURE 20.77 ■ Penetrating Abdominal Trauma. Machete wounds such as this one pose a serious risk to both solid and hollow organs. (Photo contributor: Mark Silverberg, MD.)

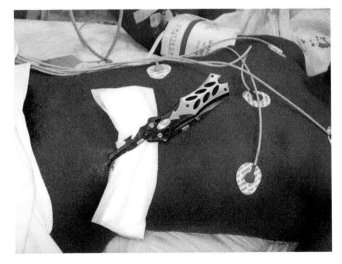

FIGURE 20.76 ■ Penetrating Abdominal Trauma. Stab wounds such as this one should be addressed in the operating room and never in the ED. The knife might be tamponading a vascular injury, and the injury could lead to exsanguination on removal of the knife if vascular control cannot be gained. (Photo contributor: Mark Silverberg, MD.)

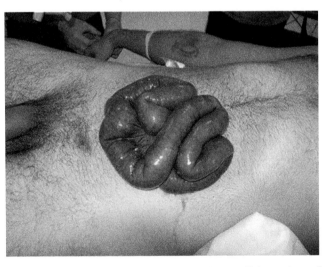

FIGURE 20.78 ■ Penetrating Abdominal Trauma. Eviscerations of the bowel need to be covered with moist sterile gauze as quickly as possible to prevent adhesions from forming later in life. (Photo contributor: Mark Silverberg, MD.)

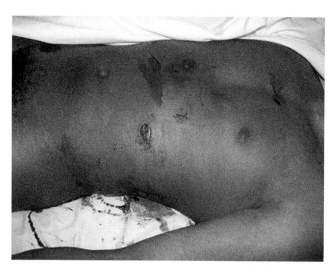

FIGURE 20.79 ■ Penetrating Abdominal Trauma. Ten bullet holes are visible in this image of a young patient who was shot with an automatic weapon during a drug deal. In the setting of penetrating trauma, holes plus bullets found on x-ray should be an even number. (Photo contributor: Mark Silverberg, MD.)

injury. Hematuria is an important sign in pediatric trauma and may indicate renal, hepatic, or splenic injuries. However, hematuria may be absent in up to 50% of patients with renal pedicle injuries and isolated ureteral injuries. Maintain a high index of suspicion for intra-abdominal trauma when there are lower rib fractures (causing splenic or hepatic injury), testicular injuries, pelvic fractures, or spinal cord injury (decreased sphincter tone, priapism, hypotension, relative bradycardia, and decreased strength/sensation).

TABLE 20.2 ■ INDICATIONS FOR LAPAROTOMY

Absolute Indications	Relative Indications
Multisystem trauma and need for craniotomy	Increasing abdominal tenderness
Persistent hemodynamic instability	Evidence of peritoneal irritation
Penetrating abdominal trauma	Transfusion of >40 mL/kg packed RBCs
Abdominal distension, hypotension	
Pneumoperitoneum with possible GI source	

Note: Delayed laparotomy is indicated when there is a delayed diagnosis of a hollow viscus injury or solid organ injury with >50% blood volume loss in 24 hours.

Emergency Department Treatment and Disposition

Stabilize airway, breathing, and circulation first and then proceed to rapidly identifying life-threatening conditions. Monitor cardiovascular status, obtain vascular access, provide fluid resuscitation, perform bladder catheterization (if no evidence of urethral injuries), and order plain films, CT, and US as needed before proceeding to definitive care. Whenever possible, obtain a history regarding the exact mechanism of injury to assist in making early and correct diagnoses. Examine the abdomen on arrival; repeat the abdominal exam serially, preferably by the same clinician. In hemodynamically stable children with blunt abdominal trauma, obtain baseline hemoglobin (Hgb), serum amylase, liver function tests (liver enzymes), urinalysis, and a type and screen or cross-match. In children who are hemodynamically stable, unsuspected injury may be identified by the presence of hematuria or elevated transaminases. With suspected pancreatic injury, consider serial serum amylase and lipase values (commonly elevated with blunt abdominal trauma, but sensitivity for pancreatic injury increases with serial values).

Plain abdominal radiographs are usually not helpful but may show an elevated hemidiaphragm, displaced gastric bubble, or free abdominal gas or help to identify and localize foreign bodies and detect pneumoperitoneum in penetrating trauma. Bedside US (the FAST exam) has demonstrated mixed evidence in its sensitivity and specificity to detect intra-abdominal fluid and organ damage in children; however, it does not accurately detect hollow viscus injury. Quality is diminished by bowel gas and fat, and the test characteristics are operator dependent. *Negative US does not exclude intra-abdominal injury in children.* Abdominal CT is the superior imaging modality in both blunt and penetrating trauma because it is both sensitive and specific in diagnosing intra-abdominal and retroperitoneal injuries. Use and type of contrast (IV, oral, or both) vary among centers (eg, oral contrast is not used by some centers because it prolongs scan time and induces vomiting without significantly aiding diagnosis). CT scan will identify (and assist in grading) most significant solid organ injuries including hepatic, splenic, adrenal, and renal injuries as well as the vast majority (~96%) of hollow viscus injuries. Emergent abdominal and pelvic CT scan should be considered with any suspected blunt abdominal trauma, significant fluid resuscitation with or without obvious source of blood loss, multisystem trauma, or an Hgb of <10 g/dL without obvious blood loss and/or hematuria. In patients with isolated microscopic hematuria, obtain renal imaging if there is another indication to obtain abdominal CT (eg, severe pain or decreasing hematocrit) or consider other modalities of imaging such as US.

The Arizona-Texas-Oklahoma-Memphis-Arkansas Consortium (ATOMAC) guidelines are an algorithm in use in many centers to guide nonoperative management. Consider peritoneal lavage for discriminating between mesenteric injury (may be missed by CT) and bowel perforation in consultation with a surgeon. Immediate clinical symptoms of mesenteric injuries include hypotension secondary to hemorrhage, abdominal distention, pain, and tenderness.

Nonoperative management is appropriate when there is hemodynamic stability despite solid organ injuries. These patients require close monitoring in a setting that is prepared for an operative intervention if needed. When transfusing these patients, a laparotomy is indicated if 40% to 50% of the patient's blood volume has been replaced in the first 24 hours. When blood products are used to resuscitate patients with any of these injuries, patients are at risk for transfusion-related coagulopathies, and a 1:1:1 ratio of packed RBCs–platelets–fresh frozen plasma should be administered. Patients with documented abdominal injuries or multiple organ system injuries should be admitted to the ICU. Consider transfer to a designated pediatric trauma center if specialty expertise is unavailable.

Pearls

1. Signs of abdominal injury include ecchymosis, abrasions, seatbelt marks, abdominal distension, tenderness, rigidity, mass, and Kehr sign (pain in left shoulder induced by palpation of left upper quadrant).

2. The most frequently injured organs in blunt trauma are spleen and liver followed by kidney, stomach, and intestines.

3. Children may maintain a normal BP even with a significant amount of blood loss (up to 25%). Persistent tachycardia can be due to blood loss or a variety of other factors (eg, fear, pain).

4. Initial Hgb/hematocrit values might be normal despite significant blood loss; serial monitoring is extremely valuable.

5. A metabolic acidosis is seen in children in hypovolemic shock. The base deficit is a useful marker for the presence of abdominal trauma requiring surgery.

SPLENIC INJURIES

Clinical Summary

The spleen is the most commonly injured organ in blunt abdominal trauma. Patients may present with diffuse abdominal tenderness, left upper quadrant pain, or referred left shoulder pain. Bruising on the left flank or abdominal wall may be present. Kehr sign, pain in the left shoulder induced by palpation of the left upper quadrant, is often found in patients with splenic injuries. The Organ Injury Scaling Committee of the American Association for the Surgery of Trauma has put forward a grading system for splenic trauma.

TABLE 20.3 ■ SPLENIC INJURY GRADING SCALE

Grade	Radiologic Findings
I	Capsular laceration <1 cm deep
	Subcapsular hematoma involving <10% of surface area
II	Laceration 1–3 cm deep, does not involve trabecular vessels
	Subcapsular hematoma from 10% to 50% of surface area
	Intraparenchymal hematoma <5 cm in diameter
III	Laceration >3 cm deep or involving trabecular vessels
	Subcapsular hematoma >50% of surface area
	Expanding hematoma
	Intraparenchymal hematoma >5 cm in diameter
	Rupture of the subcapsular or parenchymal hematoma
IV	Vessels injury with major (>25% of spleen) devascularization
V	Hilar vascular injury with devascularization of the majority of the spleen
	Shattered spleen

Emergency Department Treatment and Disposition

For a detailed approach to abdominal trauma, see page 1019. Plain abdominal films may show a medially displaced gastric bubble. A CT scan with IV contrast is more sensitive and specific for evaluation and grading the injury. Laparotomy is indicated when there is persistent hemodynamic instability or active bleeding.

The decision to proceed to surgical repair is based on hemodynamic instability. Admit patients and follow the American Pediatric Surgical Association–published guidelines for the length of hospital stay for children with splenic and hepatic injuries. A 24-hour stay in the ICU is recommended for grade IV and V spleen or liver injuries followed by 5 days in the hospital. For grade I, II, and III spleen or liver injuries, it is recommended that the patient be observed in the hospital for 2, 3, and 4 days, respectively. Restricted activities (eg, no contact sports) are recommended for 6, 5, 4, and 3 weeks for grades V/IV, III, II, and I injuries, respectively, as well.

Pearls

1. Nonoperative management is preferred if the patient is hemodynamically stable; the goal is preservation of spleen to avoid future infectious risk.
2. Less than 10% of children with spleen injuries require surgery.

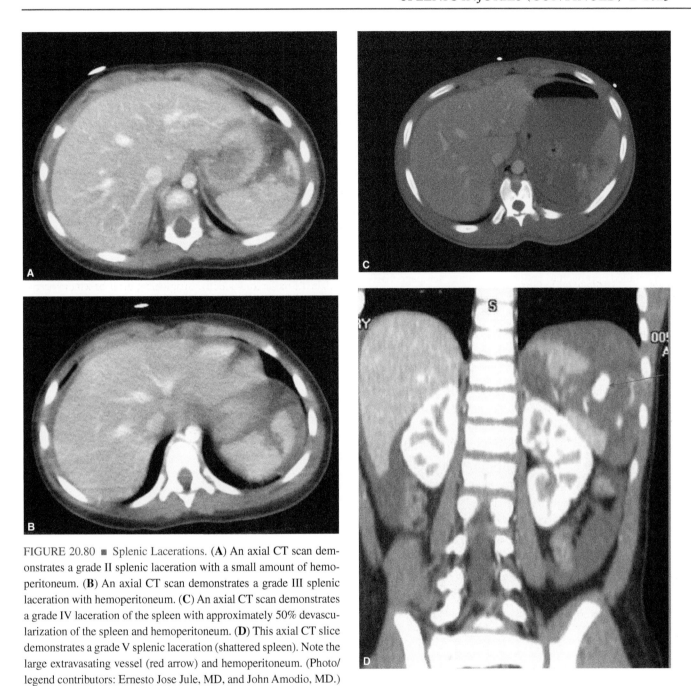

FIGURE 20.80 ▪ Splenic Lacerations. (**A**) An axial CT scan demonstrates a grade II splenic laceration with a small amount of hemoperitoneum. (**B**) An axial CT scan demonstrates a grade III splenic laceration with hemoperitoneum. (**C**) An axial CT scan demonstrates a grade IV laceration of the spleen with approximately 50% devascularization of the spleen and hemoperitoneum. (**D**) This axial CT slice demonstrates a grade V splenic laceration (shattered spleen). Note the large extravasating vessel (red arrow) and hemoperitoneum. (Photo/legend contributors: Ernesto Jose Jule, MD, and John Amodio, MD.)

Clinical Summary

The liver is the second most commonly injured organ in blunt abdominal trauma. It is the most common fatal abdominal injury in children, in whom the liver is relatively large and has decreased fibrous stroma (compared with adult liver). Patients may present with relatively nonspecific signs and symptoms or more likely will have distinct right upper quadrant (RUQ) pain and tenderness.

Emergency Department Treatment and Disposition

For a detailed approach to abdominal trauma, see page 1019. Obtain serum transaminases; any elevated aspartate amino-transferase (AST) or alanine aminotransferase (ALT) values may be significant and useful in assessing severity. Values of AST >450 IU/L and ALT >250 IU/L together have 100% sensitivity and 92% specificity for significant hepatic injury. Obtain an abdominal CT scan if the transaminases are above these values; however, RUQ tenderness in the setting of abdominal trauma should prompt an abdominal CT regardless of these values. Nonoperative management is preferred if the patient is hemodynamically stable with a liver injury. Grades IV, V, and VI liver lacerations are more likely to require surgical repair than lower grades. The indications for hospitalization of hepatic injuries (or for that matter any solid organ injuries) is any injury that is documented on CT scan because even if the level of injury is low (eg, class 1 or II minor hepatic injuries), and despite the fact that ~90% of hepatic injuries can be managed conservatively, patient is often at a risk for decompensation due to bleeding and may

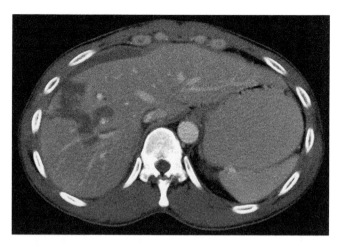

FIGURE 20.81 ■ Liver Laceration. An axial CT scan demonstrates a grade II liver laceration of the right lobe of the liver with adjacent subcapsular hematoma. (Photo/legend contributors: Shashidhar Rao Marneni, MD, and John Amodio, MD.)

have non-isolated hepatic injuries. Hence it is prudent to admit them under surgical or trauma services for close observation for at least 24-48 hours with serial clinical examinations and sequential hematocrit levels as indicated. Indeed, patient disposition decisions should be taken in consultation with pediatric surgeons.

Pearls

1. Liver injuries can be potentially fatal despite an innocuous initial physical examination with only mild RUQ pain.
2. Less than 10% of children with liver injuries require surgery.

Clinical Summary

Pancreatic injury is rare in children and caused most often by bicycle handlebars, motor vehicle accidents, and direct blows to the abdomen (child abuse). Patients may present with vomiting, abdominal pain radiating to the back, and/or persistent epigastric tenderness. The classic presentation of delayed signs or symptoms of a pancreatic pseudocyst include epigastric pain, palpable abdominal mass, and hyperamylasemia.

In children, gastrointestinal injury most often affects the jejunum and ileum. Assault and motor vehicle and bicycle crashes are the most typical causative mechanisms. Abdominal wall bruising may be seen. As peritonitis develops as a complication, fever, tachycardia, and abdominal tenderness will be present. Classically, the diagnosis is delayed because of the lack of symptoms of hollow viscus injury. Diffuse, dull abdominal pain or frank peritonitis may be the only indicators of hollow viscus injury with intestinal spill of contents.

Duodenal hematoma is rare and may occur 1 to 5 days after the original injury. Patients present with gastric distension, abdominal pain, anorexia, and progressive bilious vomiting leading to dehydration. In patients with small bowel, duodenal, or other abdominal injuries that are not consistent with the mechanism, a high clinical suspicion for child abuse should be maintained. Skeletal surveys and reporting to protective services are warranted when this situation arises.

Abdominal wall contusions and lumbar spine injuries (compression fractures and subluxation) from blunt

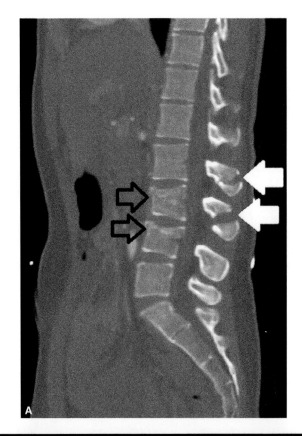

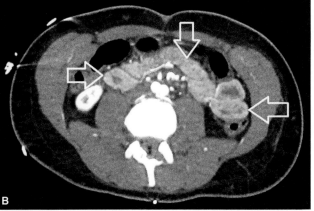

FIGURE 20.83 ■ Chance Fracture. (**A**) Sagittal view CT of the abdomen and pelvis demonstrates horizontally oriented fractures extending through the L3 and L4 vertebral bodies (black arrows) into the posterior elements of L2 and L3 (solid white arrows) compatible with Chance fractures in this 23-year-old woman after a motor vehicle accident who presented with upper abdominal pain and positive seatbelt sign without any neurologic deficits. (**B**) Axial CT image of the mid abdomen in arterial phase imaging demonstrates hyperenhancing loops of bowel (arrows) compatible with associated bowel injury, commonly seen with Chance fracture. The patient was found to have serosal tears of bowel on emergent exploratory laparotomy. (Photo contributors: Gregory N. Emmanuel, MD, and Dan Klein, MD.)

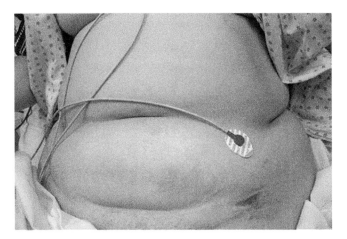

FIGURE 20.82 ■ Seatbelt Sign. This restrained passenger in a motor vehicle collision struck a parked car and sustained this seatbelt sign, noted to go across the abdomen and from the left hip up to the chest. (Photo contributor: Mark Silverberg, MD.)

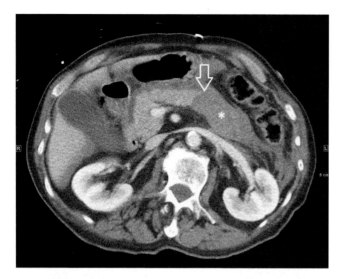

FIGURE 20.84 ▪ Acute Pancreatic Transection. Axial postcontrast CT of the abdomen demonstrates an acute pancreatic transection (arrow) with distal devitalized pancreas with associated hematoma (asterisk) in a patient who fell off a ladder, striking the end of a chair with his abdomen. (Photo contributors: Jesse Chen, MD, and Ryan Logan Webb, MD.)

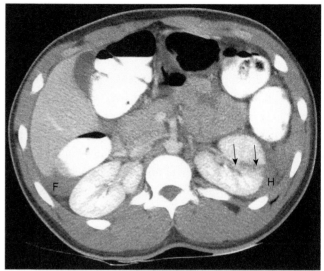

FIGURE 20.85 ▪ Kidney Laceration. CT scan demonstrates a grade II laceration (arrows) of the left kidney, extending from cortex to the collecting system. There is a perinephric hematoma (H) and free fluid (F) inferior to the liver. (Photo/legend contributors: Mark Silverberg, MD, and John Amodio, MD.)

abdominal trauma are associated with an ill-fitting child car restraint or seatbelt. This is most commonly seen in children age 5 to 9 years because of poor fit of an adult-sized lap belt in that age group.

Emergency Department Treatment and Disposition

For a detailed approach to abdominal trauma, see page 1019. Measure and monitor electrolytes and serial Hgb and hematocrit levels. An abdominal and pelvic CT scan with contrast is the imaging modality of choice. Coronal and/or sagittal reconstructions may be helpful in identifying spinal injuries. Treat pancreatic injuries conservatively, whereas intestinal

perforation almost always requires fluid resuscitation, antibiotic therapy, and rapid surgical repair.

Pearls

1. Hematuria is an important marker for serious renal and nonrenal trauma in children.
2. If you see a child who is <4 years old with duodenal injuries, think abuse!
3. Only 20% to 50% of children with pancreatic injuries require surgery.
4. The Waddell triad of pedestrian children struck by an automobile consists of a contralateral head injury, intra-abdominal injury, and midshaft femur fracture.

Clinical Summary

Due to the large external force required, pediatric pelvic fractures are more commonly seen with significant mechanisms of injury such as a fall from a significant height, a high-impact motor vehicle accident, or a pedestrian struck by a motor vehicle. There are 4 categories of pelvic fractures. In pediatrics, the type I fracture is an avulsion fracture and no pelvic ring fracture. Fracture of the iliac wing without displacement of the pelvic ring is a type II fracture. In type III fractures, there are 2 or more fractures of the pelvic ring, resulting in a free-floating segment (eg, Malgaigne and straddle fractures). Type IV fractures are acetabular fractures. Types I and II are considered stable. In pediatric patients, the stability of type III pelvic fractures will depend on the specific fracture pattern. Type IV fractures are always unstable.

Patients may present with ecchymosis over the pubis, iliac wings, scrotum, or labia. Blood at the penile meatus can indicate significant pelvic injury and should prompt concern for a urethral tear. There are often additional injuries to intraperitoneal and retroperitoneal visceral and vascular structures.

A significant amount of blood can be lost in the retroperitoneal space, and many patients with pelvic fractures require blood transfusion. The pelvic bones are large and thick with a rich vascular network, making fat emboli rare but occasional complications. Neurologic deficits can also be seen, especially with sacral fractures.

Emergency Department Treatment and Disposition

Consider pelvic fractures when high-energy mechanisms of injury have occurred. Anticipate the presence of a concurrent urologic injury in patients with pelvic fractures. Asymmetry of lower extremity pulses may suggest vascular compromise, although the presence of symmetric pulses does not rule out such injury. Begin IV resuscitation with 2 large-bore lines in all patients with suspected pelvic fractures and anticipate the need for resuscitation with blood. Obtain a portable AP radiograph of the pelvis, which may be done just after lateral cervical spine and AP chest radiographs in the polytrauma patient. Oblique, lateral, inlet, or 35-degree AP views may help detect subtle fractures. CT scan is more sensitive for acetabular and sacral fractures and for evaluating the posterior pelvis for retroperitoneal bleeding. If fractures are confirmed

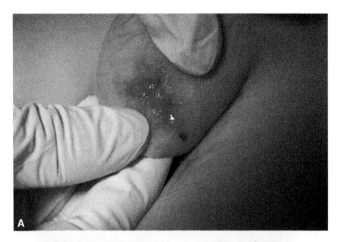

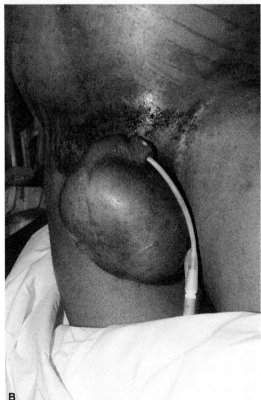

FIGURE 20.86 ■ Scrotal Injuries with Pelvic Fractures. (**A**) Scrotal laceration. (**B**) A large scrotal hematoma was noted in this patient with an open book pelvic fracture who was involved in an automobile accident. After a negative retrograde urethrogram for urethral injury, a Foley catheter was placed. (Photo contributors: Marc Baskin [A], and Michael Lucchesi, MD [B].)

on imaging, continue aggressive fluid resuscitation. If there is pain upon manipulation of the iliac wings or a pelvic ring fracture is diagnosed, avoid distraction or manipulation of the ring because this can cause increased bleeding.

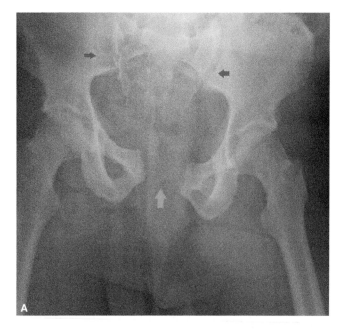

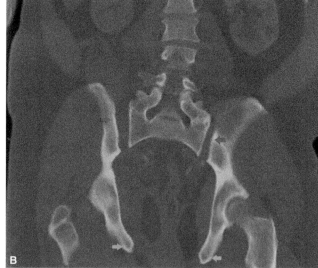

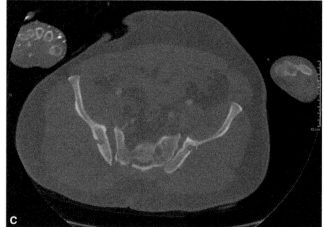

FIGURE 20.87 ■ Pelvic Fracture. (**A**) Frontal radiograph of the pelvis demonstrated widening of the pubic symphysis (blue arrows) and associated bilateral sacroiliac joint disruption (red arrows) compatible with an open book pelvic fracture seen in this patient after a motorcycle accident. (**B, C**) Coronal and axial CT images of the pelvis demonstrated widening of the pubic symphysis (blue arrows) and associated bilateral sacroiliac joint disruption (red arrows) compatible with an open book pelvic fracture. (Photo contributors: Jonathan Stern, MD, and Josh Greenstein, MD.)

Consult trauma surgery and orthopedics for surgical management of most pelvic fractures. In addition, for unstable fractures, consult orthopedics emergently to provide immobilization with an external fixation device that will limit further bony distraction and blood loss by decreasing the pelvic volume, tamponading bleeding, and promoting clot formation. The fixation device can be as simple as a sheet wrapped tightly around the pelvis and held in place with towel clips while awaiting definitive management.

Children who do not respond to blood transfusions equal to their estimated total blood volume are likely to have major vascular injuries and may require embolization.

Pearls

1. The high-energy mechanisms that result in pelvic fractures can also cause head, intra-abdominal, and long bone injuries.

2. It is rare for there to be a single fracture of the pelvic ring without a second disruption in a different location. Athletes represent the exception to this rule and can sustain an avulsion fracture due to sudden and forceful contraction of the muscle.

3. There is a high association of pelvic fracture with genitourinary injury in males. A high-riding prostate, blood at the urethral meatus, or a scrotal hematoma requires a retrograde urethrogram to further evaluate.

4. Hemorrhagic shock is the leading cause of death in patients with pelvic fractures.

Clinical Summary

Rings can be difficult to remove from edematous digits after sustained injuries or in the setting of finger infections. Swelling distal to the ring prevents it from passing over the proximal phalanx. Limited venous outflow further worsens the swelling and propagates the cycle. The digit's blood supply can become compromised and, in severe cases, can lead to ischemia and ultimately necrosis.

Emergency Department Treatment and Disposition

If the digit is only marginally swollen, use lubricants such as soap or petroleum jelly to slide the ring off the finger. If this fails, elevate the limb and/or apply cold packs to reduce swelling and attempt lubricated removal again. The ring may also be removed by winding silk suture material, umbilical tape, or straps from a non-rebreather mask around the finger, which "squeezes out the edema," allowing the end of the tape or suture to be passed under the ring and unwound to "wind the ring off."

If the above methods fail, cut the ring off the finger with a manual or electric circular blade ring cutter. Harder objects such as steel washers or nuts may require a handheld, high-speed rotary cutting instrument with a diamond-edged circular disk, which may be available from hospital engineering or dentistry. These devices generate significant heat. Avoid thermal injury by irrigating the field with running water to dissipate heat or pausing frequently to allow the object to cool. Provide eye protection for the patient and the operator during the procedure to prevent eye injuries. Other potential complications include blade injury to the underlying skin and granuloma formation from subdermally lodged metal filings. Consider restraining uncooperative patients when using electric cutting devices to prevent tissue injury from patient movement. Digital blocks may also prove helpful in such instances, although they do not allow the patient to be able to report pain from heat or direct injury.

Document digit neurovascular status before and after ring removal. Observe the patient until normal vascular and neurologic function is present, at which time the patient may be discharged.

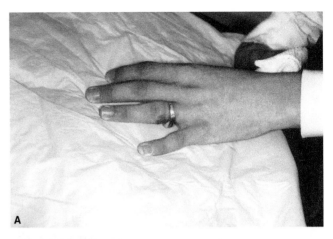

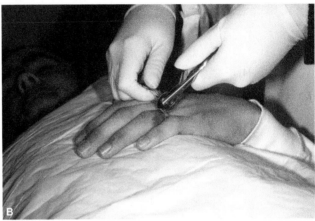

FIGURE 20.88 ■ Ring Incarceration. (**A**) Swelling of the digit associated with extreme pain was the presenting complaint of this adolescent patient who claimed that he could not remove the ring for many hours. (**B**) Unfortunately, the ring could not be slipped off of the finger so it had to be cut off using a rotary ring cutter. (Photo contributor: Binita R. Shah, MD.)

Pearls

1. Police or fire departments may assist in providing power tools for ring removal if the ring is thick or made from hardened metal, such as a washer or nut.

2. Heat generated during the ring cutting process should be dissipated using a constant stream of water. Cutting a hole at the corner of a normal saline bag may provide a stream of water for irrigation when running tap water is not readily available at bedside.

3. Rings made of material such as titanium and ceramic may not be too hard to remove using ring cutters and require removal using a technique known as cracking.

NAIL BED INJURY

Clinical Summary

Hand injuries are common. One-third of all traumatic extremity injuries affect the hands. In children, there is a bimodal distribution of hand injuries, with peaks seen in toddlers and teens. The fingertips are the most commonly injured site. Injuries to the nail bed are mostly common simple lacerations, although stellate lacerations, crush injuries, and avulsions also occur.

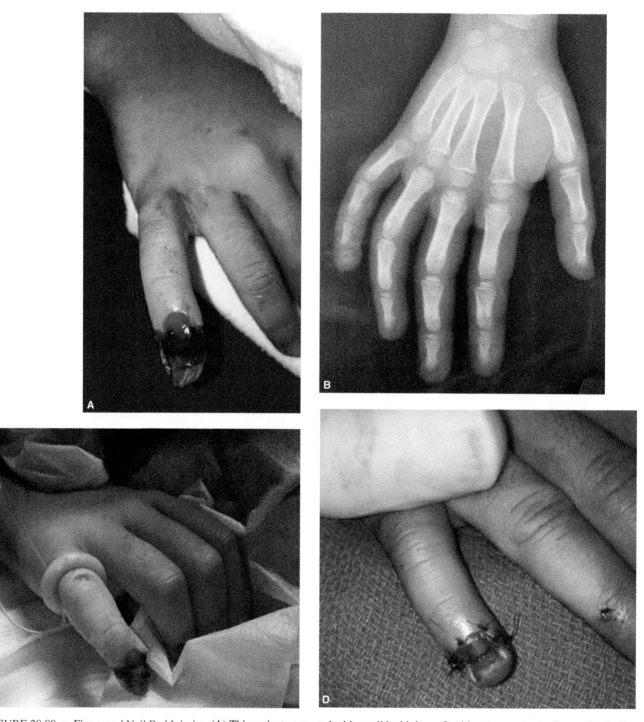

FIGURE 20.89 ■ Finger and Nail Bed Injuries. (**A**) This patient presented with a nail bed injury after blunt trauma to the finger. (**B**) Radiograph of the hand shows a fracture at the distal phalanx of the fifth digit. (**C**) Commercial tourniquet is applied to reduce bleeding during the repair. (**D**) Nail bed repaired with trimmed nail reinserted and sutured in place. (Photo contributor: Brian Labow, MD.)

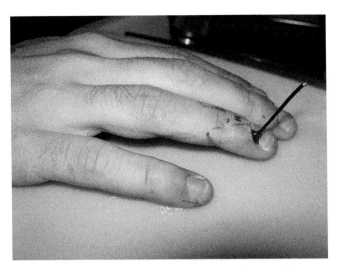

FIGURE 20.90 ■ Penetrating Injury. This patient impaled his fourth finger on his dominant hand with a bicycle spoke. It entered in the nail fold and can be seen below the skin almost back to the proximal interphalangeal joint. (Photo contributor: Mark Silverberg, MD.)

Emergency Department Treatment and Disposition

Local or regional anesthesia, with or without sedation, may be required to fully examine and treat the injured digit. If the nail is partially avulsed or loose, gently lift it and fully examine the nail bed for injuries. Order plain films because approximately 50% of nail bed lacerations have an associated fracture of the distal phalanx. If nail removal is required for examination or repair of the nail bed, prepare the entire hand with povidone-iodine and cover it with sterile drapes after a digital block has been performed and tested. Slowly advance the closed blades of a blunt-tipped hemostat or pair of iris scissors between the nail and the nail bed until they reach the nailfold. Slowly open the blades as the instrument is withdrawn, taking care to avoid causing further damage. Once the nail is sufficiently loosened, grasp it with a pair of hemostats and remove it using firm and steady distal traction. Inspect the nail carefully for attached portions of the nail bed and clean only the outer surfaces of the nail. Make a small incision or trephination in the nail to allow for drainage after it is replaced.

Repair any lacerations with 6-0 or smaller absorbable sutures. Data suggest that skin adhesive can also be used to repair nail bed injuries with equivalent outcomes as suture material. If available, reinsert the nail into the nail fold and suture it in place. If the nail is not available, splint the nail fold open with nonadherent gauze, single-thickness Adaptic, or the aluminum suture package material. Dress the finger with nonadherent gauze for easy removal during wound checks. Ensure that no nail bed is exposed.

Instruct patients to follow up 3 to 5 days after the injury to have the wound reassessed, at which time any foreign material used to hold open the nailfold should be removed. Antibiotic prophylaxis is not routinely indicated. Advise patients of potential complications from such injuries including cosmetic defects, painful nail growth, and total failure to regrow a nail if the germinal matrix of the nail bed was injured.

Pearls

1. Reducing bleeding during the repair can be accomplished with commercially available finger tourniquets or by wrapping a Penrose drain around the finger. Alternatively, cutting the fingertip off a sterile glove and rolling the glove down to the base of the finger will similarly reduce blood flow to the nail bed during the repair.

2. Nails grow at a rate of 0.1 mm per day. It may take up to 6 months for a new nail to reach the fingertip.

SUBUNGUAL HEMATOMA

Clinical Summary

Subungual hematomas usually result from blunt trauma to the nail bed. Subsequent bleeding from the underlying rich vascular blood supply accumulates under the nail. Clinically, there is pain to the digit tip and a dark red/black blood collection beneath the nail. Hematomas can be classified according to the percentage of the involved nail with blood below it.

Emergency Department Treatment and Disposition

If the fingertip is unstable or the mechanism of injury is suggestive of a significant distal phalanx injury, order plain films. If the nail is broken or the nail edges are disrupted, remove the nail and inspect the nail bed for lacerations (see page 1030 and also Figure 19.21). Significant nail bed injuries do not necessarily complicate larger hematomas, and routine nail removal for nail bed exploration is not necessary. Routine evacuation of a larger subungual hematoma (eg, >50% of the nail bed surface) is no longer recommended.

Drain (trephinate) symptomatic painful hematomas to decompress the blood collection. Digital blocks are not necessary for this procedure because it is relatively painless and there is immediate relief with decompression. First, clean the finger with Betadine and place it in a sterile field. Wear a face shield because the fluid under the nail can escape forcefully. Trephinate the nail with an 18-gauge needle or a portable hot-wire cautery device. Although a straightened and heated paperclip can be used, the risk of complications with this technique may be higher, and therefore, alternative methods are favored. If using an 18-gauge needle, rotate it between the thumb and index finger while applying gentle pressure. Proceed slowly because the "give" is less noticeable with this technique. If using thermal cautery, place the hot end of the instrument above the center of the hematoma and

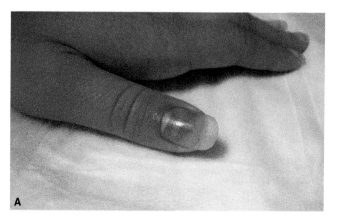

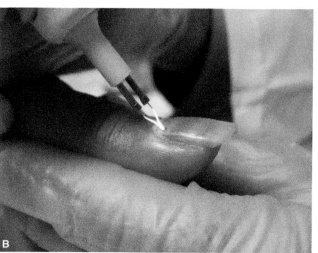

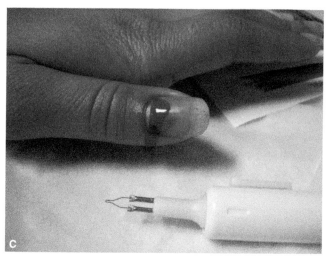

FIGURE 20.91 ■ Subungual Hematoma. (**A**) Crush injury to the thumb on the nondominant hand in a car door. Notice the subungual hematoma below approximately 50% of her nail. (**B**) Nail trephination using a battery-powered thermal cautery. It is important not to injure the nail bed after piercing the nail. (**C**) Drainage of the subungual hematoma with 2 holes in the nail results in drainage and release of pressure below the nail, alleviating pain. (Photo contributor: Mark Silverberg, MD.)

slowly advance until a "give" is felt and the nail breached. Alternatively, touch the nail gently in the same spot multiple times rather than holding the cautery in one place; this will avoid overheating the nail bed and causing additional injury. Rotate the device slowly as the nail is being penetrated to ensure an adequate-sized drainage hole is created. Note that artificial nails are quite flammable and must be removed prior to thermal trephination. Nail trephination in the presence of an underlying distal phalanx fracture technically converts the fracture to an open fracture. However, trephination is not contraindicated and oral antibiotics are not required. After decompression, apply antibacterial ointment and dress the wound with gauze or a nonadherent bandage.

Pearls

1. Avoid soaking the finger and keep it dry for 2 days after trephination.
2. Injured nails may fall off after significant hematomas.

DIGITAL AMPUTATION

Clinical Summary

Digit amputations are relatively rare, accounting for 0.1% to 1% of all hand injuries. Partial or incomplete amputations retain some interconnecting tissue between the distal segment and the limb. Reliable hand function is ultimately dependent on restored pinch and grasp function. If the index finger is removed, pinching can still be accomplished with the middle finger. An effective grip is primarily the function of the middle and fourth fingers. Functionally, the thumb is the most important digit. Loss of a thumb typically results in significant disability.

Emergency Department Treatment and Disposition

Treat patients with digit amputations as any trauma patient, first stabilizing and evaluating for life-threatening injuries. Digit amputations can bleed significantly and even result in hemorrhagic shock or exsanguination. Examine the injured area and document the neurologic, vascular, and musculotendinous status. Remove all jewelry from the injured part to avoid incarceration due to impending swelling. Provide adequate pain control with regional nerve blocks or systemic analgesia, keeping in mind that nerve blocks may compromise full evaluation by consultants.

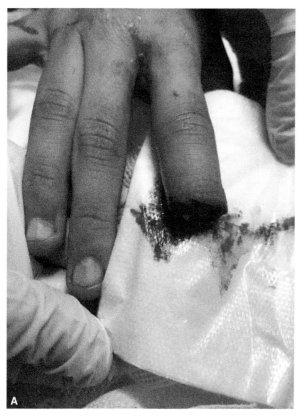

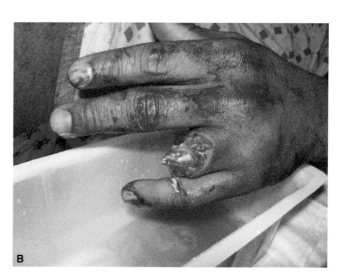

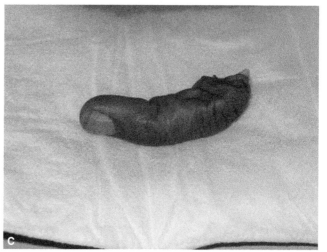

FIGURE 20.92 ■ Digit Amputation. (**A**) This patient was accidentally struck in the hand by a lawn tool. Note the bruising and swelling of the proximal portion of the digit. The avulsed digit portion of the digit should be placed in saline-soaked gauze and then sealed in a plastic bag and placed on ice until it can be reimplanted. (**B, C**) Digital amputation in a telephone repairman who slipped off of his ladder and caught his finger in one of the rungs as he was falling, avulsing it at the proximal interphalangeal joint as shown. The avulsed digit (**C**) was not brought to the ED with proper precautions. (Photo contributors: Joshua Nagler, MD [A], and Mark Silverberg, MD [B, C].)

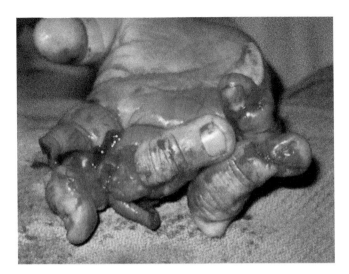

FIGURE 20.93 ▪ Multiple Partial Amputations. This school-age child sustained significant injuries to multiple digits when he placed his hand in a commercial meat grinder. (Photo contributor: Amir Taghinia, MD.)

Management goals are to (1) provide supportive care, (2) prolong viability of amputated tissues, (3) protect wounds from further injury, and (4) arrange expeditious subspecialist consultation. Replantation is indicated with complete amputations, whereas revascularization is used for partial amputations. Technical limitations to microvascular repair in vessels <0.3 mm in diameter limit the success of replantation of digits distal to the distal interphalangeal joint. Obtain radiographs of the proximal and amputated portions of the affected digit to assess the degree of bony destruction and exclude foreign bodies. For complete amputations, cleanse the stump by irrigation with normal saline. Avoid antiseptics such as peroxide and alcohol as they cause further tissue injury. Avoid manipulating the wound when possible. Do not clamp bleeding arterial vessels; instead, control bleeding with direct pressure. Cover the proximal portion of the digit with saline-soaked gauze to prevent further contamination and desiccation of the wound. Wrap the amputated part in saline-soaked gauze and place it in a sealed plastic bag and place the bag in ice water. Do not allow the amputated part to come in direct contact with ice because this can cause thermal injury.

For partial amputations, the treatment is similar. Cleanse and irrigate with normal saline and then wrap and splint the injured part. Treat with tetanus as appropriate. Most authorities recommend antibiotic prophylaxis against *Staphylococcus aureus* with a first-generation cephalosporin or other anti-staphylococcal antibiotic.

The more proximal the amputation, the less ischemia time the amputated part can tolerate. Cooling extends the viability of the amputated digit; for example, if left warm, the distal amputation is typically viable for 6 to 8 hours, but cooling to 4°C extends that time to 12 to 24 hours.

Pearls

1. Microvascular salvage should be considered for all injuries of the thumb.
2. Be aware of the limits of replantation surgery and do not encourage unrealistic expectations in patients or their families.
3. Do not discard amputated tissue if replantation is not possible because it may serve as a biologic graft.

Clinical Summary

Degloving or avulsion injuries typically result from motor vehicle collisions or industrial incidents. High-energy shearing forces separate large areas of skin and subcutaneous tissue from the underlying vascular supply, disrupting the dermal architecture and leaving it devitalized. The skin may be completely detached or partially connected. The dissecting plane is typically superficial to the deep fascia and muscle. Typically, the degloved skin cannot be reattached, but it may serve

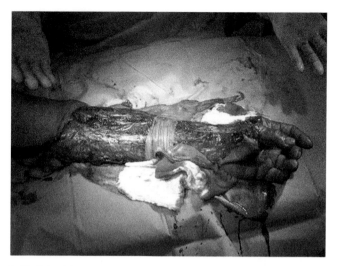

FIGURE 20.95 ■ Degloving Injury. The degloved arm was the result of riding in a car with the arm hanging out the window. In the ED, the arm was provisionally washed off with sterile saline to remove the feathers from the coat he was wearing at the time of the accident. Dry gauze was placed in the extremity as well as a splint until the patient was cleared for the operating room. (Photo contributor: Michael Stracher, MD.)

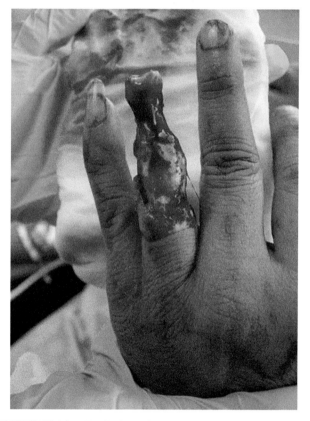

FIGURE 20.94 ■ Degloving Injury. This patient fell off of a chair with his hand on top of the refrigerator catching his wedding ring on the hinge. As he fell, the ring degloved his left fourth digit and avulsed the distal finger at the distal interphalangeal joint. (Photo contributor: Mark Silverberg, MD.)

as a skin graft. Patients often have other significant traumatic injuries that may delay expedient reconstruction by a plastic surgeon.

Emergency Department Treatment and Disposition

As with all trauma patients, stabilize the patient first and then assess the degloving injury. Obtain plain films of the degloved part to rule out fractures or retained foreign bodies. Irrigate and cleanse the flap with normal saline. Sharply debride any foreign material and obvious necrotic tissue. Carefully correct any kinks or rotations in the avulsed tissue that may further compromise vascular flow. All but the most minor degloving injuries should be taken to an operating room setting to be closed in a sterile environment following adequate irrigation.

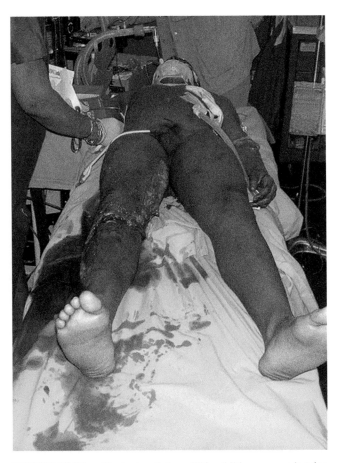

FIGURE 20.96 ■ Degloving Injury. This child was a pedestrian struck by an automobile. He had degloving injury to his right lower extremity associated with a proximal tibial physeal fracture and a hip dislocation. He underwent emergent irrigation in the ED as well as reduction of the hip dislocation and splinting. (Photo contributor: Michael Stracher, MD.)

Administer tetanus as appropriate and initiate broad-spectrum antibiotics to prevent infection in the devitalized tissue. Consult plastic surgery early.

Pearls

1. Degloving injuries are often dramatic and can easily distract providers. These patients require thorough evaluation for other associated injuries.
2. Even if the avulsed skin is not suitable for reattachment, it can be used for skin grafting.
3. Administer tetanus as appropriate and initiate broad-spectrum antibiotics.

Clinical Summary

Hand and foot injuries account for up to 5% of ED visits. Maintenance and restoration of function are the primary goals in managing hand injuries. Foreign bodies may become lodged in the soft tissues after any penetrating trauma, regardless of the size of injury. The most common foreign bodies are pieces of glass, wood, or metal.

Emergency Department Treatment and Disposition

Take a thorough history and evaluate carefully for injuries over the dorsal aspect of the metacarpal phalangeal joints, commonly known as "fight bites." Perform a thorough physical evaluation of the affected limb and document neurologic,

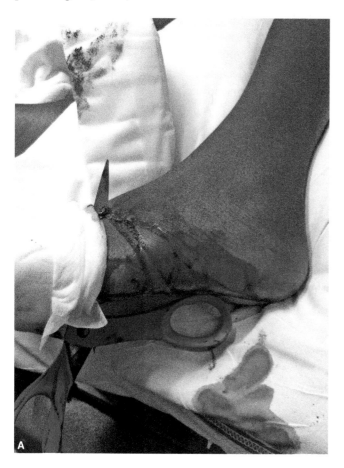

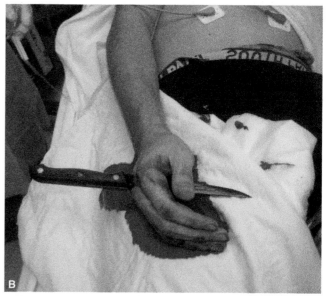

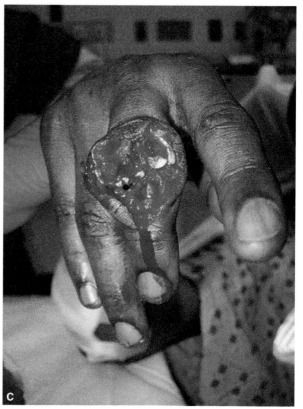

FIGURE 20.97 ■ Penetrating Injuries. (**A**) This teenager stepped on an open scissor while barefoot. The scissor blade can be seen exiting from the dorsum of the foot. Impaled objects like these must be removed in the operating room. (**B**) A teenager who was playing "5-finger fillet" ("stab between the fingers game") by placing the palm down on a table with fingers apart and using a knife to stab back and forth between the fingers (of course trying not to hit the fingers, but a dangerous game as seen here!). (**C**) This teenager got into a fight at a nightclub and was fighting over a hand gun. As he grabbed the muzzle, the owner pulled the trigger and the gun went off in his hand. (Photo contributors: Joshua Nagler, MD [A], Barry Hahn, MD [B], and Mark Silverberg, MD [C].)

vascular, and musculotendinous function. Order plain films to rule out fractures and retained radiopaque foreign bodies. If there is suspicion of a foreign body that is not seen on plain films, US or CT scan may be used. Some useful signs of a foreign body at presentation include pain with deep palpation at the injury site and pain associated with a mass. Retained foreign body may be identified by failure of an injury to heal or persistent pain with movement at the injury site.

Remove foreign bodies under direct visualization only. If that is not possible, refer the patient to a specialist. Fractures associated with foreign bodies require prompt surgical debridement to prevent osteomyelitis. Do not close penetrating injuries to the hand or foot; instead, allow them to heal via secondary intention. Administer tetanus prophylaxis as appropriate. Prescribe antibiotics if there is an associated fracture or if the injury is from an animal or human bite. Notify local health authorities of all animal bites. Instruct patients with heavily contaminated wounds to return for follow-up in 1 to 2 days for wound reevaluation.

Pearls

1. Foreign bodies that enter the foot through the sole of a shoe may be at increased risk of contamination with *Pseudomonas*, which should influence antibiotic selection as needed.

2. Foreign bodies of the sole or palm should be taken out under fluoroscopy by a specialist if they cannot be easily seen and removed in the ED.

Clinical Summary

Traumatic amputation of an extremity is a devastating event, both physically and psychologically. Traumatic amputations are classified by type of amputation, level of amputation, and mechanism and character of injury. The *type* of amputation can be classified as either partial (incomplete) or complete. The *level* of amputation is defined by the site of skeletal disruption; minor amputations are those distal to the wrist or ankle, whereas major amputations occur proximal to those joints. The typical *mechanisms* of amputation are as follows: (1) guillotine: sharp wound with minimal skin or soft tissue damage; (2) cutting: sharp wounds with a surrounding contusion zone; (3) crushing: skin and soft tissue injury zone is significant, often with comminuted fractures; and (4) avulsion: different levels of injury for bone, skin, and soft tissues.

Emergency Department Treatment and Disposition

Patients with traumatic amputations often have other significant injuries. First, stabilize the patient and then obtain radiographs of the stump and amputated part after irrigation with normal saline. Avoid antiseptics such as hydrogen peroxide and alcohol, which can cause further tissue damage. Do not clamp, tag, or tie off any portions of the stump or amputated part; apply direct pressure to control any bleeding. Wrap the stump with saline-soaked gauze, and elevate it, if possible. Wrap the amputated part in saline-soaked gauze as well and place it in a sealed plastic bag and place the bag in ice water. Direct contact with ice can cause further tissue damage. Cooling the amputated part will prolong viability and make

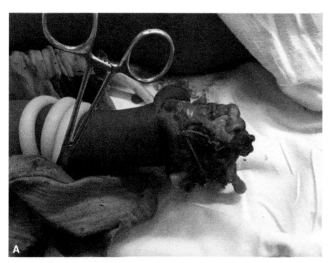

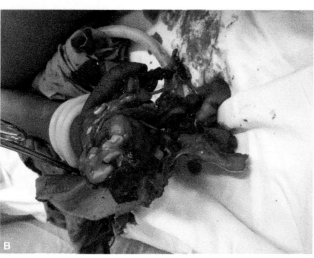

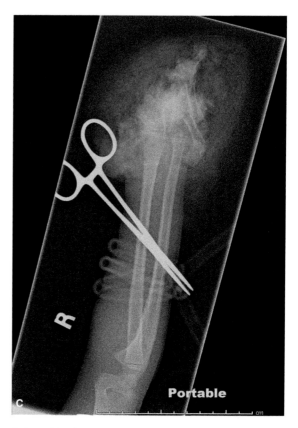

FIGURE 20.98 ■ Blast Injury. (**A, B**) This patient suffered a traumatic amputation to his hand while holding a firework during a July 4th celebration. (**C**) Radiograph of the affected extremity showing numerous, irregular disorganized bone fragments and missing bony and soft tissue in the region of the right hand. (Photo contributor: Brian Labow, MD.)

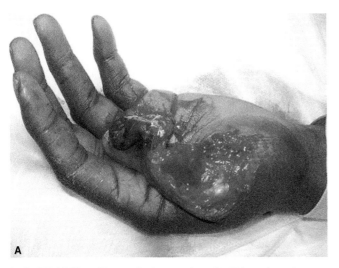
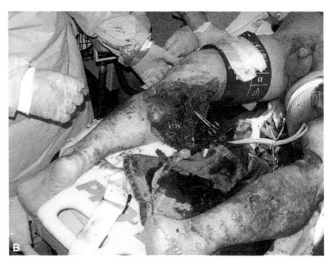

FIGURE 20.99 ■ Traumatic Amputation. (**A**) This patient almost completely amputated his nondominant thumb when operating a chainsaw while under the influence of alcohol. (**B**) This teenager was hit by a car and had his legs pinned against the bumper of his sports car by another car traveling >20 mph. Both of his legs were crushed and can be seen here facing backward. He eventually lost both limbs. (Photo contributor: Mark Silverberg, MD.)

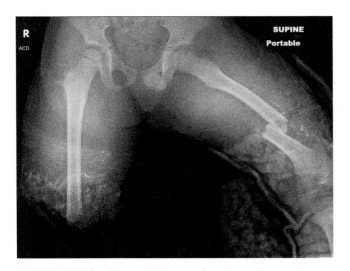

FIGURE 20.100 ■ Traumatic Amputation. Heavy farm equipment fell onto the legs of this patient. Radiographs show an above-the-knee amputation of the right leg and a displaced femur fracture of the left leg. (Photo contributor: Joshua Nagler, MD.)

successful reattachment more likely. Splint partially amputated parts to prevent further damage.

Replantation should be attempted for complete amputations, whereas revascularization is used for partial amputations. Consult the local or regional reimplantation center emergently. Administer tetanus as appropriate, and initiate antibiotic coverage for *S aureus* with a first-generation cephalosporin or other antistaphylococcal antibiotic.

Pearls

1. Patients with extremity amputations often have other significant injuries.
2. Cool the amputated part without allowing direct contact with ice to prolong viability.

Clinical Summary

Fishhooks can become embedded in soft tissues, most often in the upper extremities and head. Usually the penetration is superficial. Removal depends on the location of the injury and the type of fishhook embedded. Fishhooks can be single-barbed, multiple-barbed, or treble (multiple single-barbed in 1 hook).

Emergency Department Treatment and Disposition

Assess the location of tissue injury and type of fishhook involved. Radiologic studies are usually not necessary because most injuries are superficial. Four techniques are commonly used to remove fishhooks: retrograde, string, needle cover, and advance and cut. Provide adequate anesthesia prior to any attempt at removal. In the retrograde technique, apply downward pressure on the shank of the fishhook to disengage the

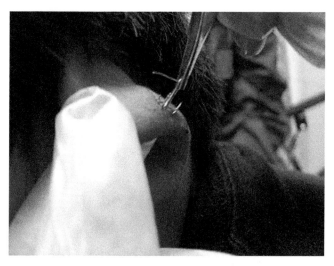

FIGURE 20.102 ■ Treble Hooks Impaction. Treble hooks are very difficult to remove because the 3 hooks face in all different directions. The skin on the back of this ear eventually had to be cut away from the hook and then reclosed. (Photo contributor: Ee Tay, MD.)

barb, while backing the hook out of the entry pathway. This method is rarely successful unless the barb is very small. In the string method, wrap a string around the bend of the hook and tug it out along the entry pathway as downward pressure is applied on the fishhook shank. In the needle cover technique, advance an 18-gauge or larger bore needle along the entry of the wound to cover the barb of the hook if possible, and then remove the hook and the needle together. In the advance and cut method, advance the fishhook through the skin using pliers or needle drivers and then cut the barb with pliers or wire cutters. Back out the remainder of the fishhook.

If a tendon or bone is involved in the injury or the patient is immunocompromised, begin prophylactic systemic antibiotic coverage. Provide tetanus prophylaxis as needed. Consult orthopedics and vascular surgery for deeper penetrations involving nerves, tendons, or vessels. Consult ophthalmology urgently for all ocular injuries.

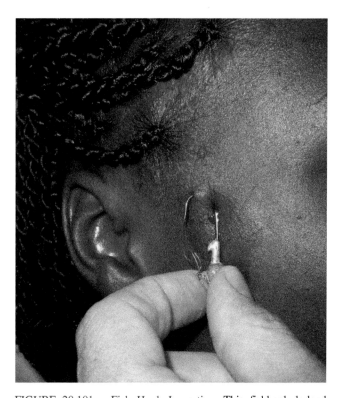

FIGURE 20.101 ■ Fish Hook Impaction. This fishhook lodged in the patient's face while someone was casting it without looking at who was behind him. It was removed by cutting off the eye and easily advancing it through the skin. (Photo contributor: Mark Silverberg, MD.)

Pearls

1. If a treble fishhook is involved, cutting the uninvolved fishhook(s) may simplify removal of the embedded fishhook.
2. Local anesthesia and either physical restraint or sedation may be necessary for removal when using any of the described removal techniques.

Clinical Summary

Zipper entrapment of penile skin occurs most commonly in uncircumcised boys during downward zipper movement. The skin can either be trapped in between the teeth of the zipper or within the zipper clasp. Skin entrapment may result in severe pain, laceration, or swelling of the skin.

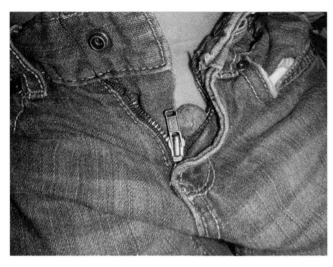

FIGURE 20.103 ■ Zipper Injury. This boy caught his foreskin in his zipper. Cutting the pants away from the zipper before attempting to remove the skin from the zipper's grip can be helpful. (Photo contributor: Jennifer Chao, MD.)

Emergency Department Treatment and Disposition

The appropriate method of zipper release depends on patient cooperation and type of entrapment. Forcibly unzipping the zipper to extract the foreskin is often unsuccessful because of the associated pain from manipulation. Physical restraint or sedation for uncooperative patients may be necessary. The most common method is to use a wire cutter or trauma shears to cut the median bar of the zipper. Other methods include cutting the zipper teeth, wedging a flat-head screwdriver between the faceplates of the zipper clasp, and soaking the area with mineral oil for 10 minutes followed by gentle traction of the foreskin. In rare cases, circumcision may be necessary to release the foreskin. Consult urology for complicated cases of foreskin entrapment or failed zipper release attempts. Apply topical antibiotic ointment or cream to any superficial lacerations or abrasions.

Pearls

1. Hospital engineers, dentists, or orthopedic surgeons may assist in providing the proper tools for cutting the median bar, such as a wire or bone cutter.
2. Zipper release may be simplified if the clothing surrounding the entrapment is trimmed.

Chapter 21

EMERGENCY ULTRASOUND

Jay Pershad
John P. Gullett

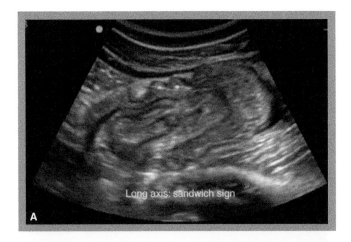

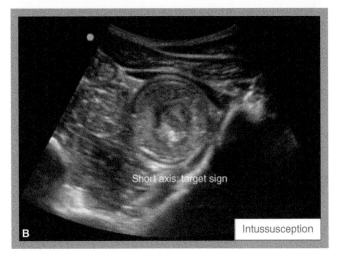

(Photo contributor: Michael Stone, MD)

The authors acknowledge the special contributions of Dimitrios Papanagnou, MD, and Michael Secko, MD, to prior editions.

Clinical Summary

Ultrasonography (US) is increasingly being applied in EDs for evaluation and management of patients with traumatic injuries and nontraumatic conditions. US is particularly useful in trauma. The extended focused assessment with sonography for trauma (eFAST) examination is a brief, repeatable, nonionizing, diagnostic exam used to detect gross blood in the abdomen, pericardium, and thorax in patients with blunt or penetrating torso trauma. The exam is limited to detecting free fluid as evidence of hemorrhage within an anatomic compartment, rather than the injury itself, because US is insensitive for visualizing solid organ injuries. Hemoperitoneum in the pediatric trauma patient is most often a result of hepatic or splenic injury and will typically appear as an anechoic (black) fluid collection on US.

Historically the focused assessment with sonography for trauma (FAST) exam, later modified to EFAST for visualization of the lungs, was intended for use in adults to detect massive hemoperitoneum in hemodynamically unstable blunt trauma patients to identify those who may need immediate laparotomy. The FAST exam includes 3 views of the abdomen (right upper quadrant [RUQ], left upper quadrant [LUQ], and pelvis) and a view of the pericardium. Later, views of the lung bases for hemothorax and pleura for pneumothorax were included to compose the EFAST exam. Furthermore, the role of the EFAST has extended to other scenarios such as penetrating trauma or undifferentiated hypotension, where EFAST can help the clinician prioritize management based on site of blood loss (chest, pericardium, or abdomen).

Technique

A low-frequency (1–5 MHz) curvilinear abdominal or phased array probe is typically used for its deeper penetration. Perform the scan with the patient in the supine position. *Direct the probe indicator toward the patient's head or the patient's right side.* When imaging the RUQ and LUQ, you may rotate the probe slightly to image in the plane of the intercostal spaces.

Obtain the following 4 views:

1. Hepatorenal space (Morison pouch) in the RUQ
2. Suprapubic view
   a. Rectovesicular pouch (males)
   b. Pouch of Douglas (females)
3. LUQ—subphrenic and splenorenal space
4. Pericardium

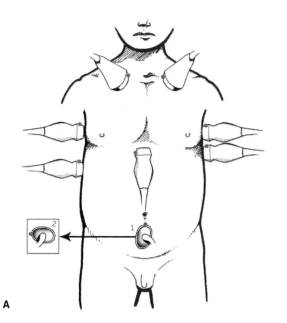
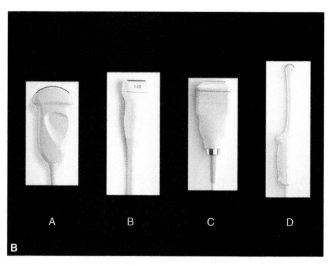

FIGURE 21.1 ■ eFAST Views with Probe Position and Probe Types. (**A**) The 5 main US windows of the eFAST exam: (1) The right upper quadrant view of the hepatorenal recess; (2) the left upper quadrant view of the splenorenal recess; (3) the subxiphoid cardiac view; (4) the suprapubic view; and (5) transthoracic lung windows. (**B**) Probes used for US. A few probes that one may use in their clinical practice are shown. A. Low-frequency curved array or convex probe. B. Low-frequency phased array or sector probe. C. High-frequency linear array probe. D. High-frequency endocavitary probe. (Photo contributors: John P. Gullett, MD [A], and Dimitrios Papanagnou, MD [B].)

In the supine pediatric patient, RUQ and pelvic views are the most dependent areas and thus the most sensitive in detecting intraperitoneal free fluid.

Ultrasound Findings

Free fluid in the RUQ appears as an anechoic collection between the liver and the right kidney. This dependent space

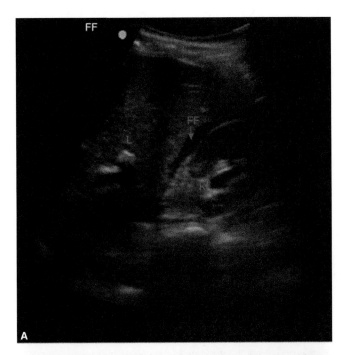

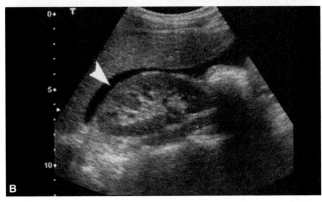

FIGURE 21.2 ■ Positive Right Upper Quadrant FAST View. (**A**) The liver (L) is visualized on the left side of the image with the right kidney (K) on the right side of the image; between the 2 organs, an anechoic stripe is visualized, representing free fluid (FF or hemoperitoneum) in a patient sustaining blunt trauma. (**B**) Positive right upper quadrant view. Arrow indicates extensive anechoic fluid in the Morison pouch. (Photo contributors: James Tsung, MD [A], and Jay Pershad, MD [B].)

is the most sensitive location to detect the hemoperitoneum, and therefore, it should be the first view obtained. In the LUQ, free fluid appears first above the spleen as an anechoic stripe between the spleen and diaphragm in the left subphrenic space. The spleen readily floats away from the diaphragm, unlike the liver. If the volume is large enough, blood will collect in the splenorenal space as well and soon flow to other dependent spaces in the abdomen (ie, hepatorenal space, suprapubic space). Note that the presence of fluid in any 1 abdominal view does not necessarily localize an injury. For example, fluid in the LUQ does not necessarily diagnose a splenic injury.

Use suprapubic imaging to visualize the bladder in both transverse and sagittal views. The bladder is a fluid-containing, anechoic structure on US and serves as an acoustic window to detect free fluid in the dependent space below it. The transducer is placed transversely over the pubic symphysis and angled downward into the pelvis. The bladder appears anechoic and roughly square shaped with rounded edges. If empty, the bladder may be quite difficult to visualize. If extremely full, it will appear more circular in shape. A sagittal view is also obtained to see fluid above the dome of the bladder or intermixed with adjacent bowel. Clinicians should look for the characteristic sharp corners in the shape of anechoic fluid pockets. The rounded edges of most intra-abdominal organs make external free fluid around them appear to have sharp angles. This helps distinguish free fluid from fluid in bowel or bladder. Suprapubic imaging also helps to assess bladder volume prior to bladder catheterization procedures.

A single view of the heart is obtained to rule out hemopericardium. This is typically done with a subxiphoid view, but other views are acceptable if a subxiphoid view is difficult and the clinical information is still obtained. This view is particularly relevant in penetrating trauma. The transducer orientation marker points to the patient's right side with the transducer just below the xiphoid process and flattened somewhat against the abdomen to aim upward and slightly to the patient's left shoulder. Pericardial fluid appears as a dark, anechoic stripe between the heart and the liver.

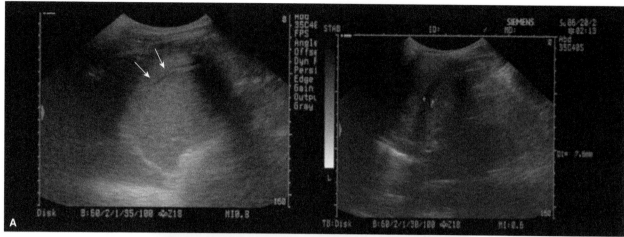

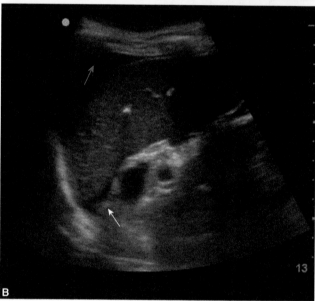

FIGURE 21.3 ■ Positive Left Upper Quadrant FAST View. (**A**) Free fluid in the left upper quadrant will first be visualized above the spleen, in the subphrenic space (double arrows). Note the hyperechoic curved diaphragm overlying the spleen on the left. Anechoic fluid is seen above the spleen (arrows) and between the spleen and the left kidney (cursors), representing free fluid. (**B**) This is an image taken from the left upper quadrant during a FAST exam. Note the anechoic fluid surrounding the spleen in the splenophrenic recess (red arrow), with a small amount of fluid at the tip of the spleen (small arrow) and no distinguishable fluid in the splenorenal recess. (Photo contributors: James Tsung, MD [A], and Michael Secko, MD, RDMS [B].)

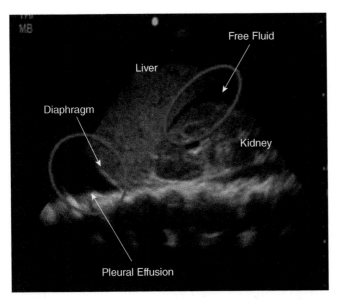

FIGURE 21.4 ■ Hemothorax. (Photo contributor: Jay Pershad, MD.)

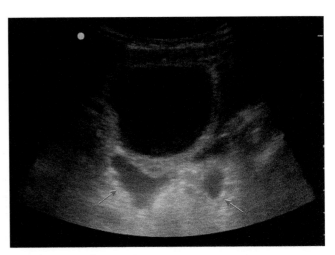

FIGURE 21.6 ■ Positive Suprapubic FAST View. Note the anechoic, urine-filled bladder (transverse view) with anechoic pockets inferior to it (arrows), representing free fluid in this pediatric patient with hemoperitoneum. (Photo contributor: Dimitrios Papanagnou, MD, MPH.)

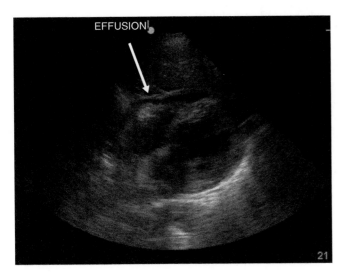

FIGURE 21.5 ■ Pericardial Fluid on Subxiphoid View. Note the echoic liver in the near field (top) of the image, with the heart in the far field (bottom) of the screen. Between the 2 organs, an anechoic stripe is visualized, representing pericardial fluid. (Photo contributor: James Tsung, MD.)

Pearls

1. Blood in the LUQ collects between the spleen and the diaphragm *first*, not between the spleen and kidney as with the Morison pouch in the RUQ.

2. With a smaller volume of hemoperitoneum, an anechoic collection may be seen first around the liver tip on the RUQ view before there is enough volume to fill the Morison pouch.

3. FAST exam does not rule out intra-abdominal solid organ injury; a CT scan should strongly be considered in patients with heightened suspicion for injury.

4. A parasternal long view of the heart can also be used to evaluate for free fluid when images of the heart cannot be obtained from the subxiphoid view.

APPENDICITIS

Clinical Summary

Consider bedside US in patients with signs and symptoms suggestive for appendicitis. US is a safe, nonionizing imaging modality in patients with moderate to high pretest probability of acute appendicitis. US is dependent on operator skill, body habitus of patient, and anatomic location of the appendix. It has lower sensitivity when compared to CT, but higher specificity. Although a normal pediatric appendix is difficult to identify, an inflamed enlarged appendix is often visualized.

The diagnosis of appendicitis in children can be difficult by history and physical alone, and the need to spare pediatric patients exposure to ionizing radiation indicates a more prominent role for US.

Technique

A high-frequency (6–12 MHz) linear probe is preferable for visualizing the appendix and most gastrointestinal pathology in children. Children tend to have lower body fat and thin habitus compared to adults; therefore, selecting a higher frequency probe is not usually an issue and provides higher resolution without compromising depth. In patients with a larger body habitus, deeper visualization of the abdomen

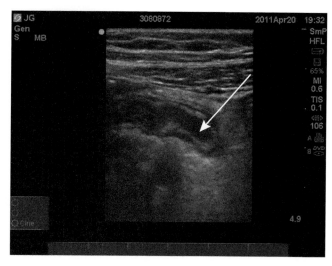

FIGURE 21.8 ■ Acute Appendicitis. A long-axis view of a dilated fluid-filled appendix (arrow). (Photo contributor: John P. Gullett, MD.)

may be required, necessitating the use of the low-frequency (2–5 MHz) curvilinear, or "abdominal," probe. It may be advisable to start with the low-frequency probe to get a larger field of view and then switch to a linear probe to focus on an object of interest. Consider using a low-frequency probe as analogous to looking through a doorway and the linear high-frequency probe as analogous to looking through a keyhole.

The best landmark to begin the exam is the point of maximum tenderness, if it can be specified. Otherwise, place the probe in the transverse orientation with the marker to the patient's right and identify the psoas muscle, which is characteristically round, and the iliac vessels. The appendix will often overlie these structures. If the appendix is retrocecal or in another atypical location, then US is unlikely to visualize it.

Use gentle pressure to displace gas from the bowel and identify a round structure with concentric layers—a "target" pattern. Observe for peristalsis; if it is seen, then the structure is the small bowel, which is easily mistaken for the appendix. Measure the diameter of the appendix in transverse axis, from outer wall to outer wall.

Ultrasound Findings

Appendicitis is identified by the following characteristics:

1. Diameter of >6 mm in transverse
2. Does not demonstrate peristalsis or pulsations
3. Blind-ended tubular structure
4. Noncompressible

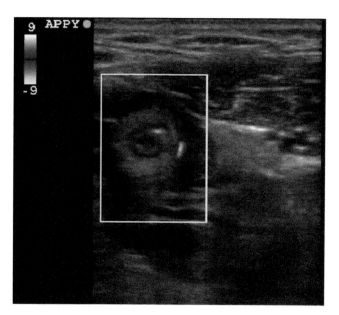

FIGURE 21.7 ■ Acute Appendicitis. A short-axis view of this inflamed, "target pattern" appendix has a diameter >6 mm and does not compress; it should not be confused with a vessel. (Photo contributor: Michael Secko, MD, RDMS.)

Other supportive findings include a fluid-filled appendix and periappendiceal fluid. A phlegmon, abscess, or perforation will often obscure the architecture of the appendix, making the diagnosis more difficult on US. Fecaliths may be seen in the appendix with posterior shadowing, however their presence is not diagnostic.

Pearls

1. Look for a target-like appearance, created by the layers of the dilated appendix wall, interior anechoic fluid, and possibly hyperechoic fecalith.

2. Because of its low sensitivity, a nondiagnostic bedside US should be followed up with an official radiologist-performed US or surgical consultation if the clinical suspicion is high.

3. If an inflamed appendix has perforated, US has a much lower sensitivity in detecting appendicitis.

4. Finding the iliac vessels adjacent to the psoas muscle in the right lower quadrant (RLQ) is a good landmark to search for the appendix.

Clinical Summary

US is highly accurate in diagnosis of intussusception, with a sensitivity of 95% to 97%, which is much greater than a 2-view plain radiograph of the abdomen. Thus, US is the preferred imaging modality for intussusception.

Technique

Use a high-frequency (6–12 MHz) linear probe or, in patients with a larger body habitus, a low-frequency (2–5 MHz) curvilinear probe for deeper penetration into the abdomen. Perform the scan with the patient comfortably in the supine position. If an abdominal mass is noted on inspection or palpation, scan the mass in at least 2 perpendicular planes. If no mass is immediately appreciated, scan the abdomen slowly along the path of the bowel, beginning from the ileocecal region (RLQ); scan in a clockwise fashion around the abdomen, keeping note of any potential mass below the abdominal wall.

Ultrasound Findings

The normal, unaffected bowel appears as a uniform, thin, hypoechoic rim around an echogenic center of variable widths and demonstrates peristaltic activity. An intussuscepted bowel appears as another "target sign" in transverse orientation (similar to but different in appearance to appendicitis), representing concentric layers of mucosa, muscularis, and serosa,

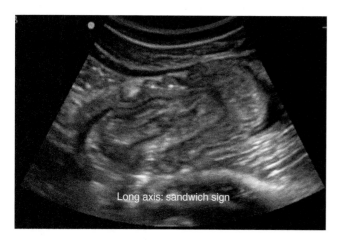

FIGURE 21.9 ■ Intussusception. A longitudinal (long axis) view of intussuscepted bowel with its alternating layers of hypoechoic bowel wall has been described as resembling a "sandwich." (Photo contributor: Michael Stone MD.)

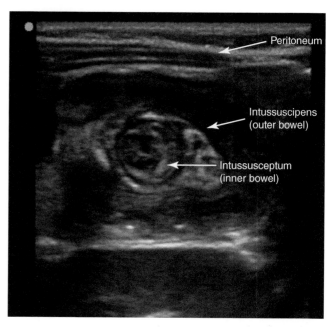

FIGURE 21.10 ■ Intussusception. A short-axis view of an intussusception. Notice its resemblance to a "target sign" representing the alternating circular layers of bowel, with the intussusceptum (inner bowel) within the intussuscipiens (outer bowel). (Photo contributor: John P. Gullett, MD.)

or as the "sandwich" or "pseudo-kidney" sign in the longitudinal view, representing "stacked" layers of bowel wall.

Intussusception is most often found in the RLQ and is ileocolic. Similar to appendicitis, it will not demonstrate peristalsis and will be target shaped in transverse axis. However, intussusception will contain more layers or rings within it, representing the multiple layers of bowel wall telescoped within one another.

Pearls

1. Intussusception also creates a "target sign" when seen in transverse orientation but is a significantly larger structure with more or thicker concentric layers and will not be filled with anechoic fluid.
2. Fecal matter in the colon can imitate intussusception on US.
3. Other pathologic causes of bowel wall thickening, including but not limited to inflammatory bowel disease, colitis, and appendicitis can resemble an intussusception on US.

Clinical Summary

Idiopathic hypertrophic pyloric stenosis is the most common surgical diagnosis in an infant and requires pyloromyotomy. Pyloric stenosis typically presents in the first month of life with *nonbilious* vomiting that may become projectile. There may be a characteristic palpable olive-sized mass in the RUQ or peristaltic wave. The high sensitivity and specificity of US and its ionization-sparing characteristics make it the initial diagnostic study of choice during the evaluation of an infant with suspected pyloric stenosis.

Technique

Use a high-frequency (6–12 MHz) linear probe because the neonatal stomach and pylorus are relatively superficial anatomic structures. Warm the US gel prior to the exam for patient comfort and cooperation. Perform the exam with the

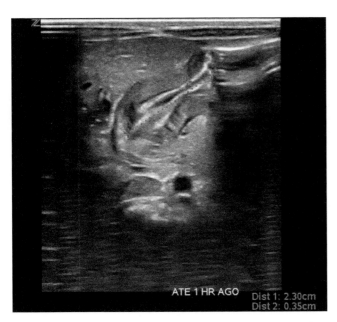

FIGURE 21.11 ■ Pyloric Stenosis (Longitudinal View). Note elongation of the pyloric channel (2.3 cm) and pyloric muscle thickening (0.35 cm). (Photo contributor: John Amodio, MD.)

patient in a supine and slightly inclined position in order to move the stomach fluid toward the pylorus. If there is still too much obscuring stomach gas, place the patient slightly on the left side. Begin the scan in the transverse plane, with the probe indicator directed toward the patient's right side in the subxiphoid region. Visualize the stomach first because it is larger and fluid filled (from the obstructing hypertrophied pylorus), appearing as a large anechoic structure; following the stomach caudally will lead to the pylorus.

Ultrasound Findings

If the stomach is overly distended, the pylorus may be displaced posteriorly, making it difficult to visualize. Once the pylorus is identified, measure the muscle wall thickness in the transverse and longitudinal planes. A transverse measurement of the pyloric muscle >3 mm or a longitudinal measurement of the pyloric channel >17 mm is consistent with pyloric stenosis. Ensure that the pylorus is visualized for ≥5 minutes to verify that the muscle wall thickness remains consistently thickened and is not merely in spasm. Visualization of the antral nipple sign—the redundant gastric mucosa that protrudes into the antral stomach—is also consistent with the diagnosis.

Pearls

1. If the stomach is completely empty or overly distended with air from crying, some oral fluid may be given to obtain a better image.
2. Pylorospasm also results in a false-positive exam. This can be avoided by observing the pylorus for at least 5 minutes; a hypertrophied pyloric wall will always remain thickened.
3. Severe dehydration secondary to vomiting and poor oral intake may affect pyloric muscle thickness; adequate fluid resuscitation is indicated in such cases with a high suspicion for pyloric stenosis.

BILIARY ULTRASOUND

Clinical Summary

Biliary pathology frequently involves adolescents, especially those with sickle cell disease and obese boys. US has high-performance characteristics for diagnosing gallstones and acute cholecystitis. The sonographic Murphy sign is a highly sensitive finding for acute cholecystitis. US is indicated in patients with suspected gallstones or acute cholecystitis.

Technique

Use a low-frequency (1–5 MHz) curvilinear or phased array probe or a high-frequency (6–12 MHz) linear probe. Place the patient in a supine position or in the left lateral decubitus position to help bring the gallbladder into view from the surrounding ribs. Instructing patients to breathe in deeply or hold their breath may assist in better gallbladder visualization. Start in the sagittal plane with the probe just subcostal in the midclavicular line. If bowel gas is obscuring the view, move to the sagittal plane in the midclavicular line, but now look through the rib cage and use the liver as a window to visualize the gallbladder. If this is unsuccessful, the third position is lateral in the coronal plane, similar to the RUQ view in the FAST exam, but angling anteriorly.

Scan the gallbladder in both long and short axes, with the probe marker directed toward the patient's head or right side,

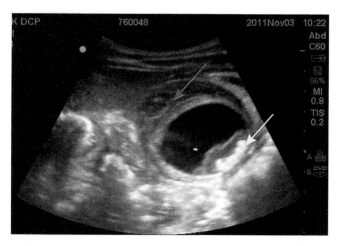

FIGURE 21.13 ■ Cholecystitis. The gallbladder wall is irregularly thickened (red arrow), and a small amount of bright stones (yellow arrow) can be seen in the dependent portion. These are covered in a layer of hypoechoic biliary sludge. (Photo contributor: John P. Gullett, MD.)

respectively. Next, scan the gallbladder from the fundus to the neck, checking for stones or pockets of pericholecystic fluid. Pay attention to a potential sonographic Murphy sign during the exam (elicited by localizing the gallbladder with the US probe and attempting to find the point of maximal pain around the gallbladder). Measure the anterior gallbladder wall (in the near field) from outer wall to outer wall; normal gallbladder wall thickness should be <3 mm. Identify and measure the common bile duct (CBD) and identify the portal triad. Use color or power Doppler to identify the CBD by appreciating the absence of color when compared to the portal vein and hepatic artery, which will demonstrate blood flow.

Ultrasound Findings

Gallstones appear as hyperechoic foci of varying sizes within the anechoic gallbladder and usually have associated shadows immediately inferior to them as the US beams are reflected back to the transducer. Gallstones lie in the most dependent part of the gallbladder, unless impacted (ie, in the gallbladder neck). Changing the position of the patient will often demonstrate movement of the gallstones. Stones in the neck should be considered possibly impacted. Repositioning the patient may demonstrate that the stone rolled freely out of the neck.

The gallbladder wall may appear falsely thick, especially when the US exam is performed postprandially. Other causes of a thick gallbladder wall in the absence of cholecystitis are hypoalbuminemia, edematous states, and adjacent inflammatory processes such as hepatitis, pancreatitis, and AIDS.

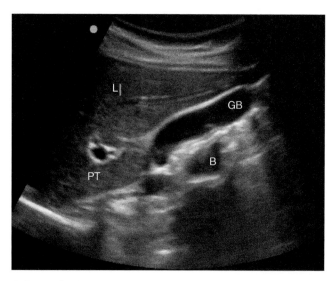

FIGURE 21.12 ■ Long-Axis View of the Gallbladder. A sagittal image of the gallbladder (GB) adjacent to the liver (L). The gallbladder is fluid filled and appears as an anechoic (black) structure on US. Portal triad (PT) and bowel (B) can also be seen. (Photo contributor: Michael Secko, MD, RDMS.)

In such cases, the wall is often thick but homogenous in appearance. The gallbladder wall of cholecystitis has a heterogeneous, layering or "onion skin" appearance.

Consider a diagnosis of cholecystitis if the anterior gallbladder wall thickness exceeds 3 mm, there is noted pericholecystic fluid, or a sonographic Murphy sign is elicited. Pericholecystic fluid is not always appreciated with acute cholecystitis but has been found to be specific for the diagnosis.

Pearls

1. Visualize the entire gallbladder from fundus to neck.
2. Gallbladder wall thickness may be caused by a number of pathologic entities (eg, ascites, hepatitis, HIV, pancreatitis) and may not necessarily imply a case of cholecystitis.
3. Measure the anterior (near-field) wall of the gallbladder for near-accurate assessment of gallbladder wall thickness as acoustic enhancement may falsely increase posterior (far-field) wall measurements.
4. Acalculous cholecystitis is rare. Therefore, just ruling out gallstones almost effectively rules out routine acute cholecystitis.
5. If the CBD is difficult to visualize, the absence of a second large tubular structure immediately anterior to the portal vein effectively rules out an enlarged CBD. Correlation with hepatic markers must be made.

Clinical Summary

ED provider–performed US is a safe, rapid, and nonionizing diagnostic imaging test for managing gynecologic and obstetric complaints and has become the standard of care for patients presenting with abdominal or pelvic pain and/or vaginal bleeding during the first trimester of pregnancy. Exclusion of ectopic pregnancy during the first trimester by visualization of an intrauterine pregnancy (IUP) is the most common application. In the hemodynamically unstable patient, FAST can allow for visualization of free fluid, allowing rapid identification of patients requiring immediate surgical intervention for suspected ruptured ectopic pregnancy. The differential diagnosis is also assisted by identification of other acute gynecologic pathologies (ie, ovarian torsion, tubo-ovarian abscess, or pelvic mass). These findings and diagnoses, however, should be approached with great caution by the bedside emergency sonographer and should be confirmed by radiology exams.

Positioning and Technique

Use a low-frequency (1–5 MHz) curvilinear or phased array probe for transabdominal imaging and a high-frequency (4–7 MHz) endocavitary probe for transvaginal imaging. With the patient in the supine position, obtain transabdominal imaging in both sagittal and transverse planes; then with the probe marker toward the head, obtain a longitudinal view

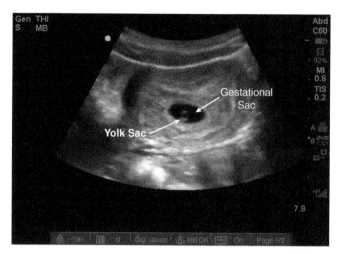

FIGURE 21.15 ■ Intrauterine Pregnancy. Yolk Sac (YS) and Gestational Sac (GS) are seen in the endometrium. Note that the fetal pole is not visible, but visualization of the YS confirms the presence of intrauterine pregnancy. (Photo contributor: John P. Gullett, MD.)

of the uterus. Rotate the probe counterclockwise, so that the probe indicator is pointed toward the patient's right side to obtain a transverse view of the uterus. If pregnancy is early and an IUP cannot be visualized well on abdominal US or if better visualization is desired, proceed to transvaginal imaging and scan completely through the uterus and adnexal regions. Obtain multiple views of the uterus beginning with the longitudinal axis (sagittal plane) looking for the endometrial stripe, and scan the entire length of the uterus from

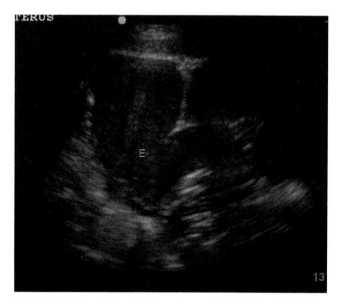

FIGURE 21.14 ■ Normal Uterus. A transabdominal sagittal image of an anteverted uterus with a normal endometrial stripe (E). (Photo contributor: Michael Secko, MD, RDMS.)

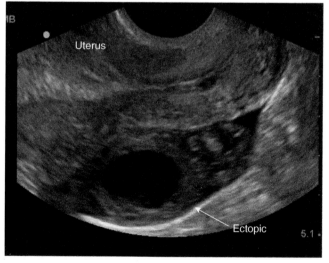

FIGURE 21.16 ■ Ectopic Pregnancy. A transvaginal sagittal image of anteverted uterus with a thickened endometrial stripe with a visible ectopic pregnancy posterior to the uterus. (Photo contributor: Tom Chi, MD, RDMS.)

left to right, as well as laterally to visualize the adnexa. Turn the probe counterclockwise with the probe indicator directed to the patient's right side to visualize the uterus in the transverse plane. Determine whether there is evidence of an IUP (ie, yolk sac or fetal pole) and correlate US findings with quantitative assessment of β-human chorionic gonadotropin (β-hCG) blood levels as follows:

1. With a β-hCG level between 1500 and 3000 mIU/mL, a yolk sac should be visualized on transvaginal US.
2. With a β-hCG level between 6000 and 6500 mIU/mL, a yolk sac should be visualized on transabdominal US.

Note that β-hCG reference values only apply to normal pregnancies.

If an IUP is appreciated, cardiac activity should be sought if a fetal pole is present. Fetal heart movement can be captured using a video clip or by using M-mode.

Ultrasound Findings

The normal prepubertal uterus has a tubular configuration on US without an apparent endometrium and a length of 3 to 4 cm with a thickness that does not exceed 10 mm. A pubertal uterus has a pear-shaped configuration with average length of 5 to 9 cm and width of 3 to 4 cm. Endometrial lining varies with the menstrual cycle. The normal prepubertal ovary measures 1 cm in length by 1 cm in height by 1 cm in depth on US. A pubertal ovary measures 3 cm in length by 2 cm in height by 2 cm in depth.

Ovarian torsion is more common with a predisposing lesion, such as an ovarian cyst or mass. An 8- to 12-mm mean gestational sac diameter should contain a yolk sac. An 18- to 22-mm mean gestational sac diameter should contain a fetal pole. A 5-mm fetal pole should contain a fetal heartbeat.

Pearls

1. Always attempt to visualize the uterus in 2 planes.
2. A full bladder provides the best acoustic windows for transabdominal visualization of the uterus and adnexa, whereas an empty bladder yields better evaluation on transvaginal sonography.
3. Identifying a yolk sac is the first reliable confirmation of an IUP.
4. If there is high suspicion for an ectopic pregnancy, examine the hepatorenal space for possible free fluid.
5. An empty uterus with a low β-hCG level should not exclude an ectopic pregnancy because close to half of ectopic pregnancies present with a β-hCG level of <1000 mIU/mL.

Clinical Summary

US is a safe, nonionizing, and repeatable method of assessing parenchymal or pleural diseases in the dyspneic or critically ill pediatric patient. US has better sensitivity than a supine CXR for detecting pneumothorax or pleural fluid, especially in the critically ill patient in whom an upright or decubitus CXR cannot be performed. Lung US is a viable alternative to CT or radiographs for evaluation of pediatric pneumonia. US can also be used in real time to assess endotracheal tube

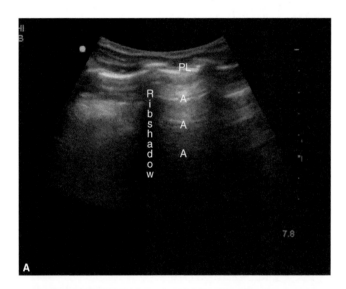

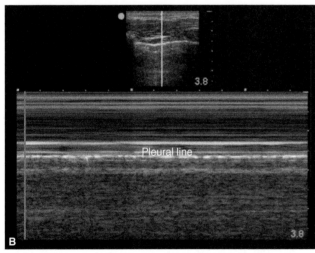

FIGURE 21.17 ■ Normal Lung. (**A**) A sagittal image of the lung using a curvilinear array probe. Note the bright hyperechoic pleural line (PL) between the ribs and the reverberation artifacts corresponding to A-lines. (**B**) An M-mode image of normal lung. Note how normal lung generates continuous laminar lines, followed by a "grainy" appearance deep to the pleural line, producing a "sandy beach" appearance. (Photo contributors: Dimitrios Papanagnou, MD, MPH, and Michael Secko, MD, RDMS.)

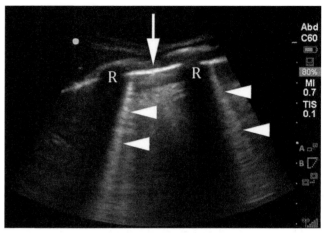

FIGURE 21.18 ■ B-Lines. Vertical white stripes that move with respirations and originate from the pleura are caused by interstitial thickening or fluid. This is often caused by pulmonary edema, but other causes include acute respiratory distress syndrome, pulmonary contusion, or interstitial pneumonia. Note the rib shadows (R) and arrow pointing to the pleural interface. (Photo contributor: Jay Pershad, MD.)

placement. The lack of lung sliding of the left hemithorax after intubation is indicative of a right mainstem intubation.

Positioning and Technique

Use a high-frequency (6–12 MHz) linear array or a high-frequency (5–8 MHz) micro-convex array with the patient in

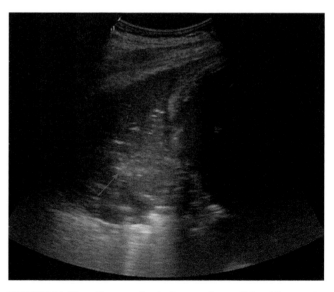

FIGURE 21.19 ■ Pneumonia. An image of consolidated lung at the right lung base taken from a pediatric patient with pneumonia. Note the multiple hyperechoic air bronchograms (arrow). (Photo contributor: Michael Secko, MD, RDMS.)

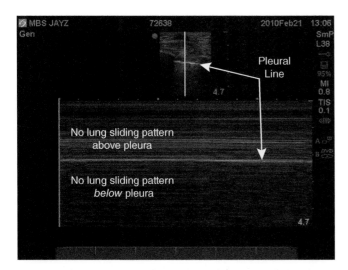

FIGURE 21.20 ■ Pneumothorax. An M-mode image of the lung consistent with a pneumothorax. Note the loss of lung sliding by the continuous laminar lines producing a "stratosphere" appearance. (Photo contributor: John P. Gullett, MD.)

the supine position and the probe indicator pointed toward the patient's head. Scan in longitudinal (sagittal) and coronal planes, moving through all rib spaces of the anterior, axillary, and posterior chest wall.

Ultrasound Findings

The pleural space is found between and slightly deep to the ribs, and a strong acoustic interface between the pleura and aerated lung produces strong posterior reverberations and a bright-appearing pleura. This allows for visualization of normal pleural sliding motion of the lung during respiration. This is caused by the visceral pleura touching and moving against the parietal pleura on the inside of the chest cavity. If there is a pneumothorax and there is air between these layers, no lung sliding is seen because air is a poor conductor of ultrasonic waves.

When there is fluid in the interstitial lung tissue (eg, pneumonia, pulmonary edema, pulmonary contusion, or acute respiratory distress syndrome), artifacts called B-lines are observed and appear as vertical white rays that start at the pleura and extend to the bottom of the screen. The number and density are proportional to the degree of interstitial edema. The presence of >3 B-lines is considered abnormal.

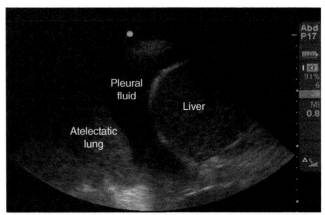

FIGURE 21.21 ■ Pleural Effusion. The bright curved line of the diaphragm is visible in the center, liver is to the left beneath the diaphragm, and above the diaphragm is a moderate to large anechoic effusion and atelectatic lung is seen on the right. (Photo contributor: John P. Gullett, MD.)

When normal aerated lung becomes consolidated or atelectatic, it becomes possible to examine the lung parenchyma with US. Airless, consolidated lung appears sonographically similar to the liver (often described as hepatization), making it possible to visualize air bronchograms as bright branching linear echogenicities.

The sonographic appearance of pleural fluid depends on its composition. The fluid may be completely anechoic from a transudative process, may be more echogenic from an infectious process or hemorrhage, or have internal septations from an empyema or an organized infection.

Pearls

1. You can only rule out a pneumothorax with lung sliding in the area directly under the probe.
2. The lung is a voluminous organ system, and the chest has much surface area. Scan all lung fields on both hemithoraces for completeness.
3. A "lung point"—the interface between sliding and non-sliding lung—is pathognomonic for a pneumothorax.
4. The anterior-superior chest below the clavicles is the best location to observe B-lines. The lung bases are the best location to see fluid, such as pleural effusions

Clinical Summary

Cellulitis can be appreciated on bedside US in most cases by identifying the accumulation of associated edematous fluid. US can aid in identifying the extent of the cellulitis surrounding an abscess and is helpful in addressing the extent of the abscess, presence of fluid, and the optimal location for incision and drainage (I&D) by identifying the "pocket" and any surrounding structures (eg, artery) that must be avoided during I&D.

Positioning and Technique

Because the skin and subcutaneous tissues are relatively superficial, the high-frequency (6–12 MHz) linear probe is often used, affording higher resolution images. In patients with a larger body habitus, deeper visualization of the tissue may be required, necessitating the use of the low-frequency (2–5 MHz) curvilinear probe. Place the patient in a comfortable position depending on the location of the cellulitis and/or abscess with the affected area readily exposed. Use gentle manipulation and pressure of the US transducer because the affected area may be sensitive and painful.

Ultrasound Findings

Compare affected tissue with normal skin and subcutaneous tissue to appreciate subtle findings. Cellulitis

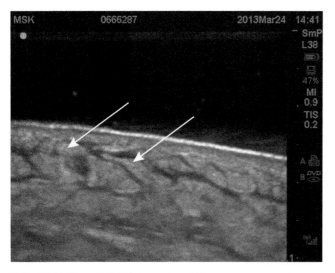

FIGURE 21.22 ■ Cellulitis. Note the cobblestone appearance (arrows) of soft tissue cellulitis. (Photo contributor: John P. Gullett, MD.)

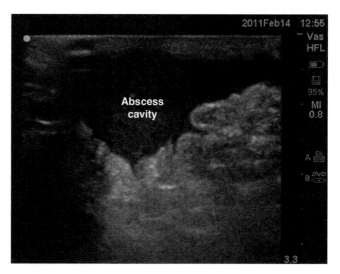

FIGURE 21.23 ■ Abscess of Soft Tissue. A soft tissue image of an abscess. Note the large pocket of hypoechoic fluid. (Photo contributor: John P. Gullett, MD.)

exhibits hyperechoic skin and a reticulated pattern of areas of hypoechoic edema, which can be seen with the probe in either longitudinal or transverse axes, with depth and gain adjustments. The lace-like appearance of the edematous tissue has been described as "cobble stoning." This is because the observed edema is fluid surrounding the subcutaneous fat globules, which gives the appearance of cobblestones. This presumably infected fluid coalesces into an actual pocket of pus. Abscesses appear as relatively hypoechoic fluid collections that are irregular in shape and often surrounded by edematous soft tissue. The (purulent) abscess cavity may contain debris or septations, which can appear as hyperechoic regions in the anechoic collection on US. Use color flow Doppler to differentiate abscesses (no color) from vascular structures (colored) and lymph nodes.

If there is doubt about the nature or content of a possible fluid pocket, perform the "squish test," wherein the gain is increased to see if echogenic material or the solid structure of a soft tissue mass or lymph node is revealed. Press down gently with the probe and look for the flow or motion of fluid.

Necrotizing fasciitis can also be visualized on US, with hyperechoic artifacts generating dirty shadowing. Hyperechoic gas bubbles and fluid may be seen tracking along the fascial planes.

Pearls

1. Identify any adjacent structures (eg, nerve, artery, or vein) that can potentially be injured before I&D of an abscess.
2. US should not supplement a good physical exam for the diagnosis of necrotizing fasciitis.
3. Cysts may also exhibit heterogeneous internal material and echoes; however, they have smooth well-circumscribed borders.

PEDIATRIC HIP ULTRASOUND

Clinical Summary

Consider bedside US for children presenting with hip pain, a painful limp, or refusal to bear weight to identify hip effusion(s) or perform US-guided hip arthrocentesis.

Positioning and Technique

Use a high-frequency (7–12 MHz) linear array transducer and place the patient comfortably in the supine position with legs in neutral position. Scan with the US transducer in a sagittal-oblique plane (toward the umbilicus), in line with the long axis of the femoral head.

Ultrasound Findings

A capsular-synovial thickness >5 mm measured at the concavity of the femoral-synovial neck, from the anterior surface of the femoral neck to the posterior surface of the iliopsoas

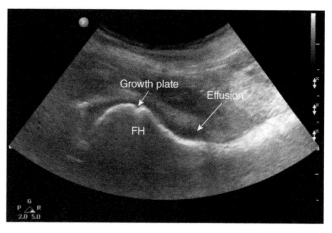

FIGURE 21.25 ■ Hip US. An image of pediatric hip effusion. Note the anechoic fluid (E) overlying the femoral neck adjacent to the femoral head (FH). (Photo contributor: John P. Gullett, MD.)

muscle, or a >2-mm difference compared to the asymptomatic contralateral hip is suggestive of hip effusion.

A septic hip may show increased echogenicity, a thick articular capsule (>2 mm), and/or increased capsular blood flow on power Doppler.

Pearls

1. US alone cannot make the distinction between infected and inflammatory effusions.
2. Real-time US-guided arthrocentesis can increase the success rate of the aspiration of hip effusions.
3. Note that cartilage is anechoic on US and may be confused with a layer of fluid. Cartilage is very regular and smooth in appearance.

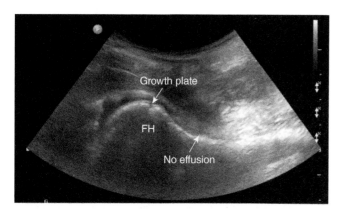

FIGURE 21.24 ■ Hip US. An image of a normal pediatric hip. Note there is no anechoic fluid adjacent to the femoral neck. Also, note the small indentation on the femoral head (FH) consistent with the growth plate, not to be mistaken for a fracture. (Photo contributor: John P. Gullett, MD.)

Clinical Summary

US is a rapid, nonionizing tool for evaluating pediatric fractures and evaluating the success of a fracture reduction, especially the forearm. The reflective acoustic properties of cortical bone make US highly specific for fractures as small as 1 mm.

Positioning and Technique

Use a high-frequency (7–12 MHz) linear array transducer and a low-frequency (2–5 MHz) curvilinear transducer for deeper structures (eg, femur). Scan the bone(s) of interest in both the longitudinal (parallel) and transverse (perpendicular) planes. Note that only the near-field cortex of bone will be identified.

Ultrasound Findings

Cortical bone is hyperechoic on US due to its strong acoustic impedance, and sharp disruption or loss of the normal

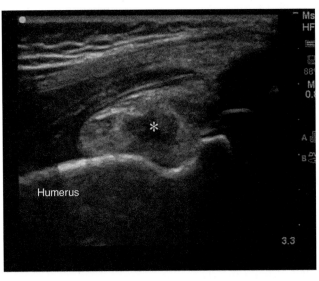

FIGURE 21.27 ■ Posterior Fat Pad Suggesting a Fracture. A sagittal image of a posterior distal humerus with olecranon fossa filled with fluid of multiple echogenicities (asterisk) consistent with a posterior fat pad. This patient was found to have a radial head fracture. (Photo contributor: John P. Gullett, MD.)

contour of the near-field cortical bone is strongly suggestive for fracture. The posterior fossa of the elbow can be identified by applying the US beam in parallel with the posterior distal humerus following the triceps insertion on the olecranon.

Pearls

1. Do not confuse growth plates or joints with fractures.
2. If the posterior fat pad of the distal humerus is elevated on US, there is a fracture about the elbow.

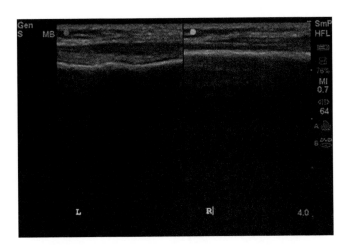

FIGURE 21.26 ■ Distal Radius Fractures US. A dual image of a buckle fracture (left image) and corresponding normal forearm (right image) of the radius in a child. (Photo contributor: Michael Secko, MD, RDMS.)

Clinical Summary

Focused cardiac sonography can be used to rapidly assess the critically ill patient for structural abnormalities, ventricular function, volume status, pericardial effusions, tamponade, chamber size, cardiomyopathy, and response to resuscitation.

Evaluating global systolic function by qualitative assessment (normal, hypercontractile, or depressed) of the ventricular squeeze may help the ED provider distinguish cardiac from other causes of hypoxia or shock.

Focused echocardiography can also assess for pericardial effusion to exclude cardiac tamponade in the traumatized patient (see FAST examination) and in nontraumatic shock.

The International Liaison Committee on Resuscitation (ILCOR) pediatric basic and advanced life support recommendations state that bedside echocardiography "may be considered to identify potentially treatable causes of a cardiac arrest (tamponade), but the benefits must be carefully weighed against the known deleterious consequences of interrupting chest compressions."

The inferior vena cava (IVC) should be included as part of the cardiac exam because it is directly related to right heart pressure and volume status. Serial point-of-care US examinations can help to gauge the patient's response to resuscitative interventions, such as fluid boluses, inotropic support, and pericardiocentesis.

It is also important to use serial US exams to assess a patient's physiologic status. In volume assessment, the provider should perform cardiac, lung, and IVC exams at the

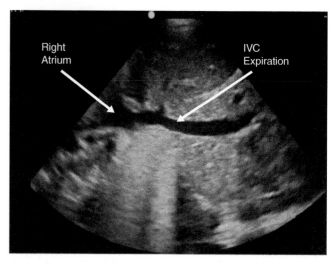

FIGURE 21.29 ■ Inferior Vena Cava (IVC). IVC visualized in longitudinal axis at end of expiration. (Photo contributor: Jay Pershad, MD.)

same time to determine the volume status. Poor systolic function is indicative of heart failure and warrants judicious use of IV fluids during resuscitation. B-lines on US imply interstitial thickening or edema and usually mean the lung is "wet," although fibrosis, acute respiratory distress syndrome,

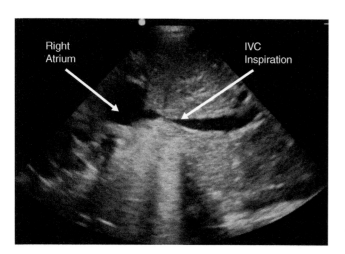

FIGURE 21.28 ■ Inferior Vena Cava (IVC). IVC visualized in longitudinal axis showing near complete collapse during quiet inspiration suggesting volume depletion. (Photo contributor: Jay Pershad, MD.)

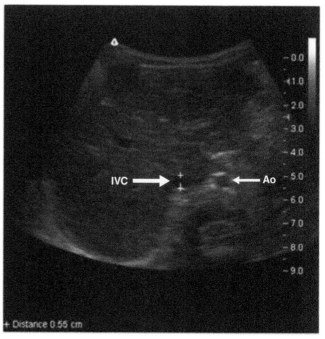

FIGURE 21.30 ■ Inferior Vena Cava (IVC) and Abdominal Aorta (Ao). IVC-to-aorta ratio can be assessed in the transverse plane (Photo contributor: Jay Pershad, MD.)

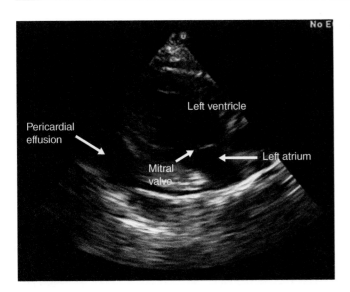

FIGURE 21.31 ■ Parasternal Long-Axis (PSLA) View of the Heart. PSLA view with the probe marker pointing to the right shoulder, obtained on a transthoracic bedside US showing moderate-size pericardial effusion. (Photo contributor: Jay Pershad, MD.)

contusion, interstitial pneumonia, and acute chest syndrome can also create B-lines.

A full IVC implies a high right heart pressure, often from volume overload. This can also be seen in large pulmonary embolism, tamponade, or other causes of increased right heart pressure. A patient with congestive heart failure from cardiomyopathy or structural heart conditions will likely reveal a large noncollapsible IVC, B-lines throughout the lungs indicating edema, and poor systolic function.

A patient in septic shock will usually present with a flat or highly collapsible IVC, a hypercontractile heart, and clear lungs with normal A-lines, or perhaps an infiltrate suggesting a pneumonia as the source of infection.

Technique

Standard cardiac assessment includes views in the subxiphoid, parasternal long axis, parasternal short axis, and apical 4-chamber windows with a high-frequency (5–8 MHz) phased array probe.

The IVC is usually assessed in a subxiphoid longitudinal plane as it travels through the liver parenchyma, crosses the diaphragm, and enters the right atrium. A transabdominal curvilinear probe or the phased array probe may be used.

Dynamic assessment of IVC collapsibility with measurements of vessel diameter during quiet spontaneous inspiration and expiration can estimate right ventricle filling. Often simply estimating the collapsibility of the IVC is sufficient without taking measurements.

Ultrasonographic Findings

IVC collapsibility of <50% suggests impaired right ventricle filling as in volume overload or congestive heart failure. Significant collapse of IVC suggests hypovolemia and decreased preload. The descending aorta is also typically viewed in its subxiphoid location, and measurements of maximum size during systole are compared to the IVC in the transverse plane, usually at the level of the renal arteries. An IVC/aorta cutoff ratio of 1.2 can help diagnose dehydration.

Pearls

1. Focused cardiac US is not primarily directed to the diagnosis or exclusion of congenital heart disease or its complications.
2. Cardiovascular assessment/windows may be limited by injuries, dressings, or body habitus (including cachexia, obesity, scoliosis, and contractures).
3. Standard measurements of the IVC and aorta are not well established for all age groups. Serial exams may be more useful to guide resuscitation than an exam at a single point in time.
4. Inotropic medications and positive-pressure ventilation may affect the size and elasticity of the IVC.
5. Serial assessments of IVC parameters are more useful in assessing a patient's volume status.
6. IVC size and collapsibility with spontaneous respirations must be interpreted in conjunction with bedside evaluation of cardiac function and presence of pulmonary edema (B-lines on lung US).

Note: Page numbers followed by "*f*" indicate figures; those followed by "*t*" indicate tables.

A

ABCs. *See* Airway, breathing, and circulation (ABCs)
Abdominal mass, 543–545, 543*f*, 544*f*, 545*f*
  with intraspinal extension, 638*f*
  Wilms tumor and, 720*f*
Abdominal pain, with sickle cell disease (SCD), 512
Abdominal trauma. *See also* Splenic injuries; Thoracoabdominal trauma
  blunt, 40*f*, 41*f*
  clinical summary for, 1019–1020
  emergency department treatment and disposition, 1020–1021
  head trauma and, 1019
  hepatic injuries, 1024, 1024*f*
  intra-abdominal, 1025–1026, 1025*f*, 1026*f*
  laparotomy indications, 1020*t*, 1021
  penetrating, 1019*f*, 1020*f*
Abdominal wall contusions, 1025–1026
ABI (ankle-brachial index), 910
Abnormal uterine bleeding (AUB), 184, 184*f*, 185*f*, 186
Abortion, incomplete, abnormal uterine bleeding (AUB) and, 184*f*
Abrasions
  child abuse, 2*f*
  corneal, 407, 407*f*
Abrin, 764, 765*f*
ABRS. *See* Acute bacterial rhinosinusitis (ABRS)
Abrus precatorius, 764–765, 765*f*
Abscesses
  anterior neck, 456*f*
  appendiceal, 476
  Bartholin gland, 177*f*, 496, 496*f*
  Bezold, 429–430
  of brain
    bacterial meningitis and, 598*f*
    subdural empyema and, 627*f*
  emergency ultrasound (US) of, 1060–1061, 1060*f*
  epidural, with spinal cord compression, 638*f*
  orbital, 449*f*
  parapharyngeal space, 456, 456*f*
  peritonsillar, 460–461, 460*f*, 461*f*
  retropharyngeal space, 456, 457*f*, 458*f*
  tubo-ovarian. *See* Tubo-ovarian abscess (TOA)
Abuse. *See* Child abuse
Abusive head trauma (AHT), 12*f*
  clinical summary for, 35
  emergency department treatment and disposition, 35–36
  epidural hematoma (EDH), 38*f*
  NAT with traumatic brain injury, 37*f*
  radiography of, 37*f*
  retinal hemorrhage and, 36*f*
  rib fractures with, 30*f*–31*f*
  shaken impact syndrome, 35, 35*f*
  skull fractures with, 34*f*
  subdural hematoma (SDH) and, 5*f*, 36*f*
AC. *See* Activated charcoal (AC)
AC (acromioclavicular) injuries, 919, 919*f*
Acanthosis nigricans (AN), 376–377, 376*f*, 377*f*, 650*f*
ACE (angiotensin-converting enzyme) inhibitors, 296
Acetaminophen (APAP) toxicity, 746–748, 746*f*, 747*f*
Acetazolamide, 854–855
Acetylcholine (ACh), 645*f*, 802
N-Acetylcysteine (NAC), 747–748
Acetylsalicylic acid (ASA) toxicity, 749–751, 749*f*, 750*f*
ACh (acetylcholine), 645*f*, 802
Achilles tendon rupture, 925–926, 925*f*
Acidic burns. *See also* Caustics
  of eyes, 422, 422*f*
ACL (anterior cruciate ligament) tear, 923, 923*f*

Acne fulminans, 317, 317*f*
Acrocyanosis, 576–577
Acromioclavicular (AC) injuries, 919, 919*f*
Acropustulosis of infancy, 360–361, 360*f*, 361*f*
ACS. *See* Acute chest syndrome (ACS)
ACTH (adrenocorticotropic hormone), Addison disease and, 654
Activated charcoal (AC)
  administration of, 739*f*, 744
  for caffeine toxicity, 804
  for castor bean ingestion, 765
  for clonidine, 793
  for cyclic antidepressants (CAs), 795
  decontamination with, 744
  for isoniazid (INH) toxicity, 771
  for nicotine toxicity, 802
  for opioids, 755
  for phenothiazine toxicity, 767
  for rosary pea ingestion, 765
  for salicylate overdose, 750
Acute acetaminophen (APAP) toxicity, 746–748, 746*f*, 747*f*
Acute appendicitis, 1050, 1050*f*
Acute bacterial rhinosinusitis (ABRS)
  clinical summary for, 447
  emergency department treatment and disposition, 447–448, 450
  intracranial complications of, 447, 450, 450*f*
  intraorbital complications of, 449*f*
  orbital abscess and, 449*f*
  orbital cellulitis with, 447, 449*f*
  ostiomeatal complex obstruction in, 448*f*
  purulent rhinorrhea, 447, 447*f*
Acute chest syndrome (ACS)
  radiography of, 516*f*
  sickle cell anemia with, 516–518, 516*f*
  sickle cell disease (SCD) and, 510, 512, 516
Acute epididymitis
  orchitis and, 487–488, 487*f*, 488*f*, 489*f*
  testicular torsion versus, 484*t*, 489*f*
Acute ethmoid sinusitis, 449*f*
Acute hemorrhagic edema of infancy (AHEI), 63–64, 63*f*
Acute invasive fungal sinusitis (AIFS), 448
Acute isoniazid toxicity, 770–771, 770*f*, 771*f*
Acute lymphoblastic leukemia (ALL), 539–540, 539*f*
Acute mountain sickness (AMS), 854–855
Acute myocarditis
  causes of, 242*t*
  clinical summary for, 239, 239*f*
  ECG changes in, 239, 240*f*–241*f*
  emergency department treatment and disposition, 239
  fulminant, 239*f*, 241*f*
  sinus tachycardia (ST) compared with, 208*f*
Acute nonperforated appendicitis
  appendicolith and, 473*f*
  clinical summary for, 473
  ectopic pregnancy compared with, 474*f*
  emergency department treatment and disposition, 474–475
  hyperemia, and 473*f*
  noncompressible appendix, 473*f*
  pearls for, 475
  periappendiceal fat in, 474*f*
  target sign of, 474*f*
Acute osteomyelitis, 930–932, 930*f*, 931*f*, 932*t*
Acute otitis externa (AOE), 432–433, 432*f*
Acute otitis media (AOM)
  clinical summary of, 426, 426*f*
  complications of, 429, 429*f*, 430*f*, 431, 431*f*, 431*t*
  emergency department treatment and disposition, 426–428

Acute otitis media (AOM) (*Cont.*):
 facial palsy and, 431*f*
 mastoiditis with, 429, 429*f*
 otorrhea and, 426–427, 426*f*, 429*f*
 pearls for, 428
 tympanic membrane perforation and, 427*f*
Acute pain, sickle cell anemia with, 512, 513*f*, 514–515, 514*f*
Acute pediatric scrotum
 cellulitis compared with, 483*f*
 differential diagnosis for, 483*t*
 hydrocele compared with, 479*f*, 483*f*
 testicular mass compared with, 482*f*
Acute pericarditis, 236–238, 236*f*, 237*f*
Acute poststreptococcal glomerulonephritis (APSGN)
 as acute hypertensive emergency, 720–721
 clinical summary for, 711–712
 congestive heart failure (CHF) and, 711*f*
 emergency department treatment and disposition, 712
 glomerulonephritis and, 703
 hematuria with, 711*f*
 impetigo with, 712*f*
Acute rheumatic fever (ARF)
 clinical summary for, 247–248
 diagnosis of, 248*t*
 emergency department treatment and disposition, 248
 erythema marginatum, 247*f*, 248
 first-degree atrioventricular (AV) block and, 193*f*
 rheumatic carditis, 247–248, 247*f*
Acute salicylate toxicity, 749–751, 749*f*, 750*f*
Acute sinusitis. *See* Acute bacterial rhinosinusitis
Acute splenic sequestration crisis (ASSC), sickle cell anemia and, 529–530, 529*f*
Acute subdural hematoma. *See* Subdural hematoma (SDH)
Acute urticaria, 294, 294*f*
AD. *See* Atopic dermatitis (AD)
Addison disease, 654–655, 654*f*, 655*f*
Adenopathy
 with incomplete Kawasaki disease (KD), 568*f*
 with Kawasaki disease (KD), 563*f*
 supraclavicular, 537
Adenosine
 for atrial flutter, 217, 218*f*
 for supraventricular tachycardia (SVT), 214, 214*f*, 215*t*
Adenotonsillar hyperplasia, 280
Adenoviral conjunctivitis, 398, 398*f*
Adrenocorticotropic hormone (ACTH), Addison disease and, 654
Advanced Trauma Life Support (ATLS), 846, 849
Adverse drug eruptions. *See* Drug reaction
AF (atrial flutter), 217, 217*f*, 218*f*
AHEI (acute hemorrhagic edema of infancy), 63–64, 63*f*
AHT. *See* Abusive head trauma (AHT)
AIFS (acute invasive fungal sinusitis), 448
Airway, breathing, and circulation (ABCs)
 abdominal trauma and, 1020
 anticholinergic toxicity and, 768
 caffeine toxicity and, 804
 caustics and, 799
 hydrocarbon toxicity and, 774
 insecticide toxicity and, 763
 isoniazid (INH) toxicity and, 771
 methemoglobinemia and, 760
 opioids and, 788
 peripheral cold injuries and, 814
 phenothiazine toxicity and, 767
 poisoning and, 743
 zygomatic complex and arch fractures and, 977
Airway obstruction, traumatic, 1013, 1013*f*
Alanine aminotransferase (ALT), 1024
Albumin, 700
Alkaline burns. *See also* Caustics
 of eyes, 422, 422*f*

ALL (acute lymphoblastic leukemia), 539–540, 539*f*
Allergic conjunctivitis, 398–399, 399*f*
Allergic contact dermatitis
 clinical summary for, 320
 emergency department treatment and disposition, 320
 Neosporin and, 320*f*
 nickel and, 321*f*
 pearls for, 322
 perichondritis and, 435*f*
 poison ivy and, 321*f*
 shoe material and, 320*f*
Allergic fungal sinusitis, 451, 452*f*
Allergic reaction, acute, 618*f*
Allergic rhinitis, 451
Allergies, urticaria and, 294
Alopecia, raccoon eye and, 70*f*, 71
Alpha-gal, 294
ALT (alanine aminotransferase), 1024
Altered mental status
 anticholinergics and, 768–769
 camphor and, 772
 clinical summary for, 605
 cocaine and, 757
 common causes of, 608*t*
 definitions of, 607*t*
 dextromethorphan and, 779
 differential diagnosis of, 608*t*
 ecstasy/molly toxicity, 776
 emergency department treatment and disposition, 605–606
 epidural hematoma (EDH) and, 605*f*
 ethanol and, 786
 etiology of, 608*t*
 global anoxic brain injury, 606*f*
 hemorrhagic stroke, 606*f*
 hydrocarbon (HC) and, 773, 775
 hypertensive encephalopathy and, 607*f*
 intussusception and, 607*f*
 with iron toxicity, 752
 isoniazid (INH) and, 771
 ketamine and, 778
 marijuana and, 780*f*, 781
 phenothiazines and, 766
 purpura and septic shock and, 605*f*
Altitude sickness, 854–855, 854*f*
Ambiguous genitalia, 656, 657*f*
Amenorrhea, 186
 congenital imperforate hymen with hematometrocolpos and, 493–494, 493*f*, 494*f*, 495*f*
Aminoglycoside antibiotics, 645*f*
Amoxicillin. *See* Penicillin
Amputation
 digital, 1034–1035, 1034*f*, 1035*f*
 extremity, 1040–1041, 1040*f*, 1041*f*
AMS (acute mountain sickness), 854–855
Amylase, 688
AN (acanthosis nigricans), 376–377, 376*f*, 377*f*, 650*f*
Anal fissure, 695
Anaphylactoid reactions, 817
Anaphylaxis
 angioedema and, 296, 297*f*
 castor bean ingestion and, 764*f*
 environmental, 817–819, 817*f*, 818*f*
 urticaria and, 294, 294*f*
Anaplasma phagocytophilum, 123*t*
Anaplasmosis, 123*t*
ANCA (antineutrophil cytoplasmic antibodies), 587
Ancylostoma sp., 153–154, 153*f*
Anemia
 hemolytic, naphthalene and, 774*f*
 sickle cell. *See* Sickle cell anemia
Angioedema, 296, 297*f*

Angiogram
    of anomalous origin of left main coronary artery, 234*f*
    of coarctation of aorta, 226*f*
    of Kawasaki disease (KD), 565*f*
    of ruptured arteriovenous malformation (AVM) and hematoma, 626*f*
    of stroke, 520*f*
Angiotensin II receptor blockers (ARBs), 296
Angiotensin-converting enzyme (ACE) inhibitors, 296
Ankle
    dislocation of, 911, 911*f*, 912*f*
    fracture and sprain of, 892–893, 892*f*, 893*f*
Ankle-brachial index (ABI), 910
Annular hymen, normal estrogenized, 161*f*
Annular plaques, 337*f*
Annular psoriasis, 330*f*
Anogenital warts. *See* Condylomata acuminata
Anomalous origin of left main coronary artery, 233*f*, 234*f*
Anopheles mosquitoes, 157
Anorectal foreign bodies, 673–674, 673*f*
Anterior cruciate ligament (ACL) tear, 923, 923*f*
Anterior drawer sign, 923
Anterior flexion fractures, 992, 992*f*, 993*f*
Anterior glenohumeral joint dislocation, 904–906, 904*f*
Anterior neck abscess, 456*f*
Anterior subluxation, 1001, 1001*f*
Anterior superior iliac spine avulsion, 915*f*
Antibiotics
    for acute bacterial rhinosinusitis (ABRS), 447–448
    acute generalized exanthematous pustulosis and, 312*f*
    for acute otitis media (AOM), 427
    for acute pericarditis, 238
    auricular foreign body (FB) and, 438
    for bacterial conjunctivitis, 398
    for bacterial meningitis, 597
    for cat bites, 831
    for cat-scratch disease (CSD), 125
    for corneal abrasion, 407
    for deep neck space infection, 459
    for dog bites, 827–828
    for ecthyma, 102
    for eczema herpeticum (EH), 328
    for epididymo-orchitis, 487
    for erysipelas, 65*f*, 67, 104
    for GABHS infection, 97
    for gonorrhea, 178
    for guttate psoriasis, 332, 334
    for hidradenitis suppurativa (HS), 379
    for human bites, 833–834
    for impetigo, 65*f*, 67, 99–100
    for intestinal malrotation and volvulus, 504–505
    for lymphadenitis, 127–128
    for meningococcemia, 119–120
    for orbital cellulitis, 390
    for osteomyelitis, 932
    for otitis externa (AOE), 433
    for pelvic inflammatory disease (PID), 182–183
    for perianal bacterial dermatitis (PBD), 84–85, 85*f*
    for perichondritis, 434–435
    for perioral dermatitis (PD), 386
    for peritonsillar abscess (PTA), 460
    for pertussis, 258
    for pneumonia, 272
    for preseptal cellulitis, 395
    for Rocky Mountain spotted fever (RMSF), 122
    for septic arthritis, 941
    for sickle cell anemia, with fever, 510–511
    for soft tissue trauma, 979
    for staphylococcal scalded skin syndrome (SSSS), 116
    for starfish and sea urchin stabs, 842
    for stingray stabs, 846
    for stonefish and scorpionfish stabs, 845

    for syphilis, 175
    for toxic shock syndrome (TSS), 113
    for urethral prolapse, 89
    for urinary tract infection, 714
Anticholinergic drug and plant toxicity, 768–769, 768*f*, 769*t*
Anticonvulsant therapy
    for febrile seizures, 609
    for seizures, 613
    for status epilepticus, 616*t*
    toxin-induced seizures and, 743
Antidotal therapy
    for acetaminophen (APAP) toxicity, 747–748, 747*f*
    for anticholinergic toxicity, 768–769
    application of, 744
    for ethylene glycol (EG) toxicity, 782
    for insecticide toxicity, 763
    for isoniazid (INH) toxicity, 770*f*, 771, 771*f*
    for methanol, 785
    for methemoglobinemia, 761, 761*f*
    for opioid toxicity, 755*t*
Antifreeze, 782, 782*f*
Antifungal agents
    for seborrheic dermatitis, 319
    for tinea corporis, 348, 349*f*
    for tinea pedis, 353
    for tinea unguium, 355
    for tinea versicolor, 342
Antihistamines
    for acropustulosis of infancy, 360
    for acute bacterial rhinosinusitis (ABRS), 448
    for allergic contact dermatitis, 320
    for anaphylaxis, 819
    for coral, sea anemone, and hydroid stings, 835–836
    for mastocytosis, 371
    for serum sickness–like reactions, 299
    for urticaria, 295
    for urticaria multiforme (UM), 300
Antihypertensive medication, 721
Antineutrophil cytoplasmic antibodies (ANCA), 587
Antivenom
    black widow spider, 823
    box jellyfish, 838
    scorpion, 825
    snake, 852, 852*f*
    stonefish, 845
Antivirals
    for chickenpox, 129
    for eczema herpeticum (EH), 328
    for erythema multiforme (EM), 302
    for genital herpes, 179
    for herpetic whitlow, 136
Antral nipple sign, 1053
Antrochoanal polyps, 451, 453*f*
AOE (acute otitis externa), 432–433, 432*f*
AOM. *See* Acute otitis media (AOM)
Aorta, coarctation of, 226, 226*f*
Aortic arch interruption, 226
Aortic disruption, 1014, 1014*f*
APAP (acetaminophen) toxicity, 746–748, 746*f*, 747*f*
Appendiceal abscesses, 476
Appendicitis
    acute, 1050, 1050*f*
    acute nonperforated. *See* Acute nonperforated appendicitis
    emergency ultrasound (US) of, 1050–1051, 1050*f*
    nephrotic syndrome (NS) and, 708
    perforated. *See* Perforated appendicitis
Appendicolith, 473*f*, 476*f*
Appendix testis torsion, 490, 490*f*
APSGN. *See* Acute poststreptococcal glomerulonephritis (APSGN)
Aqueductal stenosis leading to hydrocephalus, 632*f*–633*f*
ARBs (angiotensin II receptor blockers), 296

ARF. *See* Acute rheumatic fever (ARF)
Arizona hairy scorpion, 824*f*
Arrhythmias
   with acute myocarditis, 239
   hyperthyroidism and, 661
   hypokalemia and, 731
   infective endocarditis (IE) and, 230*t*
   syncope and, 205
Arterial blood gas
   methemoglobinemia and, 760*f*
   poisoned patient and, 740*t*
Arteriovenous malformation (AVM), 245*f*
   hematoma and ruptured, 626*f*
   with seizures, 612*f*
Arthritis
   acute rheumatic fever (ARF) and, 247
   juvenile idiopathic. *See* Juvenile idiopathic arthritis
   Lyme disease and, 591, 593*t*
   psoriatic, 583*f*, 585*t*
   septic. *See* Septic arthritis
   systemic lupus erythematosus (SLE) and, 571*f*
   temporomandibular joint (TMJ), 585
Arthrocentesis, for septic arthritis, 938*f*
Arthropod bites, bullous, 99*f*
ASA (acetylsalicylic acid) toxicity, 749–751, 749*f*, 750*f*
Ascariasis, 155–156, 155*f*
Ascites, with minimal change nephrotic syndrome (MCNS), 708*f*
Aspartate aminotransferase (AST), 1024
Aspergillosis, 452*f*, 453*f*
Aspiration. *See* Foreign body (FB) aspiration
ASSC (acute splenic sequestration crisis), sickle cell anemia and, 529–530, 529*f*
AST (aspartate aminotransferase), 1024
Asthma
   acute chest syndrome and, 517
   with air-leak syndrome, 283*f*
   bronchiolitis and, 266*f*
   clinical features of, 283, 285
   emergency department treatment and disposition, 282–283
   endobronchial tuberculosis and, 285*f*
   foreign body (FB) aspiration and, 284*f*, 285*f*
   intubation indications in, 285*t*
   with sickle cell disease (SCD), 512
   tension pneumothorax and, 284*f*
Atlanto-occipital dislocation, 994–995, 994*f*
Atlas fracture, 988, 988*f*
ATLS (Advanced Trauma Life Support), 846, 849
Atopic dermatitis (AD)
   clinical summary for, 323, 325*f*
   eczema herpeticum (EH) and, 327–328, 327*f*
   emergency department treatment and disposition, 323–324, 326
   generalized erythroderma, 325*f*
   with hand-foot-and-mouth disease (HFMD), 150*f*
   infantile, 323*f*, 324*f*
   with secondary bacterial infection, 326*f*
Atresia
   biliary, with portal hypertension, 684*f*
   tricuspid, 224*f*
Atrial ectopic tachycardia, 210*f*
   with rapid ventricular response, 211*f*
Atrial flutter (AF), 217, 217*f*, 218*f*
Atrial paced rhythm
   atrial flutter (AF) and, 217, 217*f*
   syncope and, 205*f*
Atrioventricular (AV) block
   atrial flutter (AF) and, 217, 217*f*
   first-degree, 193, 193*f*, 194*f*, 194*t*
   Lyme disease and, 591–592, 593*f*
   second-degree, 194*t*, 195–196, 195*f*, 196*f*, 196*t*
   third-degree, 194*t*, 197–198, 197*f*, 198*f*, 199*f*, 199*t*
   types of, 194*t*

Atrioventricular septal defect, complete, 244*f*
Atropine
   for insecticide toxicity, 763
   for second-degree atrioventricular (AV) block, 195
Atypical hemolytic uremic syndrome (D-HUS), 716, 720–721
AUB (abnormal uterine bleeding), 184, 184*f*, 185*f*, 186
Aura, 611
Auricular foreign body, 437–438, 437*f*, 438*f*
Auricular hematoma, 439–440, 439*f*
Auricular trauma, 978, 978*f*
Automatism, 611
AV block. *See* Atrioventricular (AV) block
Avascular necrosis, 911
AVM. *See* Arteriovenous malformation (AVM)
Avulsion fractures, 861*f*, 865*t*
   pelvic, 914, 914*f*
   tibial tubercle, 915, 915*f*
Axillary nerve injury, 904
Azithromycin, drug reaction to, 310*f*

B
Bacteremia
   endocarditis and, 229
   sickle cell anemia and, 510
Bacterial adenitis, cat-scratch disease (CSD) compared with, 124, 124*f*
Bacterial conjunctivitis, 398, 398*f*
Bacterial infection, secondary
   atopic dermatitis with, 326*f*
   with community-acquired pneumonia (CAP), 271*f*
   with eczema herpeticum (EH), 328
   with scabies, 339–340
   with tinea pedis, 352–353, 353*f*
Bacterial meningitis
   brain abscesses and, 598*f*
   bulging anterior fontanelle and, 596*f*
   cerebrospinal fluid (CSF) findings in, 599*t*
   clinical summary for, 596
   hydrocephalus and, 597*f*, 599*f*
   neurologic sequelae of, 597*f*
   with purpura, 596*f*
   signs and symptoms of, 599*t*
Bacterial pneumonia, 268–269
   chest pain and, 232*f*
   influenza A infection, 271*f*
   pneumococcal
      with empyema, 269*f*
      lobar consolidation in, 268*f*
   staphylococcal, 269*f*
   treatment for, 272
Bacterial tracheitis, 261–262, 261*f*, 262*f*
Bacterial vaginosis, management of, 167*t*
Bacteriuria, urinary tract infection and, 713*f*, 714
Bactrim, SSLR with, 298*f*
"Bagging," 773, 774*f*
BAIs (blunt aortic injuries), 1014
Baker cyst, 584
Baking soda, for coral, sea anemone, and hydroid stings, 835
Balanitis xerotica obliterans, 82
Balanoposthitis, 500*f*
Bankart lesions, 904
Bark scorpion, 824
Bartholin gland abscess, 177*f*, 496, 496*f*
Bartonella henselae, 124–125, 126, 127*t*, 128
Bartter syndrome, 731
Basilar skull fracture (BSF), 953, 953*f*, 954*f*
Bat exposure, 830
Battery ingestions, 262*f*, 675, 675*f*–676*f*, 677, 677*f*, 678*f*
Battle sign, 953, 953*f*
BBs. *See* β-Blockers (BBs)
Beet ingestion, 695*f*, 696
Bell palsy, 624–625, 624*f*, 625*f*

Bell phenomenon, 624
Bell-clapper deformity, 480, 480f
Belt marks, 10f, 11f
Bennett fracture, 871, 871f
Benzodiazepines, 767, 776, 788–789, 788f, 797, 805
    for black widow spider bites, 823
    for scorpion bites, 825
Benzolamide, 854
Berloque dermatitis, 59
β-Blockers (BBs)
    for aortic disruption, 1014
    for cocaine toxicity, 758
    epinephrine and, 817
    for infantile glaucoma, 405
    for long QT syndrome (LQTS), 202, 202f
    for thyroid storm, 664
    toxicity with, 790–791, 790f
β-Human chorionic gonadotropin (β-hCG), 1057
Bezold abscess, 429–430
Bilateral cervical lymphadenopathy, 537, 537f
Bilateral facet dislocation, 998, 998f
Biliary atresia, with portal hypertension, 684f
Biliary colic, 689, 689f
Bilirubin, 526, 526f
Bilirubinuria, 526f
Binocular diplopia, 972
Birth trauma
    epidermolysis bullosa (EB) and, 363f, 364f
    scrotal trauma and, 486f
Bismuth subsalicylate, 655f
Bites
    blue-ringed octopus, 848, 848f
    cat, 831–832, 831f, 832f
    dog, 826–828, 826f, 827f
    human, 833–834, 833f
    inflicted, 8f
    scorpion, 824–825, 824f
    snake, 850–853, 850f, 851f, 852f
    spider
        black widow spider, 823, 823f
        brown recluse spider, 820–822, 820f, 821f
Biting marine animals, blue-ringed octopus, 848, 848f
Black dot appearance of tinea capitis, 345f, 347
Black tongue, with Addison disease, 655f
Black widow spider, envenomation, 823, 823f
Blast injury, 1040f
Blebectomy, thoracoscopic, 290f
Bleeding
    abnormal uterine, 184, 184f, 185f, 186
    lower GI (rectal). See Lower GI bleeding (LGIB)
Blepharospasm, 404
B-lines, 1058f, 1059
Blood. See also Bleeding
    chocolate brown, 760, 761f
    congenital syphilis and, 171t
    hyphema and, 411–412, 411f
    intracranial pressure (ICP) elevations and, 604t
Blood pressure, poisoned patient and, 740t
Bloody stool. See Lower GI bleeding (LGIB)
Blue-gray macules of infancy, 48–49, 48f, 49f
Blue-ringed octopus, 848, 848f
Blunt aortic injuries (BAIs), 1014
Blunt trauma
    abdominal, 40f, 41f
    epidural hematoma (EDH) and, 957–958, 957f
    extension teardrop fracture and, 991
    to finger, 1030f
    flail chest and, 1008
    flexion teardrop fractures and, 992
    hemothorax and, 1012
    midfacial fractures and, 969f

    orbital fracture, 972f, 973f
    pneumothorax and, 1010
    pulmonary contusion and, 1006
    to scrotum, 485–486, 485f, 486f
    to soft tissue, 978
    subungual hematoma and, 1032
    temporomandibular joint (TMJ) dislocation and, 983
    traumatic airway obstruction and, 1013
Blurred vision, 407
"Body packing," 754, 754f, 758, 758f
"Body stuffing," 754, 758, 759f
Bohan and Peter Classification Criteria, 579
Böhler angle, 894
Bone marrow
    acute lymphoblastic leukemia (ALL) and, 539–540
    immune thrombocytopenic purpura (ITP) and, 531
    infarction of, 512, 516
Bones. See also Osteomyelitis
    acute lymphoblastic leukemia (ALL) and, 539–540
    congenital syphilis and, 171t, 173f
    emergency ultrasound (US) of, 1063, 1063f
    Ewing sarcoma, 558, 558f, 559f, 560, 560f
    fractures of. See Fractures
    lead and, 796, 796f
    osteosarcoma, 553–554, 553f–557f
    retained, 679–680, 679f, 680f
Bony lesions
    in acne fulminans, 317
    in congenital syphilis, 173f
Bordetella parapertussis, 258
Bordetella pertussis, 258, 258f
Borrelia sp., 591
Borreliosis, 591–592, 591f, 592f
Botulism, infantile, 644–645, 644f, 645f
Bow legs, 76, 77f
Bowing fractures, 859f
Box jellyfish, 837–839, 838f
Boxer's fracture, 872
Bradycardia
    causes of, 192, 192t
    clinical summary of, 190
    clonidine and, 792, 792f
    differential diagnosis of, 191f
    emergency department treatment and disposition, 190
    etiologies of, 192, 192t
    intracranial pressure (ICP) elevations and, 601
    sinus. See Sinus bradycardia
Brain
    abscesses of
        bacterial meningitis and, 598f
        subdural empyema and, 627f
    congenital syphilis and, 171t
    diabetic ketoacidosis (DKA) and, 648f
    global anoxic injury of, 606f
    intracranial pressure (ICP) elevations and, 601, 604t
    tuberculomas, 278f, 279f
Brain contusion, 959, 959f
Brain tumors
    cerebellar astrocytoma, 629–630, 630f
    clinical summary of, 629–631
    craniopharyngioma, 629f
    emergency department treatment and disposition, 631
    focal seizures and, 610f
    ganglioglioma, 629f
    intracranial pressure (ICP) elevation and, 602f
    medulloblastoma, 628f
    midbrain, 630f, 631
    pituitary gland tumors, 631, 631f
    pontine glioma, 630f
    posterior fossa tumors, 629, 630f
    supratentorial, 629f

Breast, condylomata acuminata and, 169*f*
Breath-holding spells, 204, 207*t*
Brittle bone disease, 80
Bronchiolitis
  clinical summary for, 265, 265*f*
  differential diagnosis for, 266*f*, 267*f*
  emergency department treatment and disposition, 265–267
Bronchoscopy, for foreign body (FB) aspiration, 257
Brown recluse spider, envenomation, 820–822, 820*f*, 821*f*
Brown syndrome, 585
Brown tube sponge, 840*f*
Bruises, inflicted
  acute hemorrhagic edema of infancy (AHEI) versus, 63–64, 63*f*
  child abuse, 2*f*, 4*f*, 8–9, 9*f*
  coin rubbing versus, 50*f*
  cold panniculitis versus, 53*f*, 54*f*
  congenital dermal melanocytosis and, 48*f*, 49, 49*f*
  differential for, 11*f*
  ear, 13*f*
  nevi of Ota and Ito versus, 55*f*
  oral, 15*f*
  pattern marks, 10, 10*f*, 11*f*, 12*f*
  phytophotodermatitis (PPD) versus, 59, 59*f*, 60*f*
BSF (basilar skull fracture), 953, 953*f*, 954*f*
Buccal cellulitis, 53*f*
Buckle fractures, 861*f*
Buckling forces, 961
Bullous arthropod bites, 99*f*
Bullous erysipelas, 104
Bullous impetigo, 65–67, 65*f*, 66*f*, 98–100, 98*f*, 99*f*
Bullous varicella, 130*f*
Buphthalmic eye, 404*f*
Burns
  chemical. *See* Chemical burns
  circumferential, 810, 813*f*
  inflicted, 5*f*
    abusive, 21, 22*f*
    chemical, 20*f*
    clinical summary for, 18, 21
    emergency department treatment and disposition, 21
    immersion, 19*f*, 20*f*, 21
    impetigo versus, 65–67, 65*f*, 66*f*
    iron, 21*f*
    scald, 18, 18*f*, 21
    senna contact dermatitis and, 61, 62*f*
  lightning injuries, 849
  scald, 18, 21, 808, 811*f*–812*f*
  silver nitrate, 506*f*
  thermal, 808–811, 808*t*, 809*f*–813*f*
Butterfly rash
  of erysipelas, 103*f*, 104
  of neonatal lupus (NL), 575*f*
  of systemic lupus erythematosus (SLE), 570*f*, 571*f*
Button battery ingestion, 262*f*, 675, 675*f*–676*f*, 677, 677*f*, 678*f*

C

CAA. *See* Coronary artery aneurysm (CAA)
Café-au-lait spots (CALS)
  clinical summary for, 373–374
  emergency department treatment and disposition, 374
  in McCune-Albright syndrome, 373, 374*f*
  neurofibromatosis and, 373, 373*f*, 611*f*
  segmental pigmentation disorder, 373*f*, 374
Caffeine toxicity, 804–805, 804*f*, 805*f*
CAH (congenital adrenal hyperplasia), 656–657, 656*f*, 657*f*
Caida de mollera, 51
Calcaneal fracture, 894, 894*f*
Calcitriol, 728
Calcium channel blockers (CCBs), toxicity of, 790–791, 790*f*
Calcium oxalate crystals, 782, 783*f*
CALS. *See* Café-au-lait spots (CALS)

Camphor toxicity, 772, 772*f*
Candidal diaper dermatitis, 384–385, 384*f*
Candidal onychomycosis, 354, 354*f*
Candidiasis, with diabetic ketoacidosis (DKA), 649*f*
Cannabinoids, 780–781, 780*f*, 781*f*
Cannabis, 780–781, 780*f*, 781*f*
Cantharidin, UM and, 295*f*
Cao Gio, 50, 50*f*
CAP. *See* Community-acquired pneumonia (CAP)
Carbamate toxicity, 762–763
Cardiac syncope, 204–205, 207*t*
Cardiac tamponade, 237–238
Cardiology
  acute rheumatic fever (ARF). *See* Acute rheumatic fever (ARF)
  atrial flutter (AF), 217, 217*f*, 218*f*
  bradycardia, 190, 190*f*, 191*f*, 192, 192*t*
  chest pain. *See* Chest pain
  congestive heart failure (CHF). *See* Congestive heart failure (CHF)
  ductal-dependent cardiac lesions, 226–227, 226*f*, 227*f*, 228*t*
  emergency ultrasound (US) of, 1064–1065, 1064*f*, 1065*f*
  first-degree atrioventricular (AV) block, 193, 193*f*, 194*f*, 194*t*
  hypercyanotic spell of tetralogy of Fallot, 222–223, 222*f*, 223*f*, 224*f*, 225, 225*t*
  infective endocarditis (IE), 229–231, 229*f*, 230*f*, 230*t*
  long QT syndrome (LQTS), 200, 200*f*, 201*f*, 202–203, 202*f*, 202*t*, 203*t*
  myocarditis, acute, 239, 239*f*, 240*f*, 241*f*, 242*t*
  pericarditis, acute, 236–238, 236*f*, 237*f*
  premature ventricular contractions, 219, 219*f*, 220*f*, 221, 221*f*, 221*t*
  pulmonary hypertensive crises, 249–251, 249*f*, 250*f*, 250*t*
  second-degree atrioventricular (AV) block, 194*t*, 195–196, 195*f*, 196*f*, 196*t*
  sinus tachycardia (ST), 208–209, 208*f*, 209*f*, 209*t*
  supraventricular tachycardia. *See* Supraventricular tachycardia (SVT)
  syncope, 204–207, 204*f*, 205*f*, 206*f*, 207*t*
  third-degree atrioventricular (AV) block, 194*t*, 197–198, 197*f*, 198*f*, 199*f*, 199*t*
Cardiomyopathy
  dilated, 243*f*, 244*f*
  multifocal premature ventricular contractions with, 220*f*
Cardiopulmonary resuscitation (CPR), 849
Carditis, rheumatic, 247–248, 247*f*
Carpal bone fractures, 873, 873*f*
Carrot aspiration, 255*f*
Cartilage necrosis, perichondritis and, 434–435, 435*f*
CAs (cyclic antidepressants) toxicity, 794–795, 794*f*, 795*f*
Castor bean ingestion, 764–765, 764*f*
Cat bites, 831–832, 831*f*, 832*f*
Cataract, 403*f*, 405*f*
Cat-scratch disease (CSD)
  bacterial adenitis compared with, 124, 124*f*
  clinical summary for, 124, 124*f*
  emergency department treatment and disposition, 125
  hepatosplenic, 125*f*
Cauliflower ear, 439, 439*f*
Caustics
  clinical summary for, 798
  degreaser, 800*f*
  emergency department treatment and disposition, 799, 801
  lithium hydroxide, 798*f*
  sodium hydroxide, 798, 799*f*, 801*f*
Cavitary lung nodules, 587*f*
CBD (common bile duct), 1054
CBF (cerebral blood flow), 601–602
CCBs (calcium channel blockers), toxicity of, 790–791, 790*f*
CDC (Centers for Disease Control and Prevention), 829
Cefaclor, SSLR with, 298*f*
Cefdinir–iron interaction, 695*f*, 696
Cellulitis
  acute otitis externa (AOE), 432–433, 432*f*
  deep neck space infection and, 457, 458*f*
  dog bites, 827*f*

ecthyma and, 101
emergency ultrasound (US) of, 1060–1061, 1060*f*
erysipelas and, 104, 104*f*
necrotizing. *See* Necrotizing fasciitis (NF)
nephrotic syndrome (NS) and, 708
orbital, 390, 390*f*, 391*f*, 392*f*, 393, 393*f*
with paronychia, 928*f*
preseptal, 394–395, 394*f*, 395*f*
with staphylococcal scalded skin syndrome (SSSS), 115*f*
with streptococcal toxic shock syndrome, 110*f*
testicular torsion compared with, 483*f*
Centers for Disease Control and Prevention (CDC), 829
Centruroides exilicauda, 824–825, 824*f*
Cerebellar astrocytoma, 629–630, 630*f*
Cerebellar herniation, 626
Cerebellar stroke, 619*f*
Cerebral blood flow (CBF), 601–602
Cerebral concussion, 960, 960*f*
Cerebral contusion, 959, 959*f*
Cerebral edema, shaken impact syndrome and, 35
Cerebral perfusion pressure (CPP), 601–602
Cerebrospinal fluid (CSF). *See also* Hydrocephalus
    bacterial meningitis and, 599*t*
    basilar skull fracture (BSF) and, 953
    intracranial pressure (ICP) elevations and, 604*t*
    miliary tuberculosis and, 279
    in subarachnoid hemorrhage (SAH), 620*f*
Cerebrovascular disease, sickle cell anemia and, 519, 519*f*, 520*f*, 521
Cervarix, 169
Cervical lymphadenitis, 126, 126*f*, 127*t*, 538*f*
Cervical lymphadenopathy, 537, 537*f*
Cervical spine injuries (CSI), 986–987, 986*f*
    anterior subluxation, 1001, 1001*f*
    atlanto-occipital dislocation, 994–995, 994*f*
    bilateral facet dislocation, 998, 998*f*
    extension teardrop fracture, 991, 991*f*
    flexion teardrop fractures, 992, 992*f*, 993*f*
    hangman's fracture, 37*f*, 990, 990*f*
    Jefferson burst fractures, 988, 988*f*
    odontoid fractures, 989, 989*f*
    spinal cord injury without radiographic abnormality (SCIWORA), 996–997, 996*f*
    unilateral facet dislocation, 999–1000, 999*f*
Chalazion, 396–397, 396*f*, 397*f*
Chance fracture, 1025*f*
Chancre, with syphilis, 174, 174*f*, 175*f*
CHB. *See* Complete heart block (CHB)
CHD. *See* Congenital heart disease (CHD)
Cheek trauma, 978, 978*f*
Chemical burns. *See also* Caustics
    child abuse and, 20*f*
    of eyes, 422–423, 422*f*
Chemical conjunctivitis, 400–401
Chemoprophylaxis, for meningococcemia, 120
Chemosis
    with traumatic globe rupture, 416*f*
    urticaria with, 294*f*
Chest pain
    with acute pericarditis, 237
    anomalous origin of left main coronary artery, 233*f*, 234*f*
    causes of, 234*t*
    clinical summary for, 232
    differential diagnosis of, 232*f*, 233*f*
    emergency department treatment and disposition, 232, 235
    gunshot injury, 234*f*
    with sickle cell disease (SCD), 512
Chest X-ray (CXR). *See* Radiography
Cheyne-Stokes respiration, 605
CHF. *See* Congestive heart failure (CHF)
Chicken bones, 679*f*
Chickenpox, 129–130, 129*f*, 130*f*

Chilblains, 577
Child abuse, 1
    abdominal trauma. *See* Abdominal trauma
    abusive burns, 21, 22*f*
    bites, inflicted, 8*f*
    bruises
        differential for, 11*f*
        ear, 13*f*
        inflicted, 2*f*, 4*f*, 8–9, 9*f*
        oral, 15*f*
        pattern marks, 10, 10*f*, 11*f*, 12*f*
    burns, inflicted. *See* Burns, inflicted
    chemical burns, 20*f*
    clinical summary for, 2
    conditions mistaken for. *See* Conditions mistaken for child abuse and sexual abuse
    cutaneous manifestations of. *See* Cutaneous manifestations of child abuse
    dental neglect, 15–16, 16*f*
    diagnostic examination for, 3
    emergency department treatment and disposition, 2–7
    eye injuries, 14*f*
    fractures. *See* Fractures, child abuse and
    genital injuries, 6*f*
    head trauma, abusive. *See* Abusive head trauma
    immersion burns, 19*f*, 20*f*, 21
    infanticide. *See* Infanticide versus sudden unexplained infant death syndrome
    interview for, 4
    intraoral injuries, 14*f*
    iron burns, 21*f*
    neck injuries, inflicted, 9*f*
    orofacial trauma. *See* Orofacial trauma
    physical examination for, 2–3
    ping pong fracture, 33*f*
    reporting of, 6–7
    scald burns, 18, 18*f*, 21
    sexual abuse. *See* Sexual abuse
    skeletal manifestations of. *See* Skeletal manifestations of child abuse
    subdural hematoma (SDH), 5*f*
    subgaleal hematoma, 3*f*
    sudden unexplained infant death syndrome. *See* Infanticide versus sudden unexplained infant death syndrome
Child Protective Services (CPS), 6–7, 10, 16, 31
Chironex fleckeri, 837
Chlamydia pneumoniae, sickle cell disease (SCD) and, 516
Chlamydia trachomatis
    conjunctivitis with, 400, 400*f*
    epididymo-orchitis with, 487
    management of, 167*t*
    sexual abuse and, 165*f*
Chlamydia vaginitis, 165*f*
Chlamydophila pneumoniae, pneumonia with, 269
Chlorine bleach burn, 20*f*
Chocolate brown blood, 760, 761*f*
Cholecystitis, 514*f*, 524*f*, 689
    emergency ultrasound (US) of, 1054–1055, 1054*f*
Choledocholithiasis, obstructive, 524, 526
Cholelithiasis, 689
Cholesteatoma, chronic otitis media with, 430*f*
Choriocarcinoma, 549
Chronic osteomyelitis, 933–934, 933*f*
Chronic otitis media, with cholesteatoma and mastoiditis, 430*f*
Chronic rhinosinusitis (CRS), 451, 452*f*, 453*f*
Chronic urticaria, 294–295
Chvostek sign, 726
Circle of Willis, 519*f*
Circumcision, female, 86, 87*f*
Circumferential burns, 810, 813*f*
Classic metaphyseal lesion (CML), 24, 24*f*, 25*f*, 75
Clavicle fracture, 884–885, 884*f*
Clavulanic acid, 827

Clay shoveler's fracture, 1002, 1002f
Clitoral-tourniquet syndrome, 72
CLM (cutaneous larvae migrans), 153–154, 153f
Clonidine, 721, 739f
    toxicity with, 792–793, 792f
Closed fractures, 865t
Closed-lip schizencephaly, 613f
Clostridium botulinum, 644
Clostridium difficile, 696
Cloudy urine, 713f
CML (classic metaphyseal lesion), 24, 24f, 25f
CMV (cytomegalovirus), convulsion and, 609f
Cnidocil, 835
Coagulation disorder, child abuse differential, 11f
Coarctation of aorta, 226, 226f
Coats disease, 403f
"Cobble stoning," 1060, 1060f
Cobras, 850–853, 851f
Cocaine toxicity, 757–759, 757f, 758f, 759f
Cocaine washout syndrome, 757
Codeine, sickle cell disease (SCD) and, 514
Codman triangle, 553, 559f
Coin rubbing, 50, 50f
Cold panniculitis, 53–54, 53f, 54f
Collarette scale, 335f
Colles fracture, 874
Coma, 607t, 740t
Comminuted fractures, 860f, 865t
Common bile duct (CBD), 1054
Common duct, 524f
Common skin warts, 356, 356f, 357f
Community-acquired pneumonia (CAP)
    clinical summary for, 268–271
    differential diagnosis for, 271f
    emergency department treatment and disposition, 272
    emergency ultrasound (US) of, 1058–1059, 1058f
    influenza A infection, 271f
    with parapneumonic effusion, 268f
    pneumococcal
        with empyema, 269f
        lobar consolidation in, 268f
    secondary bacterial infection, 271f
    staphylococcal, 269f, 270f
    viral pneumonia/pneumonitis, 270f
Compartment syndrome, 866t
Complete atrioventricular septal defect, 244f
Complete fractures, 859f, 865t
Complete heart block (CHB), 194t, 197–198, 197f
    characteristic features of, 199t
    with junctional escape beat, 199f
    Lyme carditis and, 591–592, 593f
    in neonatal lupus (NL), 574, 575f
    with ventricular escape beat, 198f
Complex febrile seizures, 610f, 610t
Compressive optic neuropathy visual loss, 972
Computed tomography (CT)
    of abdominal trauma, 1020–1021
    of abusive head trauma (AHT), 35, 35f, 36f, 37f, 38f
    of acute bacterial rhinosinusitis (ABRS), 448f
    of acute nonperforated appendicitis, 474f
    of acute subdural hematoma (SDH), 955f, 956f
    of anomalous origin of left main coronary artery, 233f
    of anterior neck abscess, 456f
    of anterior subluxation, 1001f
    of antrochoanal polyps, 453f
    of aortic disruption, 1014f
    of arteriovenous malformation, 612f
    of atlanto-occipital dislocation, 994f
    of bacterial meningitis, 597f
    of basilar skull fracture (BSF), 954f
    of bilateral facet dislocation, 998f

of brain tumor, 602f
of calcaneal fracture, 894f
of cat bite, 832f
of cerebral contusion, 959f
of cervical spine injuries (CSI), 986f, 987
of Chance fracture, 1025f
of chronic otitis media, 430f
of clavicle fracture/dislocation, 884f
of CMV infection, 609f
of coalescent mastoiditis, 430f
of cocaine complications, 757f
of coup and contrecoup injury, 959f
of craniopharyngioma, 629f
of deep neck abscess, 457f
of dental foreign body (FB), 1004f
of dental trauma, 1005f
of diabetic ketoacidosis (DKA), 648f
of epidural hematoma (EDH), 605f, 950f, 957f
    with herniation, 601f
of epiglottitis, 263
of ethmoid sinusitis, 449f
of Ewing sarcoma, 558f, 559f
of extension teardrop fracture, 991f
flexion teardrop fractures, 992f
of foreign body (FB) aspiration, 256f, 257
of Fournier's gangrene, 106f
of global anoxic brain injury, 606f
of granulomatosis with polyangiitis (GPA), 588f
of hangman's fracture, 990f
of hemicraniectomy, 603f
of hemorrhagic stroke, 601f, 606f
of hip dislocation, 907f
of Hodgkin lymphoma (HL), 542f
of hydrocephalus, 632f, 634–635
of hypertensive encephalopathy, 607f
of incarcerated inguinal hernia, 478f
of intestinal malrotation and volvulus, 504f
of intravaginal foreign body (FB), 185f
of intussusception, 470f
of ischemic stroke, 618f
of Jefferson burst fractures, 988f
of juvenile nasopharyngeal angiofibroma, 443f
of Le Fort fractures, 968f
of Lemierre syndrome, 457f, 462f, 463f, 464f
of liver laceration, 1024f
of mandible fractures, 965f, 966f
of mediastinal teratoma, 551f
of medulloblastoma, 628f
of Menkes disease, 74f
of 3,4-methylenedioxymethamphetamine (MDMA) toxicity, 776f
of midfacial fractures, 968f
of miliary TB, 278f
of nasal fractures, 964f
of nasoorbitoethmoid (NOE) fractures, 970f
of nephrolithiasis, 723f, 724
of neuroblastoma, 546f, 548f
of obstructive sleep apnea syndrome (OSAS), 281f
of odontoid fractures, 989f
of orbital fracture, 419, 419f, 972f, 973f
of osteosarcoma, 554f
of ovarian torsion, 501f
of pancreatic laceration, 688f
of pancreatitis, 687f
of parapharyngeal space abscess, 456f
of pelvic fracture, 1027, 1027f
of penetrating head injury, 949f
of perforated appendicitis, 476, 476f
of pneumocephalus, 949f, 970f
of pneumonia, 269f
of pneumothorax, 1010f
of polycystic kidney disease (PKD), 705f

of Pott disease, 944f, 945f
of Pott puffy tumor, 454f, 455
of primary spontaneous pneumothorax (PSP), 288f
of proptosis and fungal sinusitis, 452f
of pulmonary contusion, 1006, 1006f, 1009f
of pulmonary embolism (PE), 291f
of retinoblastoma, 403f
of retropharyngeal cellulitis, 458f
of retropharyngeal space abscess, 458f
of rhabdomyosarcoma, 545f
of rib fractures and flail chest, 1008f
of right upper quadrant (RUQ) syndrome, 514f
of ruptured arteriovenous malformation (AVM) and hematoma, 626f
of scapular fracture, 886f
of sharp object ingestion, 682f
of skull fractures, 32f, 33f, 951f
of spinal cord injury without radiographic abnormality (SCIWORA), 996f
of splenic injuries, 1023f
of splenic rupture, 145f
of stroke, 520f, 521, 619
of Sturge-Weber syndrome (SWS), 615f
of subarachnoid hemorrhage (SAH), 603f, 620f
of subgaleal hematoma, 70f
of temporomandibular joint (TMJ) dislocation, 983, 983f
of thoracoabdominal trauma, 40f, 41, 41f
of tracheobronchial tree injury (TBTI), 1017f
of traumatic diaphragm rupture, 1015f
of tuberculomas, 278f
of tuberculosis, 273f, 275f
of tubo-ovarian abscess (TOA), 182f, 183f
of unilateral facet dislocation, 999f
of vein of Galen malformation and, 245f
of VP shunt, 636f
of Wilms tumor, 544f, 703f, 720f
of zygomatic arch fractures, 975f
of zygomatic complex fractures, 976f
Conditions mistaken for child abuse and sexual abuse
acute hemorrhagic edema of infancy (AHEI), 63–64, 63f
cold panniculitis, 53–54, 53f, 54f
congenital dermal melanocytosis, 48–49, 48f, 49f
contact dermatitis from senna, 61–62, 61f, 62f
folk healing practices, 50–52, 50f, 51f, 52f
hair-tourniquet syndrome (HTS), 72–73, 72f
Henoch-Schönlein purpura (HSP), 315f
impetigo, 65–67, 65f, 66f
infantile hemangioma (IH), 166f
Jacquet diaper dermatitis, 166f
labial adhesion, 86–87, 86f, 87f
lichen sclerosus et atrophicus (LSA), 82–83, 82f
Menkes disease, 74–75, 74f
neonatal menstruation, 166f
nevi of Ota and Ito, 55–56, 55f, 56f
osteogenesis imperfecta (OI), 79–81, 79f, 80f, 81f
perianal bacterial dermatitis (PBD), 84–85, 84f, 85f
phytophotodermatitis (PPD), 59–60, 59f, 60f
port-wine stain (PWS), 56f, 57, 57f
postinflammatory hyperpigmentation, 68, 68f
raccoon eyes, 69–71, 69f, 70f, 71f
rickets, 25f, 76, 78f
straddle injury. See Straddle injury
urethral prolapse, 88–89, 88f
vitamin D insufficiency and deficiency, 76, 77f
Condylomata acuminata, 356
clinical summary for, 168–169, 168f, 169f
emergency department treatment and disposition, 169
management of, 167t
sexual abuse and, 163f
Condylomata lata, 164f, 173f, 175f
Cone shells, 847, 847f
Confusion, 607t

Congenital adrenal hyperplasia (CAH), 656–657, 656f, 657f
Congenital brain malformations, with hydrocephalus, 633f
Congenital dermal melanocytosis, 48–49, 48f, 49f
Congenital heart disease (CHD)
congestive heart failure (CHF) from, 246t
cyanotic. See Cyanotic congenital heart disease
ductal-dependent cardiac lesions as, 226
infective endocarditis (IE) and, 229, 229f, 230t
Congenital imperforate hymen with hematometrocolpos, 493–494, 493f, 494f, 495f
Congenital neuroblastoma, 547f, 548f
Congenital rubella syndrome (CRS), 142, 142f
infantile glaucoma and cataract with, 405f
Congenital syphilis, 24f
Congestive heart failure (CHF)
with acute myocarditis, 239
acute poststreptococcal glomerulonephritis (APSGN) and, 711f
atrial flutter (AF) and, 217
bronchiolitis and, 267f
causes of, 246t
clinical summary for, 243
complete atrioventricular septal defect, 244f
dilated cardiomyopathy, 243f, 244f
emergency department treatment and disposition, 243–244
hyperthyroidism and, 661
infective endocarditis (IE) and, 230t
premature ventricular contractions and, 219
supraventricular tachycardia (SVT) and, 210, 214
third-degree atrioventricular (AV) block and, 197
vein of Galen malformation and, 245f
ventriculoseptal defect (VSD) and, 243, 243f
Conjunctival edema, urticaria and, 294f
Conjunctival laceration, 417f
Conjunctival warts, 356, 397f
Conjunctivitis
allergic, 398–399, 399f
bacterial, 398, 398f
clinical summary for, 398
emergency department treatment and disposition for, 398–399
with measles, 140–141, 140f
with molluscum contagiosum, 358
newborn, 400–401, 400f, 401f
nonexudative limbic-sparing, 563f, 568f
pearls for, 399
viral, 398, 398f, 399f
Consciousness. See Altered mental status
Constipation
clinical summary for, 692, 692f
emergency department treatment and disposition, 692–693
Hirschsprung disease (HD) and, 692–693, 693f, 694f
with infantile botulism, 644, 644f
radiography of, 692f
Contact dermatitis. See also Allergic contact dermatitis
from senna, 61–62, 61f, 62f
Contact irritant dermatitis, 386f
Contrecoup injury, 959, 959f
Convulsion, 609f, 611
Copper deficiency, 74–75, 74f
Coral snake, 850–853, 851f
Corals, 835–836, 835f, 836f
Cornea
abrasion of, 407, 407f
chemical burn of, 422–423, 422f
clouding of, 405f
foreign body (FB) in, 406, 406f
laceration of, 417f
ulceration of, 408–409, 408f, 410f
Coronary artery, anomalous origin of left main, 233f, 234f
Coronary artery aneurysm (CAA)
incomplete Kawasaki disease (KD) and, 569f
Kawasaki disease (KD) and, 562, 565f

Corticosteroids
for acute pericarditis, 236–238, 236*f*, 237*f*
for allergic contact dermatitis, 321*f*
for anaphylaxis, 819
for asthma, 286
for coral, sea anemone, and hydroid stings, 836
for Henoch-Schönlein purpura (HSP), 316
for infectious mononucleosis (IM), 146
Coup injury, 959, 959*f*
Coxiella burnetii, 123*t*
Coxsackie infection
hand-foot-and-mouth disease (HFMD), 149, 149*f*, 150*f*, 151
herpangina, 152, 152*f*
pancreatitis, 687
CPP (cerebral perfusion pressure), 601–602
CPR (cardiopulmonary resuscitation), 849
CPS (Child Protective Services), 6–7, 10, 16, 31
Craniopharyngioma, 629*f*
Craniotabes, 76
Creeping eruption, 153–154, 153*f*
Crescent sign of intussusception, 467*f*
Crescentic hymen, normal unestrogenized, 161*f*
CroFab (Crotalidae polyvalent immune fab), 852
Crohn disease, 690, 691*f*
Crotalidae polyvalent immune fab (CroFab), 852
Croup, 259–260, 259*f*, 260*f*
Crowe sign, 611*f*
Crown-of-thorns starfish, 842–843, 842*f*
CRS (chronic rhinosinusitis), 451, 452*f*, 453*f*
CRS (congenital rubella syndrome), 142, 142*f*
infantile glaucoma and cataract with, 405*f*
CSD. *See* Cat-scratch disease (CSD)
CSF. *See* Cerebrospinal fluid (CSF)
CSI. *See* Cervical spine injuries (CSI)
CT. *See* Computed tomography (CT)
Cupping (ventosa), 50, 51*f*
Currant-jelly stool, 466*f*, 467, 607*f*
Cushing triad, 949–950
Cutaneous larvae migrans (CLM), 153–154, 153*f*
Cutaneous manifestations of child abuse. *See also* Child abuse
abusive head trauma (AHT), 12*f*
bites, inflicted, 8*f*
bruises, inflicted, 8–9, 9*f*
clinical summary of, 8–9
emergency department treatment and disposition, 9–10
pattern bruises, 10, 10*f*, 11*f*, 12*f*
CXR (chest X-ray). *See* Radiography
Cyanosis
airway obstruction and, 1013
with hypercyanotic spell of tetralogy of Fallot, 222, 222*f*, 224*f*
methemoglobinemia and, 760–761
Raynaud phenomenon (RP) and, 576, 576*f*, 577*t*
Cyanotic congenital heart disease
Ebstein anomaly, 227*f*
tetralogy of Fallot (TOF) and, 222, 222*f*, 223*f*, 224*f*
Cyclic antidepressants (CAs) toxicity, 794–795, 794*f*, 795*f*
Cystinuria, 722
Cystitis
hemorrhagic, 702*f*
urinary tract infection and, 713–714
Cystourethrogram, voiding. *See* Voiding cystourethrogram
Cytomegalovirus (CMV), convulsion and, 609*f*

D
Dacryoadenitis, 587*f*
Dacryocystitis
granulomatosis with polyangiitis (GPA) and, 588
preseptal cellulitis and, 395*f*
Dapsone, 820–821
Darier sign, 370, 370*f*
DCM (diffuse cutaneous mastocytosis), 370–371, 372*f*

DDAVP (desmopressin), 536
Deep neck space infection
anterior neck abscess, 456*f*
clinical summary for, 456–457
emergency department treatment and disposition, 459
Lemierre syndrome and, 456–457, 457*f*
parapharyngeal space abscess, 456, 456*f*
pearls for, 459
retropharyngeal cellulitis and, 457, 458*f*
retropharyngeal space abscess, 456, 457*f*, 458*f*
Deferoxamine, 752*f*, 753, 753*f*
Degloving injury, 1036–1037, 1036*f*, 1037*f*
Dehydration
with diabetic ketoacidosis (DKA), 649, 652*t*
with hyperosmolar hyperglycemic syndrome (HHS), 651
with hypertrophic pyloric stenosis, 472
Delirium, 607*t*
Deltoid ligament, 862
Demyelinating disorders, 638
Dens fractures, 989, 989*f*
Dental neglect, 15–16, 16*f*
Dental trauma
clinical summary for, 1003
emergency department treatment and disposition, 1003, 1005
foreign body (FB), 1004*f*
mandibular fractures and, 1003*f*, 1005*f*
subluxed teeth, 1003*f*, 1004*f*
tooth avulsion, 1003*f*, 1004*f*, 1005
Dentinogenesis imperfecta, 81*f*
Depressed skull fracture with subdural hematoma, 32*f*
Dermatitis
allergic contact. *See* Allergic contact dermatitis
atopic. *See* Atopic dermatitis
contact
irritant, 386*f*
from senna, 61–62, 61*f*, 62*f*
diaper, 166*f*
candidal, 384–385, 384*f*
eczematous, 436*f*
perianal bacterial, 84–85, 84*f*, 85*f*
perioral, 386, 386*f*
phytophotodermatitis (PPD), 59–60, 59*f*, 60*f*
seborrheic, 318–319, 318*f*, 319*f*
Dermatology
acanthosis nigricans (AN), 376–377, 376*f*, 377*f*
acne fulminans, 317, 317*f*
acropustulosis of infancy, 360–361, 360*f*, 361*f*
allergic contact dermatitis, 320, 320*f*, 321*f*, 322
angioedema, 296, 297*f*
atopic dermatitis. *See* Atopic dermatitis
café-au-lait spots (CALS). *See* Café-au-lait spots (CALS)
candidal diaper dermatitis, 384–385, 384*f*
drug reactions, 310, 310*f*, 311*f*, 312*f*, 313, 313*f*
eczema herpeticum (EH), 327–328, 327*f*, 328*f*
epidermolysis bullosa (EB), 363–365, 363*f*, 364*f*
erythema multiforme (EM). *See* Erythema multiforme (EM)
erythema nodosum (EN), 375, 375*f*
erythema toxicum neonatorum (ETN), 362, 362*f*
granuloma annulare (GA), 337–338, 337*f*
guttate psoriasis, 332, 332*f*, 333*f*, 334
Henoch-Schönlein purpura (HSP). *See* Henoch-Schönlein purpura (HSP)
hidradenitis suppurativa (HS), 378–379, 378*f*
incontinentia pigmenti (IP), 387–388, 387*f*
infantile hemangioma (IH). *See* Infantile hemangioma (IH)
mastocytosis, 370–372, 370*f*, 371*f*, 372*f*, 372*t*
molluscum contagiosum, 358–359, 358*f*, 359*f*
perioral dermatitis (PD), 386, 386*f*
pityriasis rosea (PR), 335–336, 335*f*, 336*f*
psoriasis. *See* Psoriasis
scabies, 339–341, 339*f*, 340*f*, 341*f*
seborrheic dermatitis, 318–319, 318*f*, 319*f*

serum sickness, 298
serum sickness–like reactions, 298–299, 298f, 299t
Stevens-Johnson syndrome (SJS), 305, 305f, 306f, 307, 309
subcutaneous fat necrosis (SCFN), 382–383, 382f
tinea capitis, 345–347, 345f, 346f, 347f
tinea corporis, 348, 348f, 349f
tinea cruris, 350–351, 350f, 351f
tinea pedis, 352–353, 352f, 353f
tinea unguium, 354–355, 354f
tinea versicolor, 342, 343f, 344f
toxic epidermal necrolysis (TEN), 305, 306f, 307, 307f, 308f, 309
transient neonatal pustular melanosis (TNPM), 380–381, 380f
urticaria, 294–295, 294f, 295f
urticaria multiforme (UM). See Urticaria multiforme (UM)
warts, 356–357, 356f, 357f
Dermatomyositis, juvenile (JDM), 579, 579f, 580f, 581, 581t
Dermographism
with mastocytosis, 371f, 372
with urticaria multiforme (UM), 295f
Desmopressin (DDAVP), 536
Desquamation
with congenital syphilis, 172f
drug reaction and, 313f
with guttate psoriasis, 333f
with incomplete Kawasaki disease (KD), 568f, 569f
with Kawasaki disease (KD), 564f
with scarlet fever, 94, 97f
with seborrheic dermatitis, 318–319
with staphylococcal scalded skin syndrome (SSSS), 114, 115f
with streptococcal toxic shock syndrome, 110f
Dexamethasone
acute chest syndrome and, 517
for high-altitude illness, 854
Dextromethorphan (DXM) toxicity, 779, 779f
Dextrose, 743
DGI (disseminated gonococcal infection), 177–178, 178f
D-HUS (Atypical or sporadic hemolytic uremic syndrome), 716, 720–721
D+HUS (diarrhea associated hemolytic uremic syndrome), 716
Diabetes
acute otitis externa (AOE) and, 432
obesity and, 651f
Diabetic ketoacidosis (DKA)
acanthosis nigricans (AN) and, 650f
brain swelling with, 648f
candidiasis with, 649f
clinical summary for, 648–649
dehydration with, 649, 652t
description of, 648
emergency department treatment and disposition, 649–651
fluid therapy for, 649, 653f
hyperosmolar hyperglycemic syndrome (HHS) versus, 653t
laboratory studies for, 652t
Dialysis, 717, 719, 734–735
Diaper dermatitis, 166f
candidal, 384–385, 384f
Diaphragm rupture, traumatic, 1015–1016, 1015f
Diaphragm sign, 232f
Diarrhea associated hemolytic uremic syndrome (D+HUS), 716
Diastatic skull fracture, 32f, 34f
DIC (disseminated intravascular coagulation), with meningococcemia, 118f, 119, 119f
Diffuse airspace disease, 589f
Diffuse brain swelling, with diabetic ketoacidosis, 648f
Diffuse cutaneous mastocytosis (DCM), 370–371, 372f
Digits
amputation of, 1034–1035, 1034f, 1035f
axial loading of, 869f
ring incarceration and, 1029, 1029f
Dilated cardiomyopathy, 243f, 244f
Diltiazem, 790
Dimercaptosuccinic acid (DMSA) scan, of renal scarring, 714

Dinner fork deformity, 874, 874f
Diphenhydramine, 767
Dislocations
ankle, 911, 911f, 912f
atlanto-occipital, 994–995, 994f
bilateral facet, 998, 998f
elbow, 903, 903f
Galeazzi fracture, 876, 876f
glenohumeral joint, 904–906, 904f, 905f
hip, 907–908, 907f, 908f
interphalangeal joint, 899–900, 899f
knee, 909–910, 909f, 910f
lunate, 901–902, 901f
metacarpophalangeal (MCP) joint, 900f
Monteggia fracture, 876, 876f
patella, 913, 913f
perilunate, 901–902, 902f
temporomandibular joint (TMJ), 983, 983f
testicular, 485
unilateral facet, 999–1000, 999f
Disseminated gonococcal infection (DGI), 177–178, 178f
Disseminated intravascular coagulation (DIC), with meningococcemia, 118f, 119, 119f
Disseminated zoster, 131
Distal esophagus, foreign body (FB) at, 667f
Distal subungual onychomycosis, 354, 354f
Divers Alert Network, 836, 839, 841–842, 845, 848
DKA. See Diabetic ketoacidosis (DKA)
DMSA (dimercaptosuccinic acid) scan, of renal scarring, 714
DNET (dysembryoplastic neuroepithelial tumor), 612f
Dog bites, 826–828, 826f, 827f
Donepezil, 762
Down syndrome (DS), acanthosis nigricans (AN) and, 377f
DRESS (drug reaction with eosinophilia and systemic symptoms), 310, 311f
Drug reaction
acute generalized exanthematous pustulosis, 312f
to azithromycin, 310f
clinical summary for, 310
emergency department treatment and disposition, 310
erythematous papules, 312f–313f
pearls for, 313
Drug reaction with eosinophilia and systemic symptoms (DRESS), 310, 311f
Drug-induced hypersensitivity syndrome, 310, 311f
DS (down syndrome), acanthosis nigricans (AN) and, 377f
Ductal-dependent cardiac lesions
clinical summary for, 226
coarctation of aorta, 226f
Ebstein anomaly, 227f
emergency department treatment and disposition, 227
features of, 228t
hyperoxia test for, 228t
hypoplastic left heart syndrome (HLHS), 227f
left-sided, 226f
treatment of, 228t
DUMBELS symptoms, 742t, 762
Duodenal hematoma, 1025
Duodenojejunal junction perforation, 682f
DXM (dextromethorphan) toxicity, 779, 779f
Dysembryoplastic neuroepithelial tumor (DNET), 612f
Dysfunctional uterine bleeding, 184, 184f, 185f, 186
Dysgerminoma, 549
Dystrophic epidermolysis bullosa, 363, 364f

E
EAC. See External auditory canal (EAC)
Ears. See also Otolaryngology
bruises of, 13f
cauliflower, 439, 439f
piercing of, 434f
swimmer's, 432–433, 432f
trauma of, 978, 978f, 980

EB. *See* Epidermolysis bullosa (EB)
Ebstein anomaly, 227*f*
EBV. *See* Epstein-Barr virus (EBV)
Ecchymosis
    with immune thrombocytopenic purpura (ITP), 531, 532*f*
    with pelvic fracture, 1027
    periorbital, 258*f*, 953*f*
ECG. *See* Electrocardiogram (ECG)
Echinoderms, 842–843, 842*f*
Echocardiography
    of complete atrioventricular septal defect, 244*f*
    of congestive heart failure (CHF), 244*f*
    of dilated cardiomyopathy, 244*f*
    of hypoplastic left heart syndrome (HLHS), 227*f*
    of incomplete Kawasaki disease (KD), 569*f*
    of infective endocarditis (IE), 229*f*
    of pericardial effusion (PE), 237, 237*f*, 1064
    of pulmonary embolism (PE), 292
    of pulmonary hypertension (PH), 249–250, 250*f*
    of syncope, 206*f*
Ecstasy/molly toxicity, 776–777, 776*f*, 777*f*
Ecthyma, 101–102, 101*f*, 102*f*
Ecthyma gangrenosum (EG), 108–109, 108*f*, 109*f*
Ectopic pregnancy, 187–188, 187*f*, 188*f*
    acute nonperforated appendicitis compared with, 474*f*
    emergency ultrasound (US) of, 1056–1057, 1056*f*
Eczema coxsackium, 150*f*
Eczema herpeticum (EH), 327–328, 327*f*, 328*f*
Eczematous dermatitis, 436*f*
Edema
    acute hemorrhagic edema of infancy (AHEI), 63–64, 63*f*
    cerebral. *See* Cerebral edema
    conjunctival, urticaria and, 294*f*
    with epiglottitis, 263
    with erythema infectiosum (EI), 147*f*
    facial, 707*f*
    of genitals, 708*f*
    of hypothyroidism, 659*f*
    with Kawasaki disease (KD), 564*f*
    with minimal change nephrotic syndrome (MCNS), 707–708, 707*f*, 708*f*
    nephrotic syndrome (NS) with, 700*f*
    with paraphimosis, 497, 497*f*
    penile, 499*f*
    periorbital, 707*f*
    pitting, 708*f*
    proteinuria with, 701*f*
    with streptococcal toxic shock syndrome, 110, 110*f*
EDH. *See* Epidural hematoma (EDH)
EFAST (extended focused assessment with sonography for trauma), 1046, 1046*f*
EG (ecthyma gangrenosum), 108–109, 108*f*, 109*f*
EG (ethylene glycol) toxicity, 782–783, 782*f*, 783*f*
Egg on string appearance, 223*f*
EH (eczema herpeticum), 327–328, 327*f*, 328*f*
Ehrlichia chaffeensis, 123*t*
Ehrlichiosis, 123*t*
EI (erythema infectiosum), 147–148, 147*f*
Elapidae family, 850–853, 851*f*
Elbow
    dislocation of, 903, 903*f*
    nursemaid's, 917–918, 917*f*
Electrical burns, 809*f*, 810
Electrocardiogram (ECG)
    of acute myocarditis, 239, 240*f*–241*f*
    of acute pericarditis, 236*f*
    of atrial flutter (AF), 217, 217*f*, 218*f*
    of bradycardia, 190, 190*f*, 191*f*
    of caffeine toxicity, 804–805, 804*f*, 805*f*
    of chest pain, 233*f*
    of clonidine toxicity, 739*f*
    of cyclic antidepressants (CAs), 794–795, 794*f*, 795*f*

    of first-degree atrioventricular (AV) block, 193, 193*f*, 194*f*
    of hypercalcemia, 729*f*
    of hyperkalemia, 733, 733*f*
    of hypocalcemia, 726*f*
    of hypokalemia, 731–732, 731*f*
    of hypoplastic left heart syndrome (HLHS), 226
    of hypothermia, 816*f*
    of long QT syndrome (LQTS), 200*f*, 201*f*, 202*f*
    of Lyme carditis, 593*f*
    of monomorphic ventricular tachycardia, 220*f*–221*f*
    of premature ventricular contractions, 219, 219*f*, 220*f*
    of pulmonary embolism (PE), 292
    of pulmonary hypertension (PH), 249, 249*f*
    of sinus tachycardia (ST), 208*f*, 240*f*
    of supraventricular tachycardia (SVT), 210*f*, 211*f*, 212*f*, 213*f*, 214*f*, 663*f*
    of syncope, 204*f*, 205*f*
    of third-degree atrioventricular (AV) block, 197*f*, 198*f*, 199*f*
    of tricuspid atresia, 224*f*
    of ventricular tachycardia (VT), 233*f*
    of Wolff-Parkinson-White (WPW) syndrome, 213*f*
Electrolyte abnormalities
    with congenital adrenal hyperplasia, 656
    with hypertrophic pyloric stenosis, 472
Ellis system, 1003, 1003*f*
EM. *See* Erythema multiforme (EM)
EM (erythema migrans), 591, 591*f*
Emergency ultrasound (US)
    of abscesses, 1060–1061, 1060*f*
    of appendicitis, 1050–1051, 1050*f*
    of biliary, 1054–1055, 1054*f*
    cardiac point-of-care, 1064–1065, 1064*f*, 1065*f*
    of cellulitis, 1060–1061, 1060*f*
    clinical summary for, 1046
    extended focused assessment with sonography for trauma (EFAST), 1046, 1046*f*
    of first-trimester pregnancy, 1056–1057, 1056*f*
    focused assessment with sonography for trauma (FAST) view of left upper quadrant (LUQ), 1047, 1048*f*
    focused assessment with sonography for trauma (FAST) view of right upper quadrant (RUQ), 1047, 1047*f*
    of fractures, 1063, 1063*f*
    hemothorax, 1049*f*
    of intussusception, 1052, 1052*f*
    of lung, 1058–1059, 1058*f*, 1059*f*
    of pediatric hip, 1062, 1062*f*
    pericardial fluid on subxiphoid view, 1049*f*
    positive suprapubic focused assessment with sonography for trauma (FAST) view, 1049*f*
    of pyloric stenosis, 1053, 1053*f*
    technique for, 1046–1047
Emperor scorpion, 824*f*
Empyema
    with pneumococcal pneumonia, 269*f*, 271
    subdural, 450*f*
EN (erythema nodosum), 375, 375*f*
Encephalitis, herpes, 616*f*
Encephalopathy, hypertensive, 607*f*
Endemic typhus, 123*t*
Endobronchial tuberculosis, asthma and, 285*f*
Endocarditis, infective, 229–231, 229*f*, 230*f*, 230*t*
Endocrinology
    Addison disease, 654–655, 654*f*, 655*f*
    congenital adrenal hyperplasia, 656–657, 656*f*, 657*f*
    diabetic ketoacidosis (DKA). *See* Diabetic ketoacidosis (DKA)
    hyperthyroidism, 661, 661*f*, 662*f*, 663*f*, 664
    hypothyroidism, 658–659, 658*f*, 659*f*, 660*f*
    myxedema, 658–659, 659*f*
    thyroid storm, 661, 661*f*, 662*f*, 663*f*, 664
Endodermal sinus tumors, 549
Enophthalmos, 973*f*

Enterovirus infection
    hand-foot-and-mouth disease (HFMD), 149, 149*f*, 150*f*, 151
    herpangina, 152, 152*f*
Enthesitis-related arthritis, 585*t*
Envenomation
    black widow spider, 823, 823*f*
    brown recluse spider, 820–822, 820*f*, 821*f*
    marine animals. *See* Venomous marine animals
    scorpion, 824–825, 824*f*
    snake, 850–853, 850*f*, 851*f*, 852*f*
Environmental emergencies
    anaphylaxis, 817–819, 817*f*, 818*f*
    black widow spider envenomation, 823, 823*f*
    blue-ringed octopus bites, 848, 848*f*
    box jellyfish, true jellyfish, and Portuguese man-of-war stings, 837–839, 837*f*, 838*f*, 839*f*
    brown recluse spider envenomation, 820–822, 820*f*, 821*f*
    cat bites, 831–832, 831*f*, 832*f*
    cone shell stabs, 847, 847*f*
    coral, sea anemone, hydroid, and fire coral stings, 835–836, 835*f*, 836*f*
    dog bites, 826–828, 826*f*, 827*f*
    high-altitude illness, 854–855, 854*f*
    human bites, 833–834, 833*f*
    lightning injuries, 849, 849*f*
    peripheral cold injuries, 814–816, 814*f*, 815*f*, 816*f*, 816*t*
    rabies exposure and vaccine prophylaxis, 829–830, 829*f*, 829*t*
    scorpion envenomation, 824–825, 824*f*
    snake envenomations, 850–853, 850*f*, 851*f*, 852*f*
    sponge stings, 840–841, 840*f*
    starfish and sea urchin stabs, 842–843, 842*f*
    stingray stabs, 846, 846*f*
    stonefish and scorpionfish stabs, 844–845, 844*f*, 845*f*
    thermal burns, 808–811, 808*t*, 809*f*–813*f*
Eosinophilia reaction, to drugs, 310
Epidemic typhus, 123*t*
Epidermolysis bullosa (EB)
    birth trauma and, 363*f*, 364*f*
    clinical summary for, 363
    dystrophic, 363, 364*f*
    emergency department treatment and disposition, 363–365
    impetigo versus, 66, 66*f*
    junctional, 363
Epididymitis, acute
    orchitis and, 487–488, 487*f*, 488*f*, 489*f*
    testicular torsion versus, 484*t*, 489*f*
Epididymo-orchitis, 487–488, 487*f*, 488*f*, 489*f*
Epidural abscess with spinal cord compression, 638*f*
Epidural hematoma (EDH), 38*f*
    altered mental status and, 605*f*
    head trauma and, 950*f*
    with herniation, 601*f*
    trauma and, 957–958, 957*f*
Epiglottitis, 263–264, 263*f*, 264*f*
Epilepsy, 611, 611*f*, 612*f*, 613, 613*f*. *See also* Status epilepticus
Epinephrine
    for anaphylaxis, 817–819, 817*f*
    for priapism, 522–523
Epiphora, 979
Epiphyseal fractures, 865*t*
Epistaxis
    clinical summary for, 441
    immune thrombocytopenic purpura (ITP) with, 441, 442*f*
    instruments for, 441–442, 441*f*
    juvenile nasopharyngeal angiofibroma and, 441, 443*f*
    nasal pack placement for, 442–443, 442*f*
    nasal septum arteries, 441, 441*f*
Epstein-Barr virus (EBV)
    infectious mononucleosis (IM) and, 144–145
    obstructive sleep apnea syndrome (OSAS) and, 280*f*
Erysipelas
    clinical summary for, 65–66, 65*f*, 103–104, 103*f*, 104*f*

    emergency department treatment and disposition, 66–67, 104
    necrotizing. *See* Necrotizing fasciitis (NF)
Erythema infectiosum (EI), 147–148, 147*f*
Erythema marginatum, 247*f*, 248
Erythema migrans (EM), 591, 591*f*
Erythema multiforme (EM)
    clinical summary for, 302
    emergency department treatment and disposition, 302
    herpes simplex virus (HSV) and, 134*f*
    herpes simplex virus (HSV) infection and, 302*f*
    Mycoplasma pneumoniae–induced rash and mucositis, 304*f*
    pearls for, 303
    serum sickness–like reactions and urticaria multiforme (UM) compared with, 299*t*
    target or "iris" lesions, 303*f*
    urticaria multiforme (UM) and, 295*f*
Erythema nodosum (EN), 375, 375*f*
Erythema toxicum neonatorum (ETN), 362, 362*f*
Erythematous lesions
    of acropustulosis of infancy, 360, 360*f*
    with allergic contact dermatitis, 320, 320*f*, 321*f*
    with atopic dermatitis, 323*f*, 325*f*
    with drug reactions, 312*f*
    with eczema herpeticum (EH), 327*f*
    with erythema nodosum (EN), 375, 375*f*
    with erythema toxicum neonatorum (ETN), 362, 362*f*
    with guttate psoriasis, 332*f*, 333*f*
    with Lyme disease, 591*f*
    with perichondritis, 434, 434*f*
    with perioral dermatitis (PD), 386, 386*f*
    with psoriasis, 329, 329*f*, 331*f*
    with seborrheic dermatitis, 318, 318*f*
    with Stevens-Johnson syndrome (SJS), 305*f*
    with subcutaneous fat necrosis (SCFN), 382–383, 382*f*
    with tinea corporis, 348, 349*f*
    with tinea cruris, 350, 350*f*, 351*f*
    with urticaria, 294, 294*f*
Erythematous rash
    with atopic dermatitis, 323*f*, 325*f*
    with congenital syphilis, 172*f*
    drug reaction and, 312*f*–313*f*
    with eczema herpeticum (EH), 327*f*
    with erythema infectiosum (EI), 147*f*, 148
    with guttate psoriasis, 332, 332*f*, 333*f*, 334
    with hand-foot-and-mouth disease (HFMD), 149*f*, 150*f*, 151
    with herpangina, 152, 152*f*
    with incomplete Kawasaki disease (KD), 568*f*
    with infectious mononucleosis (IM), 144, 145*f*
    with juvenile dermatomyositis, 579*f*
    with Kawasaki disease (KD), 562*f*, 564*f*
    with measles, 140–141, 140*f*
    with neonatal lupus (NL), 574, 574*f*, 575*f*
    with psoriasis, 329, 329*f*, 331*f*
    with Rocky Mountain spotted fever (RMSF), 121, 121*f*
    with roseola infantum, 138–139, 138*f*
    with rubella, 142, 142*f*
    scarlatiniform, 95*f*, 115*f*
    with staphylococcal scalded skin syndrome (SSSS), 115*f*
    with systemic lupus erythematosus (SLE), 571*f*, 572*f*
Erythroderma, with staphylococcal toxic shock syndrome, 111*f*
Erythrodermic psoriasis, with arthritis, 584*f*
Erythropoiesis, parvovirus B19 and, 527
Esmolol, 721
Esophageal foreign bodies. *See* Foreign body (FB), esophageal
Esophageal penetrating injuries, 984
Esophageal varices, 685*f*
Estrogen treatment
    for labial adhesions, 87
    for urethral prolapse, 89
Estrogenized annular hymen, 161*f*
Ethanol toxicity, 786–787, 786*f*

Ethmoid sinusitis, acute, 449f
Ethylene glycol (EG) toxicity, 782–783, 782f, 783f
ETN (erythema toxicum neonatorum), 362, 362f
Ewing sarcoma, 558, 558f, 559f, 560, 560f
Exanthem subitum, 138–139, 138f
Exanthematous reaction, to drugs, 310, 312f, 313
Exchange transfusion, 521, 761
Exercise, premature ventricular contractions and, 219
Exfoliation
    with atopic dermatitis, 325f
    with staphylococcal scalded skin syndrome (SSSS), 114, 114f, 115f, 116f
Exfoliative toxins, 114
Extended focused assessment with sonography for trauma (EFAST), 1046, 1046f
Extension teardrop fracture, 991, 991f
External auditory canal (EAC)
    auricular hematoma and, 439–440
    cellulitis of, 432–433, 432f
    foreign body (FB) in, 437–438, 437f, 438f
Extracranial hematoma, 5f
Extrapyramidal side effects, of phenothiazines, 766, 766f
Extremity amputation, 1040–1041, 1040f, 1041f
Exudative tonsillopharyngitis, 94, 94f
    with infectious mononucleosis (IM), 144, 144f, 145f
Eye injuries. See also Ophthalmology
    differential diagnosis, 14f
    raccoon eye versus, 69f
Eyelid laceration, 414, 414f–415f, 978–979
Eyes
    chemical burns of, 422–423, 422f
    congenital syphilis and, 171t

F
Facet dislocation
    bilateral, 998, 998f
    unilateral, 999–1000, 999f
Facial edema, 707f
Facial nerve injury, 978, 980
Facial nerve paralysis. See also Bell palsy
    otitis media and, 431
Facial palsy
    acute otitis media (AOM) and, 431f
    corneal ulcer with, 408f, 410f
    hypopyon with, 410f
    Lyme disease and, 591
    rhabdomyosarcoma and, 625f
    with stroke, 617f
Factor IX deficiency, 534, 536
Factor VIII deficiency, 534, 536
FAST (focused assessment with sonography for trauma), 1046–1047, 1047f
    positive suprapubic view, 1049f
Fat embolism, 866t
Fat embolization syndrome, 516–517
FB. See Foreign body (FB)
Febrile seizures, 609–610, 609f, 610f, 610t
Fecal masses, 544
Female circumcision, 86, 87f
Femur fractures, 888–889, 888f
    child abuse and, 28–29, 28f, 29f
Fenoldopam, 721
Ferric chloride reaction, 750f
Fever
    altered mental status and, 605
    sickle cell anemia with, 510–511, 510f, 511f
Fever blisters, 134f, 135
Fifth disease, 147–148, 147f
Filiform warts, 356
Finger injuries, 1030f
Finkelstein disease, 63–64, 63f
Fire coral, 835–836, 836f
First disease, 140–141, 140f, 141f

First-degree atrioventricular (AV) block, 193, 193f, 194f, 194t
First-trimester pregnancy, emergency ultrasound (US) of, 1056–1057, 1056f
Fish bones, 680f
Fishhook removal, 1042, 1042f
Flail chest, rib fractures and, 1008–1009, 1008f
Flat warts, 356, 356f
Flesh-eating bacteria syndrome. See Necrotizing fasciitis (NF)
Flexion teardrop fractures, 992, 992f, 993f
Flexor tenosynovitis, 929, 929f
Fluid therapy
    for burns, 810
    for diabetic ketoacidosis (DKA), 649, 653f
    for hemolytic uremic syndrome (HUS), 717
    for hyperosmolar hyperglycemic syndrome (HHS), 651
    for IBD, 690
Flumazenil, 755t, 789
Fluoroscopy
    of foreign body (FB) aspiration, 257
    of intussusception, 468f
Focal seizure, 611
Focused assessment with sonography for trauma (FAST), 1046–1047, 1047f
    positive suprapubic view, 1049f
Folk healing practices
    caida de mollera, 51
    coin rubbing, 50, 50f
    cupping (ventosa), 50, 51f
    garlic, 50–51, 51f, 52f
    maquas, 51
    moxibustion, 51
    spooning, 50
Food, aspiration of, 254–255, 254f, 255f
FOOSH injury, 874, 878, 880, 882
Foot penetrating injury, 1038–1039, 1038f
Forearm fractures, 874–875, 874f
Foreign body (FB)
    anorectal, 673–674, 673f
    aspiration
        asthma and, 284f, 285f
        bacterial tracheitis and, 262f
        bronchiolitis and, 266f
        clinical features of, 254–255, 257
        croup and, 259f
        emergency department treatment and disposition, 257
        by food products, 254–255, 254f, 255f
        pneumonia and, 271f
    auricular, 437–438, 437f, 438f
    battery ingestions, 262f, 675, 675f–676f, 677, 677f, 678f
    corneal, 406, 406f
    dental trauma and, 1004f
    distal to esophagus, 671–672, 671f, 672f
    esophageal
        clinical summary for, 666
        drooling and, 666f
        emergency department treatment and disposition, 666–667
        locations of, 667f
        orientation of, 668f
        radiolucent, 669f
        signs and symptoms of, 666t
        stick-pin ingestion, 669f
        tracheal FB mimicking by, 668f
    intra-articular, 927f
    intravaginal
        abnormal uterine bleeding (AUB) and, 185f
        in prepubertal child, 491, 491f, 492f
    magnet ingestion, 683, 683f
    nasal, 444, 444f, 445f, 446
    open fractures and, 866t
    penetrating injuries and, 927, 927f
    retained bones, 679–680, 679f, 680f
    retropharyngeal space abscess and, 457f

sharp objects, 681, 681f, 682f
tracheal, esophageal FB mimicking of, 668f
Fournier's gangrene, 106, 106f
Fractures
  ankle, 892–893, 892f, 893f
  atlas, 988, 988f
  avulsion. *See* Avulsion fractures
  Bennett, 871, 871f
  boxer's, 872
  calcaneal, 894, 894f
  of carpal bone, 873, 873f
  Chance, 1025f
  child abuse and
    classic metaphyseal lesion (CML), 24, 24f, 25f
    congenital syphilis and, 24f
    hemothorax with, 39f
    humerus, 883f
    inflicted versus accidental, 23–24, 23f
    multiple, 26f, 28f
    osteogenesis imperfecta (OI) and, 25f, 79
    radiography of, 23f, 24f, 25, 25f, 26f
    radionuclide bone scan for, 26f
    rickets and, 25f, 76, 78f
  clavicle, 884–885, 884f
  clinical summary for, 858
  complications of, 866t
  copper deficiency and, 75
  emergency department treatment and disposition, 858, 863
  emergency ultrasound (US) of, 1063, 1063f
  extension teardrop, 991, 991f
  femur. *See* Femur fractures
  flexion teardrop, 992, 992f, 993f
  forearm, 874–875, 874f
  frontal sinus, 970
  Galeazzi fracture dislocation, 876, 876f
  hangman's, 37f, 990, 990f
  humerus, 882–883, 882f, 883f
  Jefferson burst, 988, 988f
  Jones fracture, 895–896, 895f
  Le Fort, 968–969, 968f, 969f
  Lisfranc fracture, 897, 897f
  Maisonneuve, 891, 891f
  mallet finger, 870, 870f
  mandible, 965–967, 965f, 966f
  maxillary, 968–969, 968f, 969f
  midfacial, 968–971, 968f, 969f, 970f
  Monteggia fracture dislocation, 876, 876f
  nasal, 963–964, 963f, 963t, 964f
  nasoorbitoethmoid (NOE), 963t, 969–970, 970f
  odontoid, 989, 989f
  olecranon, 877, 877f
  orbital, 419, 419f, 972, 972f, 973f
  patella, 890, 890f
  pelvic, 1027–1028, 1027f, 1028f
  phalanx, 868–869, 868f, 869f
  pseudo-Jones fracture, 895–896, 895f
  radial head and neck, 878–879, 878f
  ribs. *See* Rib fractures
  Rolando, 871, 871f
  Salter-Harris classification of, 862f, 863f, 864f, 866t
  scapular, 886–887, 886f
  skull. *See* Skull fractures
  with special considerations, 865t
  spinal process, 1002, 1002f
  stress fracture, 898, 898f
  supracondylar, 880–881, 880f, 881f
  testicular, 485, 485f
  toddler's, 864f
  tripod, 976, 976f
  tuft, 867, 867f
  types of, 858f–861f, 865t

zygomatic arch, 975–977, 975f
zygomatic complex, 975–977, 976f
Free T$_3$, 661
Free T$_4$, 658, 661
Frogfish, 844–845, 844f
Frog-leg position, 160f, 162, 491
Frontal bone osteomyelitis, 454–455, 454f, 455f
Frontal bossing, 76
Frontal sinus fractures, 970
Frostbite, 577, 814
  first-degree, 814f, 816t
  fourth-degree, 815f, 816t
  second-degree, 814f, 816t
  third-degree, 815f, 816t
Fulminant myocarditis, acute, 239f, 241f
Fungal sinusitis, 451, 452f
Furocoumarin compound, 59–60, 59f, 60f
Fusobacterium necrophorum, 456–457, 457f, 462

G
GA (granuloma annulare), 337–338, 337f
GABHS. *See* Group A β-hemolytic *Streptococcus* (GABHS)
Galeazzi fracture dislocation, 876, 876f
Gallbladder, 525f, 689
  emergency ultrasound (US) of, 1054–1055, 1054f
Gallstone pancreatitis, 687f
Gallstones
  biliary colic and, 689, 689f
  emergency ultrasound (US) of, 1054–1055, 1054f
  sickle cell disease (SCD) and, 524
Gamekeeper's thumb, 916, 916f
Gamow bag, 854
Ganglioglioma, 629f
Gardasil, 169
Garlic, 50–51, 51f, 52f
Gartland classification, 880
Gastric lavage
  for anticholinergic toxicity, 768
  for camphor toxicity, 772
  for castor bean and rosary pea toxicity, 765
  for hydrocarbon toxicity, 774
  for insecticide toxicity, 763
  for iron toxicity, 752f
  for isoniazid (INH) toxicity, 771
  for phenothiazine toxicity, 767
Gastric outlet obstruction
  with iron toxicity, 752
  pyloric stenosis and, 471
Gastric ulcer, 685f
Gastrointestinal (GI) decontamination
  for acetaminophen (APAP), 747–748
  for β-blockers (BBs), 791
  for calcium channel blockers (CCBs), 791
  for clonidine, 793
  for cocaine toxicity, 758
  for cyclic antidepressants (CAs), 795
  for ethanol, 786
  for iron toxicity, 752f
  for isoniazid (INH) toxicity, 771
  methods for, 744
  for phenothiazine toxicity, 767
Gastrointestinal (GI) disorders. *See also* Foreign body (FB)
  anorectal foreign bodies, 673–674, 673f
  battery ingestions, 262f, 675, 675f–676f, 677, 677f, 678f
  biliary colic, 689, 689f
  constipation, 692–693, 692f, 693f, 694f
  esophageal foreign bodies, 666–667, 666f, 666t, 667f, 668f, 669f, 670
  foreign bodies distal to esophagus, 671–672, 671f, 672f
  hematemesis, 684–686, 684f, 685f
  inflammatory bowel disease (IBD), 375f, 690, 690f, 691f
  magnet ingestion, 683, 683f

Gastrointestinal (GI) disorders (*Cont.*):
pancreatitis, 524, 687–688, 687*f*, 688*f*
rectal bleeding. *See* Lower GI bleeding (LGIB)
retained bones, 679–680, 679*f*, 680*f*
sharp objects, 681, 681*f*, 682*f*
Gastrointestinal (GI) injury, 1025
GBS (Guillain-Barré syndrome), 640–641, 640*f*, 641*f*
GCS (Glasgow Coma Scale), 602, 605, 948, 960
Generalized erythroderma, atopic dermatitis and, 325*f*
Generalized pustular psoriasis, 329, 331, 331*f*
Generalized tonic-clonic seizures, 611
Genital herpes
clinical summary for, 179, 179*f*, 180*f*, 181*f*
emergency department treatment and disposition, 179
management of, 167*t*
sexual abuse and, 164*f*
Genital warts. *See* Condylomata acuminata
Genitals. *See also* Penis; Vagina
ambiguous, 656, 657*f*
edema of, 708*f*
hair-tourniquet syndrome (HTS), 72, 72*f*
injury to, 6*f*
labial adhesion, 86–87, 86*f*, 87*f*
lichen sclerosus et atrophicus (LSA), 82–83, 82*f*
straddle injury. *See* Straddle injury
Genitourinary and surgery
acute nonperforated appendicitis, 473–475, 473*f*, 474*f*
appendix testis torsion, 490, 490*f*
Bartholin gland abscess, 177*f*, 496, 496*f*
congenital imperforate hymen with hematometrocolpos, 493–494, 493*f*, 494*f*, 495*f*
epididymo-orchitis, 487–488, 487*f*, 488*f*, 489*f*
hypertrophic pyloric stenosis, 471–472, 471*f*
incarcerated inguinal hernia, 478–479, 478*f*, 479*f*
intestinal malrotation and volvulus, 504–505, 504*f*
intussusception, 466–467, 466*f*–470*f*, 469–470
ovarian torsion, 501, 501*f*, 502*f*, 503, 503*f*
paraphimosis, 497, 497*f*–500*f*, 499
perforated appendicitis, 476–477, 476*f*
testicular torsion. *See* Testicular torsion
testicular trauma, 485–486, 485*f*, 486*f*
umbilical granuloma, 506–507, 506*f*
umbilical hernia, 508, 508*f*
vaginal foreign body (FB) in prepubertal child, 491, 491*f*, 492*f*
Genu valgum, 76, 77*f*
Genu varum, 76, 77*f*
Germ cell testicular cancer, 482*f*
Germ cell tumors, mixed, 549
German measles, 142–143, 142*f*
Ghon primary complex, 277*f*
GI decontamination. *See* Gastrointestinal (GI) decontamination
GI disorders. *See* Gastrointestinal (GI) disorders
GI (gastrointestinal) injury, 1025
Gianotti Crosti syndrome, 56*f*, 150*f*
Giant molluscum contagiosum, 359*f*
Giemsa stain
of mastocytoma, 371
of molluscum contagiosum, 358
for newborn conjunctivitis, 400–401
of transient neonatal pustular melanosis (TNPM), 380
Gilbert syndrome, 526
Gingivostomatitis, herpetic, 134–135, 135*f*
Gitelman syndrome, 731–732
Glasgow Coma Scale (GCS), 602, 605, 948, 960
Glaucoma, infantile, 404–405, 404*f*, 405*f*
Glenohumeral joint
dislocations of, 904–906, 904*f*, 905*f*
intra-articular foreign body, 927*f*
Global anoxic brain injury, 606*f*
Globe rupture, traumatic, 416–417, 416*f*, 417*f*, 418*f*, 974*f*
Glomerular disease, 702

Glomerulonephritis
hematuria with, 702–703
poststreptococcal, 101
Glucose, 740*t*
Glucose-6-phosphate dehydrogenase deficiency
human parvovirus B19 and, 527
naphthalene and, 773, 774*f*
Glycosuria, 648
Goat bones, 679*f*
Goiter, 658*f*, 659*f*, 662*f*, 663*f*
Gonadoblastomas, 549
Gonococcal conjunctivitis, 398
Gonococcal infections. *See* Gonorrhea
Gonorrhea
Bartholin gland abscess and, 496*f*
child abuse and, 15
clinical summary for, 177–178, 177*f*, 178*f*
conjunctivitis with, 400, 400*f*
emergency department treatment and disposition, 178
epididymo-orchitis with, 487
management of, 167*t*
sexual abuse and, 164*f*
Gottron papules, 580*f*
Gottron sign, 579*f*
Gower signs, 579
GPA (granulomatosis with polyangiitis), 587–588, 587*f*, 588*f*
Gradenigo triad, 429, 431
Gram stain, for newborn conjunctivitis, 400–401
Granuloma
pyogenic, 397*f*
umbilical, 506–507, 506*f*
Granuloma annulare (GA), 337–338, 337*f*
Granulomatosis with polyangiitis (GPA), 587–588, 587*f*, 588*f*
Graves disease, 661, 661*f*, 662*f*
Great arteries, transposition of, 223*f*
Green mamba, 851*f*
Greenstick fractures, 861*f*, 865*t*
Gross hematuria, 702*f*
Group A β-hemolytic *Streptococcus* (GABHS)
acute rheumatic fever (ARF) and, 247
bacterial meningitis and, 596
chickenpox and, 129
deep neck space infection and, 456–457
ecthyma and, 101–102, 101*f*
epiglottitis and, 263, 264*f*
erysipelas and, 103–104
guttate psoriasis and, 332, 332*f*, 333*f*, 334
Henoch-Schönlein purpura (HSP) and, 314
impetigo and, 65, 65*f*, 67, 98
lymphadenitis and, 126, 127*t*
necrotizing fasciitis (NF) and, 106
osteomyelitis with, 932*t*
perianal bacterial dermatitis (PBD) and, 84–85, 84*f*, 85*f*
peritonsillar abscess (PTA) and, 460
pneumonia with, 269
streptococcal pharyngitis and, 94–95, 94*f*
toxic shock syndrome (TSS), 110, 110*f*, 112*t*, 113
Guillain-Barré syndrome (GBS), 640–641, 640*f*, 641*f*
Gunshot wound
abdominal trauma, 1020*f*
fatal, 46*f*
glenohumeral joint and, 927*f*
to heart, 234*f*
neck, 984, 985*f*
traumatic globe rupture with, 417*f*
Guttate psoriasis, 332, 332*f*, 333*f*, 334

H
H₁/H₂-receptor–blocking agents, 819
HACE (high-altitude cerebral edema), 854–855
Haemophilus influenzae

acute otitis media (AOM) and, 427
bacterial meningitis and, 596
cellulitis and, 104, 104*f*
epiglottitis and, 263
osteomyelitis with, 930
HAIR-AN syndrome, 376, 376*f*
Hair-tourniquet syndrome (HTS), 72–73, 72*f*, 499*f*
"Hallmark sign," 972*f*
Hand infections, paronychia, 928, 928*f*
Hand penetrating injury, 1038–1039, 1038*f*
Hand-foot-and-mouth disease (HFMD), 149, 149*f*, 150*f*, 151
Hangman's fracture, 37*f*, 990, 990*f*
HAPE (high-altitude pulmonary edema), 854–855, 854*f*
Hard coral, 835–836, 835*f*
Harrison groove, 76
Hashimoto thyroiditis, 658, 658*f*, 659*f*, 663*f*
Hashitoxicosis, 663*f*
Hb. *See* Hemoglobin (Hb)
HC (hydrocarbon) toxicity, 773–775, 773*f*, 774*f*
HD (Hirschsprung disease), 692–693, 693*f*, 694*f*
HDCV (human diploid cell vaccine), 829
Head trauma
    abdominal trauma and, 1019
    abusive. *See* Abusive head trauma
    cerebral concussion, 960, 960*f*
    cerebral contusion, 959, 959*f*
    clinical summary for, 948
    emergency department treatment and disposition, 948–950
    epidural hematoma (EDH), 950*f*. *See also* Epidural hematoma (EDH)
    inflicted, 601*f*
    lip laceration, 981, 981*f*
    mandible fractures, 965–967, 965*f*, 966*f*
    midfacial fractures, 968–971, 968*f*, 969*f*, 970*f*
    nasal fractures, 963–964, 963*f*, 963*t*, 964*f*
    nasal septal hematoma, 961–962, 961*f*
    orbital trauma, 972, 972*f*, 973*f*, 974, 974*f*
    penetrating injuries, 948*f*, 949*f*
    penetrating neck injury, 984, 984*f*, 985*f*
    pneumocephalus, 949*f*, 970*f*
    soft tissue trauma, 978–980, 978*f*, 979*f*, 980*f*
    temporomandibular joint (TMJ) dislocation, 983, 983*f*
    tongue laceration, 982, 982*f*
    zygomatic arch fractures, 975–977, 975*f*
    zygomatic complex fractures, 975–977, 976*f*
Headache, 626–627, 626*f*, 627*f*, 628*f*
Headlight sign, 324*f*
Hearing
    auricular foreign body (FB) and, 437–438
    otitis externa (AOE) and, 432
Heart block. *See* Atrioventricular (AV) block
Heimlich maneuver, 257
Hemangioma, infantile. *See* Infantile hemangioma (IH)
Hemarthrosis, 534, 535*f*, 536
Hematemesis, 684–686, 684*f*, 685*f*
Hematocele, testicular, 485
Hematocolpos, 493
Hematology
    abdominal mass, 543–545, 543*f*, 544*f*, 545*f*
    acute lymphoblastic leukemia (ALL), 539–540, 539*f*
    Ewing sarcoma, 558, 558*f*, 559*f*, 560, 560*f*
    hemophilia, 534, 534*f*, 535*f*, 536
    immune thrombocytopenia, 531–533, 531*f*, 532*f*
    lymphadenopathy. *See* Lymphadenopathy
    neuroblastoma, 546–547, 546*f*, 547*f*, 548*f*
    ovarian tumors, 549, 549*f*, 550*f*, 551*f*, 552
    sickle cell anemia
        with acute chest syndrome, 516–518, 516*f*
        with acute pain, 512, 513*f*, 514–515, 514*f*
        acute splenic sequestration crisis (ASSC) and, 529–530, 529*f*
        cerebrovascular disease and, 519, 519*f*, 520*f*, 521
        with fever, 510–511, 510*f*, 511*f*

with priapism, 522–523, 522*f*, 523*f*
with right upper quadrant (RUQ) syndrome, 524, 524*f*, 525*f*, 526, 526*f*
transient aplastic crisis (TAC) and, 527–528, 527*f*
Hematoma
    auricular, 439–440, 439*f*
    duodenal, 1025
    epidural. *See* Epidural hematoma (EDH)
    extracranial, 5*f*
    intracerebral, 959, 959*f*
    nasal septal, 961–962, 961*f*
    ruptured arteriovenous malformation (AVM) and, 626*f*
    scrotal, 92, 92*f*
    subdural. *See* Subdural hematoma (SDH)
    subgaleal. *See* Subgaleal hematoma
    subungual, 868, 868*f*, 1032–1033, 1032*f*
    testicular, 485
Hematometrocolpos, imperforate hymen with, 493–494, 493*f*, 494*f*, 495*f*
Hematuria
    with abdominal trauma, 1020
    with acute poststreptococcal glomerulonephritis (APSGN), 711*f*
    clinical summary for, 702–703
    emergency department treatment and disposition, 703, 705–706
    gross, 702*f*
    with lymphoblastic leukemia, 544
    nephrolithiasis and, 722*f*
    polycystic kidney disease (PKD) and, 705*f*
    renal cell carcinoma with, 704*f*
    schistosomiasis and, 705*f*
    sickle cell disease (SCD) and, 705*f*
    terminal, 702–703
    Wilms tumor and, 702*f*–703*f*
Hemicraniectomy, elevated intracranial pressure (ICP) and, 603*f*
Hemiparesis, sickle cell disease (SCD) and, 521
Hemiplegia, 520*f*
Hemoglobin (Hb)
    abdominal trauma and, 1020
    acute chest syndrome and, 517
    acute splenic sequestration (ASSC) and, 530
    methemoglobin, 760
    parvovirus B19 and, 527, 527*f*
Hemoglobinuria, 774*f*
Hemolytic anemia, naphthalene and, 774*f*
Hemolytic uremic syndrome (HUS), 716–717, 716*f*
Hemoperitoneum, 1046
Hemophilia, 534, 534*f*, 535*f*, 536
Hemopneumothorax, 290*f*
Hemorrhage
    intraparenchymal, 606*f*
    retinal, 36*f*
    retrobulbar, 420, 420*f*, 421*f*
    splinter, 229*f*
    subarachnoid. *See* Subarachnoid hemorrhage (SAH)
    subconjunctival, 258*f*, 413, 413*f*
    subdural. *See* Subdural hemorrhage (SDH)
Hemorrhagic cystitis, 702*f*
Hemorrhagic stroke
    altered mental status, 606*f*
    intracranial pressure (ICP) elevation and, 601*f*
Hemothorax
    emergency ultrasound (US) of, 1049*f*
    with fractures, 39*f*
    trauma and, 1012, 1012*f*
Henoch-Schönlein purpura (HSP)
    acute hemorrhagic edema of infancy (AHEI) and, 63–64
    clinical summary for, 314
    emergency department treatment and disposition, 314–316
    immune thrombocytopenic purpura (ITP) and, 532*f*
    intussusception in, 469*f*
    meningococcemia compared with, 119, 119*f*
    pearls, 316

Henoch-Schönlein purpura (HSP) (*Cont.*):
  Rocky Mountain spotted fever (RMSF) compared with, 121, 122*f*
    with vasculitis, 314–316, 315*f*
Hepatic injuries, 1024, 1024*f*
Hepatoblastoma, 543*f*, 545
Hepatopathy, sickle cell, 524, 526*f*
Hepatosplenic cat-scratch disease, 125*f*
Hepatosplenomegaly
  acute lymphoblastic leukemia (ALL) and, 539*f*, 540
  with biliary atresia, 684*f*
  immune thrombocytopenic purpura (ITP) and, 531
  macrophage activation syndrome (MAS) and, 589*f*
  miliary TB and, 278, 278*f*
Hepatotoxicity, acetaminophen (APAP), 746, 746*f*, 747*f*, 748
Herald patch, 335, 335*f*, 336*f*
Hernia
  incarcerated inguinal. *See* Incarcerated inguinal hernia
  umbilical, 508, 508*f*
Heroin, 754*f*
Herpangina, 152, 152*f*
Herpes encephalitis, 616*f*
Herpes labialis, 134*f*, 135
Herpes simplex virus (HSV)
  conjunctivitis with, 398, 399*f*, 400, 401*f*
  eczema herpeticum (EH) with, 327–328, 327*f*
  of genitals. *See* Genital herpes
  herpetic whitlow, 136, 136*f*
  management of, 167*t*
  neonatorum, 180*f*, 181*f*
  oropharyngeal, 134–135, 134*f*, 135*f*
  preseptal cellulitis and, 395*f*
Herpes zoster, 131, 131*f*, 132*f*, 133
Herpes zoster ophthalmicus, 131
Herpetic gingivostomatitis, 134–135, 135*f*
Herpetic whitlow, 136, 136*f*
HFMD (hand-foot-and-mouth disease), 149, 149*f*, 150*f*, 151
HHS (hyperosmolar hyperglycemic syndrome), 651
  diabetic ketoacidosis (DKA) versus, 653*t*
HHV-6 (human herpesvirus-6), 138–139, 138*f*
Hidradenitis suppurativa (HS), 378–379, 378*f*
High-altitude cerebral edema (HACE), 854–855
High-altitude pulmonary edema (HAPE), 854–855, 854*f*
Hilar adenopathy, 277*f*
Hill-Sachs lesions, 904, 904*f*
  reverse, 905*f*
Hip
  dislocation of, 907–908, 907*f*, 908*f*
  emergency ultrasound (US) of, 1062, 1062*f*
Hirschsprung disease (HD), 692–693, 693*f*, 694*f*
Histoplasmosis
  acute pericarditis and, 236
  pericardial effusion (PE) and, 237*f*
HIV, management of, 167*t*
Hives, 294–295, 294*f*, 295*f*
HL (Hodgkin lymphoma), 541–542, 541*f*, 542*f*
HLHS (hypoplastic left heart syndrome), 226–227, 227*f*, 228*t*
Hodgkin lymphoma (HL), 541–542, 541*f*, 542*f*
Hoffman sign, 584
Hordeolum, 396–397, 396*f*
  with preseptal cellulitis, 394*f*
Horner syndrome, 546
Hose nozzle, as foreign body (FB), 673*f*
Hospital gangrene. *See* Necrotizing fasciitis (NF)
Household products, 738*f*
HPV. *See* Human papillomavirus (HPV)
HS (hidradenitis suppurativa), 378–379, 378*f*
HSP. *See* Henoch-Schönlein purpura (HSP)
HSV. *See* Herpes simplex virus (HSV)
HTN. *See* Hypertension (HTN)
HTS (hair-tourniquet syndrome), 72–73, 72*f*
"Huffing," 773, 774*f*

Human bites, 833–834, 833*f*
Human diploid cell vaccine (HDCV), 829
Human herpesvirus-6 (HHV-6), 138–139, 138*f*
Human papillomavirus (HPV)
  child abuse and, 15
  condylomata acuminata and, 168. *See also* Condylomata acuminata
  warts with, 356–357, 356*f*, 357*f*
Human parvovirus B19
  erythema infectiosum (EI), 147–148, 147*f*
  transient aplastic crisis (TAC) and, 527
Humerus fracture, 882–883, 882*f*, 883*f*
HUS (hemolytic uremic syndrome), 716–717, 716*f*
Hydration. *See also* Fluid therapy
  acute chest syndrome and, 517
  for cocaine toxicity, 758
Hydrocarbon (HC) toxicity, 773–775, 773*f*, 774*f*
Hydrocele
  incarcerated inguinal hernia compared with, 479*f*
  testicular torsion compared with, 483*f*
Hydrocephalus
  aqueductal stenosis leading to, 632*f*–633*f*
  bacterial meningitis and, 597*f*, 599*f*
  clinical summary for, 632
  emergency department treatment and disposition, 634–636
  multiple congenital brain malformations with, 633*f*
  pituitary gland tumor and, 631*f*
  subarachnoid hemorrhage (SAH) and, 620*f*
  VP shunt
    complications with, 636*f*
    fracture of, 635*f*
    obstruction of, 635
    series of, 634*f*
Hydrocolpos, imperforate hymen with, 495*f*
Hydroids, 835–836, 835*f*
Hydromorphone, sickle cell disease (SCD) and, 512
Hydronephrosis, 543–544, 546*f*
21-Hydroxylase, 656, 657*f*
17-Hydroxyprogesterone, 656
Hymen
  examination of, 161*f*, 162
  imperforate
    with hematometrocolpos, 493–494, 493*f*, 494*f*
    with hydrocolpos, 495*f*
    labial fusion compared with, 495*f*
    normal estrogenized annular, 161*f*
    normal unestrogenized crescentic, 161*f*
Hymenotomy, 545
Hyperbilirubinemia, 524, 526
Hypercalcemia
  clinical summary for, 728, 730
  electrocardiogram of, 729*f*
  emergency department treatment and disposition, 730
  laboratory algorithm for, 728*f*
  with lymphoblastic leukemia, 544
  medullary nephrocalcinosis, 729*f*
  with subcutaneous fat necrosis (SCFN), 382
Hypercholesterolemia, with nephrotic syndrome (NS), 708
Hypercyanotic spell of tetralogy of Fallot
  clinical summary of, 222–223, 222*f*, 223*f*, 224*f*
  cyanosis with, 222*f*
  emergency department treatment and disposition, 223
  management of, 225*t*
  presenting features of, 225*t*
Hyperemia
  acute nonperforated appendicitis and, 473*f*
  Raynaud phenomenon (RP) and, 576*f*, 577*t*
Hyperextension deformity, 868
Hyperglycemia, 648
Hyperhemolysis, 527
Hyperkalemia
  with acute poststreptococcal glomerulonephritis (APSGN), 712

clinical summary for, 733
electrocardiogram of, 733, 733*f*
emergency department treatment and disposition, 733–735
with first-degree atrioventricular (AV) block, 194*f*
treatment of, 734–735, 734*f*
Hyperosmolar hyperglycemic syndrome (HHS), 651
diabetic ketoacidosis (DKA) versus, 653*t*
Hyperosmolar nonketotic coma, 651
Hyperoxaluria, 722, 722*f*
Hyperoxia, elevated intracranial pressure (ICP) and, 602
Hyperoxia test, 228*t*
Hyperparathyroidism, 728, 730
Hyperpigmentation
with Addison disease, 654, 654*f*, 655*f*
postinflammatory, 68, 68*f*
Hyperplasia
lymphoid, 537
sickle cell disease (SCD) and, 519, 521
Hyperpronation technique, 917
Hypersensitivity reactions and disorders
anaphylaxis, 817–819, 817*f*, 818*f*
angioedema as, 296
to drugs, 310, 310*f*
EM as, 302
erythema nodosum (EN) as, 375, 375*f*
scabies as, 339
serum sickness as, 298
SJS and TEN as, 305
UM as, 300
urticaria as, 294
Hypertension (HTN)
portal, with biliary atresia, 684*f*
pulmonary. *See* Pulmonary hypertension (PH)
Wilms tumor and, 720*f*
Hypertensive emergencies, 720–721, 720*f*
Hypertensive encephalopathy, 607*f*
Hypertensive urgency, 720
Hyperthyroidism, 661, 661*f*, 662*f*, 663*f*, 664
Hypertrophic pyloric stenosis, 471–472, 471*f*
emergency ultrasound (US) of, 1053, 1053*f*
Hyperventilation
for diabetic ketoacidosis (DKA), 649
elevated intracranial pressure (ICP) and, 602
Hyphema, 411–412, 411*f*
with traumatic globe rupture, 416, 417*f*
Hypoalbuminemia, 690
Hypocalcemia, 725–727, 725*f*, 726*f*
Hypokalemia, 731–732, 731*f*
caffeine and, 804, 805*f*
Hypomelanosis of Ito, 611*f*
Hyponatremia, 776
Hypopigmentation
with congenital syphilis, 173*f*
hypomelanosis of Ito, 611*f*
with neonatal lupus (NL), 575*f*
Hypoplastic left heart syndrome (HLHS), 226–227, 227*f*, 228*t*
Hypopyon, 410, 410*f*
with leukocoria, 402
Hypothalamic–pituitary–adrenal axis, congenital adrenal hyperplasia and, 656*f*
Hypothermia
altered mental status and, 605
electrocardiogram (ECG) of, 816*f*
Hypothyroidism, 658–659, 658*f*, 659*f*, 660*f*
Hypoventilation
acute chest syndrome and, 517
elevated intracranial pressure (ICP) and, 602
Hypoxemia
airway obstruction and, 1013
with sickle cell disease (SCD), 516

I

IBD (inflammatory bowel disease), 375*f*, 690, 690*f*, 691*f*
ICP. *See* Intracranial pressure (ICP)
Id reaction, of tinea capitis, 346*f*, 347
Idiopathic acute transverse myelitis, 638
IE (infective endocarditis), 229–231, 229*f*, 230*f*, 230*t*
IH. *See* Infantile hemangioma (IH)
IM. *See* Infectious mononucleosis (IM)
Immersion burns, 19*f*, 21
differential diagnosis, 20*f*
Immune thrombocytopenic purpura (ITP)
with epistaxis, 441, 442*f*
newly diagnosed, 531–533, 531*f*, 532*f*
Immunosuppression
acute bacterial rhinosinusitis (ABRS) and, 447–448
ecthyma gangrenosum (EG) and, 108
herpes zoster and, 131*f*
otitis externa (AOE) and, 433
staphylococcal scalded skin syndrome (SSSS) and, 114
transient aplastic crisis (TAC) and, 528
Impacted fractures, 865*t*
Imperforate hymen
with hematometrocolpos, 493–494, 493*f*, 494*f*
with hydrocolpos, 495*f*
labial fusion compared with, 495*f*
Impetigo
with acute poststreptococcal glomerulonephritis (APSGN), 712*f*
clinical summary for, 65–66, 98–99, 98*f*, 99*f*
emergency department treatment and disposition, 66–67, 99–100
Incarcerated inguinal hernia
clinical summary for, 478
emergency department treatment and disposition, 478
hydrocele compared with, 479*f*
in infant, 478*f*
loop of bowel, 478*f*
pearls for, 479
testicular torsion compared with, 479*f*
Incense, 781*f*
Incomplete abortion, abnormal uterine bleeding (AUB) and, 184*f*
Incomplete fractures, 865*t*
Incomplete Kawasaki disease, 567–568, 567*f*, 568*f*, 569*f*
Incontinentia pigmenti (IP), 387–388, 387*f*
Infanticide versus sudden unexplained infant death syndrome
autopsy findings for, 43*f*, 44*f*, 45*f*
clinical summary for, 43–44
emergency department management for, 44–46
fatal gunshot wound, 46*f*
multiple trauma in, 43*f*
rib fractures in, 44*f*, 45*f*
Infantile atopic dermatitis, 323*f*, 324*f*
Infantile botulism, 644–645, 644*f*, 645*f*
Infantile glaucoma, 404–405, 404*f*, 405*f*
Infantile hemangioma (IH)
chalazion and, 397*f*
clinical summary for, 366–367
emergency department treatment and disposition, 367–368
mixed, 367*f*
pearls for, 369
segmental, 366, 366*f*
sexual abuse and, 166*f*
spinal dysmorphism and, 368, 368*f*
superficial, 366*f*, 368*f*
with ulceration, 368, 368*f*
Infantile scabies, 339, 340*f*, 341*f*
Infectious diseases
ascariasis, 155–156, 155*f*
cat-scratch disease (CSD), 124–125, 124*f*, 125*f*
chickenpox, 129–130, 129*f*, 130*f*
cutaneous larvae migrans (CLM), 153–154, 153*f*
ecthyma, 101–102, 101*f*, 102*f*
ecthyma gangrenosum (EG), 108–109, 108*f*, 109*f*

Infectious diseases (*Cont.*):
erysipelas, 65–67, 65*f*, 103–104, 103*f*, 104*f*
erythema infectiosum (EI), 147–148, 147*f*
hand-foot-and-mouth disease (HFMD), 149, 149*f*, 150*f*, 151
herpangina, 152, 152*f*
herpes zoster, 131, 131*f*, 132*f*, 133
herpetic whitlow, 136, 136*f*
impetigo, 65–67, 65*f*, 66*f*, 98–100, 98*f*, 99*f*
lymphadenitis, 126–128, 126*f*, 127*f*, 127*t*
malaria, 157–158, 157*f*, 158*t*
measles, 140–141, 140*f*, 141*f*
meningococcemia, 118–120, 118*f*, 119*f*, 120*f*
mononucleosis. *See* Infectious mononucleosis (IM)
mumps, 137, 137*f*
necrotizing fasciitis (NF), 105–107, 105*f*, 106*f*
oropharyngeal herpes simplex virus (HSV), 134–135, 134*f*, 135*f*
rickettsial infections, 123*t*
Rocky Mountain spotted fever (RMSF), 121–122, 121*f*, 122*f*, 123*t*
roseola infantum, 138–139, 138*f*
rubella, 142–143, 142*f*
scarlet fever, 94–97, 95*f*, 96*f*, 97*f*
staphylococcal scalded skin syndrome (SSSS), 114–117, 114*f*, 115*f*, 116*f*, 117*f*, 117*t*
streptococcal pharyngitis, 94–97, 94*f*
toxic shock syndrome (TSS), 110, 110*f*, 111*f*, 112*t*, 113
Infectious mononucleosis (IM)
bilateral cervical lymphadenopathy, 537*f*
clinical summary of, 144–145, 144*f*, 145*f*
emergency department treatment and disposition, 145–146, 146*t*
Infective endocarditis (IE), 229–231, 229*f*, 230*f*, 230*t*
Inferior rectus muscle entrapment, 972*f*
Inferior vena cava (IVC), 1064–1065, 1064*f*
Infibulation, 86, 87*f*
Inflammatory bowel disease (IBD), 375*f*, 690, 690*f*, 691*f*
Inflammatory disorders, seborrheic dermatitis, 318–319, 318*f*, 319*f*
Inflicted bites, 8*f*
Inflicted bruises. *See* Bruises, inflicted
Inflicted burns. *See* Burns, inflicted
Inflicted head trauma, 601*f*
Inflicted neck injuries, 9*f*
Influenza A infection, 271*f*
INH (isoniazid) toxicity, 770–771, 770*f*, 771*f*
Inhalation injury, 808–809, 810*f*
Insecticide toxicity, 762–763, 762*f*
Insulin
deficiency of, 648
for diabetic ketoacidosis (DKA), 650–651
for hyperosmolar hyperglycemic syndrome (HHS), 651
Interferon-γ release assays, 274
Interphalangeal joint dislocation, 899–900, 899*f*
Intestinal malrotation and volvulus, 504–505, 504*f*
Intra-abdominal trauma, 1025–1026, 1025*f*, 1026*f*
Intra-articular foreign body, 927*f*
Intracerebral hematoma, 959, 959*f*
Intracranial complications, of acute bacterial rhinosinusitis (ABRS), 447, 450, 450*f*
Intracranial pressure (ICP), 601–603
brain tumor and, 602*f*
causes of raised, 604*t*
diabetic ketoacidosis (DKA) and, 649–650
epidural hematoma (EDH) and, 601*f*
ganglioglioma and, 629*f*
head trauma and, 950
headache and, 626
hemorrhagic stroke and, 601*f*
hydrocephalus and, 632
intraventricular drain and hemicraniectomy and, 603*f*
neurocysticercosis and, 621
subarachnoid hemorrhage (SAH) and, 603*f*
Intramedullary spinal cord tumor, 638*f*
Intraocular pressure (IOP), 404, 411

Intraparenchymal bleed, 601*f*
Intraparenchymal hemorrhage, 606*f*
Intrascrotal appendages, 490*f*
Intraspinal extension, abdominal mass with, 638*f*
Intrathoracic tuberculosis
clinical summary for, 273–274
emergency department treatment and disposition, 274–275
pearls for, 277
Intrauterine device (IUD), pelvic inflammatory disease (PID) and, 183*f*
Intrauterine pregnancy (IUP), 188
emergency ultrasound (US) of, 1056–1057, 1056*f*
Intravaginal foreign body
abnormal uterine bleeding (AUB) and, 185*f*
in prepubertal child, 491, 491*f*, 492*f*
Intraventricular drain, elevated intracranial pressure (ICP) and, 603*f*
Intubation, in asthma, 285*t*
Intussusception
as abdominal mass, 544
air reduction procedure for, 468*f*
altered mental status and, 607*f*
clinical summary for, 466–467, 469
computed tomography of, 470*f*
crescent sign of, 467*f*
currant-jelly stool with, 466*f*, 467
emergency department treatment and disposition, 469–470
in Henoch-Schönlein purpura (HSP), 469*f*
pearls for, 470
radiography of, 467*f*, 469–470, 469*f*
rectal bleeding and, 695*f*, 696–697
rectal prolapse and, 467*f*
ultrasound (US) of, 468*f*, 470
emergency, 1052, 1052*f*
Inverse form of PR, 335
Iodine deficiency, 658
IOP (intraocular pressure), 404, 411
IP (incontinentia pigmenti), 387–388, 387*f*
"Iris" lesions, 303*f*
Iron burns, 21*f*
Iron toxicity, 752–753, 752*f*, 753*f*
Ischemic stroke, 618*f*
Isoniazid (INH) toxicity, 770–771, 770*f*, 771*f*
ITP. *See* Immune thrombocytopenic purpura (ITP)
IUD (intrauterine device), pelvic inflammatory disease (PID) and, 183*f*
IUP (intrauterine pregnancy), 188
emergency ultrasound (US) of, 1056–1057, 1056*f*
IV immunoglobulin (IVIG)
for immune thrombocytopenic purpura (ITP), 531–532, 531*f*
for incomplete Kawasaki disease (KD), 569*f*
for Kawasaki disease (KD), 562, 563*f*
IVC (inferior vena cava), 1064–1065, 1064*f*
IVIG. *See* IV immunoglobulin (IVIG)

J
Jacquet diaper dermatitis, 166*f*
Janeway lesions, 230*t*
Jaundice
with biliary atresia, 684*f*
with biliary colic, 689
with sickle cell anemia, 514*f*
Jaw pain, 965
JDM (juvenile dermatomyositis), 579, 579*f*, 580*f*, 581, 581*t*
Jefferson burst fractures, 988, 988*f*
Jellyfish stings, 837–839, 838*f*, 839*f*
JIA. *See* Juvenile idiopathic arthritis (JIA)
Jimson weed, 768*f*
Jones fracture, 895–896, 895*f*
Junctional epidermolysis bullosa, 363
Juvenile dermatomyositis (JDM), 579, 579*f*, 580*f*, 581, 581*t*
Juvenile idiopathic arthritis (JIA)
clinical summary for, 582–583
emergency department treatment and disposition

for patients suspected to have, 583–585
for patients with known diagnosis of, 585
erythrodermic psoriasis with, 584*f*
oligoarticular, 582*f*
pearls for, 586
polyarticular, 582*f*
psoriatic, 583*f*
systemic-onset, 583*f*
Juvenile nasopharyngeal angiofibroma, epistaxis and, 441, 443*f*
JWH-018, 780, 780*f*

K
K2 Spice, 780, 780*f*
Kanavel signs, 929
Kawasaki disease (KD)
clinical features of, 563*f*, 566*t*
clinical summary for, 562
diagnosis of, 567*f*
differential diagnosis of, 566*t*
emergency department treatment and disposition, 562, 565
extremity changes in, 564*f*
imaging of, 565*f*
incomplete, 567–568, 567*f*, 568*f*, 569*f*
pearls for, 566
Kennel cough, 258
Kerion, 345–347, 347*f*
Ketamine toxicity, 778, 778*f*
Ketoconazole
for priapism, 523
for seborrheic dermatitis, 318*f*, 319
for tinea versicolor, 342
Ketonemia, 649–650
Ketorolac, sickle cell disease (SCD) and, 512, 514
Kidney
congenital syphilis and, 171*t*
laceration of, 1026*f*
multicystic dysplastic, 713*f*
Kidney stones, 722–724, 722*f*, 723*f*, 724*f*
Kiesselbach plexus, 441
King snake, 850, 851*f*
Kingella kingae, 937, 941
Kissing disease. *See* Infectious mononucleosis (IM)
Klinefelter syndrome, 387
Klippel-Trenaunay syndrome (KTS), 57, 58*f*
Knee dislocation, 909–910, 909*f*, 910*f*
Knee-chest position, 160*f*, 162, 491
Knock-knees, 76, 77*f*
Kocher's criteria, 937
Koebner phenomenon, 329, 333*f*
Koplik spots, 141, 141*f*
Kratom powder, 754*f*
KTS (Klippel-Trenaunay syndrome), 57, 58*f*
Kussmaul breathing, 648–649
Kussmaul respirations, 770
Kyphoscoliosis, 76, 77*f*

L
Labetalol, 721
Labia majora
Mycoplasma pneumoniae-induced rash and mucositis (MIRM) and, 304*f*
straddle injury, 90, 90*f*, 91*f*
Labial adhesion, 86–87, 86*f*, 87*f*
Labial fusion, imperforate hymen compared with, 495*f*
Labial traction, 160*f*
Labialis, herpes, 134*f*, 135
Lacerations
of cheek, 978, 978*f*
conjunctival, 417*f*
corneal, 417*f*
eyelid, 414, 414*f*–415*f*, 978–979

kidney, 1026*f*
lip, 981, 981*f*
of liver, 1024*f*
of nail bed, 1031
nasal, 979*f*, 980
pancreatic, 688*f*
scalp, 979–980, 979*f*
scrotal, 486*f*
splenic, 1022*t*, 1023*f*
straddle injury, 90, 90*f*
tongue, 982, 982*f*
Lachman test, 923
Lambert-Eaton syndrome, 645*f*
Lamotrigine, SJS/TEN with, 306*f*
Laparotomy indications, 1020*t*, 1021
Laryngeal papillomatosis, 356
croup and, 260*f*
Latrodectism, 823
Latrodectus mactans, 823, 823*f*
Laxative, contact dermatitis from, 61–62, 61*f*, 62*f*
LCPD (Legg-Calvé-Perthes disease), 922, 922*f*
Le Fort fractures, 968–969, 968*f*, 969*f*
Lead toxicity, 796–797, 796*f*, 797*f*
Left upper quadrant (LUQ), focused assessment with sonography for trauma (FAST) view of, 1047, 1048*f*
Left-sided ductal-dependent cardiac lesions, 226, 226*f*
Legg-Calvé-Perthes disease (LCPD), 922, 922*f*
Legius syndrome, 373
Lemierre syndrome
cavernous sinus thrombosis and, 462*f*
clinical summary for, 462–463
deep neck abscess and, 456–457, 457*f*
emergency department treatment and disposition, 463
epidural abscess and, 464*f*
nonocclusive thrombus of, 462*f*, 463*f*
pansinusitis and, 464*f*
pearls for, 464
septic emboli and, 463*f*
Lesser trochanter avulsion, 915*f*
Lethargy
with acute splenic sequestration (ASSC), 529, 529*f*
definition of, 607*t*
with infantile botulism, 644, 644*f*
with intussusception, 466*f*, 469, 469*f*
LETM (longitudinally extensive transverse myelitis), 637*f*, 638
Leukemia, acute lymphoblastic, 539–540, 539*f*
Leukocoria, 402, 402*f*, 403*f*
Leukocytoclastic vasculitis, 63, 63*f*
Leukocytosis, pertussis with, 258
Leukocyturia, urinary tract infection and, 713*f*, 714
Leukoerythroblastosis, 527
Level of consciousness (LOC). *See* Altered mental status
LGIB. *See* Lower GI bleeding (LGIB)
Lichen sclerosus et atrophicus (LSA), 82–83, 82*f*
Lichtenberg figures, 849
Lidocaine, for jellyfish and Portuguese man-of-war stings, 838
Ligament injury, 866*t*
Ligament of Treitz, 671
Lightning injuries, 849, 849*f*
Linear marks, abusive, 11*f*
Linear skull fracture, 33*f*
Lines of Blaschko, 387, 387*f*
Lionfish, 844–845, 844*f*
Lip laceration, 981, 981*f*
Lipase, 688
Lisfranc fracture, 897, 897*f*
Listeria monocytogenes, bacterial meningitis and, 596
Lithium hydroxide, 798*f*
Little's area, 441
Liver
acute lymphoblastic leukemia (ALL) and, 540

Liver (*Cont.*):
  congenital syphilis and, 171*t*
  laceration of, 1024*f*
LOC (level of consciousness). *See* Altered mental status
Long QT syndrome (LQTS)
  clinical summary of, 200, 203*t*
  with complete heart block (CHB), 200, 201*f*
  emergency department treatment and disposition, 200, 202–203
  polymorphic ventricular tachycardia and, 200, 202, 202*f*, 725
  prolonged QT interval, 200*f*
Longitudinally extensive transverse myelitis (LETM), 637*f*, 638
Loop and linear marks, 10*f*, 11*f*
Loop diuretic, 730, 734
"Loop marks," child abuse, 2*f*
Loop of bowel, 478*f*
Lower GI bleeding (LGIB)
  clinical summary for, 695–696
  differential diagnosis of, 697*t*
  emergency department treatment and disposition, 696–697
  etiology of, 697*t*
  melena, 696, 696*f*, 696*t*
  types of, 696*t*
Loxosceles reclusa, 820–822, 820*f*, 821*f*
Loxoscelism, 820
LQTS. *See* Long QT syndrome (LQTS)
LSA (lichen sclerosus et atrophicus), 82–83, 82*f*
Lumbar spine injuries, 1025–1026
LUMBAR syndrome, 366–367
Lunate dislocations, 901–902, 901*f*
Lung, emergency ultrasound (US) of, 1058–1059, 1058*f*, 1059*f*
Lung window algorithms, 1006*f*
Lupus
  neonatal, 574, 574*f*, 575*f*
  systemic lupus erythematosus (SLE). *See* Systemic lupus erythematosus (SLE)
LUQ (left upper quadrant), focused assessment with sonography for trauma (FAST) view of, 1047, 1048*f*
Lyell disease. *See* Staphylococcal scalded skin syndrome (SSSS)
Lyme carditis, 591–592, 593*f*
Lyme disease, 591–592, 591*f*, 592*f*, 593*t*, 624
Lymphadenitis
  with bacterial adenitis, 124*f*
  with cat-scratch disease (CSD), 124*f*
  clinical summary for, 126–127
  common causes of, 126–127, 127*t*
  emergency department treatment and disposition, 127–128
  mycobacterial cervical, 126–128, 127*f*, 127*t*, 538*f*
  suppurative cervical, 126, 126*f*, 127*t*, 537*f*
Lymphadenopathy
  acute lymphoblastic leukemia (ALL) and, 539*f*, 540
  with atopic dermatitis, 323
  bilateral cervical, 537, 537*f*
  with cat-scratch disease (CSD), 124–125, 124*f*
  clinical summary for, 537
  emergency department treatment and disposition, 537–538
  with erysipelas, 104
  Hodgkin lymphoma (HL) and, 541*f*, 542, 542*f*
  immune thrombocytopenic purpura (ITP) and, 531
  with impetigo, 99
  with infectious mononucleosis (IM), 144, 144*f*
  miliary TB and, 278
  pearls for, 538
  with roseola infantum, 138
  with rubella, 142
Lymphedema, osteosarcoma versus, 556*f*–557*f*
Lymphoblastic leukemia
  acute, 539–540, 539*f*
  hypercalcemia with, 544
Lymphocytosis, pertussis with, 258
Lymphoid hyperplasia, 537
Lymphoma

Hodgkin, 541–542, 541*f*, 542*f*
non-Hodgkin, 541*f*

M
Macrophage activation syndrome (MAS)
  clinical summary for, 589–590
  emergency department treatment and disposition, 590
  hepatosplenomegaly in, 589*f*
  juvenile idiopathic arthritis, 585
  purpura, 590*f*
  systemic lupus erythematosus (SLE) and, 570, 572
Magnet ingestion, 683, 683*f*
Magnetic resonance angiography (MRA)
  of hemarthrosis, 535*f*
  of ischemic stroke, 618*f*
  of stroke, 519*f*, 521, 619
Magnetic resonance imaging (MRI)
  of abdominal mass, 638*f*
  of acute osteomyelitis, 930f, 931*f*
  of arteriovenous malformation, 612*f*
  of brain abscess, 627*f*
  of cerebellar astrocytoma, 630*f*
  of cerebellar stroke, 619*f*
  of chronic osteomyelitis, 933*f*
  of closed-lip schizencephaly, 613*f*
  of dysembryoplastic neuroepithelial tumor (DNET), 612*f*
  of epidural abscess with spinal cord compression, 638*f*
  of Ewing sarcoma, 558*f*, 559*f*, 560*f*
  of flexion teardrop fractures, 993*f*
  of ganglioglioma, 629*f*
  of Guillain-Barré syndrome (GBS), 640*f*, 641*f*
  of hepatoblastoma, 543*f*
  of herpes encephalitis, 616*f*
  of hydrocephalus, 633*f*, 634–635
  of hypertensive encephalopathy, 607*f*
  of intramedullary spinal cord tumor, 638*f*
  of ischemic stroke, 618*f*
  of Lemierre syndrome, 462*f*
  of medulloblastoma, 628*f*
  of midbrain brain tumors, 630*f*
  of neonatal osteomyelitis, 942*f*
  of neuroblastoma, 546*f*
  of neurocysticercosis, 622, 622*f*
  of osteomyelitis in sickle cell disease (SCD), 936*f*
  of osteosarcoma, 554*f*, 557*f*
  of ovarian torsion, 502*f*
  of pontine glioma, 630*f*
  of posterior reversible leukoencephalopathy syndrome (PRES), 720*f*
  of Pott puffy tumor, 455*f*
  of renal cell carcinoma, 704*f*
  of spinal cord injury without radiographic abnormality (SCIWORA), 996*f*
  of spinal cord lesions, 637*f*
  of status epilepticus, 614*f*
  of stroke, 519*f*, 520*f*, 521, 619
  of Sturge-Weber syndrome (SWS), 615*f*
  of tuberculomas, 279*f*
  of unilateral facet dislocation, 999*f*
Maisonneuve fracture, 891, 891*f*
Malar rash
  Raynaud phenomenon (RP) and, 576*f*
  of systemic lupus erythematosus (SLE), 571*f*, 572*f*
Malaria, 157–158, 157*f*, 158*t*
Malassezia furfur, 342, 344*f*
Malignant otitis externa, 432–433
Mallet finger, 870, 870*f*
Mallory-Weiss tear, 471
Malrotation, intestinal, volvulus and, 504–505, 504*f*
Mandible fractures, 965–967, 965*f*, 966*f*
  dental trauma and, 1003*f*, 1005*f*
MAP (mean arterial pressure), 601–602

Maquas, 51
Marijuana toxicity, 780–781, 780*f*, 781*f*
Marine animals. *See* Venomous marine animals
MAS. *See* Macrophage activation syndrome (MAS)
Mast cell degranulation triggers, 370, 372*t*
Mastocytosis
 clinical summary for, 370
 Darier sign, 370, 370*f*, 371*f*
 dermographism, 371*f*, 372
 diffuse cutaneous, 370–371, 372*f*
 emergency department treatment and disposition, 370–371
 mast cell degranulation triggers, 370, 372*t*
 pearls for, 372
 urticaria pigmentosa, 370–371, 371*f*
Mastoid air cells, middle ear infection and, 429
Mastoiditis
 acute, 429, 429*f*
 chronic otitis media with, 430*f*
 coalescent, 430*f*
Matles sign, 925
Maxillary fractures, 968–969, 968*f*, 969*f*
MCA (middle cerebral artery) infarct, 618*f*
McCune-Albright syndrome, café-au-lait spots (CALS) in, 373, 374*f*
MCNS. *See* Minimal change nephrotic syndrome
MCP (metacarpophalangeal) joint dislocation, 900*f*
MDMA (3,4-methylenedioxymethamphetamine), 776–777, 776*f*, 777*f*
Mean arterial pressure (MAP), 601–602
Measles, 140–141, 140*f*, 141*f*. *See also* Rubella
Mediastinal mass, 542*f*
Mediastinal teratoma, 551*f*
Medical alert bracelet, 819
Medications, poisoning by, 738, 738*f*
Medullary nephrocalcinosis, 729*f*
Medulloblastoma, 628*f*
Melena, 696, 696*f*, 696*t*
Meningitis
 bacterial. *See* Bacterial meningitis
 TB, 278–279, 596
Meningococcemia
 clinical summary for, 118–119, 118*f*, 119*f*, 120*f*
 emergency department treatment and disposition, 119–120
 Henoch-Schönlein purpura (HSP) compared with, 119, 119*f*
 Rocky Mountain spotted fever (RMSF) compared with, 121, 122*f*
Meningoencephalitis, mumps and, 137
Menkes disease, 74–75, 74*f*
Menometrorrhagia, 186
Menorrhagia, 186, 531
Menstruation
 abnormal uterine bleeding (AUB) and, 184, 184*f*, 185*f*, 186
 neonatal, 166*f*
Metabolic disease, bones and, 26–27
Metacarpophalangeal (MCP) joint dislocation, 900*f*
Metaphysitis, congenital syphilis and, 173*f*
Metastatic neuroblastoma, 392*f*
Methamphetamine toxicity, 777*f*
Methanol toxicity, 784–785, 784*f*, 785*f*
Methemoglobin (MetHb), 760–761
Methemoglobinemia, 740*t*, 760–761, 760*f*, 761*f*
Methicillin-resistant *S aureus* (MRSA)
 deep neck space infection and, 456–457
 staphylococcal scalded skin syndrome (SSSS) and, 116
Methylene blue, 761, 761*f*
3,4-Methylenedioxymethamphetamine (MDMA), 776–777, 776*f*, 777*f*
Metrorrhagia, 186
MG (myasthenia gravis), 642–643, 642*f*, 645*f*
Micrognathia, 585
Microsporum canis, 348
Midbrain brain tumors, 630*f*, 631
Middle cerebral artery (MCA) infarct, 618*f*
Middle ear
 effusion, acute otitis media and, 426, 426*f*
 infection of
  acute otitis media (AOM) and, 429
  mastoid air cells and, 429
Mid-esophagus, foreign body (FB) at, 667*f*
Midfacial fractures, 968–971, 968*f*, 969*f*, 970*f*
Migraine, 626–627
Miliary tuberculosis, 278–279, 278*f*, 279*f*
Miller-Fisher syndrome, 640
Minimal change nephrotic syndrome (MCNS)
 ascites with, 708*f*
 clinical summary for, 707–709
 edema with, 708*f*
 emergency department treatment and disposition, 709–710
 periorbital and facial edema with, 707, 707*f*
 pleural effusion, 708*f*
 scrotal swelling and, 709*f*
MIRM (*Mycoplasma pneumoniae*-induced rash and mucositis), 304*f*, 307*f*
Mites, 339, 339*f*
Mixed germ cell tumors, 549
Mobitz type I heart block, 195, 195*f*, 196*t*
Mobitz type II heart block, 195, 196*f*, 196*t*
Modified Duke criteria, 229–230
Modified measles, 141
Molluscum contagiosum, 358–359, 358*f*, 359*f*
Molly/ecstasy toxicity, 776–777, 776*f*, 777*f*
Mongolian spots, 48–49, 48*f*, 49*f*
Monomorphic ventricular tachycardia, 220*f*–221*f*
Mononucleosis. *See* Infectious mononucleosis (IM)
Mons pubis, condylomata acuminata and, 169*f*
Monteggia fracture dislocation, 876, 876*f*
Moraxella catarrhalis, acute otitis media (AOM) and, 427
Morphine, sickle cell disease (SCD) and, 512, 514
Mosquitoes, 157
Motor seizures, 743
Moxibustion, 51
MRA. *See* Magnetic resonance angiography (MRA)
MRI. *See* Magnetic resonance imaging (MRI)
MRSA. *See* Methicillin-resistant *S aureus* (MRSA)
Mucocele, congenital imperforate hymen with, 493
Mucocutaneous lymph node syndrome. *See* Kawasaki disease
Mucous membrane warts, 356
Multicystic dysplastic kidney, 713*f*
Multifocal premature ventricular contractions, 220*f*
Mumps, 137, 137*f*
Murphy sign, 687, 689, 1054–1055
Musculoskeletal injuries
 acromioclavicular (AC) injuries, 919, 919*f*
 anterior cruciate ligament (ACL) tear, 923, 923*f*
 gamekeeper's thumb, 916, 916*f*
 nursemaid's elbow, 917–918, 917*f*
 slipped capital femoral epiphysis (SCFE), 920–921, 920*f*
Myasthenia gravis (MG), 642–643, 642*f*, 645*f*
Mycobacterial lymphadenitis, 126–128, 127*f*, 127*t*, 538*f*
Mycobacterium bovis, 944
Mycobacterium tuberculosis. *See also* Tuberculosis
 deep neck space infection and, 456–457
 miliary TB with, 278–279, 278*f*, 279*f*
 pneumonia with, 269
 Pott disease and, 944
Mycoplasma pneumoniae, sickle cell disease (SCD) and, 516
Mycoplasma pneumoniae–induced rash and mucositis (MIRM), 304*f*, 307*f*
Myocarditis. *See* Acute myocarditis
Myonecrosis, bacterial, 106
Myositis ossificans, 883*f*
Myxedema, 658–659, 659*f*

N
NAC (*N*-acetylcysteine), 747–748
Nail beds
 injury to, 1030–1031, 1030*f*
 with juvenile dermatomyositis, 580*f*

Nail beds (*Cont.*):
  subungual hematoma and, 1032
  of tetralogy of Fallot (TOF), 222*f*
  tinea unguium, 354–355, 354*f*
  tuft fractures and, 867, 867*f*
Nail ingestion, 681*f*
Nail pitting, with psoriasis, 330*f*
Naloxone, 755, 755*t*
Naphthalene toxicity, 773–775, 774*f*, 775*f*
Napkin psoriasis, 62*f*, 330*f*
Nasal foreign bodies, 444, 444*f*, 445*f*, 446
Nasal fractures, 963–964, 963*f*, 963*t*, 964*f*
Nasal lacerations, 979*f*, 980
Nasal pack, placement of, 442–443, 442*f*
Nasal polyps, 451
Nasal saline irrigation, 448
Nasal septal hematoma, 961–962, 961*f*
Nasal septum, arteries of, 441, 441*f*
Nasal warts, 356
Nasoorbitoethmoid (NOE) fractures, 963*t*, 969–970, 970*f*
Nasopharyngeal airway, 281*f*
Nasopharyngeal angiofibroma, epistaxis and, 441, 443*f*
Nasopharyngeal aspergillosis, 452*f*, 453*f*
NAT. *See* Nonaccidental trauma
Neck injuries
  child abuse, 9*f*
  penetrating, 984, 985*f*
  zones of, 984*f*
Necrotizing enterocolitis, 695
Necrotizing fasciitis (NF)
  clinical summary for, 105–106, 105*f*, 106*f*
  emergency department treatment and disposition, 106–107
  emergency ultrasound (US) of, 1060
Necrotizing otitis externa, 432–433
Needle ingestion, 682*f*
Neisseria gonorrhoeae. See Gonorrhea
Neisseria meningitidis, 118, 120. *See also* Meningococcemia
  bacterial meningitis and, 596
Nematocysts, 835
Neonatal lupus (NL), 574, 574*f*, 575*f*
Neonatal osteomyelitis, 942–943, 942*f*, 943*f*
Neonate
  herpes simplex (HSV) in, 180*f*, 181*f*
  menstruation in, 166*f*
Neosporin, allergic contact dermatitis and, 320*f*
Nephroblastoma, hematuria and, 702*f*–703*f*
Nephrocalcinosis, medullary, 729*f*
Nephrolithiasis, 722–724, 722*f*, 723*f*, 724*f*
Nephrology
  acute poststreptococcal glomerulonephritis (APSGN), 703, 711–712, 711*f*, 712*f*
  hematuria. *See* Hematuria
  hemolytic uremic syndrome (HUS), 716–717, 716*f*
  hypercalcemia. *See* Hypercalcemia
  hyperkalemia. *See* Hyperkalemia
  hypertensive emergencies, 720–721, 720*f*
  hypocalcemia, 725–727, 725*f*, 726*f*
  hypokalemia, 731–732, 731*f*
  minimal change nephrotic syndrome (MCNS). *See* Minimal change nephrotic syndrome (MCNS)
  nephrolithiasis, 722–724, 722*f*, 723*f*, 724*f*
  obstructive uropathy, 718–719, 718*f*, 719*f*
  proteinuria, 700–701, 700*f*, 701*f*
  urinary tract infection, 713–715, 713*f*, 714*f*
Nephrostogram, of obstructive uropathy, 718*f*
Nephrotic syndrome (NS)
  with edema and proteinuria, 700*f*
  minimal change. *See* Minimal change nephrotic syndrome (MCNS)
  penile edema and, 499*f*
  proteinuria and, 707
Nephrotic-range proteinuria, 701

Neuroblastoma, 546–547, 546*f*, 547*f*, 548*f*
  brain tumors. *See* Brain tumors
  metastatic, 392*f*
Neurocysticercosis, 621–622, 621*f*, 622*f*, 623*f*
Neurofibromatosis, café-au-lait spots (CALS) and, 373, 373*f*, 611*f*
Neurology
  bacterial meningitis. *See* Bacterial meningitis
  Bell palsy, 624–625, 624*f*, 625*f*
  epilepsy, 611, 611*f*, 612*f*, 613, 613*f*
  febrile seizures, 609–610, 609*f*, 610*f*, 610*t*
  Guillain-Barré syndrome (GBS), 640–641, 640*f*, 641*f*
  headache, 626–627, 626*f*, 627*f*, 628*f*
  hydrocephalus. *See* Hydrocephalus
  infantile botulism, 644–645, 644*f*, 645*f*
  myasthenia gravis (MG), 642–643, 642*f*
  neurocysticercosis, 621–622, 621*f*, 622*f*, 623*f*
  raised intracranial pressure (ICP), 601–603, 601*f*, 602*f*, 603*f*
  seizures. *See* Seizures
  spinal cord lesions, 637–639, 637*f*, 638*f*
  status epilepticus, 614, 614*f*, 615*f*, 616, 616*f*
  stroke in children. *See* Stroke
Neuromuscular transmission, 645*f*
Neuromyelitis optica (NMO), 637
Neurovascular compromise, 866*t*
Nevi of Ota and Ito, 55–56, 55*f*, 56*f*
Nevus flammeus, 56*f*, 57, 57*f*
Newborn conjunctivitis, 400–401, 400*f*, 401*f*
NF. *See* Necrotizing fasciitis (NF)
Nicardipine, 721
Nickel contact dermatitis, 321*f*
Nicotine toxicity, 802, 803*f*
Nikolsky sign
  with SJS and TEN, 305, 305*f*
  with staphylococcal scalded skin syndrome (SSSS), 114, 117
"Nipple sign," 471*f*
NL (neonatal lupus), 574, 574*f*, 575*f*
NMO (neuromyelitis optica), 637
NOE (nasoorbitoethmoid) fractures, 963*t*, 969–970, 970*f*
Nonaccidental trauma (NAT)
  linear skull fracture, 33*f*
  multiple fractures of, 28*f*, 29*f*
  straddle injury versus, 91*f*
  with traumatic brain injury (TBI), 37*f*
Nonbullous impetigo, 65, 98–99, 98*f*
Nonexudative limbic-sparing conjunctivitis, 563*f*
  with incomplete Kawasaki disease (KD), 568*f*
Non-Hodgkin lymphoma, 541*f*
Nonossifying fibroma, fracture of, 861*f*
Nonperforated appendicitis. *See* Acute nonperforated appendicitis
Nonsteroidal anti-inflammatory drugs (NSAIDs)
  for atopic dermatitis (AD), 326
  for black widow spider bites, 823
  for migraine, 627
Nontuberculous mycobacteria (NTM), lymphadenitis with, 126–128, 127*f*, 127*t*
Nonunion of fracture, 866*t*
Normal estrogenized annular hymen, 161*f*
Normal unestrogenized crescentic hymen, 161*f*
NS. *See* Nephrotic syndrome (NS)
NSAIDs. *See* Nonsteroidal anti-inflammatory drugs (NSAIDs)
NTM (nontuberculous mycobacteria), lymphadenitis with, 126–128, 127*f*, 127*t*
Nursemaid's elbow, 917–918, 917*f*

O

Obesity, diabetes and, 651*f*
Oblique fractures, 860*f*, 861*f*, 865*t*
Obstructive choledocholithiasis, 524, 526
Obstructive sleep apnea syndrome (OSAS)
  clinical summary for, 280, 280*f*

emergency department treatment and disposition, 280, 282
   laboratory tests for, 281t
   nasopharyngeal airway, 281f
   postoperative pulmonary edema, 281f
Obstructive uropathy, 718–719, 718f, 719f
Obtundation, 607t
Occult fractures, 865t
Octopus bites, 848, 848f
Ocular compartment syndrome, 420, 420f
Odontoid fractures, 989, 989f
Odor, poisoned patient and, 741t
OI. See Osteogenesis imperfecta (OI)
Oil of wintergreen, 749, 749f
Olecranon fracture, 877, 877f
Oligoanuria, 716
Oligoarthritis, 585t
Oligoarticular juvenile idiopathic arthritis, 582f
Omphalitis, 506, 506f
OMS (opsoclonus-myoclonus syndrome), 546
Oncology
   abdominal mass, 543–545, 543f, 544f, 545f
   acute lymphoblastic leukemia (ALL), 539–540, 539f
   Ewing sarcoma, 558, 558f, 559f, 560, 560f
   Hodgkin lymphoma (HL), 541–542, 541f, 542f
   lymphadenopathy. See Lymphadenopathy
   neuroblastoma, 546–547, 546f, 547f, 548f
   osteosarcoma, 553–554, 553f–557f
   ovarian tumors, 549, 549f, 550f, 551f, 552
Onychomycosis, 354–355, 354f
Open fractures, 858f, 865t
   complications with, 866t
Ophthalmia neonatorum, 400–401, 400f, 401f
Ophthalmology
   acute conjunctivitis. See Conjunctivitis
   chalazion, 396–397, 396f, 397f
   chemical burns, 422–423, 422f
   conjunctivitis. See Conjunctivitis
   corneal abrasion, 407, 407f
   corneal foreign body (FB), 406, 406f
   corneal ulcer, 408–409, 408f
   eyelid laceration, 414, 414f–415f
   hordeolum, 396–397, 396f
   hyphema, 411–412, 411f
   hypopyon, 410, 410f
   infantile glaucoma, 404–405, 404f, 405f
   leukocoria, 402, 402f, 403f
   ophthalmia neonatorum, 400–401, 400f, 401f
   orbital cellulitis, 390, 390f, 391f, 392f, 393, 393f
   orbital fracture, 419, 419f
   preseptal cellulitis, 394–395, 394f, 395f
   retrobulbar hemorrhage, 420, 420f, 421f
   subconjunctival hemorrhage, 413, 413f
   traumatic globe rupture, 416–417, 416f, 417f, 418f
Opioids
   for black widow spider bites, 823
   prescription, 788–789
   toxicity of, 754–756, 754f, 755f, 755t
Opsoclonus-myoclonus syndrome (OMS), 546
Oral injuries, differential diagnosis, 14f, 15f
Oral warts, 356
Orbit
   abscess of, 449f
   acute bacterial rhinosinusitis (ABRS) and, 447, 449f, 450
   fractures of, 419, 419f, 972, 972f, 973f
   sagittal view of, 390f
   trauma of, 972, 972f, 973f, 974, 974f
Orbital cellulitis
   acute bacterial rhinosinusitis (ABRS) with, 447, 449f
   clinical summary for, 390, 391f
   emergency department treatment and disposition, 390
   metastatic neuroblastoma and, 392f

orbit, sagittal view of, 390f
   preseptal cellulitis and, 394, 394f
   rhabdomyosarcoma and, 393f
Orbital septum, 390f
Orchitis
   epididymitis and, 487–488, 487f, 488f, 489f
   mumps and, 137
Organophosphate toxicity, 762–763, 762f
Orofacial trauma, child abuse
   clinical summary, 13–16
   dental neglect, 15–16, 16f
   ear bruises, 13f
   emergency department treatment and disposition, 16–17
   eye injuries, 14f
   intraoral injuries, 14f
   oral bruising, 15f
Oropharyngeal herpes simplex virus, 134–135, 134f, 135f
Oropharyngeal penetrating trauma, 980f
Orthopedics. See also Avulsion fractures; Dislocations
   Achilles tendon rupture, 925–926, 925f
   acromioclavicular (AC) injuries, 919, 919f
   acute osteomyelitis, 930–932, 930f, 931f, 932t
   ankle dislocation, 911, 911f, 912f
   ankle fracture and sprain, 892–893, 892f, 893f
   anterior cruciate ligament (ACL) tear, 923, 923f
   Bennett fracture, 871, 871f
   boxer's fracture, 872
   calcaneal fracture, 894, 894f
   carpal bone fractures, 873, 873f
   chronic osteomyelitis, 933–934, 933f
   clavicle fracture, 884–885, 884f
   elbow dislocation, 903, 903f
   femur fracture, 888–889, 888f
   flexor tenosynovitis, 929, 929f
   forearm fractures, 874–875, 874f
   foreign bodies and penetrating injuries, 927, 927f
   fracture types, 858f–861f, 865t
   fractures, 858, 863. See also Fractures
   Galeazzi fracture dislocation, 876, 876f
   gamekeeper's thumb, 916, 916f
   glenohumeral joint dislocations, 904–906, 904f, 905f
   hip dislocation, 907–908, 907f, 908f
   humerus fracture, 882–883, 882f, 883f
   interphalangeal joint dislocation, 899–900, 899f
   Jones fracture, 895–896, 895f
   knee dislocation, 909–910, 909f, 910f
   Legg-Calvé-Perthes disease (LCPD), 922, 922f
   Lisfranc fracture, 897, 897f
   lunate dislocations, 901–902, 901f
   Maisonneuve fracture, 891, 891f
   mallet finger, 870, 870f
   Monteggia fracture dislocation, 876, 876f
   neonatal osteomyelitis, 942–943, 942f, 943f
   nursemaid's elbow, 917–918, 917f
   olecranon fracture, 877, 877f
   Osgood-Schlatter disease, 924, 924f
   osteomyelitis in sickle cell disease (SCD), 935, 935f, 936f
   paronychia, 928, 928f
   patella dislocation, 913, 913f
   patella fractures, 890, 890f
   pelvic avulsion fractures, 914, 914f
   perilunate dislocations, 901–902, 902f
   phalanx fractures, 868–869, 868f, 869f
   Pott disease, 944–945, 944f, 945f
   radial head and neck fracture, 878–879, 878f
   Rolando fracture, 871, 871f
   Salter-Harris classification of fractures, 862f, 863f, 864f, 866t
   scapular fracture, 886–887, 886f
   septic arthritis. See Septic arthritis
   slipped capital femoral epiphysis (SCFE), 920–921, 920f
   stress fracture, 898, 898f

Orthopedics (*Cont.*):
supracondylar fracture, 880–881, 880*f*, 881*f*
tibial tubercle avulsion fracture, 915, 915*f*
tuft fractures, 867, 867*f*
Orthostatic proteinuria, 700
Orthostatic syncope, 204–205, 207*t*
OSAS. *See* Obstructive sleep apnea syndrome (OSAS)
Osgood-Schlatter disease, 924, 924*f*
Osler nodes, 229*f*, 230*t*
Osserman scale, 642
Osteoarticular tuberculosis, 944–945, 944*f*, 945*f*
Osteochondritis, congenital syphilis and, 173*f*
Osteogenesis imperfecta (OI)
blue sclera with, 79, 79*f*
clinical features of, 79
congenital fractures, 80*f*
cracked egg shell appearance, 80*f*
emergency department treatment and disposition, 79–80
fractures and, 25*f*, 79
Osteomyelitis
acute, 930–932, 930*f*, 931*f*, 932*t*
chronic, 933–934, 933*f*
frontal bone, 454–455, 454*f*, 455*f*
neonatal, 942–943, 942*f*, 943*f*
open fractures and, 866*t*, 868
pathogens of, 932*t*
with penetrating injuries, 927, 927*f*
in sickle cell disease (SCD), 935, 935*f*, 936*f*
sickle cell disease (SCD) and, 510*f*, 512
temporal bone, 432–433
Osteopenia, 79, 80*f*
Osteoporosis, 80
Osteosarcoma, 553–554, 553*f*–557*f*
Otalgia
acute otitis media (AOM) and, 426, 429
otitis externa (AOE) and, 433
Otitis externa, 432–433, 432*f*
Otitis media. *See also* Acute otitis media (AOM)
chronic, 430*f*
complications of, 429, 429*f*, 430*f*, 431, 431*f*, 431*t*
Otolaryngology
acute bacterial rhinosinusitis (ABRS). *See* Acute bacterial rhinosinusitis (ABRS)
acute otitis media (AOM). *See* Acute otitis media (AOM)
auricular foreign body (FB), 437–438, 437*f*, 438*f*
auricular hematoma, 439–440, 439*f*
chronic sinusitis, 451, 452*f*, 453*f*
complications of otitis media. *See* Acute otitis media (AOM)
deep neck space infection, 456–457, 456*f*, 457*f*, 458*f*, 459
epistaxis, 441–443, 441*f*, 442*f*, 443*f*
Lemierre syndrome. *See* Lemierre syndrome
nasal foreign bodies, 444, 444*f*, 445*f*, 446
otitis externa, 432–433, 432*f*
perichondritis, 434–435, 434*f*, 435*f*, 436*f*
peritonsillar abscess (PTA), 460–461, 460*f*, 461*f*
Pott puffy tumor, 454–455, 454*f*, 455*f*
Otorrhea
acute otitis externa (AOE) and, 432, 432*f*
acute otitis media (AOM) and, 426–427, 426*f*, 429*f*
basilar skull fracture (BSF) and, 953*f*
Ovarian teratoma, 502*f*, 503*f*, 549, 549*f*, 550*f*, 551*f*
Ovarian torsion, 501, 501*f*, 502*f*, 503, 503*f*
emergency ultrasound (US) of, 1057
Ovarian tumors, 549, 549*f*, 550*f*, 551*f*, 552
Over-the-counter preparations
with acetaminophen (APAP), 746*f*
caffeine, 804
camphor, 772
dextromethorphan, 779, 779*f*
ethanol, 786*f*
general examples of, 738, 738*f*

methanol-containing, 784*f*
with salicylates, 749*f*

P
P waves
in bradycardia, 190, 190*f*, 191*f*
caffeine and, 804, 804*f*
in first-degree atrioventricular (AV) block, 194*f*
in hyperkalemia, 733, 733*f*
in long QT syndrome (LQTS), 201*f*
in premature ventricular contractions, 219
in second-degree atrioventricular (AV) block, 195*f*
in sinus tachycardia (ST), 208, 208*f*
in supraventricular tachycardia (SVT), 211
in third-degree atrioventricular (AV) block, 197*f*, 198*f*, 199*f*
Pacemaker, syncope and, 204*f*
Pain
chest. *See* Chest pain
jaw, 965
sickle cell anemia with, 512, 513*f*, 514–515, 514*f*
Pallor
abdominal mass and, 544
abnormal uterine bleeding (AUB) and, 184*f*
acute chest syndrome and, 516*f*
acute splenic sequestration (ASSC) and, 529, 529*f*
hemolytic uremic syndrome (HUS) and, 716*f*
Raynaud phenomenon (RP) and, 577*t*
transient aplastic crisis (TAC) and, 527, 527*f*
Palmoplantar psoriasis, 329*f*
Palsy
Bell, 624–625, 624*f*, 625*f*
facial. *See* Facial palsy
peripheral seventh nerve, 592*f*, 624
Pancreas, 524*f*
injury to, 1025, 1026*f*
laceration of, 688*f*
Pancreatitis, 524, 687–688, 687*f*, 688*f*
Papilledema, 725
Papular PR, 335
Paradichlorobenzene (PDB), 773
Paramyxovirus
measles, 140–141, 140*f*, 141*f*
mumps, 137
Parapharyngeal space abscess, 456, 456*f*
Paraphimosis
balanoposthitis, 500*f*
clinical summary of, 497
differential diagnosis of, 499*f*
dorsal slit incision for, 497*f*
edema and swelling with, 497*f*
emergency department treatment and disposition, 497
manual reduction of, 497*f*, 498*f*, 499*f*
Parapneumonic effusion, with pneumonia, 268*f*
Parasternal long axis (PSLA) view of heart, 1065*f*
Parathyroid hormone (PTH), 725*f*, 726, 730
Parinaud oculoglandular syndrome, with cat-scratch disease (CSD), 124
Parkland formula, 810
Paronychia, 136*f*, 928, 928*f*
Parotid duct injury, 980
Parotid gland, 137, 137*f*
Parotitis, mumps, 137, 137*f*
Partial thromboplastin time (PTT)
hemophilia and, 534
immune thrombocytopenic purpura (ITP) and, 531
Parvovirus B19
erythema infectiosum (EI), 147–148, 147*f*
transient aplastic crisis (TAC) and, 527
Pastia sign, with scarlet fever, 94
Patch test, 320
Patella

dislocation of, 913, 913*f*
    fracture of, 890, 890*f*
Patent ductus arteriosus (PDA), 243
Pathologic fractures, 861*f*, 865*t*
Pathologic proteinuria, 700–701
Pattern bruises, 10, 10*f*, 11*f*, 12*f*
PBD (perianal bacterial dermatitis), 84–85, 84*f*, 85*f*
PCECV (purified chick embryo cell vaccine), 829–830, 829*f*
PD (perioral dermatitis), 386, 386*f*
PDA (patent ductus arteriosus), 243
PDB (paradichlorobenzene), 773
PE. *See* Pericardial effusion (PE)
PE (pulmonary embolism), 291–292, 291*f*, 292*f*
Pediatric Asthma Severity Score, 286
Pediatric poisoning
    clinical summary for, 738, 743
    emergency department treatment and disposition, 743–744
    mnemonics for, 741*t*–742*t*
    pearls for, 745
    quantitative serum concentrations and, 743*t*
    toxicologic clues and tests for, 740*t*–741*t*
Pediatric scrotum, acute. *See* Acute pediatric scrotum
Pelvic avulsion fractures, 914, 914*f*
Pelvic brim avulsion, 914*f*
Pelvic fractures, 1027–1028, 1027*f*, 1028*f*
Pelvic inflammatory disease (PID), 182–183, 182*f*, 183*f*
Pencil ingestion, 672*f*
Penetrating injuries
    abdominal, 1019*f*, 1020*f*
    to cheek, 978
    diaphragm and, 1015
    esophageal, 984
    foot, 1038–1039, 1038*f*
    foreign bodies, 927, 927*f*
    hand, 1038–1039, 1038*f*
    head, 948*f*, 949*f*
    to nail bed, 1031*f*
    neck, 984, 984*f*, 985*f*
    oropharyngeal, 980*f*
    pneumothorax and, 1010
Penicillin
    for dog bites, 827
    for GABHS infection, 97
    infectious mononucleosis (IM) and, 145*f*, 146
    for perianal bacterial dermatitis (PBD), 84–85, 85*f*
    for syphilis, 175
Penile-tourniquet syndrome, 72, 72*f*
Penis
    condylomata acuminata and, 169*f*
    constipation and, 692
    edema of, 499*f*
    genital herpes and, 179*f*
    gonorrhea and, 177*f*
    injury to, 6*f*
    paraphimosis, 497, 497*f*–500*f*, 499
    syphilis and, 174, 174*f*
    zipper injury, 1043, 1043*f*
PEP (postexposure prophylaxis), rabies, 829–830, 829*f*, 829*t*
Peptic ulcer disease, 685*f*
Perforated appendicitis, 476–477, 476*f*
Perforation of tympanic membrane (TM), 849*f*
Perianal bacterial dermatitis (PBD), 84–85, 84*f*, 85*f*
Perianal warts, 168*f*
Pericardial effusion (PE)
    acute pericarditis with, 236
    echocardiography of, 237, 237*f*, 1064
Pericardial fluid on subxiphoid view, 1049*f*
Pericardial friction rub, 237
Pericardiocentesis, 237–238, 237*f*
    emergency ultrasound (US) of, 1064
Pericarditis, acute, 236–238, 236*f*, 237*f*

Pericholecystic fluid, 1055
Perichondritis, 434–435, 434*f*, 435*f*, 436*f*
Perilunate dislocations, 901–902, 902*f*
Perioral dermatitis (PD), 386, 386*f*
Periorbital ecchymosis
    with basilar skull fracture (BSF), 953, 953*f*
    with pertussis, 258*f*
Periorbital edema, 707*f*
Periostitis, congenital syphilis and, 173*f*
Peripheral blood smear, hemolytic uremic syndrome (HUS), 716*f*
Peripheral cold injuries
    classification, 816*t*
    clinical summary, 814
    emergency department treatment and disposition, 814–815
    frostbite, 814, 814*f*, 815*f*, 816*t*
Peripheral seventh nerve palsy, 592*f*, 624
Peritonsillar abscess (PTA), 460–461, 460*f*, 461*f*
Periungual warts, 356
Perniosis, 577
Persistent hyperplastic primary vitreous (PHPV), 402
Persistent pulmonary hypertension of newborn (PPHN), 249
Pertussis, 258, 258*f*
Pesticide toxicity, 762–763, 762*f*
Petechial eruption
    abdominal mass and, 544
    with erythema infectiosum (EI), 147*f*
    with immune thrombocytopenic purpura (ITP), 531, 532*f*
    with infective endocarditis (IE), 230*f*, 230*t*
    with meningococcemia, 118*f*, 119, 120, 120*f*
    with Rocky Mountain spotted fever (RMSF), 121, 121*f*
    with systemic lupus erythematosus (SLE), 571*f*
Petrositis, 429
PF (purpura fulminans), with meningococcemia, 118*f*, 119, 119*f*
PH. *See* Pulmonary hypertension (PH)
PHACE syndrome, 366, 368–369
Phalanx fractures, 868–869, 868*f*, 869*f*
Pharyngitis, 134–135; 711
Phenobarbital, TEN and, 307, 308*f*
Phenothiazine toxicity, 766–767, 766*f*
Phenylephrine
    for caffeine toxicity, 805
    for priapism, 522*f*, 523*f*
Pheochromocytoma, 721
Phimosis, 82–83
    balanoposthitis with, 500*f*
Photophobia, 408
PHPV (persistent hyperplastic primary vitreous), 402
Physostigmine, 762, 768–769
Phytophotodermatitis (PPD), 59–60, 59*f*, 60*f*
PID (pelvic inflammatory disease), 182–183, 182*f*, 183*f*
Pigmentation. *See* Hyperpigmentation; Hypopigmentation
Ping pong fracture, 33*f*
Pitting edema, 708*f*
Pituitary gland tumors, 631, 631*f*
Pityriasis rosea (PR), 335–336, 335*f*, 336*f*
Pityrosporum ovale, 318
PKD (polycystic kidney disease), hematuria and, 705*f*
Plantar warts, 356
Plasmodium sp., 157, 157*f*, 158*t*
Pleural effusion
    emergency ultrasound (US) of, 1059, 1059*f*
    with minimal change nephrotic syndrome (MCNS), 708*f*
    pneumonia with, 268*f*, 271*f*
    primary spontaneous pneumothorax (PSP) and, 290*f*
    pulmonary tuberculosis with, 274, 276*f*
Pleural tuberculosis, 273, 275
Pneumocephalus, 949*f*, 970*f*
Pneumococcal pneumonia
    with empyema, 269*f*
    lobar consolidation in, 268*f*
Pneumococcal vaccines, 510

Pneumomediastinum
  chest pain and, 232*f*
  pneumothorax with, 1010*f*
  tracheobronchial tree injury (TBTI) and, 1017, 1017*f*
Pneumonia. *See* Community-acquired pneumonia
Pneumonitis
  hydrocarbon, 773*f*
  viral, 270*f*
Pneumopericardium, pneumothorax with, 1010*f*
Pneumothorax, 287
  emergency ultrasound (US) of, 1058–1059, 1059*f*
  primary spontaneous. *See* Primary spontaneous pneumothorax
  tension. *See* Tension pneumothorax
  tracheobronchial tree injury (TBTI) and, 1017, 1017*f*
  trauma and, 1010–1011, 1010*f*
Poison ivy dermatitis, 320, 321*f*, 322
Poisoning, pediatric. *See* Pediatric poisoning
Poisons, 738, 738*f*
Polyangiitis, granulomatosis with, 587–588, 587*f*, 588*f*
Polyarticular juvenile idiopathic arthritis, 582*f*
Polycystic kidney disease (PKD), hematuria and, 705*f*
Polyethylene glycol, 693
Polymorphic ventricular tachycardia, 200, 202, 202*f*, 725
Polymyositis, 581*t*
Polyps
  nasal, 451
  umbilical, 506
Pontine glioma, 630*f*
Popliteal artery, 910, 910*f*
Popsicle panniculitis, 53–54, 54*f*
Porifera sponges, 840–841, 840*f*
Portal hypertension, biliary atresia with, 684*f*
Portuguese man-of-war, 837–839, 837*f*
Port-wine stain (PWS), 56*f*, 57, 57*f*, 615*f*
Posterior fossa tumors, 629, 630*f*
Posterior glenohumeral joint dislocation, 904–906, 905*f*
Posterior reversible leukoencephalopathy syndrome (PRES), 607*f*, 720*f*
Posterior urethral valves (PUV), 718–719
Postexposure prophylaxis (PEP), rabies, 829–830, 829*f*, 829*t*
Postinflammatory hyperpigmentation, 68, 68*f*
Posttraumatic reflex dystrophy, 866*t*
Pott disease, 944–945, 944*f*, 945*f*
Pott puffy tumor, 454–455, 454*f*, 455*f*
PPD (phytophotodermatitis), 59–60, 59*f*, 60*f*
PPHN (persistent pulmonary hypertension of newborn), 249
PR (pityriasis rosea), 335–336, 335*f*, 336*f*
PR interval
  in first-degree atrioventricular (AV) block, 193, 193*f*
  in hyperkalemia, 733, 733*f*
  in hypokalemia, 731*f*, 732
  in long QT syndrome (LQTS), 200*f*
  in second-degree atrioventricular (AV) block, 195*f*, 196*f*, 196*t*
  in sinus tachycardia (ST), 208*f*
  in Wolff-Parkinson-White (WPW) syndrome, 213*f*
Pralidoxime, 763
Pregnancy
  congenital syphilis and, 171
  ectopic, 187–188, 187*f*, 188*f*
  emergency ultrasound (US) of, 1056–1057, 1056*f*
  herpes zoster and, 132*f*
  hyperthyroidism and, 661
  intrauterine, 188
  ovarian teratoma and, 551*f*
  syncope and, 205
Prehn sign, 480, 487
Premature ventricular contractions (PVCs), 221
  clinical summary of, 219
  differential of, 221*t*
  emergency department treatment and disposition, 219
  etiology of, 221*t*
  monomorphic ventricular tachycardia and, 220*f*–221*f*

  multifocal, 220*f*
  unifocal, 219*f*
PRES (posterior reversible leukoencephalopathy syndrome), 607*f*, 720*f*
Prescription drugs of abuse, 788–789, 788*f*
Preseptal cellulitis, 394–395, 394*f*, 395*f*
Prevnar, 510
Priapism, sickle cell anemia with, 522–523, 522*f*, 523*f*
Primary adrenal insufficiency, 654–655, 654*f*, 655*f*
Primary hyperoxaluria, 722, 722*f*
Primary spontaneous pneumothorax (PSP)
  clinical summary for, 287, 287*f*, 288*f*
  emergency department treatment and disposition, 287–288
  hemopneumothorax and thoracoscopic blebectomy, 290*f*
  tension pneumothorax from, 289*f*
Primary syphilis. *See* Syphilis
Prone position, 160*f*, 162, 491
Propoxyphene, 788*f*
Propranolol, 790*f*
Proptosis
  fungal sinusitis and, 452*f*
  granulomatosis with polyangiitis (GPA) and, 588
  neuroblastoma and, 546
  with orbital cellulitis, 391*f*, 392*f*, 393*f*
Proteinuria, 700–701, 700*f*, 701*f*
Prothrombin time (PT)
  hemophilia and, 534
  immune thrombocytopenic purpura (ITP) and, 531
Proximal esophagus, foreign body (FB) at, 667*f*
Proximal subungual onychomycosis, 354, 354*f*
Pseudo-Jones fracture, 895–896, 895*f*
"Pseudo-kidney sign," 1052, 1052*f*
Pseudomonas aeruginosa
  acute otitis externa (AOE) and, 432
  ecthyma gangrenosum (EG) and, 108, 108*f*, 109*f*
  necrotizing fasciitis (NF) and, 106
Pseudoparalysis of Parrot, 173*f*
PSLA (parasternal long axis) view of heart, 1065*f*
Psoralen compound, 59–60, 59*f*, 60*f*
Psoriasis
  annular, 330*f*
  clinical summary for, 329
  emergency department treatment and disposition, 329, 331
  erythrodermic, with arthritis, 584*f*
  generalized pustular, 329, 331, 331*f*
  guttate, 332, 332*f*, 333*f*, 334
  nail pitting with, 330*f*
  napkin, 62*f*, 330*f*
  palmoplantar, 329*f*
  pearls for, 331
Psoriatic arthritis, 583*f*, 585*t*
PSP. *See* Primary spontaneous pneumothorax (PSP)
PT. *See* Prothrombin time (PT)
PTA (peritonsillar abscess), 460–461, 460*f*, 461*f*
PTH (parathyroid hormone), 725*f*, 726, 730
PTT. *See* Partial thromboplastin time (PTT)
Pubic rami avulsion, 914*f*
Pulled elbow, 917–918, 917*f*
Pulmonary aspiration, of hydrocarbons, 773
Pulmonary contusion, 1006–1007, 1006*f*, 1009*f*
Pulmonary embolism (PE), 291–292, 291*f*, 292*f*
Pulmonary hypertension (PH)
  cardiac causes of, 250*t*
  clinical summary for, 249–250, 250*f*
  emergency department treatment and disposition, 251
  right ventricular hypertrophy with strain pattern, 249, 249*f*
Pulmonary hypertensive crisis, 250
Pulmonary tuberculosis
  active, 275*f*
  cavitary, 273*f*
  lung collapse secondary to, 276*f*
  with lymph node calcification, 277*f*

with pleural effusion, 274, 276f
reactivation, 274f
testing for, 274–275
Pulmonary venous congestion, 243
Pulse, poisoned patient and, 740t
Pulsus paradoxus, 237
Purified chick embryo cell vaccine (PCECV), 829–830, 829f
Purpura
altered mental status and, 605f
bacterial meningitis with, 596f
with ecthyma gangrenosum (EG), 108f
with Henoch-Schönlein purpura (HSP), 122f, 314, 314f–315f
with infective endocarditis (IE), 230f, 230t
macrophage activation syndrome (MAS), 590f
with systemic lupus erythematosus (SLE), 571f
Purpura fulminans (PF), with meningococcemia, 118f, 119, 119f
Purulent rhinorrhea, 447, 447f
Pustular psoriasis, 329, 331, 331f
Pustular tinea capitis, 347, 347f
PUV (posterior urethral valves), 718–719
PVCs. See Premature ventricular contractions (PVCs)
PWS (port-wine stain), 56f, 57, 57f, 615f
Pyelonephritis, 713–714
Pyloric stenosis
emergency ultrasound (US) of, 1053, 1053f
hypertrophic, 471–472, 471f
Pyoderma. See Impetigo
Pyogenic granuloma, 397f
Pyridoxine (vitamin B₆), 770f, 771, 771f
Pyuria, urinary tract infection and, 713f, 714

Q
Q angle, 913
Q fever, 123t
QRS complex
in acute myocarditis, 239
in atrial flutter (AF), 217
in bradycardia, 190, 190f, 191f
cyclic antidepressants (CAs) and, 794–795, 794f, 795f
in first-degree atrioventricular (AV) block, 193, 193f
in hyperkalemia, 733, 733f
in long QT syndrome (LQTS), 200f, 201f
in premature ventricular contractions, 219
in second-degree atrioventricular (AV) block, 195f, 196f, 196t
in sinus tachycardia (ST), 208, 208f
in supraventricular tachycardia (SVT), 211
in syncope, 204f, 205f
in third-degree atrioventricular (AV) block, 197f, 198f, 199f
in Wolff-Parkinson-White (WPW) syndrome, 213f
QT interval. See also Long QT syndrome (LQTS)
in acute myocarditis, 239
in hypercalcemia, 729f
in hyperkalemia, 733, 733f
in hypocalcemia, 725
in hypokalemia, 731f, 732
in ventricular tachycardia, 202, 202f, 203t
QTc, 200f, 201f, 202t, 203t
Quartan malaria, 158t
Quat sha, 50
Quinolones, for perichondritis, 434–435

R
RabAvert, 829–830, 829f
Rabies exposure and vaccine prophylaxis, 829–830, 829f, 829t
Rabies immune globulin (RIG), 829, 829f
Raccoon eye
with basilar skull fracture (BSF), 953, 953f
clinical summary for, 69
emergency department treatment and disposition, 69, 71
inflicted eye trauma versus, 69f

neuroblastoma and, 546
subgaleal hematoma and, 70f
Rachitic deformities, 76, 77f
Rachitic rosary, 76, 77f
Radial head and neck fracture, 878–879, 878f
emergency ultrasound (US) of, 1063, 1063f
Radial head subluxation, 917–918, 917f
Radiography
of abusive head trauma (AHT), 37f
of acromioclavicular (AC) injuries, 919f
of acute chest syndrome, 516f
of acute myocarditis, 239f
of acute osteomyelitis, 930f
of acute pericarditis, 237f
of anorectal foreign bodies, 673–674, 673f
of avulsion fractures
pelvic, 914f
tibial tubercle, 915, 915f
of bacterial pneumonia, 232f, 268f, 269f, 270f, 271f
of bacterial tracheitis, 261f
of battery ingestion, 262f, 675, 675f–676f, 677, 677f, 678f
of "body packing," 758f
of "body stuffing," 759f
of bronchiolitis, 265, 265f
of child abuse, 23f, 24f, 25, 25f, 26f
of chronic osteomyelitis, 933f
of coarctation of aorta, 226f
of cocaine complications, 757f
of congenital syphilis, 173f
of congestive heart failure (CHF), 243, 243f, 245f
of constipation, 692f, 693f
of croup, 259, 259f
of dilated cardiomyopathy, 243f
of dislocations
ankle, 911f, 912f
anterior glenohumeral joint, 904f
atlanto-occipital, 994f
elbow, 903f
hip, 907f
interphalangeal joint, 899f
knee, 909f, 910f
lunate, 901f
metacarpophalangeal (MCP) joint, 900f
patella, 913f
perilunate, 902f
posterior glenohumeral joint, 905f
of Ebstein anomaly, 227f
of endobronchial tuberculosis, 285f
of epiglottitis, 263, 263f, 264f
of esophageal foreign bodies, 666–667, 667f, 668f, 669f
of Ewing sarcoma, 558f, 559f, 560f
of finger and nail bed injuries, 1030f
of foreign body (FB)
aspiration, 255, 255f, 256f, 257, 257f, 259f, 284f, 285f
distal to esophagus, 671f, 672f
of fractures
ankle, 892f, 893f
Bennett, 871f
boxer's fracture, 872f
calcaneal, 894f
carpal bone fractures, 873f
clavicle, 884f
clay shoveler's, 1002f
femur, 28, 28f, 29f, 888f
flexion teardrop, 992f
forearm fractures, 874f
Galeazzi fracture dislocation, 876f
humerus, 882f, 883f
Jones fracture, 895f
Lisfranc fracture, 897f
Maisonneuve, 891f

Radiography, of fractures (*Cont.*):
  mallet finger, 870*f*
  mandible, 965*f*
  Monteggia fracture dislocation, 876*f*
  nasal, 964*f*
  olecranon, 877, 877*f*
  patella, 890*f*
  pelvic, 1028*f*
  phalanx, 868*f*
  pseudo-Jones fracture, 895*f*
  radial head and neck, 878*f*
  rib, 28*f*, 30*f*, 31
  Rolando, 871*f*
  scapular, 886*f*
  skull, 32, 32*f*, 33*f*, 951*f*
  supracondylar, 880*f*, 881*f*
  tuft, 867, 867*f*
  types of, 858*f*–861*f*
  zygomatic arch, 975*f*
 of gamekeeper's thumb, 916*f*
 of granulomatosis with polyangiitis (GPA), 588*f*
 of hemarthrosis, 535*f*
 of hemopneumothorax, 1012*f*
 of hemothorax, 1012*f*
 of Hodgkin lymphoma (HL), 542*f*
 of intravaginal foreign body (FB), 185*f*, 491*f*, 492*f*
 of intussusception, 467*f*, 469–470, 469*f*
 of iron toxicity, 752*f*
 of Kawasaki disease (KD), 565*f*
 of lead toxicity, 796, 796*f*
 of left-sided ductal-dependent cardiac lesions, 226*f*
 of Legg-Calvé-Perthes disease, 922*f*
 of Lemierre syndrome, 463*f*
 of macrophage activation syndrome (MAS), 589*f*
 of magnet ingestion, 683, 683*f*
 of mediastinal teratoma, 551*f*
 of miliary TB, 278*f*
 of nasal foreign bodies, 445*f*
 of neonatal osteomyelitis, 942*f*, 943*f*
 of neuroblastoma, 546*f*, 548*f*
 of obstructive sleep apnea syndrome (OSAS), 281*f*
 of Osgood-Schlatter disease, 924*f*
 of osteogenesis imperfecta (OI), 79–80, 79*f*, 80*f*, 81*f*
 of osteomyelitis in sickle cell disease (SCD), 936*f*
 of osteosarcoma, 553*f*, 555*f*, 556*f*
 of ovarian teratoma, 549*f*, 550*f*
 of ovarian torsion, 502*f*
 of penetrating injuries, 927*f*
 of pneumocephalus, 949*f*
 of pneumomediastinum, 232*f*
 of pneumonia, 268*f*, 269*f*, 270, 270*f*, 271*f*
 of Pott disease, 944*f*
 of primary spontaneous pneumothorax (PSP), 287, 287*f*, 288*f*, 289*f*
 of pulmonary contusion, 1006*f*
 of pulmonary embolism (PE), 292
 of pulmonary hypertension (PH), 249, 250*f*
 of retained bones, 679, 679*f*
 of retropharyngeal cellulitis, 458*f*
 of retropharyngeal space abscess, 457*f*, 458*f*
 of rhabdomyosarcoma, 545*f*
 of rib fractures and flail chest, 1008*f*
 of rickets, 76, 78*f*
 of septic arthritis, 937*f*
 of sharp object ingestion, 681*f*, 682*f*
 of slipped capital femoral epiphysis (SCFE), 920*f*
 of systemic lupus erythematosus (SLE), 572*f*
 of tension pneumothorax, 284*f*, 1010*f*
 of tetralogy of Fallot (TOF), 222*f*
 of thoracoabdominal trauma, 37*f*, 41*f*
 of total anomalous pulmonary venous return (TAPVR), 224*f*
 of tracheobronchial tree injury (TBTI), 1017*f*
 of traumatic airway obstruction, 1013*f*
 of traumatic diaphragm rupture, 1015*f*
 of tuberculosis (TB), 273–274, 273*f*, 274*f*, 275*f*, 276*f*, 277*f*
 of tubo-ovarian abscess (TOA), 182*f*
 of vein of Galen malformation and, 245*f*
 of viral pneumonia, 270*f*, 271*f*
 of VP shunt, 634*f*, 635*f*
 of Wilms tumor, 543*f*
Radiological rickets, 76
Radionuclide bone scan
  for child abuse, 26*f*
  of osteosarcoma, 554
Ramsay Hunt syndrome, 131, 624
Rattlesnakes, 850–853, 850*f*
Raynaud phenomenon (RP), 576–578, 576*f*, 577*f*, 577*t*
Rectal bleeding. *See* Lower GI bleeding (LGIB)
Rectal prolapse, intussusception and, 467*f*
Red strawberry tongue
  with Kawasaki disease (KD), 563*f*
  with scarlet fever, 94, 96*f*
Reflex sympathetic dystrophy, 911
Reflex tachycardia, 790
Renal cell carcinoma, with hematuria, 704*f*
Renal scarring, 714*f*
Renal stones, 722–724, 722*f*, 723*f*, 724*f*
Renal tubular acidosis, 773
Respiration, poisoned patient and, 740*t*
Respiratory disorders
  asthma. *See* Asthma
  bacterial tracheitis, 261–262, 261*f*, 262*f*
  bronchiolitis, 265–267, 265*f*, 266*f*, 267*f*
  community-acquired pneumonia (CAP), 268–272, 268*f*–271*f*
  croup, 259–260, 259*f*, 260*f*
  epiglottitis, 263–264, 263*f*, 264*f*
  intrathoracic tuberculosis, 273–275, 273*f*, 274*f*, 275*f*, 276*f*, 277, 277*f*
  miliary tuberculosis, 278–279, 278*f*, 279*f*
  obstructive sleep apnea syndrome (OSAS), 280, 280*f*, 281*f*, 281*t*, 282
  pertussis, 258, 258*f*
  primary spontaneous pneumothorax (PSP), 287–289, 287*f*, 288*f*, 289*f*, 290*f*
  pulmonary embolism (PE), 291–292, 291*f*, 292*f*
  tracheobronchial foreign bodies (FB). *See* Foreign body, aspiration
Respiratory syncytial virus (RSV)
  bronchiolitis and, 265
  pneumonia and, 269
Retained bones, 679–680, 679*f*, 680*f*
Reticulocytopenia, 527
Retinal hemorrhage, 36*f*
Retinoblastoma
  hypopyon and, 410, 410*f*
  leukocoria and, 402, 402*f*, 403*f*
Retrobulbar hemorrhage, 420, 420*f*, 421*f*
Retropharyngeal abscess, 261*f*
Retropharyngeal space abscess, 456, 457*f*, 458*f*
Reverse Hill-Sachs lesions, 905*f*
Revised Jones criteria, 247, 248*t*
Rewarming, 814–815
Rhabdomyosarcoma
  as abdominal mass, 545*f*
  epistaxis and, 441
  facial palsy and, 625*f*
  orbital cellulitis and, 393*f*
  preseptal cellulitis and, 395*f*
Rheumatic carditis, 247–248, 247*f*
Rheumatology
  granulomatosis with polyangiitis (GPA), 587–588, 587*f*, 588*f*
  incomplete Kawasaki disease (KD), 567–568, 567*f*, 568*f*, 569*f*
  juvenile dermatomyositis, 579, 579*f*, 580*f*, 581, 581*t*
  juvenile idiopathic arthritis, 582–586, 582*f*, 583*f*, 584*f*, 585*t*
  Kawasaki disease (KD), 562, 562*f*, 563*f*, 564*f*, 565–566, 565*f*, 566*t*
  Lyme disease, 591–592, 591*f*, 592*f*, 593*f*, 593*t*

macrophage activation syndrome (MAS), 589–590, 589*f*, 590*f*
neonatal lupus (NL), 574, 574*f*, 575*f*
Raynaud phenomenon (RP), 576–578, 576*f*, 577*f*, 577*t*
systemic lupus erythematosus (SLE), 570–573, 570*f*, 571*f*, 572*f*, 573*t*
Rhinitis, with congenital syphilis, 173*f*
Rhinoliths, 444
Rhinorrhea, purulent, 447, 447*f*
Rib fractures
child abuse and, 27, 28*f*, 29*f*
with abusive head trauma (AHT), 30*f*
clinical summary for, 30
with cutaneous manifestations, 12*f*
emergency department treatment and disposition, 31
infanticide versus SUIDS, 44*f*, 45*f*
inflicted versus accidental, 23*f*
radionuclide bone scan for, 26*f*
flail chest and, 1008–1009, 1008*f*
Ricin, 764, 764*f*
Ricinus communis, 764–765, 764*f*
Rickets, 25*f*, 76, 78*f*
Rickettsia prowazekii, 123*t*
Rickettsia rickettsii, 121–122
Rickettsia typhi, 123*t*
RIG (rabies immune globulin), 829, 829*f*
Right upper quadrant (RUQ)
focused assessment with sonography for trauma (FAST) view of, 1047, 1047*f*
syndrome, sickle cell anemia with, 514*f*, 524, 524*f*, 525*f*, 526, 526*f*
Right ventricular hypertrophy with strain pattern, 249, 249*f*
Right-sided ductal-dependent cardiac lesions, 226
Ring incarceration, 1029, 1029*f*
Ring of scale, 335*f*
Ringworm, 348, 348*f*, 349*f*
Rinne test, 438
Ritter disease. *See* Staphylococcal scalded skin syndrome (SSSS)
Rocky Mountain spotted fever (RMSF)
clinical summary for, 121, 121*f*, 122*f*
emergency department treatment and disposition, 122
Henoch-Schönlein purpura (HSP) compared with, 121, 122*f*
meningococcemia compared with, 121, 122*f*
Rolando fracture, 871, 871*f*
Rosary pea ingestion, 764–765, 765*f*
Roseola infantum, 138–139, 138*f*
Rotator cuff injury, 904
Roth's spots, 230*t*
Roundworm, 155–156, 155*f*
RP (Raynaud phenomenon), 576–578, 576*f*, 577*f*, 577*t*
RSV. *See* Respiratory syncytial virus (RSV)
Rubella, 142–143, 142*f*
Rubeola, 140–141, 140*f*, 141*f*
Rumack-Matthew nomogram, acetaminophen (APAP), 747*f*
Rupture
splenic, 144, 145*f*, 146
testicular, 485
traumatic globe, 416–417, 416*f*, 417*f*, 418*f*, 974*f*
Ruptured ectopic pregnancy, 188
RUQ. *See* Right upper quadrant (RUQ)

S
SABAs (short-acting β-agonists), 286
Saddle nose deformity, 587*f*
Safety-net antibiotic prescription (SNAP), for acute otitis media (AOM), 427
SAH. *See* Subarachnoid hemorrhage (SAH)
"Sail sign," 878
Salicylate toxicity, 749–751, 749*f*, 750*f*
Salmonella sp., 935, 936*f*
Salt wasting crisis, 656
Salter-Harris classification of fractures, 862*f*, 863*f*, 864*f*, 866*t*
"Sandwich sign," 1052, 1052*f*
Sandworm disease, 153–154, 153*f*

Sarcoptes scabiei, 339, 339*f*
Saturation gap, 760
Scabies
acropustulosis of infancy compared with, 360, 361*f*
clinical summary for, 339
emergency department treatment and disposition, 339–340
incognito, 339
infantile, 339, 340*f*, 341*f*
pearls for, 341
Sarcoptes scabiei, 339, 339*f*
scabetic nodules, 339, 341*f*
Scald burns, 18, 18*f*, 21, 808, 811*f*–812*f*
napkin psoriasis and, 61, 62*f*
Scalp laceration, 979–980, 979*f*
Scaphoid fracture, 873, 873*f*
Scapular fracture, 886–887, 886*f*
Scarlet fever
clinical summary for, 94–95, 94*f*–97*f*
in dark-skinned patients, 95*f*
emergency department treatment and disposition, 95, 97
Pastia sign with, 94
SCD. *See* Sickle cell disease (SCD)
SCFE (slipped capital femoral epiphysis), 920–921, 920*f*
SCFN (subcutaneous fat necrosis), 382–383, 382*f*
Schistosomiasis, hematuria and, 705*f*
Schizencephaly, closed-lip, 613*f*
SCIWORA (spinal cord injury without radiographic abnormality), 996–997, 996*f*
Scleral icterus, 526*f*
Scorpaenidae family, 844–845, 844*f*, 845*f*
Scorpion envenomation, 824–825, 824*f*
Scorpionfish, 844–845, 844*f*, 845*f*
Screw ingestion, 672*f*
Screwdriver nozzle, as foreign body (FB), 673*f*
Scrotum
acute pediatric. *See* Acute pediatric scrotum
blunt trauma to, 485–486, 485*f*, 486*f*
epididymo-orchitis, 487–488, 487*f*, 488*f*, 489*f*
hematoma of, 92, 92*f*
intrascrotal appendages, 490*f*
laceration of, 486*f*
pelvic fracture and, 1027, 1027*f*
swelling of, 709*f*
SDH. *See* Subdural hematoma (SDH); Subdural hemorrhage (SDH)
Sea anemones, 835–836, 836*f*
Sea urchins, 842–843, 842*f*
Seatbelt sign, 1025*f*, 1026
"Seatbelt sign," 1014
Seborrheic dermatitis, 318–319, 318*f*, 319*f*
Secondary bacterial infection. *See* Bacterial infection, secondary
Secondary hyperoxaluria, 722*f*
Secondary syphilis. *See* Syphilis
Second-degree atrioventricular (AV) block, 194*t*, 195–196, 195*f*, 196*f*, 196*t*
Sedative-hypnotic toxicity, 755*t*
Segmental pigmentation disorder, 373*f*, 374
Seidel test, 418*f*
Seidlmayer syndrome, 63–64, 63*f*
Seizures. *See also* Status epilepticus
arteriovenous malformation with, 612*f*
clinical summary for, 611
closed-lip schizencephaly, 613*f*
emergency department treatment and disposition, 611, 613
febrile, 609–610, 609*f*, 610*f*, 610*t*
isoniazid (INH) and, 770
motor, 743
neurocutaneous manifestations in, 611*f*
with neurocysticercosis, 621, 622*f*, 623*f*
syncope *vs.*, 207*t*
Selenium sulfide shampoo
for seborrheic dermatitis, 319
for tinea versicolor, 342

Senna, contact dermatitis from, 61–62, 61f, 62f
Septic arthritis
    arthrocentesis for, 938f
    clinical summary for, 937, 940
    diagnosis of, 937t
    elbow effusion with, 940f
    emergency department treatment and disposition, 940–941
    etiologies of, 937t
    neonatal, 942
    osteomyelitis and, 931, 931f
    ultrasound (US) of, 938f–939f, 940f
Septic shock
    altered mental status and, 605f
    emergency ultrasound (US) of, 1065
Septicemia, *Pseudomonas aeruginosa*, 108
Serotonin toxicity, 779
Serum Epstein-Barr virus antibodies, 145, 146t
Serum sickness, 298
Serum sickness–like reactions (SSLR)
    with Bactrim, 298f
    with cefaclor, 298f
    clinical summary for, 298
    emergency department treatment and disposition, 299
    urticaria multiforme (UM) and erythema multiforme (EM) compared
        with, 299t
Sexual abuse. *See also* Child abuse; Conditions mistaken for child abuse
        and sexual abuse
    clinical summary of, 160, 161f
    disclosure elements for, 160–161, 162t
    emergency department treatment and disposition, 160–162
    infantile hemangioma (IH) and, 166f
    injuries with, 165f
    intraoral trauma and, 14–15
    intravaginal foreign body (FB) in prepubertal child and, 491, 491f, 492f
    Jacquet diaper dermatitis, 166f
    labial adhesions and, 86–87
    lichen sclerosus et atrophicus (LSA) versus, 82–83, 82f
    neonatal menstruation and, 166f
    perianal bacterial dermatitis (PBD) versus, 84–85, 84f, 85f
    physical examination positions for, 160f
    sexually transmitted infections and. *See* Sexually transmitted infections
    straddle injury versus, 92
    urethral prolapse versus, 89
Sexually transmitted infections (STIs)
    abnormal uterine bleeding (AUB), 184, 184f, 185f, 186
    chlamydia vaginitis, 165f
    clinical summary for, 163, 163f, 164f, 165f, 166f
    condylomata acuminata, 163f, 167t, 168–169, 168f, 169f
    condylomata lata, 164f
    congenital syphilis, 24f, 171, 171t, 172f, 173f
    ectopic pregnancy and, 187–188, 187f, 188f
    emergency department treatment and disposition, 163, 166, 167t
    genital herpes, 164f, 167t, 179, 179f, 180f, 181, 181f
    gonococcal infections. *See* Gonorrhea
    management of, 167t
    pelvic inflammatory disease (PID), 182–183, 182f, 183f
    syphilis, 167t, 174–176, 174f, 175f
    trichomoniasis, 167t, 170, 170f
Shaken impact syndrome, 35, 35f
Sharp object ingestion, 681, 681f, 682f
Shingles. *See* Herpes zoster
Shock, septic. *See* Septic shock
Short-acting β-agonists (SABAs), 286
Shoulder joint dislocations, 904–906, 904f, 905f
SIADH (syndrome of inappropriate antidiuretic hormone) secretion, 776f
Sickle cell anemia
    with acute chest syndrome, 516–518, 516f
    with acute pain, 512, 513f, 514–515, 514f
    acute splenic sequestration crisis (ASSC) and, 529–530, 529f
    cerebrovascular disease and, 519, 519f, 520f, 521
    with fever, 510–511, 510f, 511f

    with priapism, 522–523, 522f, 523f
    with right upper quadrant (RUQ) syndrome, 514f, 524, 524f, 525f, 526,
        526f
    transient aplastic crisis (TAC) and, 511f, 527–528, 527f
Sickle cell disease (SCD), 510
    diagnosis of, 529
    gallstones and, 524
    hematuria and, 705f
    hyperplasia and, 519, 521
    hypoxemia with, 516
    infections and, 516
    osteomyelitis in, 935, 935f, 936f
    stroke and, 519–521, 519f, 520f
    tachypnea with, 512, 516
    transfusion therapy for, 516–517
    treatment for, 512, 514
    vaso-occlusive crisis (VOC) and, 510f, 513f
Sickle cell hepatopathy, 524, 526f
Sickle cell vasculopathy, 512
Silver nitrate, 506, 506f
Silver sulfadiazine, 808
Simple febrile seizures, 610t
Sinus bradycardia, 190, 190f
    clonidine toxicity and, 739f
    with junctional escape rhythm, 191f
    propranolol and, 790f
Sinus tachycardia (ST), 208–209, 208f, 209f, 209t
    acute myocarditis and, 240f
    supraventricular tachycardia (SVT) versus, 215t
Sinusitis. *See also* Acute bacterial rhinosinusitis (ABRS); Chronic
        rhinosinusitis (CRS); Pott puffy tumor
    brain abscess and subdural empyema following, 627f
Sixth disease, 138–139, 138f
Sjögren syndrome, neonatal lupus (NL) and, 574
SJS (Stevens-Johnson syndrome), 305, 305f, 306f, 307, 309
Skeletal manifestations of child abuse
    classic metaphyseal lesion (CML), 24, 24f, 25f
    clinical summary of, 23–25
    emergency department treatment and disposition, 25–27
    inflicted versus accidental fractures, 23–24, 23f
    rickets and, 25f, 76, 78f
Skin. *See also* Cutaneous manifestations of child abuse; Dermatitis;
        Dermatology
    congenital syphilis and, 171t, 172f
    poisoned patient and, 741t
Skin popping, 755f
Skin warts, 356, 356f, 357f
Skull fractures
    basilar, 953, 953f, 954f
    child abuse and, 24, 27
        clinical summary for, 32
        with cutaneous manifestations, 12f
        depressed, with subdural hematoma (SDH), 32f
        diastatic, 32f, 34f
        emergency department treatment and disposition, 32
        head trauma and, 34f
        linear, 33f
        ping pong fracture, 33f
    epidural hematoma (EDH) and, 957f
    raccoon eye and, 69, 69f, 70f, 71
    trauma and, 951–952, 951f
Slap marks, 12f
SLE. *See* Systemic lupus erythematosus (SLE)
Slipped capital femoral epiphysis (SCFE), 920–921, 920f
SMA (superior mesenteric artery), malrotation and, 504f
Small bowel obstruction, with iron toxicity, 752
SMV (superior mesenteric vein), malrotation and, 504f
Snake envenomations, 850–853, 850f, 851f, 852f
SNAP (safety-net antibiotic prescription), for acute otitis media (AOM), 427
"Sniffing," 773
Snoring, 280, 280f

Sodium hydroxide, 798, 799f, 801f
Sodium nitroprusside, 721
Soft coral, 835–836, 835f
Soft tissue trauma, 978–980, 978f, 979f, 980f
"Special K," 778, 778f
Spider bites
    black widow spider, 823, 823f
    brown recluse spider, 820–822, 820f, 821f
Spinal cord compression, epidural abscess with, 638f
Spinal cord injury without radiographic abnormality (SCIWORA),
    996–997, 996f
Spinal cord lesions, 637–639, 637f, 638f
Spinal cord tumor, intramedullary, 638f
Spinal dysmorphism, infantile hemangioma (IH) and, 368, 368f
Spinal process fracture, 1002, 1002f
Spiral fractures, 860f, 865t
Splash burns. See Scald burns
Splenectomy, 530
Splenic injuries
    infectious mononucleosis (IM) and splenic rupture, 144, 145f, 146
    traumatic, 1022, 1022t, 1023f
Splenic sequestration crisis, sickle cell anemia and, 529–530, 529f
Splinter hemorrhages, 229f
Spondylolisthesis of C2, 37f, 990, 990f
Sponges, stinging, 840–841, 840f
Spooning, 50
Sporadic hemolytic uremic syndrome (D-HUS), 716, 720–721
Sprains, ankle, 892–893, 893f
"Squish test," 1060
SSLR. See Serum sickness–like reactions (SSLR)
SSSS. See Staphylococcal scalded skin syndrome (SSSS)
ST. See Sinus tachycardia (ST)
ST segment
    in acute myocarditis, 239, 240f
    in acute pericarditis, 236f, 237
    in first-degree atrioventricular (AV) block, 194f
    in hypokalemia, 731–732, 731f
    in pulmonary embolism (PE), 292
    in pulmonary hypertension (PH), 249, 249f
    in supraventricular tachycardia (SVT), 211
St. Vitus's dance (Sydenham chorea), 248
Stab wounds
    penetrating abdominal injuries, 1019f
    penetrating head injury, 948f
    penetrating neck injuries, 984, 985f
    pneumocephalus with, 949f
    soft tissue trauma with, 978
    tracheobronchial tree injury (TBTI) and, 1017f
Stabbing marine animals
    cone shells, 847, 847f
    starfish, sea urchins, and crown-of-thorns starfish, 842–843, 842f
    stingray, 846, 846f
    stonefish and scorpionfish, 844–845, 844f, 845f
Staghorn calculus, 722f
Staphylococcal pneumonia, 269f
Staphylococcal pustulosis, 380f
Staphylococcal scalded skin syndrome (SSSS)
    clinical summary for, 114, 114f, 115f, 116f, 117f
    emergency department treatment and disposition, 115–116
    toxic epidermal necrolysis (TEN) comparison with, 117t
Staphylococcal toxic shock syndrome, 110, 111f, 112t, 113
Staphylococcus aureus. See also Methicillin-resistant *S aureus* (MRSA)
    acute otitis externa (AOE) and, 432
    bacterial tracheitis and, 261
    cellulitis and, 104f
    chickenpox and, 129, 130f
    deep neck space infection and, 456–457
    ecthyma and, 101–102, 101f
    erysipelas and, 103–104
    impetigo and, 65, 65f, 67, 98
    infective endocarditis (IE) and, 229

lymphadenitis and, 126, 127t
necrotizing fasciitis (NF) and, 106
osteomyelitis with, 932t, 942
perianal bacterial dermatitis (PBD) and, 84–85, 84f, 85f
pneumonia with, 269, 270f
staphylococcal scalded skin syndrome (SSSS) and, 114, 116, 117f
toxic shock syndrome (TSS) and, 110, 111f, 112t, 113
Starfish, 842–843, 842f
Status asthmaticus, 283
Status epilepticus, 610t, 614, 614f, 615f, 616, 616f
Stensen duct, 137
Stevens-Johnson syndrome (SJS), 305, 305f, 306f, 307, 309. *See also*
    Mycoplasma pneumoniae–induced rash and mucositis
Stimson technique, 905
Stinging marine animals
    box jellyfish, true jellyfish, and Portuguese man-of-war, 837–839, 837f,
        838f, 839f
    corals, sea anemones, hydroids, and fire coral, 835–836, 835f, 836f
    sponges, 840–841, 840f
Stingrays, 846, 846f
STIs. See Sexually transmitted infections (STIs)
Stokes-Adams attack, 197
Stonefish, 844–845, 844f, 845f
Straddle injury
    clinical summary for, 90–91
    differential diagnosis for, 90–91
    emergency department treatment and disposition, 91–92
    labia majora laceration, 90, 90f
    NAT versus, 91f
    scrotal hematoma, 92, 92f
    vaginal wall laceration, 90, 90f
Strawberry tongue, 94, 96f
Strep throat. See Streptococcal pharyngitis
Streptococcal gangrene. See Necrotizing fasciitis (NF)
Streptococcal pharyngitis
    acute rheumatic fever (ARF) and, 247
    clinical summary for, 94–95
    emergency department treatment and disposition, 95, 97
    guttate psoriasis and, 332
Streptococcal toxic shock syndrome, 110, 110f, 112t, 113
Streptococcus. See Group A β-hemolytic *Streptococcus* (GABHS)
Streptococcus pneumoniae
    acute otitis media (AOM) and, 427
    bacterial meningitis and, 596
    bacterial pneumonia and, 232f
    bacterial tracheitis and, 261
    cellulitis and, 104, 104f
    pneumonia with, 268f, 269, 269f
    sickle cell disease (SCD) and, 510
Streptococcus pyogenes. See Group A β-hemolytic *Streptococcus* (GABHS)
Streptococcus viridans, infective endocarditis (IE) and, 229
Stress fractures, 865t, 898, 898f
Stroke
    acute chest syndrome and, 517
    cerebellar, 619f
    clinical summary of, 617–618
    emergency department treatment and disposition, 618–619
    facial palsy with, 617f
    hemorrhagic
        altered mental status, 606f
        intracranial pressure (ICP) elevation and, 601f
    ischemic, 618f
    sickle cell disease (SCD) and, 519, 519f, 520f, 521
    subarachnoid hemorrhage (SAH) and, 620f
Stupor, 607t
Sturge-Weber syndrome (SWS), 57, 57f, 615f
Stuttering priapism, 522
Subarachnoid hemorrhage (SAH), 12f, 191f
    cerebrospinal fluid (CSF) examination in, 620f
    communicating hydrocephalus with, 620f
    elevated intracranial pressure (ICP) and, 603f

Subconjunctival hemorrhage, 413, 413*f*
  with pertussis, 258*f*
  with traumatic globe rupture, 416, 416*f*, 974*f*
Subcutaneous fat necrosis (SCFN), 382–383, 382*f*
Subdural empyema, 450*f*, 627*f*
Subdural hematoma (SDH)
  abusive head trauma (AHT) and, 5*f*, 36*f*
  acute, 955–956, 955*f*, 956*f*
  depressed skull fracture with, 32*f*
  shaken impact syndrome and, 35
Subdural hemorrhage (SDH)
  caida de moller and, 51
  child abuse and, 12*f*
  infanticide and, 43*f*
  Menkes disease and, 75
Subfalcine herniation, 601*f*
Subgaleal hematoma
  child abuse and, 3*f*
  computed tomography (CT) of, 70*f*
  raccoon eye and, 69, 70*f*, 71
Sublingual glands, 137
Subluxation
  anterior, 1001, 1001*f*
  radial head, 917–918, 917*f*
  tooth, 1003*f*, 1004*f*
Submaxillary glands, 137
Subungual hematoma, 868, 868*f*, 1032–1033, 1032*f*
Subxiphoid view, pericardial fluid on, 1049*f*
Sudden sniffing death, 773
Sudden unexplained infant death syndrome (SUIDS). *See* Infanticide versus
  sudden unexplained infant death syndrome
SUIDS. *See* Infanticide versus sudden unexplained infant death syndrome
Sunsetting, 626
Sunshine deficiency, 76
Superior mesenteric artery (SMA), malrotation and, 504*f*
Superior mesenteric vein (SMV), malrotation and, 504*f*
Superior vena cava syndrome (SVCS), 540, 541
Supination and flexion, 917
Supine position, 160*f*, 162, 491
Suppurative cervical lymphadenitis, 126, 126*f*, 127*t*, 537*f*
Supraclavicular adenopathy, 537
Supracondylar fracture, 880–881, 880*f*, 881*f*
Supratentorial brain tumor, 629, 629*f*
Supraventricular tachycardia (SVT)
  with aberrancy, 214*f*
  adenosine administration for, 214, 214*f*, 215*t*
  atrial ectopic tachycardia, 210*f*
    with rapid ventricular response, 211*f*
  caffeine and, 804–805, 804*f*
  clinical summary for, 210–211, 212*f*
  emergency department treatment and disposition, 212, 214–215, 214*f*,
    215*t*
  sinus tachycardia (ST) versus, 215*t*
  with thyrotoxicosis, 663*f*
  Wolff-Parkinson-White (WPW) syndrome and, 210–211, 213*f*
Surgery and genitourinary
  acute nonperforated appendicitis, 473–475, 473*f*, 474*f*
  appendix testis torsion, 490, 490*f*
  Bartholin gland abscess, 177*f*, 496, 496*f*
  congenital imperforate hymen with hematometrocolpos, 493–494, 493*f*,
    494*f*, 495*f*
  epididymo-orchitis, 487–488, 487*f*, 488*f*, 489*f*
  hypertrophic pyloric stenosis, 471–472, 471*f*
  incarcerated inguinal hernia, 478–479, 478*f*, 479*f*
  intestinal malrotation and volvulus, 504–505, 504*f*
  intussusception, 466–467, 466*f*–470*f*, 469–470
  ovarian torsion, 501, 501*f*, 502*f*, 503, 503*f*
  paraphimosis, 497, 497*f*–500*f*, 499
  perforated appendicitis, 476–477, 476*f*
  testicular torsion. *See* Testicular torsion
  testicular trauma, 485–486, 485*f*, 486*f*

  umbilical granuloma, 506–507, 506*f*
  umbilical hernia, 508, 508*f*
  vaginal foreign body (FB) in prepubertal child, 491, 491*f*, 492*f*
Surgical scarlet fever, 94
SVCS (superior vena cava syndrome), 540, 541
SVT. *See* Supraventricular tachycardia (SVT)
Swan-neck deformity, 868, 870, 870*f*
Swimmer's ear, 432–433, 432*f*
SWS (Sturge-Weber syndrome), 57, 57*f*, 615*f*
Sydenham chorea (St. Vitus's dance), 248
Sympathetic crisis, 721
Sympathomimetics, 769*t*
Symptomatic seizures, 611
Syncope
  atrial paced rhythm, 205*f*
  cardiac tumor with, 206*f*
  clinical summary for, 204
  differential diagnosis for, 207*t*
  emergency department treatment and disposition, 204–206
  etiology of, 207*t*
  seizures *vs.*, 207*t*
  ventricular paced rhythm, 204*f*
Syndrome of inappropriate antidiuretic hormone (SIADH) secretion, 776*f*
Syphilis
  clinical summary for, 174–175, 174*f*, 175*f*
  congenital, 24*f*, 171, 171*t*, 172*f*, 173*f*
  emergency department treatment and disposition, 175–176
  management of, 167*t*
Systemic arteriovenous fistula, 243
Systemic arthritis, 585*t*
Systemic lupus erythematosus (SLE)
  clinical features of, 570*f*, 573*t*
  clinical summary of, 570–571
  emergency department treatment and disposition, 571–572
  lesions of, 571*f*
  neonatal lupus (NL) and, 574
  pearls for, 573
  Raynaud phenomenon (RP) and, 576*f*, 577*f*
  with serositis, 572*f*
Systemic venous congestion, 243
Systemic-onset juvenile idiopathic arthritis, 583*f*, 590*f*

T
T waves
  in acute myocarditis, 240*f*
  in acute pericarditis, 236*f*
  in first-degree atrioventricular (AV) block, 194*f*
  in hypercalcemia, 729*f*
  in hyperkalemia, 733, 733*f*
  in hypokalemia, 731–732, 731*f*
  in pulmonary embolism (PE), 292
  in pulmonary hypertension (PH), 249, 249*f*
  in sinus tachycardia (ST), 208, 208*f*
  in supraventricular tachycardia (SVT), 211
  in ventricular tachycardia (VT), 200
TAC (transient aplastic crisis), sickle cell anemia and, 511*f*, 527–528, 527*f*
Tachycardia
  acute splenic sequestration (ASSC) and, 529, 529*f*
  atrial ectopic, 210*f*, 211*f*
  cyclic antidepressants (CAs) and, 794–795, 794*f*, 795*f*
  intracranial pressure (ICP) elevations and, 601
  as physiologic response, 208
  reflex, 790
  sinus, 208–209, 208*f*, 209*f*, 209*t*
  supraventricular. *See* Supraventricular tachycardia (SVT)
  transient aplastic crisis (TAC) and, 527
  ventricular. *See* Ventricular tachycardia (VT)
  wide-complex, 241*f*
Tachypnea
  altered mental status and, 605
  with sickle cell disease (SCD), 512, 516

Taenia solium, 621, 621*f*
Tamm-Horsfall protein, 700
Tapeworm, 621, 621*f*
TAPVR (total anomalous pulmonary venous return), 224*f*
Target lesions, 303*f*, 307*f*
"Target sign," 1052, 1052*f*
TB. *See* Tuberculosis (TB)
TBI. *See* Traumatic brain injury (TBI)
TBTI (tracheobronchial tree injury), 1017–1018, 1017*f*
TDR (traumatic diaphragm rupture), 1015–1016, 1015*f*
Teardrop fractures
    extension, 991, 991*f*
    flexion, 992, 992*f*, 993*f*
Teardrop pupil, 416, 416*f*
Telson, 824
Temperature, poisoned patient and, 740*t*
Temper-tantrum elbow, 917–918, 917*f*
Temporal bone osteomyelitis, 432–433
Temporomandibular joint (TMJ)
    arthritis, 585
    dislocation of, 983, 983*f*
TEN. *See* Toxic epidermal necrolysis (TEN)
Tenosynovitis
    flexor, 929, 929*f*
    juvenile idiopathic arthritis (JIA) and, 585
Tension pneumothorax
    asthma and, 284*f*
    from primary spontaneous pneumothorax (PSP), 289*f*
    trauma and, 1010–1011, 1010*f*
Teratomas
    mediastinal, 551*f*
    ovarian, 502*f*, 503*f*, 549, 549*f*, 550*f*, 551*f*
Terminal hematuria, 702–703
Tertian malaria, 158*t*
Testicular dislocation, 485
Testicular fracture, 485, 485*f*
Testicular hematocele, 485
Testicular hematoma, 485
Testicular mass, testicular torsion compared with, 482*f*
Testicular rupture, 485
Testicular torsion
    acute epididymitis versus, 484*t*, 489*f*
    acute pediatric scrotum, 483*t*
    bell-clapper deformity, 480, 480*f*
    cellulitis compared with, 483*f*
    clinical summary for, 480
    emergency department treatment and disposition, 481
    hydrocele compared with, 483*f*
    incarcerated inguinal hernia compared with, 479*f*
    pearls for, 484
    testicular mass compared with, 482*f*
    vascularity of, 481*f*
Testicular trauma, 485–486, 485*f*, 486*f*
Tet spells. *See* Hypercyanotic spell of tetralogy of Fallot
Tetanus, prophylaxis, 810, 826, 831, 834
Tetralogy of Fallot (TOF). *See also* Hypercyanotic spell of tetralogy of Fallot
    abnormalities of, 222, 223*f*
    boot-shaped heart of, 222*f*
    clubbing and cyanotic nail beds of, 222*f*
Tetralogy spells. *See* Hypercyanotic spell of tetralogy of Fallot
Thermal burns
    classification, 808*t*
    clinical summary, 808
    emergency department treatment and disposition, 808–810
Third-degree atrioventricular (AV) block, 194*t*, 197–198, 197*f*
    characteristic features of, 199*t*
    with junctional escape beat, 199*f*
    in neonatal lupus (NL), 574, 575*f*
    with ventricular escape beat, 198*f*
Thompson test, 925, 925*f*

Thoracoabdominal trauma, child abuse and
    blunt abdominal, 40*f*, 41*f*
    clinical summary for, 39–40
    computed tomography (CT) of, 40*f*, 41, 41*f*
    emergency department treatment and disposition, 40–41
    hemothorax with fractures, 39*f*
    radiography of, 37*f*, 41*f*
Thoracoscopic blebectomy, 290*f*
Threadlike warts, 356
3-day measles, 142–143, 142*f*
Thumbprint sign, 263, 263*f*
Thyroid antibodies, 661
Thyroid storm, 661, 661*f*, 662*f*, 663*f*, 664
Thyroid-stimulating hormone (TSH), 658, 661
Thyrotoxicosis, 661, 661*f*, 663*f*
TIAs (transient ischemic attacks), 521
Tibial tubercle
    avulsion fracture of, 915, 915*f*
    Osgood-Schlatter disease, 924, 924*f*
Tick-borne infection, 121. *See also* Lyme disease
Tinea capitis
    black dot appearance of, 345*f*, 347
    clinical summary for, 345
    emergency department treatment and disposition, 345–347
    id reaction, 346*f*, 347
    kerion, 345–347, 347*f*
    pearls for, 347
    pustular, 347, 347*f*
Tinea corporis, 348, 348*f*, 349*f*
Tinea cruris, 350–351, 350*f*, 351*f*
Tinea incognito, 349*f*
Tinea pedis, 352–353, 352*f*, 353*f*
Tinea unguium, 354–355, 354*f*
Tinea versicolor, 342, 343*f*, 344*f*
TLS (tumor lysis syndrome), 540
TM. *See* Tympanic membrane (TM)
TMJ. *See* Temporomandibular joint (TMJ)
TNPM (transient neonatal pustular melanosis), 380–381, 380*f*
TOA. *See* Tubo-ovarian abscess (TOA)
Todd phenomenon, 621
Toddler's fracture, 864*f*
TOF. *See* Tetralogy of Fallot (TOF)
Tongue laceration, 982, 982*f*
Tonsillectomy, for peritonsillar abscess (PTA), 460–461
Tonsillopharyngitis, exudative, 94, 94*f*
    with infectious mononucleosis (IM), 144, 144*f*, 145*f*
Tooth avulsion, 1003*f*, 1004*f*, 1005
Tooth subluxation, 1003*f*, 1004*f*
Torsades de pointes, 725
Torsion
    appendix testis, 490, 490*f*
    ovarian, 501, 501*f*, 502*f*, 503, 503*f*, 1057
    testicular. *See* Testicular torsion
Torticollis, 986*f*
Torus fractures, 861*f*, 865*t*
Total anomalous pulmonary venous return (TAPVR), 224*f*
Toxic epidermal necrolysis (TEN)
    clinical summary for, 305
    emergency department treatment and disposition, 307, 309
    phenobarbital and, 308*f*
    staphylococcal scalded skin syndrome (SSSS) comparison with, 117*t*
    Stevens-Johnson syndrome (SJS) overlap with, 306*f*
    trimethoprim-sulfamethoxazole and, 307*f*
Toxic shock syndrome (TSS)
    emergency department treatment and disposition, 113
    staphylococcal, 110, 111*f*, 112*t*, 113
    streptococcal, 110, 110*f*, 112*t*, 113
Toxicity nomogram, acetaminophen (APAP), 747*f*
Toxicology
    acute acetaminophen (APAP) toxicity, 746–748, 746*f*, 747*f*
    acute isoniazid (INH) toxicity, 770–771, 770*f*, 771*f*

Toxicology (*Cont.*):
    acute salicylate toxicity, 749–751, 749*f*, 750*f*
    anticholinergic drug and plant toxicity, 768–769, 768*f*, 769*t*
    β-blockers (BBs) toxicity, 790–791, 790*f*
    caffeine toxicity, 804–805, 804*f*, 805*f*
    calcium channel blockers (CCBs) toxicity, 790–791, 790*f*
    camphor toxicity, 772, 772*f*
    carbamate toxicity, 762–763, 762*f*
    castor bean ingestion, 764–765, 764*f*
    caustics, 798–799, 798*f*, 799*f*, 800*f*, 801, 801*f*, 801*t*
    clonidine toxicity, 792–793, 792*f*
    cocaine toxicity, 757–759, 757*f*, 758*f*, 759*f*
    cyclic antidepressants (CAs) toxicity, 794–795, 794*f*, 795*f*
    dextromethorphan (DXM) toxicity, 779, 779*f*
    ecstasy/molly toxicity, 776–777, 776*f*, 777*f*
    ethanol toxicity, 786–787, 786*f*
    ethylene glycol (EG) toxicity, 782–783, 782*f*, 783*f*
    hydrocarbon (HC) toxicity, 773–775, 773*f*, 774*f*
    iron toxicity, 752–753, 752*f*, 753*f*
    ketamine toxicity, 778, 778*f*
    lead toxicity, 796–797, 796*f*, 797*f*
    marijuana toxicity, 780–781, 780*f*, 781*f*
    methanol toxicity, 784–785, 784*f*, 785*f*
    methemoglobinemia, 740*t*, 760–761, 760*f*, 761*f*
    naphthalene toxicity, 773–775, 774*f*, 775*f*
    nicotine toxicity, 802, 803*f*
    opioid toxicity, 754–756, 754*f*, 755*f*, 755*t*
    organophosphate toxicity, 762–763, 762*f*
    phenothiazine toxicity, 766–767, 766*f*
    poisoning evaluation and management. *See* Pediatric poisoning
    prescription drugs of abuse, 788–789, 788*f*
    rosary pea ingestion, 764–765, 765*f*
    screening for, 743
Toxidromes, 738, 742*t*, 743
Tracheitis, bacterial, 261–262, 261*f*, 262*f*
Tracheobronchial foreign bodies. *See* Foreign body (FB), aspiration
Tracheobronchial tree injury (TBTI), 1017–1018, 1017*f*
Traction–countertraction technique, 905
Transfusion therapy
    abdominal trauma and, 1021
    for sickle cell disease (SCD), 516–517, 521
    for transient aplastic crisis (TAC), 527
Transient aplastic crisis (TAC), sickle cell anemia and, 511*f*, 527–528, 527*f*
Transient ischemic attacks (TIAs), 521
Transient neonatal pustular melanosis (TNPM), 380–381, 380*f*
Transposition of great arteries, 223*f*
Transtentorial herniation, 601*f*, 626
Transverse fractures, 859*f*, 865*t*
Transverse myelitis, 637–639, 637*f*, 641*f*
Trauma
    abdominal. *See* Abdominal trauma
    acute subdural hematoma (SDH), 955–956, 955*f*, 956*f*
    airway obstruction, 1013, 1013*f*
    anterior subluxation, 1001, 1001*f*
    aortic disruption, 1014, 1014*f*
    atlanto-occipital dislocation, 994–995, 994*f*
    basilar skull fracture (BSF), 953, 953*f*, 954*f*
    bilateral facet dislocation, 998, 998*f*
    cerebral concussion, 960, 960*f*
    cerebral contusion, 959, 959*f*
    cervical spine injuries, 986–987, 986*f*
    degloving injury, 1036–1037, 1036*f*, 1037*f*
    dental, 1003, 1003*f*, 1004*f*, 1005, 1005*f*
    diaphragm rupture, 1015–1016, 1015*f*
    digital amputation, 1034–1035, 1034*f*, 1035*f*
    epidural hematoma (EDH). *See* Epidural hematoma (EDH)
    extension teardrop fracture, 991, 991*f*
    extremity amputation, 1040–1041, 1040*f*, 1041*f*
    fishhook removal, 1042, 1042*f*
    flail chest, 1008–1009, 1008*f*

    flexion teardrop fractures, 992, 992*f*, 993*f*
    foot penetrating injury, 1038–1039, 1038*f*
    hand penetrating injury, 1038–1039, 1038*f*
    head. *See* Head trauma
        abusive. *See* Abusive head trauma (AHT)
    hemothorax, 1012, 1012*f*
    hepatic injuries, 1024, 1024*f*
    intra-abdominal, 1025–1026, 1025*f*, 1026*f*
    Jefferson burst fractures, 988, 988*f*
    lip laceration, 981, 981*f*
    mandible fractures, 965–967, 965*f*, 966*f*
    midfacial fractures, 968–971, 968*f*, 969*f*, 970*f*
    nail bed injury, 1030–1031, 1030*f*
    nasal fractures, 963–964, 963*f*, 963*t*, 964*f*
    nasal septal hematoma, 961–962, 961*f*
    odontoid fractures, 989, 989*f*
    orbital, 972, 972*f*, 973*f*, 974, 974*f*
    orofacial. *See* Orofacial trauma
    pelvic fractures, 1027–1028, 1027*f*, 1028*f*
    penetrating neck injury, 984, 984*f*, 985*f*
    pneumothorax, 1010–1011, 1010*f*
    pulmonary contusion, 1006–1007, 1006*f*, 1009*f*
    rib fractures, 1008–1009, 1008*f*
    ring incarceration, 1029, 1029*f*
    scrotal, 485–486, 485*f*, 486*f*
    skull fractures. *See* Skull fractures
    soft tissue, 978–980, 978*f*, 979*f*, 980*f*
    spinal cord injury without radiographic abnormality (SCIWORA), 996–997, 996*f*
    spinal process fracture, 1002, 1002*f*
    splenic injuries, 1022, 1022*t*, 1023*f*
    spondylolisthesis of C2, 37*f*, 990, 990*f*
    subungual hematoma, 1032–1033, 1032*f*
    temporomandibular joint (TMJ) dislocation, 983, 983*f*
    tension pneumothorax, 1010–1011, 1010*f*
    thoracoabdominal. *See* Thoracoabdominal trauma
    tongue laceration, 982, 982*f*
    tracheobronchial tree injury (TBTI), 1017–1018, 1017*f*
    unilateral facet dislocation, 999–1000, 999*f*
    zipper injury, 1043, 1043*f*
    zygomatic arch fractures, 975–977, 975*f*
    zygomatic complex fractures, 975–977, 976*f*
Traumatic airway obstruction, 1013, 1013*f*
Traumatic brain injury (TBI)
    cerebral concussion and, 960, 960*f*
    nonaccidental trauma (NAT) with, 37*f*
Traumatic diaphragm rupture (TDR), 1015–1016, 1015*f*
Traumatic extremity amputation, 1040–1041, 1040*f*, 1041*f*
Traumatic globe rupture, 416–417, 416*f*, 417*f*, 418*f*, 974*f*
Treble hooks impaction, 1042*f*
Trendelenburg signs, 579
Treponema pallidum. See Syphilis
Trichoepitheliomas, 359*f*
Trichomonas vaginalis, 167*t*, 170, 170*f*
Trichomoniasis, 167*t*, 170, 170*f*
Trichophyton rubrum, 348
Tricorporal priapism, 522
Tricuspid atresia, 224*f*
Trimethoprim-sulfamethoxazole, TEN and, 307*f*
Tripod fracture, 976, 976*f*
True jellyfish, 837–839, 838*f*, 839*f*
TSH (thyroid-stimulating hormone), 658, 661
TSS. *See* Toxic shock syndrome (TSS)
Tube thoracostomy, 984, 1017
Tuberculin skin test, 274, 277*f*
Tuberculomas, 278*f*, 279*f*
Tuberculosis (TB)
    endobronchial, asthma and, 285*f*
    intrathoracic. *See* Intrathoracic tuberculosis
    miliary, 278–279, 278*f*, 279*f*
    osteoarticular, 944–945, 944*f*, 945*f*

pleural, 273, 275
pulmonary. *See* Pulmonary tuberculosis
Tuberculous meningitis, 278–279, 596
Tuberous sclerosis, 610*f*
Tubo-ovarian abscess (TOA)
    ectopic pregnancy and, 188*f*
    pelvic inflammatory disease (PID) and, 182, 182*f*, 183*f*
Tuft fractures, 867, 867*f*
Tumor lysis syndrome (TLS), 540
Tunica vaginalis, 480
Tympanic membrane (TM)
    acute otitis media (AOM) and, 426, 426*f*, 427*f*
    auricular hematoma and, 439–440
    foreign bodies and, 437–438
    perforation of, 849*f*
    rhabdomyosarcoma and, 625*f*
Tyndall effect, 48
Typhus, 123*t*
Tzanck smear
    of erythema toxicum neonatorum (ETN), 362, 362*f*
    of herpetic infection, 135*f*

U

Ulcerative colitis, 690, 690*f*
Ulcers
    corneal, 408–409, 408*f*, 410*f*
    gastric, 685*f*
    with infantile hemangioma (IH), 368, 368*f*
    peptic ulcer disease, 685*f*
    with systemic lupus erythematosus (SLE), 571*f*, 572*f*
Ultrasound (US)
    of acute nonperforated appendicitis, 473*f*, 474*f*
    of acute osteomyelitis, 931*f*
    of acute poststreptococcal glomerulonephritis (APSGN), 711*f*
    of appendix testis torsion, 490*f*
    of cholecystitis, 524*f*–525*f*
    of congenital imperforate hymen, 493*f*, 494*f*
    of ectopic pregnancy, 187*f*, 188, 188*f*
    emergency. *See* Emergency ultrasound (US)
    of epididymo-orchitis, 487, 487*f*, 488*f*
    of flexor tenosynovitis, 929*f*
    of gallbladder, 525*f*
    of germ cell testicular cancer, 482*f*
    of hematometrocolpos, 493*f*, 494*f*
    of hematuria, 705*f*
    of hydrocele, 479*f*
    of hypertrophic pyloric stenosis, 471–472, 471*f*
    of incarcerated inguinal hernia, 478, 478*f*
    of incomplete abortion, 184*f*
    of intussusception, 468*f*, 470
    of Kawasaki disease (KD), 565*f*
    of Lemierre syndrome, 462*f*, 463*f*
    of medullary nephrocalcinosis, 729*f*
    of nephrolithiasis, 723*f*, 724
    of obstructive uropathy, 718*f*
    of ovarian teratoma, 550*f*
    of ovarian torsion, 501, 501*f*, 502*f*, 1057
    of paronychia, 928*f*
    of perforated appendicitis, 476*f*
    of peritonsillar abscess (PTA), 460, 461*f*
    of pneumonia, 268*f*, 270, 271*f*
    of pulmonary embolism (PE), 292
    of renal cell carcinoma, 704*f*
    of right upper quadrant (RUQ) syndrome, 514*f*
    of septic arthritis, 938*f*–939*f*, 940*f*
    of testicular torsion, 480*f*, 481, 481*f*
    of testicular trauma, 405, 405*f*
    of tubo-ovarian abscess (TOA), 182*f*, 183*f*
    of Wilms tumor, 544*f*, 702*f*
UM. *See* Urticaria multiforme (UM)
Umbilical granuloma, 506–507, 506*f*

Umbilical hernia, 508, 508*f*
Umbilical polyps, 506
Uncal herniation, 626
Unestrogenized crescentic hymen, 161*f*
Unicameral bone cyst, fracture of, 861*f*
Unifocal premature ventricular contractions, 219*f*
Unilateral facet dislocation, 999–1000, 999*f*
UP (urticaria pigmentosa), 370–371, 371*f*
Urethral prolapse, 88–89, 88*f*
Urinary tract infection (UTI), 713–715, 713*f*, 714*f*
Urine
    in acute poststreptococcal glomerulonephritis (APSGN), 711*f*
    cloudy, 713*f*
    in hematuria, 702, 702*f*, 704*f*, 722*f*
    hemoglobinuria, 774*f*
    poisoned patient and, 740*t*
    vin rose, 753*f*
Urobilinogen, 526*f*
Uropathy, obstructive, 718–719, 718*f*, 719*f*
Urticaria, 294–295, 294*f*, 295*f*
Urticaria multiforme (UM)
    cantharidin and, 295*f*
    clinical summary for, 300
    emergency department treatment and disposition, 300
    lesions with, 301*f*
    serum sickness–like reactions and erythema multiforme (EM) compared
        with, 299*t*
    wheals with, 300*f*
Urticaria pigmentosa (UP), 370–371, 371*f*
Urushiol, 320, 321*f*, 322
US. *See* Ultrasound (US)
Uterine bleeding, abnormal, 184, 184*f*, 185*f*, 186
UTI (urinary tract infection), 713–715, 713*f*, 714*f*
Uvulitis, acute, with streptococcal pharyngitis, 94*f*

V

Vaccines
    for HPV, 169
    for pertussis, 258
    pneumococcal, 510
    for rabies, 829–830, 829*f*, 829*t*
Vagal maneuvers, 212
Vagina
    chlamydia and, 165*f*
    condylomata acuminata and, 168, 168*f*
    examination of, 161*f*, 162
    foreign body (FB) in
        abnormal uterine bleeding (AUB) and, 185*f*
        in prepubertal child, 491, 491*f*, 492*f*
    genital herpes and, 179*f*
    gonococcal infection and, 164*f*, 177*f*
    laceration of wall of, 90, 90*f*
    sexual abuse and, 163
    trichomoniasis and, 170, 170*f*
Valsalva maneuvers, 212–213, 287
Valvulitis, infective endocarditis (IE) and, 230*t*
Varicella-zoster immune globulin (VariZIG), 129–130
Varicella-zoster virus (VZV)
    chickenpox with, 129–130
    herpes zoster and, 131
Varices, esophageal, 685*f*
VariZIG (varicella-zoster immune globulin), 129–130
Vasculitis, Henoch-Schönlein purpura (HSP) and, 314–316, 315*f*
Vasculopathy, sickle cell, 512
Vaso-occlusive crisis (VOC), sickle cell disease (SCD) and, 510*f*, 513*f*
Vasopressors, 791
Vasovagal syncope, 204–205, 207*t*
Vein of Galen malformation and, 245*f*
Venereal warts, 168*f*
Venomous marine animals
    biting, blue-ringed octopus, 848, 848*f*

Venomous marine animals (*Cont.*)
  stabbing
    cone shells, 847, 847*f*
    starfish, sea urchins, and crown-of-thorns starfish, 842–843, 842*f*
    stingray, 846, 846*f*
    stonefish and scorpionfish, 844–845, 844*f*, 845*f*
  stinging
    box jellyfish, true jellyfish, and Portuguese man-of-war, 837–839, 837*f*, 838*f*, 839*f*
    corals, sea anemones, hydroids, and fire coral, 835–836, 835*f*, 836*f*
    sponges, 840–841, 840*f*
Ventosa (cupping), 50, 51*f*
Ventricular extrasystoles, 219, 219*f*, 220*f*, 221, 221*f*, 221*t*
Ventricular fibrillation, 773
Ventricular paced rhythm
  atrial flutter (AF) and, 217, 217*f*
  syncope and, 204*f*
Ventricular premature contractions, 219, 219*f*, 220*f*, 221, 221*f*, 221*t*
Ventricular tachycardia (VT)
  acute myocarditis and, 241*f*
  chest pain and, 233*f*
  long QT syndrome (LQTS) and, 200, 202, 202*f*
  monomorphic, 220*f*–221*f*
  polymorphic, 200, 202, 202*f*, 725
Ventriculoperitoneal (VP) shunt, 634*f*, 635, 635*f*, 636*f*
Ventriculoseptal defect (VSD), 243, 243*f*
Verapamil, 790
Vermilion border, 981, 981*f*
Verruca plana, 356, 356*f*
Verruca plantaris, 356
Verruca vulgaris, 356, 356*f*, 357*f*
Vesicourethral reflux (VUR), 714*f*
Vibrators, as foreign body (FB), 673*f*
Vin rose urine, 753*f*
Vinegar
  for coral, sea anemone, and hydroid stings, 835
  for jellyfish and Portuguese man-of-war stings, 837–838
  for sponge stings, 840
Viperidae family, 850–853, 850*f*
Vipers, 850–853, 850*f*
Viral conjunctivitis, 398, 398*f*, 399*f*
Viral infection
  acute bacterial rhinosinusitis, 447
  acute myocarditis, 239
  community-acquired pneumonia (CAP), 269–270
  croup, 259
  human bites, 833
Viral pneumonia, 268–270, 270*f*, 272
Visceral dissemination, 131
Vision
  blurred, 407
  compressive optic neuropathy, 972
  corneal ulcer and, 408
  traumatic globe rupture and, 416–417, 416*f*, 417*f*, 418*f*, 974*f*
Vitamin B₆ (pyridoxine), 770*f*, 771, 771*f*
Vitamin D insufficiency and deficiency, 76, 77*f*
Vitamin K deficiency, 684
VOC (vaso-occlusive crisis), sickle cell disease (SCD) and, 510*f*, 513*f*
Voiding cystourethrogram
  of obstructive uropathy, 718*f*
  of vesicourethral reflux (VUR), 714*f*
Volkmann ischemic contracture, 866*t*

Volume overload lesions, 243
Volvulus, intestinal malrotation and, 504–505, 504*f*
von Willebrand disease, 534
VP (ventriculoperitoneal) shunt, 634*f*, 635, 635*f*, 636*f*
VSD (ventriculoseptal defect), 243, 243*f*
VT. *See* Ventricular tachycardia (VT)
Vulvar agglutination, 86–87, 86*f*, 87*f*
Vulvovaginitis
  gonococcal, 164*f*
  herpetic, 179*f*, 180*f*
VUR (vesicourethral reflux), 714*f*
VZV. *See* Varicella-zoster virus (VZV)

W
Waddell triad, 889
Warts, 356–357, 356*f*, 357*f*
  conjunctival, 397*f*
  perianal, 168*f*
  venereal, 168*f*
WBI. *See* Whole bowel irrigation (WBI)
Weber test, 438
Wegener granulomatosis, 587–588, 587*f*, 588*f*
Wenckebach block, 195, 195*f*, 196*t*
Westley score, 259
Wharton duct, 137
Wheezing. *See* Asthma; Bronchiolitis
"Whirlpool sign," 501
White pupillary reflex, 402, 402*f*, 403*f*
White strawberry tongue, 94, 96*f*
White superficial onychomycosis, 354, 354*f*
Whole bowel irrigation (WBI)
  "body packing" and, 758*f*
  for castor bean ingestion, 765
  decontamination with, 744
  for iron toxicity, 752*f*
  for lead toxicity, 796
  for rosary pea ingestion, 765
  for salicylate overdose, 750
Whooping cough, 258, 258*f*
Wide-complex tachycardia, 241*f*
Wilms tumor, 543–545, 543*f*, 544*f*
  hematuria and, 702*f*–703*f*
  with hypertension (HTN) and abdominal mass, 720*f*
Wimberger's sign, 173*f*
Wintergreen oil, 749, 749*f*
Wolff-Parkinson-White (WPW) syndrome, 210–211, 213*f*
Wong-Baker FACES scale, 512
Wound care, basic principles of, 826, 831, 833
WPW (Wolff-Parkinson-White) syndrome, 210–211, 213*f*
Wright stain
  of erythema toxicum neonatorum (ETN), 362
  of molluscum contagiosum, 358
  of transient neonatal pustular melanosis (TNPM), 380, 380*f*

Y
Yolk sac tumors, 549

Z
Zipper injury, 1043, 1043*f*
Zygomatic arch fractures, 975–977, 975*f*
Zygomatic complex fractures, 975–977, 976*f*